Past history
- Immunizations
- Major illnesses
- Allergies
- Previous surgery or hospitalization
- Injuries
- Obstetric history

Family history
- Hereditary conditions
- General physical and emotional health
- Familial tensions

- Health and hygiene habits
- Use of alcohol or tobacco
- Emotional level
- Educational status
- Occupation
- Use of health-care systems, financial support systems, family support systems

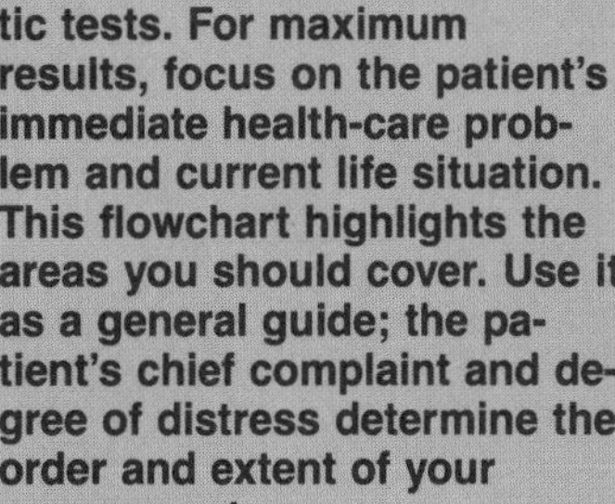

tic tests. For maximum results, focus on the patient's immediate health-care problem and current life situation. This flowchart highlights the areas you should cover. Use it as a general guide; the patient's chief complaint and degree of distress determine the order and extent of your assessment.

Skin assessment
Texture, temperature, turgor; presence of lacerations, contusions, abrasions, deep open wounds, pressure areas, pallor, cyanosis, rash, or petechiae

Respiratory assessment
Pattern, rate; shape and symmetry of chest excursion; breath sounds, exertion response, cough, sputum color and consistency; presence of pain

Cardiovascular assessment
Rate and rhythm, blood pressure, heart sounds, chest sounds, apical impulse, peripheral pulses, activity tolerance, voiding frequency, use of pillow support; presence of Homan's sign, ulcerations, jugular vein distention, edema

Gastrointestinal assessment
Condition of teeth, gums, mucous membrane; abdominal pulsations, abdominal contour and symmetry, presence of scars, visible blood vessels; appetite; bowel habits; bowel sounds; stool; special diets; nutritional status; presence of abdominal distention, nausea, vomiting, pain

THE NURSE'S REFERENCE LIBRARY®

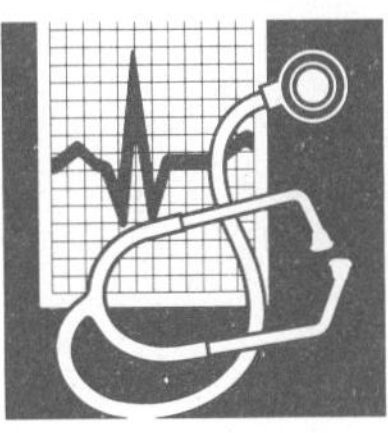

Assessment

Nursing83 Books™
Intermed Communications, Inc.
Springhouse, Pennsylvania

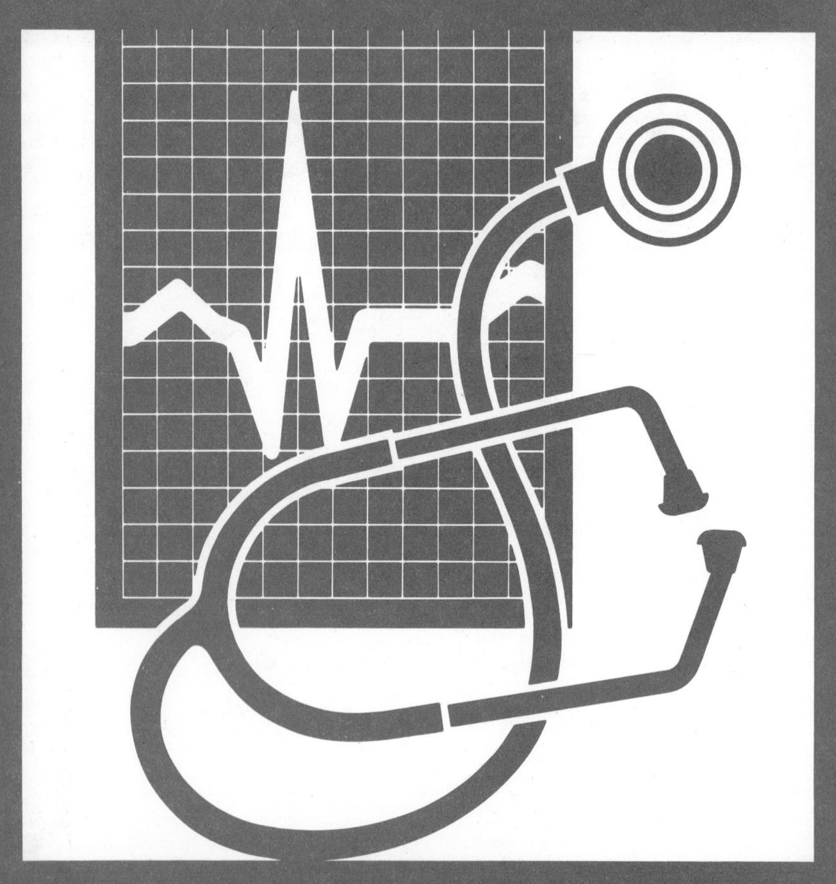

THE NURSE'S REFERENCE LIBRARY®

Assessment

Nursing83 Books™
Intermed Communications, Inc.
Springhouse, Pennsylvania

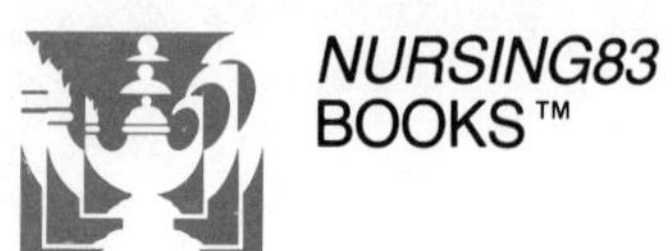

Intermed Communications Book Division

The clinical procedures described and recommended in this publication are based on research and consultation with medical and nursing authorities. To the best of our knowledge, these procedures reflect currently accepted clinical practice; nevertheless, they can't be considered absolute and universal recommendations. For individual application, recommendations must be considered in light of the patient's clinical condition and, before administration of new or infrequently used drugs, in light of latest package-insert information. The authors and the publisher disclaim responsibility for any adverse effects resulting directly or indirectly from the suggested procedures, from any undetected errors, or from the reader's misunderstanding of the text.

NRL4-020183

Library of Congress Cataloging in Publication Data
Main entry under title:

Assessment.

(The Nurse's reference library)
"Nursing82 books."
Bibliography: p.
Includes index.
1. Nursing. 2. Physical diagnosis. 3. Medical history taking. I. Intermed Communications, Inc. II. Series.
RT48.A87 1982 616.07'54'024613 82-11760
ISBN 0-916730-39-5

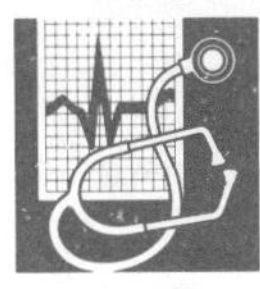

NURSE'S REFERENCE LIBRARY® SERIES

Staff for this volume

EDITORIAL DIRECTOR
Diana Odell Potter

CLINICAL DIRECTOR
Minnie Bowen Rose, RN, BSN, MEd

Editorial Managers: Martin DiCarlantonio, Thomas J. Leibrandt, Richard Samuel West
Senior Clinical Editor: Regina Daley Ford, RN, BSN, MA
Clinical Coordinator: Susan M. Glover, RN, BSN
Clinical Editors: Joanne Patzek DaCunha, RN; Judith A. Schilling McCann, RN, BSN; Anna Marie Seroka, RN, BSN, MEd; Janet C. Stolar, RN, MSN
Contributing Clinical Editors: Mary Gyetvan, RN, BSEd; Suzanna Joy Kravitz, RN, BA; Paula Stephens Okun, RN, MSN; Karen Dyer Vance, RN, BSN
Clinical Pharmacy Editor: Larry N. Gever, RPh, PharmD
Associate Editor: June F. Gomez
Assistant Editors: Holly Ann Burdick, William James Kelly, Neysa Simon Maxwell, Brenda L. Moyer, Pauline L. Wollack
Graphics Coordinator: Debra M. Rosenberg
Production Coordinator: Rebecca S. Van Dine
Copy Chief: Jill Lasker
Copy Editors: Barbara Hodgson, David R. Moreau
Contributing Copy Editors: Catherine Barr, Andrea F. Barrett
Associate Designer: Carol Cameron-Sears
Assistant Designer: Jacalyn M. Bove
Contributing Designers: Marsha Drummond, Lynn Foulk, Donna Monturo, Carol Stickles
Art Production Manager: Robert Perry
Art Assistants: Virginia Crawford, Diane Fox, Don Knauss, George Retseck, Louise Stamper, Joan Walsh, Ron Yablon
Illustrators: Michael Adams, Jack Crain, Jean Gardner, Tom Herbert, Robert Jackson, Bob Jones, Pat Macht, Cynthia Mason
Typography Manager: David C. Kosten
Typography Assistants: Nancy Merz Ballner, Janice Auch Haber, Ethel Halle, Diane Paluba, Nancy Wirs
Production Manager: Wilbur D. Davidson
Quality Control Manager: Robert L. Dean
Editorial Assistants: Maree E. DeRosa, Bernadette M. Glenn, Sally Johnson
Indexer: Rosemarie Klimowicz
Researcher: Vonda Heller

Special thanks to Jean Robinson and Edward J. Quigley for their editorial assistance.

Contents

Chapter 9: Respiratory System

Chapter 10: Cardiovascular System

Chapter 11: Gastrointestinal System

Conducting the physical examination

Formulating a diagnostic impression

Assessing pediatric patients

Assessing geriatric patients

Chapter 12: Urinary System

Introduction

Chapter 14: Female Reproductive System

Atlas of 100 Common Abnormalities

Chapter 15: Nervous System

Chapter 16: Musculoskeletal System

Introduction

Reviewing anatomy and physiology

Collecting appropriate history data

Conducting the physical examination

Formulating a diagnostic impression

Assessing pediatric patients

Chapter 17: Blood-forming and Immune Systems

Chapter 18: Endocrine System

Chapter 19: The Pregnant Patient

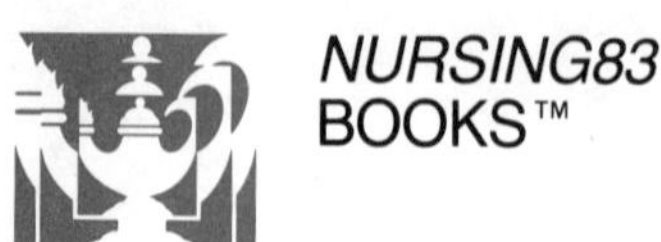

NURSE'S REFERENCE LIBRARY® SERIES

This volume is part of a new series conceived by the publishers of *Nursing83®* magazine and written by hundreds of nursing and medical specialists. This series, the NURSE'S REFERENCE LIBRARY, is the most comprehensive reference set ever created exclusively for the nursing profession. Each volume brings together the most up-to-date clinical information and related nursing practice. Each volume informs, explains, alerts, guides, educates. Taken together, the NURSE'S REFERENCE LIBRARY provides today's nurse with the knowledge and the skills that she needs to be effective in her daily practice and to advance in her career.

Other volumes in the series:

Diseases
Diagnostics
Drugs
Procedures

Other publications:

NURSING SKILLBOOK® SERIES

Reading EKGs Correctly
Dealing with Death and Dying
Managing Diabetics Properly
Assessing Vital Functions Accurately
Helping Cancer Patients Effectively
Giving Cardiovascular Drugs Safely
Giving Emergency Care Competently
Monitoring Fluid and Electrolytes Precisely
Documenting Patient Care Responsibly
Combatting Cardiovascular Diseases Skillfully
Coping with Neurologic Problems Proficiently
Using Crisis Intervention Wisely
Nursing Critically Ill Patients Confidently

NURSING PHOTOBOOK™ SERIES

Providing Respiratory Care
Managing I.V. Therapy
Dealing with Emergencies
Giving Medications
Assessing Your Patients
Using Monitors
Providing Early Mobility
Giving Cardiac Care
Performing GI Procedures
Implementing Urologic Procedures
Controlling Infection
Ensuring Intensive Care
Coping with Neurologic Disorders
Caring for Surgical Patients
Working with Orthopedic Patients
Nursing Pediatric Patients
Helping Geriatric Patients
Attending Ob/Gyn Patients
Aiding Ambulatory Patients
Carrying Out Special Procedures

***Nursing83* DRUG HANDBOOK™**

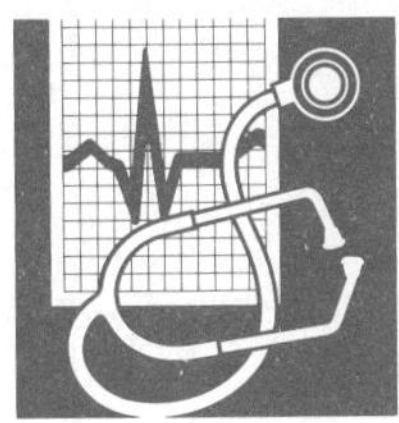

Advisory Board

At the time of original publication, the advisors, clinical consultants, and contributors held the following positions:

Lillian S. Brunner, RN, MSN, ScD, FAAN, Consultant in Nursing, Presbyterian–University of Pennsylvania Medical Center, Philadelphia.

Donald C. Cannon, MD, PhD, Professor, Pathology and Laboratory Medicine, the Medical School, University of Texas Health Science Center, Houston.

Luther Christman, RN, PhD, Dean, Rush College of Nursing; Vice-President, Nursing Affairs, Rush University, Chicago, Ill.

Kathleen A. Dracup, RN, MN, CCRN, Research Fellow, Medicine/Cardiology, University of California at Los Angeles.

Stanley J. Dudrick, MD, Professor, Department of Surgery, University of Texas Medical School at Houston; St. Luke's Episcopal Hospital, Houston.

Halbert E. Fillinger, MD, Assistant Medical Examiner, Philadelphia County, Philadelphia, Pa.

M. Josephine Flaherty, RN, PhD, Principal Nursing Officer, Department of National Health and Welfare, Ottawa, Ont.

Joyce LeFever Kee, RN, MSN, Associate Professor, College of Nursing, University of Delaware, Newark.

Dennis E. Leavelle, MD, Director, Mayo Medical Laboratories, Department of Laboratory Medicine, Mayo Clinic, Rochester, Minn.

Roger M. Morrell, MD, PhD, FACP, Professor, Neurology and Immunology/Microbiology, Wayne State University, School of Medicine, Detroit, Mich.; Chief, Neurology Service, Veterans Administration Medical Center, Allen Park, Mich.

Ara G. Paul, PhD, Dean, College of Pharmacy, University of Michigan, Ann Arbor.

Rose Pinneo, RN, MS, Associate Professor of Nursing and Clinician II, University of Rochester, N.Y.

Thomas E. Rubbert, JD, LLB, BSL, Attorney-at-Law, Los Angeles, Calif.

Maryanne Schreiber, RN, BA, Product Manager, Patient Monitoring, Hewlett Packard Co., Waltham Division, Waltham, Mass.

Frances J. Storlie, RN, PhD, ANP, Adult Nurse Practitioner, Vancouver, Wash.

Claire L. Watson, RN, Supervisor, Systems Support Department, IVAC Corporation, San Diego, Calif.

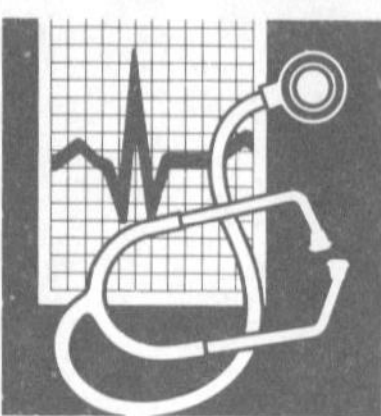

Contributors

Kathleen Gainor Andreoli, RN, DSN, FAAN, Executive Director of Academic Affairs, University of Texas Health Science Center at Houston.

Beverly A. Baldwin, RN, MA, PhD, Assistant Professor, School of Nursing, University of Maryland, Baltimore.

Margaret Hamilton Birney, RN, MSN, Assistant Professor, College of Nursing, University of Delaware, Newark.

Judith K. Bobb, RN, BSN, Nurse Coordinator, Maryland Institute for Emergency Medical Services Systems, Baltimore.

Marie Scott Brown, RN, PhD, Professor of Nursing, University of Oregon Health Sciences Center School of Nursing, Portland.

Janice L. Clark, RN, BSN, Kidney Transplant Coordinator, University of Mississippi Medical Center, Jackson.

Leonard V. Crowley, MD, Pathologist, St. Mary's Hospital, Minneapolis, Minn.; Clinical Assistant Professor of Laboratory Medicine and Pathology, University of Minnesota, Minneapolis; Staff Physician, West Side Community Health Center, St. Paul, Minn.; Clinical Assistant Professor of Family Practice and Community Health, University of Minnesota.

Nancy B. Davis, RN, BSN, FNP, Nurse Practitioner; Non-physician Surgical Assistant, Cardiovascular and Chest Surgical Associates, Boise, Idaho.

Charlotte M. Dienhart, PhD, Assistant Professor of Anatomy and Associate Professor of Community Health, Emory University School of Medicine, Atlanta, Ga.

Colleen Jane Dunwoody, RN, BA, Head Nurse-Adult Orthopedics, Presbyterian University Hospital, Pittsburgh, Pa.

Carol A. Eggleston, RN, BSN, Neurosurgical Nurse Clinician, Saint Louis University, Missouri.

Margaret J. Giragosian, RN, MSN, Medical-Surgical Clinical Specialist, Anne Arundel General Hospital, Annapolis, Md.

Mary Chapman Gyetvan, RN, BSEd, Clinical Consultant, Intermed Communications, Inc., Springhouse, Pa.

Catherine L. Hawkes, RN, MSN, Instructor, University of Pennsylvania School of Nursing, Philadelphia.

Mary C. Holderman, RN, BSN, Dermatology Nurse Specialist, Permanente Medical Group, Santa Teresa Community Medical Center, San Jose, Calif.

Andrea O. Hollingsworth, RN, MSN, Instructor, Health Care of Women and the Childbearing Family, School of Nursing, University of Pennsylvania, Philadelphia.

Karen M. Kleeman, RN, MS, Assistant Professor, Graduate Medical-Surgical Nursing, University of Maryland at Baltimore.

Mary Beth Lyman-Pais, RN, BSN, MNEd, Head Nurse-Orthopedics and Arthritis Rehabilitation, Presbyterian University Hospital, Pittsburgh, Pa.

Robert J. Merklin, PhD, Professor of Anatomy, Jefferson Medical College, Philadelphia, Pa.

Jacqueline K. Miller, RN, BSN, Pediatric Nurse, Hospice of Louisville, Kentucky.

Richard L. Miller, DDS, PhD, Professor and Chairman, Department of Oral Pathology/Pathology, University of Louisville School of Dentistry, Kentucky.

Barbara A. Mlynczak, RN, BSN, CCRN, Division of Clinical Nursing Education Coordinator, Anne Arundel General Hospital, Annapolis, Md.

Wendy Nelson, BA, BSN, MPH, Epidemiology Research Specialist, University of Pennsylvania School of Medicine, Philadelphia.

William Yale Reifman, RN, BS, FNP-ENP, Ear, Nose and Throat Nurse Practitioner, Associates of Otolaryngology, Denver, Colo.

Catherine Stewart Sackett, RN, BS, CANP, Ophthalmological Nurse Practitioner, Wilmer Institute, Johns Hopkins Hospital, Baltimore, Md.

Karen Wielgosz St. Marie, RN, MSN, CANP, Adult Nurse Practitioner, Department of Medicine, Children's Hospital of Buffalo, New York.

Lawrence K. Schneider, PhD, Professor and Chairman, Departments of Anatomy and Pathology, University of Nevada School of Medicine, Reno.

H. Joanne Schwartzberg, RN, MEd, Nursing Faculty, Medical College School of Nursing; Coordinator, Baccalaureate Nursing Program, University of Toledo, Ohio; Clinical Nurse Specialist, Gerontology; Assistant Professor of Nursing, Medical College of Ohio, Toledo.

Barbara Gorham Slaymaker, RN, BSN, CRNP, Adult Nurse Practitioner, Doylestown, Pa.

Carol E. Smith, RN, MSN, Assistant Professor of Nursing, Winona State University, Rochester, Minn.

Mary Lillian Smith, RN, MSN, Director of Nursing, Burlington County Memorial Hospital, Mount Holly, N.J.

Carolyn G. Smith-Marker, RN, MSN, CNA, Faculty Consultant, Resource Applications, Inc., Baltimore, Md. (formerly Assistant Director, Critical Care, Anne Arundel General Hospital, Annapolis, Md.)

Sharon Spilker, RD, BS, Clinical Dietitian, Thomas Jefferson University Hospital, Philadelphia, Pa.

Frances J. Storlie, RN, PhD, ANP, Adult Nurse Practitioner, Vancouver, Wash.

Karen Sweet, RN, LLB, Student-At-Law, Gottlieb, Hoffman, and Chaiton, Willowdale, Ontario.

Julia Lyon Tanis, RN, MSN, Instructor, Health Care of Women and the Childbearing Family, School of Nursing, University of Pennsylvania, Philadelphia.

Janice M. Vitello, RN, MSN, CANP, Adult Nurse Practitioner, Department of Medicine, Children's Hospital of Buffalo, New York.

Anne M. Riordan Warwick, RN, MSN, Assistant Director of Nursing, Wilmer Institute, Johns Hopkins Hospital, Baltimore, Md.

Phyllis d'Entremont Welch, RN, MS, Senior Nursing Instructor, Lankenau Hospital School of Nursing, Philadelphia, Pa.

Rebecca A.D. Zechman, RN, MSN, Assistant Professor/Clinical Nurse Specialist, Medical College of Ohio, Toledo.

Bernadette M. Zorio, RN, MSN, CS, Psychiatric Clinical Nurse Specialist, Edgewater, Md.

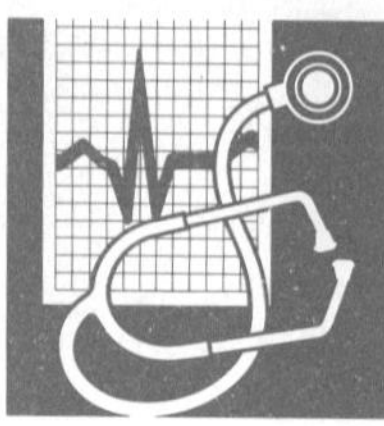

Clinical Consultants

Katherine Green Baker, RN, MN, Clinical Nurse Specialist, Department of Nursing, Center for the Health Sciences, University of California at Los Angeles.

Edmund Martin Barbour, MD, Clinical Assistant, Professor of Medicine, Wayne State University, Detroit, Mich.

Nancy Bergstrom, RN, MSN, PhD, Graduate Medical-Surgical Nursing Faculty—Associate Professor, University of Nebraska Medical Center, Omaha.

Robert Biern, MD, Director, Coronary Care Unit, Anne Arundel General Hospital, Annapolis, Md.

Gregory P. Blair, MD, Senior Pulmonary Fellow, University of California, Irvine Medical Center, Orange.

Ellen K. Boyda, RN, MS, CCRN, Instructor, Critical Care, Clinical Specialist in Pulmonary Nursing, Crozer-Chester Medical Center, Chester, Pa.

William F. Bruther, MD, Chief, Ophthalmology Service, Anne Arundel General Hospital, Annapolis, Md.

Carla J. Burton, RN, BS, Dermatology Nurse Clinician, Beth Israel Hospital, Boston, Mass.

Jeffrey P. Callen, MD, FACP, Associate Clinical Professor of Medicine (Dermatology), University of Louisville School of Medicine, Kentucky.

Constance Carino, RN, DNSc, Clinical Director, Psychiatric/Mental Health Nursing, Hospital of the University of Pennsylvania, Philadelphia.

Carolyn Ann Clyde, RN, BSN, Assistant Head Nurse, Haverford Dialysis Unit, Bryn Mawr, Pa.

Sandra Galloway Crandall, RN, C, MSN, Coordinator, Continuing Education, Montgomery County Community College, Blue Bell, Pa., and Bucks County Community College, Newtown, Pa.; Family Nurse Clinician, Pennswood Village, Warminster, Pa.

John M. Daly, MD, Associate Professor of Surgery, Memorial Sloan-Kettering Cancer Center, New York, N.Y.

Helen Hahler D'Angelo, RN, MSN, Clinical Consultant, Intermed Communications, Inc., Springhouse, Pa.

Catherine Davis, RN, MSN, Instructor, Psychiatric Nursing, and Assistant Professor of Nursing, Hahnemann College of Allied Health Professions, Philadelphia, Pa.

Judy Donlen, RN, C, MSN, Perinatal Nursing Instructor, University of Pennsylvania School of Nursing, Philadelphia.

Brian Doyle, MD, Associate Clinical Professor, Psychiatry, George Washington University School of Medicine, Washington, D.C.

Barbara Boyd Egoville, RN, MSN, Former Instructor, Critical Care Nursing, Lankenau Hospital School of Nursing, Philadelphia, Pa.

Bruce N. Garrett, MD, Assistant Professor of Medicine, George Washington University Medical Center, Washington, D.C.

Carol Hart Harris, RN, BSN, Primary Staff Nurse, Haverford Dialysis Unit, Bryn Mawr, Pa.

Alene Bender Herman, RN, MSN, Clinical Instructor, Maternal-Infant Nursing, Temple University College of Allied Health Professions, Philadelphia, Pa.

Rebecca Umbower Hones, RN, BSN, MS, Staff Nurse, Sacred Heart Hospital, Norristown, Pa.

Charlotte D. Kain, RN, BSN, MAEd, Assistant Professor of Nursing and

Curricular Coordinator, Department of Nursing, Montgomery County Community College, Blue Bell, Pa.

Howard M. Kandell, MD, FAAP, Medical Director and Vice President, INA Healthplan of Miami, Fla.

Lois R. Kimble, RN, BSN, MEd, Associate Professor, Department of Nursing, Bucks County Community College, Newtown, Pa.

Leonard J. Kryston, MD, Head, Endocrine Section, Pennsylvania Hospital, Philadelphia; Assistant Professor of Clinical Medicine, University of Pennsylvania School of Medicine, Philadelphia, and Pennsylvania Hospital.

Martha Lipshitz, RN, BSN, Senior Staff Clinic Nurse, Cardiac Outpatient Department, Children's Hospital Medical Center, Boston, Mass.

Melvina J. Lohmann, RN, C, MEd, ANP, Assistant Professor of Community Health Nursing, Department of Nursing, Cedar Crest College, Allentown, Pa.

Judith Lower, RN, CCRN, CNRN, Head Nurse, Neurosciences Critical Care Unit, Johns Hopkins Hospital, Baltimore, Md.

Donald McNellis, MD, Obstetric Medical Officer, National Institute of Child Health and Human Development, Bethesda, Md.

Roger M. Morrell, MD, PhD, FACP, Professor, Neurology and Immunology/ Microbiology, Wayne State University, School of Medicine, Detroit, Mich.; Chief, Neurology Service, Veterans Administration Medical Center, Allen Park, Mich.

Patrice M. Nasielski, RN, Staff, Los Robles Regional Medical Center, Thousand Oaks, Calif.

Lawrence Charles Parish, MD, Associate Clinical Professor of Dermatology, Jefferson Medical College, Philadelphia, Pa.

Richard T. Payton, RN, AD, Clinical RN, Department of Urology, University Hospital, Boston University Medical Center, Massachusetts.

Shaukat M. Quereshi, MD, FRCS, Chief Urology Resident, Thomas Jefferson University Hospital, Philadelphia, Pa.

Frank C. Riggall, MD, Associate Professor and Head, Division of Reproductive Endocrinology, Department of Obstetrics and Gynecology, University of Florida School of Medicine, Gainesville.

Estelle H. Rosenblum, RN, PhD, Associate Professor of Nursing, College of Nursing, University of New Mexico, Albuquerque.

Elaine D. Schultz, RN, MEd, Assistant Professor of Nursing, Department of Nursing, Montgomery County Community College, Blue Bell, Pa.

C. Richard Scipione, MD, Chairman, Department of Otorhinolaryngology, Graduate Hospital; Assistant Professor, University of Pennsylvania, Philadelphia.

Denise McFadden Semands, RN, BSN, Instructor, Nursing Staff Development, Hermann Hospital, Houston, Tex.

Barbara Gorham Slaymaker, RN, BSN, CRNP, Adult Nurse Practitioner, Doylestown, Pa.

Sandra Small, RN, MSN, CCRN, Director, Medical Intensive Care Units, University Hospital, Indiana University Medical Center, Indianapolis.

Linda J. Smith, RN, BSN, MAEd, Nursing Supervisor, Haverford Dialysis Unit, Bryn Mawr, Pa.

Maryann Burman Thayer, RN, MSN, CPNP, Pediatric Nurse Practitioner, Child Care Counseling, Virginia Beach Pediatric Center, Virginia.

D. Jane Turan-MacKinnis, RN, COGNP, Nurse Practitioner Doctor's Office, Ob-Gyn Nurse Practitioner, Women's Health Care of Tidewater, Norfolk, Va.

Susan Vigeant, RN, BSN, Staff Nurse, Department of Corrections, Bucks County (Pa.) Prison; Public Health Nurse, Neshaminy Manor, Warrington, Pa.

Madeline Musante Wake, RN, MSN, Director, Continuing Education in Nursing, Marquette University College of Nursing, Milwaukee, Wis.

Cheryl A. Walker, RN, MSN, CANP, PNP, Assistant Professor, Clinical Coordinator, University of Colorado Health Science Center, Denver.

Gail Zeigler, RN, Senior Research Assistant, University of Pittsburgh School of Medicine, Division of Rheumatology and Clinical Immunology, Pennsylvania.

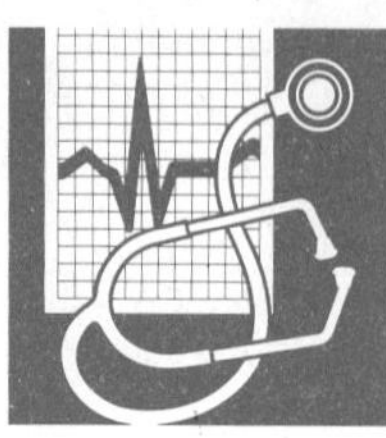

Foreword

The past 20 years have seen an explosion in biomedical information and technology. In response to this, nursing responsibilities have grown as well, particularly in the area of patient assessment. To meet this new challenge of decision-making in patient care, the nurse needs a comprehensive data base. This is a prerequisite for nursing diagnoses and individualized intervention strategies, making assessment the essential first phase in the nursing process. But where can the nurse turn for the accurate and comprehensive information she needs to guide her through this essential phase?

The answer is ASSESSMENT. This new volume in the Nurse's Reference Library, written and edited by nurses, fills the void between theory and practice. It tells you what you need to know to perform patient assessments with confidence.

ASSESSMENT is divided into four parts, covering:
- foundations of assessment (Chapters 1 to 3)
- psychological and nutritional assessment (Chapters 4 and 5)
- assessment of body systems (Chapters 6 to 18)
- assessment of the pregnant patient and the neonate (Chapters 19 and 20).

Chapters 1 to 3 cover the fundamentals of assessment—its place in the nursing process, the critical technique of history-taking, and methods for conducting the physical examination. I think you'll find these chapters so valuable you'll return to them again and again.

Chapters 4 to 20 begin with brief introductions. In Chapter 4, the next section is devoted to understanding psychological theory. In Chapter 5, this second section deals with the physiology of nutrition. In Chapters 6 to 20, it covers relevant anatomy and physiology. The third and fourth sections of Chapters 4 to 20 discuss the important points of collecting appropriate history data and conducting the physical examination. Helpful illustrations, diagrams, tables, charts, and supplementary pieces of text augment all these chapter sections. In the history section, for example, you'll find a chart listing some medications that can affect the body system you're assessing. And a special feature in some chapters, "Emergency Assessment," alerts you to ominous signs and symptoms in your patient that preclude routine history-taking and demand immediate intervention. The fifth section in Chapters 4 to 20, called "Formulating a Diagnostic Impression," takes you through the process of arriving at a nursing diagnosis. (For more information on this important section, see "How to Use This Book.") Pediatric and geriatric sections—unique to this book—round out Chapters 4 through 18. Here you'll learn about significant variations in assessment techniques and findings in children and the elderly. Finally, the appendices provide important information to underscore your knowledge of assessment. Included here are the main points of postoperative assessment as well as valuable listings of accepted nursing diagnoses and standard laboratory values.

The organization and scope of ASSESSMENT make it a suitable text for all nurses: the student, the graduate, the nurse returning to the profession, the seasoned practicing nurse. You may read it in sequence or in selected segments. And because of its easy-to-use format, it can serve both as a source of new knowledge and as a means to reinforce what you've already learned.

ASSESSMENT is an indispensable text. I recommend it highly. Don't let it gather dust on your library shelf; instead use it frequently to help you fulfill your role as a contemporary professional nurse.

KATHLEEN ANDREOLI, RN, DSN, FAAN
Executive Director of Academic Affairs
The University of Texas Health Science Center
Houston, Texas

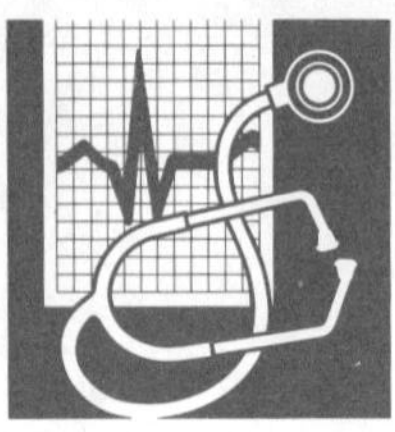

Overview

The role of the registered nurse has changed dramatically since Cherry Ames and Sue Barton first won the hearts of little girls more than 50 years ago. While women have been making important social gains throughout society, a new generation of nurses has arisen. These nurses, knowledgeable and proficient, consider themselves full colleagues with other members of the health-care team. The nurse-as-handmaiden image has faded like the once-bright colors on the covers of those old nursing storybooks.

In the mid-60s, a logical outgrowth of this changing role—a four-phase problem-solving procedure called the *nursing process*—was identified and incorporated into nursing. Actually, this procedure is just a more sophisticated way of classifying what nurses have always done—assessed the patient and identified his problem, planned his care, implemented that care, and evaluated the result—*except* that the nursing process provides for an expanded view of assessment. Physical assessment of patients presents nursing with its most significant new challenge. How we meet this challenge will in large part determine our future as independently accountable members of the health-care team.

Of course, physical assessment by nurses is controversial, primarily because it requires skills that were once regarded as exclusively medical. Ironically, those who most oppose this shift in nurses' responsibilities are not doctors or administrators or patients—they are nurses. The debate is most heated *within* our ranks. Some nurses perform physical assessment routinely and consider it rightfully within their province. But other nurses see it as a dangerous departure from traditional nursing practice.

In my opinion, every registered nurse *should* perform physical examinations. Why? Because good patient care requires it. This is my premise: As a nurse, you generally spend more time with each patient than any other caregiver. Your judgment about whether or not to call the doctor about a patient's changing signs and symptoms may be critical. Making appropriate decisions in this situation requires that you have the confidence and the authority to examine that patient thoroughly—using practiced inspection, palpation, percussion, and auscultation skills.

Of course, a nurse must be properly prepared for this new responsibility. Competence is paramount. Fortunately, nursing education is becoming increasingly sophisticated—and such books as ASSESSMENT provide the information you need. So the competence of nurses to do patient assessment is becoming less and less of an issue.

Other aspects of this development, however, are still being debated: Exactly how much education is necessary for this expanded nursing role? Where do you draw the line between medical and nursing practice? Are the distinctions between the two realistic or arbitrary? These questions are difficult to answer, but one thing's certain: We can't expect others to recognize the nurse's expanded role if we ourselves can't agree on what that role is. The first order of business for the nursing profession in the 1980s is to resolve this controversy.

As nurses, we've always prided ourselves on our ability to communicate. What a tragedy it would be if our failure to do so among ourselves and resolve our differences resulted in an irreconcilable division within our ranks.

This book can serve as a starting point for the nurse who wonders how she can contribute to and support nursing's role in patient assessment. Even the skeptical nurse will find that ASSESSMENT argues persuasively for this new responsibility's place in nursing. Organized by body systems, ASSESSMENT provides a wealth of detailed information, easy to understand and appealingly illustrated. It tells how you can move step by step through history-taking and physical examination to a complete nursing diagnosis. In fact, it should be your indispensable companion in any patient-care situation.

I urge every nurse who reads this book to practice her assessment skills with an attitude that fosters mutual understanding and compromise among members of the health-care team. For all today's controversy, nursing has never been at a more exciting juncture. By performing physical examinations and making nursing diagnoses, we're expanding the scope of our practice and making important contributions to the quest for better patient care.

FRANCES J. STORLIE, RN, PhD, ANP

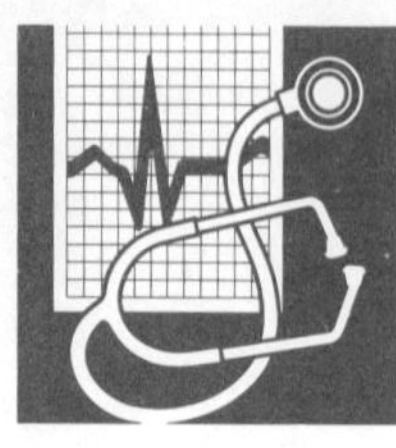

How to Use This Book

In ASSESSMENT, you'll discover distinctive features that give you instant access to this book's wealth of practical information. Foremost among these is the book's numbered-entry format. The information in each chapter is grouped into self-contained entries, each covering a single important topic. (The entry numbers also help you locate cross-referenced information quickly.) You can use ASSESSMENT as a learning or teaching tool, a resource for reviewing your assessment knowledge, or a quick reference. In all these situations, the numbered entries will help you find the information you want easily and quickly. For instance, to brush up on auscultating heart sounds, you needn't thumb through the entire "Conducting the Physical Examination" section in Chapter 10. Just consult ASSESSMENT's table of contents and turn to the appropriate numbered entry.

In Chapters 6 through 19, each "Reviewing Anatomy and Physiology" section features an *anatomic illustration* that shows you the system's location in the body and gross structure at a glance. When appropriate (as in Chapter 9, RESPIRATORY SYSTEM), the anatomic illustration also depicts the relationship of underlying organs to surface landmarks.

Each chapter section "Collecting Appropriate History Data" contains a *chief complaint entry* that lists the most common signs and symptoms for disorders of that particular body system. You'll find that, throughout each chapter, important diagnostic tools are organized around these lists. Also in this section, an entry on history of present illness features a *mnemonic (memory-assisting) device* based on the letters *PQRST,* to help you recall standard questions for preliminary analysis of each chief complaint. Then, each chief complaint is listed in the text together with a series of specific follow-up questions that help you explore the patient's chief complaint comprehensively. Use them to expand your knowledge of the patient's chief complaint.

Most ASSESSMENT chapters have *assessment tips* sprinkled throughout the text, particularly in the "Formulating a Diagnostic Impression" section. Highlighted by a nurse's cap symbol, these tips provide special hints for performing examination techniques and evaluating your findings.

The "Formulating a Diagnostic Impression" section, which appears in most chapters, helps you interpret the patient assessment information you've recorded. The first entry broadly *classifies common disorders* of the body system discussed, usually according to the body functions the disorders affect. This approach helps you make nursing diagnoses based on your patient's actual or potential health problems. The accompanying entries explain the physiology of the most common chief complaints and provide rationales for appropriate nursing diagnoses. Also in this section, *special charts* describe the possible medical significance of pertinent signs and symptoms. These charts aren't intended as aids to medical diagnosis; they're convenient references to help you, as a nurse, recognize patients' signs and symptoms and respond to them appropriately within the legal scope of nursing practice. Another feature in this section, a *case history flowchart,* will help you understand the nursing diagnosis process better through its concise clinical examples.

To provide comprehensive assessment coverage, this book also includes *information on some advanced assessment techniques and tests.* Remember that only some nurses, with specialized training, may perform these procedures. The specific assessment techniques you'll use depend on your level of nursing education and experience, the laws of your state, and the standards, policies, and regulations of your institution.

ASSESSMENT's appendices include a valuable *list of accepted nursing diagnoses* you can use when compiling your patient's assessment data. Also included is a *list of laboratory values* that will come in handy when you're interpreting the doctor's orders and charting your patient's progress. Finally, a special *postoperative complications section* prepares you for the assessment challenge posed by the surgical patient. Use these charts to help minimize or avert postoperative problems in your patients, whatever their surgical problems may be.

1

KEY POINTS IN THIS CHAPTER

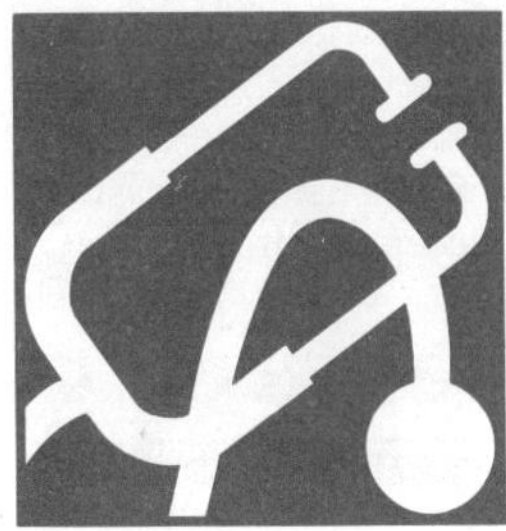

Approach to Assessment

Introduction

1 Assessment: The nurse's changing role

Patient assessment—history, physical examination, and laboratory data—is the vital first phase in the nursing process. Assessment skills are essential for *all* nurses, not just nurse practitioners and clinical specialists. Indeed, planning patient care on the basis of accurate assessment is the foundation of current nursing practice. This is why nursing books and journals emphasize assessment, and why it's a popular continuing-education topic. Yet, many staff nurses feel so ambivalent about using assessment that they undervalue its importance in their daily practice.

In many cases, the hospital staff nurse feels a need to justify using assessment. Why? The history of nursing provides a clue. In the past, nursing education stressed doing what one was told. For example, a nurse was expected to follow the doctor's orders: collect blood, urine, and drainage specimens for laboratory studies; give medications; secure prescribed diets; provide comfort; and monitor vital signs. After carrying out an order, she was expected to report what she had done. These were the acknowledged limits of her responsibilities. The doctor's unwritten expectation, however, was that she would also recognize and report any change in the patient's condition, and encourage the patient to take part in his own recovery. Thus, even before the nursing process was identified and put into practice, nurses were expected to assess patients. But recognition of assessment as a nursing skill and a nursing responsibility was yet to come.

This picture changed slowly as nurses became more capable listeners and observers, and as their contributions to patient care were recognized. The recent explosion in health-care science and technology paralleled this growth in nurses' professional self-assurance: New and complex patient-care procedures created an expanded role for nurses who were professionally mature and equal to the challenge. Independent accountability for many nursing services followed, as sophisticated and capable nurses moved into new positions of patient-care responsibility.

When the nursing process was recognized as the framework for patient care, nursing education started to incorporate these new trends. In most professional nursing programs, educators now teach students to conduct patient assessments, emphasizing the importance of physical assessment as an integral part of day-to-day nursing care. Students gather assessment information, analyze it, and learn to make patient-care decisions based on their findings. They also learn that the other nursing process phases—patient-care planning, intervention, and evaluation—depend on the quality of the assessment data for their effectiveness.

Today, many practicing nurses are skilled in assessment and in making a nursing diagnosis. And those that still feel uncertain about using assessment are gradually accepting it.

Understanding the nursing process

2 The nursing process: Framework for assessment

Quality nursing care results from deliberate decision-making and action. Your guide to quality care is the nursing process: a systematic problem-solving method illustrated on the opposite page. As you can see, the first phase of the nursing process is assessment—data gathering, identification, description, and analysis of a patient's problem(s). The other nursing process phases are development of a care plan, implementation of the plan, and evaluation of the results. In actual practice, the nursing process is continuous. The four phases overlap and recur as a patient's needs, and appropriate nursing responses, change.

The nursing process is based on the scientific method, involving the recognition and statement of a problem, the collection of data about the problem through observation and experiment, and the creation and testing of hypotheses to solve the problem.

Your initial patient assessment creates the foundation (a defined data base) for the remaining nursing process phases. It begins with the collection of data (patient history, physical examination data, laboratory data) and ends with a statement of the patient's problem(s)—your nursing diagnosis.

3 Styles of thinking in the nursing process

The nursing process is often defined as the application of critical thinking to patient-care activities. In addition, because nursing is a human, caring discipline, other styles of thinking influence your nursing decisions. You use four ways of thinking—ritual, random, and appreciative, as well as critical—to solve your patients' problems.

Ritual thinking underlies the development of habits—actions we perform so often or regularly (such as getting dressed or driving to work) that we do them automatically, without a conscious decision. You can't practice effective nursing without some ritual thinking, because you habitually follow standard nursing protocols in caring for patients; for example, providing routine preoperative care to a patient scheduled for a particular type of surgery. (Such protocols, of course, were originally devised and tested using critical thinking.)

Here's another example: A patient admitted to the hospital with a medical diagnosis of congestive heart failure must have his fluid intake and output recorded regularly. You don't perform this procedure because it's hospital routine, however. You do it because you know, without stopping to think, that fluid accumulation in body tissues resulting from cardiac insufficiency can lead to respiratory distress. Measuring the patient's fluid intake and output indirectly monitors the fluid balance in his whole body, providing an indication of potential fluid accumulation in his lungs.

Ritual thinking saves you time and effort in caring for patients. But use it only in appropriate situations and when you know the reasons behind its application.

Random thinking is the free association of ideas at the unconscious level. Although it can lead to impulsive im-

PHASES OF THE NURSING PROCESS

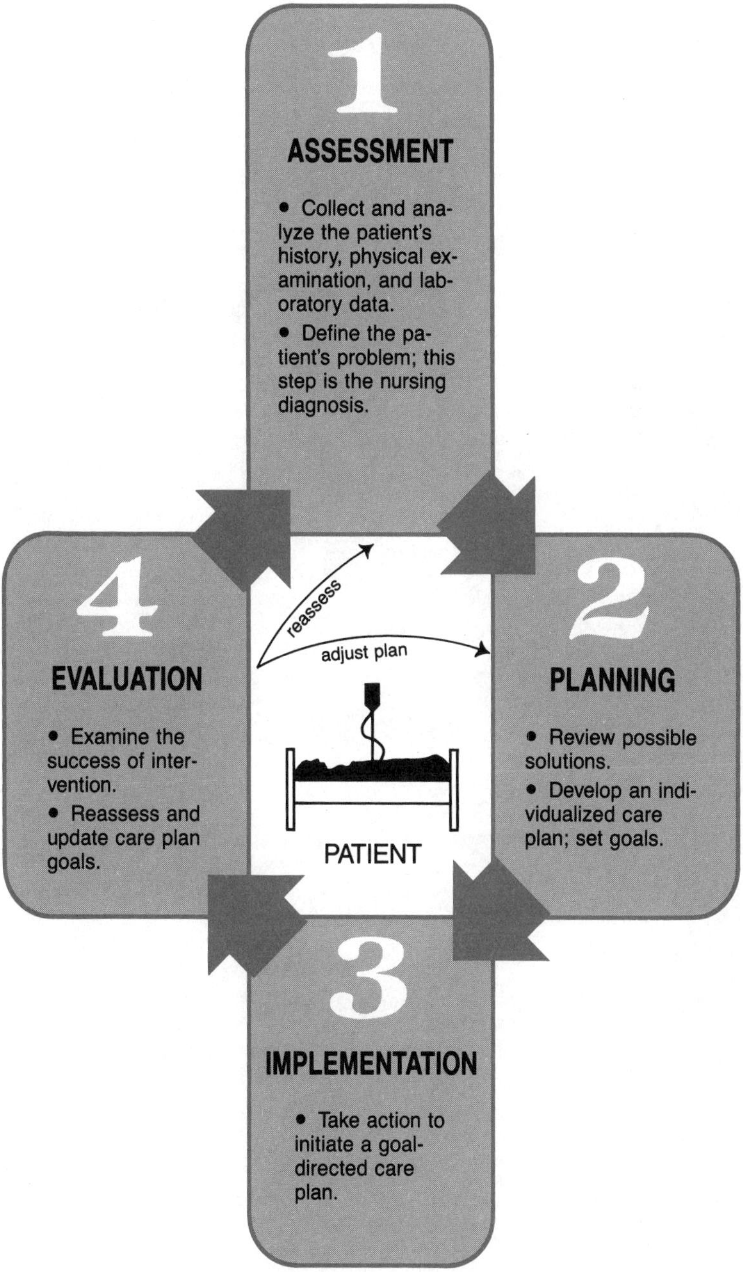

USING DIFFERENT STYLES OF THINKING IN PATIENT CARE

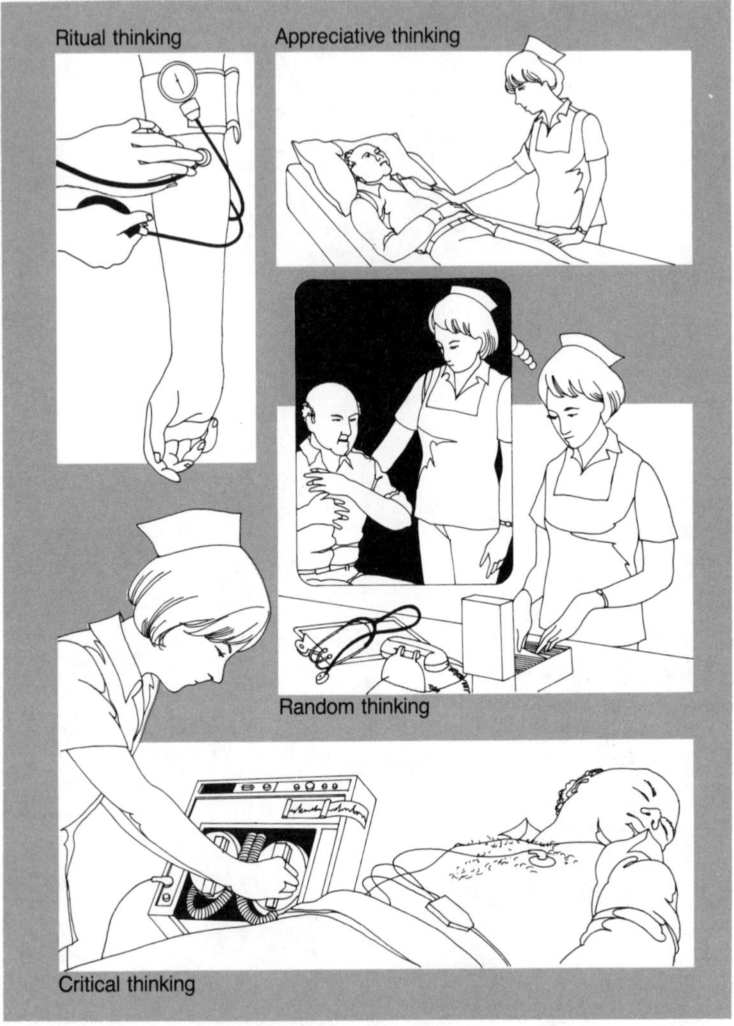

A patient complaining of chest pain is admitted to the emergency department. Directed by *ritual thinking,* you follow standard nursing protocol—you check his pulse rate and blood pressure.

Sensing his apprehension, you reassure him and briefly explain the situation. Through *appreciative thinking,* you ease his worry.

On reviewing the patient's signs and symptoms, you decide—using *critical thinking*—to prepare for possible defibrillation.

After the patient's left your care, you review the procedure you followed. How could you have performed the assessment process more efficiently? You have an idea. *Random thinking* promotes such innovations.

plementation of the first problem-solving solution that comes to mind, it also can be the creative source of new problem-solving ideas and approaches. For example, the nurse who first thought of devising Montgomery straps—rather than repeatedly traumatizing her patients' skin by removing and reapplying tape with every dressing change—used innovative, or random, thinking.

Random thinking isn't systematic, however, so you can't always trace the sequence of thoughts leading to an action. Making decisions solely by random thinking doesn't allow you to repeat your successes and to avoid repeating your failures. Analyze your patient-care hunches critically before acting on them.

Appreciative thinking reflects your awareness of human values and respect for your patients' individual needs. However, overemphasizing appreciative thinking in caring for a patient—as when you base your nursing decisions entirely on the patient's wishes—may cause you to neglect some necessary therapeutic actions. For example, if you allowed a patient to remain in one position all day because he felt most comfortable that way, he'd probably develop a decubitus ulcer. Such a nursing action, instead of solving your patient's problem(s), would have created additional ones.

Critical thinking is based on the scientific method—the deliberate and systematic use of rational, informed thought processes in problem-finding and problem-solving. It's the keystone of sensible decision-making using the nursing process and it yields predictable, repeatable results. Overemphasis on critical thinking, however, can cause problems for you if you respond to your patient's needs in rigidly patterned, coldly scientific ways. To give him the full benefit of your nursing skills, balance your critical analysis of his needs with considerations based on the other thinking styles already described.

Defining your assessment data base

4 The defined data base in assessment

The information you collect in taking your patient's history, performing his physical examination, and identifying necessary laboratory tests is your assessment data base. Make your patient history as comprehensive as you can while choosing your data carefully. You can't collect or use *all* the information that exists about your patient. Your goal is to gather information that will be most helpful to you in assessing your patient. To define, or limit, your data base appropriately, ask yourself these questions: What data do I want to collect? How should I collect the information? How should I organize it to make decisions, before I intervene as a nurse?

Your answers will help you to be selective in collecting meaningful data during patient assessment.

The well-defined data base for a patient may begin with his admission signs and symptoms, chief complaint, or medical diagnosis. It also may center on the type of patient care given in a specific nursing unit, such as the intensive care unit or the emergency department (ED). For example, you wouldn't ask a trauma victim in the ED if she has a family history of breast cancer, and you wouldn't perform a routine breast examination on her either. You would, however, do these types of assessment during a comprehensive health checkup in an ambulatory-care setting.

If you work in a setting where patients with similar diagnoses are treated, choose your data base from information pertinent to this specific patient population. Ask yourself these questions:

DEFINING THE PATIENT POPULATION: YOUR DATA BASE

SETTING	PATIENT POPULATION	SPECIFIC DATA REQUIRED
Orthopedic clinic	Patients with musculoskeletal disorders	• Ease of motion (observation) • Range of motion—including amount of resistance and muscle contraction • Condition of muscles, tendons, and joints
Pediatric unit	Children (under age 18)	• Birth history, immunization record, and growth/development factors • Play history • Eating and snacking habits • Behavior and discipline patterns
Obstetric unit	Women during pregnancy, labor, and postpartum	• Uterine contractions (strength, duration, intervals) or membrane rupture • Position of uterus • Condition of cervix • Date and findings of last pelvic examination • Position, presentation, and engagement of fetus • Fetal heart rate

• *What is my defined patient population?* Begin by describing the typical patient you care for in your practice. What common problems do your patients experience or risk experiencing? For example, if many of your patients are immobilized and risk hypostatic pneumonia, your defined assessment data base should include a careful physical examination of the respiratory system. Perhaps many of them are insulin-dependent diabetics. Then the defined data base should include information about the knowledge and skill of the person giving the injections, as well as examination of the patient's skin at the injection sites *and* at pressure points on his arms and legs.

• *What are the standards for nursing care of the people in my defined patient population?* Consider both the standards set by nursing experts and those set by your hospital. For example, cardiology specialists tell us that a proper assessment of a patient with heart disease includes checking his heart rate and rhythm. You palpate his radial artery for 1 minute, then auscultate his apical pulse for 1 minute, then compare the two findings. Therefore, these techniques should be included in your data base for a cardiac population. Another example: Most hospitals require that you monitor a patient's vital signs when he's admitted, so assessment of vital signs must be included in your data base.

• *How can I provide good care to the specified patient population?* Typically, a patient enters your sphere of influence in one condition and leaves it in a different (you hope improved) condition. The information you collect according to your defined data base should be sufficient to plan, implement, and complete all the nursing care needed between these two points in time. For example, in an ED, where patients enter with life-threatening problems and are transferred to other units when stabilized, your data base must include assessing respiratory, cardiac, and central neurologic function. Long-term–care considerations and discharge planning need not be included. Or, suppose a patient enters a screening clinic to find out if he has hypertension. Taking his blood pressure is appro-

DOCUMENTING

GATHERING SUBJECTIVE AND OBJECTIVE DATA

A form like this is an integral part of a complete data base. Note the type of information that goes into each part. The health history contains subjective data (in colored type), data the patient supplies; the physical examination contains objective data, data you supply.

HEALTH HISTORY

Section I: Date 3/1/81 Time 1:30pm Name Beth Tanner

Mode Ambulatory Age 52

T 99⁶ P 90 R 18 BP 140/90 Ht 5'3" Wt 156

Diet: 1,800 cal. ADA Bloodwork: Yes ✓ No ___ Urinalysis: Yes ✓ No ___

Prosthesis: Glasses none Contact lenses none

Dentures none Other none

General orientation to hospital environment by:

Signature M. Adams, RN Date 3/1/81

Section II: Date 3/1/81 Time 2:00pm

Reason for hospitalization or chief complaint: vaginal bleeding-postmenopausal

Duration of this problem/onset: 2 months 1/81

PHYSICAL EXAMINATION FINDINGS

Eyes: Vision: 20/20 O.U., Snellen; lids, conjunctiva, cornea, and iris s̄ lesions or defects. PERRLA, EOM intact bilaterally s̄ nystagmus; gross visual fields normal by confrontation. Funduscopic exam: red reflex present; arteries and veins appear normal—no hemorrhages or exudates.

Ears: Gross hearing: watch tick heard in both ears at 15". External ears: structure normal. Canal: no lesions, discharges; wax-soft, yellow, moderate amount. Weber and Rinne: bilaterally normal. Otoscopic exam: TM intact, pearly gray, landmarks visualized.

priately included in your defined data base, but a rectal examination would be inappropriate and not included.

• *What are my available nursing-care resources?* Your physical assessment can only be as complete as your knowledge and skill, and the time and equipment available, allow it to be. If the nurses on your unit can't perform the palpation component of an abdominal examination, the defined data base shouldn't include it—until the nurses develop the necessary skills. Similarly, if an otoscope is unavailable, tympanic membrane inspection has no significance in the defined data base.

A practical defined data base results when you ask and answer these questions before doing a patient assessment. This data base, when used to guide data collection in assessment, produces the essential information for planning and delivering appropriate patient care.

5 Collect subjective and objective data

The three types of data you'll collect and analyze in the assessment decision-making process—history, physical examination, and laboratory data—fall into two important categories, subjective and objective. Here's how they differ:

Your patient's *history* consists of the subjective data you collect from him, using interviewing skills that help him describe his biologic, social, and psychological responses to the particular anatomic, physiologic, and chemical processes involved in his illness or injury. In addition, he may recall events in his own or relatives' lives that place him at increased risk for certain pathologic processes to occur. The subjective data collected in your history include his chief complaint or concern, history of present illness (current health status), past history, family history, psychosocial history, activities of daily living, and review of systems.

The patient's history, embodying his *personal perspective* of his problems, is your most important source of assessment data. In fact, some clinicians claim that approximately 80% of the information on which they base their nursing diagnoses and patient management decisions comes from the history. It remains the most subjective source of patient information, however, and must be carefully interpreted.

In the *physical examination* of a patient—involving inspection, palpation, percussion, and auscultation—you collect objective data about your patient's health status, or about the pathologic processes that may be related to his illness or injury. Besides adding to your patient data base, this information helps you interpret the patient's history more accurately by providing another source of information for comparison. Use it to validate and amplify the historical data. However, don't allow the physical examination of your patient to assume undue importance—even though it's an exciting new aspect of nursing practice.

Laboratory test results are the most objective form of assessment data. They provide another source of patient data for validation and amplification of your history and physical examination findings. The advanced technology involved in laboratory tests lets you measure anatomic, physiologic, and chemical processes that your and your patient's senses aren't capable of measuring. For example, if your patient complains of feeling tired (history) and you observe conjunctival pallor (physical examination), check his hemoglobin and hematocrit (laboratory data).

You need both subjective and objective data for comprehensive patient assessment. They're complementary, too, in that they validate each other and together provide more data than either could provide alone. For example, *subjective data* for a patient with an apparent respiratory disorder might include his description of having difficulty breathing, while the *objective data* would include finding rales by auscultation, tibial edema by palpation, and cardiomegaly on the

CASE IN POINT: MR. JOHN JAY

ASSESSMENT

Subjective data
- Occipital headache every morning for 3 weeks
- Difficulty sleeping
- Nosebleeds 3 times a week, lasting about 15 minutes each time
- Stopped taking antihypertensive medication because blood pressure was normal on last visit 1 month ago and "thought he was cured"

Objective data (cardiovascular system)
- Inspection: precordial apical thrust
- Palpation: precordial apical thrust
- Auscultation: blood pressure 180/110, both arms, recumbent accentuated A_2. No rales, murmurs, or gallops
- Laboratory: elevated serum cholesterol and triglycerides
- X-ray: normal, without cardiomegaly

Nursing diagnosis
- Cardiovascular stress secondary to hypertensive episode, related to lack of knowledge regarding appropriate use of antihypertensives and lack of self-care monitoring practices.

PLAN

- Eliminate headache, nosebleeds, insomnia.
- Maintain normal apical impulse.
- Maintain normal heart sounds.
- Lower systolic blood pressure to less than 150; diastolic to less than 90.

IMPLEMENTATION

- Monitor vital signs twice daily.
- Measure intake and output.
- Record daily weight.
- Administer antihypertensive medications.
- Explain hypertensive episode to patient.
- Teach appropriate use of medication, diet, and self-monitoring techniques.

EVALUATION

Subjective data
- Patient states he "feels better."
- Patient reports no episode of headache or nosebleed.
- Patient describes appropriate use of medication and self-monitoring practices.

Objective data
- Apical impulse in fifth intercostal space, at midclavicular line, 1 cm in diameter
- S_1 and S_2 normal, rate 89/minute, rhythm regular
- Blood pressure 148/90, both arms, sitting

Analysis
- Hypertensive episode resolved. Patient asks many questions and repeats information learned. Likely to take medication secondary to increased knowledge.

Plan
- Patient to return to hypertension clinic after 1 month.
- Patient to call clinic doctor if problems develop.
- Patient to leave hospital with prescriptions for medications and self-monitoring blood pressure equipment.

X-ray film. Similarly, a patient's report of abdominal pain might be the *subjective* finding that correlates with a palpable enlarged liver or hyperresonant bowel sounds found *objectively* on physical examination.

Respect the value of both subjective and objective data when assessing a patient. And consider all three types of assessment information—history, physical examination, and laboratory data—in their appropriate relationship to one another. Performing an accurate physical examination requires technical skill that in itself is valuable. It becomes even more valuable, however, when you place the examination findings in perspective. Use them to validate historical and laboratory data, and recognize that the physical examination is only one aspect of total patient assessment. This and other considerations are part of the discipline you need for learning and using assessment skills.

Here's something else to remember: During the data collection phase of assessment, don't *interpret* your findings. Describe what you see, hear, and find when you take your patient's history and examine him, but guard against any tendency to write what you think statements, sounds, or lumps may mean. A lump may be a malignant tumor but, of course, it may not be. Are your patient's tears caused by depression? Maybe—or perhaps he has hay fever. Because each assessment observation can represent any of a number of possible causes, *suspend* decision-making related to your patient's problem(s) until you've collected *all* the subjective and the objective data and have created your assessment data base.

Using nursing diagnosis

6 Make your nursing diagnosis

Translating your history, physical examination, and laboratory data about a patient into a nursing diagnosis involves organizing the data into clusters and interpreting what the clusters reveal about your patient's ability to meet his basic needs. In addition to identifying his needs in terms of how he's coping with the effects of his condition, consider what assistance he requires to grow and develop to his highest potential.

Specifically, your nursing diagnosis (or problem statement) describes the cluster of symptoms and signs indicating an actual or potential health problem you can identify—and your nursing care can resolve. In writing your nursing diagnosis, state only the patient's problem(s) and their probable origins. Omit references to possible solutions to the problem(s). (Your solutions will derive from your nursing diagnosis but aren't part of it.) For example, rather than say, "Need to administer medications to relieve pain, as ordered," say instead, "Alterations in comfort, related to pain." (The words *related to, secondary to,* or *due to* are usually used in your written nursing diagnosis.)

Creating your nursing diagnosis is a logical extension of collecting assessment data. In your patient assessment, you asked each history question, performed each physical examination technique, and considered each laboratory result because it provided evidence of how your patient could be helped by your care, or because the data could affect nursing care.

The case of Mr. John Jay (page 9) demonstrates how to make and write a nursing diagnosis after collecting assessment data. Here are the main points to remember:

• Examine the data collected, and ask yourself if, on the basis of your assessment information, the patient is having difficulty meeting a basic need or cop-

MEDICAL DIAGNOSIS VERSUS NURSING DIAGNOSIS

To understand the difference between the medical diagnosis and the nursing diagnosis, study the examples below. The medical diagnosis describes a disorder or injury and directs the doctor toward medical treatment. The nursing diagnosis, a statement of actual or potential health problems, directs the nurse to those problems she's licensed to treat.

SITUATION

Frank Smith, age 67, complains of "stubborn, old muscles." He has difficulty walking, as you can see by his shuffling gait. During the interview, Mr. Smith speaks in a monotone and seems very depressed. Physical examination shows pill-rolling hand tremor. Laboratory tests reveal a decrease in dopamine level.

MEDICAL DIAGNOSIS

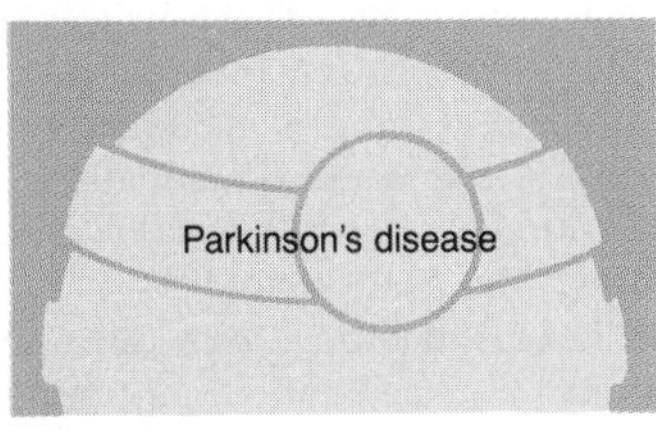

NURSING DIAGNOSIS

- Mobility impairment due to decreased muscle control
- Disturbance in self-concept due to physical alterations
- Knowledge deficit, related to lack of information about progressive nature of illness

SITUATION

For 5 consecutive days Judy Wilson, age 26, has had sporadic abdominal cramps of increasing intensity. Most recently, the pain has been accompanied by vomiting and a slight fever. Your examination reveals rebound tenderness and muscular guarding.

MEDICAL DIAGNOSIS

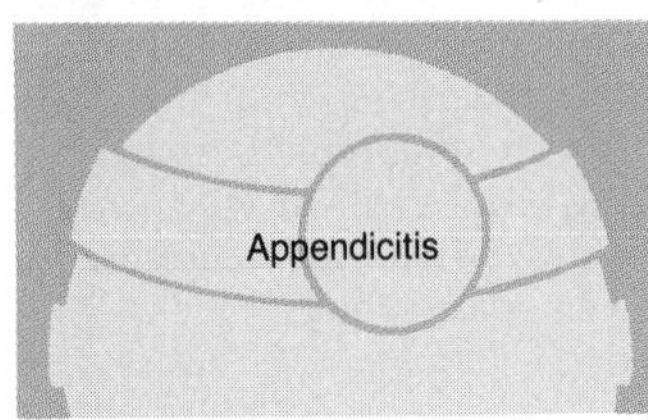

NURSING DIAGNOSIS

- Alterations in comfort; pain due to sporadic abdominal cramps
- Alterations in fluid and electrolyte balance—less than body requirements due to vomiting

SITUATION

During an extensive bout with respiratory tract infections, Tom Bradley, age 7, complains of throbbing ear pain. Tom's mother notes his hearing difficulty and his fear of the pain and possible hearing loss. On inspection, his tympanic membrane appears red and bulging.

MEDICAL DIAGNOSIS

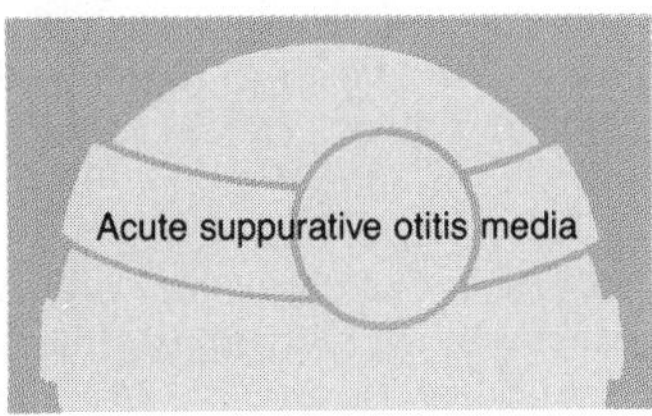

NURSING DIAGNOSIS

- Alterations in comfort; pain due to swollen tympanic membrane
- Fear due to progressive hearing loss
- Sensory perceptual alterations (hearing loss) due to related obstructed middle ear

ing with an altered health state. In the case of Mr. Jay, his subjective and objective data show that he's experiencing cardiovascular stress secondary to a hypertensive episode.

• Now, examine the data again to try to identify *why* this patient is having difficulty meeting the need(s) you've identified, or coping with his altered health state. Review of Mr. Jay's subjective data indicates that the probable cause of his problem is that he stopped taking his medication, thinking his hypertension was cured. He also lacked an understanding of hypertension and its management—or perhaps wished to deny its seriousness. The nursing diagnosis states Mr. Jay's problems in terms of their probable origin. The resulting nursing actions are designed to modify or resolve these problems.

7 How nursing and medical diagnoses differ

You assess your patient to obtain data for making a nursing diagnosis, just as the doctor examines him to establish a medical diagnosis. Learn the differences between the two, and remember that sometimes they overlap. You do a complete patient assessment to identify patient problems that your nursing intervention can help resolve. Your nursing diagnosis states these problems. (Some may occur secondary to medical treatment.) If you plan your care of a patient around only the medical aspects of his illness, you'll probably overlook other significant problems.

For example, suppose your patient's medical diagnosis is a fractured femur. In your assessment, take a careful history. Include questions to determine if he has adequate financial resources to cope with prolonged disability. Gather data about his previous life-style, too; this information will help you assess his capacity to adjust to the physical restrictions of his disability.

Let's presume your physical examination of this patient—in addition to uncovering signs and symptoms pertaining to his medical diagnosis—reveals actual or potential skin breakdown secondary to his immobility.

Your nursing diagnoses, then, will state such problems as difficulty in home management and lack of recreational activity (because of prolonged immobility) and include alteration or impairment in skin integrity.

The care plan you prepare for this patient should include the nursing interventions suggested by your nursing diagnoses, as well as the nursing actions necessary to fulfill the patient's medical treatment plan. Together, the nursing and medical diagnoses and care plans describe the complete nursing care your patient needs.

Completing the nursing process

8 After assessment: Planning

Relevant and accurate assessment data make your nursing care purposeful and direct you toward meeting stated patient goals. In the planning phase of the nursing process, you and your patient, through interaction and agreement, set mutual goals. Then, you decide what nursing actions are necessary to achieve your patient's goals, as in Mr. Jay's case.

To identify and write a patient goal, follow these steps:

• Translate the problem statement (nursing diagnosis) into a positive health statement. (Mr. Jay and his nurse decide that the goal is to decrease Mr. Jay's cardiovascular stress.)

• Establish criteria—the positive changes you'll look for in your patient's condition—by which you and the patient will know the goal has been met. To do this, modify the subjective and objective findings drawn from your initial assessment data to reflect potential for positive change. (Mr. Jay's criteria are to have at least one less sign or symptom, as well as a systolic pressure less than 150 mm Hg and a diastolic pressure less than 90 mm Hg.)

To identify appropriate nursing interventions, review the probable cause or origin of the problem. Then, design and implement nursing interventions that you think will resolve your patient's problem(s) by removing or modifying the cause.

9 After planning: Intervention

During the intervention phase, put your nursing-care plan into action. Your plan may require any (or all four) of the following essential nursing interventions:

- *therapeutic interventions* (such as administering antihypertensive medications to Mr. Jay)
- *teaching/counseling interventions* (such as teaching Mr. Jay how to perform self-monitoring procedures, how to take his medication, and how to reduce his sodium intake)
- *monitoring/assessment* interventions (such as recording Mr. Jay's vital signs, checking his fluid intake and output, monitoring his weight, and explaining to him the meaning of the hypertensive episode)
- *referral interventions* (such as instructing Mr. Jay to return to the clinic in 1 month, and to call anytime if problems develop).

10 After intervention: Evaluation/reassessment

The final phase of the nursing process is evaluation. You've completed your planned intervention, and now you must evaluate the results. How effective was your intervention? Did the patient get better or worse, or show no change? Have his goals for care been met? The nurse who took care of Mr. Jay evaluated his condition after her intervention, using the following steps. Use these steps in your own evaluations:

- Examine the results of your intervention, including whether or not you met the subjective and objective criteria established during the planning phase. (For Mr. Jay, the subjective criterion was that he would have at least one less sign or symptom; the objective criterion was that his blood pressure would be lowered.)
- Assess your patient for possible side effects and/or adverse effects of the nursing intervention.
- Analyze the results: Is your patient better? Why? Is your patient worse? Why? Is your patient the same? Why? Then, make a nursing judgment based on the data. This statement of your patient's current problem(s)—if any remain—is a *new nursing diagnosis.*
- Modify the care plan accordingly. If your data indicate that the problem is resolved, discontinue your intervention. If the data indicate improvement—to the extent that was anticipated—continue your intervention. But if the data show that the patient's condition is unchanged or has deteriorated, begin your investigative work again, with a new patient assessment. Your new nursing diagnosis indicates how you'll set new patient goals and what nursing actions you'll take to achieve them.

Selected References

Gordon, M., et al., "Nursing Diagnosis: Looking at Its Use in the Clinical Area," *American Journal of Nursing.* 80:4, April 1980.

Price, M.R., "Nursing Diagnosis: Making a Concept Come Alive," *American Journal of Nursing.* 80:4, April 1980.

Yura, Helen, and Mary B. Walsh, *The Nursing Process*, 3rd ed. New York: Appleton-Century-Crofts, 1978.

2

KEY POINTS IN THIS CHAPTER

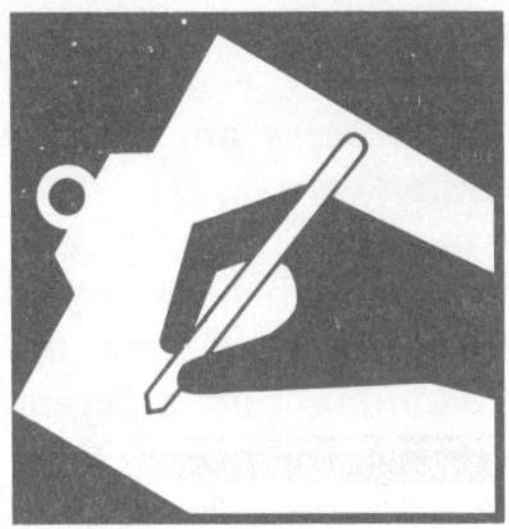

The Health History

Introduction

11 The importance of the health history

The health history is an organized body of information that tells what you need to know about a patient to examine him competently. It tells his age, present and past medical (and other) problems, and health-related activities. Obtain this information by interviewing the patient in a comfortable environment and recording his answers to your questions.

The health history is *the patient's story*. It provides the *subjective* data base for your assessment, to be supplemented by the objective data gathered during your physical examination of him. Your own observations and opinions shouldn't intrude in this assessment phase. Ideally, a health history tells the reader a great deal about your patient and nothing about you—except that you've mastered the skills necessary to be a good interviewer.

12 How the health history guides assessment

A thorough health history provides about 80% of the information you use in assessing a patient. Health history data not only describe the current state of a patient's health but also guide you in structuring the physical examination. For example, knowing a patient's chief complaint allows you to focus your examination on the involved body region. This information also helps you decide which of the four classic assessment skills—inspection, palpation, percussion, or auscultation—you'll use during the physical examination. Sometimes the physical examination serves merely to confirm the information that was obtained during the health history interview.

You can also use the health history interview to help your patient gain insight into his condition. Do this by asking questions that suggest relationships he may have overlooked. For example, let's say a patient tells you his chief complaint is that he's having trouble swallowing during meals. Later in the interview, he says his father died of throat cancer 2 years ago. Without dismissing the possibility that the patient's problem may be caused by the same condition, try to get him to explore the possible connection between these two facts. Ask if his difficulty in swallowing started (or got worse) around the time of his father's death. In this way, history-taking can be therapeutic in itself.

Your patient will cooperate with your history-taking efforts if your attitude during the interview promises help and support. Approach him considerately; then listen carefully and phrase your questions thoughtfully.

Mastering interviewing skills

13 The therapeutic nurse-patient relationship

You need empathy, compassion, self-awareness, and objectivity to promote a trusting relationship with your patient. Your behavior should demonstrate dependability and reliability, as well as respect for the confidential nature of the interview. Remember, the best way to establish a therapeutic nurse-patient relationship is to communicate to the patient that his thoughts and behavior are important to you.

Trust, the basis of all health-care relationships, takes time to develop—but the health history interview usually signals the *start* of your relationship with your patient. How can you gain his trust quickly, so the interview can proceed? First, be on time for the interview. To begin your conversation, ask the patient what name he prefers you to use in addressing him; use this name consistently throughout the interview. As the interview progresses, be sensitive to areas of information your patient seems reluctant to share, and respect his privacy concerning them.

14 How your attitudes can affect the interview

Your personal values and biases influence the course of your relationships with your patient—and sometimes create communication barriers (see diagram on page 17). During the health history interview, you need to recognize the ways in which your values and your reactions to the patient are influencing the interviewing process. For example, consider the nurse who, because of her personal values, can't understand or accept her patient's decision to have an abortion. She may become impatient, rude, and abrupt with the patient because of this. She then impedes the interviewing process and blocks appropriate nursing care.

As a nurse, you needn't give up your personal attitudes and beliefs to understand a patient's point of view. Instead, your recognition of his different perceptions as the interview progresses helps you explore every significant area of his experience objectively.

15 Understanding silence

Talking with another person involves silence as well as speech. Learn how and when to be silent during the health history interview. Listen carefully to what the patient says in response to your questions. Don't rush him or attempt to figure out what he's going to say before he says it. Sometimes accepting a few moments of silence until you or the patient feels like talking again can be therapeutic. Interpreting silences thoughtfully can greatly increase the effectiveness of your health history interviews.

To use silence effectively when interviewing a patient, imagine yourself in the patient's situation, keeping in mind the circumstances for his seeking health care. Of course, some people are normally less talkative than others. Or, the patient's lapse into silence may indicate that he's thinking carefully about how to answer your question. Give him time. But when your patient is unresponsive to your questions—whether throughout the discussion or just at a single point—you need to understand what's happening so the interview can continue.

In considering how you'll handle such situations, examine your own responses to silence—how *you* react when a patient doesn't reply to your questions. You probably feel anxious about how the interview is progressing. To relieve your anxiety, analyze the situation in terms of how the *patient* may be feeling, and respond to his need for reassurance. Perhaps you need to restate the question in a less threatening way. Keep your anxiety under control, and don't think of your patient's silence as a vacuum you must rush to fill. In addition, avoid labeling the patient as uncooperative, or otherwise interpreting his silence negatively.

Other reasons for a patient's silence do exist, of course. Maybe he's angry, fearful, or suspicious about the need for the interview, or about the kinds of questions you're asking. Help him relax by speaking calmly and reassuringly, and be sure you explain fully why the interview questions are important.

16 Understanding your patient's verbosity

Like the silent patient, the individual who is extremely talkative during the interview may be trying to avoid confronting anxiety by keeping you and your questions at a distance. As long as he's talking, he remains in control of the interview. When dealing with a talkative patient, strive to decrease his anxiety. Provide him gentle feedback about his talkativeness. Say something like: "I feel concerned that you haven't heard me, because you seem to be thinking about what to say next. It's

CONSIDERING COMMUNICATION BARRIERS

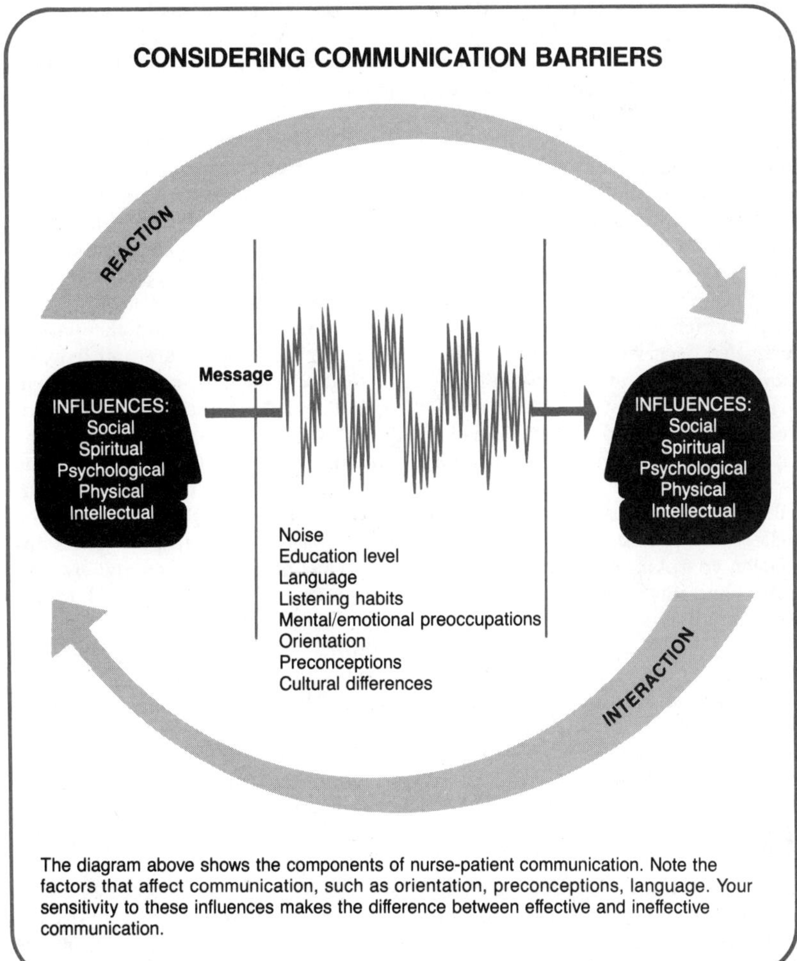

The diagram above shows the components of nurse-patient communication. Note the factors that affect communication, such as orientation, preconceptions, language. Your sensitivity to these influences makes the difference between effective and ineffective communication.

important to me that we understand each other." In addition to reminding him that you need to have his answers to your questions, this direct statement of the problem shows you're really interested in him and his responses.

Sometimes a patient who talks on and on can irritate you and frustrate your efforts to take a comprehensive health history. Be direct with him (without being offensive), and keep the discussion going so you can obtain the history information you need.

17 The fundamentals of successful interviewing

A sound knowledge of therapeutic interviewing skills can help you get a clear picture of your patient that can lead, in turn, to a complete and accurate physical assessment. During the health history interview you'll gather information about your patient's past and present health status. Straightforward questioning usually succeeds in eliciting most of this information. At times, however, you'll have to explore your patient's concerns about his condition, which can call for more sophisticated interviewing skills. In either situation, asking the right questions during the interview, listening attentively, and interpreting your patient's responses objectively and accurately are important.

Taking a health history involves both intellectual and motor skills. With your intellect, you plan and conduct the interview and interpret the results. Your motor activities consist of recording the data, as well as speaking, listening, and gesturing (to emphasize what you say). Coordinating these skills during an interview is difficult, but with experience you'll gain confidence in your interviewing technique.

18 Plan your approach to the interview

Your sense of timing is crucial to a successful interview, especially if your patient is hospitalized. A time convenient for you may not be convenient for your patient. Show him you're willing to let him have some control over his schedule. To enlist his cooperation, for example, say, "I'd like to spend some time talking with you about your health history. Is this a good time for you?" If the patient says no, find another time that's convenient for both of you.

Think about your patient's probable frame of mind, too, before approaching him for a health history interview. For example, if he just received distressing news from his doctor, postpone the interview until he has had time to absorb what he has learned. Keep your schedule flexible. If necessary, plan more than one interview session with your patient, especially if his history is detailed or if he's critically ill or debilitated.

19 The proper interview environment

Both you and the patient must be comfortable to communicate with each other effectively. If he's in pain, try to alleviate as much of his discomfort as possible before attempting to interview him. Make sure you and the patient agree on the temperature and lighting in the room. If the room is too warm or too cool, have the temperature adjusted (if possible), after asking the patient's permission; or, provide the patient with extra blankets or ventilation as necessary. If the room is too dark, you may have trouble maintaining eye contact with your patient and observing his gestures and facial expressions. Before you change the lighting, ask the patient's permission to do so. He may want the room dark because he has a headache or irritated eyes, or because he feels depressed. Explain why you want to change the lighting, too. For example, you might say something like: "I'd like to adjust the shades because sunlight is causing glare in your room. Is that all right with you?"

Make an effort to create a private environment for your talk with the patient. Try to avoid interruptions during the time you've set aside for the interview. If the patient is in a semiprivate room but ambulatory, you can take him to a quiet area outside the room. If the patient isn't ambulatory but his roommate is, you might ask the roommate to leave you alone with the patient for the length of time you need for the interview. If you can't achieve privacy with your patient in or outside his room, draw the curtains around the bed and speak in a low tone to convey respect for his privacy.

The interview setting should be quiet as well as private. If a television or radio is on in the room, ask the patient if you may turn it off or lower the volume. If the corridor or neighboring rooms are noisy and you can't move the patient to a quieter area, ask the noisy persons if they would mind keeping their voices down. Then close the patient's door.

By creating a comfortable, private, and quiet environment for the health history interview, you let your patient know you're interested in what he tells you, and that you respect the confidentiality of the information he shares with you.

20 Hospitalization anxiety and your patient

During a stay in the hospital, a patient passes through stages of adjustment—from denial to anger, to depression, to helplessness. To obtain the necessary history information from a patient whose attitude is blocking communication, accept and work with his particular emotional and behavioral responses. Try to determine the meaning of his behavior by looking at the interview through his eyes (see *Understanding the Patient's Point of View).* Then decide what verbal and nonverbal responses would be therapeutic.

In addition to the emotional responses a hospitalized patient has to his medical problems, he may feel dehumanized by the health-care system's rapid pace and advanced technology. Hospitalization can shut off his usual means of maintaining self-esteem. Furthermore, he may be frightened by loss of control over his body and his environment, because of illness. Forfeiting his normal daily routine and adapting to the hospital's schedule also may cause him anxiety.

If you sincerely communicate that you

UNDERSTANDING THE PATIENT'S POINT OF VIEW

You're not the only person gathering data when you perform a patient interview. Your patient is gathering data on you and—from his impression of you—on the whole health-care team. As you interview him, he's probably asking himself the following questions:

- What information does this nurse want?
- Does she care about me as a person or is she just filling out another form?
- Is she really listening to me? Can I confide in her?
- Will these people respond quickly when I need them? Are they competent?

How can you create a favorable impression on your patient? Follow these suggestions:

- Come to the interview well organized. Hunting for forms or for a working pen may cause the patient to doubt the quality of your hospital's management.
- Give the patient your undivided attention. Taking phone calls or frequently interrupting the interview for other reasons will lead the patient to think the interview —and his problems—aren't important to you.
- Be professional but friendly. Don't act so formally with the patient that he thinks you're not interested in his problems.
- Be nonjudgmental and open. You'll discourage the patient from talking if you avoid eye contact, adopt a cool tone, move about restlessly, or tap your pen impatiently.

By being sensitive to your patient's point of view, you'll not only compile a better interview, but you'll also make the patient more at ease.

care about your patient and his well-being, and respect his individual needs, you can reduce the dehumanizing effects of his hospital stay.

Strategies you can employ in helping your patient cope with hospitalization anxiety include obtaining his permission to perform certain procedures at particular times, discussing his food preferences with him, adjusting his sleeping schedule—and periods of rest and privacy—to reflect his wishes, and asking him how he wants to schedule visitors. Don't be afraid to discuss the patient's anxiety with him to help him understand its cause. The direct approach often works best. You might say something like: "Many times hospitalization and illness produce a lot of anxiety. These situations are often difficult, but I'll be glad to assist you in any way I can that will make this time easier for you."

21 Explain the importance of health history data

After introducing yourself to the patient, begin the interview by explaining the history's purpose so the patient understands why you'll be asking him personal questions. Remember, your attitude about history-taking is important. Be calm, relaxed, and unhurried. The patient who sees these qualities in you and also understands the purpose and importance of the history will be more apt to provide the information you need.

22 Conversational interviewing techniques

Communication is a continuous process by which we relate to our environment and other persons in it. All kinds of behavior that you use to interact with patients—verbal and nonverbal, consciously and unconsciously motivated—are forms of communication. In the health history interview, the way you direct the conversation can enhance the communication process—or hinder it. For example, the patient shouldn't have to defend himself. Use nonjudgmental and nonthreatening language. Say, "Tell me about..." or "What happened after..." "What was the experience like for you?" Don't say, "Why did you do that?" or "Explain your behavior."

Another conversational technique you can use is *reflecting*—repeating the patient's words back to him in an inquiring way. By using his words, you avoid adding your personal viewpoint to what he's said. And he's encouraged to continue his story.

Try *restating* or *summarizing* what the patient has just told you. If he confirms that you've understood him correctly, you can confidently move on to the next history question.

Mannerisms such as nodding to acknowledge what your patient's just said, saying "Yes" or "I see" when the patient pauses briefly, and maintaining eye contact with the patient are called *facilitation.* They let the patient know you're listening to him and want him to continue.

When you have to ask your patient for additional clarification about some point, don't make him feel he hasn't presented his story clearly. Preface your request for more information with "I'm not quite sure about..." or a similar approach. In this way you assume responsibility for not fully understanding what the patient said; you don't arouse defensive feelings.

In all these conversational techniques, the key element is *listening;* the more conscientiously you listen, the more skillfully you will interpret what your patient tells you and respond appropriately (see the chart on page 21). Listening attentively also allows you to identify recurring themes in your patient's history and to clarify any statements or issues you don't understand. Above all, you must let the patient know you care about him and want to know his problems.

23 How to communicate without words

The verbal and nonverbal exchanges

RESPONDING TO YOUR PATIENT APPROPRIATELY

How you direct the interview determines its fruitfulness. Your first step—listen effectively; your second step—respond appropriately. Phrase your statements to allow for the patient's response. Remember the interview's purpose: you're interested in *his* feelings, not your reactions to or judgments of these feelings. The responses outlined below encourage the patient to continue and elaborate on his story.

USING THE BEST RESPONSE

Patient's statement	Nurse's response	Purpose of response
"I just haven't felt comfortable since I went on this new treatment schedule."	"How are you handling your new treatment routine?"	*Open-ended questions* allow the patient to clarify and elaborate on his thoughts and feelings.
"I had a battery of tests done at my last doctor's appointment."	"When was your last doctor's visit?"	*Closed questions* direct the patient toward providing specific information.
"Right after New Year's Day, I went in for tests. At that time they found the cause of my abdominal pain immediately. I followed my medication very carefully, but I had to go back to the hospital again last month because the gastritis had started up again."	"So, this is your third visit this year. You were admitted in January and again in May, each time for gastritis."	*Restatement* (summarizing) clarifies meaning for your understanding as well as the patient's.
"My folks have gone out of their way recently to care for me and I'm grateful to them. But I find myself thinking back to just a month ago when I was completely on my own."	"It must be hard to be dependent on your parents after being independent for so long."	*Communicating support* (empathy) encourages the patient to continue and reflects your concern.
"I don't know... My family is so upset by my illness that I guess I've tried to ignore other treatment possibilities."	"You say your family has been so upset by your illness that you haven't explored alternative treatments."	*Reflecting* (echoing) allows the patient to evaluate his thoughts and feelings through your restatement of them.
"I guess what it comes down to is that I felt too guilty about being a burden."		*Silence* allows the patient to collect his thoughts and reflect on the conversation.

that occur between you and your patient during the first few minutes set the tone for the entire interview, and usually affect how much he'll cooperate with you. During the health history interview, you and the patient communicate on many levels simultaneously. Along with your careful choice of words, you communicate with your eyes, gestures, and facial expressions. Even the distance between you and the patient affects your ability to communicate.

Maintaining *eye contact* with your patient during the interview—without staring—can help close the physical and the psychological distance between you. Intermittent eye contact suffices to show your interest in the patient and your respect for his privacy. Suppose your patient refuses to make eye contact. He may feel embarrassed or hesitant about talking with you, or he may simply want to avoid the interview. When your patient won't look you in the eye, use conversational interviewing techniques, such as reflecting and restating, to involve him in the discussion. Examine your own willingness to make eye contact, too. You may need to practice this technique with patients. As your confidence increases, so will the effectiveness of your interviewing technique.

Gestures often speak louder than words. When your patient says he'll put his belongings in "that closet" and points to the closet, the meaning of his gesture is clear. But sometimes a patient's gestures express feelings he's unaware of—or doesn't want to reveal. If he taps his fingers continuously on the table while you're questioning him, crosses and uncrosses his legs, sighs deeply, or coughs repeatedly, he's probably tense, anxious, or bored. Your interpretation of such gestures can help you assess your patient's mood and structure the interview accordingly. Be sure you've interpreted his gestures correctly before you respond. If you're not sure what his gesture means (or whether it has any particular significance), make the patient aware of it and explore the matter further, if necessary.

Your patient's *facial expressions* can also tell you a lot about him. Like gestures, facial expressions can have direct or indirect meaning. They're probably the most common form of nonverbal communication. A smile, for instance, may be a happy greeting, or it may be a mask for sadness or pain. Some people need to present themselves as strong and always in control; they may use a smile to cover up their pain or anxiety.

Listen closely. Sometimes a patient's words don't match his facial expression; this is called *incongruency*. If he says, "I'm fine, no problems" but looks sad and tearful, he needs your encouragement to talk about his feelings. To help, say something like: "I'm concerned about you. You say you're fine, but you look unhappy. How can I help?"

Be aware of *your* facial expression, too. A patient usually notices it before he notices anything else about you. Keep this in mind when you approach a patient to interview him.

Posture and *body appearance* are additional ways in which you communicate with patients. Your positive self-image gives the patient confidence and also shows your concern for what he may think of you. In turn, observation of your patient's appearance can give you important clues about his body image, self-esteem, and hygienic practices.

The *space* or *distance* you put between yourself and others affects your ability to communicate. On the one hand, if you attempt to interview your patient while standing or sitting too near to him, he'll probably feel uncomfortable and react accordingly. On the other hand, if you talk with a patient who's in bed while you're standing in the doorway of his room, he'll be reluctant to communicate; he can't be sure you really want to make contact. Many people feel more comfortable sitting at an angle with respect to another person, perhaps with a small table or stand between them, which gives each person a sense of his own space.

Of course, the most comfortable distance between you and your patient during the history interview varies with individual patients and interviewing situations. Let your awareness of your own comfort and sensitivity to your patient's wishes guide you.

24 Interviewing the family and extended family

A family usually consists of a husband, wife, and children; this unit is known as the *nuclear* family. *Extended-family* members (also called *significant others*) include grandparents and other relatives. A person's family gives him his strongest sense of community and generally lends stability and security to his life.

Your patient's hospitalization has

great impact on the well-being and functioning of his family. By sharing information about his condition with his family, you can decrease their anxiety and increase their cooperation.

Of course, you interview the patient himself to record his health history, if possible. If he is too ill, or if you suspect his history information isn't completely reliable, talk with a family member or friend—after obtaining the patient's permission to do so. Reassure the patient and his family that you'll keep this information confidential.

Family members often help you validate, clarify, and elaborate on the patient's history, especially his daily activities. For example, you may learn that the patient frequently overindulges in alcoholic beverages, or that he hasn't told you of recent stressful events. In addition, observing the interaction between the patient and family members may give you clues to his role and responsibilities in the family, and to the strength and character of his relationships with family members.

Of course, the basic principles of interviewing patients apply when you interview your patient's relatives and friends. Never give a family member information without your patient's permission or you risk undermining his trust in you. For example, a husband and wife in the process of getting a divorce may not want to share personal information with each other. You wouldn't disclose information to either one without the other's consent.

When you interview someone close to the patient who isn't part of his family, be sure to note the nature of the relationship and the length of time the individual has known the patient. For instance, in your documentation, write something like this: *Information received from John Jones, a friend, who has lived with the patient for 3 years.*

Taking and recording the health history

25 Develop effective history-taking methods

Health history data must be recorded in an organized fashion, so the information will be meaningful to everyone involved in a patient's care. Some hospitals provide patient questionnaires or computerized checklists for gathering history data. These forms make history-taking easier, but they're not always available. Therefore, you must know how to take a comprehensive health history without them. This is easy to do if you develop an orderly and systematic method of interviewing. Ask the history questions in the same order every time. With experience, you'll know which types of questions to ask in specific patient situations.

No matter which format you use, be sure to record negative findings as well as positive ones. Note the absence of symptoms that other history data indicate could be present. For example, if a patient reports pain and burning in his abdomen, ask him if he has experienced nausea and vomiting, or noticed blood in his stool. Record the presence *or* absence of these symptoms.

26 How to record precise history data

While recording history data, remember that the information will be used by others who'll also care for the patient. It may even be used as a legal document in a liability case, malpractice suit, or insurance disability claim. With these considerations in mind, record history data precisely. Continue your questioning until you're satisfied you've recorded sufficient detail. Don't be satisfied with inadequate answers, such as *a lot* or *a little.* These words mean different things to different people and must be explained to be meaningful. If the patient seems anxious about your note-taking at any point during the interview, explain the importance of it so he'll feel more at ease. To facilitate accurate recording of your patient's answers, familiarize yourself with standard history data abbreviations.

27 The parts of a complete health history

A complete health history provides the following information about a patient:
- biographical data
- chief complaint (or concern)
- history of present illness (or current health status)
- past history
- family history
- psychosocial history
- activities of daily living
- review of systems.

Follow this orderly format in taking your patient's history, but allow for modifications on the basis of your patient's chief complaint or concern. For example, the health history of a patient with a localized allergic reaction will be much shorter than that of a patient who complains vaguely of mental confusion and severe headaches.

A patient may not even have a chief complaint; he may be feeling fine and simply seeking a complete physical checkup. Such a patient's health history would be comprehensive, with detailed information about his life-style, self-image, family and other interpersonal relationships, and degree of satisfaction with his current health.

The health history of a patient who has a chief complaint must provide information to help you decide if your patient's problems are from physical pathology or psychophysiologic maladaptation, as well as how your nursing care can help him. The depth of such a history depends on the patient's cooperation and your skill in asking insightful questions.

ELICITING THE CHIEF COMPLAINT

Here are several tips you can use to elicit your patient's chief complaint:
- Ask open-ended questions. This lets the patient explain the problem in his own words. Closed questions may affect the patient's word choice and discourage him from elaborating. For example, don't say, "Do you feel all right today?" Instead, say, "What can we do to help you?"
- Emphasize the positive when questioning, and avoid making assumptions, so the patient feels less threatened. If you act negatively, or as if you already know what his problem is, you'll put him on the defensive and discourage him from continuing. For example, don't say: "What's wrong now?" Instead, say, "Can I help you in any way?"
- Help the patient who's confused or noncommittal to clarify his feelings by gradually using more directed questions. Avoid abrupt or embarrassing questions. Here's an example of how you can tactfully clarify the patient's answer to one of your questions:

NURSE: "What brought you here today?"
PATIENT: "I just don't feel right."
NURSE: "You don't feel like your usual self?"
PATIENT: "That's for sure!"
NURSE: "In what ways don't you feel like you usually feel?"
PATIENT: "I'm awful tired and dizzy lately."
NURSE: "You say you feel tired and dizzy. When do you feel that way?"

28 Biographical data

Begin the health history interview by collecting biographical data about your patient. This includes the following information: full name, address, telephone number, sex, age, date of birth, race, marital status, nationality, religion (optional), occupation, and source of referral. If any of this information is available in the patient's medical record, hospital admission form, or some other document in his file, don't ask him for it again. Just ask him if the information you have is correct.

Aside from the obvious purpose of identifying the patient, this part of the health history helps you assess the patient's reliability as an informant, since

ANALYZING THE HISTORY OF PRESENT ILLNESS

When discussing the history of present illness with your patient, make sure he describes his problems fully. To do this, ask him the following questions about each complaint:

- *Time of onset.* When was the first date (the problem) happened? What time did it begin?
- *Type of onset.* How did (the problem) start: suddenly? gradually?
- *Original source.* What were you doing when you first experienced or noticed (the problem)? What seems to trigger it: stress? position? certain activities? arguments? If describing a discharge: thick? runny? clear? colored? If describing a psychological problem: Do the voices drown out other sounds? Whose voice does it sound like?
- *Severity.* How bad is (the problem) when it's at its worst? Does it interfere with your normal activities? Does it force you to lie down, sit down, slow down?
- *Radiation.* In the case of pain, does it travel down your back or arms, up your neck, or down your legs?
- *Time relationship.* How often do you experience (the problem): hourly? daily? weekly? monthly? When do you usually experience it: daytime? at night? in the early morning? Are you ever awakened by it? Does it ever occur before, during, or after meals? Does it occur seasonally?
- *Duration.* How long does an episode of (the problem) last?
- *Course.* Does (the problem) seem to be getting better, to be getting worse, or does it remain the same?
- *Associations.* Does (the problem) lead to anything else? Is it accompanied by other signs and symptoms?
- *Source of relief.* What relieves (the problem): changing diet? changing position? taking medications? being active?
- *Source of aggravation.* What makes (the problem) worse?

You can remember *all* these questions using the letters PQRST:

P — *Provocative/Palliative*
What causes it? What makes it better? What makes it worse?

Q — *Quality/Quantity*
How does it feel, look, or sound, and how much of it is there?

R — *Region/Radiation*
Where is it? Does it spread?

S — *Severity scale*
Does it interfere with activities? How does it rate on a severity scale of 1 to 10?

T — *Timing*
When did it begin? How often does it occur? Is it sudden or gradual?

his chart usually already contains correct biographical data. If you can't obtain this information from the patient, or if you're not certain about the patient's reliability as an informant, try to interview a friend or relative. Be sure to identify the informant in the health history.

29 Chief complaint (or concern)

For this part of the health history, ask the patient to briefly describe his reason for seeking health care. The best way to prompt a patient to identify his chief complaint or concern is to ask him an open-ended question (see *Eliciting the Chief Complaint,* page 24). Record his response, in his own words, using quotation marks.

Don't elaborate on the chief complaint or concern in this section of the history. If the patient has more than one complaint, record each one separately; if he doesn't have a chief complaint, record his reason for requesting a physical examination.

30 History of present illness

This is probably the most challenging part of the health history and requires adept questioning and an adequate knowledge base. Begin by asking your patient to describe the progression of his chief complaint or concern, from the time it started to the present. Skillful questioning will clarify the clinical ramifications of the chief complaint and provide the framework for your nursing diagnosis. Ask general questions about the chief complaint at first, to give the patient direction in describing it chronologically. To do this effectively, ask only open-ended questions. You might say, "Tell me about your problem, from when it first began until now." Don't suggest answers or interrupt the patient while he's talking.

When the patient finishes recalling the history of his illness and associated symptoms, you may need to ask questions that will elicit further essential information. Question him directly about each symptom, using the PQRST mnemonic device (see *Analyzing the History of Present Illness,* page 25). Record negative findings if they help to clarify the significance of symptom clusters. Such findings are often critical in completing an accurate clinical picture.

31 Past history

A comprehensive survey of a patient's past history provides you with information about his previous major health problems, his experiences with the health-care system, and his attitude toward it. This part of the health history (see sample form on page 27) usually yields important clues about the patient's present condition. It also helps determine the treatment plan and may suggest the patient's prognosis.

Ask your patient about the following elements of his past history:

• *Childhood and infectious diseases.* Concentrate your questioning on diseases with sequelae. For example, if a patient reports he had rheumatic fever, determine if the disease was diagnosed by a doctor, how old the patient was when he contracted it, and whether he is taking antistreptococcal drugs prophylactically.

• *Immunizations.* Vaccinations for poliomyelitis and rubella are especially important, since these diseases can affect unvaccinated adults and pose serious risks for women of childbearing age. Don't forget to ask about vaccinations your patient may have received in the armed forces or before a recent trip to a foreign country.

• *Accidents.* Consider your patient's history of accidents apart from his history of illnesses. Does he appear to be accident-prone? If injuries suffered in an accident have potential legal implications, record as many details about the accident as your patient can provide. Don't forget to ask specifically about fractures, since patients frequently forget to mention broken bones from childhood accidents. A good way to elicit this information is to ask the patient if he was ever treated in an emergency department.

• *Surgical procedures and hospitalizations.* For this part of the past history, ask the patient if he's had any major illnesses that required hospitalization or surgery. His chief complaint may be associated with a previous illness. When

DOCUMENTING

RECORDING THE PATIENT'S PAST HISTORY

Childhood and infectious diseases: Measles, German Measles, Chickenpox

Immunizations: DPT, TOPV, Can't remember others

Surgical procedures/hospitalizations: 1976 - Tonsillectomy and Adenoidectomy
1981 - Appendectomy, uncomplicated

Accidents: 1965 - Broken arm, uncomplicated

Allergies: None known

Current medications: ASA gr. X 3-4 times daily

asking your patient about such previous surgery, include mention of common procedures like tonsillectomy and appendectomy. Record information in this section chronologically, listing events by date or by the patient's age at the time of hospitalization or surgery.

• *Allergies.* To determine the cause of an allergic reaction, ask the patient for precise details of the precipitating circumstances. Inquire about allergies to foods, medications, substances (such as soap), and textiles. Asking about medications is especially important, since patients often confuse drug side effects with true allergic reactions.

• *Current medications.* Knowing the medications a patient is taking provides helpful information about a chronic illness. It can also help explain a medical condition that may have occurred secondary to drug toxicity or overdose. Be sure to ask your patient about over-the-counter *and* prescription drugs. Use brand names and nonmedical terms so he understands your questions. And be alert for clues that suggest he needs patient teaching. For example, if you suspect that your patient's condition stems from a drug interaction, discuss it with him so he'll be aware of this danger in the future. Also, notify the doctor. Knowing all you can about your patient's current medications can prevent drug interactions and also help identify drugs that may affect laboratory tests.

32 Family history

A brief description of the medical history of the patient's family helps to identify familial patterns common to some illnesses. For example, diabetes mellitus, migraine headaches, heart disease, and hypercholesterolemia all have hereditary tendencies. Ask your patient if anyone in his family had allergies, asthma, tuberculosis, hypertension, heart disease, or a stroke. Inquire about anemia, hemophilia, ar-

CHARTING THE FAMILY HISTORY

An easy way to keep track of your patient's family history is by using a genogram. The three-tiered genogram shown here displays three generations.

First, draw a family tree. Enter the age and major medical problems of each family member who is living. Then, enter the age at death and cause of death of each deceased relative. This system readily displays illnesses common to several family members.

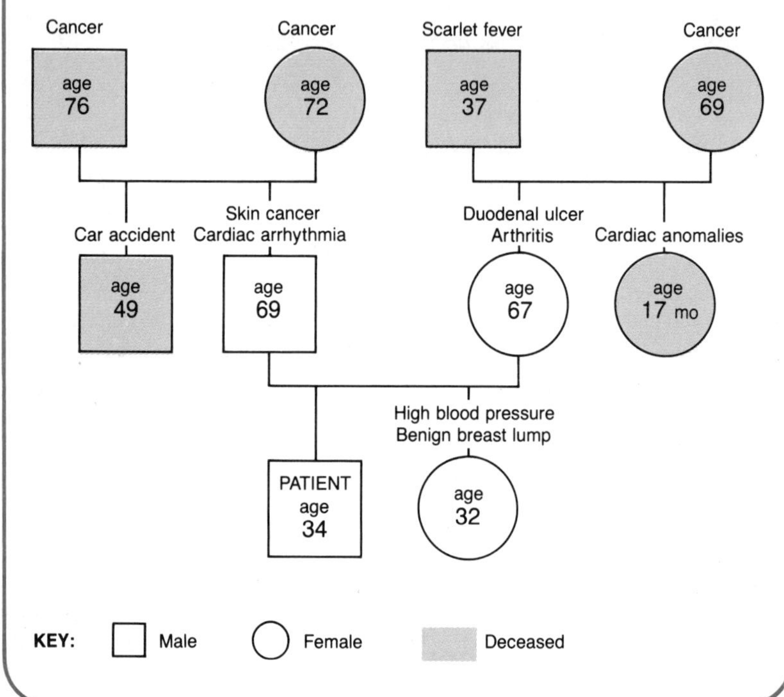

thritis, migraine headaches, diabetes, cancer, and emotional problems. As in the portion of the history dealing with present illness, record negative findings as well as positive ones.

You can use a written statement and a diagram to record and depict your patient's family history. A family tree diagram showing the age and general health of each living family member, and the cause of death of each deceased family member, can help you trace hereditary disease patterns (see *Charting the Family History*).

Knowing something about the general physical and emotional health of the patient's family may help you to better understand his illness. A patient's family, for example, can be a source of stress, which may underlie the chief complaint. When appropriate, explore your patient's family relationships. With whom does he live? What are his family relationships like? Inquire about previous and current marriages, and find out if your patient has any children. If remarried, how does he compare his present family with his original family? Ask, too, how far away extended-family members live, and how important they are to your patient as sources of physical, emotional, and economic support. Can he describe the family members with whom he has the closest relationships?

Determine if the patient's illness has affected the way the family lives. Does the patient have concerns about his family? Ask if there have been other major family changes recently besides his illness. Is the family financially able to cope with crises?

Have there been family conflicts over money, sex, childbearing, religion? Which topics are openly discussed among family members? Which are never discussed? Don't forget to ask about positive factors in the patient's family, the sources of harmony as well as discord.

Unless your questions uncover strong indications of a possible hereditary cause of your patient's problems, ask only about the immediate family's health. Where possibilities of hereditary factors do exist, follow up with further questioning in these areas.

33 Psychosocial history

To formulate an effective nursing diagnosis, you often have to know a lot more than just the status of the patient's physical health; you have to consider certain aspects of his personal life as well. The psychosocial history serves this purpose. Here you're seeking to define the patient in terms of his place in society, relationships with others, and satisfaction with self.

The patient's reason for seeking health care determines the kinds of questions you ask in this part of the health history interview. For example, if the patient's illness requires him to change activities of daily living significantly, then asking about his *place of residence* is appropriate. Ask where he lives, and in what kind of house or apartment. How are the rooms and furniture arranged? How many flights of stairs does he have to climb? Does the layout of the house pose any health hazards?

Inquire whether there are shops near your patient's house. Does he have a way of getting to them? Does the community provide adequate recreational opportunities? If so, does he take advantage of them? Explain to your patient that all this information will be used to help him adjust to his illness after returning home from the hospital.

If your patient expresses concern about being able to cope with financial pressures, ask about his *economic situation.* Before asking these questions, explain that this type of information helps you to identify patients who need referral for financial assistance.

Is his annual income adequate for his needs and the standard of living he prefers? What kind of insurance (if any) does he have? If he seems to be preoccupied with financial matters, help him determine how much income goes toward maintaining his standard of living and how much toward paying medical bills.

If a patient's chief complaint seems related to his work, record further *occupational information.* Appropriate queries include the following: How long have you held your present job? How would you describe the responsibilities of your position? Does the job entail any health hazards, such as exposure to chemicals, heavy metals, or excessive dust or noise levels?

Explore the patient's feelings about his job. Is it satisfying, or a source of constant frustration? Does his present condition interfere with the performance of his usual duties? Your patient's past occupational history and military service record may be helpful here, too.

Questions relating to the patient's social life may also be pertinent. Does the patient have friends whom he sees regularly? If so, how often does he see them? Do they provide emotional support in times of trouble? Does he have one friend who is closer to him than anyone else?

The patient's methods of coping with past *medical* or *emotional* crises may be revealing. Ask what worked best for him during these difficult times. What

SURVEYING THE ACTIVITIES OF DAILY LIVING

Recording daily activities can provide you with a comprehensive view of your patient's history. To learn as much as possible, ask the patient all these questions:

Diet/Elimination
- How would you describe your appetite?
- What do you normally eat in a 24-hour period?
- What do you like and dislike to eat? Is your diet restricted in any way?
- How much fluid do you drink during an average day?
- Are you allergic to any foods?
- When do you usually go to the bathroom? Has this pattern changed in any way recently?
- Do you take any foods, fluids, or drugs to help you maintain your normal bowel and urination pattern?

Exercise/Sleep
- Do you have any special exercise program? What kind? How long have you been following it? How do you feel after exercising?
- How many hours do you sleep each day? When? Do you feel rested afterward?
- Do you fall asleep easily?
- Do you take any drugs or do anything special to help you fall asleep?
- What do you do when you can't sleep?
- Do you awake during the night?
- Do you have sleepy spells during the day? When?
- Do you take naps routinely?

Recreation
- What do you do when you're working?
- What kind of nonpaid work do you do for enjoyment?
- How much leisure time do you have?
- Are you satisfied with what you can do in your leisure time?
- Do you and your family share leisure time?
- How do your weekends differ from your weekdays?

Tobacco/Alcohol/Drugs
- Do you use tobacco? What kind do you use? How much do you use each day? Each week? For how long have you used it? Have you ever tried to stop?
- Do you drink any alcoholic beverages?
- How much alcohol do you drink each day? Each week? What time of day do you drink, usually?
- What kind (beer, wine, whiskey) do you drink?
- Do you usually drink alone or with others?
- Do you drink more when you're under stress?
- Has drinking ever hampered your job performance?
- Do you or your family worry about your drinking?
- Do you feel dependent on alcohol, coffee, tea, or soft drinks? How much of these other beverages do you drink in an average day?
- Do you take any drugs not prescribed by a doctor (marijuana, sleeping pills, tranquilizers)?

proved least effective or did more harm than good?

One of the most difficult parts of taking a psychosocial history may be asking your patient questions about his *sex life.* Effective communication about this delicate subject depends on how comfortably you can discuss the subject and how well you choose appropriate words and phrases. Questions about a patient's sex life are necessary whenever the patient's illness appears related to sexual function. Before you proceed, bear in mind that the patient may never have discussed his sex life with a health-care professional before. Try to put him at ease by using words you think he'll be comfortable with. Phrase your questions in such a way that you encourage the patient to discuss this part of his life without putting undue pressure on him. You might begin by saying, "Are you having any problems with your sexual functioning that you'd care to discuss?" Point out the importance of this information in your assessment of his illness.

As you proceed with this line of questioning, observe the patient's nonverbal behavior carefully. He may become uneasy or uncommunicative. Remind him several times during the

REVIEW OF SYSTEMS: AREAS TO COVER

Use this review of systems as a guide. Ask the patient, in your own words, if he has experienced or noticed any of the following:

General: Overall state of health, ability to carry out ADL, weight changes, fatigue, exercise tolerance, fever, night sweats, repeated infections

Skin: Changes in color, pigmentation, temperature, moisture, or hair distribution; eruptions; pruritus; scaling; bruising; bleeding; dryness; excess oiliness; growths; moles; scars; rashes; scalp lesions; brittle, soft, or abnormally formed nails; cyanotic nail beds

Head: Trauma, lumps, alopecia, headaches

Eyes: Near-sightedness, far-sightedness, glaucoma, cataracts, blurring of vision, double vision, problem with tearing, burning, itching, photophobia, pain, inflammation, swelling, color blindness, injuries. Also ask about use of glasses and date of last checkup.

Ears: Deafness, tinnitus, vertigo, discharge, pain, tenderness behind the ears, mastoiditis, otitis or other ear infections, earaches, ear surgery.

Nose: Sinusitis, discharge, colds, coryza more than four times a year; rhinitis, trauma, sneezing, loss of sense of smell, obstruction, breathing problems, epistaxis

Mouth/throat: Sores on tongue, dental caries, loss of teeth, toothaches, bleeding gums, lesions, loss of taste, hoarseness, sore throats (streptococcal), tonsillitis, voice changes, dysphagia. Also ask about date of last checkup, use of dentures or bridges.

Neck: Pain, stiffness, swelling, limited movement

Breasts: Change in development or lactation pattern, trauma, lumps, pain, discharge from nipples, gynecomastia, changes in contour or in nipples, mastectomy

Cardiovascular: Palpitations, tachycardia, or other irregularities; pain in chest; dyspnea on exertion; paroxysmal nocturnal dyspnea; orthopnea; cough; cyanosis; edema, ascites; intermittent claudication; cold extremities; phlebitis; postural hypotension; hypertension; rheumatic fever. Also ask if EKG has been performed recently.

Respiratory: Dyspnea, shortness of breath, pain, wheezing, paroxysmal nocturnal dyspnea, orthopnea (number of pillows used), cough, sputum, hemoptysis, night sweats, emphysema, pleurisy, bronchitis, tuberculosis (contacts), pneumonia, asthma, other upper respiratory tract infections. Also ask about results of chest X-ray and tuberculin skin test.

Gastrointestinal: Changes in appetite or weight, dysphagia, nausea, vomiting, heartburn, eructation, flatulence, abdominal pain, colic, hematemesis, jaundice (pain, fever, intensity, duration, color of urine), stools (color, frequency, consistency, odor, frequent use of laxatives), hemorrhoids, rectal bleeding, changes in bowel habits

Renal-genitourinary: Color of urine, polyuria, oliguria, nocturia (number of times per night), dysuria, frequency, urgency, problem with stream, dribbling, pyuria, retention, passage of stones or gravel, venereal disease (discharge), infections, perineal rashes and irritations. Also ask if protein or sugar is present in urine.

Reproductive: male–Lesions, impotency, prostate problems. Also ask about use of contraceptives; **female**–Irregular bleeding, discharge, pruritus, pain on intercourse (dyspareunia), protrusions, dysmenorrhea, vaginal infections. Also ask about number of pregnancies; dates of deliveries; complications; abortions; about onset, regularity, and amount of flow during menarch; last normal period; use of contraceptives; date of menopause; last Pap test.

Nervous: Headaches, convulsions, fits, seizures, fainting spells, dizziness, tremors, twitches, aphasia, loss of sensation, weakness, paralysis, balance problems

Psychiatric: Changes in mood, anxiety, depression, inability to concentrate

Musculoskeletal: Muscle pain, swelling, redness, pain in joints, back problems, injuries (i.e., broken bones, pulled tendons), numbness, tingling, balance problems, gait problems, weakness, paralysis, deformities, limited motion

Hematopoietic: Anemia (type, degree, treatment, response), bleeding, fatigue, bruising. Also ask patient if he's receiving anticoagulant therapy.

Endocrine, metabolism: Polyuria, polydipsia, polyphagia, thyroid problem, heat-cold intolerance, excessive sweating, changes in hair distribution and amount, nervousness, swelling neck (goiter), sugar in urine.

discussion that if any question makes him uncomfortable, he doesn't have to answer it. If he doesn't want to discuss his sex life at all, don't persist. Say you'll be available to discuss the topic at another time, if he wishes. Just note his discomfort and that he chooses not to discuss his sex life.

If the patient's chief complaint seems directly related to his sex life, ask him if he is currently sexually active. If so, tactfully ask whether he's satisfied with his sex life. Does he use any form of contraception? How does he protect against contracting a sexually transmitted disease? Other possible lines of questioning include asking the patient if there's anything he would like to change about his sex life.

34 Activities of daily living

This part of the health history describes your patient's activities during the course of a normal day. Your questions help determine how his personal habits affect his health. Ease your way into this series of questions by asking the patient to describe a normal day. What does he usually do? Where does he go? Whom does he see? Then ask specific questions (see *Surveying the Activities of Daily Living*, page 30) about each of these four categories:

- diet and elimination
- exercise and sleep
- recreation
- tobacco, alcohol, and drug use.

The answers to these questions will help you better understand the patient's problems and plan appropriate nursing interventions. They may also indicate a need for patient teaching. For example, if your patient says he can't sleep without first having an alcoholic drink, explore this point and discuss other means of ensuring a good night's sleep.

35 Review of systems

For this part of the health history, review the major body systems (and certain body regions) to find out if your patient is having (or has had) cardinal signs and symptoms of systemic disorders. You may use a prepared checklist or a standard form for this part of the health history, to facilitate recording and to serve as a memory aid (see chart on page 31). Although medical terminology is used on these checklists or forms, substitute or add simpler terms, when necessary, to help the patient understand exactly what you're asking. Remember that the information you record, like the rest of the health history, must be subjective data. The patient *tells* you whether he's had any of these signs or symptoms.

If the patient reports a sign or symptom that seems to be related to his present illness, explore it further with questions like those asked during the *history of present illness* part of the health history. (Don't forget to record all pertinent negative signs and symptoms.) Your notes from this part of the history should adequately review the body system affected by your patient's chief complaint. Don't ask the patient to repeat this information during the review of body systems unless something remains unclear or you feel you need more specific information. When your discussion gets to the affected system, refer in your notes to the earlier information.

36 The health history: A perspective

Once you complete your patient's health history, it becomes part of his permanent written record. It will serve as a subjective data base with which you and other health-care professionals can monitor the patient's progress. Remember that history data must be specific and precise. Avoid vague generalities. Instead, provide pertinent, concise, detailed information that will help determine the direction and sequence of the physical examination—the next phase in your patient assessment. When finished, your patient's complete health history may resemble the sample on the opposite page.

DOCUMENTING

CASE IN POINT: HISTORY OF AN ILL ADULT

Patient: Marian Miller

Address: 2654 N. 76th Street

Vital statistics:

Age 35 Wt 130 lbs. P 78

Ht 64" BP 126/78 R 18

Chief complaint: 1. Dizziness 2. Fatigue 3. Joint pain

HISTORY OF PRESENT ILLNESS

light-headed, loses balance 4-5 times per day for last 2 years. Diagnosed 2/15/76. NOT related to any special activity, but is hungry after "attack." Takes candy, which relieves symptoms.

PAST HISTORY

Major illnesses, operations, and hospitalizations (include dates): 1972-Delivered male child, 1975-Delivered female child Rheumatoid Arthritis 1976 to present

Treatment: Occasional use of dry heat to painful knees.

Medication: Aspirin 600 mg with meals and @ bedtime

Allergies: Food None Drug None Other None

FAMILY HISTORY

Hereditary illnesses: None

Family members in home:

Name	Age	Health	Occupation
Husband	36 years	good	sales
daughter	2 years	good	—
son	5 years	good	—

Changes in family routine, employment, relationships, or prior goals/values: None

PSYCHOSOCIAL HISTORY

Present mental status:

Alert ✓ confused ___ forgetful ___ disoriented ___ lethargic ___

Comments: Oriented to time, place, and person

Present behavior:

Cooperative ✓ anxious ___ depressed ✓ demanding ___

CASE IN POINT: HISTORY OF AN ILL ADULT *(continued)*

distrustful ______ lethargic ______ talkative ✓ withdrawn ______

Comments: worries about further disability from RA

Mental status and behavior prior to illness: good

Environment:

Adequate space ✓ cleanliness yes safety hazards no

Comments: house is all on one level with few stairs

Financial status:

Family concerned about income no present job none education college (2 years)

Employment:

Interruption for patient due to illness ______ interruption for family to give care ______

emotional reaction ______ Comments: housewife

ACTIVITIES OF DAILY LIVING

Needs assistance in:

Mobility ✓ hygiene ______ dressing ✓ feeding ______ shopping ______

meal preparation ______ housework ✓ laundry ✓ banking ______

Comments: needs more assistance in morning

Sleep:

Hours 7-8 naps sometimes aids no insomnia no due to: ______

Comments: ______

Activities:

Reading ✓ TV ✓ games ______ cards ✓ handwork ✓

Limitations imposed by illness: handwork, housework, child care

Visitors: ______ Comments: Has person come into house to help with child care and housework

Habits:

Alcohol no tobacco no drugs no Comments: ______

REVIEW OF SYSTEMS

Skin:

Description (dryness, color, turgor): oily, good color, firm

rashes none location ______ lesions none location ______

lotions or aids Hand lotion Comments: ______

Vision:

No difference ✓ glasses ______ last examination ______ blurring ______

diplopia ______ pain ______ inflammation ______ cataracts ______ glaucoma ______

Comments: ______

Hearing:

No difference ✓ limitations ______ aid ______ pain ______ tinnitus ______

discharge ______ Comments: ______

Respiratory:

No difference ✓ pain ______ dyspnea ______ cough ______ sputum ______

sinusitis ______ epistaxis ______ frequent colds ______ last chest X-ray ______

results ______ Comments: ______

Circulatory:

No difference ✓ edema ______ numbness ______ syncope ______

dizziness ______ cyanosis ______ anemia ______ bruising ______ chest pain ______

palpitations ______ congenital defect ______

Comments: ______

Gastrointestinal:

Nutrition:

No difference ✓ steady appetite good proper diet ______

adequate fluid 6-7 glasses difficulty chewing no dental status good due to: ______

meal/snack pattern 3 meals 4/5 snacks dysphagia no nausea no vomiting no

Comments: ______

Elimination:

No difference ✓ elimination pattern 1-2 days constipation ______ diarrhea ______

incontinence ______ ileostomy ______ colostomy ______ who cares for: ______

Comments: ______

Urinary:

No difference ✓ urine color clear, amber incontinence ______ nocturia ______

hematuria ______ UTI ______ stones ______ dribbling ______ catheter type ______

size ______ reason ______ date inserted ______ removed ______

Comments: ______

Nervous:

No difference ✓ incoordination ______ convulsions ______ paralysis ______

parasthesias ______ weakness ______

Comments: ______

Musculoskeletal:

No difference ______ deformities ______ pain ✓ stiffness ✓ on arising

contractures none arthritis see PH exercises 3Xday done by self

Comments: takes rests between exercises

Reproductive:

No difference ✓ menses problem ______ last Pap test 1/15

results Neg. menopause ______ breast self-examination monthly

infection ______ prostate problems ______ Comments: ______

Managing communication problems

37 Patients' attitudes toward health and illness

Most of your patients' backgrounds and health beliefs vary somewhat from yours. In the health history interview, explore your patient's background, lifestyle, values, norms, and experiences with the health-care system. Try to identify major influences that might affect his adaptation to hospital care. For example, suppose your patient is a 70-year-old woman who is an Orthodox Jew and lives alone. She enters the hospital, for the first time in her life, for exploratory surgery to rule out colorectal cancer.

Several factors may influence this woman's adjustment to hospitalization. Her age, first of all, is an obvious factor, since elderly people experience a great deal of stress on entering a hospital. Second, her religious beliefs, especially as they relate to dietary restrictions, will have to be taken into consideration. The fact that this is her first hospitalization—for an unknown and possibly fatal illness—will significantly affect her ability to adapt to hospitalization. Lastly, the fact that this woman, who is used to being independent, may now become dependent on others will have considerable bearing on her hospital stay.

Consider, too, that certain types of questions and behaviors considered inappropriate in one culture may be sanctioned in another. For example, in some cultures, loud and prolonged weeping and wailing when someone dies is part of the grieving experience. In our culture, we usually mourn quietly and try to control our emotions.

Everyone has a right to his own social, political, religious, and economic beliefs. Try to assess every patient's cultural values and health beliefs accurately. Be careful about interpreting his behavior until you've explored his cultural background and determined its influence on his behavior.

38 Obtain a translator when you need one

Make every effort to find a translator for a patient who speaks a language that's foreign to you. If the translator is clearly instructed to translate and not to interpret or summarize, he can add the dimension of objectivity. Friends and relatives may also be helpful in such cases, but they may distort the patient's meaning by adding their own interpretation of what has been said, based on their knowledge of the patient.

39 The terminally ill patient

If you have to interview a dying patient for a health history, try to determine how he feels about his impending death. His attitude will have been shaped partly by his own health and personal history and partly by his reactions to the deaths of family members and friends. Listen carefully for any references to death the patient may make, directly or indirectly. Integrate the topic into the conversation when you think he's ready to talk about it.

The attitudes of your patient's friends and family members toward death will affect how much help they can give him. Talk with them, and describe in your notes their potential for helping the patient accept his condition.

The dying patient experiences various emotional responses, all related to the grieving process: shock and disbelief, denial, anger, bargaining, depression, and finally acceptance (see the chart on page 37). Knowing about this process helps you understand the adaptation maneuvers and emotional reactions he's experiencing, so you can control the interview. *Bargaining* is essentially a private state that doesn't affect your patient's behavior during the interview. And *acceptance* represents a tranquillity that your questions won't disrupt. But shock and disbelief, anger, depression, and denial can impede the interview's progress.

If your patient's in the initial stage of *shock and disbelief,* postpone the interview until he's calmer. Entries 45 and 46 provide guidelines for you in responding to your patient's *anger* or *depression.* Interviewing a patient who's *denying* his terminal condition presents a paradoxical situation: You need to discuss the reality of his present condition, but he's not acknowledging this condition. Important: Remember that his denial, by suppressing awareness of his impending death, is helping him maintain his emotional equilibrium. Don't try to force him to admit his condition, but don't hold out false hope for his recovery either. Instead, gently ask your questions at a pace your patient can tolerate. Use your awareness of verbal and nonverbal forms of communication to guide you.

Remember that most patients don't progress in an orderly manner from one phase of this grieving process to the next. For example, a dying patient experiencing anger about his impending death may displace it onto someone or something else, while denying being terminally ill.

40 The patient with multiple symptoms

You usually have to modify the history-taking process when interviewing patients with multiple symptoms. Cover each symptom in detail; then correlate your findings in one system with your findings in another. This requires a sound knowledge of compensatory mechanisms and of the relationships between body systems. If your patient has numerous symptoms, involving

RECOGNIZING THE FIVE STAGES OF GRIEF

When interviewing a terminally ill patient, try to determine how he feels about his illness. Has he accepted the reality of his physical condition, or is he still working through the grieving process? He may move through the grieving stages in a mixed and overlapping pattern. Note the particular stage he's currently experiencing and his attitudes toward his illness.

SHOCK/DENIAL	ANGER	BARGAINING	DEPRESSION	ACCEPTANCE
Patient displays:	**Patient displays:**	**Patient displays:**	**Patient displays:**	**Patient displays:**
• overwhelming shock and disbelief • rejection of reality • possible physical changes, such as sweating, pallor, faintness, nausea, confusion	• impatience • uncooperativeness • bitterness • jealousy • helplessness • increasing awareness	• depression and exhaustion • final attempt to avoid reality • possible physical changes, such as shortness of breath and weakness	• quietness and withdrawal • melancholy • gradual acceptance of reality	• contemplativeness and serenity • ability to talk about his condition

many body systems, but you can't find any obvious organic reason for them, investigate the possibility that he has serious emotional problems by taking a detailed psychosocial history (see Entry 122).

41 When a patient can't communicate well

If your patient's intellectual capacity is limited, you'll certainly have to use different history-taking methods. Your first consideration is whether he's capable of understanding your questions. Then, does he have the language skills to answer them?

You can estimate the limits of a patient's intelligence by the vocabulary he uses, the amount of detail with which he describes his illness, and how well he recalls past events. In addition, assess his understanding and compliance with past medical-care instructions. Note the extent of his schooling, such as highest grade completed and courses of study taken, and what type of job he has. Use validation procedures to determine if the patient understands what you're saying. The patient's responses to questions involving general knowledge may give additional data.

A retarded patient may not be able to give you a reliable history. You may have to refer him for formal psychological testing to determine the extent of the deficit, and rely on family members or friends for the history information. This procedure is also useful when you interview a patient you suspect has organic brain syndrome. Don't try to obtain a detailed history from him.

Your patient's apparently limited intellectual functioning may be caused by a diminished level of consciousness. Of course, a patient who is critically ill or has a language barrier may also be unable to supply the history information you need. Here again, family members and friends can help.

DEALING WITH THE ANXIOUS PATIENT

Interviewing an anxious patient may make you anxious as well. If you plan how you'll manage this situation, you can keep your composure and help your patient, too. Here are some tips and suggestions you can follow:

- Approach the patient in a quiet, reassuring manner.
- Help the patient identify the cause of his anxiety. Then, see if you can minimize or relieve it.
- Contact the doctor of a patient who's having an acute anxiety attack. The doctor may order a tranquilizer.
- Check your own anxiety level periodically, and get support from your co-workers, if necessary.
- Encourage your patient to relax by practicing deep breathing. If he begins to hyperventilate, have him breathe into a paper bag.

42 The sensory-impaired patient

When interviewing a patient with *impaired hearing,* try the following techniques: Face the patient, so he has a direct view of your eyes and mouth; use common words; make your questions simple, short, and direct. Don't shout. Also, check whether the patient is wearing a hearing aid. If so, is it turned on? With an elderly patient who is hard of hearing, speaking in a low tone of voice will help you communicate, because his ability to hear high-pitched tones has deteriorated first. For a patient whose impairment is severe, you may have to conduct the history totally in writing or through family or friends, asking only the most essential questions. (Obtain additional data in subsequent contacts and interviews with him.) If the patient knows sign language, try to find a sign language translator who can also speak, hear, and therefore communicate with you, too.

A *visually impaired* patient may be slow to respond to your questioning or may have difficulty following directions. Be patient with him, and remember to respond to him by speaking rather than gesturing. He'll be less con-

COPING WITH THE AGGRESSIVE PATIENT

Your most effective way to deal with the patient who exhibits aggressive behavior is by intervening to prevent it—before he becomes combative. You can identify the potentially combative patient by asking yourself these questions:

- Does he seem elated, restless, agitated?
- Does he demand constant attention from everyone?
- Does he talk loudly or boisterously?
- Does he tease and bait others with sarcasm?
- Does he use vulgar language?
- Does he show a limited attention span?

If you answer yes to several or all these questions, don't try to control or suppress the patient's behavior. Instead, give him room to express his feelings so he can get them out of his system.

As you talk to the potentially aggressive patient, remember these points:

- Listen to him, but don't respond to provocative remarks or abusive language.
- Try not to show disapproval of his words or actions.
- Speak in short sentences. Avoid complex ideas or involved explanations.
- Make firm decisions, and don't feel obligated to explain them.
- Try to remain relaxed. Don't appear aggressive or defensive.
- Use gestures and other nonverbal messages carefully. Smiling, nodding, and other positive messages may communicate the opposite of what you intend. The agitated patient may misinterpret your smile and think you're laughing at him.

Suppose, despite your best efforts, the patient becomes combative. Now the patient—not you—is in control. To protect yourself and others in the area, act quickly using these guidelines:

- Call for assistance. However, ask the others to stay out of sight or in the background. Make sure they know what you're doing at all times.
- Protect yourself. Observe your position in relation to the door, to possible alternative escape routes, and to any potential weapons in the room. *Never* turn your back on the patient.
- Don't sound authoritarian when you speak to him. Avoid making threats or raising your voice.
- Test your progress at resolving the situation. Move closer to the patient and watch his reaction. If the patient gets more combative, back off *immediately.* Be sensitive to his need for personal space.
- Continue to communicate. Listen and respond with empathy. Bargain with the patient, but don't make promises you can't keep.
- Be prepared to use restraints. If this step is necessary, you'll need an order from a doctor and help from co-workers.

Afterward, document the entire episode in your nurse's notes.

fused if the lighting in the interviewing area is strong but not glaring, and doesn't vary in intensity.

43 The patient who is tired or in pain

Fatigued patients and those in pain may find it difficult or impossible to respond fully to your history questions. If interviewing a patient who's in pain proves difficult, obtain an order for an analgesic and allow time for it to take effect. When you're ready to resume history-taking, approach the patient calmly. During the interview, pause now and then to give him a rest. You may need to take his history over the course of several interviews. Start by taking essential information, and ask questions that minimize your patient's requirement to respond. Take noncritical parts of the history in subsequent interviews.

44 Patients who are anxious or fearful

A patient may feel uneasy or anxious about the information he discloses during the health history interview. Signs of anxiety or fear that you may observe include blushing or pallor, restlessness, hyperventilation, and lassitude. In addition, your patient may report muscle cramps or tenseness, headache, nausea, diarrhea, excessive perspiration, dry mouth, rapid heartbeat, or insomnia—also suggestive, among other possibilities, that he's feeling anxious or afraid. (Make sure the patient isn't in a physical crisis demanding prompt medical attention.) To help relieve these feelings, reassure your patient that no one will see his health history except those involved in his care. Your challenge during the interview is to determine whether these signs are related to fear and anxiety, to the symptoms of his illness, or to a physiologic problem that may be developing.

Anxiety is an extremely contagious emotion. Don't allow your patient's anxiety to disturb your composure during the interview (see *Dealing with the Anxious Patient,* page 38). To manage an anxious or fearful patient most effectively, discuss the situation openly with him. Ask him if he's feeling anxious, and encourage him to describe his feelings. Usually he'll relax somewhat, and you'll proceed more comfortably with the interview. If the patient denies anxious feelings, make sure your own anxiety isn't interfering with the progress of the interview.

45 The angry or aggressive patient

The patient who directly or indirectly expresses anger or aggression during the health history interview needs special attention (see *Coping with the Aggressive Patient,* page 39). Anger, like silence, can be healthy, but it can also be destructive. If your patient becomes angry during the interview, remain calm and show that you accept his emotional response as an expression of important feelings. Then try to help the patient find out why he's angry. Anxiety, frustration, and helplessness are the most common causes. You might say, "Obviously, you're upset. Would you like to talk about it?" Don't say, "You look angry. Why?" (Generally, this approach only increases the patient's defensiveness and anger.)

46 The depressed patient

Interviewing a depressed patient for a health history can be especially difficult. The patient may be sullen, and refuse to answer your questions. He may also be an unreliable historian, since his depression can cause him to exaggerate his symptoms' severity.

A depressed patient may look older than his stated age, with a sullen facial expression. Suspect depression, too, if he's experienced weight loss or gain over a short period. He may complain of insomnia or difficulty in concentrating. Disinterest in personal hygiene and physical appearance is also common. His posture may be poor, his gait slow and dragging.

Basically, an individual's body functions slow down in response to depression. Some examples of this are slowed respirations, a constant feeling of fullness, belching, and constipation from decreased alimentary tract motility. Remember that illness other than depression may also manifest itself in this way. Don't be misled into "labeling" depression. Many depressed patients turn out to have serious physical illnesses, such as ulcers or cancer, as well. So always explore the reasons for a patient's depression, using such communication skills as direct questioning, clarification, feedback, and expressions of support. Describe this part of the health history interview in detail in your notes to ensure thoughtful planning for your patient's care.

When dealing with depressed patients, be sure to consider their suicidal potential (see the chart on page 116). Not every depressed person is suicidal, but the possibility always exists. You can help by empathizing with his despair, then trying to get him to recognize his strengths as well as the alternative choices he can make to improve the situation.

If you suspect your patient has suicidal or self-destructive feelings, try to get him to acknowledge them. If you succeed, the power and anxiety your patient associates with these feelings will diminish. Never agree to keep suicidal feelings confidential. You have a responsibility to communicate these feelings to the patient's doctor immediately and to take proper precautions.

Taking a pediatric health history

47 Pediatric considerations

A pediatric health history is a modified version of an adult health history, with special emphasis on such areas as childhood diseases and, if the patient is still an infant, the mother's health during pregnancy. Usually you'll obtain information about the child's present health from one of his parents (note this on the health history). If someone other than the child's mother or father—such as a relative or guardian—gives you the information, mention this in the history, and state how much everyday contact this person has with the child. Sometimes the child himself will give you history information.

Take advantage of the opportunity to observe parent-child interactions when a parent is present during a child's health history interview. (Usually the child's mother brings him in.) Your observations may prove as enlightening as their answers to your questions. Don't overlook the chance to observe the apparent level of the young child's motor abilities and coordination. When appropriate, take the time to teach good health habits as related points are discussed during the interview. Above all, let the child and the parents get to know you so they'll trust you and confide in you as a friend.

Some children, especially those age 10 and older, may not wish to have a parent present during the interview. If your patient's an adolescent, you'll probably want to ask questions about sexual development; in this situation, the presence of a parent may inhibit your patient's responses. Be particularly sensitive to an adolescent's request for confidentiality. If you must share an adolescent's history information with a parent, get the patient's permission first.

The way you approach a child and phrase your questions can determine the success of the interview. Avoid a condescending manner; a child can sense this easily. To lessen a child's

INTERVIEWING A SICK CHILD

What do you do when you're interviewing a sick child whose verbal skills aren't adequate to describe how she feels? Here's a possible solution: Give the child crayons and paper. Ask her to draw how she feels, or how she feels that's different from usual. Especially revealing: what the drawing says about her body image, what's the size of her drawing, and what colors she chooses. The drawing pictured here clearly shows that the child is experiencing abdominal pain. Leave the paper and crayons with her, and ask her to note any changes as they occur. In this way, even the least verbal child can give you a continuous record of her condition.

This technique can also be adopted for adults with speech impairments or language difficulties. Many patients who can't express themselves well verbally will be reassured having a pencil and paper nearby as an aid to communication.

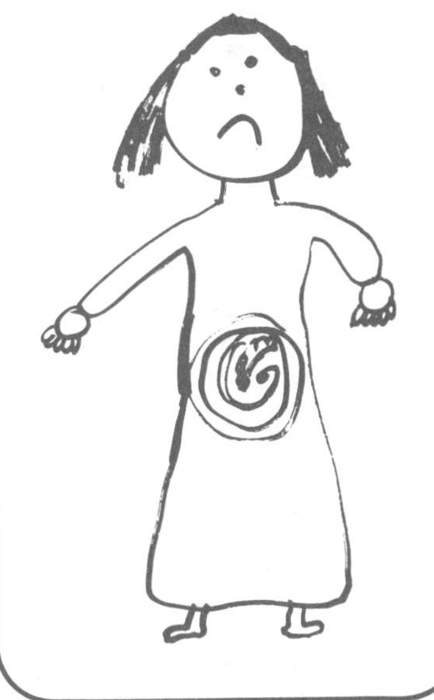

anxiety, you may want to wear casual dress instead of your uniform (if this is possible where you work). A child's personality and age also influence the way you phrase your questions, as well as the information you can expect to obtain.

State your questions simply, in a friendly manner. Be patient; let the child take his time responding. You may want to ask a very young child to draw how he feels (see *Interviewing a Sick Child*, page 41).

48 Young children's limited communication skills

Children younger than age 7 are limited in their ability to understand and answer questions. They can't always understand things from another person's point of view. They're egocentric—that is, interested chiefly in themselves—so don't expect to obtain history information that doesn't pertain to their own experience. In addition, a child under age 7 can usually focus on only one perception at a time. When recalling an illness, for example, he may relate only its most vivid characteristic, such as a rash, even though the illness had more serious manifestations.

A child in this age-group may not be able to discuss hypothetical situations. For example, he may not be able to answer if you ask what he'd do if he cut his hand and couldn't stop the bleeding. Instead, he may reply simply that he didn't cut his hand. Similarly, he may not be able to understand or talk about events from another time. If he can't comprehend that his parents were children at one time, he won't be able to tell you clearly about his past history. Concepts of time and its duration are vague to young children, although most have some understanding of past, present, and future. For example, if your young patient tells you he had a stomachache *yesterday*, you may find that *yesterday* was actually several months ago. A cold that lasted 2 days may seem no different to him than a cold that lingered for a month.

A young child's ability to reason logically isn't fully developed. He usually can't generalize from specific instances or understand a specific consequence of a general statement. Rather, the child usually reasons from instance to instance. For example, he will say Johnny couldn't go to school when he had measles, so Alice can't go to school when she has measles. But he may not be able to reason that no children with measles can go to school. And if you told him only this, he could possibly not realize that *he* couldn't go to school if he had measles.

The child under age 7 also has difficulty categorizing illnesses according to anything but obvious qualities. For example, he'll assume that diseases with similar characteristics, such as a rash, are the same disease. A young child may also have trouble understanding a complex cause-and-effect relationship. He may understand that germs cause illness but would have trouble understanding that germs are more likely to cause illness when a person's resistance is lowered.

49 Children ages 7 to 12

Many cognitive skills—seeing things from another's point of view, being able to focus thought on more than one perception simultaneously, imagining hypothetical situations, understanding time concepts, and reasoning logically—develop gradually in children between ages 7 and 12. You'll be able to communicate more easily with children in this age-group and obtain more accurate information from them. Remember, though, that each child differs in his rate of development.

50 The adolescent's special concerns

When a child reaches adolescence, beginning at about age 12, his cognitive development is nearly complete. He is likely to have a fully developed ability to see another person's viewpoint. But his accelerated development, as well as self-consciousness about his personal appearance, may cloud his reasoning ability. In the health history interview, he may ask you about health measures to enhance appearance—for example, personal hygiene measures that will improve his acne. These concerns can cause your adolescent patient a great deal of anxiety. When appropriate, reassure him that he's developing normally. And let him know that you accept him as he is.

51 Recording a child's chief complaint

If the child can describe his chief complaint (or concern) well enough, quote his exact words in your notes. Otherwise, record what the parents tell you. Frequently, the parents simply want the child to have a checkup. If the child has a chief complaint that suggests he may have a communicable disease, ask whether the child or anyone in the family has been exposed to a contagious disease within the past 3 weeks.

Always listen carefully to what a parent tells you. Sometimes you may be able to discern an underlying reason for bringing a child to be examined. For example, if a mother is anxious about her child's social development, she may view this concern as less legitimate—in terms of seeking care for the child—than an illness. The subconscious goal of exploring this concern may be her reason for bringing the child for a checkup or treatment of a minor injury.

52 The child's past history

In addition to recording the same kinds of information for a child as you would for an adult, you'll also note details of the child's birth and development. Keep the birth history brief unless your patient is under age 2 or you suspect he has a developmental deficiency. For these exceptions, obtain information about prenatal, natal, and postnatal events (see *Recording the Child's Birth History*).

If your patient has any siblings, ask his mother how she would compare this child's development to theirs. Was this child quicker or slower to arrive at developmental milestones? How does the child interact with his siblings?

RECORDING THE CHILD'S BIRTH HISTORY

If your patient is under age 2, or if you suspect a developmental deficiency, obtain a detailed birth history as follows:

Prenatal

Ask the mother where and when she received medical care during her pregnancy. Find out if she had any vaginal bleeding, illnesses, infections, prolonged nausea or vomiting, fever, or rashes. Was she injured in any way or hospitalized while pregnant? Was she exposed to X-rays? If so, was a lead shield used to protect her? Was she taking medications at any time during this period? What diet did she follow, and how much weight did she gain?

Ask her if the infant was full-term, premature, or postmature. Has she had any other children, or any stillbirths, abortions, or miscarriages? What is her blood group and that of the child's father?

Natal

Find out in which city and hospital the mother gave birth. How long and difficult was her labor? What type of delivery did she have? Did she receive an anesthetic? What was the infant's weight and physical condition at birth?

Postnatal

Ask about the child's condition during the first 28 days after birth. Did he have any problems in the nursery, such as jaundice, cyanosis, rashes, feeding problems, or unusual weight gain or loss? Did he leave the hospital with his mother? With a high-risk infant, learn as many details as possible about his problem and duration of hospitalization.

Next, question the parent about the child's development. At what age did the child first hold his head up, roll over, sit up, stand, walk, and talk? When did he start speaking in complete sentences? At what age did he achieve control of his bladder and bowels, both during the day and at night?

Record other aspects of the child's past history as you would for an adult patient. Be sure to ask about all childhood diseases, and whether the child has frequent colds (more than four a year) or ear infections. Be alert for speech problems that may reflect hearing loss, especially in children with frequent ear infections. Ask about accidents, including whether the child has ever ingested any toxic substances. When discussing immunizations, ask about booster inoculations the child has received.

53 Family and psychosocial histories

When taking a child's family history, pay special attention to hereditary tendencies toward blood dyscrasias, mental retardation, and other familial conditions that can surface during childhood.

When exploring the child's psychosocial history, remember that the physical and the emotional aspects of a child's home life can affect his health and well-being. Does he live in a house or an apartment? In an urban, suburban, or rural community? How large is the home? Is it near his school and a playground? Does he have his own room, his own bed? Does the home have stairs that might be hazardous to the child? Where are poisonous substances stored? Does the child have a yard in which to play?

Ask about the parents' marital situation. Are there marital problems that might affect the child? Do his parents live together, or does he live with one or the other—or with someone else? Is life at home happy and cooperative, or antagonistic and chaotic? Who usually cares for the child? If the parents work, who stays with the child when they're not home? Does he go to a day-care center? Explore the financial, occupational, and other psychosocial aspects of the parents' or guardians' life-style

SURVEYING THE CHILD'S DAILY ACTIVITIES

To learn about a child's activities of daily living (ADL), you'll probably want to interview his parents instead of the child himself. But even though you're talking to an adult, you'll want to ask some questions different from the adult ADL survey. Here are questions you should ask to compile an ADL survey for a child:

Diet/Elimination

- How is the child's appetite?
- Is he on a formula? What type?
- When are his usual mealtimes?
- Does he eat with family members?
- Does someone help him eat?
- Does he use utensils?
- Does he have any difficulty eating? What sort?
- What are his favorite foods and beverages?
- Does he snack? What does he usually snack on?
- Does he take daily vitamins?
- Is he toilet trained? At what age did he learn?
- What are his usual bowel habits?
- Does he wet the bed?

Exercise/Sleep

- Does his daily schedule include play?
- Does he participate in sports?
- Does he have any special exercises he performs regularly?
- What is his normal amount of sleep? From when to when?
- Does he take naps?
- Does he have a routine before going to sleep (drinking a bottle, playing, being read to)?
- Does he sleep with other siblings or alone?
- What is his favorite sleeping position?
- Does he have any sleeping problems? Nightmares?
- Is he tired during the day?

Recreation

- How much time does he get for recreation each day?
- Does he have a group of friends with whom he plays?
- What are his favorite play activities?

REVIEW OF SYSTEMS: AREAS TO COVER WITH THE PEDIATRIC PATIENT

Ask the parent of the child you're interviewing if the child has complained (or the parents have been aware) of any of the following problems:

Eyes: Vision difficulties, problem with tearing, crossed eyes

Ears: Hearing difficulties, earaches

Nose: Nosebleeds, sinus infections

Throat: Sore throats (streptococcal), pneumonia, colds (more than four a year)

Cardiovascular: Coloring (bluish), fatigue

Respiratory: Breathing difficulties, shortness of breath, frequent exhaustion

Gastrointestinal: Changes in bowel habits, diarrhea, constipation, bleeding, pain, vomiting

Renal: Frequency of urination, pain, bleeding on urination; males—straight urinary flow

Reproductive: Female—menstrual cycle onset

Nervous: Headaches, convulsions, fainting spells, tremors, twitches, blackouts, dizziness

Musculoskeletal: Painful joints, redness around joints, swelling, sprains, broken bones, coordination difficulties

if you need this information to care for your patient.

54 Pediatric activities of daily living

In most cases, the topics to investigate in this portion of a child's history are similar to those for an adult patient. You'll need information on diet, elimination, exercise, sleep, and recreational activities. For an adolescent, ask about tobacco, alcohol, and drug use, too, but try to reserve such questions until you're alone with the patient; the presence of a parent may prevent your patient from answering freely.

Don't forget to inquire about the child's school activities. Does the child go to school? If so, ask what grade he is in and whether he likes school. Is his schoolwork good? Does he have friends at school? What does he enjoy most about school? Question the child about after-school activities, too.

At this point in the history, discuss with the parents any concerns they may have about their child's habits. This is also a good time to find out if temper tantrums, masturbation, thumb-sucking, nail-biting, and bed-wetting are part of your patient's history—and how his parents manage such incidents (see Entry 141).

55 Pediatric review of systems

Use your standard format for the review of systems when your patient is a child, but be sure to include additional questions appropriate for his age. For example, you'd probably ask the parent of a 1-year-old child whether any teeth are erupting—and whether they're causing any problems.

For all children, ask about any recent significant weight loss or gain. Does the child have trouble gaining weight? Is he irritable or nervous? Are there any problems with the child's growth or personality? Have there been any changes or deformities in his posture or gait?

For adolescents, your review of systems should also include questions about sexual development. If your patient is female, ask if she has begun to menstruate. If she has, find out how often she menstruates and if she has any problems with menstruation.

Taking a geriatric patient's health history

56 Your elderly patient's special needs

Approaching an elderly patient for a health history and conducting the interview needn't be difficult if you anticipate his special needs. If possible, plan to talk with an elderly patient early in the day, when he's likely to be most alert. (Many elderly people experience the so-called *sundown syndrome,* which means their capacity for clear thinking diminishes by late afternoon or early evening. Some of these patients may even become disoriented or confused late in the day.)

Have a comfortable chair available for your elderly patient (if he isn't on bed rest), especially if the interview might be lengthy. Arthritis and other orthopedic disabilities may make sitting in one position for a long time uncomfortable. Encourage your patient to change his position in the bed or chair and to move around as much as he wants during the interview.

A geriatric patient may have some hearing and vision loss, so sit close to him and face him. Speak slowly in a low-pitched voice. Don't shout at a patient who has a hearing problem. Shouting raises the pitch of your voice and may make understanding you more difficult, not easier. (Hearing loss from aging affects perception of high-pitched tones first.)

Try to evaluate your patient's ability to communicate, and his reliability as an historian, early in the interview. If you have any doubts about these matters before the interview begins, ask him if a family member or a close friend can be present.

Don't be surprised if your elderly patient *requests* that someone accompany him—he too may have concerns about getting through the interview on his own. Having another person present during the interview gives you an opportunity to observe your patient's interaction with this person and provides more data for the history. However, this may prevent the patient from speaking freely, so plan to talk with him privately sometime during your assessment.

57 Attitudes toward aging

Communicating with an elderly patient may challenge you to confront your personal attitudes and prejudices about aging. Examine these feelings before taking the patient's history, and decide in advance how you'll handle them. Any prejudices you reveal will probably interfere with your efforts to communicate, since elderly patients are especially sensitive to others' reactions and can easily detect negative attitudes and impatience.

Then consider your *patient's* attitude toward his body and health. An elderly patient may have a distorted perception of his health problems; he may dwell on them needlessly or dismiss them as normal signs of aging. A patient may ignore a serious problem because he doesn't want his fears confirmed. If your elderly patient is seriously ill, the subjects of dying (discussed in Entry 39) and death may come up during the health history interview. Listen carefully to any remarks your patient makes about dying. Be sure to ask about his religious affiliation and spiritual needs; many elderly patients find comfort in their religious beliefs and practices. You should also inquire tactfully about the matter of a living will (see *Understanding the Living Will,* page 47).

58 Obtaining an elderly patient's cooperation

Patience is the key to communicating with an elderly patient. He may respond slowly to your questions. Don't confuse patience with patronizing behavior. Your patient will easily perceive such behavior and may interpret it as lack of geniune concern for him. Keep your questions concise, rephrase those he doesn't understand, and use nonverbal techniques in a meaningful way.

To further foster your elderly patient's cooperation, take a little extra time to help him see the relevance of your questions. You may need to repeat this explanation several times as the interview progresses. But don't repeat questions unnecessarily. Ask only for information that is relevant to his condition. For example, you wouldn't obtain a detailed obstetric history from a 75-year-old woman who doesn't have a gynecologic problem.

Once you have obtained an elderly patient's cooperation, you may have some trouble getting him to keep his story brief. He has a lot of history to relate and may reminisce during the interview. Try to find time for this. Let the patient talk. You may obtain valuable clues about his current physical, mental, and spiritual health. If you must keep the history brief, let him know before the interview how much time you've set aside for it. Offer to come back another time to chat with him informally.

59 Past history: Longer than usual

A geriatric patient's past medical history is likely to be extensive. His detailed recall of all major illnesses, surgical procedures, and injuries is necessary for you to complete the history. Fractures the patient may have experienced early in life, for example, may figure significantly now in osteoporosis. As you record his past history, try to get an idea of the amount of stress he has had recently and the way he has handled previous health problems. Don't be concerned if he can't relate this medical history chronologically; just be sure to record his age at the time each medical condition occurred.

Pay special attention to your elderly patient's medication history, since he probably takes medication routinely. Find out what medications—over-the-counter and prescription—he's now taking and has taken in the past, and the dosage for each. Ask him to show you samples, if possible, of all the medications he currently takes.

60 The elderly patient's psychosocial history

Make it a point to talk with your elderly patient about his family and friends. With whom does he live? How does he spend his time? Find out what significant relationships he has. If your patient is hospitalized and seriously ill, or must transfer to another type of institution (such as a nursing home), he'll need the emotional support of family and friends. If he's returning

UNDERSTANDING THE LIVING WILL

A living will legally documents the patient's wishes regarding to what extent heroic measures should be performed to save the patient's life if he has suffered extreme physical or mental disability. Clarifying the patient's wishes on this matter before a crisis situation occurs makes terminal illness easier to deal with—for the patient's family and for hospital personnel.

Once the dying patient has reached the stage when he can discuss his condition, you may wish to tactfully broach the subject of a living will with him and his family. If the patient is already extremely disabled and cannot communicate, discuss the matter of a living will with the patient's family.

If the patient or his family chooses to have a living will, it must be scrupulously respected. You and other hospital staff members are obliged to follow the will's instructions to the letter. If, for example, the patient or his family expresses the desire that no heroic measures be taken in a crisis situation, the doctor must record a *no-code* order in his progress notes and on his order sheet. You should transfer this order to the patient's chart or Kardex. Inform hospital personnel on other shifts of the no-code order, so no one misunderstands the patient's or his family's wishes.

home after an illness, he may need their assistance.

If your patient doesn't have a family or any friends on whom he can depend for support, record this in the psychosocial history for possible later referral of the patient to a social agency. Record the names of his next of kin. Without your intervention here, loneliness may discourage an elderly patient from getting well.

If your patient is employed, inquire about his job to find out if his health problems will interfere with his returning to work. Talk with him about his plans for retirement, if he has any, and his attitude toward this phase of his life.

If your patient expresses financial concerns, explore them further in a financial history. Remember to ask your elderly patient if he receives any pensions or Social Security payments.

When appropriate, inquire about the patient's sex life. Don't ignore it because of the patient's age. Approach this aspect of the psychosocial history with the same sensitivity and respect for privacy that you would show with younger patients. If the patient is reluctant to discuss his sex life, don't press him for the information.

SURVEYING THE ELDERLY PATIENT'S ADL

When questioning an elderly patient about his daily activities, use general questions that will inform you of his usual habits and whether he has any problems performing them. An elderly patient may also have personal concerns, such as financial worries or transportation problems, that keep him from going about his daily routine. Structure your questions as outlined here.

Diet/Elimination

- What do you eat on a typical day?
- Do you feel hungry between meals?
- Do you prepare your own meals?
- With whom do you eat?
- What types of food do you enjoy most?
- Do you have any specific problems eating?
- Have you noted any change in your sense of taste?
- Do you snack? When are your snack times? What do you have for a snack?
- What are your usual bowel habits? Have you noticed any changes in them?

Exercise/Sleep

- Do you take daily walks?
- Do you do your own housework?
- Do you have any difficulty moving about?
- Has your doctor restricted your exercise or suggested a special exercise program?
- What time do you go to bed at night?
- What time do you awake?
- Do you follow a routine that helps you sleep?
- Do you sleep soundly or awake often?
- Do you take a nap during the day? How often and for how long?

Recreation

- Do you belong to any social groups, such as senior citizen clubs or church groups?
- What do you enjoy doing in your leisure time?
- How many hours a day do you watch television?
- Do you share leisure time with your family?

Tobacco/Alcohol

- Do you use tobacco? If so, do you smoke cigarettes, cigars, or a pipe? How long have you smoked? How much do you smoke each day? If you quit smoking, when did you quit?
- Do you drink alcohol? How often do you drink? Do you drink with friends or alone? How much do you normally drink? Has your drinking increased recently?

Personal concerns

- Do you wear dentures? Are they a hindrance when eating or talking?
- Do you wear glasses? Do you have any problems with your vision when wearing your glasses?
- Do you hear those around you with no difficulty? Does poor hearing hinder any of your activities?
- What is your source of income?
- Do you shop for your own groceries? If not, who does this for you?

REVIEW OF SYSTEMS: FOR THE ELDERLY PATIENT

Certain disorders commonly affect the elderly. When reviewing your elderly patient's systems, note the following possibly pathologic signs:

Skin: Delayed wound healing, change in texture

Nails: Brittleness, clubbing, pitting

Head: Facial pain or numbness

Eyes: Diplopia, tunnel vision, halo effect, glaucoma, cataracts

Ears: Excessive wax formation, use of wax softeners

Nose: Epistaxis, allergic rhinitis

Mouth/throat: Sore tongue, problems with teeth or gums, gums bleeding at night, hoarseness

Neck: Pain, swelling, restricted range of motion

Respiratory: Tuberculosis, difficulty or painful breathing, excessive cough producing excessive or blood-streaked sputum

Breasts: Discharge, change in contour, change in nipples, gynecomastia, lumps

Cardiovascular: Chest pain on exertion, orthopnea, cyanosis, syncope, fatigue, murmur, leg cramps, varicosities, coldness or numbness of extremities, hypertension, heart attack

Gastrointestinal: Difficulty swallowing, epigastric pain, abdominal pain, intolerance to certain foods, increased thirst, dysphagia, change in bowel habits, rectal bleeding

Renal: Flank pain, dysuria, polyuria, nocturia, incontinence, enuresis, hematuria, renal or bladder infections or stones

Reproductive: Male—hernia, testicular pain, prostatic problems; female—postmenopausal problems (bleeding, hot flashes, painful intercourse)

Endocrine: Goiter, tremor

Musculoskeletal: Pain, joint swelling, crepitus, restricted joint movement, arthritis, gout, rheumatism, lumbago, amputations

Nervous: Memory loss, loss of consciousness, nervousness, nightmares, insomnia, changes in emotional state, tremors, muscle weakness, paralysis, aphasia, speech difficulty, pain or numbness

61 The elderly patient's activities of daily living

Your geriatric patient's activities of daily living may affect his health, and his health problems may, in turn, threaten his independence. Ask him to describe a typical day at home, including activities, sleep patterns, and eating habits. Because his eating habits may suggest other significant lines of questioning, find out how much of an appetite he usually has, how he prepares his food (does he use a lot of salt?), and how much fluid he normally consumes. You can put this information into a chart, showing which foods the patient eats at which times during the day.

Ask about matters related to the patient's mobility. Is he able to move around at home easily and safely? Can he supply the basic needs—food, clothing, and shelter? Does he drive to the supermarket, or does a friend or relative drive him? Does he use public transportation? Ask if he expects to be able to continue with his routine after he is discharged from the hospital. If necessary, consult with a social worker to discuss what you've learned about the patient's activities of daily living.

62 Geriatric review of systems

The review of systems for an elderly patient involves keeping in mind the following physiologic changes, considered normal in the aging process, and the common pathologic disorders described in the chart on page 49.

• *Skin, hair, and nails.* Skin color and texture commonly change as a person ages (see Entries 224 to 231). Your patient may report that his skin seems thinner and looser—less elastic—than before, and that he perspires less. Hair thins, grays, and coarsens. Distribution of hair on the scalp, face, and body may also change, and the patient may tell you his scalp feels dry. Fingernails may thicken and change color slightly. Find out if the patient can take care of his own nails.

• *Eyes and vision.* Your patient may report increased tearing, or he may have presbyopia (diminished near vision due to a normal decrease in lens elasticity; see Entry 283). Ask if he's experienced changes in his vision, especially night vision. Does he need more light than usual when reading?

• *Ears and hearing.* Your elderly patient's hearing may be affected by gradual irreversible hearing loss of no specific pathologic origin (presbycusis)—common among elderly persons (see Entry 325).

• *Respiratory system.* Remember, shortness of breath during physical activity is normal, even if this tendency has increased recently, but sudden trouble with breathing is not (see Entry 363). If your patient has trouble breathing, explore the precipitating circumstances. Does he cough excessively? Does the cough produce a lot of sputum, perhaps blood? Aging can also affect the *nose.* Your patient may report sneezing, a runny nose, a decreased sense of smell, or bleeding from mucous-membrane atrophy.

• *Cardiovascular system.* More than half of all elderly people suffer from some degree of congestive heart failure (see Entry 405). Ask your patient whether he's gained weight recently and if his belts or rings feel tight. In addition, find out if he tires more easily now than previously, if he has trouble breathing, and if he becomes dizzy when he rises from a chair or bed.

• *Gastrointestinal system.* An elderly patient may complain about problems related to his mouth and his sense of taste (see Entry 472). For example, he may experience a foul taste in his mouth because his saliva production has decreased and his mucous membranes have atrophied. If he wears dentures, find out how comfortable they are and how well they work. An elderly person's sense of taste decreases gradually. This may be why your patient reports that his appetite has decreased, or that he craves sweeter or spicier foods.

An elderly patient may also have nonspecific difficulty in swallowing (see Entry 473). Carefully assess the possible causes of regurgitation or heartburn. Ask if he has the same degree of difficulty swallowing both solid foods and liquids, or if food lodges in his throat. Does he experience pain after eating, or while lying flat? Also question him about weight loss, rectal bleeding, and altered bowel habits.

• *Urinary system.* Investigate any pattern or incontinence the patient reports (see Entry 511). When incontinence occurs, does he feel that he has lost control, or does he not sense the urge to urinate? If he says he gets up to urinate in the middle of the night, find out if the urge awakens him.

• *Female reproductive system.* Include questions about menopause in your review of an elderly female patient (see Entry 584). Ask her when menopause began and ended (if it has), what symptoms she experienced, and how she feels about it. Ask whether she is receiving estrogen replacement therapy now, or has received it in the past (for how long?). Be sure to question an elderly female patient about symptoms of breast disease. Find out if she regularly performs a breast self-examination (and if she is physically capable of doing so).

• *Nervous system.* Inquire about changes in coordination, strength, or sensory perception (see Entry 651).

Does the patient have headaches or seizures, or any temporary losses of consciousness? Has he had any difficulty controlling his bowels or his bladder?

• *Blood-forming and immune system.* Remember that anemia is common in older people and may cause fatigue or weakness (see Entry 737).

Selected References

Alexander, Mary, and Brown, Marie S. *Pediatric Physical Diagnosis for Nurses,* 2nd ed. New York: McGraw-Hill Book Co., 1979.

Bates, Barbara. *A Guide to Physical Examination,* 2nd ed. Philadelphia: J.B. Lippincott Co., 1979.

Campbell, Claire. *Nursing Diagnosis and Intervention in Nursing Practice.* New York: John Wiley & Sons, 1978.

Carter, E.A., and McGoldrick, M. *The Family Life Cycle: A Framework for Family Therapy.* New York: Gardner Press, Inc., 1980.

DeGowin, E.L., and DeGowin, R.L. *Bedside Diagnostic Examination.* New York: Macmillan Co., 1976.

Delp, Mahlon H., and Manning, Robert T. *Major's Physical Diagnosis,* 8th ed. Philadelphia: W.B. Saunders Co., 1975.

Diekelmann, Nancy. *Primary Health Care of the Well Adult.* New York: McGraw-Hill Book Co., 1977.

Enelow, Allen J., and Swisher, Scott. *Interviewing and Patient Care.* New York: Oxford University Press, 1972.

Eriksen, K. *Communications Skills for the Human Services.* Reston, Va.: Reston Publishing Co., 1979.

Flynn, Patricia A. *Holistic Health: The Art and Science of Care.* Bowie, Md.: Robert J. Brady Co., 1980.

Fowkes, W.C., and Hunn, V.K. *Clinical Assessment for the Nurse Practitioner.* St. Louis: C.V. Mosby Co., 1973.

Froelich, Robert E., and Bishop, F. Marian. *Clinical Interviewing Skills,* 3rd ed. St. Louis: C.V. Mosby Co., 1977.

Gillies, Dee Ann, and Alyn, Irene B. *Patient Assessment and Management by the Nurse Practitioner.* Philadelphia: W.B. Saunders Co., 1976.

GI Series: Physical Examination of the Abdomen. Richmond, Va.: A.H. Robins Co., 1975.

Hillman, Robert S., et al. *Clinical Skills.* New York: McGraw-Hill Book Co., 1981.

Hudak, C.M., et al. *Clinical Protocols: A Guide for Nurses and Physicians.* Philadelphia: J.B. Lippincott Co., 1976.

Judge, Richard D., and Zuidema, George D., eds. *Methods of Clinical Examination: A Physiologic Approach,* 3rd ed. Boston: Little, Brown & Co., 1974.

Kinlein, M. Lucille. *Independent Nursing Practice with Clients.* Philadelphia: J.B. Lippincott Co., 1977.

Kraytown, Maurice. *The Complete Patient History.* New York: McGraw-Hill Book Co., 1979.

Kubler-Ross, Elisabeth. *Questions and Answers on Death and Dying.* New York: Macmillan Co., 1974.

Leininger, Madeleine. *Transcultural Nursing Concepts, Theories and Practices.* New York: John Wiley & Sons, 1978.

Leitch, Cynthia J., and Tinker, Richard V. *Primary Care.* Philadelphia: F.A. Davis & Co., 1978.

Long, L., and Prophit, P. *Understanding/Responding: A Communication Manual for Nurses.* Belmont, Calif.: Wadsworth Publishing Co., 1981.

Miller, Jean R., and Janosik, Ellen H. *Family Focused Care.* New York: McGraw-Hill Book Co., 1980.

Pearson, Linda J., and Kotthoff, M. Ernestine. *Geriatric Clinical Protocols.* Philadelphia: J.B. Lippincott Co., 1979.

Prior, John A., and Silberstein, Jack S. *Physical Diagnosis: The History and Examination of the Patient,* 5th ed. St. Louis: C.V. Mosby Co., 1977.

Sana, Josephine, and Judge, Richard D., eds. *Physical Appraisal Methods in Nursing Practice.* Boston: Little, Brown & Co., 1975.

Seedor, Marie M. *The Physical Assessment: A Programmed Unit of Study for Nurses.* New York: Teachers College Press, 1981.

Selye, Hans. *The Stress of Life,* 2nd ed. New York: McGraw-Hill Book Co., 1978.

Sherman, Jacques L., Jr., and Fields, Sylvia K., eds. *Guide to Patient Evaluation,* 2nd ed. Garden City, N.Y.: Medical Examination Publishing Co., 1976.

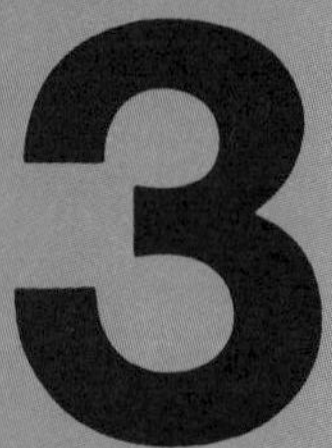

KEY POINTS IN THIS CHAPTER

KEY CHARTS IN THIS CHAPTER

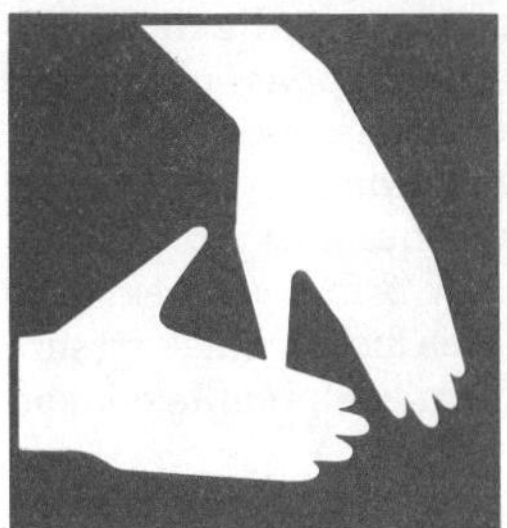

The Physical Examination

Introduction

63 Importance of the physical examination

After taking your patient's health history to obtain the subjective data on which to base clinical decisions, the next step in the assessment process is the *physical examination.* During this assessment phase you obtain objective data that usually confirm or rule out suspicions raised during the health history interview.

You use four basic techniques to perform a physical examination: *inspection, palpation, percussion,* and *auscultation* (IPPA). These skills require you to use your senses of sight, hearing, touch, and smell—all necessary for an accurate appraisal of the structures and functions of body systems. If you learn to use IPPA skills effectively, then—after much careful study and practice—the chance that you'll overlook something important during the physical examination will be reduced. In addition, each examination technique collects data that validate and amplify data collected through other IPPA techniques.

Accurate and complete physical assessments depend on two interrelated elements. One is the critical act of sensory perception, by which you receive and perceive external stimuli. The other element is the conceptual, or cognitive, process by which you relate these stimuli to your knowledge base. This two-step process gives meaning to your assessment data.

You need to develop a system for assessing patients that identifies their problem areas in priority order. By performing physical assessments systematically and efficiently instead of in a random or indiscriminate manner, you save time and identify priority problems quickly.

64 Methods for conducting a physical examination

The most commonly used methods for completing a total systematic physical assessment are *head to toe* and *major body systems.*

Using the head-to-toe method, you systematically assess your patient—as the name suggests—beginning at the head and working toward the toes. Examine all parts of one body region before progressing to the next region, to save time and energy for yourself and your patient. Proceed from left to right within each region, so you can make symmetrical comparisons. Don't examine the patient's left side from head to toe, then his right side.

The major-body-systems method involves systematically assessing your patient by examining each body system in priority order or a predesignated sequence.

Both methods are systematic and provide a logical, organized framework to help you collect physical assessment data. They also provide the same information; therefore, neither is more correct than the other. So choose the method (or a variation of it) that works well for you and is appropriate for your patient population. Follow this routine whenever you assess a patient and try not to deviate from it.

65 Equipment needed for a physical examination

Before you conduct a physical examination, collect and organize all the equipment you'll need—or make sure it's already in the examining room or at the patient's bedside. (Interrupting an examination to obtain a forgotten piece of equipment increases your patient's anxiety and weakens his trust in your competence.) Certain pieces of equipment are essential to a complete physical examination and should always be available (see *Gathering the Essential Equipment*). You may also need additional specialized equipment—such as a Doppler ultrasound or an EKG machine—depending on the extent of the examination. In any case, determine what equipment you'll need, and have it ready before you begin the examination. This includes making sure the room is warm, well ventilated, and well lighted.

66 How to relieve your patient's anxiety

When you approach your patient to perform a physical examination, one of your first priorities should be to relieve the anxiety he's probably experiencing. Almost every patient you examine will be anxious about his health problems. His worry may be severe; for example, he may suspect he has a fatal illness or that extensive surgery or treatment will strain his finances. To help your patient relax, tell him what procedures you plan to perform during the examination. Then explain the procedures as you do them. Use words he can understand.

GATHERING THE ESSENTIAL EQUIPMENT

Here's a list of equipment you'll need to perform a basic physical examination. To make the examination run more smoothly, gather all the equipment beforehand.

- Thermometer
- Scale for measuring height and weight
- Wristwatch (with sweep second-hand)
- Stethoscope (with diaphragm and bell)
- Sphygmomanometer and blood pressure cuff
- Ophthalmoscope
- Otoscope (with assorted specula)
- Nasoscope, nasal speculum, or nasal tip for otoscope
- Eye chart (Snellen) and newspaper clipping for close reading assessment
- Opaque card or eye cover
- Penlight or flashlight
- 2" x 2" and 4" x 4" sterile gauze pads and cotton swabs
- Tuning forks (512 to 1,024 cycles/second to test hearing acuity)
- Tongue depressors
- Laryngeal mirror
- Examination gloves and water-soluble lubricant
- Vaginal specula and slides
- Reflex or percussion hammer
- Safety pin
- Cloth tape measure (indicating centimeter measurements)
- Hemoculture test slides
- Urine specimen container

PREPARING YOUR PATIENT: GUIDELINES TO POSITIONING AND DRAPING

Requirements for patient positioning and draping vary according to which body systems or regions you plan to examine. These illustrations show the primary positioning and draping arrangements you'll use during a routine assessment.

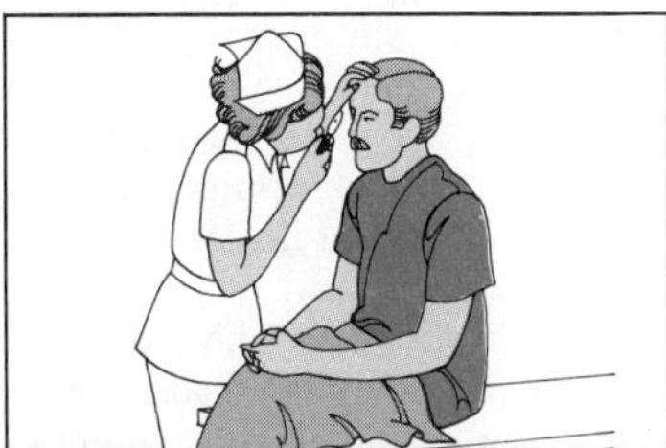

To examine the patient's head, neck, and anterior and posterior thorax and lungs, have him sit on the edge of the examining table.

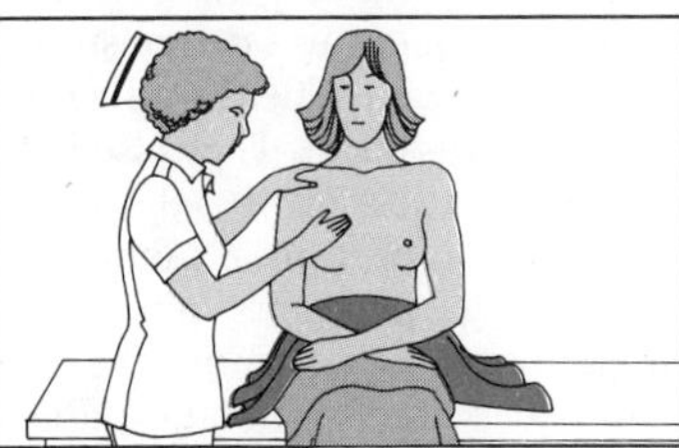

To begin examining the female patient's breasts, place her in a seated position. For the second part of the examination, ask her to lie down. When she does, place a small pillow or folded towel beneath her shoulder on the side being examined, to spread her breast more evenly over the chest.

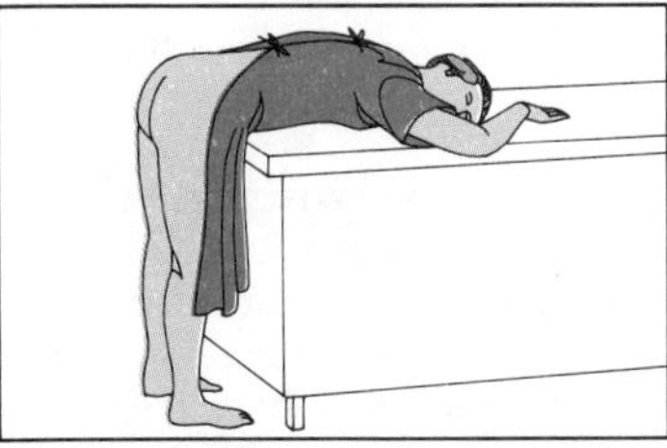

To perform a rectal examination, position the male patient so he's leaning across the examining table. If he can't stand upright, perform the examination with the patient lying on his left side, with his right hip and knee slightly flexed and his buttocks close to the edge of the examining table.

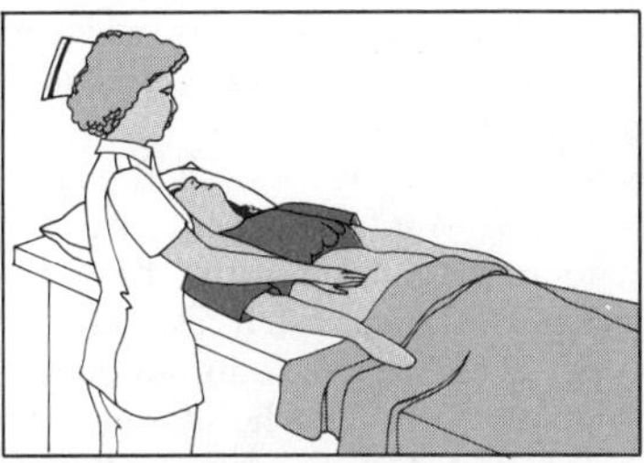

To examine the cardiovascular system and the abdomen, place the patient in supine position. To ensure privacy for a female patient during abdominal assessment, place a towel over her breasts and upper thorax. Pull down the sheet only as far as, but not exposing, her pubic symphysis.

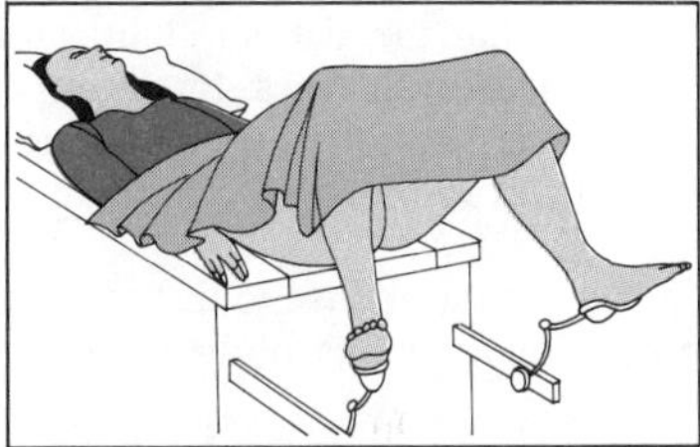

To examine the female patient's reproductive system, place her in lithotomy position. Drape a sheet diagonally over her chest and knees and between her legs. Her buttocks should be close to the edge of the table and her feet in the stirrups.

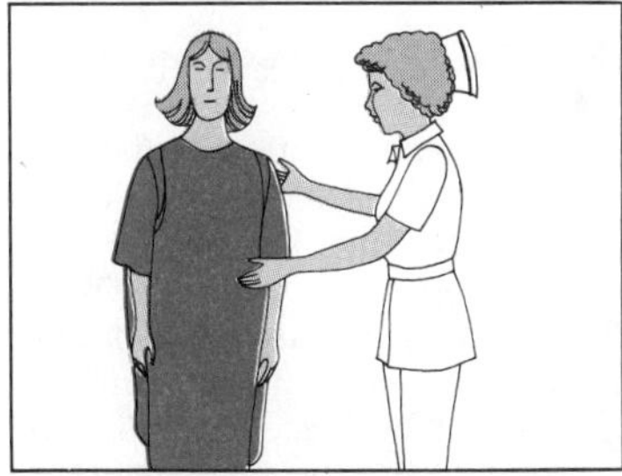

To perform some parts of the neurologic and musculoskeletal examinations, have the patient stand, when feasible, or sit.

Professional courtesy dictates that you be reassuring and gentle to help ease your patient's fears. Perhaps less obvious is your patient's need to feel that you know what you're doing. Demonstrate professionalism by approaching him in an unhurried manner. Never display negative reactions, such as surprise, alarm, distaste, or annoyance, in response to his physical appearance or anything he says.

Before you begin a physical examination, give your patient an opportunity to urinate. Tell him about the different positions you'll ask him to assume. The physical examination will probably require that he assume several positions. For example, he'll need to sit up while you examine his head, neck, chest, and back. Then he'll have to lie supine so you can examine his heart, abdomen, genitalia, extremities, and—in a female—the breasts. Certain phases of the neurologic examination necessitate that the patient stand and move in a variety of ways. By organizing the examination sequence carefully, you can minimize the number of position changes.

Your patient will have to undress for examination of most body systems. Provide a gown, and drape him appropriately for examination of the particular body area you'll assess (see *Preparing Your Patient: Guidelines to Positioning and Draping*, page 55). Explain to the patient why it is necessary for him to undress, since he may be confused or embarrassed. A female patient, for example, may not understand the importance of removing her bra. Many women, particularly teenagers and young adults, are embarrassed by this but are reluctant to ask for an explanation.

Be sure, too, that you've arranged for privacy. If you must perform the physical examination at your patient's bedside, close the door, draw the curtains around his bed, ask visitors to leave the room, and take any other necessary steps to safeguard your patient's privacy. These measures demonstrate your respect for the patient and minimize his embarrassment. They also enhance his cooperation during the examination. Remember: Your manner while conducting a physical examination can strengthen or undermine the rapport you've developed with the patient, as well as the degree of relaxation you've helped him attain.

Performing the general survey

67 The general survey

The physical examination actually begins with the general observations you make during the first few minutes with the patient—perhaps while you're introducing yourself or assisting him into a hospital gown. This information, supplemented by basic statistical information—such as height, weight, and the status of vital signs—constitutes the *general survey.*

Conduct the general survey no matter which examination method you plan to follow—head to toe or major body systems. Some initial survey observations you may make are outlined in *Your First Impression: What's Your Patient's Condition?*.

68 Vital signs: Indicators of physical status

Your patient's age, activity level, and physical and emotional status can affect his vital signs. In fact, even changing the time of day when you routinely measure his *body temperature, pulse rate, respirations,* and *blood pressure* can result in variations from the previous to the current determinations. You should keep these considerations in mind when you assess your patient's vital signs.

YOUR FIRST IMPRESSION: WHAT'S YOUR PATIENT'S CONDITION?

Ask yourself the following questions about your patient when you observe him for the first time:

- What is this patient's sex? What is his race? (As you know, some diseases are sexually or racially linked.)
- What's this patient's state of awareness? Is he alert and aware of what's going on around him, or is he inattentive and disoriented?
- Does this patient show signs of distress? For instance, is he sweating excessively or having trouble breathing? Is he moaning, or protecting a painful area? Are his hands cold and moist? Is he moving about restlessly?
- Does this patient look his age, or does he look older or younger than his actual age?
- What does his facial expression communicate? For example, does he look relaxed, apathetic, fearful, depressed?
- What attitude do his manner and mood portray? For instance, is he cooperative, hostile, tearful?
- Is this patient's speech unusually slow or fast? Is his speech thick or accented? Is his voice hoarse? Does he suffer from aphasia?
- What's this patient's skin color? For instance, is he flushed, pale, cyanotic, jaundiced?
- Do this patient's body size and shape appear normal for his age? Or is he under- or overdeveloped? Does he have any obvious deformities?
- Does this patient seem nutritionally healthy, or obese or malnourished?
- How has this patient dressed and cared for himself? Is he dressed adequately? Is he dressed appropriately? Does he look disheveled or show signs of poor personal hygiene (dull hair, uncleanliness, body odor)?
- What does this patient's posture communicate? (Consider also a body position that may reflect physiologic disturbance, such as severe respiratory distress.) For example, is he leaning, slumped, or hunched forward? Does he sit with his knees drawn up?

Taking a patient's vital signs allows you to:
- determine the relative status of vital organs, including the heart, blood vessels, and lungs
- monitor response to treatment
- establish baseline measurements that can be compared with future readings
- determine the need for further diagnostic testing.

69 Understanding body temperature

Body temperature is the difference between the amount of heat the body produces and the amount of heat it loses. Heat-producing processes within the body—for example, metabolism, disease, exercise, shivering, unconscious tensing of muscles, and increased thyroid activity—sometimes produce more heat than is necessary to maintain a normal body temperature of 97.7° to 99.5° F. (36.5° to 37.5° C.). To offset excessive heat production and restore normal temperature, the body uses some or all of these four processes: *radiation, conduction, convection,* and *evaporation* (see *Four Processes that Help Regulate Body Temperature,* page 58).

A *negative feedback system* allows the body to maintain a fairly constant temperature. Receptor cells in the skin, sensitive to heat and cold, respond to changes in cutaneous temperature. The cells' response to such alterations triggers nerve impulses, which are transmitted through the cerebral cortex to the hypothalamus—the brain's thermoregulatory center. The hypothalamus integrates the responses of the receptor cells in the skin with its own responses to blood temperature and arrives at a new *sensed* temperature. The hypothalamus then compares the sensed temperature to the body's *set point,* or *reference temperature.*

If a variation exists, the hypothala-

HOW TO CONVERT TEMPERATURE MEASUREMENTS

Formula for converting centigrade to Fahrenheit:

(C.° x 9/5) + 32 = F.°

Formula for converting Fahrenheit to centigrade:

(F.° − 32) x 5/9 = C.°

mus signals the appropriate heat-regulating mechanism to raise or lower body temperature. For example, when heat reduction is necessary, the hypothalamus sends out impulses that dilate cutaneous blood vessels and stimulate sweat glands. Radiation from the large volume of blood brought to the skin's surface, together with evaporation of the resulting perspiration, eliminates heat from the body and restores normal body temperature. The hypothalamus can also send out impulses that increase heat production and reduce heat elimination when decreased body heat threatens to drop body temperature below normal. These impulses inhibit secretion of sweat, increase the basal metabolic rate, and constrict superficial blood vessels to meet the body's demands for internal temperature regulation.

70 Routes for taking body temperature

You can take a patient's body temperature *orally* or *rectally*, or by using the *axillary* method. Before deciding which method to use for a particular patient, consider the patient's overall condition and age. The oral route is probably most convenient, and reflects arterial temperature more accurately than a rectal or axillary reading. If your patient is unconscious, confused, or disoriented, is unable to keep his mouth closed, or is receiving oxygen by face mask, take a rectal or axillary temperature. The rectal or axillary route should also be used to measure the body temperature of infants and young children.

FOUR PROCESSES THAT HELP REGULATE BODY TEMPERATURE

Four processes—radiation, conduction, convection, and evaporation—help the body eliminate excess heat. This illustration demonstrates how each process works.

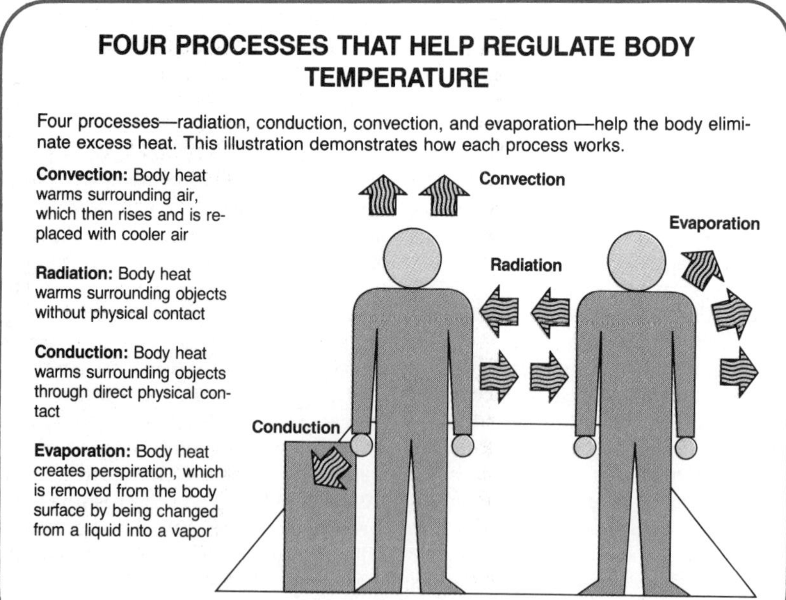

FACTORS AFFECTING BODY TEMPERATURE

When you check your patient's body temperature, keep in mind the factors listed below that can affect this temperature reading.

FACTOR	POSSIBLE RISE IN TEMPERATURE	POSSIBLE DROP IN TEMPERATURE
Time of day	99.5° F. (37.5° C.) during 4 to 8 p.m., with increased activity	97.7° F. (36.5° C.) during 4 to 6 a.m., with decreased activity
Age	100° F. (37.8° C.) in infants and 98.9° F. (37.2° C.) in children because of increased growth, metabolic rate, and activity	95° F. (35° C.) in the elderly because of slower metabolic rate and decreased muscular activity
Exercise	100° F. (37.8° C.) with exertion, and then returns to normal within 30 minutes	97.7° F. (36.5° C.) during sleep because of decreased metabolic rate and muscular activity, and increased heat loss
Menstrual cycle	99.6° F. (37.6° C.) during ovulation because of increased progesterone level	97.7° F. (36.5° C.) in early morning just before onset of menstruation
Pregnancy	100.4° F. (38° C.) during first 4 months	97° F. (36° C.) during last 5 months

For adults who won't cooperate by having their temperatures taken rectally, use the axillary route when the oral route is contraindicated.

If you use a glass thermometer to take a patient's temperature orally, leave it in place for 3 to 5 minutes. If the patient recently smoked, ate, or drank, wait 15 minutes before taking an oral temperature reading. For an accurate axillary temperature reading, leave the thermometer in place for 9 to 11 minutes. For a rectal reading, lubricate the thermometer and insert it 1½" (4 cm) into the rectum. Then keep it in place for 2 to 4 minutes.

71 Normal and abnormal body temperatures

A normal temperature reading varies with the route selected for taking the temperature (see *How Body Temperature Differs by Route,* page 60) and the time of day. Rectal temperatures register 1° F. higher than oral temperatures. All temperature readings are 1° to 2° F. lower in the early morning than in the late afternoon. Variations from normal body temperature can indicate *hypothermia* or *hyperthermia.* Hypothermia is below-normal body temperature, which slows down metabolic processes. The hypothermic patient may be drowsy or even comatose because of impaired central nervous system (CNS) functioning. His circulation rate may be slow and his heart rate irregular. If body temperature drops to 94.6° F. (34.8° C.), functioning of the hypothalamus is impaired; at 84.9° F. (29.4° C.), the hypothalamus stops functioning.

In hyperthermia (fever), certain processes cause body temperature to rise. The hypothalamus resets the set point, or reference temperature, at a higher level than normal. Causes of the malfunctioning include CNS disease or injury and infectious states. Regardless of the cause, the hypothalamus, responding to a blood (surface) temperature that is lower than the abnormally high level of the reference temperature, activates autonomic responses to elevate body temperature. When body heat reaches the hypothalamus' new set point, frank signs of fever will be exhibited.

When the disease process stops, the hypothalamus receives stimuli that allow it to reset the reference temperature at a lower (normal) level. Then the body's heat-loss mechanisms initiate vasodilation, stimulation of sweat glands, and muscle relaxation—at which point the fever usually breaks.

72 Understanding pulse rate

During systole, the heart ejects blood from the left ventricle into a full aorta. This produces a flaring of the aorta and a resultant wave or pulsation throughout the arterial system, palpable as your patient's *pulse.* Each pulse beat corresponds to a heartbeat and results from the impact of the ejected blood on arterial walls.

The heart of a normal adult at rest beats an average of 60 to 100 times per minute, pumping 5.3 qt (5 liters) of blood per minute through the body. To calculate *cardiac output,* multiply the *heart rate* per minute times the *stroke volume* (the volume of blood ejected with each beat).

A decrease in heart rate—such as *bradycardia* (a rate below 60 beats per minute)—without a compensatory increase in stroke volume causes diminished cardiac output. Bradycardia occurs with stimulation of the parasympathetic nervous system. This may result, for example, from injection of certain drugs.

Conversely, an increase in heart rate can occur when stroke volume lessens, keeping cardiac output constant. A heart rate of more than 100 beats per minute is called *tachycardia.* Pain, fear, anxiety, or anger can cause stimulation of the sympathetic nervous system, causing heart rate acceleration. Other conditions associated with tachycardia include thyroid problems, fever, anemia, hypoxia, and shock.

HOW BODY TEMPERATURE DIFFERS BY ROUTE

ROUTE	NORMAL RANGES
Oral	97.7° to 99.5° F. (36.5° to 37.5° C.)
Rectal	98.7° to 100.5° F. (37.1° to 38.1° C.)
Axilla	96.7° to 98.5° F. (35.9° to 36.9° C.)

73 Selecting an appropriate pulse site

The most accessible and commonly used artery for measuring a patient's pulse rate is the *radial artery,* which you compress against the radius to take the *radial pulse.* You can palpate other pulse sites when your patient's radial artery is inaccessible, or when testing circulation at a specific site (see *Locating Peripheral Pulse Sites*).

To palpate a *pulse,* lightly place the pads of your index and middle fingers over the pulse point. Then compress the pulse point until you detect maximum pulsation. (Never use your thumb to take a patient's pulse because the pulsations from the radial artery in your thumb can interfere with an accurate reading.)

Assess all peripheral pulses in a patient scheduled for surgery (especially cardiac or peripheral vascular surgery) or in a patient admitted for a diabetic or arterial occlusive condition. If you have difficulty palpating a peripheral pulse, mark its location on the patient's skin with a pen or marker for future reference. Document what you've done.

74 Assessing your patient's pulse rate and quality

Although the normal *pulse rate* of a resting adult is 60 to 100 beats per minute, the rate is slightly faster in women than in men, and faster still in infants and children (see *How Age Affects Arterial Pulse Rates,* page 62). If your patient's pulse rate seems abnormally fast or slow, or irregular, count the number of radial pulsations for 60 seconds, then auscultate the apical heartbeat for 60 seconds. The difference between the radial rate and the apical rate is called the *pulse deficit.* A pulse deficit means that some heartbeats aren't strong enough to produce a palpable peripheral pulsation. Thus, the radial pulse would be slower than the apical pulse (never the reverse).

Moderate exercise usually causes the pulse rate to increase by about 20 to 30 beats per minute. The rate should return to normal within 2 minutes after cessation of exercise.

When you take a patient's pulse, you must know how to assess the quality of the pulse as well as its rate. *Quality* refers to a pulse's amplitude, rhythm, and contour.

- *Amplitude* is the force of the pulse, which can be bounding or full, normal, weak, or thready.
- *Rhythm* refers to the relative equality of the intervals between beats. Bigeminal rhythm, for example, is a pattern of two beats—the first usually stronger than the second—followed by a pause.
- *Contour* describes the wavelike flow of a pulse as it rises, crests, and then collapses.

Note any change in the quality of a patient's pulse, whether in amplitude, rhythm, or contour, so that appropriate diagnostic tests can be ordered.

75 Evaluating respiration

When assessing respirations routinely with other vital signs, focus on the rate, depth, and pattern of respirations. Note the patient's general physical appearance, especially his color, as well as the ease and regularity of his breathing and chest wall movements.

LOCATING PERIPHERAL PULSE SITES

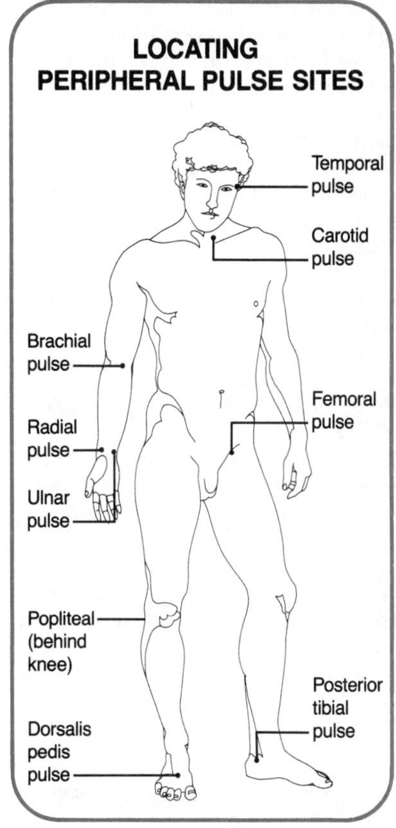

Throughout the respiratory process, the lungs maintain homeostasis of arterial blood by supplying it with inhaled oxygen. They also maintain the blood's pH by retaining carbon dioxide or disposing of it. If the major respiratory muscles—the diaphragm and the external intercostal muscles—weaken and fail to provide sufficient ventilation to meet the body's oxygen demands, then accessory muscles, such as the scalene, sternocleidomastoid, trapezius, and latissimus dorsi, attempt to compensate. If your patient relies on accessory muscles for respiration but has no history of chronic pulmonary disease, include this information in your nursing notes.

The body's normal mechanisms for stimulating respiration may break down as a result of brain trauma, a chronic increase in PCO_2 in patients with chronic obstructive lung disease, or the use of drugs such as barbiturates and narcotics. Closely observe the respiratory status of patients with acute cardiac problems, evidence of increased intracranial pressure, or acute or chronic pulmonary disease, and of patients in shock.

76 Determining respiratory rate

To determine your patient's *respiratory rate,* unobtrusively count his respirations for 60 seconds. Try to count respirations immediately after you take a pulse, *without his knowledge,* while you continue to hold his radial pulse (or, with the stethoscope still in place on the chest wall). Remember, a patient who knows his respirations are being observed tends involuntarily to alter his breathing.

The normal respiratory rate for a resting adult (male or female) is 12 to 20 breaths per minute; a faster rate is normal in infants and children. A slower than normal respiratory rate (less than 12 breaths per minute) may occur with conditions such as CNS depression that results from use of certain drugs, administration of anesthetics, or carbon dioxide narcosis. Both psychological and physical conditions—fear, pain, anxiety, fever, hypoxia, diabetic coma, and midbrain lesions, for example—can accelerate respiratory rate to more than 20 breaths per minute in an adult.

HOW AGE AFFECTS ARTERIAL PULSE RATES

AGE	PULSE RATE (beats per minute)
Under 1 month	90 to 170
Under age 1	80 to 160
Age 2	80 to 120
Age 6	75 to 115
Age 10	70 to 110
Age 14	65 to 100
Over age 14	60 to 100

77 Classify the depth of respiration

Depth of respiration is the volume of air—or *tidal volume*—moving in and out of the patient's mouth or nose with each breath. A healthy adult normally inhales and exhales 500 cc of air per breath, which provides adequate ventilation. Ideally, the depth of respiration should be constant with each breath. To approximate the depth of a patient's respiration, observe his chest movement for adequate and symmetrical chest expansion. (If he's unconscious, place the back of your hand close to his mouth and nose to feel the air he exhales.) Depth of respiration is characterized as *normal, shallow,* or *deep.* Remember that respirations in men are usually abdominal, whereas respirations in women are chiefly thoracic.

78 Normal and abnormal respiratory patterns

The rate and depth of a patient's respirations influence the respiratory *pattern* or *rhythm.* Normal respirations follow one another evenly, with little variation from one breath to another. Generally, the respiratory process follows a four-step pattern: a fairly rapid inspiration, a slight pause, then a slightly longer expiration, followed by a longer pause.

Variations in respiratory pattern can be associated with specific disease processes. Metabolic acidosis and alkalosis, for example, can adversely affect the pattern or rhythm. Severe metabolic alkalosis causes a distinctive pattern of respirations, characterized by 5- to 30-second periods of apnea.

79 Understanding arterial blood pressure

Blood pressure reading is an indirect measurement of the fluctuating pressures that blood exerts laterally on arterial walls as the heart contracts and relaxes. Arterial blood pressure reflects cardiac output, vascular resistance to circulating blood, blood viscosity and volume, and the ability of arterial walls to expand and constrict. Measuring arterial blood pressure aids the evaluation of a patient's circulatory status and fluid balance—two important indicators of overall physical status. A series of blood pressure readings, which may show the development of a trend, is nearly always more significant than a single reading.

The hemodynamics of blood pressure begins with contraction of the left ventricle, which sends blood flowing from the aorta to other arteries, and then to capillaries and veins. The pressure blood exerts against arterial walls as a result of contraction of the left ventricle (systole) is the *systolic pressure.* It indicates arterial pressure at the peak of pulsation. *Diastolic pressure* is arterial pressure at its ebb, during left ventricular relaxation (diastole), and is thus a measure of the minimum pressure being exerted on arterial walls. The difference between systolic and diastolic pressures is called *pulse pressure,* an important diagnostic indicator in such conditions as increased intracranial pressure, hypertension, and shock.

Many factors affect arterial blood pressure. The time of day, for example, can make a difference in blood pressure readings. A person's blood pressure is usually lowest in the early morning and rises when the person begins to move about. Body position also affects blood pressure; readings taken while a person is lying down will be lower than when he's sitting or standing. Another significant factor is the presence of fatty deposits lining the vessels. These deposits reduce the vessels' interior capacity and increase blood pressure, since greater force is required to propel blood through the narrowed passages.

80 How to measure arterial blood pressure

In most cases, you'll measure your patient's arterial blood pressure in millimeters of mercury (mm Hg), using three pieces of equipment: a sphygmomanometer, an inflatable cuff, and a stethoscope. Two types of sphygmomanometers are available to measure blood pressure: one has a calibrated column of mercury, the other a compact aneroid dial that gives direct readings.

Before taking your patient's blood pressure, make sure he's relaxed; for example, make sure he hasn't exercised or eaten within the past 30 minutes. When you take his blood pressure, he can be sitting, standing, or lying down. If this is the first time you've examined him, you may want to obtain baseline readings by taking his blood pressure twice in each arm—when he's lying down, then when he's sitting or standing. Remember, always wait 30 seconds before taking another reading, to allow the blood pressure to normalize.

Make sure the bladder of the inflatable cuff is about 20% wider than the diameter of the patient's arm or leg. Too narrow a cuff will produce a false high reading because of the greater pressure required to compress the artery. Conversely, a false low reading results from using a cuff that is too wide, since only minimal pressure is required for arterial compression.

To take a routine arterial blood pressure reading, keep the patient's arm level with his heart. Center the cuff over the brachial artery, and wrap it smoothly and evenly around the upper arm. The isometric contraction that occurs when a patient uses his own muscle strength to raise and straighten his arm can elevate systolic pressure about 10 mm Hg and distort the blood pressure reading. To prevent this, support his arm with your hand as you adjust the cuff. Then palpate the radial artery and rapidly inflate the cuff, until the radial pulse disappears. Continue inflating the cuff until the pressure has risen an additional 20 to 30 mm Hg.

Place the stethoscope's diaphragm over the brachial artery, about an inch below the cuff, and release the air in the cuff at the rate of 2 mm Hg per heartbeat. If you deflate the cuff too slowly, the blood vessels in the patient's arm may become congested and cause a false high reading. If you deflate the cuff too quickly, you won't have enough time to assess diastolic pressure accurately. As soon as you hear blood begin to pulse through the brachial artery again, note the height of the sphygmomanometer's mercury column—reading it at eye level—or read the sphygmomanometer's aneroid dial. This is your patient's systolic blood pressure.

Continue to deflate the cuff until the pulsations diminish or become muffled. This reading on the sphygmomanometer indicates his diastolic blood pressure. Until recently, the point at which sound *disappeared* was recorded as the diastolic pressure. But current studies have shown that the muffling of sound is closer to the true intraarterial pressure. (The American Heart Association recommends recording blood pressures as systolic/muffling/disappearance—for example, 126/70/66.)

HOW AGE AFFECTS ARTERIAL BLOOD PRESSURE READINGS

AGE	AVERAGE READING
Under 1 year	63 mean
Age 2	96/30
Age 4	98/60
Age 6	105/60
Age 10	112/64
Ages 11 to 18	120/75
Over age 18	130/80

81 Normal and abnormal blood pressure readings

Normal arterial blood pressure varies greatly among individuals. Generally, systolic blood pressure in a healthy adult ranges from 100 to 135 mm Hg; diastolic pressure usually ranges from 60 to 80 mm Hg. If your patient has been relaxed for 5 to 10 minutes, and hasn't eaten or exercised for 30 minutes, expect to obtain blood pressure readings within these ranges. A rise or fall of 10 to 20 mm Hg, with no apparent reason for the fluctuation (such as a change in the patient's position or activity level), necessitates further investigation, especially if the patient has no history of such an irregularity. Naturally, all factors that can affect blood pressure, such as age (see *How Age Affects Arterial Blood Pressure Readings*), must be ruled out.

Consistently low blood pressure may be normal in some persons. Abnormally low blood pressure (below 95/60 mm Hg) indicates *hypotension*. This condition can result from acute myocardial infarction, which decreases cardiac output, or from any other condition that reduces the patient's total blood volume. (Examples are addisonian crisis; severe burns; dehydration from decreased oral intake in an elderly person, an infant, or a severely depressed person; diarrhea; vomiting; heat exhaustion; metabolic acidosis; and hypovolemic shock.) Signs of hypotension include increased pulse rate, diaphoresis, dizziness, confusion, weakness, lethargy, cool and clammy skin, and blurred vision.

Hypertension is persistently elevated blood pressure (above 140/90 mm Hg), which occurs when blood exerts excessive pressure against arterial walls. Hypertension usually reflects an underlying disorder, such as kidney disease, but you may encounter patients with *essential*, or *idiopathic*, hypertension, in whom no cause for elevated blood pressure can be found. Some disorders, such as aortic insufficiency, increase only systolic blood pressure—diastolic pressure remains normal. This is also classified as hypertension.

Performing inspection, palpation, percussion, and auscultation

82 Inspection: Informed observation

Of the four physical assessment skills, inspection is unquestionably paramount. It appears simple and so is often taken for granted. But this skill involves more than just looking at your patient. Inspection is *informed observation*, or looking with a purpose—keenly, intently, with an eye for relevant detail. This skill goes beyond what you see with your eyes, to encompass your senses of smell, touch, and hearing. For example, your nose may detect the odor of necrotic tissue. By touch, you assess your patient's temperature or the texture of his skin. Your ears can hear noisy respirations.

For some types of inspection, you may need to use equipment, such as an ophthalmoscope, an otoscope, or a speculum, to enhance your vision or gain access to an area.

Lighting is important when you're inspecting a patient. Take advantage of daylight, if possible. In most modern hospital rooms, a broad panel of lights extends over the patient's bed, and some even have fixtures that let you direct the light to where you want it. If this kind of an arrangement isn't available, be prepared with a flashlight or portable lamp suitable for examining purposes.

Your personal data base of clinical nursing knowledge helps you to recognize the significance of inspection findings. This impression grows stronger or weaker after you analyze the information you've already gathered about your patient—particularly during the health history interview. What this means is that inspection requires you to look for physical findings similar to those you've found in the past, under similar clinical circumstances. At the same time you're looking for predictable physical findings, keep your eyes and mind open to the unexpected. Balance these two approaches to a patient and you'll be well on your way to mastering the difficult skill of inspection.

Be careful to maintain your objectivity. Don't distort your findings with preconceived ideas. (Sometimes knowledge of what *should be* distorts what *is*.) If what you expect to find isn't apparent, you shouldn't invent it.

83 What inspection is

Inspection draws on your most acute faculties. You need keen physical senses, adequate clinical knowledge, an agile mind that can quickly recall past clinical experiences, and the ability to draw accurate conclusions quickly. You can be sure of one thing: You'll never lack opportunities to practice inspection. By far the most frequently performed assessment skill, inspection comes into play every time you see a patient. As an astute observer, you'll notice changes in your patient that may signal deterioration or improvement in his condition, or the appearance of a new sign. Inspection is an ongoing process; it begins during the health history interview, continues through the physical examination, and shouldn't end until the day your patient's discharged.

84 Use a general-to-specific inspection technique

After your general survey, move on to more specific inspections. Focus on problem areas that the patient or your general survey has identified. For each body area, use the general-to-specific approach. First, note the area's general appearance; then, observe and record distinctive details, such as the normal or abnormal size, shape, location, color, texture, and motion of structures. If appropriate, record the absence or presence of common landmarks, and compare the area you're inspecting with its counterpart on the other side of your patient's body.

To be sure you're inspecting each patient accurately and thoroughly, develop a systematic inspection method that you can follow routinely, but can also adjust for individual patients.

Base your initial inspection on what you already know about the patient—his age, general physical status, and reason for seeking health care. For example, suppose you notice a rash during your initial inspection. After completing your general observations, return to the rash, inspect it more closely, and describe all its observable characteristics. Your note might read: *Erythematous, flat, circumscribed lesions, less than 1 mm in diameter, scattered randomly over entire face, becoming very dense and merging in the periauricular regions.*

85 Palpation: Touch tells you more

Generally, you'll perform palpation as the second step in assessing your patient, to rule out—or possibly confirm—suspicions raised during inspection. Sometimes you may inspect and palpate a patient simultaneously. For example, when your inspection of a patient reveals an enlarged scrotum, your palpation may detect a unilateral, nontender mass that feels like a bag of worms—a finding that suggests varicocele.

Palpation involves the trained and skillful use of your sense of touch to obtain clinical information about your patient. With your hands and fingers, you can determine the size, shape, and position of structures as well as their temperature, texture, moisture content, and movement. You can palpate all parts of your patient's body, including tissues, bones, muscles, glands, organs, hair, and skin. Palpation also helps you check for growths, swelling, muscle spasm or rigidity, pain and tenderness, and crepitus. You'll perform abdominal palpation often, to detect such problems as a distended bladder, a palpable spleen, an umbilical hernia, an enlarged liver, a prominent upper abdominal pulsation with lateral expansion—even the position of a fetus.

Like inspection, palpation relies on a sense that's important but often undervalued. Theoretically, anyone can touch or probe a human body with his hand to feel for a lump or some other abnormal sign. Only a knowledgeable and experienced health-care professional can perform such an examination thoroughly and systematically, while causing the patient as little discomfort as possible.

86 How to palpate your patient

Remember that touching a patient is apt to elicit fear, embarrassment, and other strong emotions. Be sure to explain what you're doing and why, as well as what he can expect—such as

PALPATING EFFECTIVELY: HOW TO USE YOUR HANDS AND FINGERS

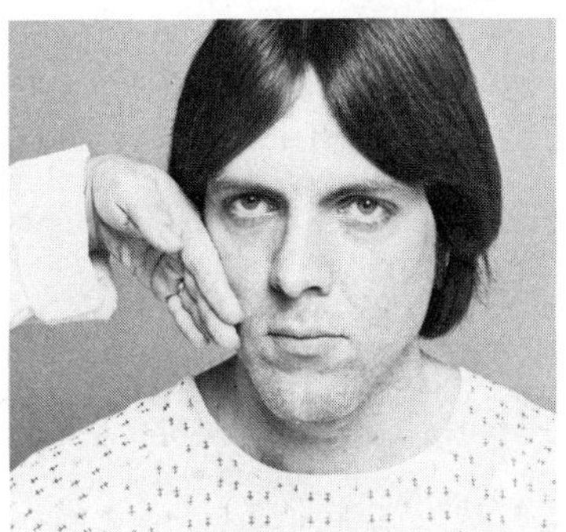

To assess your patient's skin temperature, use the backs of your fingers and hands to palpate the face, inflamed areas, and the hands and feet.

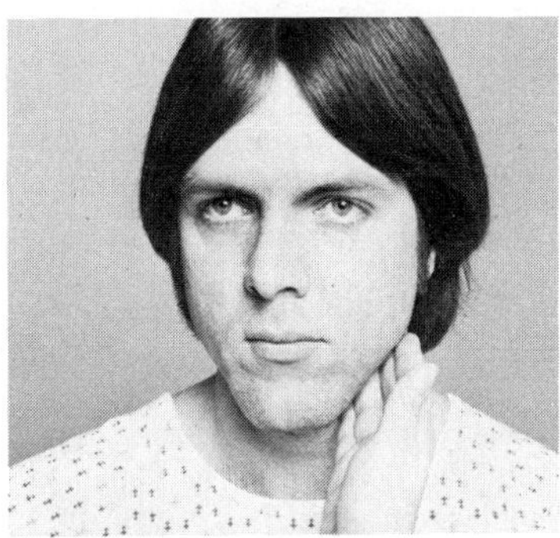

To determine size and position of lymph nodes or growths, palpate with the pads of your fingers.

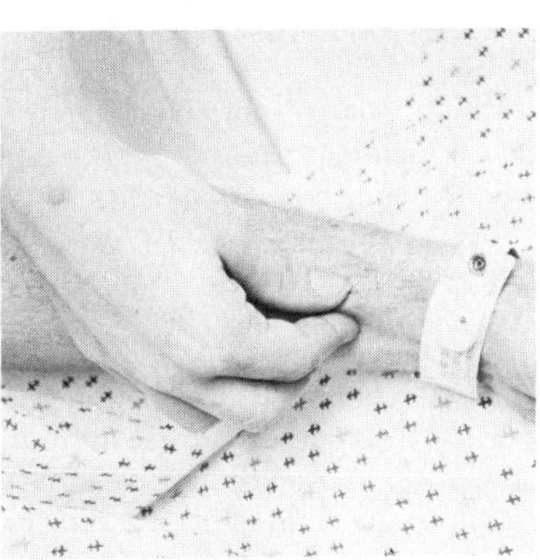

To determine muscle and tissue consistency and joint position, palpate with your thumb and index finger.

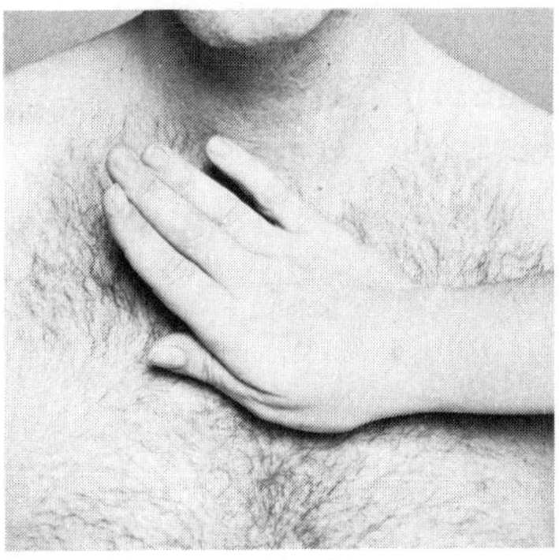

To assess for fremitus, palpate with the ball of your hand.

discomfort. Make sure your hands are warm. Try to get your patient to relax, because muscular tension or guarding can interfere with the performance and results of palpation. Instruct the patient to breathe deeply, through his mouth. If you've identified tender areas, palpate them last.

Part of the skill of palpation is in knowing which areas of your hands and fingers to use (see *Palpating Effectively: How to Use Your Hands and Fingers*). Why is this important? Because your hands and fingers are not equally sensitive to all sensations—such as temperature. For example, you might suspect that your patient has an elevated surface temperature over a sprained ankle, or a lowered surface temperature in his hands from poor circulation. To investigate these and similar suspicions, use the *back of your hand or fingers,* because the skin there is thinner and more sensitive to temperature. You may find it helpful to palpate the suspect area with the back of one hand, while palpating an unaffected area with the back of the other hand. Then switch hands to confirm the differences you perceive between the two areas. For discriminating skin surface textures, first use your fingertips, to detect general differences, then use the backs of your hands and fingers for finer distinctions. Use the *pads of your fingertips* to determine the position, form, and consistency of structures—to palpate lymph nodes, for example. For determining muscle and tissue firmness, as well as joint positions, use your *thumb and index finger* to grasp the body part. To detect vibrations (such as thrills or fremitus), use the palmar surface of the metacarpophalangeal joints—the *ball of the hand.*

87 Light and deep palpation

To begin palpation (after making sure your hands are warm), apply slow, gentle pressure. Start with light palpation and progress to deep palpation (see *Performing Light and Deep Palpation*). Be sure to palpate painful or hypersensitive areas last. You're palpating to identify tender areas, the presence of masses, organ changes, and abnormal fluid collections.

Light palpation probes to a depth of 1 to 2 cm from the body surface. Used principally to detect slight tenderness and to assess muscle tone, this technique requires a gentle dipping and circular motion. With your hand parallel to the body surface being examined, extend your fingers, keeping them together; then, gently depress them.

To use light palpation on a patient's abdomen, for example, place your palm on the abdomen, extend your fingers, and then press them into the area. (This is known as *scouting;* it allows you to detect any areas of tenderness or guarding.)

Deep palpation locates abdominal masses and organs. Using this technique, apply greater pressure than you'd use for light palpation, pressing down from the body surface to a depth of 4 to 5 cm. You can use one or both hands for deep palpation. To perform *single-handed* deep palpation, place the palm of your hand on the abdomen, extend your fingers, and press in with your fingertips at a slight angle. This causes the underlying tissues to slide back and forth against the pads of your fingertips. To perform palpation using both hands—*bimanual* palpation—place one hand on the abdomen in the usual manner. Then place your other hand—palm down—on top of it. The top hand exerts pressure on the bottom hand's relaxed distal phalangeal joints, and guides the bottom hand to detect and delineate underlying organs or masses. Use this method to apply the additional pressure needed to reach deep organs or masses, or to overcome resistance of excess body tissues, if your patient is obese.

During palpation, watch your patient's facial expressions continuously for any sign of pain, since both types of deep palpation may normally cause him some discomfort. Keeping your eyes on the patient's face while palpating also enhances your sense of touch and trains you to palpate accurately. If palpation causes the patient obvious pain, don't continue, since you could injure him. For example, palpation may cause an enlarged spleen to rupture.

Using deep palpation, you can check for rebound tenderness directly over the affected site (if your patient doesn't have too much pain) by slowly and firmly depressing the tender area with your fingers, and then rapidly removing the pressure. Be sure to note whether the patient experiences pain when you withdraw your fingers. To confirm true rebound tenderness, palpate a neighboring region—for example, palpate the lower right abdominal quadrant if you suspect rebound tenderness in the lower left quadrant. The sudden release of pressure in the unaffected area will cause a sharp pain in the suspect site if true rebound tenderness exists.

PERFORMING LIGHT AND DEEP PALPATION

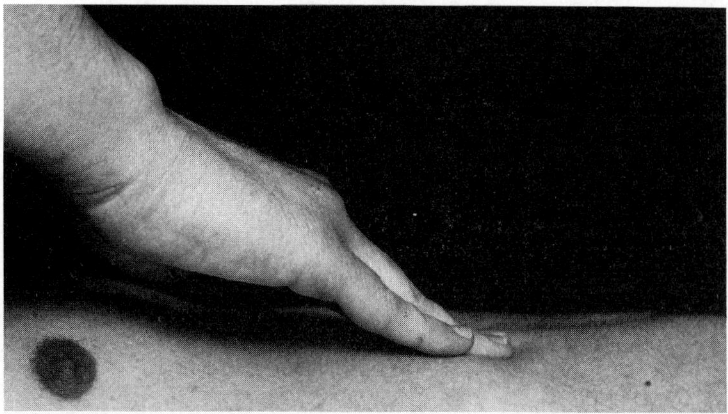

To perform light palpation, press gently on your patient's skin, indenting about 1 to 2 cm. Move your hand in a circular motion.

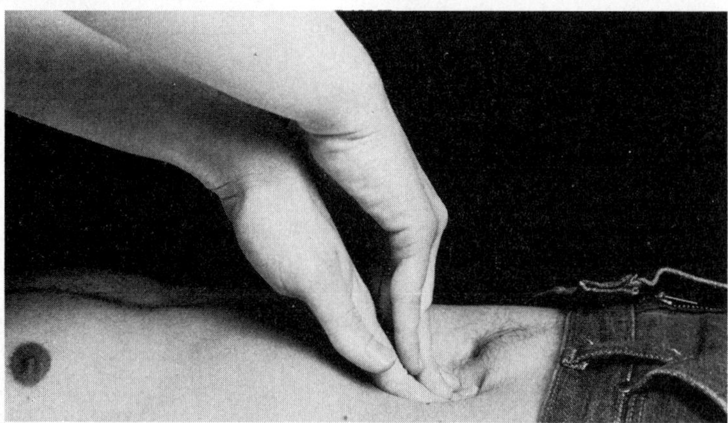

To perform deep palpation, increase your fingertip pressure, indenting about 4 cm. The nurse shown here is using both hands to perform *bimanual* deep palpation.

88 Performing ballottement

Ballottement (from the French for *tossing about*) is a palpation technique you use to determine if a freely movable mass is present beneath the abdominal wall. You'll be able to detect it with *light ballottement* because the light, rapid pressure causes solid tissue to bounce upward, toward your fingertips (see *Performing Ballottement*, page 70). You should also be able to feel a lively bounce in the upper right quadrant of the abdomen, caused by resistance from dense liver tissue.

To begin abdominal light ballottement, start low on your patient's abdomen, bouncing your fingertips lightly and rapidly upward. Besides detecting evidence of a mass (if present), this technique also demonstrates any tendency toward guarding—a sign of possible underlying inflammation.

If fluid or ascites are present in your patient's abdomen, you'll need to use a more forceful motion to feel the enlarged liver—a special palpation technique in which you exert sudden deep pressure. (This is done mainly to detect the presence of true fluid in a body cavity, as in ascites, or the presence of masses underlying collections of fluid.) To perform *deep ballottement* on the abdomen, position your hand with your fingertips perpendicular to the patient's abdominal wall. Keeping your fingers together, push inward suddenly and deeply. Then, release this pressure but keep your fingertips in contact with the abdominal surface. This will allow

PERFORMING BALLOTTEMENT

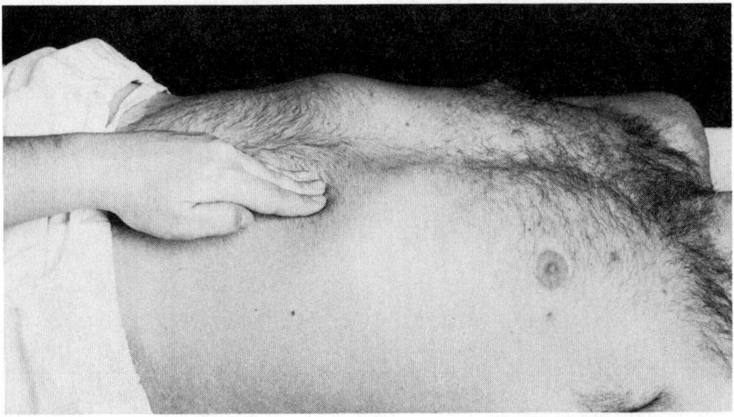

To perform light ballottement, apply light, rapid pressure, from quadrant to quadrant, on your patient's abdomen. Keep your hand on the skin surface throughout to feel tissue rebound.

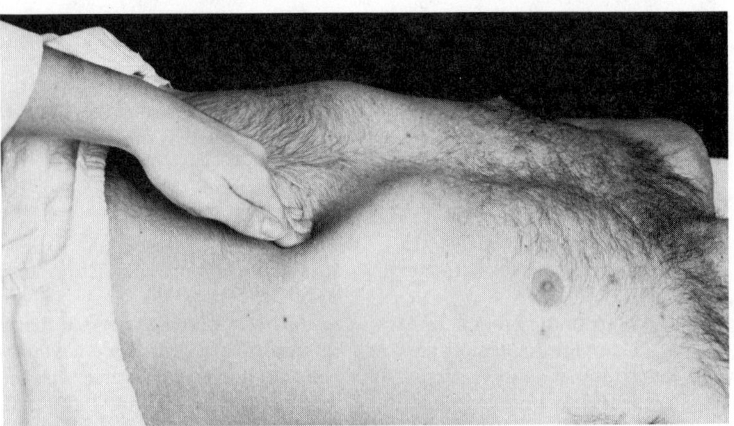

Exert abrupt, deep pressure when performing deep ballottement. Note that you should release pressure completely but maintain fingertip contact with the skin.

you to feel any movement of an organ or mass provided the mass is freely movable.

89 Why practicing palpation is important

Palpation is a sophisticated skill that you can perfect only through repeated practice. It requires more than manual dexterity; you must also be able to interpret your findings correctly. Organs and other body structures that can be palpated vary greatly in size and shape. Only through practice can you become familiar with normal findings and readily identify pathologic variations.

The skill you develop with practice will enable you to deal with difficult palpation situations. For example, if you localize a mass through palpation, next palpate it systematically to delineate its essential characteristics: size, shape, consistency, mobility, tenderness, and pulsation.

Obesity presents another challenge. Palpating the abdominal organs of an obese patient may be difficult because of the intervening excess adipose tissue. With such a patient, you may have to modify your technique, perhaps by using both hands to perform palpation adequately and applying greater pressure.

90 What percussion is

Percussion involves tapping the body surface lightly—with a sharp, quick motion—to produce sounds that help determine the size, shape, position, and density of underlying organs and tissues. This technique seems to be the physical assessment skill with which nurses are least familiar. Here's how it works: Percussion drives sound into the body by causing the body surface to vibrate. The examiner then listens and feels for various characteristics of the returning sound, which will reflect the nature of the body cavity's contents.

This technique, used most commonly over the chest and abdomen, may validate or clarify data you've obtained by history-taking, inspection, or palpation. Percussion reveals density by signaling the presence of air or solid material—to a depth of 5 to 7 cm—in a body cavity or organ. It helps you determine the size, shape, and position of internal organs by outlining their borders and approximating their depth.

91 Mediate, immediate, and fist percussion

Depending on the body region you're examining, you may use any of three types of percussion: mediate, immediate, and fist (see *Percussion: Using Three Methods,* page 72).

In the most widely used percussion method—*mediate* percussion, most frequently used to percuss the thorax and abdomen—you strike the middle finger of one hand with the middle or index finger of the other hand. The finger that does the striking is called the *plexor;* the finger that is struck is called the *pleximeter.* To perform mediate percussion, place the distal phalanx of the pleximeter (not the entire finger) against the body surface. (Keep the palm and other fingers of this hand raised off the skin.) Then strike the base of the pleximeter's distal interphalangeal joint with the tip (not the fat pad) of the plexor (see illustration).

To perform *immediate* percussion—an older technique used mainly to percuss an infant's thorax or adult sinuses—simply strike the body surface with one or more fingers of one hand. (The other hand is not involved.)

To perform *fist* percussion, place one hand flat against your patient's body surface, then strike the back of this hand with your other hand, clenched in a fist. This form of percussion, used most commonly over the lower back, helps determine the presence of pain or tenderness from kidney, liver, or gallbladder inflammation or disease.

92 Details of mediate percussion technique

The key to eliciting clear percussion notes is a quick snap of the wrist. Your

PERCUSSION: USING THREE METHODS

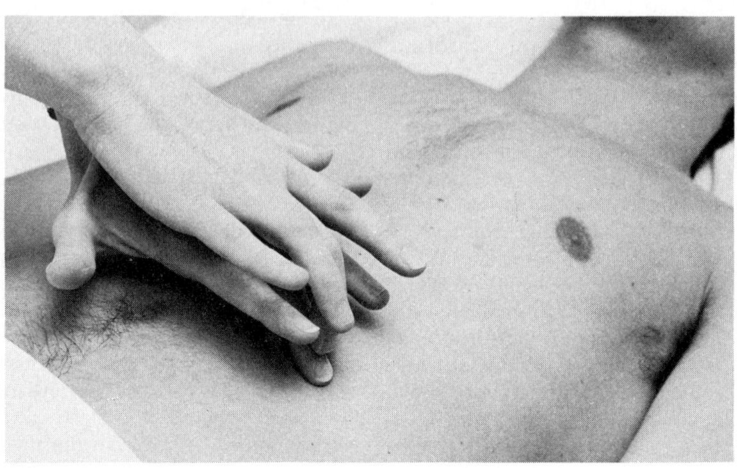

Mediate percussion
To perform mediate percussion, position your hands as the nurse is doing here. Note that her left hand is poised above, not touching, the skin. Remember, after tapping, to withdraw your right hand so you don't damp the vibrations.

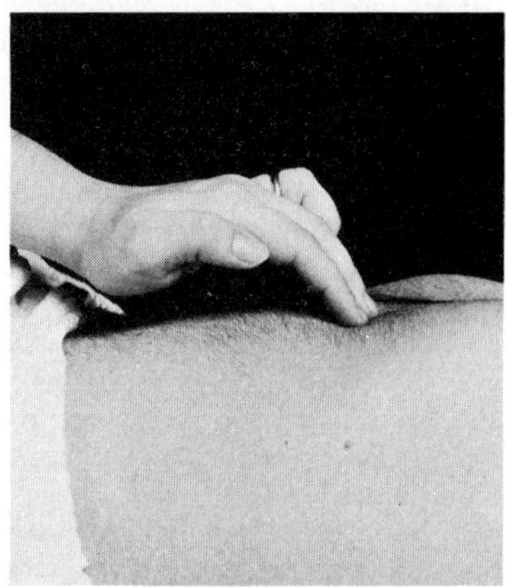

Immediate percussion
To perform immediate percussion, use only one hand, as shown here. Again, remember to keep the rest of your hand poised above, but not touching, the skin.

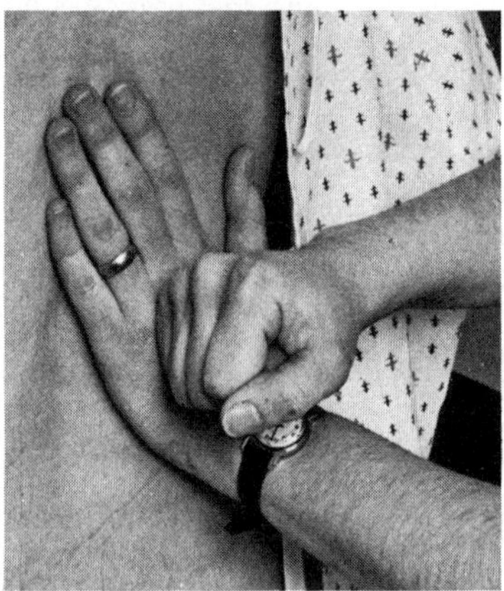

Fist percussion
To perform fist percussion, place the palm of one hand on the patient's back, as the nurse is doing here. Form a fist with the other hand and hit the back of the first hand with it.

forearm shouldn't move at all; your wrist generates all the force. Don't drive the plexor into the pleximeter as though playing a piano, and don't use your elbow and shoulder as though hammering a nail—two common mistakes in mediate percussion. Keeping your hand relaxed and using only your wrist to supply power assure percussion strokes of equal force.

Place only the distal phalanx of the pleximeter *firmly* in contact with the patient's body. Maintain this contact after the tap by the plexor, but remove the plexor immediately. If the plexor remains there for even a second or two after striking the pleximeter, the resulting sound will be muffled.

A light tap generally produces the best percussion note. A too-forceful blow may obliterate the sound, besides making the pleximeter sore. (Keep the fingernail of your plexor trimmed to prevent damage to the pleximeter.) Percussion notes needn't be loud to be useful; equally important are the pitch, duration, and quality of a note, for which lighter percussion is often superior. (Excess adipose tissue may dampen a normal percussion note. You may have to be more forceful in examining patients who are obese or who have large muscle mass.)

You shouldn't have to percuss an area more than two or three times before moving to another area. If you have to percuss the same area repeatedly to produce a meaningful note, check your technique. Needless to say, keep external noise at a minimum so you can detect changes in percussion notes. Remove all of your jewelry, too—such as rings, bracelets, or a loosely fitting watch—that might make noise while you're percussing.

93 The correct percussion sequence

Organize the percussion sequence so you move from more resonant body regions to less resonant ones. (You can perceive a change from resonance to dullness more easily than a change from dullness to resonance.) For example, when percussing to identify the lower border of liver dullness, start over the tympanic regions of the abdomen and then move up toward the dull area over the liver. To identify the liver's upper dullness border, begin over the lungs and percuss downward.

94 Characteristics of percussion sounds

Depending on the density of the organs and overlying tissues in the body region you're percussing, you'll hear percussion notes that have specific characteristics. The different qualities of the sounds are termed *resonance, hyperresonance, tympany, dullness,* and *flatness.* With practice, you'll be able to identify internal structures (such as the liver) and abnormalities (such as a gas-filled bowel from paralytic ileus) by the sounds they produce.

Sounds, of course, are difficult to describe in writing so as to be immediately identifiable when heard. The following guidelines may help you identify percussion sounds:

- *Intensity.* Is the sound loud or soft? You should hear loud tones when percussing over a normal lung and softer tones over the heart and liver.
- *Pitch.* Thinking in terms of a music scale, ask yourself if the note you hear is high or low. Dense structures emit a greater number of vibrations than less-dense structures, and so produce higher-pitched sounds. Normal bowel sounds are high pitched. A normal lung isn't dense, and so has a lower pitch than a consolidated lung.
- *Duration.* How long does the sound last?

95 What auscultation is

One of the most difficult physical examination skills to master, auscultation involves listening (with the ear or a stethoscope) to sounds produced in the body—primarily by the lungs, heart, blood vessels, stomach, and intestines. This technique can detect turbulence in the flow of air or fluid, such as that produced by a bruit at the site of an aneurysm. It can also detect almost any other kind of sound that may occur in the body, such as the cracking of a joint.

Although you can perform auscultation directly over a body surface, using only your ear, the preferred method is *indirect* auscultation with an acoustic stethoscope. This instrument conducts sound to the ears (but does *not* amplify it) while blocking out environmental noise (see *The Acoustic Stethoscope*).

96 Proper auscultation technique

Before beginning auscultation, make sure your stethoscope is in working order. Air leaks from a damaged bell or diaphragm, or from cracked eartips or tubing, are common. Don't overlook these leaks. They can let external noise into the stethoscope, decreasing sound volume by as much as 10 to 15 decibels.

Remove all sources of potentially interfering sounds. Close the door, turn off the television or radio, and ask the patient not to talk. Warm your hands and the stethoscope heads before auscultating, so your patient doesn't shiver—which can produce ralelike sounds. *Make sure the stethoscope is open to the listening end (bell or diaphragm), which is against the patient's body.* Which end you use depends on whether you're assessing high- or low-frequency sounds (see *Using the Stethoscope Heads Effectively*). Hold the bell or diaphragm firmly, without moving; otherwise, sounds from the movement of intercostal muscles, joints, or skin may occur, possibly mimicking a friction rub.

Most significant body organ sounds are of low intensity. As in percussion, the sounds auscultation produces are classified by frequency, intensity, quality, and duration. Concentrate on one sound at a time, intently and exclusively. Focus on normal sounds first,

THE ACOUSTIC STETHOSCOPE

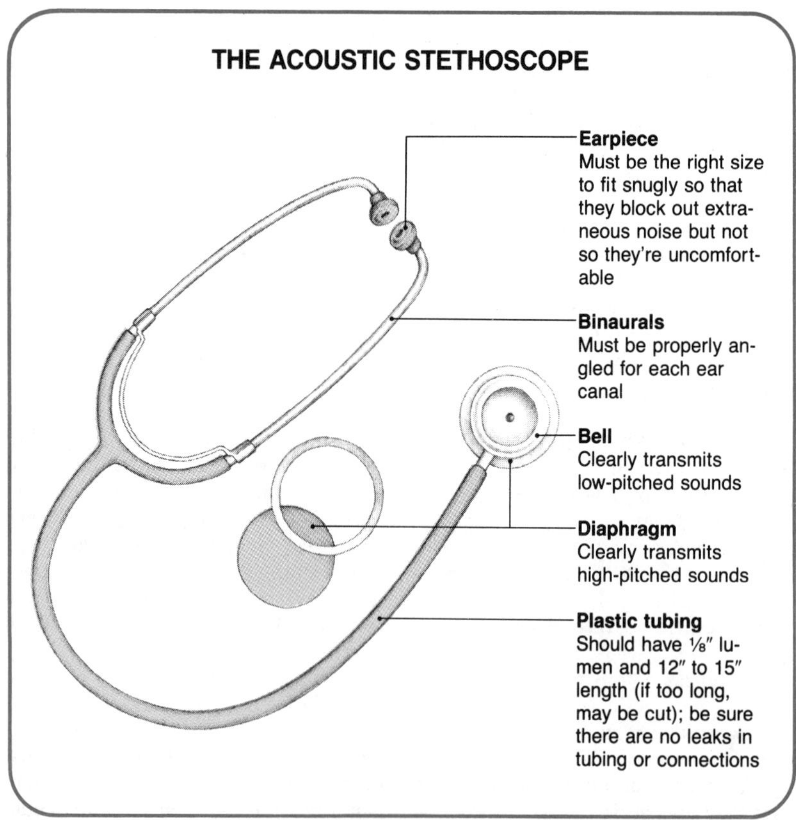

USING THE STETHOSCOPE HEADS EFFECTIVELY

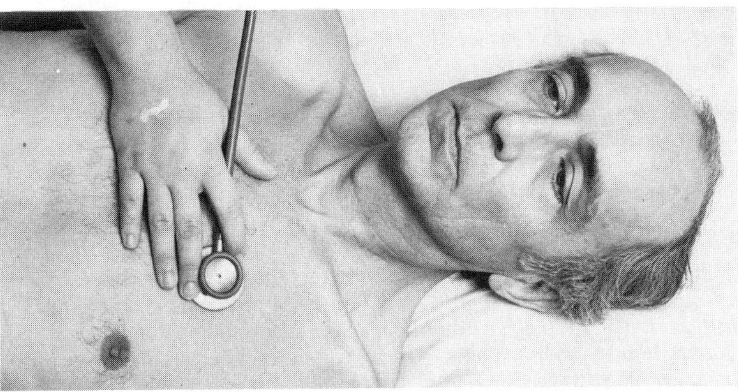

To properly assess high-frequency sounds, such as breath sounds and first and second heart sounds, use the diaphragm side of the stethoscope's chest piece. Make sure the entire surface of the diaphragm is positioned firmly on your patient's skin. If there is much hair on the chest, reduce extraneous noise and improve diaphragm contact by applying water or water-soluble jelly to your patient's chest before auscultating.

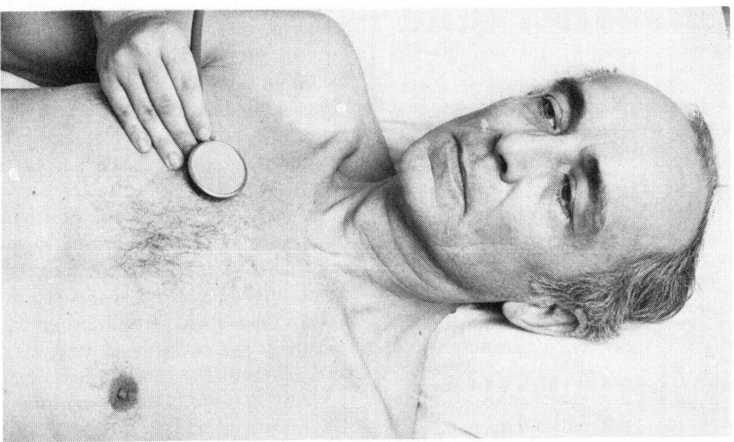

To assess low-frequency sounds, such as heart murmurs and third and fourth heart sounds, lightly place the stethoscope's bell on the appropriate skin area. Don't exert pressure. If you do, your patient's chest will act as a diaphragm, and you'll miss low-frequency sounds. If your patient is extremely thin or emaciated, use a stethoscope with a pediatric chest-piece.

to make subsequent detection of abnormal sounds easier. Keep such items as clothing, jewelry, and bedsheets from rubbing against the tubing and interfering with the transmission of sound. Sliding your fingers along the tubing or breathing on it may also cause confusing sounds. Be careful when you auscultate a body surface that is covered with hair; moving the bell or diaphragm over hair causes a sound that could be mistaken for rales.

Conducting the physical examination

97 Choosing an examination method

You need to consider several factors before deciding on the examination method—head to toe or major body systems—you'll use for a patient (see *Guidelines for a Head-to-Toe Physical Examination,* pages 77 to 87, and *Guidelines for a Physical Examination by Major Body Systems,* pages 88 to 90). (Remember, both methods of examination produce equally valid results.)

First, determine whether his condition is life-threatening. Identifying the *priority* problems of a patient suffering from life-threatening illness or injury—for example, severe trauma, heart attack, or gastrointestinal hemorrhage—is essential to preserve his life and function and to prevent compounded damage.

Next, identify the *patient population* to which the patient belongs, and take the common characteristics of that population into account in choosing an examination method. For example, elderly or debilitated patients tire easily; for a patient in either category, you'd select a method that necessitates minimal position changes. Also, you'd probably defer parts of the examination, to avoid tiring your patient.

Try to view your patient as an integrated whole rather than as a collection of parts, regardless of the examination method you use. Remember, the integrity of a body *region* may reflect adequate functioning of many body *systems,* both inside and outside this particular region. For example, the integrity of the chest region may provide important clues about the functioning of the cardiovascular and respiratory systems. Similarly, the integrity of a body *system* may reflect adequate functioning of many body *regions* and of the various systems within these regions.

98 The chief complaint guides the examination

You may want to plan your physical examination around your patient's chief complaint, or concern. To do this, begin by examining the body system or region that corresponds to the chief complaint. This allows you to identify priority problems promptly and reassures your patient that his primary reason for seeking health care is receiving proper attention.

Consider the following example. Your patient, Sarah Clemson, is a 65-year-old, well-developed, well-nourished woman who appears younger than her chronologic age. She complains of having difficulty breathing on exertion; she also has a dry, frequent, painful cough. Intermittent chills have persisted for 3 days. You'd record her vital signs: temperature, 103° F. (39.4° C.); pulse rate, 106/minute; respiratory rate, 29 to 30/minute; blood pressure, 128/82.

Because Mrs. Clemson's chief complaints are difficulty breathing, a cough, and chills, your physical examination would first focus on her *respiratory* system. You'd examine the patency of her airway, observe the color of her lips and extremities, and systematically palpate her lung fields for symmetry of expansion, crepitus, increased or decreased fremitus, and areas of tenderness. Then, after auscultating her lung fields for abnormal or adventitious sounds (such as rales, rhonchi, or wheezing), you'd percuss her lung fields for increased or decreased resonance.

Next, you'd examine Mrs. Clemson's *cardiovascular* system, looking for further clues to the cause of her signs and symptoms. You'd inspect her neck veins for distention and her extremities for edema, venous engorgement, and pigmented areas. Then, you'd palpate her chest to see if you could feel the heart's apical impulse at the fifth intercostal space, in the midclavicular line. You'd also palpate for a precordial heave and for valvular thrills. After determining her apical pulse rate, you'd auscultate for any abnormal heart sounds.

At this point in the examination, you would probably be aware of Mrs. Clemson's level of consciousness, motor ability, and ability to use her muscles and joints. You probably wouldn't need to perform a more thorough musculoskeletal and neurologic examination. You would, however, proceed with an examination of her gastrointestinal, genitourinary, and integumentary systems, modifying or shortening the examination sequences depending on your findings and Mrs. Clemson's tolerance. If her signs and symptoms worsened during the examination, you'd interrupt the procedure to report her condition to her doctor. Then you'd plan to come back and finish the examination after her condition is stabilized.

99 Recording physical examination results

Physical examination findings are crucial to arriving at a nursing diagnosis and, ultimately to developing a sound nursing-care plan. Record your examination results thoroughly, accurately, and clearly. Properly recorded information serves the following purposes:

- It identifies baseline parameters for future comparisons.
- It helps define patient problems through data analysis, synthesis of priority data, and problem identification.
- It communicates patient information to other members of the health-care team.
- It substantiates the adequacy of patient care for legal purposes or before audit committees.

While some examiners don't like to

GUIDELINES FOR A HEAD-TO-TOE PHYSICAL EXAMINATION

The guidelines in this chart show you how to proceed, and what to assess for each body system, when you perform a head-to-toe physical examination.

BODY REGION	HOW TO PROCEED	WHAT TO ASSESS	SAMPLE NORMAL DOCUMENTATION
Entire body	• Identify sex and race.		• White male
	• Observe general physical appearance.	• General state of health; signs of distress	• Follows instructions; is attentive and alert; displays no acute distress.
		• Appearance in relation to chronologic age	• Appears stated age.
		• Facial expression, mood, speech, and memory	• Alert, oriented, interested, and amiable; maintains eye contact; speech easily understood, with clear enunciation; responds appropriately; remote and recent memory intact.
		• Skin color	• Skin color uniform.

(continued)

GUIDELINES FOR A HEAD-TO-TOE PHYSICAL EXAMINATION *(continued)*

BODY REGION	HOW TO PROCEED	WHAT TO ASSESS	SAMPLE NORMAL DOCUMENTATION
Entire body *(continued)*		• Body development and nutritional state	• Extremities symmetrical and well proportioned. Skin smooth and turgor normal. Arm span equals height; distance from head to pubis nearly equals distance from pubis to feet. Muscles moderate to well developed. • Hair evenly distributed over scalp, extremities, eyebrows, and eyelashes; hair growth normal for age.
		• Dress and personal hygiene	• Neat, clean, and appropriately dressed.
		• Stature, posture, motor activity, and gait	• Body aligned, with shoulders back and relaxed; arms at sides, feet on floor, body relaxed; movements coordinated, deliberate, and smooth. Can sit and stand with smooth, even motion. Can sit motionless for brief time. Gait is even, steady, and smooth; arms swing at sides. When patient turns, his body follows his face and head. Easily performs heel strike midstance, push off and swing phases.
	• Assess vital signs.	• Temperature (oral, rectal, or axillary)	• Oral temperature is 98.6° F. (37° C.).
		• Pulse rate	• Pulse 84/minute, strong and regular.
		• Respiratory rate	• Respiratory rate 18/minute
		• Blood pressure in both arms	• Blood pressure when standing: right—126/72/64, Left—122/74/68; when lying down: right—116/68/62, left—114/64/60.
	• Measure height and weight.		• Weight 126 lb (56.7 kg) unclothed; height 5′5″ (165 cm).
	• Identify equipment being used for hospitalized patient (for example, I.V. line, nasogastric tube, chest tube, oxygen, ventilator, and urinary drainage tubes).		• I.V. infusing well at 30 gtts/minute; nasogastric tube draining thick, brown liquid; O_2 via cannula at 2 liters/minute.

GUIDELINES FOR A HEAD-TO-TOE PHYSICAL EXAMINATION *(continued)*

BODY REGION	HOW TO PROCEED	WHAT TO ASSESS	SAMPLE NORMAL DOCUMENTATION
Upper extremities	• Identify presence of cast, contractures, or traction.		• No cast, contracture, or traction noted.
	• Inspect hands and arms.	• Muscle mass and skeletal configuration	• Muscle mass and development normal for age; no deformities noted. Arms and hands symmetrical.
		• Skin color and lesions (if any)	• Normal coloring; smooth skin, no lesions or swelling
		• Nail color and condition	• Nail beds pink and clean; nail bases firm on palpation; uniform thickness; nail edges smooth and rounded; normal dorsal curvature.
	• Palpate hands and arms.	• Skin temperature, texture, and turgor	• Warm to touch; smooth and even texture; skin moves easily and immediately returns to place on release.
		• Joint swelling, stiffness, bogginess, or bony enlargement	• No swelling or enlargements noted; smooth and even movement with no apparent discomfort.
		• Radial and brachial pulses, noting rate, quality, equality	• Radial and brachial pulses easily palpable; rate 80/minute, strong and regular.
	• Assess motor strength of small and large muscle groups.		• Muscle groups tested were strong and equal bilaterally.
	• Assess range of motion of patient's elbow, wrist, and metacarpal joints.		• Full range of motion in elbows, wrist, and metacarpals; smooth movement, equal bilaterally, with no pain or tenderness.
	•Assess neural reflexes.	• Decreased or hyperactive reflex	• Reflexes normal (2^+)
	• Assess sensory response.		• Light touch, pain, and vibration to upper extremities normal and symmetrical.
Head	• Measure level of consciousness (using Glasgow coma scale or other appropriate test).	• Eye response	• Normal consciousness; scores 14 on Glasgow coma scale.

(continued)

GUIDELINES FOR A HEAD-TO-TOE PHYSICAL EXAMINATION *(continued)*

BODY REGION	HOW TO PROCEED	WHAT TO ASSESS	SAMPLE NORMAL DOCUMENTATION
Head *(continued)*		• Verbal response	
		• Motor response	
	• Examine scalp and face.	• Symmetry, size, and contour of skull	• Rounded, symmetrical appearance; skull size falls within normal limits.
		• Facial skin color, lesions, periorbital edema, masses, abnormal movements, or abnormal hair growth (in females)	• Normal pigmentation; no periorbital edema, masses, abnormal movements, or abnormal hair growth noted.
		• Hair color, quantity, distribution, and texture	• Hair is brown, thick, shiny, and smooth; evenly distributed over scalp.
		• Scaliness, lumps, lesions, or parasites on scalp	• Smooth scalp; no lumps, lesions, or parasites.
	• Assess facial sensory response.		• Light touch, pain, and vibration to face normal and symmetrical.
	• Examine eyes.	• Pupillary reaction	• Pupils equal, round, react to light and accommodation (PERRLA).
		• Conjugate gaze	
		• Redness or jaundice	• Sclera is white; bulbar conjunctiva clear, with some tiny, red vessels; palpebral conjunctiva pink, with no discharge, jaundice, or redness.
		• Visual acuity, visual field (blurring, diplopia, field cuts, photophobia, or decreased vision)—R/L glasses, R/L contact lenses	• Focuses on objects. Visual fields full. Can read newspaper smoothly and without hesitation at 18″. R/L vision measures 20/20 using Snellen chart.
	• Examine ears.	• Size, shape, and presence of any deformities,	• Symmetrical; size and shape normal; skin smooth; free of deformities, lumps, nodules, and lesions.

GUIDELINES FOR A HEAD-TO-TOE PHYSICAL EXAMINATION *(continued)*

BODY REGION	HOW TO PROCEED	WHAT TO ASSESS	SAMPLE NORMAL DOCUMENTATION
Head *(continued)*		lumps, or skin lesions	
		• Drainage or pain on manipulation; objective tinnitus	• Cerumen present; no drainage or discomfort with manipulation.
		• Decreased hearing; R/L deafness; R/L hearing aid	• Hearing equal bilaterally. Hears whisper 1′ to 2′ from ear; hears watch ticking 1″ to 2″ from ear. Rinne and Weber tests normal, AC 2x > BC.
		• Balance and equilibrium	• Normal results for Romberg test—sways but can maintain position.
	• Examine nose.	• Deformity, symmetry, and inflammation	• Nostrils are symmetrical, dry, and patent.
		• Drainage or epistasis	• Normally red nasal mucosa, with no drainage.
		• Sneezing or obstruction	• No evidence of swelling or other obstruction. Air exchange through nostrils is free and noiseless.
	• Examine lips.	• Color and moisture	• Lips are pink, smooth, and moist.
		• Lumps, ulcers, and cracking	• Symmetrical at rest and when moving; slight vertical, linear markings; otherwise, no cracking, ulcers, or lumps noted.
	• Examine oral cavity.	• Movement, color, and smoothness of tongue and papillae	• Tongue pink, with papillae; moves strongly and symmetrically.
		• Color and pigmentation of buccal mucosa; presence of ulcers and nodules	• Pale pink-to-pink pigmentation; smooth surface; no ulcers or nodules; clear saliva covers the surface.
		• Inflamed, swollen, bleeding, retracted, or discolored gums	• Pink and slightly stippled, with defined, tight margins at teeth; no swelling or inflammation; no bleeding when slight pressure applied.
		• Position, shape, and sturdiness of teeth; presence of	• Teeth present: 32. Upper incisors override lower teeth. Top back teeth rest directly on lower teeth. Dental

(continued)

GUIDELINES FOR A HEAD-TO-TOE PHYSICAL EXAMINATION *(continued)*

BODY REGION	HOW TO PROCEED	WHAT TO ASSESS	SAMPLE NORMAL DOCUMENTATION
Head *(continued)*		caries; missing teeth	work evident. No caries noted. Little movement on manipulation.
		• Color and shape of hard and soft palates	• Hard palate pale and stationary; soft palate pink, movable, and smooth, with symmetrical elevation.
		• White areas, nodules, or ulcerations in U-shaped area under tongue	• U-shaped area under tongue is pink and smooth, with large veins. Frenulum and submaxillary duct opening are present.
	• Test reflexes.	• Gag reflex	• Gag occurs with stimulation of posterior of tongue and pharynx.
		• Swallowing reflex	• Water swallowed without difficulty.
		• Corneal reflex	• Blinks bilaterally when cornea is touched.
Neck	• Inspect neck.	• Asymmetry, abnormal pulsations, enlarged thyroid or lymph glands	• Head centered on neck. Trapezius and sternocleidomastoid muscles symmetrical. Thyroid gland not palpable. No palpable masses or nodes present.
		• Involuntary movements of head and neck	• Controlled, smooth movements; no involuntary movements noted.
	• Test range of motion.		• Full range of motion possible with no discomfort or limitations.
	• Palpate lymph nodes.		• Lymph nodes not palpable.
	• Gently palpate carotid arteries (one at a time).	• Rate, quality, and equality of pulses	• Carotid pulses symmetrical, 70 beats/minute, strong and regular.
		• Thrills	• No thrills noted.
	• Palpate trachea.	• Deviation	• Trachea midline.
	• Auscultate carotid arteries.	• Bruits	• No bruits noted.
		• Referred cardiac murmurs	• No murmurs noted.
	• Auscultate thyroid gland.	• Bruits	• No bruits noted.

GUIDELINES FOR A HEAD-TO-TOE PHYSICAL EXAMINATION *(continued)*

BODY REGION	HOW TO PROCEED	WHAT TO ASSESS	SAMPLE NORMAL DOCUMENTATION
Posterior thorax	• Inspect and palpate musculoskeletal structure of back.	• Skin color and thoracic configuration	• Skin color normal; no lesions, masses, or tenderness; thorax symmetrical, without deformities. Anteroposterior diameter normal.
		• Tenderness of vertebral spine	
		• Tenderness of costovertebral areas	
	• Palpate, percuss, and auscultate posterior, and lateral lung fields.	• Thoracic expansion, tactile fremitus, and crepitus	• Respiratory excursion symmetrical; tactile fremitus bilaterally equal; lung fields resonant throughout on percussion.
		• Diaphragmatic excursion	• Normal vesicular breath sounds in bilateral peripheral lung fields. No adventitious sounds.
		• Presence of normal and adventitious lung sounds	
Anterior thorax	• Inspect and palpate musculoskeletal structure of anterior chest.	• Skin color and thoracic configuration	• Skin color normal; thorax symmetrical, without deformities.
		• Tenderness of costovertebral areas	• No tenderness of costovertebral areas noted on palpation.
	• Inspect, palpate, percuss, and auscultate anterior lung fields.	• Rate, rhythm, depth of respirations, and breathing patterns	• Respiratory rate 16 to 20 beats/minute; regular rhythm and depth
		• Tactile fremitus, crepitus, and thoracic expansion	• Fremitus normal; felt most intensely at second intercostal space at sternal border, near area of bronchial bifurcation. No crepitus noted; thoracic expansion symmetrical. Lung fields resonant throughout; flat sounds heard over sternum; tympany over stomach. Normal vesicular breath sounds over anterior lung field. Normal bronchial breath sounds heard over large bronchioles.
	• Inspect and palpate breasts (in females).	• Size, shape, symmetry, and position	• Breasts within normal size limits. R breast slightly larger than L breast, otherwise, symmetrical. Both are firm.

(continued)

GUIDELINES FOR A HEAD-TO-TOE PHYSICAL EXAMINATION *(continued)*

BODY REGION	HOW TO PROCEED	WHAT TO ASSESS	SAMPLE NORMAL DOCUMENTATION
Anterior thorax *(continued)*		• Localized redness, inflammation, skin retraction, and dimpling	• Even skin coloring throughout; no redness, skin retractions, or dimpling noted.
		• In nipples, pigment change, erosion, crusting, scaling, discharge, edema, and inversion	• Areolar area is round; area bilaterally similar. Nipples erect and equal in size and shape; color even and skin smooth; no crusting, scaling, discharge, or edema.
		• Nipple secretion	• No nipple discharge on palpation.
		• In axillary and supraclavicular regions, retractions, bulging, discoloration, rashes, and edema	• Skin is smooth, with no bulging or retractions. Normal skin color; no sign of rash. On palpation, tissue is smooth, elastic, nontender, with no masses. Lymph nodes not palpable.
	• Inspect and palpate precordium.	• Precordial heave or lift and jugular vein distention	• Chest is symmetrical; respiratory movements even, with no lift or heaves. With patient elevated 45°, jugular veins are partially filled. Jugular venous pulsations are biphasic.
		• Apical impulse, sternal lift, and thrills	• Apical impulse located at fifth, left intercostal space medial to midclavicular line. No abnormal pulsations palpated.
	• Auscultate precordium.	• Ausculatory areas—aortic, pulmonic, tricuspid, and mitral.	• Rate strong and regular, 78 to 84/minute. S_1 louder than S_2 at the apex. S_2 louder than S_1 at the base. Normal physiologic splitting of S_2 on inspiration heard at pulmonic area. No S_3 or S_4 sounds heard. No murmurs heard.
		• Abnormal intensity or splitting of S_1 and S_2, presence of S_3 or S_4, presence of murmurs	
		• Presence of physiologic splitting of S_2 at pulmonic area	
Abdomen	• Inspect abdomen.	• Color, lesions, surgical scars,	• Abdominal skin is smooth and soft, with normal coloring. No surgical

GUIDELINES FOR A HEAD-TO-TOE PHYSICAL EXAMINATION *(continued)*

BODY REGION	HOW TO PROCEED	WHAT TO ASSESS	SAMPLE NORMAL DOCUMENTATION
Abdomen *(continued)*		rashes, striae, hair distribution, and dilated vessels	scars, rashes, or dilated vessels. Small amount of white hair distributed over abdomen.
		• Color of umbilicus, contour, herniation, and drainage	• Umbilicus is centrally located and sunken. Skin is smooth, with normal coloring. No herniation or drainage noted.
		• Abdominal contour: flat, scaphoid, rounded, distended, or protuberant; and symmetrical	• Contour is flat and symmetrical.
		• Abdominal movements caused by peristalsis or arterial pulsation	• Peristaltic movement and arterial pulsation *not* visible.
	• Auscultate abdomen.	• Bowel sounds in each abdominal quadrant	• High-pitched, irregular bowel sounds, occurring 5 to 10/minute.
		• Presence of vascular bruits or murmurs	• No bruits or murmurs heard.
	• Percuss abdomen.	• Presence of solids, fluids, or gas	• Generalized tympany throughout abdomen.
	• Palpate abdominal quadrants.	• Softness, firmness, or tenderness; skin temperature; masses	• Abdomen feels smooth, soft, and warm. Muscle tension uniform throughout. No tenderness or masses. Liver and spleen not palpable. Kidneys palpable with deep palpation; contour smooth and firm, with no tenderness.
		• Assess skin turgor.	• Skin turgor normal.
Genitalia and area nodes	• Inspect and palpate male genitalia.	• Size of penis, urethral opening, and scrotum; lesions, edema, or swelling	• Urethral opening centrally located at distal tip of penis. No lesions, edema, or swelling.
		• Scrotal masses or tumors	• Scrotum hairless; rugae present; no tenderness, pitting, or masses.

(continued)

GUIDELINES FOR A HEAD-TO-TOE PHYSICAL EXAMINATION *(continued)*

BODY REGION	HOW TO PROCEED	WHAT TO ASSESS	SAMPLE NORMAL DOCUMENTATION
Genitalia and area nodes *(continued)*		• Inguinal hernias and enlarged inguinal nodes	• No inguinal hernias. Inguinal lymph nodes not palpable.
	• Inspect and palpate female genitalia.	• Lesions, varicosities, hernias, tumor masses, edema, or swelling of urethral, vaginal, or rectal openings	• Inguinal and mons pubis skin is smooth, clear, and slightly darker than rest of body. Labia majora are closed and full. Labia minora appear normal in size and color. Clitoris is approximately 0.5 cm wide by 1.5 cm long. Urethral opening is in midline, with slitlike opening. Vaginal opening is thin and slitlike, with no discharge. Rectal opening is normal; skin darker and coarser than surrounding area. No abnormalities noted.
		• Enlarged inguinal nodes	• Inguinal nodes are small, mobile, and nontender. Inguinal areas soft, with no tenderness or discharge.
	• Perform vaginal speculum examination.		• Cervix is pink, approximately 1" (2.5 cm), and pointed in anterior direction. Thin, odorless, clear discharge from cervix. No lesions noted. Vagina appears pink, smooth, and moist, with transverse rugae. No tenderness, inflammation, or lesions.
	• Take smears and cultures.		• Pap test and gonorrheal culture specimens taken.
	• Examine urine.	• Color, concentration, odor, and quantity	• Urine is pale yellow. Specific gravity is 1.018, pH 5.0. Normal odor. Quantity sufficient.
Rectal area	• Inspect anal area.	• Presence of lesions, fissures, hemorrhoids, tenderness; sphincter tone	• Skin clean; no lesions, hemorrhoids, masses noted. Sphincter tone good.
	• Examine stool.	• Color, consistency, and presence of occult blood	• Stool is brown, soft, and well formed. Negative for occult blood.
Lower extremities	• Identify presence of cast, traction, or contractures.		
	• Inspect feet and legs.	• Mass and skeletal configuration	• Muscular development and mass normal for age. No swelling or deformities present. Legs, knees, and feet bilaterally symmetrical.

GUIDELINES FOR A HEAD-TO-TOE PHYSICAL EXAMINATION *(continued)*

BODY REGION	HOW TO PROCEED	WHAT TO ASSESS	SAMPLE NORMAL DOCUMENTATION
Lower extremities *(continued)*		• Skin color, lesions, edema, or varicosities	• Skin color is normal; smooth; no lesions, varicosities, or swelling.
		• Pattern of hair distribution	• Light-colored hair distributed over legs and feet in normal pattern.
		• Nail color and condition	• Toenails intact, of uniform thickness, with normal curvature. Nail beds firm on palpation.
	• Palpate legs and feet.	• Skin temperature, texture, and turgor	• Skin is warm and smooth. Turgor is normal. Skin moves easily and returns to place on release.
		• Muscle mass, tenderness, or lumps	• No swelling, masses, or tenderness.
		• Edema	
		• Joint swelling, stiffness, bogginess, tenderness, or bony enlargement	• Joints are normal, with full range of motion. No stiffness, tenderness, or enlargement noted.
		• Femoral, popliteal, posterior tibial, and dorsalis pedis pulse rates, qualities, and equalities	• Pulses palpable, strong, regular, and equal at 78 to 84 beats/minute.
	• Check for calf pain by dorsiflexing foot.		• Negative Homans' sign
	• Assess motor strength of small and large muscle groups.		• Small and large muscle groups strong and equal bilaterally.
	• Assess joint range of motion of ankle, and metatarsal joints.		• Hips, knees, ankles, and metatarsals have complete range of motion. Movement is smooth, strong, and equal bilaterally.
	• Assess neural reflexes.	• Decreased or hyperactive reflex	• Reflexes normal (2+).
	• Assess sensory response.		• Light touch, pain, and vibration to lower extremities normal and symmetrical.

GUIDELINES FOR A PHYSICAL EXAMINATION BY MAJOR BODY SYSTEMS

GENERAL INFORMATION

- Identify the patient's sex and race.
- Observe overall physical appearance.
  Apparent state of health, mental status, and signs of distress
  Appearance in relation to chronologic age
  Facial expression, mood, and speech
  Skin color
  Body development and apparent nutritional state
  Dress, and personal hygiene
  Stature, posture, motor activity, and gait
- Monitor vital signs.
  Temperature (oral, rectal, or axillary)
  Pulse rate
  Respiratory rate
  Blood pressure
- Measure height and weight.
- Identify accessory equipment used for hospitalized patient (for example, I.V. line, nasogastric tube, chest tubes, oxygen, ventilator, or cardiac monitor).

SKIN

- Examine facial skin for abnormal color, lesions, periorbital edema, masses, or abnormal hair growth (in females).
- Assess quantity, distribution, texture, and color of hair.
- Inspect scalp for scaliness, lumps, lesions, or parasites.
- Inspect for overall color, texture, and turgor.

EYES

- Test pupillary reaction.
  Pupil size
  Reaction to light
  Consensual movement
- Observe conjugate gaze.
- Inspect for redness, jaundice, or discharge.
- Test for blurring, diplopia, field cuts, photophobia, or decreased vision (R/L blindness, R/L glasses, R/L contact lens).

EARS

- Inspect for size, shape, and any deformities, lumps, or skin lesions.
- Check for drainage, pain on manipulation, and objective tinnitus.
- Test for decreased hearing (R/L deaf, R/L hearing aid).

RESPIRATORY

- Assess rate, rhythm, and depth of respirations, and identify abnormal breathing patterns.
- Look for signs of respiratory distress.
  Lips and nail beds, noting color
  Fingers, noting any clubbing
- Inspect nasal airway for deformity, asymmetry, or inflammation; drainage or nosebleed; sneezing or obstruction
- Palpate neck, checking for asymmetry and enlargement.
  Lymph nodes (preauricular, posterior auricular, occipital, tonsillar, submaxillary, submental, anterior cervical, supraclavicular, and infraclavicular)
  Trachea
  Thyroid gland
- Inspect posterior and anterior thorax for configuration and skin integrity.
- Palpate, percuss, and auscultate lung fields, noting tenderness, thoracic expansion, tactile fremitus, crepitus, and diaphragmatic excursion

CARDIOVASCULAR

- Inspect, palpate, and auscultate thorax.
  Precordium, noting any heave or lift
  Jugular vein, noting distention
  Apical impulse, noting any sternal lift or thrills
  Heart sounds, noting rate, rhythm, and any abnormalities.
    Auscultate at apical impulse and at mitral, tricuspid, aortic, and pulmonic areas.
- Examine peripheral vascular system.
  Carotid vessels
    Palpate each carotid artery, noting rate, quality, and equality of pulses, as well as presence of thrills.
    Auscultate over carotid arteries for bruits or referred cardiac murmurs.
  Arms and hands
    Inspect skin color, noting any lesions or swelling.
    Inspect nail color and condition, noting any clubbing.
    Check skin temperature, texture, and turgor.
    Take radial and brachial pulses, noting rate, quality, and equality.
  Legs and feet
    Inspect skin color, noting lesions, edema, or varicosities.
    Note pattern of hair distribution.
    Inspect nail color and condition.
    Check skin temperature, texture, and turgor.
    Check the femoral, popliteal, posterior tibial, and dorsalis pedis pulses, noting rate, quality, and equality.
    Test for Homans' sign (possible indication of phlebitis).

GASTROINTESTINAL

- Examine lips, for color and moisture, noting lumps, ulcers, and cracking
- Examine oral cavity.
  Tongue and papillae for color and smoothness
  Buccal mucosa for color and pigmentation, noting any ulcers or nodules
  Gums for condition and color, noting any retraction, bleeding, or inflammation
  Teeth for position, shape, and sturdiness, noting any caries
  Hard and soft palates for color and shape
  U-shaped area under tongue for color and condition, noting any white areas, nodules, or ulcerations
  Salivation, noting excessiveness
- Inspect, auscultate, percuss, and palpate abdomen.
  Skin for color, color symmetry, hair distribution, and presence of lesions, surgical scars, rashes, striae, and dilated vessels
  Umbilicus for color and contour, noting any herniation and drainage
  Abdominal contour, noting whether its flat, scaphoid, rounded, or distended (protuberant)
  Abdominal movements caused by respiration, peristalsis, or arterial pulsation
  Bowel sounds in each quadrant (beginning in lower left quadrant and working clockwise)
  Presence of vascular bruits
  Presence of solid, fluid, or gas
    Auscultate from thorax down, following right and left midclavicular lines.
  Abdomen, noting firmness or tenderness and the presence of any large masses
  Stool for color and consistency
    Test for occult blood.
  Aspirate, if nasogastric tube is in place, for color, odor, consistency, and volume.

URINARY

- Check for urinary drainage tubes (Foley, cystostomy, or urethral catheter).
- Examine urine color, concentration, odor, and quantity.

(continued)

GUIDELINES FOR A PHYSICAL EXAMINATION BY MAJOR BODY SYSTEMS *(continued)*

REPRODUCTIVE

- Inspect and palpate male genitalia.
  Penis, urethral opening, and scrotum, noting size, as well as any lesions, edema, or swelling
  Scrotal contents for any masses or tumors
  External inguinal ring for any hernias or enlarged nodes
- Examine female genitalia.
  Urethral, vaginal, and rectal openings, noting any lesions, varicosities, hernias, tumor masses, edema, or swelling
  Examine with vaginal speculum. Note color, consistency, and odor of discharge. Take smears and cultures.
  Inguinal nodes, noting enlargement
- Inspect and palpate breasts.
  Breasts for size, shape, symmetry, and position, noting any localized redness, inflammation, skin retraction, and dimpling
  Nipples, noting any pigment change, erosions, crusting, scaling, discharge, edema, or inversion
  Nipple secretion
  Axillary and supraclavicular regions, noting any retractions, bulging, discoloration, rashes, and edema
  Breasts and lymph nodes in axillary and supraclavicular regions
  Palpate systematically, in clockwise fashion, from nipple to periphery.

NERVOUS

- Assess level of consciousness (using Glasgow coma scale or other appropriate tests).
  Eye response
  Verbal response
  Motor response
- Test reflexes.
  Gag reflex
  Swallowing reflex
  Corneal reflex
  Neural reflexes
  Sensory reflexes

MUSCULOSKELETAL

- Examine head and neck.
  Skull for symmetry, size, and contour
  Head and neck for involuntary movements
  Neck for range of motion
- Examine spine for contour, position, motion, and tenderness.
- Assess peripheral motor function and strength.
  Upper extremities
  Note contractures, cast, or traction.
  Inspect arms and hands for muscle mass and skeletal configuration.
  Palpate joints for any swelling, stiffness, tenderness, or bony enlargement.
  Assess motor strength of both small and large muscle groups.
  Test joint range of motion by passively flexing and extending elbow, wrist, and metacarpal joints.
  Lower extremities
  Note contractures, cast, or traction.
  Inspect legs and feet for muscle mass and skeletal configuration.
  Palpate joints for any swelling, stiffness, boggyness, tenderness, or bony enlargement.
  Assess motor strength of both small and large muscle groups.
  Test joint range of motion by passively flexing and extending knee, ankle, and metatarsal joints.

use a printed form to record physical assessment findings, preferring to work with a blank paper, others feel that standardized data collection forms can make recording physical examination results easier. These forms simplify comprehensive data collection and documentation by providing a concise format for outlining and recording pertinent information. They also remind you to include all essential assessment data.

When documenting, describe exactly what you've inspected, palpated, percussed, or auscultated. Don't use general terms, such as *normal, abnormal, good,* or *poor.* Instead, be specific. Include positive and negative findings. Try to document as soon as possible after completing your assessment. Remember that abbreviations aid conciseness.

100 Determining the nursing diagnosis

Throughout the physical examination, you must draw on your knowledge of basic anatomy and physiology, normal ranges for findings in each body region or system that you examine, and the pathophysiology of common disease processes. This knowledge base helps you to analyze the subjective and objective data that you collect, as well as to differentiate between normal and abnormal findings. To arrive at a nursing diagnosis, you use the results of this data analysis to associate various signs and symptoms with particular body systems, and to recognize certain patterns of signs and symptoms as indicative of specific problems (see Entry 6).

For example, to continue the case history of Mrs. Clemson (see Entry 98), let's assume you identified the following priority data during your analysis of the examination findings:

- Temperature, 103° F. (39.4° C.); pulse rate, 106/minute and regular; respiratory rate, 29 to 30/minute.
- On palpation, left lower lung field reveals increased vocal fremitus; on percussion, dull sounds; and on auscultation, tubular breath sounds with increased intensity, and medium rales over the base.
- Apical impulse is palpable at the fifth intercostal space, midclavicular line.
- No neck vein distention, dependent edema, or abnormal heart sounds are present.

Analysis of these results, in connection with Mrs. Clemson's chief complaints—difficulty breathing on exertion; dry, frequent, painful cough; intermittent chills of 3 days' duration—would lead you to the following nursing diagnosis: *ineffective airway clearance possibly related to left lower lobe infiltrate.* You'd verify your nursing diagnosis by consulting with Mrs. Clemson's doctor, reading her chart, and reviewing her chest X-ray and laboratory findings. Other than the slight increase in heart rate, which is probably related to her elevated temperature and increased anxiety level, Mrs. Clemson shows no signs or symptoms to indicate that her problem is related to altered cardiac function.

Perfecting physical examination skills

101 Mastering examination skills

Mastering physical examination skills is a challenging task but also a rewarding one, in light of the benefits an accurate and thorough examination can bring a patient. As you build and refine your skills, keep the following guidelines in mind:

- *Choose one body system,* and focus on a specific skill essential to assessing this system until you master it. Select one step in the physical examination—such as auscultating heart sounds, palpating the abdomen, or percussing the lungs—and perfect your skill by practicing this procedure on each patient you assess. Concentrate on improving your technique each time you perform the procedure.

• *Learn to identify normal findings first.* Individual differences in physical examination findings vary greatly. Assess healthy persons repeatedly until you're familiar with the diversity of normal findings. Besides assessing patients while you're on duty, practice your skills on family members and friends.

• *Once you're familiar with normal findings, move on to study abnormal conditions, using the same disciplined approach.* Perhaps you don't often see patients with disorders related to the assessment technique you're practicing. For example, suppose all patients admitted to your unit have normal chest findings, and you want to master auscultation of abnormal heart sounds. One solution: Try to arrange for study time on your hospital's coronary care unit.

102 Working with others to develop your skills

Working with one or more colleagues skilled in performing physical examinations can facilitate your learning and make it more interesting. Consider the following suggestions:

• *Work with a preceptor.* Find a professional associate willing to share her knowledge of physical examination skills. You may even be able to negotiate so that each of you benefits from the other's expertise. For example, if you work in a public health department, you could teach discharge planning and patient-teaching skills to nurses in a local hospital's coronary care unit (CCU). In exchange, the CCU staff could validate your physical examination findings. If you work in a nursing home, you could provide additional assistance to the visiting geriatric nurse practitioner in exchange for instruction and advice on performing physical examinations.

• *Learn physical examination skills with a friend or colleague.* Choose someone whose skill in performing physical examination is about equal to your own. Plan a regular time when you can perform examinations together. Criticize each other's technique and compare your findings. Then check them against the data recorded on the patient's chart.

• *Read about physical examination skills.* Research the subject of physical assessment in reference books and other texts. Study the material until you can label and interpret your findings accurately. Check your hospital or nursing school library for tape recordings, videotapes, and slide series that may help you validate and interpret your findings.

• *Organize physical examination nursing rounds.* This is particularly helpful if many people in your institution are attempting to master physical examination skills. Each week a different nursing unit could present an assessment of the body system (or systems) of special concern to that unit.

• *Seek help from medical or nursing school faculty.* If you work in a teaching institution, don't hesitate to request instruction—perhaps on a regular basis. Seek out faculty members, in-service personnel, clinical specialists, and supervisors who are skilled in performing physical examinations and capable of validating your examination findings.

103 Finding time to use examination skills

Clearly, the physical examination is an integral part of professional nursing practice, but you may feel that it takes too much time from your other nursing responsibilities. Once you've mastered the physical examination skills, however, you'll be able to perform assessments quickly and efficiently. In addition, several procedures can help you find the time to use these skills:

• *Use a questionnaire to collect initial history data.* Take advantage of a patient's *down time*—the time between admission to the hospital and assignment to a nursing unit or service—by asking him to complete a history questionnaire while he's waiting. You can also mail a history form to a patient before admission. (Make sure he is functionally literate.) With the history form already complete, you can devote the time you'd normally spend interviewing the patient on admission to using your physical examination skills.

• *Combine some segments of the history, such as the review of systems, with the physical examination.* A word of caution here: If you use this approach, don't allow the physical examination to take precedence over the health history.

• *Schedule time in your patient's day for a physical examination.* Negotiate with your employer for assistance from support services to free you from nonclinical functions, so you'll have more time to conduct physical examinations. For example, other staff members could help your patients complete their lists of personal articles.

In an acute-care setting, determine the number of patients likely to be admitted during a given time, then negotiate for staggered admission scheduling. For example, one patient could be admitted at noon, another at 1 p.m., a third at 2 p.m.—based on nursing needs and resources. Of course, your request must also consider doctors' needs and those of support groups, including admissions, laboratory, and dietary services.

104 The rewards of using examination skills

If you make a commitment to use physical examination skills consistently during your daily routine, you'll ensure quality care for your patients and professional satisfaction for yourself. By providing you with a systematic approach to collecting physical examination data, these skills can help you identify patient problems accurately. As a result, you'll be able to establish nursing priorities more quickly and formulate more effective nursing-care plans. Each nursing intervention you perform—even routine nursing care—will become more meaningful because you'll be able to see it as a means to achieving your ultimate goal: restoring or maintaining your patient's health.

As you become more comfortable with physical examination skills and begin to realize their importance in the nursing process, you'll find yourself assessing your patients in a more confident and composed manner. When you can concentrate on the results of your examination rather than on the skills, when you can clearly label and accurately differentiate normal and abnormal findings, then you'll have mastered the techniques of physical examination.

Selected References

Alexander, Mary M., and Brown, Marie S. "Physical Examination: Part 13, Examining the Abdomen," *Nursing76* 6:1, 1976.

Bates, Barbara. *A Guide to Physical Examination,* 2nd ed. Philadelphia: J.B. Lippincott Co., 1979.

Ford, L. "Head to Toe: A Straightforward Approach to Patient Assessment and Charting," *The Canadian Nurse,* September 1976.

Gillies, Dee Ann, and Alyn, Irene B. *Patient Assessment and Management by the Nurse Practitioner.* Philadelphia: W.B. Saunders Co., 1976.

Malasanos, Lois, et al. *Health Assessment.* St. Louis: C.V. Mosby Co., 1977.

Sana, J., and Judge, R.D., eds. *Physical Appraisal Methods in Nursing Practice.* Boston: Little, Brown & Co., 1975.

Sherman, Jacques L., and Fields, Sylvia K. *Guide to Patient Evaluation,* 2nd ed. Garden City, N.Y.: Medical Examination Publishing Co., 1976.

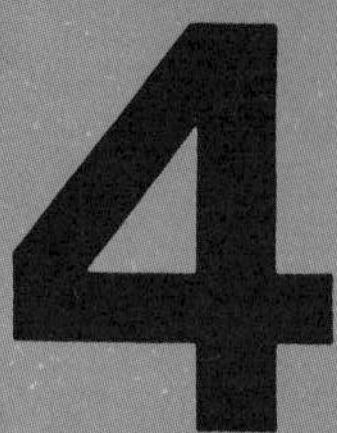

KEY POINTS IN THIS CHAPTER

KEY CHARTS IN THIS CHAPTER

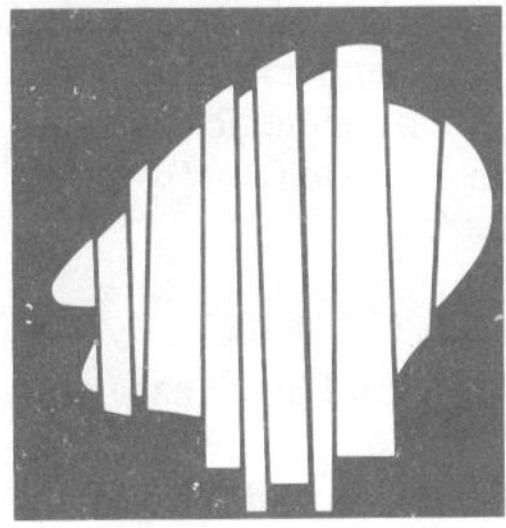

Assessing Psychological Status

Introduction

105 Identifying psychological problems

The mental status examination, part of the general survey for physical assessment (see Entry 67), helps you screen for signs and symptoms of psychological problems, as well as for the patient's emotional needs. If the subjective or objective data from this examination indicate possible emotional difficulties, perform a comprehensive psychological assessment, as described in this chapter.

You'll rely on various kinds of information to complete a psychological profile of your patient's problems and needs. Psychological assessment consists of the patient's health history, mental status examination (including your observations about his appearance, hygiene habits, coping mechanisms, and ability to relate to others), laboratory data, intelligence tests, and projective personality tests (such as the Rorschach series).

106 Challenges in psychological assessment

A patient who enters the hospital because of possible mental illness may challenge your assessment skills. For example, a patient who requests hospitalization for psychological assessment may have some insight into his problem. In contrast, the patient brought by someone else for treatment may be difficult to deal with, because he may not agree with the other person's perception of what his problem is—or even that a problem exists.

A problem you'll sometimes encounter is a patient's inability or unwillingness to verbalize all the information you need to complete his health history. For example, the patient brought in by a family member for uncontrollable behavior, talking to himself, or refusing to eat food prepared by others may be suffering from paranoia. Because of the psychotic process, he may not trust you, or anyone, enough to expose his thoughts or feelings. Such factors influence your nursing diagnosis and subsequent intervention.

As a nurse, you may be the first to notice patterns of behavior that indicate a psychological problem. For example, if you enter a patient's room and find him complaining angrily about something for the first time, you don't usually consider this a sign of a psychological disturbance. The patient could be upset for a good reason and reacting appropriately. But the patient who's *always* complaining and angry could be signaling an underlying problem that needs to be addressed.

Changes in a patient's behavior may herald a new development that's affecting his mental status. For example, if a patient who previously was oriented suddenly becomes confused, it could mean that coping mechanisms that worked adequately for him in the past are breaking down. It could also mean the patient is experiencing acute stress or possibly a physiologic change—such as from drug toxicity.

Understanding psychological theory

107 The brain and behavior

Human behavior—both normal and abnormal—depends primarily on the functioning of the central nervous system (CNS) and its masterful centerpiece, the brain. Through the perpetual flow of nervous impulses to and from the brain, by way of the spinal cord, the CNS integrates, coordinates, and controls the body's activities. The precise mechanism by which this phenomenal process takes place has been intensely studied, but not yet fully explained.

The brain's ability to function depends on its oxygen supply, hydration, electrolyte balance, temperature, blood supply, body fluid pH, and other physiochemical conditions. For example, changes in behavior may result from altered levels of neurotransmitters—chemicals in the brain that help transmit messages between brain cells. Altered levels of one or more of these chemicals (such as dopamine, norepinephrine, and serotonin) occur in such disorders as mania, depression, and schizophrenia.

108 Two levels of brain function

In terms of function, the human brain is divided into a *lower brain* and a *higher brain.* The lower brain consists of the brain stem; limbic system; sensory, auditory, visual, and motor cortices; spinal cord; and peripheral nerves. Lower brain functions include conscious awareness and the ability to react and adapt, through instincts and emotions, to internal and external stimuli.

The higher brain consists primarily of the temporal, parietal, and frontal lobes of the cerebral cortex. This part of the brain controls faculties such as intelligence, judgment, and willpower. Using the higher brain, we think, remember, understand and reason, solve problems, make decisions, and integrate and classify perceptual impressions and factual information. Psychological defenses, such as projection, displacement, suppression, and repression, also originate in the higher brain.

The two types of brain functions interact with and influence each other. An example is when the lower and higher brain coordinate so that you hear a sound *and* identify it. The lower brain—in this case, the auditory cortex—relays the sensory signal (sound) to the higher brain, to be analyzed and identified.

109 Personality development

Since a person's childhood experiences determine his adult personality to such a great extent, you need a working knowledge of developmental theory to perform an accurate psychological assessment. How successfully a person passed through earlier developmental stages can affect his ability to cope with internal and external stresses. An unsuccessful transition from one developmental stage to another can cause a person to develop abnormal coping mechanisms. The more thoroughly you understand your patient's psychosocial development, the more likely you are to recognize the stage of development at which he may have experienced such difficulties.

110 Freud's theory

Sigmund Freud was the first modern thinker to formulate a theory of personality development. Freud's ideas provided a basis for understanding how the mind influences behavior. He described the workings of the unconscious mind, the dynamics of personality development, and the tripartite structure of personality.

According to Freud, *personality* consists of three elements:
- *Id.* This unconscious realm harbors deep-seated instincts and impulses and initiates sexual and aggressive drives not under the control of reason.
- *Ego.* This part of the personality assesses reality through the five physical senses, appraises environmental and bodily changes, and directs behavior accordingly.
- *Superego.* To this aspect of personality, Freud assigned the dictates of conscience—the moral judgments that affect behavior and often oppose the urgings of the id.

Freud considered sexual energy (libido)—which arises from the id—a primary motivator of behavior. Libidinal energy, he theorized, is focused in any of various body zones (oral, anal, and genital), depending on the person's physiologic level of maturation (see *Nurse's Guide to Developmental Stages,* pages 98 to 101).

111 Piaget and cognition

Jean Piaget, like Freud, viewed personality development as a series of stages (see *Nurse's Guide to Developmental Stages,* pages 98 to 101). His theories concentrate on the development of *cognition*—the process by which the mind becomes aware of its thoughts and perceptions—as it is affected by these factors:
- biologic maturation
- experience with the physical world
- social experience
- equilibration (integration and balance of new and old experiences).

112 Erikson's eight developmental stages

Erik Erikson maintained that each of the eight developmental stages presents particular tasks a person must master to progress successfully to the next stage (see *Nurse's Guide to Developmental Stages,* pages 98 to 101). A period of stress or a crisis can cause regression to an earlier stage of development, where the person must again face the positive and negative conflicts of this stage. In Erikson's theory, an individual's personality changes as it acquires new characteristics from coping with new situations. In a healthy environment, a person should develop and maintain emotional balance.

113 Sullivan's interpersonal theory

Harry Stack Sullivan believed that the critical aspects of an individual's personality result from his ability to communicate in interpersonal relationships, not from the unconscious—as Freudian theory maintains. Sullivan's major theoretical concepts include:
- Acculturation results from man's psychological and physiologic dependence, which impels him toward the development of interpersonal relationships. The capacity for tenderness, for interest in others, and for corresponding self-interest increases in response to positive interpersonal contacts.
- Anxiety occurs in all people. A normally functioning person is neither free of anxiety nor completely consumed by it.

The two major goals of human behavior, according to Sullivan, are fulfillment of biologic needs (to feel satisfied) and the need for status and relationships (to feel secure). When a child's biologic needs aren't met, he weakens and dies. When his security needs aren't met, anxiety develops. Sullivan viewed anxiety as an interpersonal phenomenon that occurs in response to feelings of disapproval from significant others. If a person learns to handle anxiety through positive coping

NURSE'S GUIDE TO DEVELOPMENTAL STAGES

FREUD'S THEORY

ORAL STAGE
(ages 0 to 18 months)
- Uses mouth as source of satisfaction
- **Passive phase:** Is helpless, narcissistic, and egocentric. Operates on pleasure principle, feels omnipotent, wants to satisfy hunger, sucking, and security needs
- **Active phase:** Bites as a mode of pleasure, experiments and associates continuously, exhibits sensory discrimination, differentiates between mental images and reality, differentiates between others, discovers self

ANAL STAGE
(ages 1½ to 3)
- Learns muscular control of urination and defecation *(toilet-training period)*
- Exhibits increasing self-control (walks, talks, dresses, and undresses)
- Asserts independence by learning to say *no (negativism)*
- Delays gratification until proper time *(reality principle)*
- Begins ego and superego development
- Engages in parallel play

PHALLIC STAGE
(ages 3 to 6)
- Focuses libidinal energy on genitalia
- Learns sexual identity
- Experiences internalization of superego
- Engages in sibling rivalry
- Manipulates parents
- Experiences refinement of intellectual and motor activities
- Increases socialization and associative play

LATENCY STAGE
(ages 6 to 12)
- Enters quiet stage: sexual development lies dormant; emotional tension eases
- Experiences normal homosexual phase: boys join gangs and girls form cliques
- Increases intellectual capacity
- Starts school
- Identifies with teachers and peers
- Weakens home ties
- Recognizes authority figures outside home *(hero worship)*

SULLIVAN'S THEORY

INFANCY STAGE
(ages 0 to 18 months)
- Uses mouth as source of satisfaction; sucks, bites, spits out objects introduced by others; cries, babbles, and coos to call attention to self
- Has biologic needs met and experiences feelings of contentment and fulfillment *(satisfaction response)*
- Perceives others' feelings as his own immediate feelings *(empathic observation)*
- Feels he's master of all he surveys *(autistic invention)*
- Experiments, explores, and manipulates to acquaint self with environment

CHILDHOOD STAGE
(ages 1½ to 6)
- Has capacity for communicating through speech
- Uses language as tool to communicate wishes and needs
- Uses bowel control to manipulate parents by giving or withholding a part of self (feces)
- Experiences emerging concept of self and integrates it with appraisals of significant persons
- Knows that postponement of own wishes may bring satisfaction
- Begins to understand limits to experimentation, exploration, and manipulation
- Becomes more aggressive
- Uses play and curiosity to explore environment
- Uses masturbation and exhibitionism to get acquainted with self and others
- Demonstrates beginning ability to think abstractly
- Experiences beginning need for peer association

JUVENILE STAGE
(ages 6 to 9)
- Forms satisfactory relationship with peers
- Begins to assign more value to peer norms
- Competes, experiments, explores, and manipulates
- Cooperates and compromises
- Demonstrates capacity to love
- Distinguishes fantasy from reality
- Exerts internal control over behavior

ERIKSON'S THEORY	PIAGET'S THEORY
OROSENSORY STAGE **(ages 0 to 12 months)** • Develops basic attitudes of trust vs. mistrust (through mother's reaction to infant needs) • Uses mouth as source of satisfaction and means of dealing with anxiety-producing situations	**SENSORIMOTOR STAGE** **(ages 0 to 12 months)** • Experiences preverbal intellectual development • Learns relationships with external objects • Develops physically and experiences gradual increase in thought and language ability
ANAL-MUSCULAR STAGE **(ages 1 to 3)** • Focuses on development of basic attitudes of autonomy vs. shame and doubt • Learns limits of ability to affect the environment by direct manipulation • Exerts self-control and willpower	**PREOPERATIONAL STAGE** **(ages 2 to 7)** • Learns to use symbols and language • Learns to imitate and play • Displays egocentricity • Endows objects with power and ability *(animistic thinking)*
GENITOLOCOMOTOR STAGE **(ages 3 to 6)** • Experiences development of basic attitudes of initiative vs. guilt • Learns limits of ability to affect the environment through assertiveness • Explores the world through senses, thoughts, and imagination • Demonstrates direction and purpose through activities • Engages in first real social contacts through cooperative play • Develops conscience	
LATENCY STAGE **(ages 6 to 12)** • Experiences development of basic attitudes of industry vs. inferiority • Creates, develops, and manipulates • Initiates and completes tasks • Understands rules and regulations • Displays competence and productivity	**CONCRETE OPERATIONS STAGE** **(ages 7 to 11)** • Deals with visible concrete objects and relationships • Experiences increased intellectual and conceptual development; uses logic and reasoning • Becomes more socialized and rule-conscious

(continued)

NURSE'S GUIDE TO DEVELOPMENTAL STAGES *(continued)*

FREUD'S THEORY	SULLIVAN'S THEORY
	PREADOLESCENT STAGE (ages 9 to 12) • Relates to friend of same sex *(chum relationship)* • Participates in and derives satisfaction from group accomplishment • Shows signs of rebellion—restlessness, hostility, and irritability • Assumes less responsibility for own actions • Moves from egocentricity to a fuller social state • Experiments, explores, and manipulates • Seeks peer confirmation of reality *(consensual validation)*
GENITAL STAGE (ages 12 to young adult) • Develops secondary sex characteristics and experiences reawakened sex drives • Exhibits increased concern over physical appearance • Strives toward independence • Exhibits sexual maturity • Identifies member of opposite sex as love object • Matures intellectually • Plans future • Experiences identity crisis	**EARLY ADOLESCENT STAGE (ages 12 to 14)** • Experiences physiologic changes • Rebels to gain independence • Fantasizes and overidentifies with heroes • Discovers and begins relationships with opposite sex • Demonstrates higher anxiety levels in most interpersonal relationships **LATE ADOLESCENT STAGE (ages 14 to 21)** • Establishes an enduring intimate relationship • Experiences a stabilized self-concept • Attains physical maturity • Uses logic and abstract concepts **ADULT STAGE (ages 21 and older)** • Assumes responsibility relevant to station in life • Maintains balance and involvement between self, family, and community • Develops creativity further • Reaffirms values

ERIKSON'S THEORY	PIAGET'S THEORY
PUBERTY AND ADOLESCENT STAGE (ages 12 to 18) • Experiences development of basic attitudes of identity vs. role diffusion • Integrates life experiences • Seeks partner of opposite sex • Begins to establish identity and place in society	**FORMAL OPERATIONS STAGE (ages 11 to 15)** • Develops true abstract thought • Formulates hypotheses and applies logical tests • Exhibits imaginative thinking and explores ideas about own experiences *(conceptual independence)*
YOUNG ADULTHOOD STAGE (ages 18 to 25) • Experiences development of basic attitudes of intimacy vs. isolation • Wants to develop an intimate relationship with another adult	
ADULT STAGE (ages 25 to 45) • Experiences development of basic attitudes of generativity vs. stagnation • Wants to establish and maintain a family • Displays a marked degree of creativity • Adjusts to middle-age circumstances • Reevaluates life's accomplishments and goals	
MATURITY STAGE (ages 45 and older) • Experiences development of basic attitudes of ego integrity vs. despair • Accepts life-style as meaningful and fulfilling • Remains optimistic • Continues personal growth • Adjusts to limitations • Adjusts to retirement • Adjusts to reorganized family patterns • Adjusts to losses • Accepts death with serenity	

From Kreigh and Perko, *Psychiatric and Mental Health Nursing*, 1979. Reprinted with permission of Reston Publishing Co., a Prentice-Hall Co., 11480 Sunset Hills Rd., Reston, Va. 22090

STAGES OF THE FAMILY LIFE CYCLE

SINGLE YOUNG ADULT

Accepts parent-child separation

NEWLY MARRIED COUPLE

Committed to new family system

FAMILY WITH YOUNG CHILDREN

Accepts new members into family system

FAMILY WITH ADOLESCENT CHILDREN

Provides flexible boundaries to accommodate adolescents' independence; couple shifts focus to midlife issues

PARENTS RELEASE GROWN CHILDREN

Parents and children accept family additions and subtractions; couple renegotiates commitment to each other

FAMILY IN LATER LIFE

Accepts shifts and changes in parent-child roles; couple maintains functioning in old age and prepares for death (of spouse or self)

mechanisms, he develops a healthy personality. If he uses negative coping patterns to manage his anxiety, his personality development will be impaired—and so will his ability to form healthy relationships with others.

Personality is described as the principle that helps explain human behavior. Sullivan divided its development into six stages (see *Nurse's Guide to Developmental Stages,* pages 98 to 101). The concept of personality allows you to understand the relationship between a person's subjective experiences and his behavior toward others.

114 Personal identity: Three components

The basic components of personal identity are self-concept, body image, and sexual image. Each of these consists of an *ideal self* (the image a person has of what he'd like to be) and a *real self* (the view one has of what he is). In a healthy person, the ideal self and the real self are similar. None of these three identity components remains static: Relationships and experiences may alter any or all of them.

Self-concept first forms during childhood. When a child begins to act independently, he also starts interpreting his parents' responses to these actions. If the child does something that causes them anxiety, he feels anxiety, too. At this early stage, he begins to view himself as a good or a bad person, according to his parents' reactions to his behavior.

If the child views himself as good, he'll develop self-esteem—a feeling of self-confidence and self-respect. A child who sees himself as bad feels anxiety and develops defense mechanisms to cope with his feelings and thereby maintain an acceptable self-concept.

For a summary of the psychological defenses that your patient may employ, see *Understanding Defense Mechanisms,* pages 104 to 107.

Body image is a person's perception of his body and its physical capabilities. It affects both the way he treats his body and his anxiety level when dealing with others. Body image, of course, changes as each stage of life brings new physical changes. Severe anxiety can result from failure to adjust one's body image when natural development, or disease or injury, changes the body. For example, if a man who's spent years exercising and bodybuilding suffers a massive heart attack at age 60, he needs to adjust his body image to accommodate his new physical limitations. If he can't do this, he'll suffer continual anxiety and possibly depression.

Sexual image, which is closely related to self-concept and body image, is the perception one has of his own sexuality. This perception begins forming early in life, as the child explores his body and observes his parents' reactions. During adolescence, coping with sexual identity becomes a major developmental task. Parental and societal attitudes strongly affect how comfortable an adolescent feels with his sexual identity. If an adolescent develops a positive feeling about his sexuality, he's unlikely to experience severe anxiety with sexual activity.

115 Evaluating and adapting to stress

Stress is a combination of specific physiologic responses to a perceived threat to personal well-being. The threat (stressor) may be environmental, physiologic, or psychological in origin.

Hans Selye identified the stages the body experiences in trying to adapt to a stressor (see *How the Body Reacts to Stress,* page 108). In the initial stage (alarm reaction), hormone levels, blood pressure, pulse rate, and respirations increase as the body prepares to fight or flee. Then the body defends itself against stress (resistance stage) and tries to return to a normal balanced state (adaptation). If the body does not adapt and the stressor is not removed, chronic stress results. If not relieved, this condition wears out the body's resistance mechanisms, and the body ultimately surrenders (exhaustion). Exhaustion may be reversible if it affects only part of the body and the stressor is eliminated. However, if the entire body is affected and the stressor remains, total exhaustion and even death may result.

116 The family life cycle

Each person develops as a member of a family of some kind, and the positive

STAGES OF THE DISRUPTED FAMILY LIFE CYCLE

MARRIED COUPLE IN UNSUCCESSFUL MARRIAGE

Accepts inability to resolve marital tensions and decides to divorce

COUPLE PLANS FOR FAMILY BREAKUP

Supports viable arrangements for all family members

SEPARATED COUPLE

Works to continue coparental relationship and resolves mutual attachments

DIVORCED COUPLE

Works to overcome emotional upheaval of divorce

SINGLE PARENT LIVING WITH CHILDREN, LIVING WITHOUT CHILDREN

Works to continue parental contact and support the other's contact with children

POSSIBLY FOLLOWED BY

DIVORCED SPOUSE IN NEW RELATIONSHIP

Recovers emotionally from first marriage

NEW COUPLE MARRY

Remarried spouse accepts family's fears and adjustment needs about remarriage and stepfamily

REMARRIED SPOUSE WITH NEW FAMILY FORMATION

Former spouse resolves attachment to former mate and ideal of intact family. Accepts new family model with first- and second-marriage family members

UNDERSTANDING DEFENSE MECHANISMS

Study this chart to identify defense mechanisms your patient may be using, consciously or unconsciously, to deal with stress. These mechanisms protect him from anxiety by altering, concealing, or falsifying the threat posed by a stressful event.

As you know, all defense mechanisms aren't destructive. Some are normal, necessary

DEFENSE MECHANISM	CONSCIOUS OR UNCONSCIOUS USE	HEALTHY USE
Repression	Unconscious	• Keeps from awareness the drives and memories that might evoke guilt, shame, or a lower self-esteem
Suppression	Conscious	• Keeps from awareness the drives and memories that might evoke guilt, shame, or a lower self-esteem
Identification	Unconscious	• Takes on attitudes and behaviors of admired elder or peer • Empathizes with others (a limited and temporary form of identification)
Reaction formation	Unconscious	• Turns undesirable traits and tendencies into their opposite characteristics • Helps cope with anxiety when used within rational limits
Compensation	Mostly unconscious	• Maintains prestige and self-esteem (basic personality needs) even when real or imagined handicaps exist
Rationalization	Unconscious	• Maintains self-respect and prevents guilt feelings
Substitution	Unconscious	• Substitutes a similar real or symbolic goal for an unreachable goal (a useful method in preventing frustration and depression)
Displacement	Unconscious	• Displaces feelings and attitudes (such as love and hate) from original object to another; maintains repression of unacceptable feelings
Restitution	Unconscious	• Compensates for repressed guilty feelings

ways to adapt to particular situations. Consider defense mechanisms pathologic only when they interfere with your patient's daily functioning. If he isn't using defense mechanisms appropriately, he'll probably require professional guidance to help him to cope with his stress.

UNHEALTHY USE	EVIDENCE OF USE	ADDITIONAL CONSIDERATIONS
• Uses more extreme methods when repression is insufficient • Is anxious	• Prejudice and bias • Intolerance of others' improper behavior	• Cornerstone of dynamic psychotherapy
• Uses more extreme methods when suppression is insufficient • Is anxious	• Awareness of subject suppressed	• Usually precedes repression
• Exhibits open feelings of aggression toward person identified with • Doesn't truly make the traits of admired person part of self	• Inability to see the totality of admired person • Assumption of only certain traits	• Important in self-growth
• Disturbed general adjustment when this method is used extensively	• Perfectionism • Scrupulous politeness • Excessive gratitude • Other exaggerated and sometimes inappropriate traits	• Important in character establishment
• May overcompensate and sacrifice sense of reality • Imagines handicaps (real handicaps are less common)	• Pretentiousness • Concentration on development of unaffected senses, talents, or abilities	• Important in character establishment • Often results in qualities of great social use
• Maintains self-respect and prevents guilt feelings	• Devaluation of importance of task unqualified for • Belief that behavior results from unbiased deliberation done in full awareness	• Usually defended with great intensity
• Substitutes a similar real or symbolic goal for an unreachable goal (a useful method in preventing frustration and depression)	• Usually not detectable except during thorough history or insight-oriented therapy	• Used in widely varying degrees • Allows expression of repressed feelings
• Operates as in healthy purpose but object of displaced feelings may become phobia target (fear of cats instead of fear of women) or compulsion (handwashing instead of feeling morally unclean)	• Excessive emotional response	• Allows expression of repressed feelings
• Compensates for repressed guilty feelings	• Untiring goodwill	• Allows expression of repressed feelings • Used extensively by those with much unconscious guilt • Plays a part in creativity

(continued)

UNDERSTANDING DEFENSE MECHANISMS *(continued)*

DEFENSE MECHANISM	CONSCIOUS OR UNCONSCIOUS USE	HEALTHY USE
Projection	Unconscious	• Provides outlet for repressed tendencies by attributing these tendencies to others and then criticizing them for these tendencies
Symbolization	Conscious and unconscious	• Expresses repressed feelings through another idea or object • Attaches repressed feelings to the other idea or object
Regression	Mostly unconscious	• Returns to an earlier developmental level (for example, a passive dependent posture) to adjust to and avoid anxiety in certain situations, such as in the patient who must endure prolonged bed rest
Dissociation	Unconscious (one dissociated part of the personality may be aware of the other's presence; rarely, both parts are aware of each other)	• Rarely uses dissociation, although its use may never be detected • May sleep-walk (somnambulism), a form of dissociation
Resistance	Unconscious	• Uses resistance to avoid expressing a repressed thought or feeling
Denial	Unconscious	• Disowns intolerable thoughts, wishes, deeds, and facts (seen commonly in physical illness, such as when the dying patient says and believes he's fine)
Sublimation	Unconscious	• Transforms repressed, unacceptable impulses into socially useful and acceptable goals
Fantasizing and dreaming	Unconscious, but patient may be partly aware of the process	• Used frequently; important in maintaining balance and personality integrity

Adapted from A. James Morgan and Mary D. Morgan, *Manual of Primary Mental Health Care* (New York: Lippincott/Harper & Row, 1980) with permission of the publisher.

UNHEALTHY USE	EVIDENCE OF USE	ADDITIONAL CONSIDERATIONS
• Provides outlet for repressed tendencies by attributing them to others and then criticizing others for these tendencies • May hallucinate projection • Often overly critical, pessimistic, sarcastic, cynical, prejudiced, intolerant, and hateful • May have delusions	• Minimization of guilt by making another feel guilty • Blame of others for own problems • Cynical outlook	• Tends to distort view of world
• Expresses repressed feelings through another idea or object • Attaches repressed feelings to the other idea or object • Chooses obvious, bizarre symbols, if thought processes are disorganized • May have hallucinations and delusions	• Symbolic or bizarre gait, speech, or dress	• Forms basis of language, dreams, and most art (extremely important)
• Regresses excessively in extreme personality disorganization; abandons adult role and embraces child or infant role	• Highest functioning level indicates whether patient has regressed or has never advanced beyond a certain stage of development (fixation)	• Important in certain situations but not generally considered a healthy and viable method of coping
• Exhibits dual or multiple personality • Sleep-walks • Experiences fugue states	• Signs and symptoms of dual or multiple personality • Sleep-walking • Signs and symptoms of fugue states	• Repressed material becomes an expressed, separate personality (saving the primary ego from the pain of knowing this repressed material)
• Uses resistance to avoid expressing a repressed thought or feeling	• Blocking • Blushing • Embarrassment • Anxiety • Silence during therapy	• Dynamic psychotherapy attempts to achieve realization of repressed material
• Disowns intolerable thoughts, wishes, deeds, and facts (seen commonly in physical illness, such as when the dying patient says and believes he's fine)	• Denial of known fact or of reality	• Protects person from painful reality through unconscious nonawareness
• Same as in healthy purpose, except with extreme personality disorganization, when sublimation ability may be impaired	• Difficult to detect	• Types of sublimated feelings and use of sublimation differ in various cultures.
• Same as in healthy purpose, but fantasy may become satisfying enough to replace reality thinking or effective action	• Dreaming • Fantasizing	• Defends against anxiety • Expresses repressed material in symbolic form

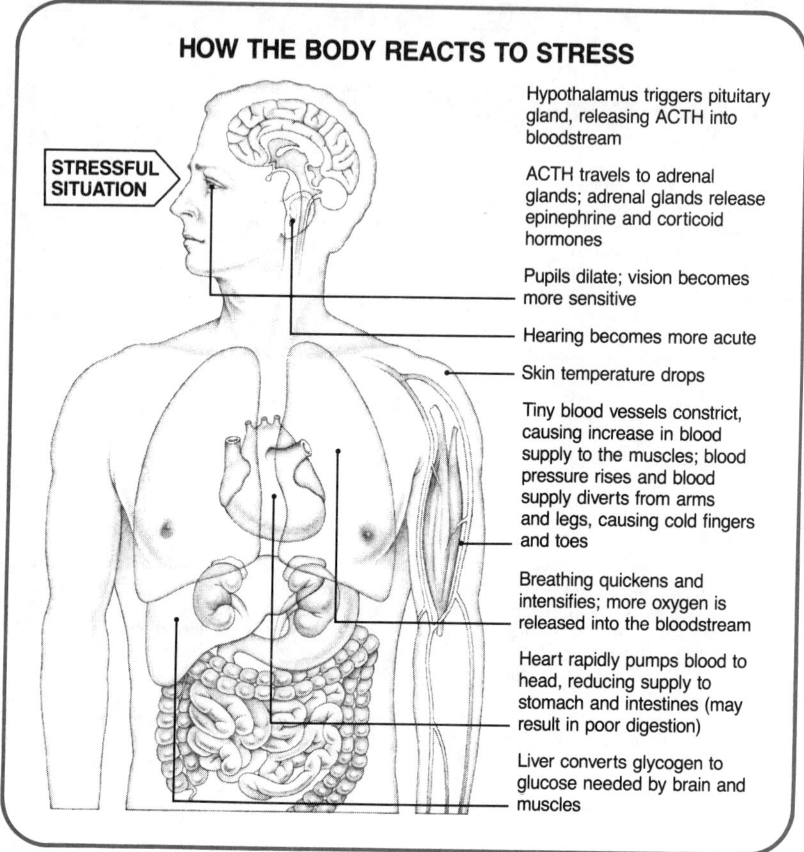

and negative values within this family affect him and his development. A family has a changing structure: When one member changes, compensatory changes occur in other members and in relationships within the family.

Carter and McGoldrick define the family as an emotional system comprising at least three generations—children, parents, and grandparents. (Although members of different generations of a nuclear family may live apart, their influence is still felt.) The family develops in stages and at each stage has specific goals to meet (see *Stages of the Family Life Cycle,* page 102).

Anxiety affecting the family system originates from above (grandparents), from the middle (parents), or from below (children). Understanding the family's life cycle can help you identify the causes of stress, anxiety, and possible dysfunction within it. For example, a family can experience anxiety from two directions: One involves the pressures of family attitudes, expectations, and taboos; the other involves stress generated by a family member during a particular developmental phase. When the family faces both sources of anxiety at the same time, dysfunction is more likely to occur.

Note that when family life is disrupted by such events as separation, divorce, and, possibly, remarriage of one or both of the parents, this process also follows stages with accompanying specific goals (see *Stages of the Disrupted Family Life Cycle,* page 103.)

Collecting appropriate history data

117 Biographical data

Keep in mind the following considerations when recording a patient's biographical data:
• ***Age.*** Organic brain syndrome occurs most often in elderly patients, who also have a high incidence of such psychological disturbances as depression, paranoia, and substance abuse disorders.
• ***Sex.*** Depression is more common in women but more often leads to suicide in men.
• ***Culture.*** Cultural values are significant because they determine a patient's concepts of normal and abnormal behavior and influence family relationships.

118 Chief complaint

One or more of the following psychiatric symptoms occur to some degree in nearly every patient with mental illness:
• anxiety
• depression
• anger or aggression
• difficulties relating to others
• thought disturbances.

119 History of present illness

Using the PQRST mnemonic device (below), ask your patient for more details about his chief complaint. Then, depending on the nature of the complaint, explore the history of his present illness by asking the following types of questions:
• ***Anxiety.*** *How would you describe this feeling?* A patient usually describes anxiety as a general uneasiness, often associated with such physical symptoms as palpitations or tight neck muscles. He may also describe his anxiety as a feeling of impending doom. *What precipitates this feeling?* The patient may attribute his anxiety to one or more specific causes, or he may be unable to pinpoint the source *(free-*

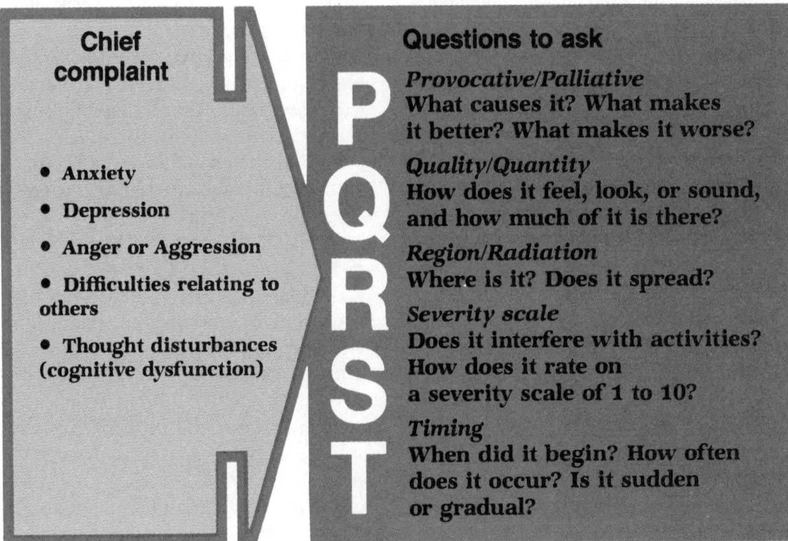

floating anxiety). If it results from an unresolved emotional conflict, it can cause maladaptive responses, such as phobias, obsessions, and conversion reactions.

- ***Depression.*** *Can you describe how you feel?* Depression can range from general unhappiness to complete despair. *Do you often experience periods of depression?* Depression may occur in reaction to a specific event, such as the loss of a loved one *(exogenous or reactive depression),* or it may take the form of a pervasive sadness unrelated to any particular circumstance *(endogenous depression).* Depression also can result from anger turned inward. *Have you ever contemplated suicide?* Carefully assess the potential for suicide in depressed patients (see Entry 46).
- ***Anger or aggression.*** Anger that causes the patient to lose control can result from deep-seated anxiety and frustration, as well as from real or imagined threats. Often the angry patient has dependency needs that he refuses to acknowledge. *How do you express your anger?* Showing aggressive behavior (such as shouting at family members, or hitting walls or people) may result from the patient's inability to relieve his anger and frustration through acceptable outlets (see Entry 36).
- ***Difficulties relating to others.*** *Can you talk about what you're feeling?* Shy, suspicious, and withdrawn patients usually fear (and avoid) close personal relationships. Difficulties relating to others may be the result of unsatisfactory emotional experiences early in life. When you ask such personal questions, remember that a patient with this type of problem may become anxious and refuse to answer.
- ***Thought disturbances.*** *Do you have trouble thinking? Recently, has it been more difficult to concentrate?* Inability to think logically and to learn abstract concepts may occur in the anxious, depressed, or aggressive patient, as well as in those with physiologic problems.

120 Past history

Ask your patient if he's ever had serious emotional problems. Also, you'll want to know if he's ever attempted suicide or been hospitalized (or undergone treatment) for psychological disturbances. Dysfunction in any body system can change mental status, so note any of the following:

- ***Serious illness.*** Life-threatening illnesses, such as heart disease or cancer, may cause severe depression or anxiety and increase suicide potential.
- ***Circulatory disorders.*** Arteriosclerosis, transient ischemic attack, or cerebral hemorrhage may interfere with the brain's nutrient supply and cause thought disturbances.
- ***Tumors and trauma.*** These conditions may alter brain tissue structure, causing cognitive dysfunction.
- ***Metabolic disorders.*** Such conditions as chronic renal disease, hypoglycemia, or vitamin deficiency can cause affective and thought disorders.
- ***Medications.*** Psychological disturbances may develop after taking certain medications (see *Nurse's Guide to Possible Psychological Effects of Selected Medications,* page 112).
- ***Food reactions.*** Food additives or sugar may produce hyperactivity or even violent behavior.
- ***Toxic or infectious agents.*** Thought disturbances may result from infection or toxicity. High fever caused by infection, for example, can make a patient delusional or cause him to hallucinate. Digitalis toxicity can cause a patient to become confused.

121 Family history

Focus your questions concerning family history on the following areas:

- ***Psychiatric problems.*** *Has anyone in your family ever had a psychiatric problem or a stress-related disorder, such as coronary artery disease or peptic ulcers?* You're looking for information about the kind of household the person grew up in, its emotional tone, and his parents' coping ability and possibly the way they related to their children. Some mental illnesses are familial; incidence is higher in an individual with a positive family history for the illness or disorder.

• ***Personal relationships.*** *Do your family and friends provide you with emotional support?* An unstable family can cause a patient to be withdrawn, depressed, dependent, suspicious, or manipulative.

• ***Recent personal loss.*** *Have you recently been separated from someone you love?* Grieving can cause changes in sleeping, eating, and elimination patterns, as well as in libido and activity level.

• ***Childhood traumas.*** Failure in early social and educational activities may lead to low self-esteem and excessive feelings of guilt. Loss of a parent may predispose a child to depression as an adult. Intense fears early in life can result in unspecified anxiety during adulthood. A history of child abuse can predispose the victim to behave aggressively as an adult.

• ***Parent-to-parent aggression.*** Observing such behavior can cause a child to behave aggressively later in life.

• ***Parental control.*** If a parent inhibits a child's efforts to become independent, the child may develop excessively dependent relationships as an adult. Setting inconsistent limits for a child may lead to an inability to understand the needs and rights of others, which may reduce his capacity for intimacy later in life.

• ***Family responsibilities.*** *How will your present problems affect the responsibilities of other family members?* (For example, will the wife have to provide for the family, or will the husband have to keep house? Who'll care for the children?) The answers to these questions may indicate the extent to which the patient's mental illness is disrupting the family. Indirectly, you may learn how much support the family will be able to give the patient, how amenable the patient will be to long-term treatment or hospitalization, and how much stress the illness is causing within the family.

122 Psychosocial history

When you explore your patient's psychosocial history, one or more of the following areas may prove to be related to his present problems:

• ***Values.*** A conflict between parental and community values, perceived during childhood and later incorporated into the adult self, may interfere with the patient's ability to make decisions and can lead to antisocial behavior.

• ***Goals.*** Interference in achieving goals can cause anxiety.

• ***Stress.*** *How do you deal with stress?* When not managed successfully, stressful events, such as a marital or occupational crisis, can cause anxiety or depression, which the patient may try to relieve with cigarettes, alcohol, or drugs.

• ***Life-style.*** Frequent changes in life-style may produce anxiety. Social isolation may result in confusion.

• ***Environment.*** *Do you consider your home environment comfortable and stable? Have you just moved to a new home (new neighborhood, new town)?*

• ***Sexual activity.*** *Are you satisfied with the nature and frequency of your sexual activity? Has it recently changed?* Here you should also note whether the patient calls attention to his or her sexuality—by wearing tight, seductive clothing, for example.

• ***Financial concerns.*** *Are you worried about your finances? Will you be able to return to your job after you're discharged from the hospital?*

123 Activities of daily living

A patient's daily activities are especially pertinent to an accurate psychological assessment, because they can readily reflect underlying emotional problems. Explore the following areas with your patient:

• ***Physical activity.*** *How do you re-*

DRUGS

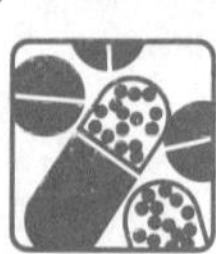

NURSE'S GUIDE TO POSSIBLE PSYCHOLOGICAL EFFECTS OF SELECTED MEDICATIONS

CLASSIFICATION	POSSIBLE SIDE EFFECTS
Anticonvulsants carbamazepine (Tegretol*) mephenytoin (Mesantoin*)	• Disorientation, depression, psychosis
Antidepressants amitriptyline hydrochloride (Elavil*) desipramine hydrochloride (Norpramin*)	• Confusion, hallucinations, diminished concentration
Antihistamines diphenhydramine hydrochloride (Benadryl*)	• Confusion
Antihypertensives reserpine (Serpasil*)	• Depression, confusion
Antipsychotics fluphenazine decanoate (Prolixin Decanoate) haloperidol (Haldol*)	• Depression, anxiety, confusion
Cardiotonic glycosides digitoxin (Purodigin*) digoxin (Lanoxin*)	• *In toxic amounts:* insomnia, agitation, stupor, disorientation, depression, memory impairment, delirium, and hallucinations
Cerebral stimulants amphetamine sulfate (Benzedrine*) caffeine (Nodoz, Vivarin)	• Hyperactivity, delirium, paradoxical sedation, euphoria
Cholinergic blockers (parasympatholytics) atropine sulfate	• Confusion or excitement, insomnia
Miscellaneous psychotherapeutic agents lithium salts (Lithane*)	• *In serum levels greater than 1.5 mEq/liter:* psychomotor retardation, confusion
Narcotic analgesics meperidine hydrochloride (Demerol*) morphine sulfate	• Disorientation, euphoria
Sedatives/hypnotics barbital (Barbital sodium) flurazepam hydrochloride (Dalmane*)	• Depression or paradoxical excitement
Tranquilizers chlordiazepoxide hydrochloride (Librium*) diazepam (Valium*)	• Confusion, depression, insomnia

*Available in U.S. and Canada. All other products (no symbol) available in U.S. only.

lax? Do you often feel fatigued?
• ***Sleeping.*** *Do you have difficulty falling asleep? Do you use medication to help you sleep? How long have you had a problem sleeping?*
• ***Appetite.*** *Have your eating patterns changed recently? Have you experienced an unusual weight loss or gain? What are your favorite foods?*

124 Review of systems

Ask about the following signs and symptoms, which may be related to psychological disorders (psychophysiologic responses):
• ***Skin.*** Skin disorders may result from prolonged stress. And recent changes in facial appearance can precipitate feelings of worthlessness or guilt.
• ***Cardiovascular.*** Hypertension may also reflect prolonged stress.
• ***Respiratory.*** Asthma attacks can be precipitated by stress.
• ***Gastrointestinal.*** Overeating may be a method of coping with anxiety, anger, or stress. (Heartburn from hydrochloric acid may be another consequence of long-standing stress.) Diarrhea or constipation also may be a symptom of either anxiety or depression.
• ***Endocrine.*** Recent changes in body size or shape can result in feelings of worthlessness or guilt.
• ***Female reproductive.*** Dysmenorrhea, amenorrhea, or menorrhagia can be caused by stress, anxiety, or depression.

The mental status examination

125 Observing your patient

As you collect health history data for a psychological assessment, conduct a mental status examination by observing the following characteristics of your patient: general appearance and behavior, motor activity, affective reactions, thought flow and content, perceptions, orientation and level of consciousness, memory, intelligence and fund of information, and judgment and insight. (For a summary of psychological tests, see *Guide to Psychological Tests*, page 114.)

126 General appearance and behavior

Note whether your patient is well groomed and cooperative. Are his clothes neat and clean? Is his clothing appropriate to place, age, and weather conditions? If the patient is female, is her makeup applied properly?

Observe the patient's facial expressions, which can be important indicators of emotional status. Look for signs of anxiety, such as sweaty palms and a moist brow. Note whether the patient looks his stated age. Is he standing erect, or slumped over? Does he maintain eye contact? Is he communicative, or withdrawn and evasive? Are his actions flirtatious or exhibitionistic?

127 Motor activity

Carefully observe your patient's motor activity. Does he pace, or move about restlessly? These can be signs of anxiety. Does he use peculiar gestures, or mannerisms? Are his movements slow, or sudden and jerky? Is he agitated, impulsive, or assaultive? Is he physically handicapped?

128 Affective reactions

Evaluate the appropriateness of your patient's emotional responses. (When assessing a patient's anxiety level, remember that the interview normally causes some tension.) Is he breathing heavily, laughing inappropriately, or wringing his hands? Does he appear sad, angry, or euphoric? Does he vac-

GUIDE TO PSYCHOLOGICAL TESTS

TEST	TYPE	TO ASSESS	AGE-GROUP
Bender Visual-Motor Gestalt Test	Projective visual/motor development	• Personality conflicts • Ego function and structure • Organic brain damage	Ages 5 to adult
Benton Visual Retention Test	Objective performance	• Organic brain damage	Adult
Draw-a-Person (DAP) Test **Draw-a-Family (DAF)-House-Tree-Person Test**	Projective	• Personality conflicts • Ego functions • Visual/motor coordination • Self-image (DAP) • Intellectual functioning (DAP) • Family perception (DAF)	Ages 2 to adult
Gesell Developmental Schedules	Preschool development	• Cognitive, motor, language, and social development	Ages 1 month to 5 years
Minnesota Multiphasic Personality Inventory (MMPI)	Paper-and-pencil personality inventory	• Personality structure • Diagnostic classification	Adolescent to adult
Rorschach Test	Projective	• Personality conflicts • Ego function and structure • Defensive structure • Thought processes • Affective integration	Ages 3 to adult
Stanford-Binet Test	Intelligence	• Intellectual functioning	Ages 2 to adult
Thematic Apperception Test (TAT) **Child's Apperception Test (CAT)**	Projective	• Personality conflicts • Defensive structure	Child to adult
Vineland Social Maturity Scale	Social maturity	• Capacity for independent functioning	Birth to adult
Wechsler Adult Intelligence Scale (WAIS)	Intelligence	• Intellectual functioning • Thought processes • Ego functioning	Ages 16 to adult
Wechsler Intelligence Scale for Children (WISC)	Intelligence	• Intellectual functioning • Thought processes • Ego functioning	Ages 5 to 15

Adapted from A. James Morgan and Mary D. Morgan, *Manual of Primary Mental Health Care* (New York: Lippincott/Harper & Row, 1980) with permission of the publisher.

illate between crying and laughing? Is he unresponsive, or easily moved? Is his affect appropriate to the thoughts he expresses?

Investigate the patient's perception of his affect and mood. Ask questions such as, "How are your spirits?"

129 Thought flow and content

Assess the patient's speech patterns, the topics he discusses, and the coherence of his thoughts. Is his speech volume normal, soft, or loud—or is he mute? Is his speech slurred? Does he blurt out his answers to your questions? Does he talk excessively, or give short, incomplete answers? Does he repeat your words or phrases (echolalia)? Does he respond to different questions with the same answer (perseveration)?

Is his thought flow extremely slow or rapid? Does he move abruptly from one topic to another (flight of ideas), or are his thoughts logical and relevant? Does he use nonsensical words (neologisms)? Does he stop in midsentence, seemingly unable to recall what he was saying (blocking)?

What does the patient talk about? Does his conversation suggest that he's delusional? (For example, does he think he's God?) Does he express somatic complaints, feelings of hopelessness or worthlessness, or suicidal intent? (See *Is Your Patient Suicidal?*, page 116.)

130 Perceptions

Evaluate your patient's perceptions to determine if he's hallucinating. Does he feel safe, or threatened, in his environment? What does he perceive his problem to be? Are his perceptions realistic? Is he experiencing auditory or visual hallucinations? Does he grimace, or smile inappropriately?

131 Orientation and level of consciousness

Determine if your patient is oriented to time, place, and person. Does he know his name and where he is? Does he know today's date? Is he alert, confused, or unresponsive? Does he respond to your questions, or touch? Does he respond to noxious stimulation, such as pain?

132 Memory

Assess your patient's memory by noting his attention span and recall of the immediate, recent, and remote past.

• *Immediate past.* Can he repeat a name or series of numbers immediately after you say it? Can he repeat it 5 minutes later?

• *Recent past.* Does he know why he's in the hospital? If he shows impairment of recent memory, does he try to fill in the gaps with imaginary details (confabulation)? Does he make up obviously false stories?

• *Remote past.* Can he name the town in which he grew up? Ask him to give a chronologic account of his life, with important dates.

133 Intelligence and fund of information

In assessing a patient's intelligence, consider his ability to comprehend and evaluate information and to think abstractly. Does he understand your questions and simple information? Can he do simple calculations?

Does he understand abstract concepts, or is his thinking strictly literal (concrete thinking)? For instance, ask him to explain "People who live in glass houses shouldn't throw stones." Does he interpret it correctly, or does he discuss it literally? Be careful not to overinterpret his answer. Keep in mind the patient's socioeconomic status and formal education level, which will influence his ability to think abstractly.

Test his fund of general information on such subjects as important current events and geography, making sure your questions are appropriate for his education and experience. Common questions you may use for most patients include: *What do we celebrate on the*

IS YOUR PATIENT SUICIDAL?

MISCONCEPTION	FACT
People who talk about suicide don't commit suicide.	Eight out of ten people who commit suicide have given definite warnings of their intentions. Almost no one commits suicide without first letting others know how he feels.
You can't stop a person who is suicidal. He's fully intent on dying.	Most people who are suicidal can't decide whether to live or die. Neither wish is necessarily stronger.
Once a person is suicidal, he's suicidal forever.	People who want to kill themselves are only suicidal for a limited time. If they're saved from feelings of self-destruction, they often can go on to lead normal lives.
Improvement after severe depression means that the suicidal risk is over.	Most persons commit suicide within about 3 months after the beginning of "improvement," when they have the energy to carry out suidical intentions. They also can show signs of apparent improvement because their ambivalence is gone—they've made the decision to kill themselves.
If a person has attempted suicide, he won't do it again.	More than 50% of those who commit suicide have previously attempted to do so.

ASSESSING LETHALITY

Age and sex: Incidence of suicide is highest in adolescents (ages 15 to 24) and in persons age 50 and over. Men succeed at suicide more often than women.

Plan: Remember these points:
Does the patient have a plan? Is it well thought out?
Is it easy to carry out (and be successful)?
Are the means available? (For example, does the patient have pills collected, or a gun?)
A detailed plan with availability of means carries maximum lethality potential.

Symptoms: What is the patient thinking and feeling?
Is he in control of his behavior? (Being out of control carries higher risk.)
Alcoholics and psychotics are at higher risk.
Depressed people are most at risk at onset and at decline of depression.

Relationships with significant others: Does the patient have any positive supports? Family, friends, therapist? Has he suffered any recent losses? Is he still in contact with people? Is he telling his family he's made his will? Is he giving away prized possessions?

Medical history: People with chronic illnesses are more likely to commit suicide than those with terminal illnesses. Incidence of suicide rises whenever a patient's body image is severely threatened—for example, after surgery or childbirth.

Fourth of July? Can you name the last four Presidents?

134 Judgment and insight

A patient's judgment involves his ability to form a reasonable opinion by analyzing a situation or idea. For example, ask him what he would do if he saw a fire start in a crowded movie theater. Then test his insight (his ability to perceive cause-effect relationships, especially those concerning his own problems). Does he know he has problems, or that he's ill? Does he know what to do about his problems? Does he understand why he behaves the way he does?

135 Substantiating your findings

Thorough physical and neurologic examinations are required to substantiate findings that suggest a mental disorder (see Chapter 3, THE PHYSICAL EXAMINATION, and Chapter 15, ASSESSING NEUROLOGIC STATUS).

To rule out such organic causes of psychological symptoms as tumors or temporal lobe epilepsy, the doctor may order a skull X-ray or special diagnostic tests, such as electroencephalography or computerized axial tomography (CT scan). Laboratory tests may detect such conditions as electrolyte imbalance, thyroid abnormalities, and the presence of excessive levels of alcohol in the blood.

Formulating a diagnostic impression

136 Diagnostic considerations

The five most common chief complaints of patients with psychological disorders occur to some degree in all psychiatric illnesses (see *Nurse's Guide to Psychological Disorders*, pages 118 to 123). A symptom's intensity, particular manifestations, and effect on the patient's functioning help determine the diagnosis. For example, nonpsychotic symptoms don't cause the severe alterations in behavior that psychotic coping measures do.

137 Mental illness classification

Traditionally, the major psychiatric illnesses were classified as personality disorders, neuroses, psychoses, organic brain syndromes, alcohol or drug dependence, and psychophysiologic disorders. Recently, the American Psychiatric Association developed a method of classificiation more reflective of the underlying dynamics of a patient's illness. Under this new method of classification, differential medical diagnosis of a psychological disorder depends on predominant symptoms—more so than before. In organic disorders, for example, a deterioration in the patient's intellectual ability—evidenced by confusion, disorientation, poor concentration, and concrete abstract reasoning—could suggest organic brain syndrome. A predominance of hallucinatory activity could mean alcohol hallucinosis, or other drug-induced hallucinoses.

Schizophrenic disorders manifest through characteristic signs and symptoms of a psychosis, including gross cognitive, perceptual, or behavioral deviations. Patients who are schizophrenic have bland affect and disorganized thoughts, as well as bizarre delusions and hallucinations.

Affective disorders manifest primarily through a mood disturbance. The degree of illness can range from mild to severe *without* psychosis, or severe *with* psychosis. If the patient presents with a depressed mood, loss of interest or pleasure, sleep disturbances, psychomotor changes (such as agitation or retardation), and feelings of worthlessness, suspect a major depressive disorder. The psychotically depressed patient can also present with delusions or hallucinations, underlying feelings of nihilism (a feeling that nothing is real and that existence is useless), or deserved persecution.

The patient with a *bipolar affective disorder* (manic-depressive illness) has episodes of manic behavior. During these episodes he'll be in an elated, expansive mood marked by increased activity, pressured speech, flight of ideas, distractibility, and a decreased need for sleep. These episodes alternate with periods of depressed behavior, when the patient displays sadness, hopelessness, sleep disturbance, and psychomotor retardation. Psychotic features of a bipolar affective disorder include feelings of inflated power,

NURSE'S GUIDE TO PSYCHOLOGICAL DISORDERS

	ANXIETY	DEPRESSION
DRUG USE DISORDERS		
Drug abuse	• Moderate to severe; uses drugs or alcohol to relieve anxiety	• Moderate to severe
SCHIZOPHRENIC DISORDERS		
Catatonic schizophrenia	• Severe; possibly manifested by rapid pulse rate and darting eyes (suggesting fear) • *In catatonic excitement:* severe; manifested by ceaseless activity	• Severe; manifested by decreased motor activity, a blank look, and waxy flexibility (arms and legs remain in whatever position they're placed • *In catatonic excitement:* patient wards off depression through overactivity, according to some theorists
Paranoid schizophrenia	• Severe; reduced through delusions	• May be present
Disorganized schizophrenia (hebephrenic)	• Severe	• May be present; flat affect
Undifferentiated schizophrenia	• May be severe—reduced through delusions	• May be present; manifested by decreased motor activity; flat affect
AFFECTIVE DISORDERS		
Depressive disorder (mild-severe but not psychotic)	• Mild, moderate, or severe	• May be mild, moderate, or severe

	PROBLEMS IN RELATING TO OTHERS	ANGER/AGGRESSION/ HOSTILITY	DISRUPTION IN THOUGHT PROCESS
	• Can't decrease or stop use; tries without success • Exhibits impaired social and occupational functioning • Becomes involved in repeated legal difficulties	• Directed inward (misuse of substance) and toward others (verbal or physical)	• Exhibits mild-to-severe interference with perceptions and cognitive processes (caused by drugs or alcohol)
	• Permits direction of self • Exhibits personality disorganization • Experiences loosening of ego boundaries (confused over depersonalization or gender identity) • Withdraws from reality	• May be present • *In catatonic excitement:* patient thrashes wildly for no apparent reason and with no apparent target	• Exhibits negativism • Experiences delusions • Hallucinates • Imitates speech (echolalia) • Imitates movement (echophaxia) • Connects thoughts illogically (loose associations)
	• Uses projection and denial pathologically • Acts suspicious • Exhibits inappropriate affect • Experiences loosening of ego boundaries • Withdraws from reality	• Patient may lash out physically or verbally in response to directions of auditory hallucinations	• Experiences systematized delusions (persecutory, grandiose, or somatic) • Connects thoughts illogically (loose associations) • Hallucinates
	• Regresses to a primitive, childlike state • Exhibits bizarre facial grimaces • Behaves in a silly manner • Exhibits inappropriate affect • Experiences loosening of ego boundaries • Withdraws from reality	• Patient exhibits angry outbursts	• Experiences delusions (bizarre and fragmentary) • Hallucinates • Giggles • Connects thoughts illogically (loose associations) • Exhibits garbled speech
	• May exhibit characteristics of catatonic, paranoid, and disorganized schizophrenia	• Patient may exhibit angry outbursts in response to voices	• Experiences delusions, hallucinations, loose associations
	• Is dependent on others • Marginally able to meet commitments	• Mild to severe; turned inward • Patient contemplates and may attempt suicide	• Remains in contact with reality (aware of behavior but can't stop it) • Can't concentrate

(continued)

NURSE'S GUIDE TO PSYCHOLOGICAL DISORDERS *(continued)*

	ANXIETY	DEPRESSION	
AFFECTIVE DISORDERS *(continued)* **Depressive disorder (severe and psychotic)**	• Severe, especially in agitated form	• Severe; may or may not have precipitating environmental factors • Worst in early morning • Flat affect • Patient inactive, hopeless; acts helpless	
Bipolar affective disorder (manic phase)	• Severe; manifested by increased activity	• Patient exhibits symptoms of mania to ward off depression • Patient exhibits labile affect (one moment happy, the next moment tearful)	
Bipolar affective disorder (depressive phase)	• Variable	• Severe • Patient may exhibit signs and symptoms of other depressions.	
ANXIETY DISORDERS **Anxiety disorder (chronic or acute)**	• Symptoms function to ward off free-floating anxiety. • Both psychological and physiologic responses occur in anxiety reaction	• May be present	
Phobias	• Anxiety is diffused by being transferred to an environmental object (anxiety changed into fear). • Patient uses displacement as defense mechanism.	• May be present	
Obsessive compulsive disorder	• Mild to moderate • Signs and symptoms function to ward off intolerable anxiety.	• Patient may experience depression.	

	PROBLEMS IN RELATING TO OTHERS	ANGER/AGGRESSION/ HOSTILITY	DISRUPTION IN THOUGHT PROCESS
	• Speaks infrequently when in groups • Has poor self-image • Becomes severely withdrawn	• Patient feels anger toward self but usually doesn't have energy to act on feelings	• Experiences delusions of sinfulness, disease, or impending doom • Suffers from severely impaired judgment
	• Overinvolved in the activities of others; manipulative • Dresses and uses makeup inappropriately and bizarrely • Lacks normal inhibitions; may become sexually indiscreet and vulgar	• Patient may be angry and irritable, especially when behavior is controlled. • Patient may become violent.	• Rhymes, plays with words • Exhibits pressured speech • Exhibits delusions of grandeur and of persecution • Exhibits flight of ideas
	• Loses interest in activities • Becomes isolated • May exhibit signs and symptoms of other depressions	• Patient hates self; thinks frequently of death and may attempt suicide. • Patient may exhibit signs and symptoms of other depressions.	• Exhibits delusions • Shows decreased thinking ability • May show signs and symptoms of other depressions
	• Remains in contact with reality (aware behavior occurs but can't stop it) • Is dependent on others • Feels impending doom • Doubts self • Displays indecision	• Usually not present	• Shows little or no impairment in intellectual function • Can't concentrate • Shows decreased ability to perceive and communicate as anxiety increases
	• Remains in contact with reality (aware behavior occurs but can't stop it) • Is dependent on others • May derive secondary gain from others' attention	• Patient displaces angry feeling to phobia target.	• Exhibits no thought disorder
	• Exhibits compulsion (repetitious performance of ritualistic acts to control anxiety) • Is obsessed (has thoughts that recur despite attempts to stop them) • Becomes anxious or panicky when acts or thoughts are interrupted • Domineering, yet detached	• Centers around aggressive or sexual thoughts or impulses (unacceptable to society) • Patient exhibits behavior that may have sadistic or masochistic elements. • Patient turns anger inward.	• May feel guilty and inadequate • Intellectualizes rigid thoughts (hampers creativity and alternatives) • May have difficulty concentrating • Has difficulty following directions that interfere with ritualistic activities

(continued)

NURSE'S GUIDE TO PSYCHOLOGICAL DISORDERS *(continued)*

	ANXIETY	DEPRESSION	
SOMATOFORM DISORDERS			
Hypochondriasis	• Mild to moderate • Patient displaces anxiety to body organ.	• Patient exhibits affective elements of depression.	
Conversion disorder	• Anxiety not observable (la belle indifference)	• Usually not observable	
DISSOCIATIVE DISORDERS			
Amnesia, fugue states, somnambulism, and multiple personality	• Mild to moderate • Patient exhibits no observable hysterical reactions. • Patient uses repression as primary defense mechanism.	• Usually not observable	
PERSONALITY DISORDERS			
Antisocial personality	• Usually lacking	• Not usually present	
Borderline personality organization	• Moderate to severe • Patient lacks tolerance to anxiety; uses projection as primary defense mechanism.	• Moderate to severe	

	PROBLEMS IN RELATING TO OTHERS	ANGER/AGGRESSION/ HOSTILITY	DISRUPTION IN THOUGHT PROCESS
	• Is dependent on others • Domineering, yet detached	• Patient is apathetic against aggressiveness.	• Tries to reason away signs and symptoms that may cause increased anxiety and new signs and symptoms • Uses illness to escape responsibilities • Is morbidly preoccupied with personal health
	• Converts conflict into an observable symptom (conversion reaction) • Doesn't have voluntary control of symptom (it can't be explained by pathophysiologic mechanism) • Is dependent on others • Derives secondary gain from others' attention	• May be caused by underlying conflict centering around depression	• Shows little or no impairment in intellectual function; usually sees problem but can't stop behavior • Insight into signs and symptoms may create overwhelming anxiety, producing new symptoms. • Memory functions in impressions instead of specifics.
	• Is dependent on others • May act childishly or impulsively • Usually appears quite calm • Suffers amnesia	• Usually not observable	• Displays normal intellectual functioning that's unrelated to amnesia • Remains in contact with reality (aware of behavior but can't stop it)
	• Appears superficially charming • Exhibits behavior patterns that cause repeated conflict with society • Acts impulsively and irresponsibly • Feels guilt infrequently • Doesn't learn from experience	• Patient can't tolerate frustration. • Patient may engage in delinquent or violent behavior.	• Lacks insight and uses poor judgment, despite great intelligence • Does not suffer delusions or irrational thoughts
	• Acts impulsively and unpredictably • Engages in patterns of intense interpersonal relationships • Displays ongoing impaired social or occupational functioning • Exhibits identity disturbance	• Patient exhibits intense rage (anger/hostility is underlying cause). • Patient engages in self-harming acts (substance abuse; physical self-abuse).	• Uses poor judgment; shows lack of insight • Exhibits impaired intelligence • May exhibit brief episodes of psychosis

knowledge, or self-worth, and perhaps belief in a personal relationship with God or a famous person.

Disorders that used to be classified as neuroses are now categorized by each disorder's major presenting symptom. *Anxiety disorders,* for example, comprise all conditions in which anxiety and its relief are the patient's major concern. These include:

- *phobias*—the persistent avoidance or fear of a specific object, activity, or situation
- *anxiety*—generalized, free-floating anxiety
- *obsessive-compulsive disorders*—recurrent and persistent ideas, or thoughts (obsessions); senseless behaviors (compulsions) that the patient, against his will, can't resist doing.

Disorders that present with physiologic symptoms can be factitious or somatoform. In a *factitious* disorder, the patient has some control over the signs and symptoms, the purpose of which is to maintain his perceived role as a patient. (A factitious disorder can also involve psychological signs and symptoms, as in a factitious psychosis.) In a *somatoform* disorder, the patient doesn't have voluntary control of his physical sign or symptom. Paralysis, blindness, or loss of sensation, for example, may occur with no organic cause. Physical examination will not identify a cause, but the presence of the sign or symptom is undeniable. Somatoform conditions include *conversion disorders* and *hypochondriasis.*

Dissociative disorders, which used to be classified as a type of hysterical neurosis, are characterized by alterations in normally integrated functions. Defects can occur in consciousness (previous events can't be recalled), identity (new identities are added to the real one), and motor behavior (the patient may wander or sleepwalk). Also included in this category of disorders are amnesia and depersonalization.

Personality disorders affect a person's long-term functioning. Patients with these disorders don't have episodes of active illness and periods of remission; the effects of the disorder are continuous. These disorders usually arise during childhood or adolescence. A patient with an *antisocial personality,* for example, may have a history of truancy, thefts, drug use, and poor school grades. *Unstable personality disorders* are marked by impulsiveness and unpredictability, inappropriately intense anger, identity problems, and physically self-damaging acts.

138 Making appropriate nursing diagnoses

To formulate a nursing diagnosis for a patient with psychological problems, carefully assess his reactions to his signs and symptoms. Your assessment must be thorough and your nursing diagnosis explicitly stated.

Anxiety can precipitate a wide range of physiologic and behavioral responses. For example, your physiologic findings may include *alterations in bowel elimination,* (such as diarrhea), *disturbances in sleep patterns,* and *alterations in nutrition (less than body requirements).* Behavioral responses to anxiety may cause *impaired ability to maintain a home* (such as when anxiety prevents a housewife from cooking meals for her family). Anxiety can also cause *alterations in parenting*—for example, disinterest in a child that leads to allowing him to play outside without adequate supervision. Since anxious patients usually express feelings of vulnerability and low self-esteem, a nursing diagnosis of *disturbance in self-concept* may also be appropriate. Severe anxiety may produce *self-care deficits* (such as inappropriate or deficient grooming) and *alterations in thought processes,* which you may notice in the patient's illogical conversation or his expression of phobias.

Depression, like anxiety, has many possible physiologic and behavioral effects, and the nursing diagnoses for an anxious patient also may apply to a depressed patient. Since the de-

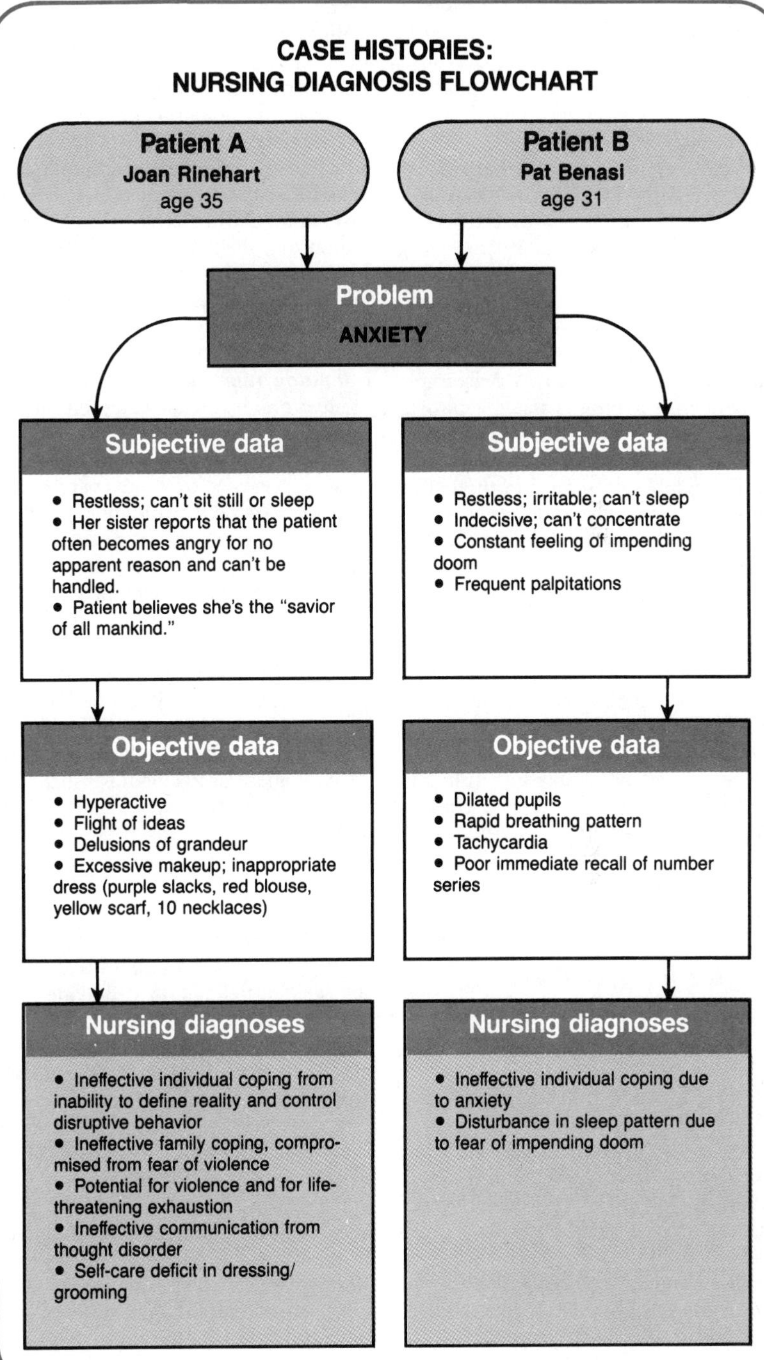
CASE HISTORIES:
NURSING DIAGNOSIS FLOWCHART
Patient A
Joan Rinehart
age 35
Patient B
Pat Benasi
age 31
Problem
ANXIETY
Subjective data
• Restless; can't sit still or sleep
• Her sister reports that the patient often becomes angry for no apparent reason and can't be handled.
• Patient believes she's the "savior of all mankind."
Subjective data
• Restless; irritable; can't sleep
• Indecisive; can't concentrate
• Constant feeling of impending doom
• Frequent palpitations
Objective data
• Hyperactive
• Flight of ideas
• Delusions of grandeur
• Excessive makeup; inappropriate dress (purple slacks, red blouse, yellow scarf, 10 necklaces)
Objective data
• Dilated pupils
• Rapid breathing pattern
• Tachycardia
• Poor immediate recall of number series
Nursing diagnoses
• Ineffective individual coping from inability to define reality and control disruptive behavior
• Ineffective family coping, compromised from fear of violence
• Potential for violence and for life-threatening exhaustion
• Ineffective communication from thought disorder
• Self-care deficit in dressing/grooming
Nursing diagnoses
• Ineffective individual coping due to anxiety
• Disturbance in sleep pattern due to fear of impending doom

pressed patient turns his anger inward, suppressing rather than expressing it, he may also have a nursing diagnosis of *potential for self-injury*, possibly manifested by suicidal intent. (See Entry 46.)

The angry or aggressive patient has a *potential for violence* and may fear *loss of self-control related to overwhelming anger*. Skillful interviewing techniques can help you determine the anger's focus and whether the anger is a realistic response or a sign of *ineffective individual coping* related to his situation (see Entry 45). An example of ineffective coping is when a patient becomes physically violent in response to the news of the sudden death of a family member. You must evaluate this behavioral response and analyze its potential effect on this patient's ability to resolve the loss. For instance, *dysfunctional grieving* frequently takes the form of anger or depression and can cause a wide range of physiologic responses. For such patients, the associated nursing diagnoses will be the same as those used to describe anxious and depressed patients.

The patient who's having difficulty relating to others may have a nursing diagnosis of *ineffective individual coping* or *fear of intimate relationships*. Determining the duration of signs and symptoms often provides clues about their causes. For example, a lifelong history of unsatisfactory relationships suggests the potential for overwhelming anxiety in relating to others and subsequent avoidance of interpersonal relationships. Recent concern with problems relating to others may reflect temporary feelings of inadequacy or low self-esteem.

The frankly psychotic patient usually has difficulty with social interactions, related to *impaired verbal communication* as indicated by flight of ideas and inconsistencies in thoughts or speech.

Evaluate *alterations in thought processes* in terms of type (perceptual, retentive, reflective, judgmental, decisional, content) and effect on the patient's behavior. These alterations may be mild and related to temporary physiologic imbalance, such as fatigue. Or the imbalance may be severe enough to threaten essential physiologic processes, such as in digitalis toxicity. Since any severe disease causes *alterations in thought processes,* a careful psychological assessment can help you differentiate true psychogenic alterations from those caused by reversible physiologic events.

Assessing a child's psychological status

139 Recognizing normal variations

To assess a child's psychological status, you need to understand the theories of childhood development, particularly those formulated by Freud, Sullivan, and Erikson. This will help you to recognize normal variations in behavior that can occur during childhood (see *Understanding Childhood Psychological Development,* pages 128 and 129).

Parents sometimes mistake normal psychological variations in their child for serious behavioral problems. This can have unfortunate repercussions for the child later in life. For example, a small child's appetite may diminish from time to time; this is perfectly normal. However, if the concerned parent force-feeds the child, real psychological problems may develop later.

Of course, parents should consider the possibility that unusual behavior in their child *is* a sign of serious emotional problems. For example, the child who doesn't regain his appetite may be depressed. In the case of such a child, psychological assessment would be in order.

140 The anxious child

When taking a pediatric health history for a psychological assessment, examine both the parents' *and* the child's perceptions. A child's responses—or lack of response—may be revealing. For example, if the child refuses to give answers to questions, he may be feeling extreme anxiety. This could be caused by a lack of trust, inability to relate to others, or fear of being punished. To help him deal with this anxiety, phrase your questions so they convey empathy and understanding, yet still define the problem. You might say, "Your parents have brought you here because they're worried about you. It sounds like there may be a problem. What's going on?" You may be able to put an anxious young child at ease by relating a story about other children in similar circumstances. You might begin with, "Sometimes when children are unhappy, they...." As the child becomes involved in the story, ask him specific questions about his particular situation. (See Entries 47 and 48.)

141 The parent-child relationship

While you're assessing the psychological status of a pediatric patient, evaluate the parents' relationship to the child—especially their understanding of his needs and their ability to meet these needs. Observe how they react when the child's upset. Do they try to comfort him? Do they comfort him effectively?

Observe how an infant's parents hold him and respond (verbally and nonverbally) to his body, when dressing him or changing his diaper. Pay careful attention to their responses to the less pleasant aspects of parenting, such as handling stool and vomitus. If they feel positive about their child, they won't be upset about these things.

Observe the parents' reaction to a toddler's normal developmental behavior. How do the parents of a 2-year-old respond to his temper tantrums? Do the parents of a 4-year-old respond appropriately to the child's interruptions and frequent demands for attention?

Also note if the parents show affection for the child and pride in his achievements. Most parents—even those who are having problems with their child—enjoy the positive elements of their relationship with him. If you observe no positive feelings at all, strongly

RECOGNIZING CHILD ABUSE

Parent, child, and environment—all generally contribute to child abuse situations. The checklists below detail some observable characteristics of abusive parents and abused children. Of course, the presence of any of these factors doesn't automatically indicate child abuse, but it does suggest that you should investigate further.

Because child abuse occurs more frequently in high-crime areas and crowded urban communities, many people associate it only with poorly educated, socioeconomically disadvantaged families. Don't be blinded by this stereotype—it's increasingly yielding to evidence that child abuse also occurs in middle- and upper-income families, among seemingly well-adjusted parents and children.

Characteristics the abusive parent may exhibit:

- Lacks knowledge of infant developmental skills
- Has unrealistic expectations of the child's behavior
- Feels intensely anxious about the child's behavior
- Feels guilty and angry about inability to provide for the child
- Feels extremely lonely and isolated
- Relates poorly with spouse and own parents
- Has also been a victim of child abuse
- Believes physical punishment is the best discipline
- Lacks a strong emotional attachment to the child (for example, a mother who hasn't bonded well with her child).

Characteristics the abused child may exhibit:

- Has a history of behavior problems
- Is overactive, demanding, defiant
- Refuses to eat, violates rules, destroys parent's property and the property of others.

UNDERSTANDING CHILDHOOD PSYCHOLOGICAL DEVELOPMENT

AGE	MINOR PROBLEMS	NORMAL VARIATIONS
Infant and toddler	• *Crying:* A normal activity (but may provoke child abuse; observe parents for angry reaction to crying) • *Self-comforting measures:* Infant sucks finger, thumb, or pacifier; clings to favorite toy or blanket; masturbates.	• *Hair-pulling, head-banging, and body-rocking:* Signs of mild or serious anxiety • *Temper tantrums:* Common, usually benign (overreaction to the tantrums may create long-term problems) • *Colic:* Probably caused by incomplete myelinization of the nervous system; usually ends by 4th month • *Toilet training:* May turn into a battle between parents and children
Preschooler	• *Nightmares, sleep-walking, sleep-talking:* Preschooler wakes up frightened after 2 or 3 hours of sleep, usually can recall the dream (dream may represent attempts to deal with unacceptable monstrous feelings or a daytime problem). • *Nose-picking, masturbating:* If excessive, may indicate high stress. • *Stuttering:* Normal phase is usually outgrown; long-term stuttering may result from overattention to the child's speech.	• *Encopresis:* May indicate psychological problems or organic disease; begins after years of bowel control; also occurs in daytime. • *Bruxism* (teeth-grinding): Possibly related to daytime tension; may also begin at toddler or school-age stage. • *Extreme emotions:* Especially anger, fear, anxiety, shyness, or antisocial behavior; preschooler needs further evaluation. • *Enuresis:* May be normal, but may want to start treatment.
School-age child	• Normal developmental occurrences seldom appear as signs of problems.	• *Cheating:* May reflect child's view of adult culture or indicate attempt to handle poor self-image. • *Lying:* Motives similar to cheating. Pathologic lying may indicate serious coping problems. • *Fighting:* May result from a lack of self-control or from imitating adult behavior: may also indicate deep-seated feelings of hostility or unhappiness • *Scatology:* Common in this age-group; can result from an attempt to irritate adults or be part of a group. • *Psychosomatic symptoms:* Headache, upset stomach, vomiting, and occasionally, psychogenic cough; may result from stress. • *Enuresis:* May result from or cause psychological problems.
Adolescent	• *Peer group behavior:* Compliance with previous standards; represents normal behavior. • *Dating and social life:* Emphasis on social life represents normal development.	• *Conflict with parents:* Common sources of disagreements include driving the car, dating, smoking, homework habits, choice of friends. • *Sexual experimentation:* Fear of being unattractive, homosexual, oversexed, or undersexed; problems and confusion commonly occur during search for sexual identity.

SEVERE PROBLEMS

- *Autism:* Infant can't relate to other people but may be attached to inanimate objects.
- *Failure to thrive:* Infant doesn't grow, shows minimal development, is unresponsive and lethargic; may result from an organic cause but usually caused by lack of love and contact with surroundings; serious, even life-threatening problem.
- *Anaclitic depression:* Infant ignores adults and surroundings, doesn't sleep well, becomes more susceptible to infections, and exhibits developmental decline; becomes expressionless and, apparently, unaware of his surroundings approximately 3 months after signs and symptoms appear. Condition occurs in infants with strong maternal attachment who are separated from their mothers between 10th and 12th month.
- *Indiscriminant attachment:* Infant appears starved for affection and willingly goes to examiner, even after parents leave, instead of exhibiting separation anxiety; indicates poor attachment.
- *Extreme emotions:* Infant exhibits fear and anger; requires further evaluation.

- *Hyperactivity:* Preschooler displays short attention span, low frustration tolerance, frequent emotional outbursts; peaks during late preschool and early school years, and should decrease during adolescence.
- *Accident prone:* Preschooler displays impulsiveness, hyperactivity, restlessness, immaturity, and resentment of authority; more prevalent in boys.
- *Hair-pulling:* Preschooler has obvious bald patches, indicating severe stress.

- *School phobia:* Child fears school and refuses to attend; problem relates to mother's ambivalent feelings toward separation from child.
- *Learning disabilities:* May be related to intelligence or to emotional or perceptual problems; requires further evaluation and treatment.
- *Schizophrenia:* Child loses interest in surroundings; exhibits blank expression, and poor appearance and hygiene; becomes withdrawn and isolated; develops special preoccupation, phobia, and anxiety; gradually becomes schizophrenic.

- *Severe acting out:* Adolescent uses behavior to express unconscious emotions, including sexual acting out, delinquency, running away, social withdrawal, and failure in school.
- *Depression:* May be accompanied by suicidal thoughts or actions.
- *Drug abuse:* Indicates poor adjustment (alcohol is the most common substance of abuse).
- *Hysteria:* Occurs occasionally; most common in girls.
- *Anorexia nervosa:* Adolescent shows excessive weight loss; potentially fatal problem.
- *Obesity:* May result from or cause psychological problems.
- *Pregnancy:* May be a symptom of a psychological problem, such as rebellion against parents; may represent need to escape an unpleasant home situation.

suspect severe disturbance in the parent-child relationship.

Is the parents' behavior consistent with all their children (if the child has siblings)? Inquire about the parents' relationship with them. Ask about their ages, how well they behave, whether they get along well with the patient. What's the parents' biggest problem with the patient, and with his siblings? Parents who treat one or some of their children differently from the others will generally give some indication of this when answering your questions.

142 Evaluating the child's mental status

Behavioral problems in a child may result from nutritional deficits, medications, visual or auditory impairments, or sudden changes in the child's home life—such as the mother's return to work or the birth of a sibling. Other problems require further psychological evaluation. You can conduct the same mental status examination that you use for an adult, rewording the questions according to each child's age and developmental level.

Also, keep in mind that certain behavioral variations considered to be abnormal for an adult are normal for a child. For example, the guilt felt by a 4-year-old who, after wishing his mother ill, learns that she's actually sick is in keeping with his typical belief that his thoughts are responsible for subsequent events.

During the pediatric mental status examination, evaluate the child's fine and gross motor activities, visual perception, hand-eye coordination, right-left discrimination, and symmetry of movement. You might suggest games for the child (hopping on one foot, or finger-thumb movements, for example) that test these abilities. If you note any gross sensorimotor difficulties, perform a complete neurologic assessment (see Entries 639 to 646).

Observing the child at play helps you assess his perceptions, concerns, self-concept, and preoccupations. When possible, provide games and toys (such as puppets, drawing material, or throwing games), and give the child time to play freely. Does the child initiate the play spontaneously or need direction? Notice whether he includes you or his parents in the games, or prefers to play alone. An abused child may act out his family situation when playing with dolls.

After the free-play period, suggest more structured activities, such as drawing pictures. Encourage the child to talk as much as he wants. For example, you might say, "Tell me about your drawing" or "What's going on in this picture?" To further assess how he relates to family members, suggest he draw a picture of himself and his family.

During these structured activities, assess the child's concepts of cause and effect, logic, and morality. You might ask him, "What would happen if a child were playing with his mother's vase and accidentally broke it?"

Identify sensitive issues. The child will let you know about these verbally (such as by not wanting to discuss certain issues) or nonverbally (such as by squirming, looking away, or playing with toys to cover his refusal to answer).

To overcome the child's resistance to discussing sensitive issues, you may want to use such communication techniques as fables, wishes, and projective questions. For example, ask the child what he'd wish for if he had three wishes. You may also find that wording your questions in the third person is an effective communication device. "How should a good mother act?" is an easier question for the child to answer than, "How do you feel about your mother?"

These techniques allow the child to tell you what he's feeling without fear of punishment or of betraying his parents. Remember, a child will usually protect his parents regardless of their behavior—even if they abuse him (see *Recognizing Child Abuse,* page 127).

Assessing an elderly patient's psychological status

143 Coping with aging

When you assess the psychological status of an elderly patient, remember that he's probably dealing with complex and important changes at a time in his life when his ability to solve problems may be diminishing. If he tends to cope well with stress and views aging as a normal part of life, he should be able to adjust smoothly to the changes aging brings.

Common psychological problems among elderly patients include organic brain syndrome, depression, grieving, substance abuse, adverse drug reactions, paranoia, and anxiety. Of course, these problems aren't limited to elderly persons. Their incidence, however, is much higher in this age-group than in others.

144 Organic brain syndrome

Organic brain syndrome is the most common form of mental illness in elderly people. It occurs in both an acute form (reversible cerebral dysfunction) and a chronic form (irreversible cerebral cellular destruction). Characteristics of both types include impaired memory (especially recent memory), disorientation, confusion, and poor comprehension.

In the elderly patient, *acute organic brain syndrome* may result from malnutrition, cerebrovascular accident, drugs, alcohol, or head trauma. Restlessness and a fluctuating level of awareness, ranging from mild confusion to stupor, may signal this condition.

The causes of *chronic organic brain syndrome* are unknown. The major signs of this disorder include impaired intellectual functioning, poor attention span, memory loss using confabulation, and varying moods, including irritability and lability.

145 An elderly patient's depression

Depression is the most common psychogenic problem found in elderly patients. Since the symptoms of depression span a wide range, consider it as a possibility in any elderly patient. Depression may appear as changes in behavior (apathy, self-deprecation, anger, inertia); changes in thought processes (confusion, disorientation, poor judgment), or somatic complaints (appetite loss, constipation, insomnia).

If you observe any of these signs, question your patient in detail about recent losses—as discussed in Entry 146—and find out how he's coping with them. Assess his feelings carefully. Remember that an elderly patient's attitude toward his own aging and death—and toward death and dying in general—will affect his chances for successful treatment of depression.

146 Adjusting to loss

A common difficulty elderly patients face is adapting to loss, since the grieving process regularly intrudes on their lives. Your patient may have to deal with losing his job, income, friends, family, health, or even his home. These losses and the associated feelings of isolation and loneliness can cause stress that has physiologic and psychological consequences. For example, the loss of a spouse or other loved one can trigger profound sorrow, and resolution may be difficult. Unsuccessful resolution of grief can cause a pathologic grief reaction, which may take the form of physical or mental illness.

147 Substance abuse

Many elderly people today are turning to substance abuse and suicide in response to severe stress. Suspect possible substance abuse or thoughts of suicide if your patient is taking an unusual number or amount of medications, or if you note such signs of alcohol abuse as jaundice and tremor.

148 Adverse drug reactions

When you assess an elderly patient, consider that his psychological problems may result from undetected adverse drug reactions. The incidence of

DRUGS

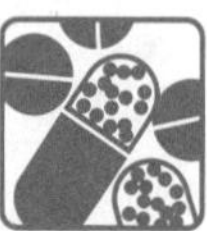

COMMON DRUGS THAT CAUSE CONFUSION IN ELDERLY PATIENTS

CLASSIFICATION	POSSIBLE SIDE EFFECTS
CNS depressants and other psychotropic drugs	
secobarbital (Seconal), phenobarbital (Luminal, Eskabarb*), and other barbiturates chlordiazepoxide (Librium*), diazepam (Valium*), flurazepam (Dalmane*), and other benzodiazepines salicylates, propoxyphene hydrochloride (Darvon, Depronal**), and other nonnarcotic analgesics hydromorphone hydrochloride (Dilaudid*) and other narcotic analgesics alcohol intake alone, or with any of these CNS depressants (lethal dose of barbiturates drops almost 50% when taken with alcohol)	• Bizarre perceptual disturbances, delusions, thought disorders, panic, memory disorders
chlorpromazine (Thorazine, Chlorprom**), thioridazine (Mellaril*), and other phenothiazines; haloperidol (Haldol*)	• Hypotension side effect causes impaired mental ability; possibly leads to syncope if blood pressure drops too low for brain perfusion
amitriptyline (Elavil*), imipramine (Tofranil*), and other tricyclic antidepressants	• Hypotension from phenothiazines is common and very serious. Dosage is adjusted for the elderly.
Anticholinergic or atropine-like drugs and other gastrointestinal drugs	
atropine, scopolamine (included in many nonprescription sleep-producing preparations), and other belladonna alkaloids diphenhydramine (Benadryl*), trihexyphenidyl (Artane*), benztropine mesylate (Cogentin*), and other anti-Parkinson agents propantheline bromide (Pro-Banthine*) cimetidine (Tagamet*)	• Disorientation, delusions, recent memory impairment, agitation, confusion (cimetidine)
Antihypertensive drugs	
guanethidine (Ismelin*), reserpine (Serpasil*), methyldopa (Aldomet*), and other sympatholytics	• Hypotension impairs mental ability; may lead to syncope if blood pressure drops too low for brain perfusion

*Available in U.S. and Canada. **Available in Canada only. All other products (no symbol) available in U.S. only.

these reactions increases in older people because they use more drugs and may not take medication in the prescribed manner. Physiologic changes related to the aging process also may alter a patient's reaction to a drug. Such routinely prescribed medications as tranquilizers and barbiturates can cause or increase depression. Other medications, including anticholinergics and diuretics, may cause confusion in elderly patients (see *Common Drugs That Cause Confusion in Elderly Patients*). Always include a detailed drug history in your psychological assessment.

149 Paranoia in an elderly patient

If you detect signs of paranoia during the mental status examination, try to determine whether they are a result of sensory-loss problems (which may be corrected by glasses or a hearing aid), psychological problems, or a realistic fear of attack or robbery.

Signs of possible paranoia include expressions of feeling alone and afraid; unpredictable behavior, affect, and thinking; difficulty relating to others; and feelings of being watched or threatened, especially by family members.

150 The effects of anxiety

In an elderly patient, the need to adjust to physical, emotional, and socioeconomic changes (such as hospitalization, loneliness, or moving to a new neighborhood) can cause acute anxiety reactions. These changes may raise his anxiety level to the point of temporary confusion and disorientation. Often an elderly person's condition is mislabeled senility or organic brain syndrome, when it should be considered a psychogenic disorder.

Selected References

American Psychiatric Association, Committee on Nomenclature and Statistics. *Diagnostic and Statistical Manual of Mental Disorders,* 3rd ed. Washington, D.C.: American Psychiatric Association, 1980.

Burnside, Irene M., and Ebersole, Patricia, eds. *Psychosocial Caring Throughout the Life Span.* New York: McGraw-Hill Book Co., 1979.

Carter, E.A., and McGoldrick, M. *The Family Life Cycle: A Framework for Family Therapy.* New York: Gardner Press, 1980.

Erikson, Erik H. *Childhood and Society.* New York: W.W. Norton & Co., 1964.

Flynn, Patricia A. *Holistic Health: The Art and Science of Care.* Bowie, Md.: Robert J. Brady Co., 1980.

Freedman, Alfred M., et al. *Modern Synopsis of Comprehensive Textbook of Psychiatry,* 2nd ed. Baltimore: Williams & Wilkins, 1976.

Hackett, Thomas P., and Cassem, Ned H. *Massachusetts General Hospital Handbook of General Hospital Psychiatry.* St. Louis: C.V. Mosby Co., 1978.

Kreigh, Helen Z., and Perko, Joanne E. *Psychiatric and Mental Health Nursing: Commitment to Care and Concern.* Reston, Va.: Reston Pub. Co., 1979.

Kyes, Joan J., and Hofling, Charles R. *Basic Psychiatric Concepts in Nursing,* 4th ed. Philadelphia: J.B. Lippincott Co., 1980.

Leininger, Madeleine. *Transcultural Nursing: Concepts, Theories, and Practices.* New York: John Wiley & Sons, 1977.

Lewis, Garland K. *Nurse-Patient Communication,* 3rd ed. Dubuque, Iowa: William C. Brown Co., 1978.

Pasquali, Elaine A., et al. *Mental Health Nursing: A Bio-Psycho-Cultural Approach.* St. Louis: C.V. Mosby Co., 1981.

Robinson, Lisa. *Psychiatric Nursing As a Human Experience.* Philadelphia: W.B. Saunders Co., 1977.

Selye, Hans. *The Stress of Life,* 2nd ed. New York: McGraw-Hill Book Co., 1978.

Wolanin, Mary O., and Phillips, Linda R. *Confusion: Prevention and Care.* St. Louis: C.V. Mosby Co., 1980.

5

KEY POINTS IN THIS CHAPTER

KEY CHARTS IN THIS CHAPTER

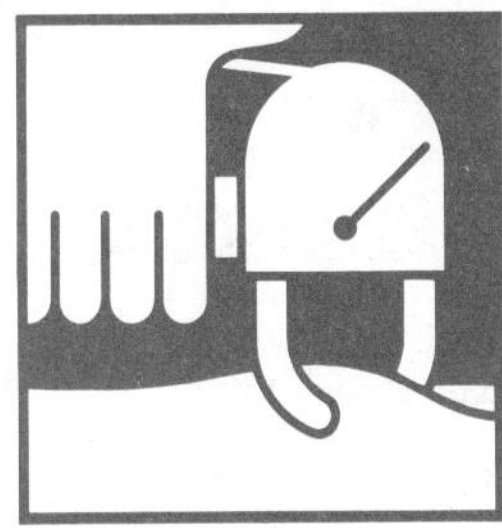

Assessing Nutritional Status

Introduction

151 Nursing and nutrition

Despite its obvious relationship to health, nutritional status is often evaluated superficially or completely overlooked in patient assessment. How often have you seen *well developed; well nourished* written next to *general appearance* on the physical examination form and wondered how this evaluation was made? As a nurse, you're responsible for the total needs of your patient. Nutritional assessment, an integral part of patient care, is essential to developing an effective care plan to meet these needs. Complete nutritional assessment includes taking your patient's nutritional and health history, inspecting for signs of obvious malnutrition, performing anthropometric measurements, and evaluating results of laboratory tests, including those for immunocompetence.

152 World malnutrition

Worldwide, the most common form of malnutrition is protein-calorie malnutrition (PCM). Many people assume that PCM occurs widely only in underdeveloped countries. Unfortunately, this isn't so: Undernutrition affects approximately two thirds of the world's population and occurs in every country, race, and age-group.

In the United States, the Ten-State Nutrition Survey and the Health and Nutrition Examination Survey, which were conducted in low-income areas, indicate that a significant portion of this population is malnourished or at high risk of developing nutritional deficiencies. The high-risk groups include children, adolescents, pregnant and lactating women, and persons over age 60. The most common nutritional deficiency found in these studies was iron deficiency anemia; others included protein deficiencies in pregnant and lactating women, and deficiencies of vitamins A, B_6, and C. Retarded growth in children (ages 1 to 3), poor dental health, and obesity also appeared in high-risk groups.

These studies underscore the importance of assessing all patients to detect malnutrition. Assessment also helps you differentiate primary malnutrition (insufficient nutrient intake) from malnutrition secondary to conditions that impair digestion, absorption, and utilization of nutrients or to conditions that increase nutrient requirements or excretion.

153 Inpatient nutrition

Provision of adequate nourishment involves much more than assuring that your patient receives sufficient vitamins

LEARNING ABOUT COMMON I.V. ADDITIVES

The components of hyperalimentation solutions usually include 50% dextrose in water, amino acids, and specific additives ordered by the doctor to prevent metabolic deficiencies or to treat deficiencies the patient already has. The specific additives may include:

- **Potassium**: needed for cellular activity and tissue synthesis
- **Folic acid**: necessary for DNA formation; promotes growth and development
- **Vitamin D**: essential for bone metabolism and maintenance of serum calcium levels
- **Trace elements** (i.e., zinc, manganese, cobalt): help in wound healing and red blood cell synthesis
- **Sodium**: helps control water distribution and maintain a normal fluid balance
- **Chloride**: regulates the acid-base equilibrium and maintains osmotic pressure
- **Vitamin B complex**: helps in final absorption of carbohydrates and protein
- **Calcium**: needed for bone and teeth development; aids in blood clotting
- **Phosphate**: minimizes the threat of peripheral paresthesias
- **Magnesium**: helps metabolize carbohydrates and protein
- **Acetate**: added to prevent metabolic acidosis
- **Vitamin K**: helps prevent bleeding disorders
- **Vitamin C**: helps in wound healing

and minerals. Because the body needs large amounts of protein and calories to maintain or restore good nutritional status, your patient must ingest large amounts of protein- and calorie-rich foods (or total-feeding formulas) to meet protein and calorie needs. Vitamin and mineral requirements, on the other hand, may be met by oral supplements. Over the past decade or so, greater attention to the nutritional status of the hospitalized patient has led to the development of sophisticated feeding techniques, including both enteral and parenteral methods. A severely malnourished patient may not recover even if these techniques are used.

154 Nurse and dietitian

The role and responsibilities of the nurse in nutritional assessment vary from institution to institution, as do policies and procedures regarding patient nutrition. In some hospitals, the nurse may be primarily responsible for evaluation of the patient's nutritional status as well as subsequent nutritional care; in some larger institutions, the specially trained, registered dietitian usually fulfills this role. In still other hospitals or institutions, a doctor, nurse, dietitian, pharmacist, social worker, and physical or occupational therapist work together as a team to provide *nutrition support services.*

Physiology of nutrition

155 Factors in nutrition

Many interrelated factors affect your patient's nutritional status. Obviously, both quantity and quality of food can significantly affect body structure and function. In developing nations, a large part of the population suffers malnutrition secondary to limited quantities and poor quality of available foodstuffs. In nations with abundant food supplies, a number of other factors affect the population's nutrition: Cultural, social, psychological, and economic considerations determine food selection and meal patterns. Even the availability of an ideal diet doesn't guarantee optimum nutrition.

Every person's nourishment depends

on his ability to ingest and transport food through the gastrointestinal tract: the adequacy of his digestive processes, which break down foodstuffs in the stomach and small intestine in preparation for absorption, and his ability to absorb nutrients from the small intestine and excrete waste products. After nutrients are absorbed, they must be efficiently processed in the liver or other organs, or used directly by the cells. The complex biochemical transformation of nutrients into energy and tissue can be disrupted by abnormalities in absorption, transport, or metabolism, or by drug interference. Deficiencies in cellular nutrition may occur secondary to increased demand or excessive excretion.

During a person's life span, nutritional requirements (proteins, fats, carbohydrates, water, vitamins, and minerals) fluctuate in response to external and internal changes. Conditions that increase the body's need for nutrients include periods of rapid growth (infancy through adolescence) and periods of stress (trauma, disease, pregnancy, and lactation). Conversely, metabolic demand for certain substances decreases with age (for example, the need for iron after menopause). Caloric requirements, too, diminish gradually after age 25, with decreased physical activity and reduced energy demands.

156 Digestion

Digestion of the three major dietary components—carbohydrates, fats, and proteins—requires that these complex substances be broken down into simpler compounds for absorption through the intestinal mucosa. This process, mainly chemical, is also partly mechanical. In the chemical digestive process, more than a dozen enzymes act to produce the simpler compounds for gastrointestinal absorption. The mechanical process begins with chewing and continues, in the stomach and small intestine, with the mixing movements that produce the homogenous semiliquid chyme.

Carbohydrate digestion begins with the action of ptyalin (a salivary enzyme), which catalyzes the breakdown of starch into maltose, a disaccharide. Carbohydrates are ultimately hydrolyzed into three monosaccharides: glucose, fructose, and galactose. Similarly, fats—with the aid of bile acids and gastric, pancreatic, and intestinal lipases—are broken down into free fatty acids, glycerol, and monoglycerides. Pepsin, pancreatic enzymes (primarily trypsin, chymotrypsin, and carboxypolypeptidase), and dipeptidases in the epithelium of the small intestine ultimately hydrolyze proteins into their constituent amino acids.

Throughout the large absorptive surface of the small intestine, monosaccharides, amino acids, and fats (as bile salts) are absorbed into the blood and lymph, primarily through the mechanisms of diffusion and active transport. They're then distributed to the cells for further chemical processing, which releases the energy necessary for bodily function.

157 Cellular metabolism

Metabolism, the physical and chemical process of cell nutrition, converts nutrients into chemical forms that produce energy and rebuild body tissue. Metabolism consists of two phases: anabolism and catabolism. *Anabolism* builds tissue by transforming simple substances into more complex ones; *catabolism* produces energy by changing complex substances into simpler compounds.

158 Carbohydrate metabolism

Carbohydrate (particularly glucose) metabolism furnishes most of the energy necessary for bodily function. In *glycolysis*—the first step of glucose metabolism—glucose molecules are broken down into pyruvic acid. Then, pyruvic acid is converted to acetylcoenzyme A and enters the *citric acid cycle.* In the citric acid cycle, ionized hydrogen ions are removed from various substances and form carbon dioxide, a byproduct. In *oxidative phosphorylation,* energy from the hydrogen electrons is trapped, forming adenosine triphosphate, the energy storage compound of cells. Finally, the electrons and hydrogen ions combine with oxygen to form water.

Carbohydrate metabolism also involves the processes of glycogenesis, glycogenolysis, and gluconeogenesis to ensure ample supplies of glucose for cellular energy. *Glycogenesis* is the formation of glycogen (a polysaccharide in which glucose is stored) from carbohydrates. This process results from saturation of the cells with glucose-6-phosphate. *Glycogenolysis* is the conversion of glycogen into glucose-6-phosphate and the liberation of free glucose in the liver. *Gluconeogenesis* is the formation of glucose from noncarbohydrates, such as fat glycerols or protein amino acids. Insulin stimulates glycolysis and glycogenesis; glucagon, catecholamines, and glucocorticoids stimulate glycogenolysis and gluconeogenesis.

159 Fat metabolism

Two processes are involved in fat metabolism: lipolysis and lipogenesis. In *lipolysis,* triglycerides are hydrolyzed into fatty acids and glycerol. Beta-oxidation further reduces fatty acids into acetylcoenzyme A, which enters the citric acid cycle, releasing energy and heat. Glucose is produced from glycerol through the process of gluconeogenesis.

In the opposite reaction, *lipogenesis,* the body converts excess carbohydrates and proteins, or fatty acids and glycerol (products of lipolysis), into fat, usually for storage in the adipose tissue. Like carbohydrates, such fat stores are primarily sources of energy for cellular metabolic processes during periods of starvation. The body can synthesize nonessential fatty acids from other substances. But linoleic acid, an essential unsaturated fatty acid necessary for synthesis of vital body compounds, can't be synthesized by the body; so it must be provided through diet. Insulin stimulates lipogenesis and fatty acid synthesis; glucagon, catecholamines, and glucocorticoids stimulate lipolysis.

160 Protein metabolism

Unlike carbohydrate and fat metabolism, protein metabolism is mainly anabolic. This process provides the body with substances necessary for cellular growth, reproduction, and repair. Protein anabolism also supplies substances necessary for life itself—such as plasma proteins. When the carbohydrate or fat supply is insufficient, or the body's energy demands are very high, the body may switch to protein as its energy source.

Protein synthesis requires an adequate supply of calories and essential and nonessential amino acids. The body can't synthesize the nine essential amino acids—valine, lysine, leucine, isoleucine, methionine, phenylalanine, threonine, tryptophan, and histidine—so diet must provide them. The body does synthesize nonessential amino acids.

Protein metabolism consists of three processes: *deamination* (the catabolic removal of the amino group from the amino acid compound, forming ammonia and a keto acid), *transamination* (anabolic conversion of keto acids to amino acids), and *urea formation* (the final catabolic step, producing the nitrogenous substance urea from ammonia compounds and amino acids).

Insulin, growth hormone, and testosterone stimulate protein anabolism; adrenocorticotropic hormone facilitates protein catabolism through the secretion of glucocorticoids. Because the nitrogen ingested usually equals the nitrogen excreted, the rate of protein anabolism usually equals the rate of protein catabolism (nitrogen balance). Anabolism (for example, during pregnancy or periods of rapid growth) will result in protein conservation, so the amount of nitrogen ingested exceeds the amount excreted (positive nitrogen balance). Conversely, excessive catabolism (for example, during calorie protein deficiency) can cause the amount of nitrogen excreted to exceed the amount ingested (negative nitrogen balance).

161 Vitamins and minerals

The body needs only minute amounts of these nutrients, which aren't synthesized by the body (except vitamins D and K) and don't provide calories or contribute to tissue mass.

Vitamins are organic compounds; their functions include helping convert fat and carbohydrates into energy, assisting in bone and teeth formation, and helping to regulate metabolism. Vitamins are classified as water-soluble (B-complex and C), which aren't stored in the body, or fat-soluble (A, D, E, and K), which are stored in the body.

Minerals are inorganic elements that, in ionic form, are distributed throughout the body fluids. They help maintain osmotic pressure, acid-base balance, and nerve and muscle irritability; participate in the membrane transfer of chemical compounds; and regulate enzyme metabolism. In combination, minerals contribute to growth and also function as fixed-salt constituents of teeth and bone.

162 Water and electrolytes

The largest component of body mass is water, the body's most essential substance after oxygen. The body needs both intracellular and extracellular water, as solvent and catalyst. Water's main functions include transporting nutrients and the waste products of metabolism, lubricating the body, and helping maintain body temperature.

Electrolytes—the dissociated ions of salts, acids, and bases—are dissolved in intracellular and extracellular fluids. Carefully proportioned concentrations of electrolytes are essential in maintaining osmotic pressure, water balance and distribution, and muscle irritability, and for regulating acid-base balance.

163 Using recommended dietary allowances

The recommended dietary allowances (RDAs) for essential nutrients are revised every 6 years. Current RDAs (revised in 1980) specify the recommended daily consumption for the following essential nutrients: protein, thiamine, riboflavin, niacin, folic acid, calcium, phosphorus, magnesium, iron, zinc, iodine, and vitamins A, C, D, E, B_6, and B_{12}. As yet, RDAs haven't been established for certain essential nutrients. When you interpret and use them properly, the RDA guidelines can help you evaluate and plan your patient's nutrient consumption.

Nutritional requirements vary according to age, sex, and body size; RDAs are grouped accordingly. The differences in the RDAs for males and females are based on differences in growth rate, body weight, and body composition except for the dietary iron requirement, which is higher in females because of blood losses during menstruation. During periods of growth, pregnancy, and lactation, the nutrient requirements per unit of body weight increase. Although the RDAs take these changed requirements into account, they don't account for altered nutritional requirements secondary to metabolic disorders, chronic diseases, trauma, burns, sepsis, or drug-nutrient reactions. RDAs estimate energy needs, including caloric requirements, for all age-groups and both sexes. However, they're intended only as guidelines.

Note that RDAs are intended to evaluate only the nutrient intake of population groups in the United States who are in *good health.* Failure to meet an RDA doesn't indicate a specific nutrient

RECOMMENDED DIETARY ALLOWANCES OF PROTEINS, VITAMINS, AND MINERALS

The recommended dietary allowances listed here are levels that will maintain good nutrition in most healthy Americans.

	MALE			FEMALE		
ELEMENT	AGES 19 TO 22 154 lb (70 kg) 70" (177 cm)	AGES 23 TO 50 154 lb (70 kg) 70" (177 cm)	AGE 51 + 154 lb (70 kg) 70" (177 cm)	AGES 19 TO 22 120 lb (55 kg) 64" (163 cm)	AGES 23 TO 50 120 lb (55 kg) 64" (163 cm)	AGE 51 + 120 lb (55 kg) 64" (163 cm)
Protein (g)	56	56	56	44	44	44
Vitamin A (mcg RE)	1,000	1,000	1,000	800	800	800
Vitamin D (mcg)	7.5	5	5	7.5	5	5
Vitamin E (mg or TE)	10	10	10	8	8	8
Vitamin C (mg)	60	60	60	60	60	60
Thiamine (mg)	1.5	1.4	1.2	1.1	1	1
Riboflavin (mg)	1.7	1.6	1.4	1.3	1.2	1.2
Niacin (mg NE)	19	18	16	14	13	13
Vitamin B_6 (mg)	2.2	2.2	2.2	2	2	2
Folacin (mcg)	400	400	400	400	400	400
Vitamin B_{12} (mcg)	3	3	3	3	3	3
Calcium (mg)	800	800	800	800	800	800
Phosphorus (mg)	800	800	800	800	800	800
Magnesium (mg)	350	350	350	300	300	300
Iron (mg)	10	10	10	18	18	18
Zinc (mg)	15	15	15	15	15	15
Iodine (mcg)	150	150	150	150	150	150

Courtesy National Research Council.

deficiency or malnutrition. However, such a dietary deficiency, over a prolonged period, will result in a nutrient deficiency.

164 The four food groups

The four food groups provide criteria for the selection of a nutritionally adequate diet. Foods included in these groups are nutrient dense (providing maximal nutritional benefit with minimal wasted calories) and are categorized by similar nutrient content and recommended number of daily servings:

- *the milk group:* contains milk and milk products; major nutrients include protein, calcium, riboflavin, vitamin D, and vitamin A (when the food is fortified)
- *the meat group:* contains meat (including poultry), fish, and eggs; dried peas and beans; and soy extenders and nuts when combined with complementary protein, iron, niacin, and thiamine
- *the fruit and vegetable group:* contains fruits and vegetables; major nutrients are vitamins A and C

• *the grain group:* contains enriched or whole grain breads, cereals, and crackers; major nutrients include thiamine, niacin, riboflavin, iron, and carbohydrates.

Although the four food groups concept is very useful, it has some limitations. Many foods, such as butter, oil, margarine, sugar, and condiments don't fit into these categories. These foods make the diet more palatable but add little nutrition. How much of these foods a person's diet should include depends on his remaining caloric requirement *after* he's eaten the recommended number of servings from each of the four food groups.

The four food groups relate only to *leader nutrients* including carbohydrates, proteins, fats, thiamine, riboflavin, niacin, vitamins A and C, calcium, and iron; no recommendation is made for other nutrients. Presumably, eating a variety of foods rich in the leader nutrients will supply the required amounts of these other nutrients.

Also, foods in the same group don't supply the same number of calories per a specific quantity; for example, 8 oz of whole milk provide approximately 170 calories, but 8 oz of skim milk supply approximately 80 calories. Yet, they have equal value (one serving) in the milk group. This means that a person selecting foods from the four groups must carefully adjust his intake to meet his caloric requirements.

Remember: A daily diet that includes the minimum number of servings from each of the four groups supplies about 1,200 calories and meets the RDAs for protein, riboflavin, calcium, and vitamins A and C. The amounts of thiamine and niacin supplied may be only marginal, and the iron supplied is about half the daily requirement for a premenopausal adult woman.

165 Tables of food composition

Another method of measuring the nutritional content of your patient's diet is through tables of food composition as determined by chemical analysis of the food. These tables list foods in either common household measures or in 100-g portions, and according to their nutrient analysis.

To use these tables, compare the amounts of nutrients consumed to the RDAs specified for healthy patients, or to the nutritional requirements specified for ill patients.

Collecting appropriate history data

166 Biographical data

Biographical data (especially your patient's age and sex) can help identify special nutritional risk factors. For example, elderly people need the same amounts of proteins, vitamins, and minerals as younger adults, but when their activity decreases, they require fewer calories. Also, iron deficiency anemia is more common in adolescent girls (because of their increased need for iron) than in adolescent boys.

167 Chief complaint

Your patient's problems concerning nutrition will probably involve one or more of the following chief complaints: *weight loss, weight gain, asthenia* (weakness), *gastrointestinal disturbances, skin changes,* and *musculoskeletal impairment.*

168 History of present condition

Using the PQRST mnemonic device, ask your patient to elaborate on his chief complaint. Then, depending on

Chief complaint		Questions to ask
• Weight loss • Weight gain • Asthenia (weakness) • Gastrointestinal disturbances • Skin changes • Musculoskeletal impairment	P	*Provocative/Palliative* What causes it? What makes it better? What makes it worse?
	Q	*Quality/Quantity* How does it feel, look, or sound, and how much of it is there?
	R	*Region/Radiation* Where is it? Does it spread?
	S	*Severity scale* Does it interfere with activities? How does it rate on a severity scale of 1 to 10?
	T	*Timing* When did it begin? How often does it occur? Is it sudden or gradual?

the complaint, explore the history of his present condition by asking the following questions:

• ***Weight loss*** (weight 20% or more below normal for height). *Was the weight loss intentional or unintentional? Has your appetite decreased lately? Have any changes occurred in your sense of taste or sense of smell?* (Obviously, diminished sense of taste makes food less appetizing; loss of sense of smell also affects the ability to taste.) Weight loss can accompany emotional disturbances, such as anxiety or depression, and pathologic disorders, such as cancer, hyperactive thyroid, infectious diseases, diabetes mellitus, chronic gastrointestinal (GI) disease, and renal failure. *Are you able to chew properly and comfortably?*

• ***Weight gain*** (20% or more above normal for height). *Was the weight gain intentional or unintentional? Has your appetite increased recently?*

• ***Asthenia.*** *Have you noticed any recent weakness or diminished strength or energy?* Asthenia may result from various nutritional deficiencies or from protein/calorie deficiency. Patients with emotional disorders and chronic illnesses may report asthenia. Further compromising of the patient's nutritional status may occur if his condition impairs his ability to prepare or obtain nutritious meals.

• ***GI disturbances.*** *Have you experienced loss of appetite, nausea, vomiting, dyspepsia, flatulence, diarrhea, or constipation lately? After eating? How often? Do you have this type of problem after you eat certain types of foods?*

Some specific physiologic and psychological conditions may produce GI disturbances that lead to nutritional deficiencies. For example, anorexia, nausea, and vomiting in the hypermetabolic patient with cancer can result in decreased intake, leading to cachexia. (For more information on GI disturbances, see Entry 453.)

• ***Skin changes.*** *Have you noticed any recent skin changes?* Be sure to inspect the skin as well (see Entries 224 and 226).

• ***Musculoskeletal impairment.*** *Have you recently noticed muscle weakness or a change in muscle size?* Inquire about other nutritionally related deformities. For example, vitamin D deficiency can result in rickets and other bone deformities.

169 Past history

When reviewing your patient's past history, focus on the following problems:

- ***Increased metabolic demand.*** This may result from *infection, cancer, trauma, pregnancy, surgery, long bone fractures,* and *major body burns,* as well as *regularly increased activity.*
- ***Decreased metabolic requirements.*** Examples are *decreased physical activity* and disorders such as *hypothyroidism.*
- ***Chewing difficulty.*** This may result from *trauma, lack of teeth, malocclusion,* or *improperly fitting dentures.*
- ***Difficulty swallowing.*** Many conditions may cause this symptom, including *cancer of the esophagus, neurologic impairment* (such as paralysis or Parkinson's disease), *esophageal stricture,* or *radiation therapy* to the head and neck. (See Entry 426.)
- ***Increased nutritional loss.*** Examples are *diarrhea, draining wounds, abscesses, gastrointestinal (GI) fistulas,* and *dialysis.*
- ***Maldigestion or nutrient malabsorption.*** These conditions may include *GI disease* (such as Crohn's disease, cancer, or ulcerative ileocolitis) or *GI surgery* (especially gastrectomy followed by dumping syndrome, massive small bowel resection that results in decreased absorptive surface, or pancreatectomy with resulting pancreatic insufficiency).
- ***Decreased nutritional intake.*** Prolonged use of *I.V. fluids* or *withholding oral food and fluids* from a hospitalized patient for more than 10 days can severely compromise his nutritional status.
- ***Chronic illnesses.*** Examples are *cirrhosis, diabetes mellitus, chronic obstructive lung disease,* and *renal disease.*
- ***Radiation therapy.*** Radiation to any part of your patient's body may cause loss of appetite, nausea, and/or vomiting.
- ***Allergy or intolerance.*** Allergic reactions or intolerance to foods or drugs may cause your patient to experience symptoms, such as diarrhea, and to change his diet.
- ***Medication interference.*** Because many drugs adversely affect the bioavailability of nutrients, be sure to take an accurate drug and vitamin history.
- ***Excessive alcohol use.*** Excessive intake of alcoholic beverages increases magnesium excretion and interferes with utilization of folic acid, thiamine, vitamin B_6, and fats. Severe alcoholism may cause malnutrition, because many alcoholics don't eat properly.

170 Family history

Your patient's risk of becoming obese increases if *obesity* has affected members of his family. *Diabetes mellitus,* which tends to recur in families, causes disturbances in carbohydrate, protein, and fat metabolism.

171 Psychosocial history

Your review of the patient's psychosocial history should cover the following areas:

- ***Financial status.*** Limited income affects nutritional status if the person lacks the money to buy the type and quantity of food he needs. For instance, elderly people on fixed incomes, faced with rising food prices, often must buy cheap food that doesn't provide sufficient nourishment. The number of family members also determines the amount of money available per person for food.
- ***Inadequate housing.*** Insufficient cooking or plumbing facilities, especially lack of running water or of proper food storage facilities, affect food quality and thus nutritional status.
- ***Cultural background.*** Religious preferences may affect food selection and preparation.
- ***Living and work arrangements.*** A person living alone may not bother to prepare nutritious meals for himself. Eating more than half the total meals away from home can affect nutrition,

too. For example, a person with a busy schedule is apt to eat on the run or to skip meals entirely, and thus compromise his nutritional status.

• ***Fad dieting.*** Fad diets and quick-weight-loss methods are usually unsafe and nutritionally unsound. Besides possibly causing nutrient imbalance or toxicity, such a diet may cause a patient to delay seeking proper treatment for an illness, or terminate prescribed treatment.

• ***Psychological conditions.*** Both increased and decreased food intake may have a psychological stimulus. For example, in some persons, depression and anxiety cause disinterest in food; others may eat more to allay their anxiety or depression.

172 Activities of daily living

To review the patient's activities of daily living include these questions:

• ***Impaired mobility.*** *Arthritis* may interfere with self-feeding or with your patient's ability to obtain or cook food.

• ***Lack of regular exercise.*** Decreased energy requirements reduce nutritional requirements accordingly.

173 Typical daily intake and 24-hour recall

You can determine how your patient's eating habits may affect his nutrition by using the 24-hour recall or recording his typical daily intake. When taking the 24-hour recall, ask the patient to describe all of the food and beverage he has consumed in the past 24 hours (including amounts), how it was prepared, and when and where he ate it. This method describes the patient's intake only over the past 24 hours; to learn more about his usual eating habits, ask him about his typical daily intake: what food and beverage types he consumes and in what amounts, how the food is usually prepared, and when and where he usually eats. Also assess the degree to which your patient's answers may reflect his desire to please you or to appear affluent enough to eat well.

174 Food intake records (calorie counts)

Through food intake records, you can determine the protein, calorie, and other nutrient intake of malnourished patients or those at nutritional risk while hospitalized. You can then compare this information with each patient's basic nutritional requirements to assess his ability to maintain adequate nutrition. These records also help determine your patient's need for enteral/parenteral hyperalimentation, or let you monitor intake when weaning a patient from a tube feeding or a parenteral hyperalimentation regimen.

To compile a food intake record for your patient, record the types and amounts of all foods and beverages he consumes in a 24-hour period; calculate the consumed amounts of calories and proteins (and other nutrients, if warranted).

Examining your patient

175 Using inspection

Of the four assessment techniques—inspection, percussion, palpation, and auscultation—you'll use inspection most often in nutritional assessment, although its uses are limited. The signs and symptoms of nutritional deficiency (such as weight loss, asthenia, skin changes, musculoskeletal impairment, and gastrointestinal disturbances) are nonspecific for particular deficiencies, because obvious abnormalities appear only in advanced nutritional deficiency states. (For a listing of typical signs and symptoms, see *Nurse's Guide to Nutritional Deficiencies,* pages 154 to 157.)

176 Using palpation

Although not as important as inspection in assessing nutritional status, palpation can be useful. For example, this technique can help you detect thyroid, parotid, liver, spleen, or other glandular enlargement, which may indicate a nutrition-compromising condition. Thyroid enlargement, for instance, is characteristic of iodine deficiency. (For more information on palpating for glandular enlargement, see Entry 761.)

177 Measuring height

Considering your patient's height together with his weight may give you clues to undernutrition or overeating.

Measure your patient's height yourself when possible; by having him remove his shoes and stand on the height scale facing forward, with his back and heels against the bar and his head held erect. Measure and record his height to the nearest ¼″ (0.5 cm).

178 Classifying body frame

A person's body frame type—small, medium, or large—relates directly to his weight. For example, a large-framed patient may weigh more than a patient of the same height with a smaller frame and still be at his ideal weight.

To determine your patient's body frame type, measure his wrist at the smallest circumference distal to the styloid processes of the radius and the ulna. Then measure his height (without shoes), and compare his wrist circumference with his height on the body frame chart (see *Determining Body Frame Type,* page 146).

179 Weigh your patient

Body weight is the total weight of lean body mass (extracellular fluid, protoplasm, and bone) and fat. When you compare your patient's weight, height, and body frame with standards and find he's above or below standard, investigate further to find out if he's obese or undernourished. Measured daily, your patient's weight reflects changes in hydration status, which can help you assess fluid retention or the effectiveness of diuretic therapy or dialysis.

Weigh your patient yourself, if possible, to obtain an accurate baseline for comparison of ideal body weight, usual weight, and future weight. If you rely on information from the patient, you may fail to identify significant weight changes.

If possible, weigh the patient at the same time each day. Make sure he's wearing lightweight clothing and no shoes. Use a beam or a lever scale, and record his weight to the nearest ½ lb (1.1 kg).

Sometimes a patient being admitted

RECOMMENDED CALORIC INTAKE FOR ADULTS

Here's a list of recommended caloric intake based on sex and age. Caloric need is measured in Kcals, or kilocalories, a laboratory value that denotes how much heat is needed to raise the temperature of 1 kg of water 1° centigrade.

Energy needs for young adults are based on light work. Energy needs for older adults decrease in proportion to their presumed general decrease in activity. Pregnant women need an additional 300 Kcals per day, and lactating women need an additional 500 Kcals per day.

	AGE	CALORIC NEEDS (Kcal)
Men (average: 154 lb [69.3 kg]; 70″ [177.8 cm])	19 to 22	(2,500-3,000)
	23 to 50	(2,300-3,100)
	51 to 75	(2,000-2,800)
	over 75	(1,650-2,450)
Women (average: 120 lb [54 kg]; 64″ [162.6 cm])	19 to 22	(1,700-2,500)
	23 to 50	(1,600-2,400)
	51 to 75	(1,400-2,200)
	over 75	(1,200-2,000)

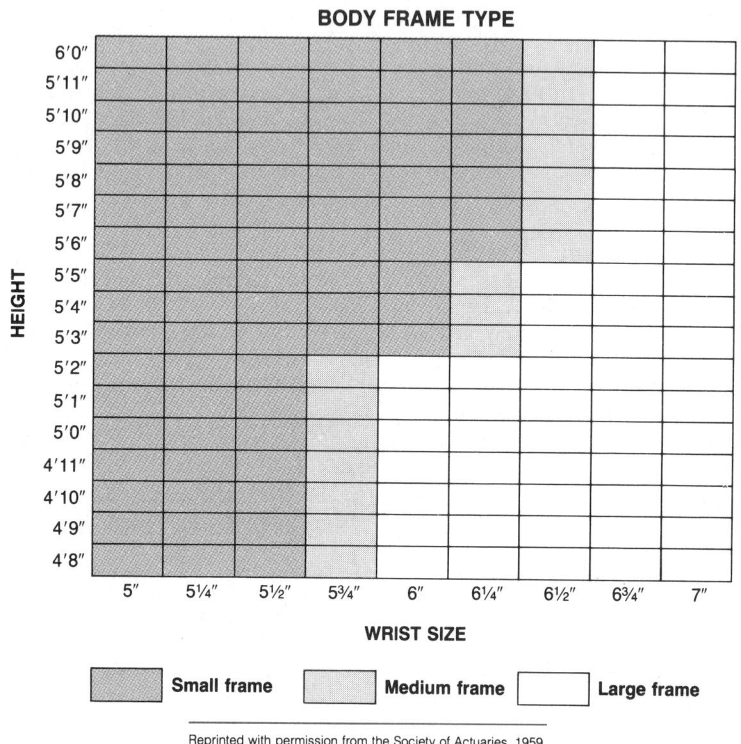

is too ill to be weighed or requires immediate medical care. In such circumstances, record what the patient tells you he weighs (always documented as *stated weight*) until you're able to weigh him. If accurate weight is essential to therapy and the patient can't stand up, weigh him using a bed scale.

The current standard of ideal body weight—for comparison with actual weight according to height, age, and frame size—is based on Society of Actuaries data (see *Assessing Body Weight*). While these guidelines are helpful in assessing your patient, you should be aware of the following limitations on their usefulness and validity:

- Ideal body weight for health maintenance has never been defined, so no such chart is completely authoritative.
- Body frame size, clothing weight, and heel height aren't defined.
- These figures were obtained at the turn of this century and may not represent current U.S. population standards.

The formula to express actual weight versus ideal weight as a percentage is *actual weight/ideal body weight multiplied by 100.* A weight-to-height ratio of about 80% or less usually indicates a significant deficit of protein and cal-

ASSESSING BODY WEIGHT

To assess your patient's weight accurately, you must know both his height and body frame type. Using the charts below, find what the ideal weight is for his height and body frame type. Then, compare this range with what he actually weighs. If he falls within this range, consider his body weight normal. If he falls above or below this range, consider him underweight or overweight.

WEIGHTS FOR WOMEN AGE 25 AND OVER

Height	Weight		
	Small frame	Medium frame	Large frame
4'8"	92-98	96-107	104-119
4'9"	94-101	98-110	106-122
4'10"	96-104	101-113	109-125
4'11"	99-107	104-116	112-128
5'0"	102-110	107-119	115-131
5'1"	105-113	110-122	118-134
5'2"	108-116	113-126	121-138
5'3"	111-119	116-130	125-142
5'4"	114-123	120-135	129-146
5'5"	118-127	124-139	133-150
5'6"	122-131	128-143	137-154
5'7"	126-135	132-147	141-158
5'8"	130-140	136-151	145-163
5'9"	134-144	140-155	149-168
5'10"	138-148	144-159	153-173

WEIGHTS FOR MEN AGE 25 AND OVER

Height	Weight		
	Small frame	Medium frame	Large frame
5'1"	112-120	118-129	126-141
5'2"	115-123	121-133	129-144
5'3"	118-126	124-136	132-148
5'4"	121-129	127-139	135-152
5'5"	124-133	130-143	138-156
5'6"	128-137	134-147	142-161
5'7"	132-141	138-152	147-166
5'8"	136-145	142-156	151-170
5'9"	140-150	146-160	155-174
5'10"	144-154	150-165	159-179
5'11"	148-158	154-170	164-184
6'0"	152-162	158-175	168-189
6'1"	156-167	162-180	173-194
6'2"	160-171	167-185	178-199
6'3"	164-175	172-190	182-204

Reprinted with permission from Metropolitan Life Insurance Company. Based on Society of Actuaries data, 1959.

orie reserves; a ratio of about 120% or more indicates obesity.

Assessment tip: Interpret these values carefully; edema may mask protein-calorie depletion or obesity.

Although weight loss can indicate loss of body cell mass or fluid, if your patient has experienced a recent unintentional loss of about 10% or more of his preillness weight, this usually indicates a decrease in body cell mass corresponding to a loss of protein or calorie reserves. A more useful measurement of nutritional status is the percentage of weight loss: *usual weight minus actual weight/usual weight, the result multiplied by 100.* For example, a patient who weighs 155 lb (70.5 kg) on admission may appear to be at an ideal weight for his height, but comparison with his usual weight of 200 lb (90.9 kg) indicates that he's lost about 22.5% of his body cell mass.

180 Triceps skinfold thickness

Measuring your patient's triceps skinfold (TSF) thickness with calipers helps you evaluate his subcutaneous fat stores, the main form in which energy is stored in the body. Although most widely used in assessing obesity, skinfold thickness measurements have recently proved helpful in assessing fat stores in undernourished hospitalized patients. The triceps area is most accessible for measurement (see *Taking Common Arm Measurements*).

You can compare the TSF thickness measurement with standard measurements (adult standards for TSF thickness are 16.5 mm for women and 12.5 mm for men) and express them as a percentage of standard: *actual measurement/standard measurement multiplied by 100.* You can also compare these measurements with stan-

TAKING COMMON ARM MEASUREMENTS

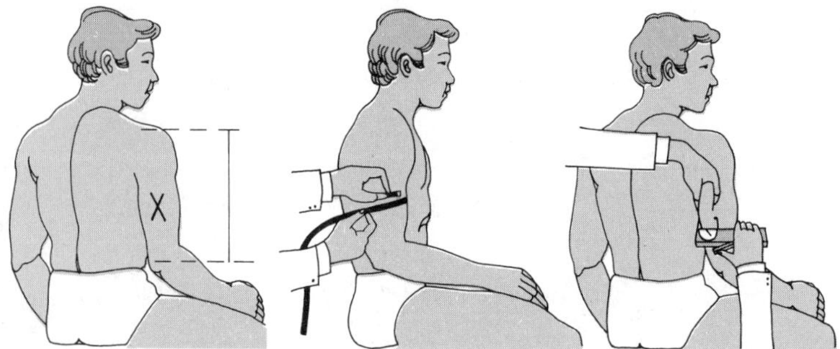

1 To take arm measurements, first locate the midpoint on your patient's upper arm using a nonstretch tape measure. Mark the midpoint with a felt-tip pen.

2 Then, measuring at the midpoint, use the tape measure to determine the patient's midarm circumference.

3 Next, determine the triceps skinfold thickness by grasping the patient's skin with your thumb and forefinger approximately 1 cm above the midpoint. Place the calipers at the midpoint and squeeze the calipers for about 3 seconds. Record the measurement registered on the handle gauge to the nearest 0.5 mm. Take two more readings, and average all three to compensate for any measurement error. Finally, calculate the midarm muscle circumference by multiplying the triceps skinfold thickness (in centimeters) by 3.143 and subtracting this figure from the midarm circumference.

NORMAL ARM MEASUREMENT VALUES

When you measure your patient's triceps skinfold thickness, midarm circumference, and midarm muscle circumference, record them as percentages of the standard measurements listed here. Use this formula: actual measurement/standard measurement multiplied by 100. A measurement that's less than 90% of the standard indicates caloric deprivation; a measurement over 90% indicates adequate or more than adequate energy reserves.

TEST	STANDARD		PERCENTILE OF POPULATION 90%	80%	70%	60%
Triceps skinfold	Men	12.5 mm	11.3	10.0	8.8	7.5
	Women	16.5 mm	11.9	13.2	11.6	9.9
Midarm circumference	Men	29.3 cm	26.3	23.4	20.5	17.6
	Women	28.5 cm	25.7	22.8	20.0	17.1
Midarm muscle circumference	Men	25.3 cm	22.8	20.2	17.7	15.2
	Women	23.2 cm	20.9	18.6	16.2	13.9

Reprinted from G. Blackburn et al., *Manual for Nutritional/Metabolic Assessment* (Chicago: American College of Surgeons, 1976). Used with permission.

dards for obesity, which provide the minimum TSF measurement of obesity for males and females by age (see *Standards for Interpreting Obesity,* page 151).

Interpret these measurements cautiously; a measurement may indicate overabundant subcutaneous fat stores, but the fat may not be readily available as an energy source. (Metabolic aberrations secondary to stress, such as trauma and sepsis, may limit the availability of adipose stores for energy use.) Although skinfold thickness and midarm muscle circumference (another assessment technique) are important tools in assessment, they have the following limitations:

- Measurements assume that humeral size is the same for everybody.
- Measurements assume that bodily distribution of adipose and skeletal protein stores doesn't vary from one person to another.
- Edema may interfere with measuring skeletal protein (muscle mass) and adipose tissues.
- Measurements may not reflect acute body changes for 3 to 4 weeks after those changes take place.

181 Subscapular skinfold thickness

This measurement, which is more reliable but less accessible than the measurement of triceps skinfold (TSF) thickness, also evaluates subcutaneous fat stores.

To measure your patient's subscapular skinfold thickness, position him so that he's sitting up or lying prone, with his arms and shoulders relaxed. With your thumb and forefinger, grasp the skinfold just below the angle of the right scapula, in line with the natural cleavage of the skin. (Note that the exact location of the measurement for subscapular skinfold thickness isn't as important as it is for a triceps measurement, since subcutaneous fat is evenly distributed in the subscapular area.) Apply the calipers and proceed as you would when you measure for TSF thickness.

Compare the subscapular skinfold thickness measurement directly with a chart, and express it as a percentage of standard according to the same formula used for TSF thickness measurement—and with the same limitations in mind.

182 Midarm circumference

Midarm circumference—also called *mid–upper-arm circumference*—reflects skeletal muscle and adipose tissue amounts and therefore helps indicate the extent of your patient's protein and calorie reserves. However, it doesn't differentiate the amount of muscle from the amount of fat present. (See *Taking Common Arm Measurements*, page 148.)

Compare the actual measurement with a standard measurement (see *Normal Arm Measurement Values*, page 149). You may also express the actual measurements as a percentage of standard: *actual measurement/standard measurement multiplied by 100.* Normal adult measurements are 29.3 cm for men and 28.5 cm for women. A measurement less than 90% of standard indicates caloric deprivation; if the measurement is greater than 90% of the standard, your patient has adequate or more than adequate muscle and fat.

183 Midarm muscle circumference

Midarm muscle circumference, also called *mid–upper-arm muscle circumference,* reflects the body's skeletal protein (muscle mass) reserves. Determine your patient's midarm muscle circumference by multiplying the triceps skinfold thickness (in centimeters) by 3.1413, then subtracting the resulting figure from the midarm circumference (in centimeters). Then, compare the midarm muscle circumference with a standard as both an actual measurement and as a percentage of standard: *actual measurement/standard measurement multiplied by 100.* Normal adult measurements are 25.3 cm for men and 23.2 cm for women. A measurement less than 90% of standard indicates protein depletion; a measurement greater than 90% indicates adequate or more than adequate protein reserves. Remember: Findings don't always correspond to actual protein stores available for energy. Interpret findings cautiously.

Formulating a diagnostic impression

184 Identify poor nutrition

You need all your assessment skills to detect nutrition problems. (Remember, the patient with a nutritional problem may not be aware of it.) For example, you'll need to monitor the nutritional intake of depressed patients, who are unlikely to tell you they don't feel like eating. Similarly, many patients with nutritional deficiencies have symptoms you can't immediately identify as nutritionally related. For instance, a school-age child's symptoms of lassitude and learning difficulties, as reported by the school nurse, may actually be caused by the iron deficiency the nutritional assessment reveals. Or a chronically ill patient with repeated infections may be suffering from protein-calorie malnutrition. So perform comprehensive nutritional assessment on *every* patient.

185 Assessing obesity

Obesity may be defined as an overabundance of body fat resulting in body weight 20% or more above normal. In the United States, obesity affects an estimated 25% to 45% of the population. In metabolic terms, obesity results from a caloric intake greater than your patient's body needs for energy metabolism.

Subjective information on typical dietary habits, related psychosocial factors, and past medical history is essential in your assessment of an obese patient. Establishing when the patient's obesity began helps you judge how well your patient will respond to treatment. A relatively fixed number of fat cells in subcutaneous tissue is established during two developmental stages—the first years of life and adolescence. Overeating during these periods results in an increase in the size and number of fat cells. This type of obesity is called *hyperplastic* obesity.

Obesity beginning in adulthood, called *hypertrophic,* is characterized by an increase in fat cell size but *not* in the number of fat cells. Both types—particularly hyperplastic obesity—are difficult to treat.

Although obesity may result from overeating in response to emotional, familial, and/or genetic stimuli, specific types of obesity are caused by endocrine and metabolic disorders, such as Cushing's syndrome, hypothyroidism, and Prader-Willi syndrome.

Your objective assessment will include weight and height measurements. *Normal* weight for a particular patient's height and body frame is difficult to determine. Growth grids are used to compare normal weight and height in children. Tables that list standard height and weight according to age are usually used to compare normal adult heights and weights, but these tables aren't consistently reliable. You also need to consider your patient's body frame size, musculature, and skinfold measurements.

Weight gain can result from factors other than obesity. For example, athletes' strenuous exercise increases the amount of their lean body mass, so their weight increases. Weight gain may also result from fluid accumulation—usually indicated in your patient's dietary history by rapid weight gain, such as (6 lb [2.7 kg] in 2 days).

Because weight gain is often an inconclusive determinant of obesity, be sure to include triceps skinfold (TSF) thickness measurements in your objective assessment. A TSF thickness measurement, described in Entry 180, is a simple and reliable method of detecting obesity. Compare your patient's measurements with standard minimum TSF thickness measurements that indicate obesity (see *Standards for Interpreting Obesity*). Although they're not currently available in common clinical situations, the following techniques (which are more precise than TSF thickness measurements) also can indicate obesity:

- *Water displacement:* determines the total amount of body fat content.
- *Radioactive potassium count:* determines the amount of lean body tissue.
- *X-ray diffraction (shadows):* determines the amount of fat that surrounds organs, as well as minimal fat deposits.

Assessment tip: Don't let an obese patient's excessive body fat mask pro-

STANDARDS FOR INTERPRETING OBESITY

How can you tell if your patient's clinically obese? One way is to compare his triceps skinfold measurement to this chart. If his skinfold measurement is equal to or greater than the one indicated for his age, consider him clinically obese. *Note:* Use metal calipers, because plastic calipers generally won't have a large enough jaw face to measure an obese patient's skinfold.

TRICEPS SKINFOLD MEASUREMENTS (MILLIMETERS)

Age	Women	Men
18	27	15
19	27	15
20	28	16
21	28	17
22	28	18
23	28	18
24	28	19
25	29	20
26	29	20
27	29	21
28	29	22
29	29	23
30 +	30	23

USING LABORATORY TESTS IN NUTRITIONAL ASSESSMENT

Laboratory tests help assess visceral protein status, cell-mediated immunocompetency, lean body mass, vitamin and mineral nutritional balance, and the effectiveness of nutritional support. In fact, laboratory tests often reveal nutritional problems before they're clinically apparent. The list below explains some laboratory tests and what their results may indicate.

- *Nitrogen balance.* Nitrogen balance reflects the difference between nitrogen intake and nitrogen output. It's used to determine the effectiveness of the nutritional support the patient's receiving. A negative nitrogen balance indicates an inadequate intake of protein and/or calories.
- *Hemoglobin and hematocrit.* Low hemoglobin and hematocrit values may occur in PCM. However, low values also occur in overhydrated states, regardless of nutritional status. Normal or above normal values may occur in underhydrated states, masking possible nutritional implications. Hemorrhage and hemolytic diseases result in low values despite nutritional status.
- *Serum iron.* Decreased serum iron—combined with findings of elevated iron-binding capacity, decreased hemoglobin and hematocrit, and the presence of hypochromatic and microcytic cells—may indicate iron deficiency.
- *Serum albumin.* Decreased serum albumin values may indicate visceral protein depletion, a possible result of gastrointestinal disease, liver disease, or nephrotic syndrome. Overhydration causes decreased values. Underhydration causes normal or increased values. Both mask true nutritional implications.
- *Serum transferrin (ST)/Total iron-binding capacity (TIBC).* Decreased levels of transferrin may indicate visceral protein depletion. Transferrin reflects acute changes in visceral protein status better than albumin, because of the two, transferrin has a much shorter half-life. Decreased ST and TIBC values appear in such protein-losing conditions as nephrotic syndrome, protein-losing enteropathy, and iron overload. Increased TIBC appears with iron deficiency alone.
- *Total lymphocyte count (TLC).* TLC tests cell-mediated immunocompetency. Decreased levels occur in protein-calorie malnutrition and represent an impaired immune response. This test is invalid in patients with inherited immunodeficiency diseases and some hematologic malignancies, patients receiving immunosuppressive drugs, or in patients who are septic.
- *Delayed hypersensitivity skin testing.* This test also assesses cell-mediated immunocompetency. It's used in assessing nutritional status because protein-calorie malnutrition slows the synthesis and response of antibodies to stimulation. One or more positive responses in 24 to 48 hours to intradermally injected common recall antigens indicate intact cell-mediated immunity; a negative response, a delayed response, or no response may indicate protein-calorie malnutrition. Trauma, sepsis, and chemotherapy may also suppress the cellular immune response.
- *Creatinine height index (CHI).* This calculated value, based on creatinine clearance and the patient's height, is used to assess nutritional status.A decreased CHI may indicate protein-calorie deficiency; however, it may also indicate impaired renal function.

tein deficits. Excessive body fat doesn't mean all bodily stores of nutrients are excessive. *Remember: The obese patient is at nutritional risk.*

186 Assessing protein-calorie malnutrition

Protein-calorie malnutrition (PCM) mainly results from a prolonged or chronic inadequate intake of calories and/or protein. The body responds by breaking down its protein and fat stores into calories needed for energy.

In a hospitalized patient, secondary PCM can result from any interference in ability to ingest and digest food or to absorb and utilize nutrients. Increased nutrient requirements that aren't met, or unchecked increased nutrient losses, also can cause PCM.

Findings in a patient with PCM include weight loss, asthenia, muscle weakness, gastrointestinal disturbances (such as diarrhea), impaired growth and development, and poor wound healing.

Inspection of a patient with PCM may reveal:
• slow-growing, brittle nails containing transverse ridges (in later PCM stages, fingernails thicken)
• excessive shedding of hair (check the patient's comb or brush)
• liver enlargement, ascites, swollen ankles
• sunken eyes, hollow temples and cheeks, and an unusually angular appearance of the nose.

A child with PCM may have muscle atrophy, poor muscle tone, a protuberant abdomen, and flat buttocks, and his cheeks may appear to be sucked in. His response to stimuli may be slow.

Weigh the patient with PCM (or potential PCM) daily. Compare his actual weight, usual weight, and ideal weight (according to his age, sex, and height) to determine the daily percentage of weight change. (A patient with PCM may lose about 10% or more of body weight in 1 month.) Be sure to ask the patient whether he dieted to lose weight.

Next, estimate the patient's muscle mass and fat stores by measuring triceps skinfold thickness or subscapular skinfold thickness, midarm circumference, and midarm muscle circumference. A patient with PCM usually will have less than 85% of normal measurements.

Other techniques for detecting patients at risk for PCM include the following:
• monitoring nutritional intake and documenting inadequacies
• estimating nutritional losses by measuring such high-protein fluid losses as wound drainage
• measuring indications of increased metabolic requirements—for example, fever.

187 Vitamin disorders

A patient's vitamin requirements depend on age, diet, activity level, metabolic rate, and factors that affect vitamin absorption, utilization, and excretion. Because the early clinical features of vitamin deficiency are typically vague and mild, they're easy to overlook or misinterpret. The time at which signs of vitamin deficiency appear, and the form they take, depend on the particular deficiency, its degree, and the patient's reserves of the vitamin. For example, if ascorbic acid is excluded from the diet of a healthy adult, lesions characteristic of scurvy appear on his skin in 3 to 6 months; such lesions occur sooner in an adult with marginal reserves of ascorbic acid. In an adult with normal vitamin reserves who's deprived of vitamin A, lesions might not appear for a year or longer. Although your patient may show signs and symptoms characteristic of a particular vitamin deficiency, usually deficiency of more than one vitamin is involved.

Be sure to inspect your patient's skin, hair, eyes, lips, tongue, mouth, teeth, and nails for changes. Note any musculoskeletal impairments and any neurologic symptoms.

Subjective information gathered for the diet history may provide early indications of a vitamin deficiency. Be sure to question your patient about drug therapy. Long-term therapy with any of a number of drugs may alter vitamin synthesis, increase vitamin requirements, or cause vitamin depletion. For example, oral antibiotic therapy may result in vitamin K deficiency; chronic alcoholism and long-term use of oral contraceptives may cause folic acid deficiency. Other conditions that may lead to vitamin or other nutrient deficiencies include:
• a bizarre or monotonous diet: for example, mainly eating canned soups or take-out foods, or feeding infants only processed cow's milk
• psychological or pathologic factors that limit nutrient intake
• conditions that cause intestinal malabsorption of vitamins or that, like pregnancy, increase demand.

Vitamin deficiencies are common in

NURSE'S GUIDE TO NUTRITIONAL DISORDERS

	CHIEF COMPLAINT
Marasmus (calorie deficiency)	• *Weight change:* Loss may be profound • *Skin changes:* Dryness • *Asthenia:* Usually present; if severe, can result in profound weakness • *Gastrointestinal problems:* Frequent diarrhea • *Musculoskeletal impairment:* Growth retardation in children; muscular wasting
Obesity	• *Weight change:* Significant gain over time • *Skin changes:* Thickness, pale striae • *Asthenia:* May be present • *Gastrointestinal problems:* None obviously related • *Musculoskeletal impairment:* Possible joint strain or pain
Vitamin A deficiency	• *Weight change:* None • *Skin changes:* Dry, scaly, roughness with follicular hyperkeratosis; shrinking and hardening of mucous membranes • *Asthenia:* Vague apathy may be present • *Gastrointestinal problems:* None directly related • *Musculoskeletal impairment:* Possible failure to thrive
Thiamine (B_1) deficiency	• *Weight change:* Emaciated appearance in dry form • *Skin changes:* Pallor may occur, especially in infants; subcutaneous edema in extremities may occur in wet form • *Asthenia:* Apathy and confusion, loss of memory, • *Gastrointestinal problems:* Anorexia, vomiting, constipation, abdominal pain may occur • *Musculoskeletal impairment:* Muscle cramps, paresthesias, polyneuritis; in severe cases, convulsions, paralysis of extremities, muscular atrophy
Riboflavin (B_2) deficiency	• *Weight change:* Less common • *Skin changes:* Seborrheic dermatitis in the nasolabial folds, scrotum, and vulva; generalized dermatitis • *Asthenia:* Usually present • *Gastrointestinal problems:* Not common • *Musculoskeletal impairment:* Possible growth retardation
Niacin deficiency	• *Weight change:* Loss possible, even in early stages • *Skin changes:* Mild eruptions in early stage, progressing to scaly dermatitis resembling severe sunburn • *Asthenia:* Present; fatigue even in early stages • *Gastrointestinal problems:* Anorexia, indigestion, nausea, vomiting, diarrhea possible • *Musculoskeletal impairment:* Muscle weakness in early stages; growth retardation in children in late-stage deficiency

	HISTORY	PHYSICAL EXAMINATION	DIAGNOSTIC STUDIES
	• Inadequate intake of proteins and calories; may occur in hospitalized patients with conditions such as cancer, Crohn's disease, and cirrhosis	• Weight/height ratio 60% to 90% below standard; triceps skinfold thickness usually 60% below standard; mid–upper-arm circumference and mid–upper-arm muscle circumference, usually 60% to 90% below normal	• Creatinine height index decreased, possibly to 60% below normal; serum levels of albumin and transferrin are normal; one or more positive reactions to skin tests
	• Commonly, pattern of overeating accompanied by decreased energy expenditure; less commonly, endocrine abnormality	• Weight/height ratio 20% or more above normal, triceps skinfold measurement indicating obesity	• None significant
	• Night blindness that may progress to permanent blindness; diet lacking in leafy green and yellow fruits and vegetables; fat malabsorption	• Dryness, roughness of conjunctiva; swelling and redness of lids; clouded cornea; ulcerations possible	• Serum values for vitamin A below 20 mcg/100 ml confirm deficiency
	• Increased need for B_1 during fever, pregnancy, etc.; infants on low-protein diets; inadequate intake, especially of whole or enriched breads or cereals, pork, beans, and nuts; malabsorption syndrome; chronic alcoholism	• In wet form, edema begins in legs and progresses upward. Cardiomegaly with tachycardia, dyspnea may occur; nystagmus possible; hyperactive knee-jerk reflex, followed by hypoactivity	• Serum values for thiamine less than 5 mcg/100 ml; elevated levels of pyruvic and lactic acid; low urine values for thiamine; nonspecific EKG changes
	• Inadequate intake of milk, meat, fish, leafy green and yellow vegetables; chronic alcoholism; use of oral contraceptives	• Cheilosis, conjunctivitis in mild form; in late stages, moderate edema, neuropathy	• Riboflavin serum level less than 2 mcg/100 ml; prolonged diarrhea; complaints of photophobia and itching, burning, tearing eyes
	• Inadequate intake, especially where corn is staple food; secondary to carcinoid syndrome or Hartnup disease, chronic alcoholism	• Mouth, tongue, and lips become reddened; atrophy of papillae; in late stages, confusion and disorientation	• Serum niacin levels less than 30 mcg/100 ml; headache, backache, sore mouth

(continued)

NURSE'S GUIDE TO NUTRITIONAL DISORDERS *(continued)*

	CHIEF COMPLAINT
Vitamin C deficiency	• *Weight change:* Loss possible • *Skin changes:* Drying roughness and dingy brown color change; petechiae, ecchymosis, follicular hyperkeratosis • *Asthenia:* May be present • *Gastrointestinal problems:* Anorexia, diarrhea, vomiting possible in children • *Musculoskeletal impairment:* Limb and joint pain and swelling
Vitamin D deficiency	• *Weight change:* None • *Skin changes:* None • *Asthenia:* Not present • *Gastrointestinal problems:* None • *Musculoskeletal impairment:* Chronic deficiency causes bone malformations from bone softening and retarded growth
Vitamin K deficiency	• *Weight change:* None • *Skin changes:* Petechiae and ecchymosis possible • *Asthenia:* Present; may be related to blood loss • *Gastrointestinal problems:* Gastrointestinal bleeding, which can include massive hemorrhage, possible. • *Musculoskeletal impairment:* Hemorrhaging in muscles, joints
Iron deficiency	• *Weight change:* None • *Skin changes:* Pallor • *Asthenia:* Present; may be extreme in severe cases • *Gastrointestinal problems:* Anorexia, flatulence, epigastric distress, constipation • *Musculoskeletal impairment:* Numbness, tingling of extremities; neuralgic pain possible
Iodine deficiency	• *Weight change:* None • *Skin changes:* Dry, cold skin in severe stages • *Asthenia:* Present; may occur even in mild deficiency • *Gastrointestinal problems:* Anorexia • *Musculoskeletal impairment:* None
Folic acid deficiency	• *Weight change:* Loss common • *Skin changes:* Severe pallor • *Asthenia:* Present • *Gastrointestinal problems:* Diarrhea • *Musculoskeletal impairment:* Absent
Vitamin B_{12} deficiency	• *Weight change:* Loss possible • *Skin changes:* Lemon-yellow pallor • *Asthenia:* Present • *Gastrointestinal problems:* Anorexia, vomiting, diarrhea • *Musculoskeletal impairment:* Hand and foot paresthesia; degeneration of spinal cord, decreased musculoskeletal innervation

	HISTORY	PHYSICAL EXAMINATION	DIAGNOSTIC STUDIES
	• Inadequate intake of fresh fruits and vegetables; overcooking; marginal intake during periods of stress. Groups at risk include infants fed processed cow's milk only, those on limited diets, and those with bizarre eating habits.	• Swollen and/or bleeding gums (early sign), loosening of teeth, pallor, ocular hemorrhages in the bulbar conjunctivas; delayed wound healing and tissue repair	• Serum ascorbic acid levels less than 0.4 mg/100 ml and WBC ascorbic acid levels less than 25 mg/100 ml (help confirm); poor wound healing; psychologic disturbances, such as hysteria, depression, anemia
	• Inadequate dietary intake of vitamin D; malabsorption; inadequate exposure to sunlight; hepatic or renal disease	• Characteristic bone malformations	• Plasma calcium levels less than 7.5 mg/100 ml; inorganic phosphorus serum levels less than 3 mg/ 100 ml; serum citrate levels less than 2.5 mg/100 ml.
	• Prolonged use of such drugs as anticoagulants and antibiotics; malabsorption of vitamin K (as in sprue, bowel resection, ulcerative colitis), biliary obstruction	• Bleeding tendencies	• Prolonged prothrombin time (25% longer than control)
	• Inadequate dietary intake of iron as prolonged unsupplemented breast- or bottle-feeding or in periods of stress; iron malabsorption, such as in diarrhea, gastrectomy, celiac disease; blood loss	• In chronic form: nails become brittle spoon-shaped; corners of the mouth crack, tongue becomes smooth; in severe cases: tachycardia, dyspnea on exertion, listlessness, irritability; liver and spleen enlargement possible	• Low hemoglobin, less than 12 g/100 ml for males, less than 10 g/100 ml for females; low hematocrit, less than 47 ml/100 ml for males, less than 42 ml/100 for females; low serum iron levels with high binding capacity; low serum ferritin levels
	• Insufficient intake (table salt, seafood); increased metabolic demands (growth, pregnancy, lactation) • Poor memory, chills, menorrhagia, amenorrhea	• Hoarseness, hearing loss, thick tongue bradycardia, lowered blood pressure, delayed relaxation phase in deep tendon reflexes	• Low T_4 with high ^{131}I uptake, low 24-hour urine iodine, and high TSH. T_3 or T_4 resin uptake test shows values 25% below normal.
	• Inadequate intake of leafy vegetables, organ meats, beef, wheat. Most common in infants, pregnant women, chronic alcoholics, and patients with malabsorption	• Glossitis, cardiac enlargement, macrocytic megaloblastic anemia	• Serum value less than 100 ng/ml
	• Strict vegetarian; malabsorption resulting from gastrectomy or ileal resection	• Macrocytic megaloblastic anemia, bright red tongue, cardiovascular changes, dyspnea, chest pain, chronic congestive heart failure	• Serum value less than 100 pg/ml; resembles folic acid deficiency, with additional neural and mental changes

CASE HISTORIES: NURSING DIAGNOSIS FLOWCHART

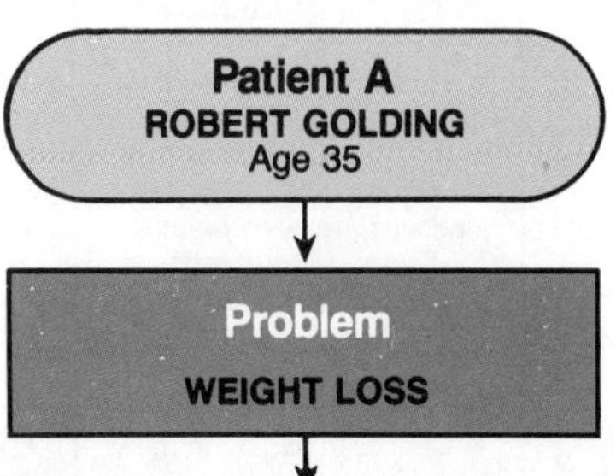

Subjective data

- Increased work pressures
- Increased hours spent working (approximately 15 hours per day)
- Decreased ability to sleep
- Upset over recent divorce; lives alone with no experience in food planning or preparation
- Weight loss of 10 lb (4.5 kg) over past 2 months
- No complaints of nausea, vomiting, diarrhea, or constipation
- Frequently anorexic
- Preillness weight: 164 to 166 lb (73.8 to 74.7 kg)

Objective data

- Weight 155 lb (69.8 kg), height 5′9″ (175.3 cm)
- Percent of IBW: 94.5%
- Percent of preillness weight: 94.5%
- Percent of weight change: 5.5%
- Triceps skinfold thickness 12.1 mm (96.8% standard)
- Arm muscle circumference: 23.4 cm (92.5% standard)
- TPR, BP (normal values): T. 98.4; P. 82; R. 18; BP 126/82
- Hemoglobin: 13.6 mg/ml
- Hematocrit: 40%

Nursing diagnoses

- Knowledge deficit concerning principles of sound nutrition and meal preparation
- Ineffective coping with life-style changes and career demands
- Alteration in nutrition: less than body requirements
- Ineffective rest/activity pattern related to excessive work hours and emotional upset over divorce

low-income areas of the United States; and institutionalized persons also are at risk. Some vitamins (such as vitamins A, D, K, and niacin) are toxic when taken in large amounts over long periods. For example, parents who mistakenly think large doses of vitamins are beneficial may administer

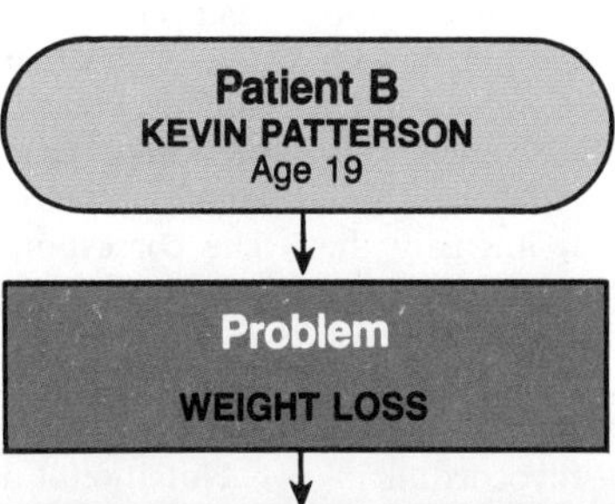

Subjective data

- Severe diarrhea (up to eight episodes per day), including passage of some blood in stools for past 4 days
- Anorexic for past 2 months, resulting in decreased intake
- Weight loss of 25 lb (11.3 kg) over past 2 months
- Worried over loss of school time (college freshman); also worried over academic standing, because it affects his scholarship
- Complains of fatigue; doesn't have the energy to wash or cook
- Preillness weight 163 lb (73.4 kg)

Objective data

- Weight 138 lb (62.1 kg), height 5′11″ (180.3 cm)
- Percent of IBW: 83%
- Percent of preillness weight: 83%
- Percent of weight change: 16%
- Arm muscle circumference: 21.3 cm (84.1% standard)
- T. 99.2; P. 100; R. 24; BP 94/60
- Hemoglobin: 10 mg/ml
- Hematocrit: 34%

Nursing diagnoses

- Alteration in nutrition: less than body requirements related to anorexia, and diarrhea with blood loss
- Fluid volume deficit related to diarrhea and insufficient fluid intake
- Fear of academic failure, resulting in severe anxiety
- Alteration in bowel elimination due to diarrhea
- Self-care deficit; cooking, washing, and grooming related to asthenia

toxic doses to their children.

In your patient's diet history, identify particular vitamins he takes, dosages, and how long he's taken them.

188 Diagnosing the effects

An adolescent who is obese will have an obvious nursing diagnosis related to his weight gain (over 20% above normal): *alteration in nutrition: more than body requirements.* Less obvious, but perhaps more crucial, may be a nursing diagnosis related to his impaired psychosocial development, such as *disturbance in self-concept related to poor body image* or even *social isolation related to peer ridicule.* These problems may, in turn, intensify the eating compulsion, completing an unfortunate cycle. An adult who is obese may also have nursing diagnoses related to psychosocial factors, such as fear of experiencing a myocardial infarction or fear of job discrimination because of his weight. Even though such fears may be realistic, they usually don't stimulate the patient to combat the problem but instead compound it. You'll probably deal with obese patients who fail to follow medical advice regarding weight loss (a nursing diagnosis of *noncompliance with therapeutic weight loss program*). To help such a patient, you'll need to do further assessment to determine the reason for the noncompliance.

Obesity is difficult to treat, so try to prevent its development by identifying the patient at risk. Such a patient may have a nursing diagnosis of *alteration in nutrition: potential for more than body requirements.* Such patients include those whose adult history reveals childhood obesity (although current triceps skinfold thickness and weight-to-height ratios may be just slightly above normal) or those whose caloric intake hasn't been adjusted after a recent change in activity levels. For example, a patient used to physical labor and recreational athletics who turns to a sedentary occupation uses less energy and should adjust his food intake accordingly.

The patient with protein-calorie malnutrition (PCM) and/or vitamin deficiencies also has an obvious nursing diagnosis: *alteration in nutrition: less than body requirements.* Other nursing diagnoses vary, depending on the particular patient or family. For example, malnutrition may be related to poverty, with a nursing diagnosis of *ineffective family coping: compromised due to loss of father's job, resulting in inadequate food purchases.*

In some instances, childhood malnutrition may be accompanied by complete deprivation—lack of physical and emotional care as well as lack of food. The corresponding nursing diagnosis may be *physical-care deficit of child (feeding, hygiene, grooming, toileting) related to reduced parental involvement.*

Nutritional deficits with weight loss are often accompanied by fluid volume deficits. An appropriate nursing diagnosis may be *actual or potential fluid volume deficit related to intestinal fistula,* for example. For a patient who's ingested toxic doses of vitamins, a nursing diagnosis of *alteration in nutrition: more than body requirements* would be appropriate; a nursing diagnosis of *knowledge deficit related to ingestion of toxic doses of vitamins* might also apply.

Musculoskeletal changes can occur in protein-calorie malnutrition. Nursing diagnoses may relate to *impaired physical mobility due to growth retardation* or even to *disturbance in self-concept due to obvious bone deformities. Alteration in comfort* may be related to joint pain.

Asthenia commonly occurs in patients with generalized undernourishment. If severe, it may interfere with the patient's ability to perform activities of daily living. Extreme weakness may result in *potential for injury due to falling.* Or you may indicate *ineffective rest activity pattern related to lack of exercise and prolonged rest/sleep need.*

Malnourished patients may also experience gastrointestinal disturbances, possibly affecting bowel activity and causing diarrhea or constipation. *Alteration in comfort* related to dyspepsia, abdominal cramping, or painful swallowing may compound nutritional problems.

Assessing a child's nutritional status

189 Children's nutrition

A child who deviates from expected growth rates and patterns requires further assessment. Assessment enables you to define nutritional problems, identify possible causes, and, possibly, obtain early intervention. Perform a complete nutritional assessment on any child at nutritional risk, especially one who's failed to thrive or has undergone surgery, in the same way you would for an adult. Additional techniques for

RECOMMENDED DIETARY ALLOWANCES FOR CHILDREN AND ADOLESCENTS

	MALE AND FEMALE			MALE	FEMALE	MALE	FEMALE
ELEMENT	AGES 1 TO 3 29 lb (13 kg) 35" (90 cm)	AGES 4 TO 6 44 lb (20 kg) 44" (110 cm)	AGES 7 TO 10 66 lb (30 kg) 54" (135 cm)	AGES 11 TO 14 97 lb (44 kg) 63" (158 cm)	AGES 11 TO 14 97 lb (44 kg) 62" (155 cm)	AGES 15 TO 18 134 lb (61 kg) 68" (172.7 cm)	AGES 15 TO 18 119 lb (54 kg) 68" (172.7 cm)
K calorie	1,300	1,700	2,400	2,700	2,200	2,800	2,100
Protein (g)	23	30	34	45	46	56	46
Vitamin A (mcg RE)	400	500	700	1,000	800	1,000	800
Vitamin A (IU)	2,000	2,500	3,300	5,000	4,000	5,000	4,000
Vitamin D (IU)	400	400	400	400	400	400	400
Vitamin E (mg or TE)	5	6.0	7.0	8.0	8.0	10	8.0
Ascorbic acid (Vitamin C) (mg)	45	45	45	50	50	60	60
Folacin (mcg)	100	200	300	400	400	400	400
Niacin (mg)	9	12	16	18	15	18	14
Riboflavin (B_2) (mg)	0.8	1.1	1.4	1.5	1.3	1.8	1.4
Thiamine (B_1) (mg)	0.7	0.9	1.2	1.4	1.1	1.4	1.1
Vitamin B_6 (mg)	0.9	1.3	1.6	1.8	1.8	2.0	2.0
Vitamin B_{12} (mcg)	2	2.5	3.0	3.0	3.0	3.0	3.0
Calcium (mg)	800	800	800	1,200	1,200	1,200	1,200
Phosphorus (mg)	800	800	800	1,200	1,200	1,200	1,200
Iodine (mcg)	70	90	120	150	150	150	150
Iron (mg)	15	10	10	18	18	18	18
Magnesium (mg)	150	200	250	350	300	400	300
Zinc (mg)	10	10	10	15	15	15	15

Courtesy National Research Council, 1980.

assessing a child include plotting his development on a growth grid and, in infants, measuring head circumference.

190 The infant: Normal growth

The average full-term neonate weighs 7 lb (3.15 kg), is 20″ (50.8 cm) long, and has a head circumference of 13½″ to 14″ (34 to 36 cm). After birth, the neonate usually loses weight but regains it within 10 days. Most full-term infants double their weight within 5 months after birth and triple it within the first year. During the first year, an infant's length increases by 10 to 12″ (25 to 30 cm). Head circumference increases about 5″ (13 cm) by the end of the first year. Keep nutritional guidelines in mind in your assessment, which should include the type of nourishment the infant is receiving.

191 Assessing a toddler's nutrition

To adequately assess a toddler's nutrition, you should be familiar with normal growth and development changes in the first 3 years of life. Don't confuse normal changes with nutritional problems. For example, during a child's second year, his growth rate slows. Decreased appetite, which often begins about age 10 months, continues into the second year and results in decreased subcutaneous fat, giving the child a thinner, more muscular appearance. The second and third years of life are characterized by abdominal protuberance and mild lordosis, apparent when the child stands.

192 The preschool child

Throughout the preschool period, a child continues to grow and gain weight. By the fourth year, the abdominal protuberance and mild lordosis characteristic of the toddler's development usually disappear. The preschool child, therefore, develops a leaner appearance.

193 The school-age child

The school-age child's energy requirements, appetite and food intake increase as he grows. Consequently, he has few apparent feeding problems. Feeding problems that do occur may result from inattention to the child's food preferences, activities that interfere with mealtimes, and excessive discipline concerning table manners.

194 The adolescent

Adolescence is the second major period of rapid growth affecting every body system. This is also a time of major

COMPOSITION OF COMMON TAKEOUT FOODS

Adolescents usually eat more takeout foods than persons in other age-groups do. You should know the composition of common fast foods to help you assess the nutritional adequacy of an adolescent's diet. Similar items from different chains have comparable composition figures; for example, a McDonald's hamburger and a Burger King hamburger contain roughly the same amount of calories and grams of protein.

	BRAND
Apple pie	McDonald's
Burrito, combination	Taco Bell
Chicken, fried drumstick	Kentucky Fried
Chicken, fried wing	Kentucky Fried
Chocolate sundae, med.	Dairy Queen
Dairy Queen cone, med.	Dairy Queen
Filet-o-Fish	McDonald's
Hamburger	McDonald's
Hot dog	Burger King
Onion rings (Brazier)	Dairy Queen
Taco	Taco Bell
Vanilla shake	McDonald's
Whopper	Burger King

psychosocial and mental growth.

In your assessment of an adolescent's nutrition, look for indications of undernutrition, overeating, need to adjust his food intake to meet changing nutritional requirements, or nutritional problems resulting from the psychosocial pressures of adolescence. For example, adolescents' busy life-style and new independence often produce irregular eating patterns, such as skipping meals and increased snacking.

As a group, 10- to 16-year-olds have the most unsatisfactory nutrition. Common nutritional deficiencies among adolescents involve iron, calcium, and vitamins A and C.

195 Pediatric diet history

Obtain a child's diet history from the person who feeds him or from the child himself (if he's old enough) or from both. Because many parents may feel threatened by questions about their child's nutrition, explain the purpose of the interview beforehand. Be sure to ask how much milk an *infant* drinks. Is he breast-fed or bottle-fed? Is a bottle left in the crib at night? Does the child take vitamin supplements? Be sure to ascertain the type and dosage. How old was he when he began eating solid foods? Many authorities currently believe that introduction of semisolids

	WEIGHT(g)	FOOD ENERGY (Kcal)	PROTEIN (g)	FAT (g)	CARBOHYDRATE (g)	CALCIUM (mg)	IRON (mg)	POTASSIUM (mg)	SODIUM (mg)	VITAMIN A VALUE (IU)	THIAMINE (mg)	RIBOFLAVIN (mg)	NIACIN (mg)	ASCORBIC ACID (mg)
	91	300	2	19	31	12	0.6	39	414	<69	0.02	0.03	1.3	3
	175	404	21	16	43	91	3.7	278	300	1,666	0.34	0.31	4.6	15
	54	136	14	8	2	20	0.9	*	†	30	0.04	0.12	2.7	0
	45	151	11	10	4	*	0.6	*	†	*	0.03	0.07	*	0
	184	300	6	7	53	200	1.1	*	†	300	0.06	0.26	0	0
	142	230	6	7	35	200	0	*	†	300	0.09	0.26	0	0
	131	402	15	23	34	105	1.8	293	709	152	0.28	0.28	3.9	4
	99	257	13	9	30	63	3	234	526	231	0.23	0.23	5.1	2
	*	291	11	17	23	40	2	170	841	0	0.04	0.02	2	0
	85	300	6	17	33	20	0.4	16	†	0	0.09	0	0.4	2
	83	186	15	8	14	120	2.5	143	79	120	0.09	0.16	2.9	0
	289	323	10	8	52	346	0.2	499	250	346	0.12	0.66	0.6	<3
	*	606	29	32	32	37	6	653	909	641	0.02	0.03	5.2	13

Adapted from Eleanor Young et al., "Perspectives on Fast Foods," *Dietetic Currents* 5:5:24, 1978, with permission from the publisher Ross Laboratories, Columbus, Ohio.

*Data unavailable
†Content varies

USING PEDIATRIC GROWTH GRIDS

When you perform a dietary pediatric assessment, you should include a growth grid. Correlate the child's height with his age and his weight with his age. Consider the child's growth normal if he falls between the 5th and 95th percentiles; consider his growth abnor-

GIRLS: AGES 2 TO 18 PHYSICAL GROWTH PERCENTILES

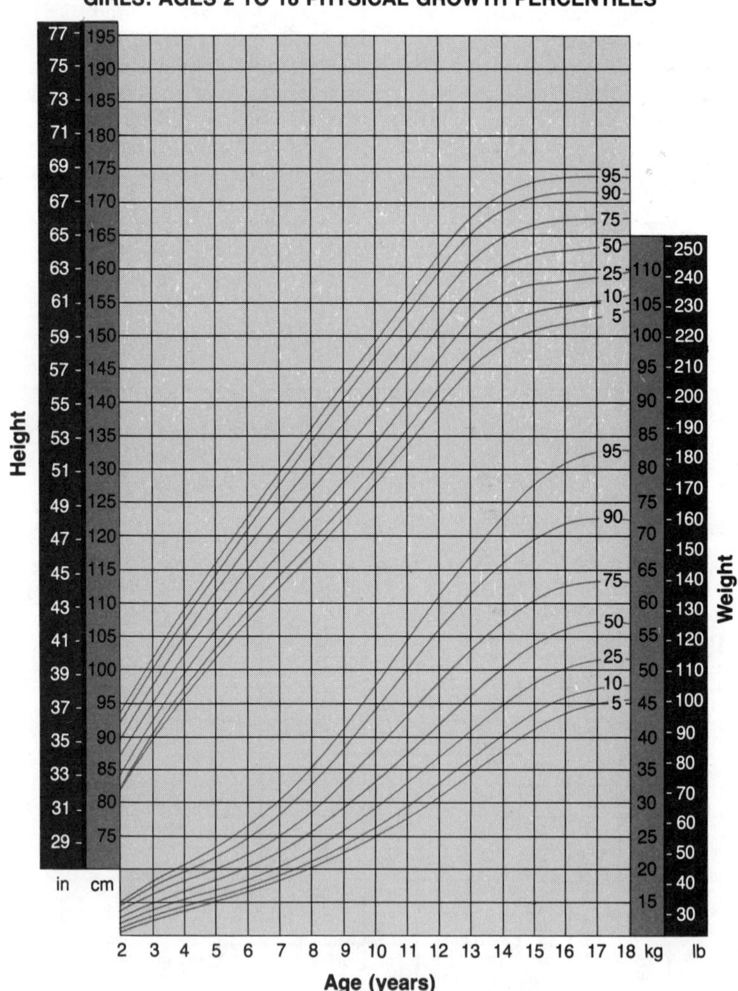

mal if he falls below the 5th or above the 95th percentile. Also consider abnormal any sharp, sudden deviation from the child's usual percentile. Abnormal results indicate the need for further evaluation.

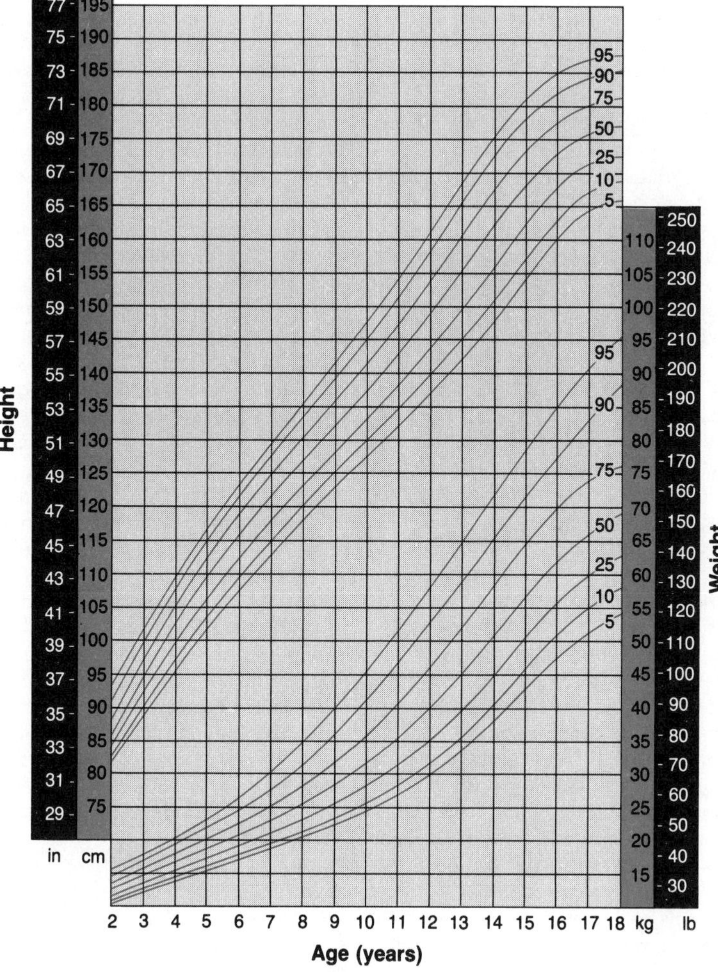

Courtesy National Center for Health Statistics, Department of Health and Human Services.

before age 4 to 6 months predisposes a child to allergy and obesity. Does the infant have any problems sucking, swallowing, or chewing? Ask how often your pediatric patient eats snack foods and what kinds he likes.

In all pediatric age-groups, special considerations in a dietary history include:
• typical daily nutritional plan (number and types of meals and snacks)
• any special or modified diet
• behavioral peculiarities associated with mealtimes or any feeding problems
• stress of illness or trauma, which can rapidly deplete nutrient stores
• sugar intake, because sugar is an *empty-calorie* food related to dental caries and obesity
• iron intake, since iron deficiency anemia is a major childhood problem
• protein intake, since it's essential for growth.

196 Growth grids

Growth grids allow you to screen for early signs of nutritional deficiencies. Include them in each young patient's chart.

Measure the child's height and weight, and plot your findings on a grid for comparison by age and sex. (Growth grids for children up to age 18, developed by the National Center for Health Statistics, are probably the most accurate source for evaluating these data.) (See *Using Pediatric Growth Grids*, pages 164-165.) These grids use percentiles rather than ideal weight for height. The 50th percentile represents average growth rates; consider findings below the 5th percentile or above the 95th percentile abnormal. Serial measurements can provide information that one measurement may not. For example, a child usually remains in the same percentile throughout his growth period, so you should consider a large deviation (such as a decrease from the 50th percentile to the 5th percentile) abnormal.

197 Skinfold thickness in children

Skinfold thickness (usually triceps skinfold thickness) measurements are useful for children older than age 3. Measure and express a child's skinfold thickness as you would an adult's.

198 Undernutrition

In any child, undernutrition can impair normal growth and development, affect body function, and (without proper intervention) have long-term deleterious effects. Undernutrition during the critical period for rapid brain growth—the prenatal period and the first 9 months of life—may cause permanent retardation. Possible clues that a child is undernourished include listlessness, apathy, pallor, dental caries, and decreased resistance to infection.

Undernutrition resulting from child neglect or abuse may accompany other signs, such as bruises, burns, and welts. The parents may act evasive or provide an implausible or contradictory explanation of the child's condition; this also makes accurate history-taking difficult.

Other factors that may cause, perpetuate, or complicate childhood undernutrition include:
• illnesses that impair digestion, absorption, or utilization of nutrients
• increased demand for nutrients due to growth
• presence of stress—such as from illness, trauma, surgery, or emotional upset.

199 Childhood obesity

Obesity is a major nutritional problem affecting children in all age-groups, including infancy. Because longstanding childhood obesity is less responsive to therapy than adult obesity, early detection and treatment are imperative. Also, psychological problems are more likely to trouble an obese child than an obese adult. Perhaps most important, childhood obesity may foreshadow adult obesity.

Obesity standards in children are the same as in adults: weight-to-height ratio greater than 120% and triceps skinfold measurement indicating obesity.

Factors that may cause childhood obesity include:

• inactivity, or chronic illnesses that impair mobility
• overfeeding, common in bottle-fed infants and in situations where parents use food as a pacifier or insist that their child clean his plate
• genetic predisposition to obesity, although children may become obese by imitating their obese parents' eating patterns
• metabolic, endocrine, or neurologic abnormalities (rare).

200 Iron deficiency anemia

In the United States, iron deficiency anemia is the most common nutritional disorder in young children. This disorder may affect a child's attention span and intellectual performance; if severe, the child may become irritable and lethargic.

Factors that may cause iron deficiency anemia include:

• limited iron reserves (at birth) in premature and low–birth-weight infants
• ingestion of large amounts of milk instead of solid foods (whole milk is a poor source of dietary iron, and the phosphate in milk combines with dietary iron and removes it). Human milk, although low in iron, is absorbed more efficiently.
• high-bulk diet (decreases iron absorption); inadequate dietary intake of iron
• hemorrhage, or occult blood loss in stools (in some infants, gastrointestinal bleeding may result from protein in homogenized cow's milk; menstrual blood losses in adolescent girls
• increased iron requirements during growth periods, such as infancy and adolescence.

Characteristic clinical features of iron deficiency anemia include dyspnea on exertion, fatigue, listlessness, pallor, inability to concentrate, irritability, headache, and susceptibility to infection. Chronic iron deficiency anemia may cause spoon-shaped brittle nails, smooth tongue, dysphagia, cracked corners of the mouth, neuromuscular effects (such as numbness and tingling of the extremities), neurologic pain, and vasomotor disturbances. Elevated serum transferrin levels occur in severe iron deficiency; hemoglobin levels less than 11 g/100 ml and hematocrit less than 33% confirm anemia.

201 Food allergies

Food allergies occur most frequently during early childhood but seldom persist into adulthood. True allergies usually result from production of antibodies to specific antigens; in food allergies, these are particular proteins in ingested food. Food allergies can result nonimmunologically, from enzyme deficiency. Food allergies can produce respiratory, gastrointestinal, and dermatologic signs and symptoms; excessive psychological or physiologic stress may exacerbate the allergic reaction.

Any food may cause an allergic reaction; some of the common reaction-producing foods are milk, eggs, chocolate, fish, shellfish, chicken, pork, beef, and wheat.

Testing for food allergies includes skin testing (with prepared food antigens to reveal IgE antibodies) and provocation and elimination testing (elimination of suspected food from the diet for 7 to 10 days; if signs and symptoms reappear after reintroduction of the food into the patient's diet, the food is confirmed as an allergen). Sometimes clinically irrelevant reactions lead to needless imposition of restricted diets. Misdiagnosis of food allergy may also lead to malnutrition in infants and children—and to anxiety and depression in their parents who may find that providing severely restricted diets is difficult.

Assessing the elderly patient's nutritional status

202 Normal aging changes

Aging is characterized by the loss of some body cells, and reduced metabolism in others. These conditions cause loss of bodily function and changes in body composition. Adipose tissue stores usually increase with age; lean body mass and bone mineral contents usually decrease.

A person's protein, vitamin, and mineral requirements usually remain the same as he ages, whereas caloric needs are lessened. Decreased activity may lower energy requirements about 200 calories/day for men and women aged 51 to 75, 400 calories/day for women over age 75, and 500 calories/day for men over age 75.

Other physiologic changes that can affect nutrition in an elderly patient include:

- decreased renal function, causing greater susceptibility to dehydration and formation of renal calculi
- loss of calcium and nitrogen (in patients who aren't ambulatory)
- decreased enzyme activity and gastric secretions
- decreased salivary flow and diminished sense of taste, which may reduce the person's appetite and increase his consumption of sweet and spicy foods
- decreased intestinal motility.

203 Patient history

Disabilities, chronic diseases, and surgical procedures (for example, gastrectomy) commonly affect an elderly patient's nutritional status, so be sure to record them in your patient history. Drugs or substances taken by your patient for his medical problem may also affect his nutritional requirements; for example, mineral oil, which many elderly persons use to correct constipation, may impair gastrointestinal (GI) absorption of vitamin A.

Some common conditions found in elderly persons, such as degenerative joint disease, paralysis, and impaired vision (from cataracts or glaucoma), can affect nutritional status by limiting the patient's mobility and therefore his ability to obtain and prepare food or feed himself.

GI complaints, especially constipation and stool incontinence, commonly occur in older patients. A decrease in intestinal motility characteristically accompanies aging; constipation may also be related to poor dietary intake, physical inactivity, or emotional stress or may occur as a side effect of certain drugs. Elderly patients often consume nutritionally inadequate diets consisting of soft, refined foods that are low in residue and dietary fiber. Laxative abuse, another common problem in elderly patients, results in the rapid transport of food through the GI tract and subsequent decreased periods of digestion and absorption (see Entries 475 and 476).

Socioeconomic and psychological factors that affect nutritional status include loneliness, decline of the elderly person's importance in the family, susceptibility to nutritional quackery, and lack of money to purchase nutritionally beneficial foods.

204 Assessment techniques

Currently, the adult standards for nutritional assessment are used for the elderly, although they're not as reliable for this age-group. Further research is needed to develop tools for assessing the nutritional requirements of elderly persons. Measures you can use to assess such a patient's nutritional status include common sense, consideration of factors that place any patient at nutritional risk, the dietary history, your objective data (keeping their limitations in mind), and monitoring of the patient's intake (if he's hospitalized). Remember, protein-calorie malnutrition is a major nutritional problem in patients over age 75 and contributes significantly to this age-group's mortality.

Selected References

American Academy of Pediatrics. *Pediatric Nutrition Handbook.* Evanston, Ill.: 1979.

Blackburn, G.L., et al. "Nutritional and Metabolic Assessment of the Hospitalized Patient," *Journal of Parenteral and Enteral Nutrition,* 1:11, 1977.

Bower, Fay L. *Nutrition in Nursing.* New York: John Wiley & Sons, 1979.

Boykin, Lorraine S. *Nutrition in Nursing.* Garden City, N.Y.: Medical Examination Publishing Co., 1975.

Butterworth, C.E., and Blackburn, G.L. *Nutrition Today,* 10:8, 1975.

Caliendo, Mary A. *Nutrition and Preventative Health Care.* New York: Macmillan Pub., Co., 1981.

Christakis, G. *Nutritional Assessment in Health Programs.* Washington, D.C.: American Public Health Assoc., Inc., 1974.

Dietary Allowances Committee, and Food and Nutrition Board. *Recommended Dietary Allowances,* 9th ed. Washington, D.C.: National Academy of Sciences, 1980.

Diseases. Springhouse, Pa.: Intermed Communications, 1981.

Guyton, Arthur C. *Textbook of Medical Physiology,* 5th ed. Philadelphia: W.B. Saunders Co., 1976.

Jensen, David, *The Principles of Physiology,* 2nd ed. New York: Appleton-Century-Crofts, 1980.

Keithley, Joyce K. "Proper Nutritional Assessment Can Prevent Hospital Malnutrition," *Nursing79,* February 1979, p. 68.

Krupp, Marcus A., and Chatton, Milton J., eds. *Current Medical Diagnosis and Treatment.* Los Altos, Calif.: Lange Medical, 1980.

Lewis, Clara M. *Nutritional Considerations for the Elderly.* Philadelphia: F.A. Davis Co., 1978.

Malasanos, Lois. *Health Assessment,* 2nd ed. St. Louis: C.V. Mosby Co., 1981.

Murray, Ruth B., and Zentner, Judith P. *Nursing Assessment and Health Promotion through the Life Span,* 2nd ed. Englewood Cliffs, N.J.: Prentice-Hall, 1979.

Pipes, Peggy L. *Nutrition in Infancy and Childhood,* 2nd ed. St. Louis: C.V. Mosby Co., 1981.

"Roundtable Geriatrics: Assess Nutrition and Digestive Impairment," *Patient Care,* Oct. 30, 1979.

Salmond, S.W. "How to Assess the Nutritional Status of Acutely Ill Patients," *American Journal of Nursing,* May 1980, p. 922.

Shafer, Kathleen. *Shafer's Medical-Surgical Nursing,* 7th ed. St. Louis: C.V. Mosby Co., 1980.

Slattery, Jill, Pearson, Gayle A., and Torre, Carolyn T., eds. *Maternal and Child Nutrition: Assessment and Counseling.* New York: Appleton-Century-Crofts, 1979.

Taylor, Robert B. *A Primer of Clinical Symptoms.* New York: Harper & Row, 1973.

United States Department of Agriculture. *Nutritive Values of American Foods in Common Units,* Agriculture Handbook No. 456. Washington, D.C.: 1976.

Vaughn, Victor C., III, et al. eds. *Nelson Textbook of Pediatrics,* 11th ed. Philadelphia: W.B. Saunders Co., 1979.

Weinsier, R.L., et al. "Hospital Malnutrition: A Prospective Evaluation of General Medical Patient During the Course of Hospitalization," *American Journal of Clinical Nutrition,* 32:418, 1979.

Williams, Emily J. "Food for Thought: Meeting the Nutritional Needs of the Elderly," *Nursing80,* September 1980, p. 60.

Williams, Sue R. *Essentials of Nutrition and Diet Therapy,* 2nd ed. St. Louis: C.V. Mosby Co., 1978.

Worthington, Bonnie, ed. "Symposium on Nutrition," *Nursing Clinics of North America,* June 1979, p. 197.

Yen, P.K. "What Is an Adequate Diet for an Older Adult?" *Geriatric Nursing,* May-June 1980, p. 64.

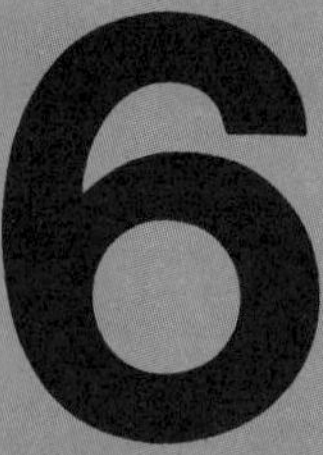

KEY POINTS IN THIS CHAPTER

KEY CHARTS IN THIS CHAPTER

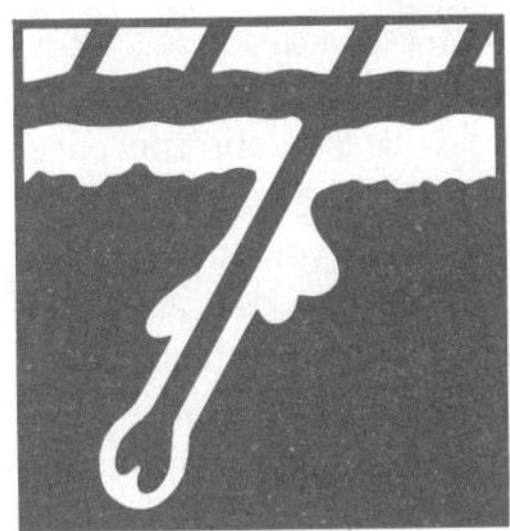

Skin, Hair, and Nails

Introduction

205 Your role in assessing skin, hair, and nails

In the entire health-care system, probably no one has a better opportunity than you, as a nurse, to observe and evaluate a patient's skin, hair, and nails. Because fingernails and head hair are usually exposed, they're easily accessible to inspection, as are portions of your patient's skin during such routine nursing procedures as bathing and repositioning, changing dressings, and giving medications. Often you can perform these brief inspections without your patient's knowledge and spare him possible discomfort or self-consciousness.

Always use tact, understanding, and reassurance when assessing any patient with a skin disorder. Even an apparently mild skin problem may cause a patient emotional distress if he considers it cosmetically unattractive.

206 Importance of skin assessment

Skin conditions may occur as primary disorders (resulting from changes in normal skin) or as secondary manifestations of dysfunction in other body systems. Two examples of secondary skin disorders are the skin infections commonly seen in patients with diabetes mellitus and the hair loss experienced by patients receiving chemotherapy. Remember this important point: Primary and secondary skin changes often exhibit a similar morphology and pattern. For example, the butterfly pattern characterizing the rash of systemic lupus erythematosus can resemble that of the facial rash of rosacea.

Skin disorders are important in themselves (because they're so closely related to the patient's body image) and as indicators of other, possibly more serious, systemic dysfunctions. Skin assessment helps you to recognize these problems, determine your patient's needs, and plan most effectively to meet them.

The skill you need to assess the integumentary system proficiently comes mainly from your experience with patients, since this system isn't covered in detail in most nursing curricula. One reason for this is that skin assessment usually takes place during assessment of other body systems. Another reason is that you don't see many patients admitted primarily for the treatment of skin disorders, unless you work in the dermatologic inpatient unit of a large medical center.

Nevertheless, whenever you see a patient with a skin disorder, give the problem your full attention as you determine his nursing needs—even if the disorder has low priority in your overall assessment.

Anatomy and physiology

207 The skin as a system

The skin (or integument) is the largest organ in the body, making up about 15% of total body weight and receiving about one third of the body's blood supply. The skin consists of two layers—the epidermis and dermis—resting on subcutaneous tissue. Skin thickness varies, ranging from 0.5 mm over the eyelids and eardrums to 5 mm on the soles and the upper back. The skin system also comprises the appendages: the sebaceous, eccrine, and apocrine glands, and the hair and nails.

In its main roles of protecting the body (acting as a physical barrier) and maintaining homeostasis, the skin functions in the following ways:

- regulating body temperature (thermoregulation) through evaporation of sweat and through cutaneous vasodilation (to cool the body) and vasoconstriction (to conserve body heat)
- preserving the wet environment of all living cells by providing a barrier to water and electrolyte loss
- protecting internal tissues from the harmful effects of microorganisms and other injurious agents the skin contacts
- sensing touch, temperature of external objects, and pain
- synthesizing vitamin D_3
- secreting sebum and sweat.

208 Epidermis

The epidermis—the outermost and regenerative layer of the skin—consists of stratified or layered squamous epithelium that produces keratin (the protective protein in the skin that also makes up hair and nails) and melanin (pigment). Except for persons with albinism, all people have pigment; darker-skinned persons have more active pigment-producing cells (melanocytes), not more of them. On exposure to ultraviolet light, these cells increase melanin production and transfer melanin to the keratin-producing cells (keratinocytes). This process gives the skin its color and protects it from penetrating ultraviolet rays. Vitamin D_3 also is synthesized in the epidermis after exposure to ultraviolet light. Because the epidermis is avascular, it depends on diffusion for nutrient distribution and for waste removal.

209 Dermis

The dermis (corium)—the inner skin layer—consists of connective tissue, cellular elements, and ground substance. The dermis contains lymphatics, blood vessels, and nerve endings. Hair follicles and three types of glands also are located in this layer. The dermis stores a significant amount of water, contributes to the support and elasticity of the skin, and provides nourishment for the avascular epidermis. It's also where infections are combated and where wound-healing and foreign-body expulsion occur.

210 Subcutaneous tissue

The subcutaneous tissue lies beneath the dermis and varies in thickness and consistency. It comprises areolar (loose) connective tissue, dense connective tissue, or adipose (fatty) tissue—depending on its location in the body. Its functions include anchoring the dermis and epidermis, insulating the body from extreme temperatures, and cushioning certain areas of the body.

211 Sebaceous glands

Sebaceous (sebum-producing) glands are located in the dermis as part of the pilosebaceous apparatus, which also contains the hair follicle and arrector pili muscle. These glands are simple, branched acinar glands connected to the follicle by a short duct.

The glandular epithelial cells slough off and disintegrate, becoming the oily sebum that contains cholesterol, fats, salts, and proteins. Sebum empties into ducts that lead to the necks of the hair follicles, keeping the hair and skin surface pliant and preventing excess water loss from the skin surface.

Sebaceous glands are usually stimulated by increased hormone levels at puberty.

212 Sweat glands

The dermis contains the apocrine and eccrine sudoriferous (sweat) glands. Apocrine glands are associated with hair follicles; eccrine glands aren't.

The eccrine glands occur over most of the body (except the lips) and help regulate body heat by secreting sweat through long tubular ducts and skin pores.

Apocrine glands occur primarily in the axilla, the areolae of the breasts, the periumbilical area, and the anogenital areas, and respond to stress and sexual stimulation. These glands empty relatively small amounts of sweat into follicles just above the opening of the sebaceous glands. There the sweat mixes with sebum and is excreted.

213 Hair

The distribution, thickness, and coarseness of a person's body hair depend on age, sex, and race. After puberty, pubic and axillary hair and (in men only) facial and chest hair gradually coarsen. Scalp hair grows at the rate of about 10 mm/month.

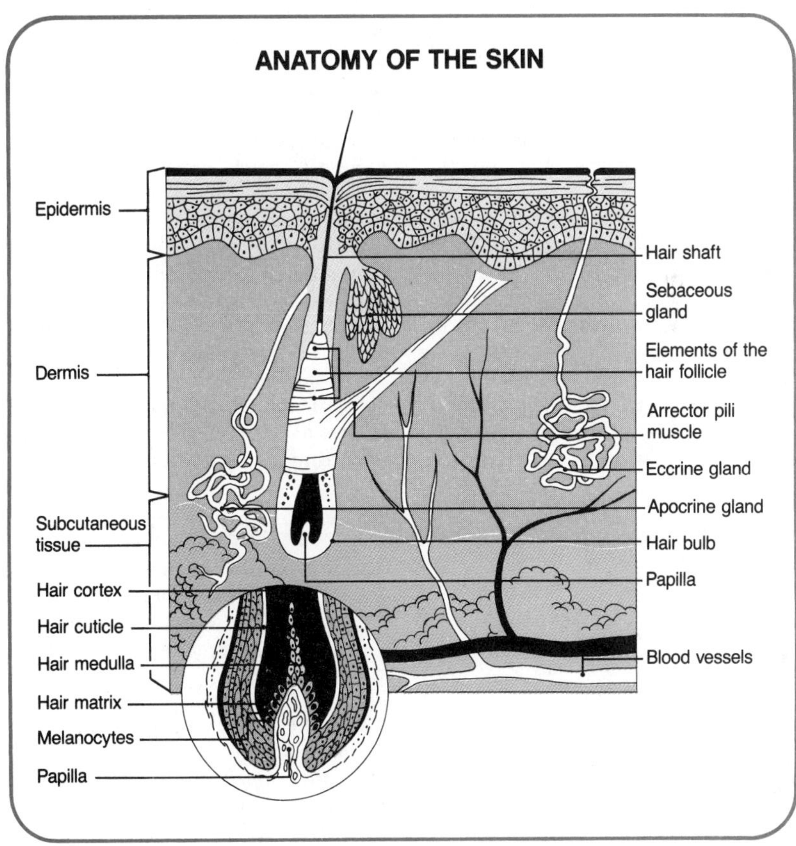

ANATOMY OF THE NAIL

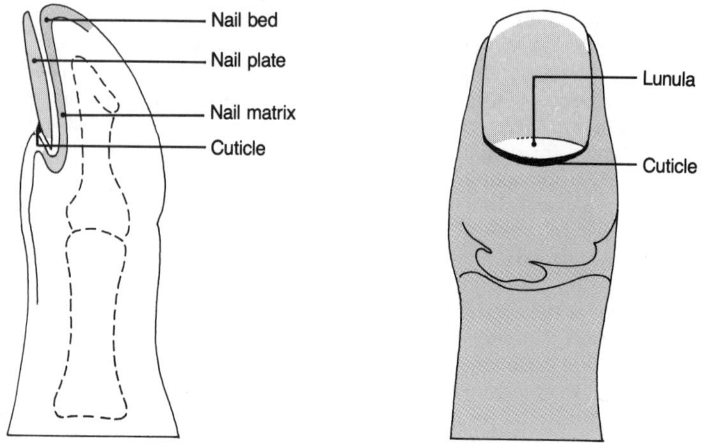

Nail bed
Nail plate
Nail matrix
Cuticle
Lunula
Cuticle

Specialized cells at the base of the hair follicles make keratin, which forms hair by first dying and then dehydrating and condensing.

Depending on the density of the keratin, the hair shaft forms three layers: the thin cuticle (outer layer), the cortex (middle layer), and the softer medulla (in the center). The melanocytes in the bulb determine hair color. After attaching to the smooth arrector pili muscle part way down the follicular sheath, the follicle slants upward and attaches to the papillary dermis. Contraction of the arrector pili muscle (for example, in response to cold) causes erection of the hair follicle (gooseflesh).

214 Nails

Nails are hard keratin that develops from specialized epidermal cells in the nail matrix. The *nail plate* overlies the nail bed; its pink color is derived from the underlying blood vessels. The *nail groove* contains the root, the only part capable of producing the visible portion of the nail. The *lunula* is the half-moon–shaped white structure near the root. It may be covered completely by the cuticle (keratinized tissue, adhering to the nail surface). At the end of the nail, the *hyponychium* (thickened epidermis) underlies the nail bed and is continuous with the nail.

Collecting appropriate history data

215 Biographical data

Biographical data can indicate whether your patient is likely to develop a particular type of skin disorder. For example, rosacea is more common in women than in men, and keloid formation is more common in blacks than in whites.

216 Chief complaint

The most common chief complaints associated with skin disorders are *itching, rashes,* and *lesions.*

217 History of present illness

Using the PQRST mnemonic device as a guide, ask the patient to elaborate on his chief complaint. Then, depending on the complaint, explore the history of his present illness by asking the following questions.

• ***Itching:*** *When did the itching begin?* If it started, for example, within 2 days after the patient began using a new dishwashing soap, this may indicate allergic contact dermatitis. *Has the itching spread? Does it get worse at a particular time of day?* Itching caused by scabies often worsens at night as the parasites become more active in the warm bedding. Itching from other disorders may also worsen at night. *Have you come in contact with anyone who has an itching problem?* Scabies can spread quickly, especially in places like dormitories or hospitals.

Have you tried creams, lotions, or special shampoos to relieve the itching? If so, which ones? Did they help, or make it worse? Some over-the-counter medicated shampoos relieve seborrheic dermatitis itching.

• ***Rash:*** *Where did the rash start? Have you had direct skin contact with known allergens? Is it spreading?* Both allergic reactions and viral exanthemas spread. *Does the rash burn or hurt?* Burning is characteristic of some vesicles, such as herpes zoster (shingles) and herpes simplex. *Have you ever had a similar rash? Do other signs and symptoms accompany the rash?* Fever and malaise may suggest that the rash has a viral origin.

• ***Lesions*** (see *Nurse's Guide to Primary and Secondary Skin Lesions,* pages 182 to 185): *How long have you had this lesion? Has the color, size, or any other characteristic of the lesion changed? How long has it been changing?* Some lesions change in appearance over time. Herpes simplex, for example, changes from red papules to vesicles to a crust. Some nevi may rise above the skin and enlarge. Always note the sequence of such changes. *Does anything irritate the lesion, for instance, clothing rubbing against it? Does the lesion limit or prevent activity?* For example, deep plantar warts can make walking painful.

218 Past history

Explore the following areas when re-

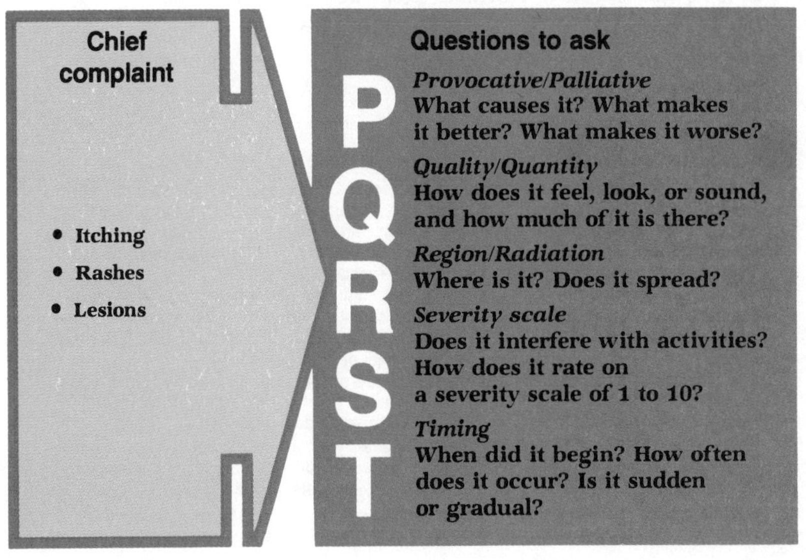

EMERGENCY

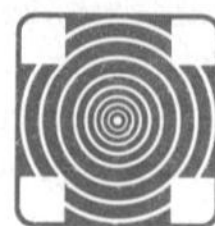

ASSESSING THE BURN PATIENT

To assess the patient who's been burned, you must first obtain complete information about the accident. If the patient can't communicate, see if the family or rescue personnel can supply the information you need. Why is this information important? If, for example, the fire occurred indoors, or if the patient's clothing was burned, you should suspect smoke inhalation as well.

Airway: Whether your patient suffered smoke inhalation or not, examine his airway closely. Suspect airway injury if the patient's nose hairs are singed, if you find soot particles in his mouth and pharynx or in his sputum, or if he drools or salivates excessively. Look for signs of laryngeal stridor and upper airway irritation and inflammation.

Respirations: Next, assess his respirations. Observe him for signs of alveolar collapse, pulmonary edema, hypoxemia, and pneumonia. You may hear rales, rhonchi, or wheezes on auscultation. Estimate his level of ventilation (rate and depth of expansion). Note any cough, and describe his sputum. If the patient's suffered circumferential chest burns, his chest expansion may be impaired because of eschar formation, and he may require escharotomy. You should also draw blood for arterial blood gas analysis of carbon dioxide, partial pressures, and pH.

Vital signs: You'll need to take the patient's vital signs and monitor urinary output to establish a baseline for assessing fluid loss. With burn wounds, fluid moves from the intravascular area into the interstitium. This may cause hypovolemia and shock.

Level of consciousness: Determine the patient's level of consciousness. Watch for symptoms of carbon monoxide poisoning: headache, weakness, dizziness, nausea, vomiting, and in severe poisoning, syncope and collapse. Elevated carboxyhemoglobin levels may also indicate carbon monoxide poisoning.

Burn size: Estimate the size of the burn wound. To do this, use the assessment method known as the Rule of Nines, discussed on the opposite page.

Burn depth: Estimating burn depth is difficult in the first few hours after the accident. Once this time has elapsed, you can determine burn depth by answering these questions:

- Is the burned area pink or red, with minimal edema?
- Is it sensitive to temperature change?

If the answers are yes, your patient has a first-degree burn, involving one or two skin layers.

- Is the burned area pink or red, and does it blanch when touched?
- Does the patient have large, thick-walled blisters, with subcutaneous edema?
- Is the burned area firm or leathery?
- Does touching the burn cause the patient severe pain?

If the answers are yes, your patient has a second-degree burn, involving at least two skin layers.

- Is the burned area waxy white, red, brown, or black?
- If red, does it remain red and not blanch when touched?
- Is it leathery, with extensive subcutaneous edema?
- Is it insensitive to touch?

If the answers are yes, your patient has a third-degree burn, involving all skin layers.

Electrical burns: If your patient has suffered an electrical burn, follow the same basic procedure outlined above. Note these special considerations:

- If an electrical current has passed through the brain or the heart, the patient will probably be unconscious or in cardiac and respiratory arrest.
- If the current passed through an extremity, assess pulses—peripheral and distal—and extremity color and temperature. Intravascular coagulation may impair his circulation.
- If your patient's in shock, note that the condition may not result from fluid loss; it may be caused by the injury or by accompanying abdominal or thoracic injury.
- If, on auscultation, your patient's bowel sounds are absent, suspect paralytic ileus. Look for an exit wound from the electrical current. If present, it can give you a general idea of the current's pathway and the blood vessels and nerves it damaged.

Chemical burns: If your patient has suffered a chemical burn, he'll probably have a localized lesion (unless other systems are injured simultaneously). You can define the injury's extent by assessing erythema, blistering, ulceration, necrosis, and sloughing.

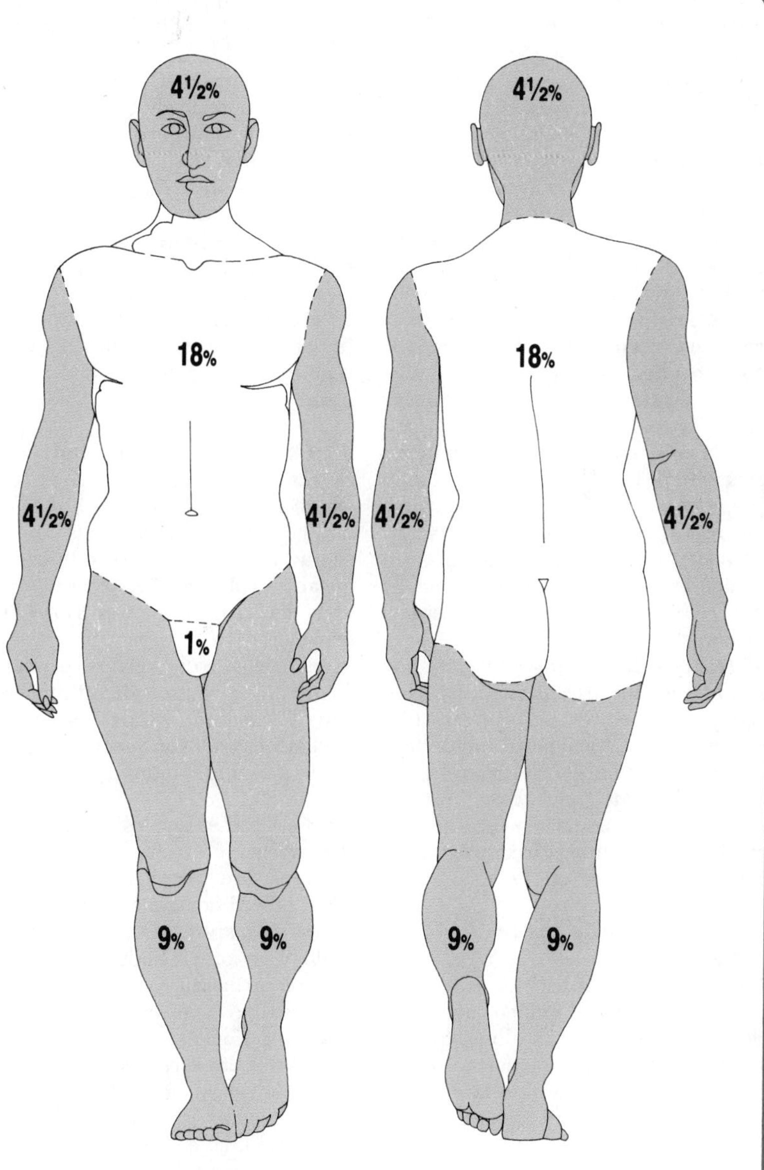

The Rule of Nines divides body surface area into percentages that, when totaled, equal 100%. To use this technique, mentally transfer your patient's burn to the body chart shown here. Add the percentages assigned to the sections in which the burn falls. This total is a rough estimate of the burn size and serves as a guide in initial fluid replacement. In non-emergency situations, you'll use more involved methods to assess burn size.

viewing the past history of a patient with a skin disorder:

• ***Related systemic conditions.*** A skin disorder may signal the onset of a systemic disorder, such as systemic lupus erythematosus, or occur as a result of prolonged illness, such as malaria, syphilis, pulmonary tuberculosis, or coronary disease.

• ***Immunosuppression therapy.*** Such therapy—for cancer or collagen diseases, for example—may reduce the patient's resistance to herpes zoster. Alopecia often results from use of steroids and chemotherapeutic agents.

• ***Allergens.*** Common allergens that may cause skin disorders include plants (such as poison ivy, oak, sumac), pollens, foods, cosmetics and perfumes, soaps and laundry detergents, and preparations containing benzocaine, neomycin, or vitamin E. Skin conditions may also be precipitated by such metals as nickel and chrome, and by rubber (especially in elastic undergarments).

• ***Medications.*** Skin eruptions may result from the use of vitamins, cold remedies, laxatives, and prescription drugs, such as penicillin and sulfonamides (for more information, see *Nurse's Guide to Some Drugs That Affect the Skin*). Some topical and systemic drugs can indirectly cause a photosensitivity reaction.

219 Family history

Certain skin disorders (such as psoriasis, acne vulgaris, vitiligo, and atopic dermatitis), as well as alopecia, may be hereditary. Atopic dermatitis is strongly associated with a family history of allergies, such as asthma and hay fever.

220 Psychosocial history

In your review of the patient's psychosocial history, include questions about the following:

• ***Occupation and hobbies.*** Exposure to chemicals containing a strong base or acid, like those used at some manufacturing plants and in some hobbies, may predispose the patient to skin eruptions.

• ***Recent travel.*** Certain skin disorders are more likely to occur in particular geographic areas—for instance, parasitic diseases, such as cutaneous larva migrans, are more prevalent in tropical climates.

• ***Housing.*** A patient is more likely to contract pediculosis corporis in an unclean or crowded home.

• ***Personal contact.*** Pediculosis capitis and pediculosis pubis, as well as scabies, may be transmitted through close personal contact.

221 Activities of daily living

Outdoor activities in very hot or cold weather may cause skin disorders or aggravate an existing condition. For instance, cold weather usually aggravates dry skin. Known as *winter itch,* this condition is especially prevalent in elderly persons. Overexposure to sunlight can cause a direct photosensitivity reaction, which may be immediate (as in sunburn) or delayed (as in premature aging).

222 Review of systems

Primary skin disorders don't usually affect other body systems, but secondary skin eruptions may indicate pathology in other body systems. For example, skin symptoms (such as rashes and itching) may appear during allergic reactions, along with symptoms (such as itchy eyes and dyspnea) related to other systems. The respiratory, cardiovascular, gastrointestinal, urinary, immune, and endocrine systems may be affected.

Pigmentation and nevi may change during pregnancy, and reversible hair loss is common after delivery. Stretch marks (striae) from distention of the skin (especially of the abdomen) may result from pregnancy, obesity, ascites, tumors, or subcutaneous edema.

NURSE'S GUIDE TO SOME DRUGS THAT AFFECT THE SKIN

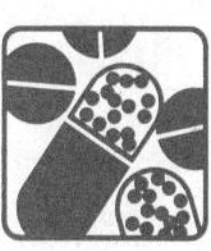

CLASSIFICATION	POSSIBLE SIDE EFFECTS
Pituitary hormones	
corticotropin (ACTH)	• Impaired wound healing, thin fragile skin, petechiae, ecchymoses, facial erythema, increased sweating, acne, hyperpigmentation, hirsutism, purpura
Antipsychotics	
chlorpromazine hydrochloride (Thorazine)	• Mild photosensitivity, dermal allergic reactions (such as exfoliative dermatitis)
haloperidol (Haldol*)	• Rash
Barbiturates	
pentobarbital sodium (Nembutal sodium*)	• Rash, urticaria
Antidiarrheals	
diphenoxylate with atropine (Lomotil*)	• Pruritus, urticaria, rash
Antiarrhythmics	
phenytoin sodium (Dilantin*)	• Scarlatiniform or morbilliform rash, exfoliative or purpuric dermatitis, erythema multiforme (Stevens-Johnson syndrome), lupus erythematosus
propranolol hydrochloride (Inderal*)	• Rash
Sulfonamides	
sulfadiazine (Microsulfon)	• Erythema multiforme (Stevens-Johnson syndrome), generalized skin eruption, epidermal necrolysis, exfoliative dermatitis, photosensitivity, urticaria, pruritus
Estrogens	
dienestrol (AVC/Dienestrol Creme)	• Erythema multiforme, chloasma, melasma
Tetracyclines	
tetracycline hydrochloride (Achromycin*, Sumycin*)	• Maculopapular and erythematous rashes, urticaria, photosensitivity, increased pigmentation
Anticonvulsants	
bromides (Lanabrom, Neurosine)	• Acneiform, morbilliform, and granulomatous eruptions; erythema nodosom; Stevens-Johnson syndrome
diazepam (Valium*)	• Rash; Urticaria

(continued)

NURSE'S GUIDE TO SOME DRUGS THAT AFFECT THE SKIN *(continued)*

DRUG	POSSIBLE SIDE EFFECT
Anticonvulsants *(continued)*	
trimethadione (Tridione)	• Acneiform and morbilliform rash, exfoliative dermatitis, erythema multiforme, petechiae, alopecia
Antituberculars	
isoniazid [INH] (Hyzyd)	• Eruptions (types vary)
Tranquilizers	
meprobamate (Equanil, Miltown*)	• Pruritus, urticaria, erythematous maculopapular rash
Oral contraceptives	
estrogen with progestogen (Brevicon, Enovid)	• Rash, chloasma or melasma, acne, seborrhea, oily skin
Penicillins	
penicillin G potassium (Pentids)	• Rash, urticaria, maculopapular eruptions, exfoliative dermatitis
Nonnarcotic analgesics	
phenolphthalein (Azolid, Butazolidin*)	• Petechiae, pruritus, purpura, various dermatoses from rash to toxic necrotizing epidermolysis
Expectorants	
codeine	• Pruritus
Anticoagulants	
dicumarol (Dufalone**)	• Dermatitis, urticaria, rash, alopecia
Skeletal muscle relaxants	
dantrolene sodium (Dantrium*)	• Eczematoid eruption, pruritus, urticaria
Antifungals	
griseofulvin (Fulvicin, Grifulvin V)	• Rash, urticaria, photosensitive reactions (may aggravate lupus erythematosus)
Gold compounds	
gold sodium thiomalate (Myochrysine*)	• Rash and dermatitis
Diuretics	
chlorothiazide (Diuril)	• Dermatitis, photosensitivity, rash
Uncategorized agents	
allopurinol (Zyloprim*)	• Rash, usually maculopapular; exfoliative, urticarial, and purpuric lesions; erythema multiforme; severe furunculosis of nose; ichthyosis; toxic epidermal necrolysis

*Available in U.S. and Canada. **Available in Canada only. All other products (no symbol) available in U.S. only.

Conducting the physical examination

223 Preparation and positioning

For skin inspection, overhead fluorescent lighting or strong natural light is best. Avoid using incandescent lighting, because it may produce a transilluminating effect. Check that the room isn't too cold (which may cause cyanosis or blanching) or too hot (which may cause flushing).

Have the patient stand or sit for the examination unless he's ill or injured, when you should place him in the supine or prone position.

224 Inspecting skin color and pigmentation

Observe the general color and pigmentation of the skin. The characteristics of normal skin vary with the patient's racial, ethnic, and familial background. Note any paleness, jaundice, or cyanosis.

Also, note the location of any *hypopigmentation:* Is the lack of color partial or total? Hypopigmentation usually occurs in patches, especially on the face and arms. Dry skin commonly causes patches of peeling hypopigmented skin, especially on the legs.

Darkened areas of skin *(hyperpigmentation)* may occur on any part of the patient's body. Note the location of any hyperpigmented areas you find on inspection.

Trauma is a common cause of *postinflammatory discoloration.*

225 Assessing skin hydration

Inspection and palpation readily identify dry skin. Skin dryness can vary from mild to the rare, severe form known as *ichthyosis.* Persons of all ages can have dry skin; you'll usually see more patients with this condition during cold weather. Almost all elderly patients have dry skin.

If your patient's skin looks oily, inspect his body for acne, especially on areas where the sebaceous glands are concentrated—the face, neck, back, chest, and buttocks.

Exertion, anxiety, or fear can cause increased perspiration (hyperhidrosis). In some persons, however, excessive perspiration has no demonstrable relationship to stress. Inspect the areas most commonly affected: the patient's palms, soles, and axillary and groin areas.

226 Examining skin texture and thickness

Feel your patient's skin. Is it rough or smooth? If you see scaling, note whether it occurs in large patches or as individual lesions. Also observe the general thickness of your patient's skin—whether it looks and feels normal or whether it's thin and fragile, as in the elderly or in patients with debilitating diseases. Check for the thickened plaques of chronic eczema and psoriasis. Inspect palms and soles for calluses.

227 Turgor, elasticity, and mobility

Test turgor and elasticity by picking up a fold of the patient's skin over a bony prominence and then releasing it. Normal skin immediately returns to its previous state. Elasticity is greatly reduced in scleroderma. To test for mobility, see if the skin moves back and forth smoothly over the same bony prominence.

228 Assessing vascularity, erythema, and edema

Observe your patient's skin for vascular abnormalities, such as *purpuric disorders,* characterized by purple or brown-red petechiae (pinpoint lesions) or *bruises (ecchymoses),* caused by hemorrhage into the cutaneous tis-

NURSE'S GUIDE TO PRIMARY AND SECONDARY SKIN LESIONS

	TYPE	DESCRIPTION	EXAMPLE
PRIMARY LESION 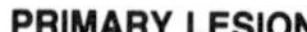			
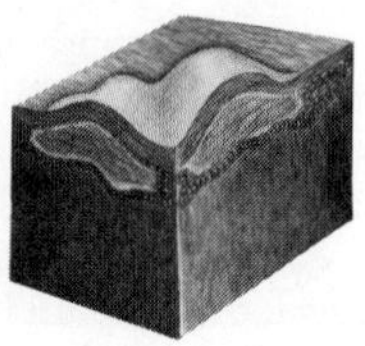	**Bulla**	Fluid-containing lesion, greater than 2 cm in diameter	Severe poison oak or ivy, dermatitis, bullous pemphigoid
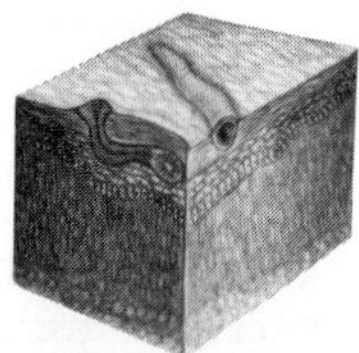	**Burrow**	Linear or zigzag, slightly raised lesion produced by a parasite	Scabies
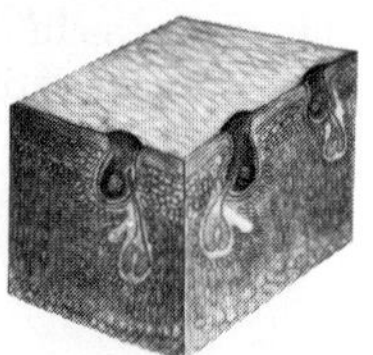	**Comedo**	Plugged pilosebaceous duct found in acne, exfoliative in nature, formed from sebum and keratin	Blackhead (open comedo), whitehead (closed comedo)
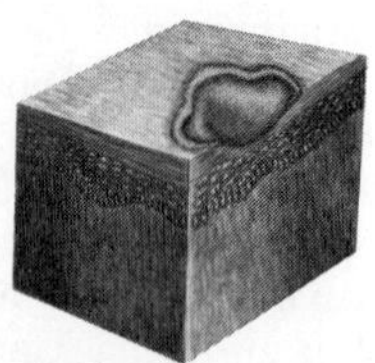 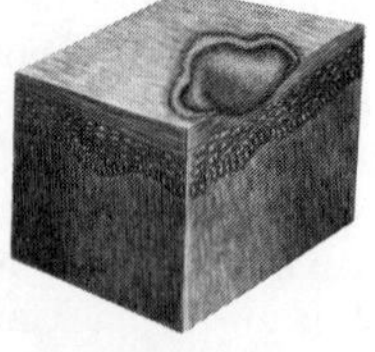	**Erosion**	Circumscribed lesion involving destruction of epidermal tissue	Granular erosion
	Macule	Flat, pigmented, circumscribed area	Freckle

NURSE'S GUIDE TO PRIMARY AND SECONDARY SKIN LESIONS *(continued)*

TYPE	DESCRIPTION	EXAMPLE
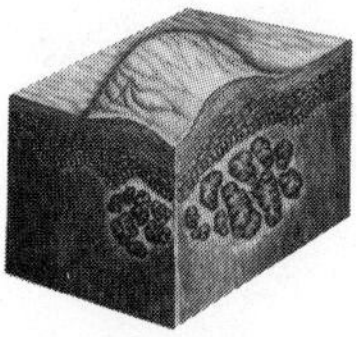 **Nodule**	Firm, raised lesion; deeper than a papule	Intradermal nevus
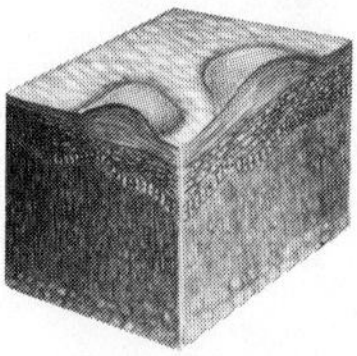 **Papule**	Firm, inflammatory, raised lesion up to 1 cm in diameter	Acne papule, lichen planus
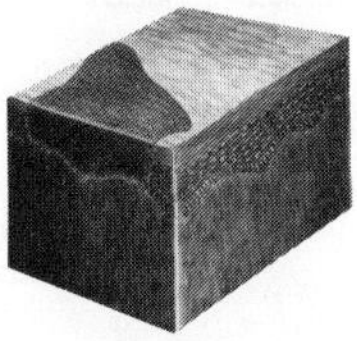 **Patch**	Flat, pigmented, circumscribed area greater than 1 cm in diameter	Herald patch (pityriasis rosea)
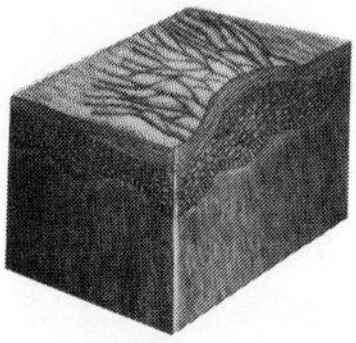 **Plaque**	Circumscribed, solid, elevated lesion greater than 1 cm in diameter. Elevation above skin surface occupies larger surface area in comparison with height.	Psoriasis
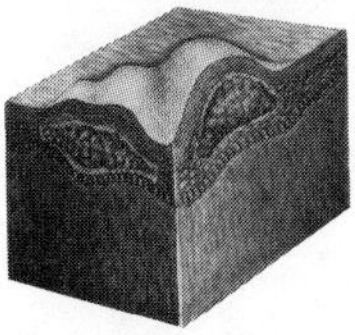 **Pustule**	Raised, circumscribed lesion, usually less than 1 cm in diameter, that contains purulent material	Acne pustule

(continued)

NURSE'S GUIDE TO PRIMARY AND SECONDARY SKIN LESIONS *(continued)*

	TYPE	DESCRIPTION	EXAMPLE
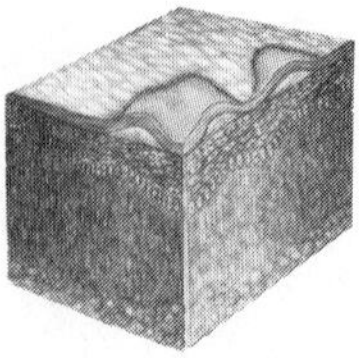	**Vesicle**	Raised, circumscribed, fluid-containing lesion less than 0.5 cm in diameter	Chicken pox, herpes simplex
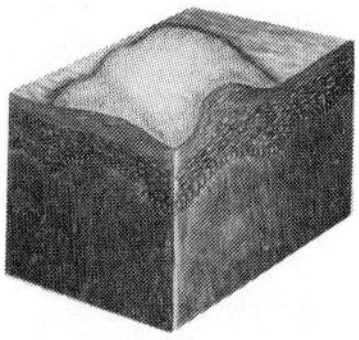	**Wheal**	Raised, firm lesion with intense localized skin edema, varying in size and shape, and transient in occurrence.Disappears in hours.	Hive
SECONDARY LESION			
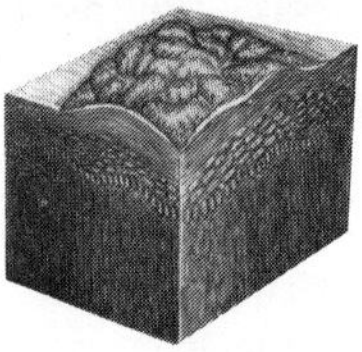	**Crust**	Dried serous or purulent exudate	Impetigo
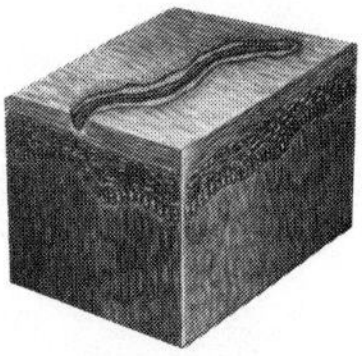	**Excoriation**	Scratched or abraded areas, often self-induced	Abraded acne lesions, eczema
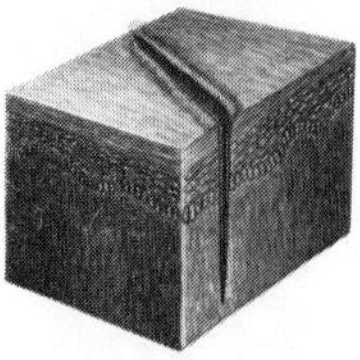	**Fissure**	Linear cracking of the skin	Hand dermatitis

NURSE'S GUIDE TO PRIMARY AND SECONDARY SKIN LESIONS *(continued)*

TYPE	DESCRIPTION	EXAMPLE
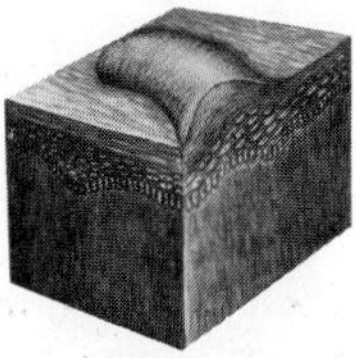 **Keloid**	Thick, red, firm scar formation that usually develops following surgery	Surgical incision
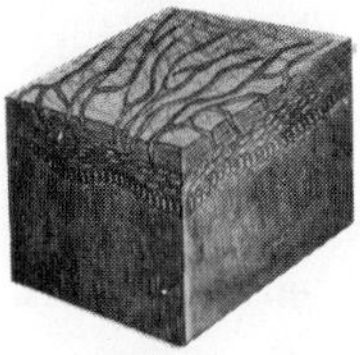 **Lichenification**	Thickening prominent skin markings caused by constant rubbing	Chronic atopic dermatitis
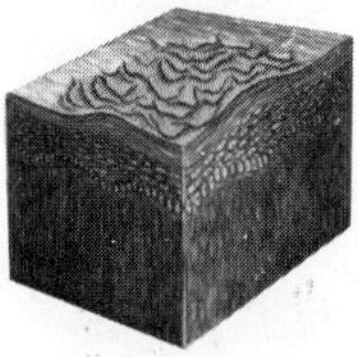 **Scale**	Thin, dry flakes of shedding skin	Psoriasis
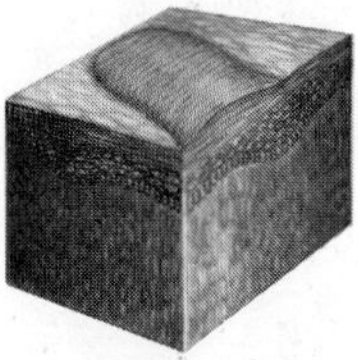 **Scar**	Formation of fibrous tissue caused by trauma or deep inflammation	Cicatrix
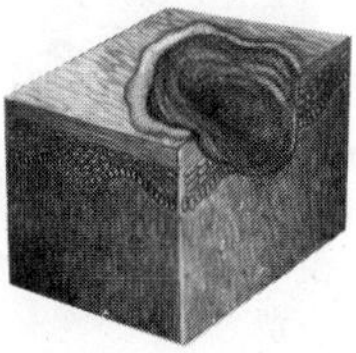 **Ulcer**	Epidermal and dermal destruction	Decubitus ulcer

sues. *Telangiectasias* (formed by the dilatation of small blood vessels) are also common.

Assessment tip: Telangiectasias blanch when pressure is applied; petechiae do not.

Note whether your patient's skin has any red areas (erythema) and whether the erythema is generalized, localized, or diffuse. (Erythema is the outstanding symptom of some systemic diseases, especially measles, rubella, and scarlet fever, and numerous dermatologic conditions.) Also note the erythema's distribution pattern because certain dermatologic conditions characteristically occur in specific anatomic areas (see *Distribution Patterns of Common Skin Disorders,* page 198). To observe overall distribution of your patient's skin lesions (for instance, the Christmas-tree pattern of pityriasis rosea), view him from a distance of 2′ to 3′ (0.6 to 0.9 m). Finally, check for any local lymphadenopathy (see Entry 725).

If you note any edema, record its location and whether it's associated with erythema, rash, or any type of lesion.

229 Inspecting hair

The color of your patient's hair has no relationship to his health status except when the color has changed suddenly.

Note any dryness, brittleness, or fragility, which may be the result of trauma (usually from cosmetic causes) or a body system dysfunction. Examine the quantity, quality, and distribution of the hair, and observe the pattern (generalized or patchy) of any hair loss. (Keep in mind that a person normally loses up to 100 head hairs a day.) If

TESTING FOR DERMATOLOGIC DISEASE

To properly assess your patient's dermatologic condition, you or the doctor (depending on the test) may need to perform one or more of the following tests:

TEST	PURPOSE	METHOD	FINDINGS
Biopsy	To confirm initial diagnostic impression; to provide additional information when diagnosis is uncertain	Punch or shave biopsy, or excision	Changes in cells consistent with disease process indicate disease.
Potassium hydroxide (KOH) wet mount	To determine fungal or monilial invasion	Skin scrapings or pulled hairs from suspect lesions, placed on a glass slide with 10% KOH, then covered and gently heated over an alcohol flame	Spores and branching hyphae indicate yeast or fungus.
Microbial culture	To determine fungal, bacterial, or viral invasion	Specimen placed in appropriate medium and sent to laboratory for examination	Presence of organism (identified by its characteristic growth pattern) confirms test.
Patch tests	To identify the cause of allergic dermatitis	Test material applied to normal skin and covered with special tape; removed after 48 hours and reaction noted	Redness or vesiculation indicates a positive reaction.

RECOGNIZING COMMON DERMATOSES

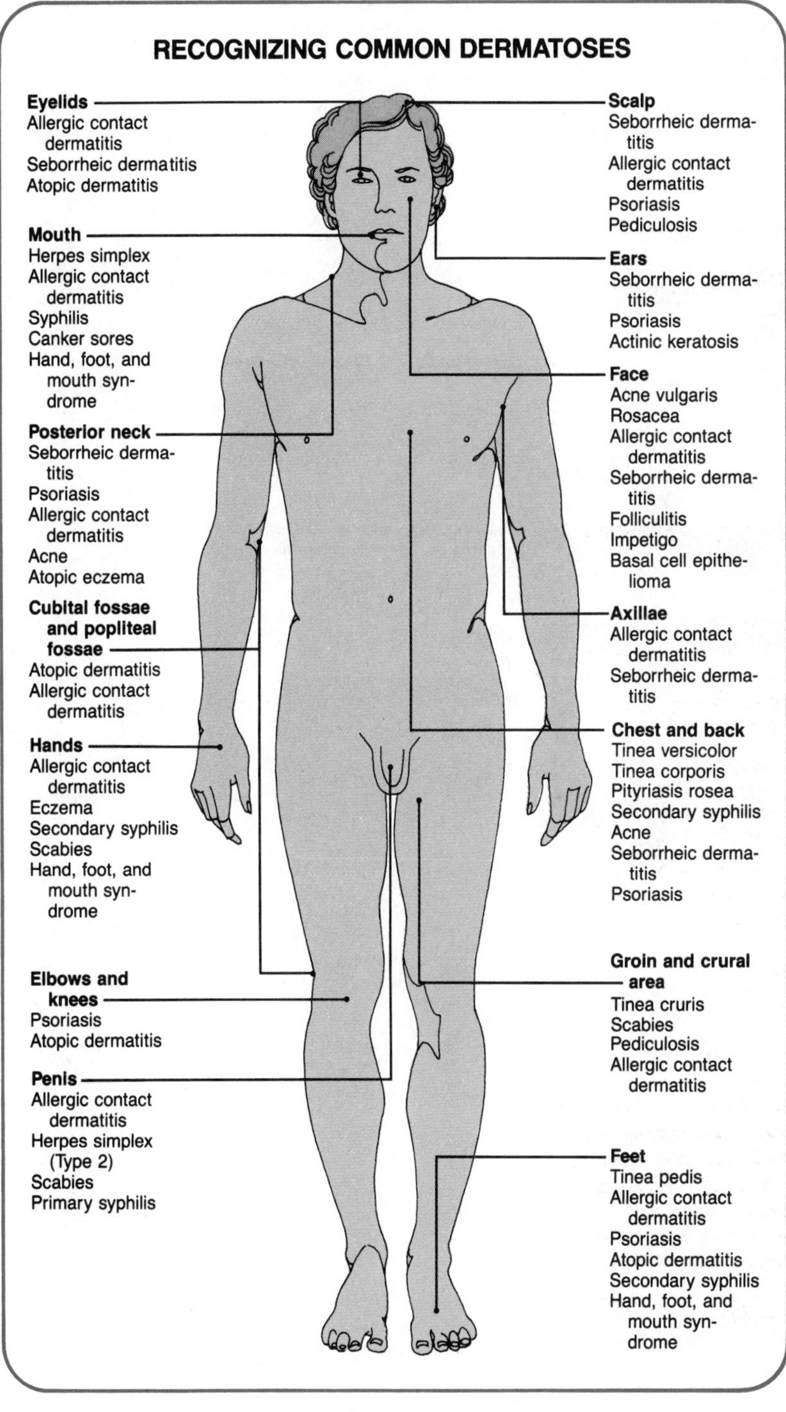

hair loss seems excessive, gently pull on the patient's hair to see if it comes out easily. Look for regrowth in patchy hair-loss areas. If you see any erythema, scaling, or crusting on the patient's scalp, along with excessive hair loss, darken the room and examine the patient's scalp under a Wood's light (a specially filtered ultraviolet light). Certain dermatophytes, such as those causing tinea capitis (ringworm), appear fluorescent green under a Wood's

UNDERSTANDING NAIL ABNORMALITIES

DISORDER	DESCRIPTION	POSSIBLE ASSOCIATED DISORDERS
Beau's lines	Transverse depressions in all nails	Severe acute illness, malnutrition, anemia
Clubbing of the nails	Early clubbing: soft, cushiony nail base; late clubbing: swollen nail base	Cardiopulmonary disorders
Koilonychia	Concave nail curve (spoon nails)	Chronic eczema, tumor of the nail bed, various systemic diseases, anemia
Leukonychia	Transverse white bands with rough borders that do not extend the entire nail width	Trauma
Mees' lines	Crescent-shaped transverse lines in the nail plate	Arsenic poisoning
Onycholysis	Partial separation of distal nail edge	Heart disease, chronic diseases

light. This may be a sign of ringworm infestation.

An excess of body and facial hair (hypertrichosis) or sparsity of such hair (hypotrichosis) is not necessarily abnormal; neither is hair in moles or birthmarks (evaluate such areas for malignancy).

230 Examining the scalp

If you see inflammation or pustular

	DISORDER	DESCRIPTION	POSSIBLE ASSOCIATED DISORDERS
	Paronychia	Erythema, swelling, and thickening of skin surrounding the nail edges, with possible severe pain and infection	Monilia (most common), diabetes, bacterial infections, third-stage syphilis, leprosy
	Pigment band	Line of discoloration in the nail plate	Junction nevus
	Pterygium	Inflammatory lesion involving the nail matrix, accompanied by fusing of the proximal nail fold to the nail bed	Peripheral vascular disease, trauma, lichen planus
	Splinter hemorrhage	Small, stripelike, brown discoloration of the nail plate	Subacute bacterial endocarditis, minor trauma
	Striated nails	Longitudinal ridges, usually accompanied by fragile nails	Variable
	Subungual hematoma	Mass of blood under the nail necessitating biopsy to rule out possible melanoma	Trauma, jogger's toe

eruption on your patient's scalp, observe whether the condition occurs only around hair follicles or is more widespread. Also observe for other lesions that can occur on the scalp, such as cysts, warts, moles, and bites.

Distinguish between the mild flaking of ordinary dandruff; heavy scaling, as in psoriasis; and the greasy scaling of seborrheic dermatitis. Seborrheic dermatitis is commonly accompanied by scaling in the eyebrows, in creases (such as the nasolabial and postauricular folds), and in hairy areas, such as a man's chest.

If the patient is scratching his head and you suspect pediculosis, wear gloves when examining his scalp or use two tongue depressors to separate the hairs for inspection. You can usually see the live adult lice. If you don't see them but still suspect pediculosis, ask the patient to bend over a large piece of white paper or a sheet and to shake his head vigorously; the lice should fall onto the paper or sheet. Also check clothing seams, especially near the collar, for nits (louse ova) or lice. Then check for erythematous papules on the nape of the neck. Detecting nits is harder than detecting lice, because the nits resemble dandruff.

Assessment tip: Nits exude a sticky substance that fastens them to the hair shaft, so you can't pull them off as you can dandruff flakes.

To estimate how long your patient's been infested with lice, measure the distance between the nits and the base of the hair shaft. Because nits are laid on the scalp, and hair grows approximately 10 mm/month, the distance indicates when the infestation began.

231 Inspecting the nails

Observe the color of your patient's nails. Normally, they're pink in Caucasians and black and brown (possibly with a pattern of longitudinal lines) in blacks. Note if the nails appear blue-black or purple, brown or yellow-gray.

Inspect the shape and texture of his nails, noting any irregularities, such as brittleness, cracking, or peeling. If any nails are missing, note whether the loss is partial or total. If the nail and its nail bed have separated (onycholysis), examine the nail for discoloration, debris accumulated under the nail, and thickening. (Remember, onycholysis is often a sign of psoriasis.)

Your inspection of the patient's nails may also reveal striations, vertical or horizontal ridges, or tiny depressions (*thimble pits*). The paronychial tissue folds around the nail may be swollen, erythematous, or oozing pus or serous fluid. Paronychial warts and ingrown nails (especially ingrown toenails) are also common. (See *Understanding Nail Abnormalities,* pages 188-189.)

Formulating a diagnostic impression

232 Assessing skin, hair, and nail disorders

The affected area in skin, hair, and nail disorders can be small (as with nail changes), large (as with psoriasis), very visible (as with acne), or easily hidden (as with pityriasis rosea). Regardless of the size or visibility of the affected area, usually your patient will be concerned about possible disfigurement and anxious for rapid diagnosis and effective treatment of his problem. Unfortunately, this may take longer than he would like it to take, because dermatoses often present complex and confusing clinical pictures.

233 Inflammatory skin disorders

Contact dermatitis, an inflammatory condition, is one of the most common skin disorders. You can identify it by its distribution pattern and the location of its usually erythematous lesions. Symmetrical distribution suggests that the allergic reaction may be due to clothing, perhaps elastic or the metal fasteners on a slip or bra. A symmetrical rash on both sides of the neck may be caused by the application of perfume. Deodorants, or the dry cleaning agents used on clothes, may cause a rash in the axillae. Dermatitis in areas where jewelry or other metal is worn suggests an allergy to metal. Dermatitis on the feet is commonly caused by the rubber toecap (or the rubber cement) used in sneakers.

Scattered linear lesions with erythema, edema, and often vesiculation usually indicate *plant dermatitis*—probably the most common type of contact dermatitis. The signs and symptoms are similar regardless of the plant involved.

Allergic contact dermatitis may appear at any time up to 2 weeks after exposure to an offending substance, but it usually appears within 24 to 48 hours after contact. The patient must have been exposed to the substance (which later becomes an allergen) at least once to have developed the disorder. When trying to identify the offensive agent, don't rule out a cosmetic that a patient says she's "used for years" as a possible cause of the allergic reaction. Manufacturers sometimes change the formula for a cosmetic or laundry product without informing consumers—some of whom may then become allergic to a previously benign product.

Atopic dermatitis, also common, results from an inherited skin characteristic that makes certain individuals more sensitive to irritants and allergens. In an adult, the chronic form occurs as dry, thickened, and potentially scarring lesions, which may develop anywhere on the body and usually itch. As the patient scratches the lesions to relieve the itch, they may become lichenified. A strong family history of asthma, eczema, or hay fever is an important diagnostic clue. Some patients are never totally free of this condition, and dry weather and emotional stress may aggravate it.

Inflammatory eruptions can also result from an allergic reaction to virtually any systemic drug. The rash (erythematous, pruritic eruptions) usually appears within a few days after the patient begins treatment but may appear up to 10 days after the patient stops taking the medication. The rash usually disappears within a week or two. (See *Nurse's Guide to Common Skin Disorders,* pages 192 to 197.)

234 Sebaceous gland dysfunctions

Sebaceous gland dysfunctions are common and include acne vulgaris, seborrheic dermatitis, and rosacea. *Acne vulgaris* most often affects young people. Its severity ranges from very mild, with only a few blackheads, through the whole scope of acne lesions including papules, inflammation, pustules, cysts, and—in severe cases—disfiguring scars. Acne may be confined to the face or may also appear on the neck, upper chest, back, and occasionally the buttocks.

Because androgen stimulates sebum secretion, boys and men usually have more severe and more frequent cases of acne. However, girls and women with endocrine imbalance may develop cystic acne, and the use of oral contraceptives with high levels of androgenic potency exacerbates the disease. Systemic corticosteroid therapy can cause steroid acne.

Inflamed, greasy, and scaling lesions characterize *seborrheic dermatitis,* which commonly occurs on body areas, such as the scalp, with large concentrations of sebaceous glands. Pruritus commonly accompanies seborrheic dermatitis. *Hair loss* may occur if the scalp becomes grossly infected secondarily.

Rosacea causes erythematous pustular eruptions across the patient's cheek

NURSE'S GUIDE TO COMMON SKIN DISORDERS

	CHIEF COMPLAINT	
BACTERIAL DISEASES		
Scarlet fever	• *Itching:* absent • *Rash:* present; bright red, finely papular in skin creases of axillae, groin, and neck; spreads rapidly to trunk, extremities, and face; lasts 1 or 2 days • *Lesion:* absent	
Impetigo	• *Itching:* present • *Rash:* rarely present; small, very fragile vesicles; when broken, exudes liquid that dries and forms honey-colored crusts; usually occurs on face but may occur anywhere on body • *Lesion:* absent	
Folliculitis	• *Itching:* present in hairy areas; accompanied by burning • *Rash:* present; tiny papules and pustules around hair follicles of scalp, beard, eyelids, upper arms, buttocks, and thighs • *Lesion:* absent	
VIRAL DISEASES		
Herpes simplex Type 1 (fever blister)	• *Itching:* absent • *Rash:* present; single group of vesicles ruptures, leaving a painful ulcer, followed by a yellow crust; usually occurs around mouth or nose but may occur anywhere on body; healing begins 7 to 10 days after initial onset, is complete within 3 weeks • *Lesion:* absent	
Herpes progenitalis Type 2 (herpes simplex)	• *Itching:* absent • *Rash:* present; small grouped vesicles around genital and mouth areas • *Lesion:* absent	
Viral herpes zoster (shingles)	• *Itching:* absent • *Rash:* present; grouped vesicles or crusted lesions along nerve root, usually unilateral • *Lesion:* absent	
Verrucae (warts)	• *Itching:* absent • *Rash:* absent • *Lesion:* present; slightly raised papules, with fingerlike projections; usually on hands or feet but may occur anywhere on body; black specks that appear within warts are coagulated blood, the result of wart abrasion and subsequent bleeding.	

	HISTORY	PHYSICAL EXAMINATION AND DIAGNOSTIC STUDIES
	• Exposure to infected person 1 or 2 days previously • Accompanied by sore throat, headache, vomiting	• Red pharynx, with exudate • Strawberry-red tongue • Fever • Peeling skin on hands and feet possible after several days.
	• Most common in children during hot weather • Predisposing factors: overcrowded living quarters, poor skin hygiene, anemia, malnutrition, minor skin trauma	• No other physical characteristics • Culture and sensitivity tests show *Streptococcus pyogenes* and *Staphylococcus aureus*
	• Excessive use of hair oils and lotions • Use of hot tub or sauna	• Stye, in deep folliculitis • Stiff eyelid hair indicates condition caused by *Staphylococcus aureus* or *Pseudomonas.*
	• Cold, fever, trauma, menstruation, or overexposure to sunlight may occur prior to sores. • Recurrences common	• No other physical characteristics
	• *In infants:* delivered vaginally with infected mother • *In adolescents and adults:* sexual contact with infected person	• No other physical characteristics
	• Chicken pox (condition caused by reactivation of chicken pox virus) • Persistent postherpetic neuralgia possible	• No other physical characteristics
	• Previous history of warts	• No other physical characteristics

(continued)

NURSE'S GUIDE TO COMMON SKIN DISORDERS *(continued)*

	CHIEF COMPLAINT	
Rubeola (measles)	• *Itching:* absent • *Rash:* present; begins with faint macules on hairline, neck, and cheeks; increases to maculopapular rash on entire face, neck, and upper arms; spreads to back, abdomen, arms, thighs, and lower legs; appears 2 to 4 days after onset of other symptoms; lasts 4 or 5 days • *Lesion:* absent	
Rubella (German measles)	• *Itching:* absent • *Rash:* present; begins with maculopapular rash on face, which spreads to trunk • *Lesion:* absent	
Exanthema subitum (roseola infantum)	• *Itching:* absent • *Rash:* present; begins with macular or maculopapular eruption on trunk; *rarely* spreads to arms, neck, face, and legs; fades within 24 hours • *Lesion:* absent	
Varicella (chicken pox)	• *Itching:* present; urticaria around vesicle • *Rash:* present; begins with crops of small red papules and clear vesicles on red base; vesicles break and then dry, causing crust formation; begins on trunk and spreads to face and scalp • *Lesion:* present; may leave scars	
FUNGAL DISEASES		
Tinea pedis (athlete's foot)	• *Itching:* present in interdigital webs, palms, and soles; accompanied by burning, stinging • *Rash:* absent • *Lesion:* present; in acute form, blisters; in chronic form, dry, scaly skin	
Tinea cruris (jock itch)	• *Itching:* present; more severe than in seborrheic dermatitis • *Rash:* absent • *Lesion:* present; bilateral, fan-shaped red scaly patches, with slightly raised borders in groin, upper thighs, and gluteal folds	
Tinea corporis (smooth skin ringworm)	• *Itching:* present; intense • *Rash:* absent • *Lesion:* present; round, red, scaly lesions, with slightly raised borders; central area heals while lesion continues outward; may be anywhere on body	

HISTORY	PHYSICAL EXAMINATION AND DIAGNOSTIC STUDIES
• Exposure to infected person 10 to 14 days previously • Cold, conjunctivitis, fever, and cough prior to rash • Greatest communicability 11 days after exposure, lasting 4 or 5 days	• Koplick's spots (white patches on oral mucosa) • Generalized lymphadenopathy, conjunctivitis
• Exposure to infected person 14 to 21 days previously • *In children:* usually no symptoms prior to rash • *In adolescents:* headache, malaise, anorexia may occur prior to rash	• *In adolescents and adults:* conjunctivitis, low-grade fever, posterior cervical and postauricular lymphadenopathy, joint pain
• Exposure to infected person 7 to 17 days previously • Sudden high fever 3 or 4 days prior to rash • Usually affects infants and children age 6 months to 3 years	• Inflamed pharynx
• Exposure to infected person 13 to 21 days previously • Malaise, anorexia prior to rash • In temperate areas, higher incidence in late fall, winter, and spring	• Slight fever
• Previous history of tinea pedis • Males more susceptible than females	• Blisters or scaly skin on feet and between toes • Potassium hydroxide diagnoses condition. • Skin scrapings examined microscopically may reveal fungus.
• Males more susceptible than females • Previous history of tinea cruris, obesity, chafing • Usually occurs concurrently with tinea pedis	• No other physical characteristics • Potassium hydroxide diagnoses condition.
• Exposure to infected animals or people • Most common in children	• No other physical characteristics • Potassium hydroxide diagnoses condition. • Hyphae can be seen with a microscope

(continued)

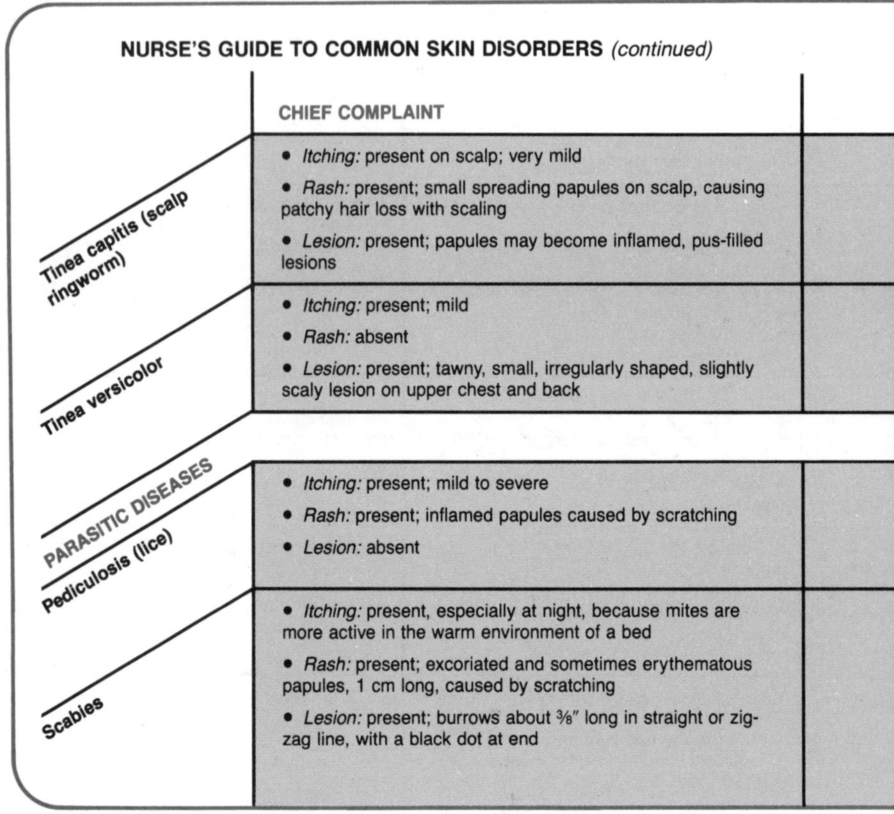

NURSE'S GUIDE TO COMMON SKIN DISORDERS *(continued)*

	CHIEF COMPLAINT
Tinea capitis (scalp ringworm)	• *Itching:* present on scalp; very mild • *Rash:* present; small spreading papules on scalp, causing patchy hair loss with scaling • *Lesion:* present; papules may become inflamed, pus-filled lesions
Tinea versicolor	• *Itching:* present; mild • *Rash:* absent • *Lesion:* present; tawny, small, irregularly shaped, slightly scaly lesion on upper chest and back
PARASITIC DISEASES	
Pediculosis (lice)	• *Itching:* present; mild to severe • *Rash:* present; inflamed papules caused by scratching • *Lesion:* absent
Scabies	• *Itching:* present, especially at night, because mites are more active in the warm environment of a bed • *Rash:* present; excoriated and sometimes erythematous papules, 1 cm long, caused by scratching • *Lesion:* present; burrows about 3/8" long in straight or zig-zag line, with a black dot at end

and nose that may be confused with the typical butterfly rash of lupus erythematosus. Rosacea occurs in adults (most commonly women) over age 30. Its occurrence in men is usually severe. If untreated, rosacea can lead to *rhinophyma*—an oily, greasy hypertrophy of the nose.

235 Papulosquamous skin dysfunctions

Two examples of papulosquamous skin dysfunctions are psoriasis and pityriasis rosea. *Psoriasis* is a chronic disease in which skin cell maturation and exfoliation accelerate, producing marked epidermal thickening. It usually occurs during adulthood but may also affect children. Psoriatic plaques are generally circumscribed, symmetrical, and erythematous, with silvery scales. Although plaques can appear anywhere and sometimes spread widely over the body, commonly affected areas include the scalp, elbows, knees, external ear canals, and the perianal and vaginal regions. Plaques sometimes appear at the site of skin injury *(Koebner's phenomenon),* such as a surgical wound, scratch, or sunburn. Most patients with psoriasis don't have pruritus.

The oval or round patches of *pityriasis rosea,* can be pink, salmon, tan, or light brown. The condition typically begins with one erythematous, scaly patch (the *herald patch*), several centimeters in diameter, that usually appears on the trunk. The hallmark of the disease—a Christmas-tree pattern of distribution on the trunk, neck, and arms—follows within a few days to a week. The lesions usually develop along

HISTORY	PHYSICAL EXAMINATION AND DIAGNOSTIC STUDIES
• Exposure to infected people	• Patchy hair loss • Infected areas sometimes appear green under Wood's light. • Hyphae can be seen with a microscope.
• Previous history of tinea versicolor • More common in summer	• No associated discomfort • White patches on tanned body • Spots prominent under Wood's light • Hyphae can be seen with a microscope.
• Exposure to infected persons • Predisposing factor: overcrowded living conditions	• Lice sometimes observable • *Pediculosis capitis:* on scalp • *Pediculosis pubis:* primarily found in pubic hairs but may extend to eyebrows, eyelashes, or axillary or body hairs
• Exposure to affected person	• May affect interdigital webs on hands, wrists, elbows, breasts, buttocks, and penis • Mites and nits can be seen with a microscope in scraping from intact lesion. • Resembles contact dermatitis, atopic dermatitis

the skin lines and are most noticeable on the back.

The number of lesions and the severity of itching in pityriasis rosea vary greatly. The disease lasts about 6 to 12 weeks, and recurrence is uncommon. Because secondary syphilis produces a similar rash, testing should include a serologic test for syphilis. The syphilitic rash rarely itches.

Papulosquamous skin lesions can also result from various types of infections: fungal (tineas), parasitic (pediculosis, scabies), and syphilitic (secondary).

236 Benign skin tumors

The most common skin tumors are moles (fleshy, pigmented *nevi*), which are usually benign. Common moles may be hairy or hairless, flat or raised, flesh-colored or pigmented (colors range from pink or tan to dark brown and even blue), and congenital or acquired. Moles may appear soon after puberty, but some don't appear until adulthood. An increase in the size or elevation of a mole over many years is common. But be sure to evaluate any mole that changes rapidly, bleeds without trauma, has pigmentary irregularities within its border, or has an irregular border.

Seborrheic keratoses are rough, elevated, tan or brown lesions that appear to be stuck on the patient's skin. These benign lesions occur mainly on the back and chest, and sometimes on the face. They most commonly affect middle-aged or elderly persons.

Small, tumor-like cysts also appear on the chest, back, face, and scalp. Of

DISTRIBUTION PATTERNS OF COMMON SKIN DISORDERS

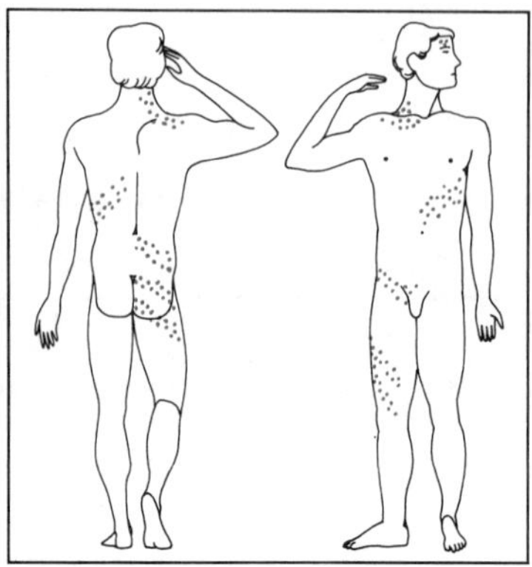
Herpes zoster

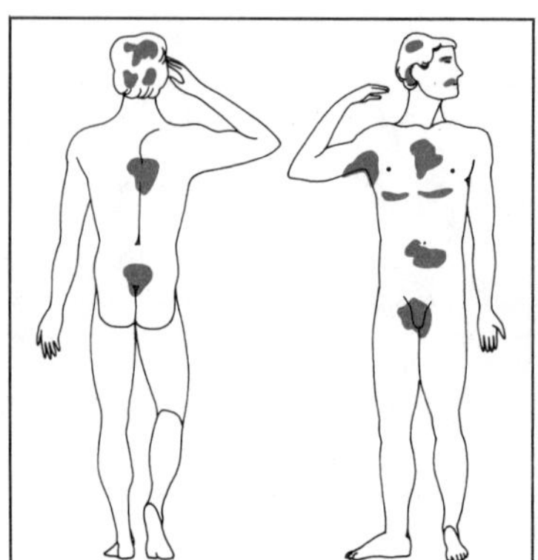
Seborrheic dermatitis

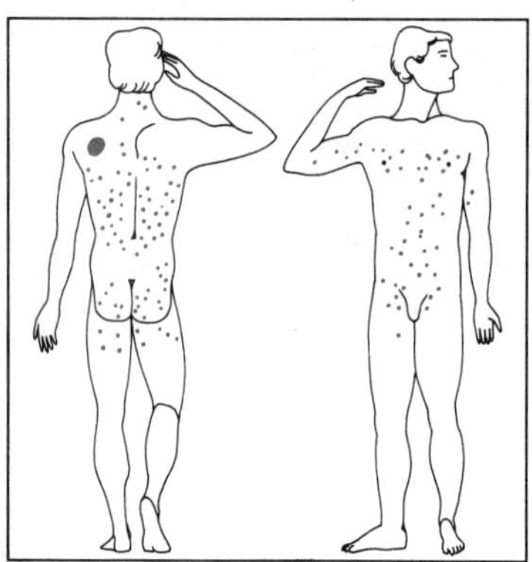
Pityriasis rosea

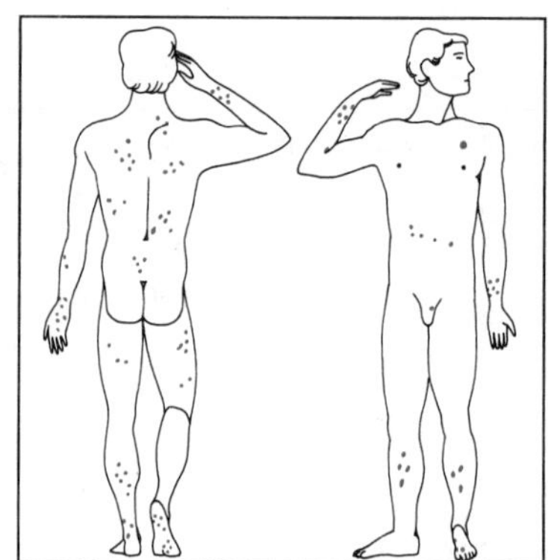
Lichen planus

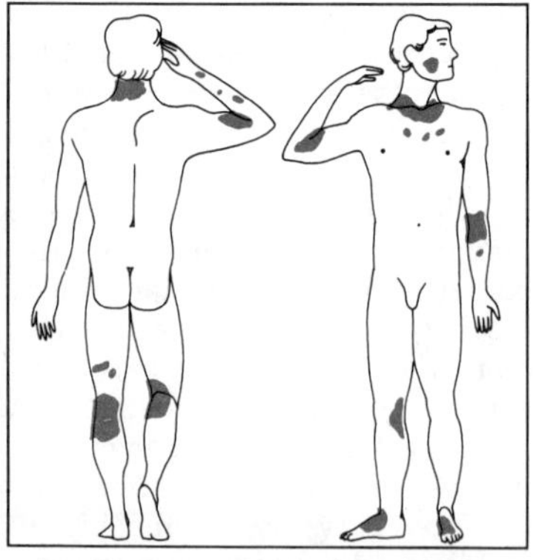
Atopic dermatitis (in young adults)

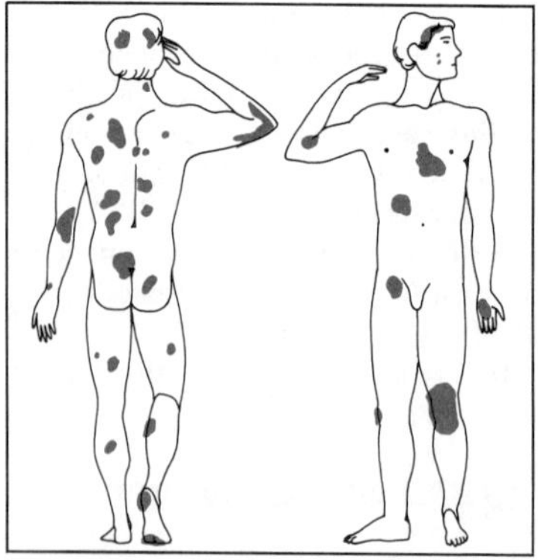
Psoriasis

the many types of cutaneous cysts, probably the most common is the *epidermoid cyst,* a palpable, saclike structure filled with sebum. Cutaneous cysts are usually benign, but they can become inflamed or tender.

The *acne cyst,* also common, is usually red or purple. It can grow to be large and even confluent with other acne cysts. If untreated, these cysts can cause scarring.

Unlike cysts with fairly regular shapes, *keloids* may have unusual configurations. Black skin is particularly susceptible to keloid development. Common sites of keloid formation are the face and upper chest.

Dermatofibromas are firm nodules of fibrous skin deposits. Usually you'll find that these single, flat (or slightly elevated) nodules occur on the legs and are tan, red, or brown. Suspect a dermatofibroma if, on palpation, you detect a firm, buttonlike mass in your patient's skin.

237 Malignant skin tumors

Potentially malignant *actinic keratoses* result from prolonged overexposure to the sun. They appear most commonly on the face, arms, and backs of the hands, and on bald areas or the scalp. Most likely to develop in fair-skinned adults, these lesions are scaly, discrete (flesh-colored or pink), and slightly raised. When an actinic keratosis becomes malignant, it evolves into a squamous cell carcinoma. This transition is heralded both by induration and by movement of the abnormal cells into the dermis.

The most common malignant skin lesion affecting Caucasions is *basal cell epithelioma.* This lesion grows slowly and doesn't metastasize, but if neglected, it can invade adjacent structures. Basal cell epithelioma most often affects skin areas exposed to the sun, such as the face.

The most common of the several types of basal cell epitheliomas usually appears as a small, raised lesion with shiny, almost translucent borders. It often contains telangiectasias. Because it grows slowly, over months or sometimes even years, a central depression may form.

Usually seen on the head or hands, *squamous cell carcinoma* is an opaque mass that may be large and funguslike in appearance, or elevated and nodular. It can spread rapidly.

Malignant melanoma usually involves a mole, wart, or birthmark—but can occur anywhere on the body. A lesion less than 1.5 cm in diameter may be blue, gray, or black; crusted or ulcerated; flat or raised. It changes form as it spreads: It may be flat, or flat with a palpable border, or nodular—entirely palpable. Malignant melanoma is the fastest-metastasizing skin cancer and also accounts for most skin-cancer deaths.

238 Making appropriate nursing diagnoses

Nursing diagnoses for patients with skin disorders reflect the patient's ability to cope with his altered appearance and discomfort.

Perhaps the major problem faced by a patient with any type of dermatosis is *alteration in self-concept.* Many patients go to great lengths to hide a skin condition. The teenager with acne vulgaris, for example, may withdraw from his peers into *social isolation.*

Your nursing diagnoses for a patient with pruritus (from contact dermatitis, for example, or seborrheic dermatitis) may include *disturbance in sleep patterns, due to increased itching at night,* and *alterations in comfort due to itching.* Pruritic skin disorders may also require these nursing diagnoses: *impairment of skin integrity,* including *actual impairment due to inflammatory response* and *potential impairment due to scratching* (which may cause a secondary infection); and including *noncompliance, due to inability to avoid scratching* or *due to abandonment of therapy because of delayed relief.*

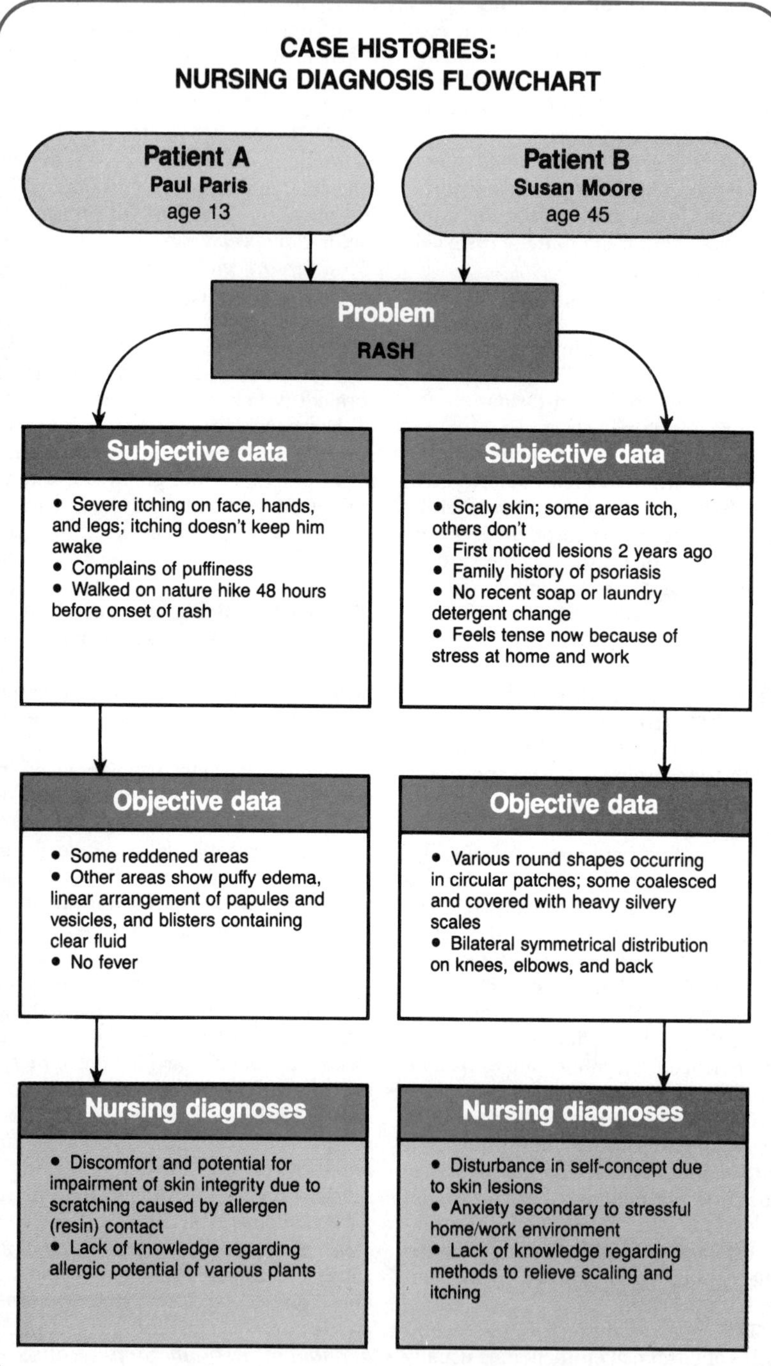
CASE HISTORIES:
NURSING DIAGNOSIS FLOWCHART
Patient A
Paul Paris
age 13
Patient B
Susan Moore
age 45
Problem
RASH
Subjective data
• Severe itching on face, hands, and legs; itching doesn't keep him awake
• Complains of puffiness
• Walked on nature hike 48 hours before onset of rash
Subjective data
• Scaly skin; some areas itch, others don't
• First noticed lesions 2 years ago
• Family history of psoriasis
• No recent soap or laundry detergent change
• Feels tense now because of stress at home and work
Objective data
• Some reddened areas
• Other areas show puffy edema, linear arrangement of papules and vesicles, and blisters containing clear fluid
• No fever
Objective data
• Various round shapes occurring in circular patches; some coalesced and covered with heavy silvery scales
• Bilateral symmetrical distribution on knees, elbows, and back
Nursing diagnoses
• Discomfort and potential for impairment of skin integrity due to scratching caused by allergen (resin) contact
• Lack of knowledge regarding allergic potential of various plants
Nursing diagnoses
• Disturbance in self-concept due to skin lesions
• Anxiety secondary to stressful home/work environment
• Lack of knowledge regarding methods to relieve scaling and itching

Assessing pediatric patients

239 Skin problems in newborns and infants

Common infant skin problems are diaper rash, cradle cap, newborn rash (erythema neonatorum toxicum), infant acne, impetigo, and roseola. If you see diaper rash, ask the patient's parents about the diaper-changing procedures they use. Do they wash the diaper-covered area with each change? Keeping the rash area clean and dry usually helps healing; if it doesn't, suspect monilial dermatitis.

Bacterial or monilial infection may occur with diaper rash: Check for papules, pustules, or vesicles. Monilial rashes are severely erythematous and pustular, with vesicular and satellite lesions. Culturing is recommended to identify the infectious agent.

The scaling and crusting of cradle cap may cover an infant's entire scalp. Ask about a family history of atopic dermatitis, which is inherited. Check for accumulations of soap residue and hair that's been shed. If an infant has severe cradle cap with diaper rash just to the diaper borders, he may have true seborrheic dermatitis.

For any skin problem, ask the parents how often they bathe the infant since excessive bathing can dry an infant's skin, and what kinds of soap, lotions, powders, and oils they use since some may produce a skin reaction.

240 Preschool and school-age children's skin

Preschool and school-age children are susceptible to such common skin disorders as allergic contact dermatitis (from poison ivy, oak, or sumac, or rubber in shoes or clothing), atopic dermatitis, warts (especially on the hands), viral exanthemas, impetigo, ringworm, scabies, and skin reactions to food allergies.

For the child with any kind of rash, obtain a thorough history. Asking about how and where the rash began, its evolution pattern, and its preceding symptoms may help differentiate between rubella, rubeola, scarlet fever, viral exanthemas, and drug reactions. (See *Distribution Patterns of Common Pediatric Skin Disorders.)*

DISTRIBUTION PATTERNS OF COMMON PEDIATRIC SKIN DISORDERS

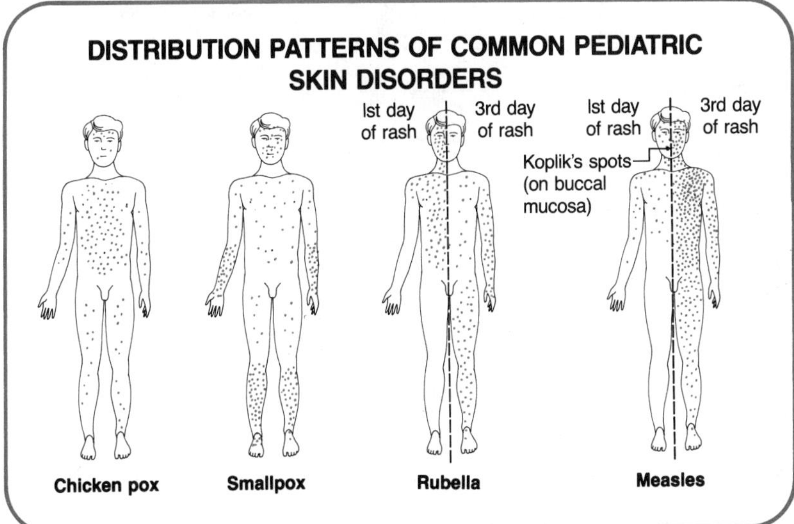

241 Adolescent skin disorders

When a child enters puberty, hormonal changes affect his skin and hair. Androgen levels increase, causing sebaceous glands to secrete large amounts of sebum, which can clog hair follicle openings. Pubic and axillary hair begin to grow. Common dermatoses occurring during adolescence include acne, warts, sunburn, scabies, atopic dermatitis, and pityriasis rosea. Also common in adolescents are allergic contact dermatitis (especially from jewelry and cosmetics) and fungal infections (especially tinea pedis, tinea cruris, and tinea versicolor). Examine an adolescent for these disorders, using the same procedures as for an adult.

If an adolescent has severe acne, observe his speech and behavior for possible signs of depression (see Entry 137). Remember, an adolescent is usually very concerned with his appearance, so skin problems can affect his self-image.

Assessing geriatric patients

242 How aging affects the skin, hair, and nails

Skin changes are the most visible signs of aging. One of the obvious changes in aging skin is the development of facial lines (crow's feet) around the eyes, mouth, and nose. These lines result from subcutaneous fat loss, dermal thinning, decreasing collagen, and increasing elastin. The skin of other body areas also shows signs of aging: increased prominence of the supraclavicular and axillary regions, the knuckles, and the hand tendons and vessels, as well as fat pads over bony

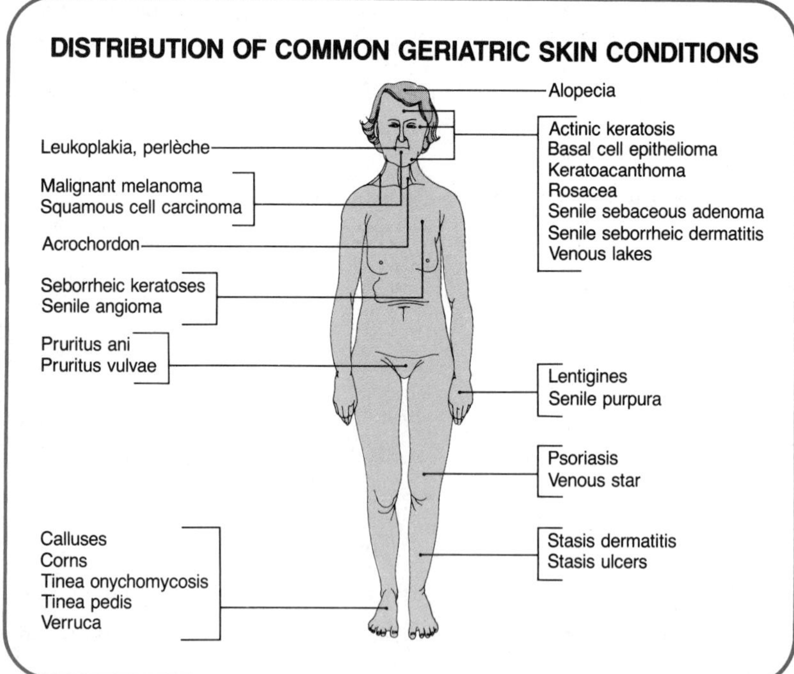

prominences. Mucous membranes become dry, and sweat gland output lessens as the number of active eccrine sweat glands is reduced. Very elderly persons' skin loses its elasticity until it may seem almost transparent. Although melanocyte production decreases as a person ages, localized melanocyte proliferations are common and cause brown spots to appear, especially in areas regularly exposed to the sun.

Hair pigment decreases with aging, so a person's hair turns gray or white (and also thins as he ages). Hormonal changes cause pubic hair loss. Facial hair often increases in postmenopausal women and decreases in aging men.

Many people's nails change significantly with aging. They may grow at different rates, and longitudinal ridges, flaking, brittleness, and alterations in form may increase. Toenails may discolor.

243 Common geriatric skin disorders

As a person ages, susceptibility to certain skin disorders increases. For example, actinic keratoses and basal cell epitheliomas from past sun exposure commonly occur in elderly persons. Xerosis, capillary hemangiomas, pedunculated fibromas, and seborrheic keratoses are extremely common. Other characteristic geriatric skin conditions include xanthelasma, plantar keratosis, seborrheic dermatitis, and pigmented nevi. If your elderly patient's mobility has decreased and his circulation is impaired, he may develop stasis dermatitis and possibly stasis ulcers. (See *Distribution of Common Geriatric Skin Conditions*.)

Selected References

Arndt, Kenneth A. *Manual of Dermatologic Therapeutics*, 2nd ed. Boston: Little, Brown and Co., 1978.

Bates, Barbara. *A Guide to Physical Examination*, 2nd ed. New York: J.B. Lippincott, Co., 1979.

Beeson, Paul B., McDermott, Walsh, and Wyngaarden, James B., eds. *Cecil Textbook of Medicine*, 15th ed. Philadelphia: W.B. Saunders Co., 1979.

Braverman, Irwin M. *Skin Signs of Systemic Disease*. Philadelphia: W.B. Saunders Co., 1970.

Carotenuto, Rosine, and Bullock, John. *Physical Assessment of the Gerontological Client for Nurses*. Philadelphia: F.A. Davis Co., 1980.

Coleman, William P., III, and McBurney, Elizabeth I. *Pediatric Dermatology*. Garden City, N.Y.: Medical Examination Publishing Co., 1981.

DeGowin, Elmer L., and DeGowin, Richard L. *Bedside Diagnostic Examination*, 2nd ed. New York: Macmillan Pub. Co., 1969.

Fisher, Alexander A. *Contact Dermatitis*, 2nd ed. Philadelphia: Lea & Febiger, 1973.

Fitzpatrick, T.B., et al. *Dermatology in General Medicine*, 2nd ed. New York: McGraw-Hill Book Co., 1979.

Isselbacher, Kurt J., et al., eds. *Harrison's Principles of Internal Medicine*, 9th ed. New York: McGraw-Hill Book Co., 1980.

Symposium on Cutaneous Signs of Systemic Disease, vol. 64, no. 5 in *The Medical Clinics of North America*. Philadelphia: W.B. Saunders Co., 1980.

Moschella, Samuel L., et al. *Dermatology*, vols. 1 and 2, 2nd ed. Philadelphia: W.B. Saunders Co., 1975.

Rook, A., et al. *Textbook of Dermatology*, 2 vols., 3rd ed. St. Louis: C.V. Mosby Co., 1979.

Sauer, Gordon C. *Manual of Skin Diseases*, 4th ed. Philadelphia: J.B. Lippincott Co., 1980.

Stewart, William D., et al. *Dermatology: Diagnosis and Treatment of Cutaneous Disorders*, 4th ed. St. Louis: C.V. Mosby Co., 1978.

Vaughan, Victor C., III, et al. eds. *Nelson Textbook of Pediatrics*, 11th ed. Philadelphia: W.B. Saunders Co., 1979.

Weinberg, Samuel, and Hoekelman, Robert A. *Pediatric Dermatology for the Primary Care Practitioner*. New York: McGraw-Hill Book Co., 1978.

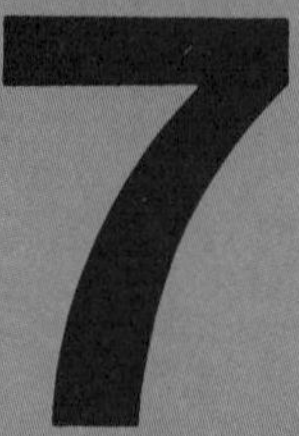

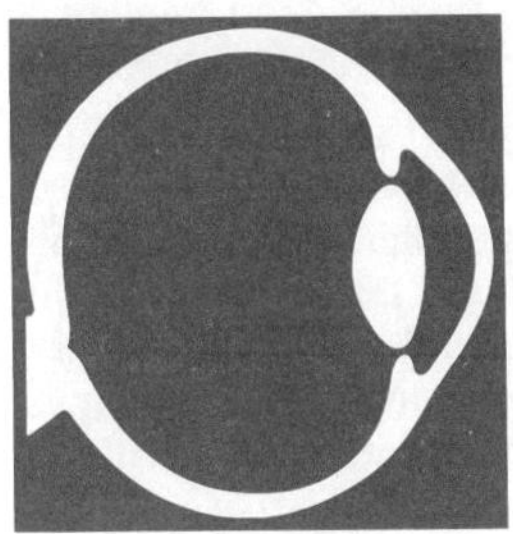

Eyes and Vision

Introduction

244 The priceless sense of sight

People rely mainly on vision to give them accurate information about their environment. It has been estimated that about 90% of the information sent to a person's brain enters the nervous system through his eyes. Because of this, sight is the physical sense the majority of people value most. What does this mean to you as a nurse? For one thing, a person who is experiencing changes or disturbances in his vision can feel a great deal of anxiety. You need to approach assessment of a patient's eyes and vision with extreme care and heightened sensitivity for his state of mind.

Don't let your respect for the delicate nature of the eye intimidate you into thinking that only an ophthalmologist is qualified to assess the visual system. As a nurse, you should be able to accurately and confidently assess a patient's eyes and vision—not only to recognize signs and symptoms of primary ophthalmologic disorders but also of disorders in other body systems that may have eye manifestations. For example, a jaundiced sclera may be the first sign of liver disease, ptosis can indicate a cerebrovascular accident, and subtle changes on a patient's retina can signal the onset of visual changes from diabetes mellitus or the beginning of retinopathy from hypertension.

With your assessment data in hand, you can arrive at meaningful nursing diagnoses. (An effective care plan, too, depends on your assessment data.) You also can be instrumental in the following ways:

- clarifying patients' and families' misconceptions about eye disorders and their treatment. Patients often get their information about the implications of a disorder from family and friends—and misinformation can cause a patient to experience extreme anxiety.
- preventing a patient's social withdrawal and isolation from decreased sensory input
- helping the patient adjust to temporary or permanent physical limitations
- helping the patient and his family plan for the future with realistic expectations.

You can also teach your patients about prevention of eye disease and accidents, the importance of regular eye examinations, and the need for prompt treatment of eye disorders. The National Society for the Prevention of Blindness has estimated that at least 50% of all cases of sight loss are preventable. As a health-care provider who has frequent and easy access to patients, you can play a key role in helping people preserve this vital physical sense.

Reviewing anatomy and physiology

245 Bony orbit

Each of the two *bony orbits* that contain the eyeballs is a space in the skull that resembles a pyramid with the apex pointing back and the base lying forward and laterally. Each has four walls—a medial wall, a lateral wall, a roof, and a floor—formed by parts of seven bones. The walls of each orbit also form the lateral wall of the nose, the floor for the cerebrum's frontal lobes, and the roof of the maxillary sinus.

The orbits' medial walls, each about 2″ (5 cm) long, run parallel to each other, approximately 1″ (2.5 cm) apart. The lateral walls, each of which is also about 2″ (5 cm) long, extend at a 90° angle to each other. Their structure allows for greater lateral gaze and increased peripheral vision.

Each orbit contains seven openings, at the junctions of its walls, that conduct nerves and blood vessels through the orbit: the optic, oculomotor, trochlear, ophthalmic (part of the trigeminal), and abducens cranial nerves, and the ophthalmic artery and veins.

One of the internal carotid artery's 10 branches, the *ophthalmic artery,* alone provides blood to the orbital structures. It also supplies arterial blood to the eyelids and parts of the nose and forehead. The *central retinal artery,* a branch of the ophthalmic artery, pierces the optic nerve's center and travels through the nerve to nourish the retina. The *superior* and *inferior*

ANATOMY OF THE EYE

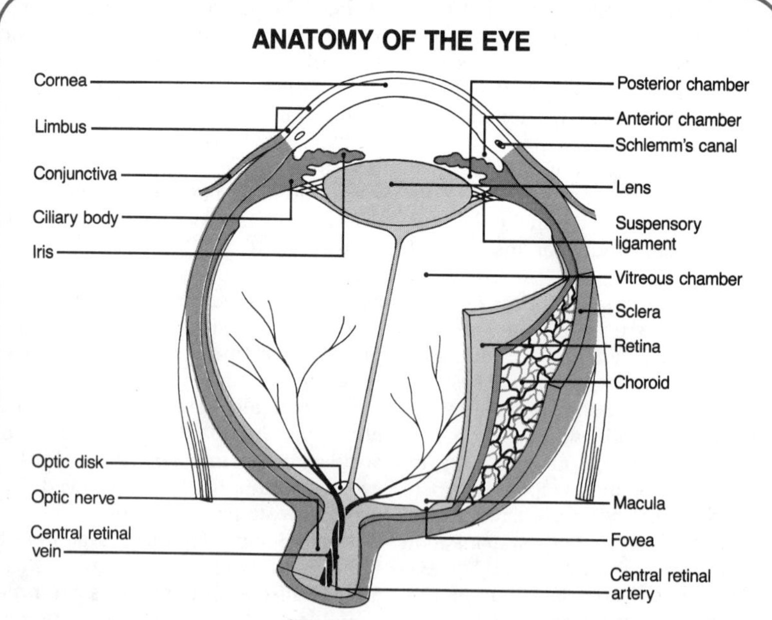

This lateral cross section shows the three layers of the eye: the external or *fibrous* layer, which contains the sclera and cornea; the middle or *vascular* layer, which contains the choroid, ciliary body, and iris; and the internal or *nervous* layer, which contains the retina.

UNDERSTANDING VISUAL PATHWAYS

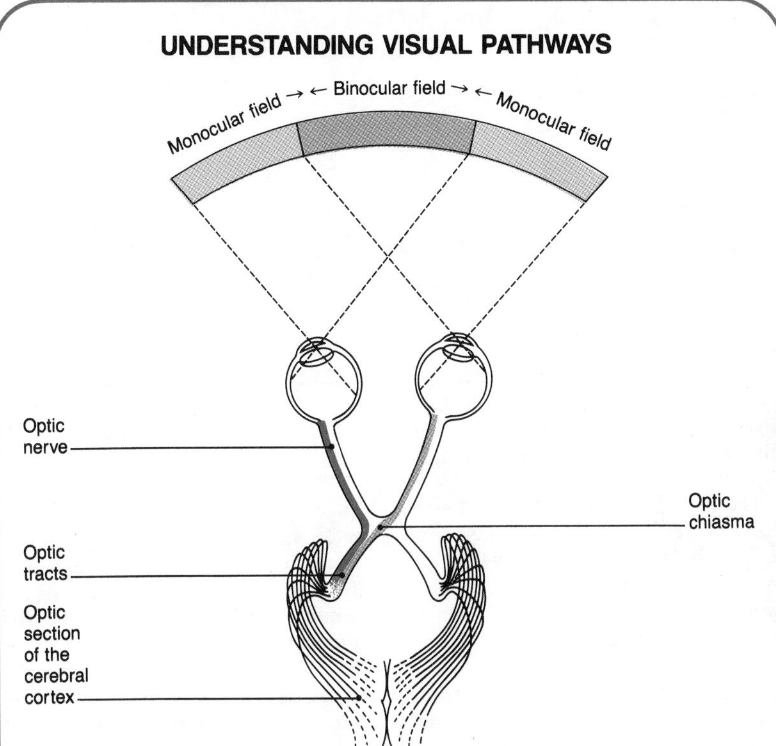

Vision and ocular reflexes depend on the visual pathway. Normally, vision is *binocular*, involving the overlap of each eye's monocular field. Binocular vision allows for a larger visual field and for depth perception. Because both eyes are involved, they move identically so that images fall on the same point of each retina; if they don't, double vision results. The image projected on each retina is inverted and reversed.

The visual pathway begins with the rods and cones of the retina, which turn the projected image into an impulse and transmit it to the *optic nerve.* The impulse then travels to the *optic chiasma,* where the two optic nerves unite, split again into two *optic tracts,* and then continue into the optic section of the cerebral cortex. This is where the inverted and reversed image on the retina is changed back to its original form.

In the optic chiasma, fibers from the nasal aspects of both retinas cross to opposite sides; fibers from the temporal portions remain uncrossed. Both crossed and uncrossed fibers form the optic tracts. Whereas injury to one of the optic nerves results in total blindness in the corresponding eye, an injury or lesion in the optic chiasma results in a partial visual loss; for example, loss of the two temporal visual fields.

ophthalmic veins drain blood from the orbit. These veins don't contain valves, so blood flows through them in either direction.

246 Eyelids and accessory structures

The *eyelids* (palpebrae) are two movable folds that protect the exposed portion of the eyeball and keep the cornea moist with tears. The upper lid is larger than the lower lid. It contains a levator muscle that also makes it more mobile. The oval opening between the eyelids is called the *palpebral fissure.*

Where the eyelids meet at the corners of the eye, they form the *medial canthus* and *lateral canthus.* Four small open-

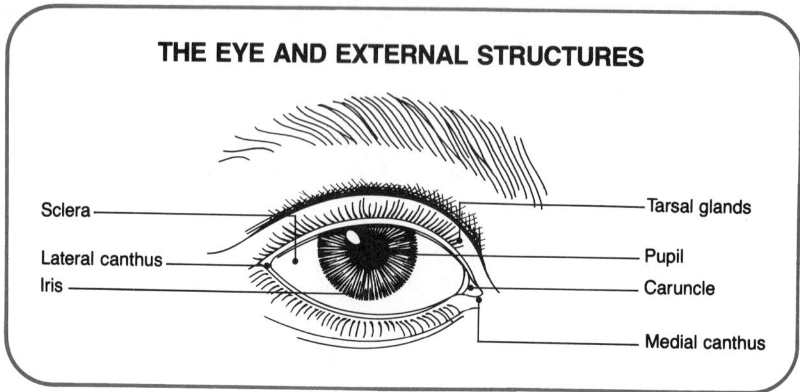

ings called *puncta,* located at the medial end of each eyelid, open into the canaliculi.

The innermost layer of eyelid tissue, the *conjunctiva,* is a thin, transparent membrane that lines the eyelids and the anterior surface of the eyeball. *Eyelashes* are short, thick hairs attached to the lid margins.

The eyelids contain three types of glands, which open on the lid margins. The *tarsal glands* (also known as *meibomian glands*) are modified sebaceous glands. They secrete an oily substance that helps prevent tears from evaporating rapidly. The *glands of Zeis* also secrete an oily layer of the tear film. *Moll's glands* are modified sweat glands that lie between the eyelashes.

247 Lacrimal apparatus

The lacrimal apparatus is composed of lacrimal glands, lacrimal canaliculi, lacrimal sac, and nasolacrimal duct. Its primary function is to produce and excrete tears, which maintain the wet epithelium covering the eyeball's exposed surface. Tears have bactericidal properties and also flush foreign bodies from the eye.

The larger portion of the lacrimal gland lies in the upper, outer portion of the bony orbit. The smaller portion is in the upper eyelid. These glands produce and excrete tears, which are spread over the cornea and conjunctiva by blinking, and then drain into the nose.

248 Sclera and cornea

The eyeball is a sphere embedded in fat within the bony orbit. It consists of an outer fibrous layer, a middle vascular layer, and an inner nervous layer. The outer fibrous layer is made up of the sclera and the cornea. The white, opaque *sclera* covers the posterior five sixths of the eyeball, continuing back to the dural sheath surrounding the optic nerve. The *cornea* is the transparent anterior part of the fibrous coat that bulges forward. Although it has no blood vessels, the cornea contains many sensory nerve fibers, making it highly sensitive to pain. At the limbus (the junction of the sclera and the cornea), the sinus venosus sclerae (Schlemm's canal) encircles the eyeball and drains aqueous humor from the anterior chamber into the bloodstream to maintain intraocular pressure. It also supplies oxygen and nutrients to the anterior segment of the eye.

249 Choroid, ciliary body, and iris

The eyeball's middle vascular layer (uveal tract) comprises the choroid, the ciliary body, and the iris. The *choroid* lines the recessed part of the eyeball beneath the sclera and contains many small arteries and veins, connected to a rich capillary plexus. This vascular system nourishes the retina and channels blood to other portions of the eye.

The *ciliary body* is the anterior continuation of the choroid. It consists of bundles of smooth muscle attached to fibers of the *suspensory ligament* that suspends the lens and facilitates accommodation. The ciliary body also contains from 60 to 80 *ciliary processes* that produce aqueous humor.

The *iris,* the colored part of the anterior eyeball, is made of smooth-muscle fibers. Its color, determined by the amount and distribution of its melanin pigment, ranges from light blue to dark brown. Within the iris, the muscle fibers control the size of the *pupil*—the iris' central opening—by expansion and contraction of the iris in response to the amount of light entering the eye.

250 Retina

The function of the *retina,* the eyeball's innermost coat, is to receive visual stimuli, partly analyze these images, and send the information to the brain. The retina consists of ten layers. Of these, the outer layer contains pigmented epithelium; the inner layer is light-sensitive and contains photoreceptor cells called *rods* and *cones.* The axons of the ganglionic layer of these cells form the *optic nerve,* which exits the retina at the *optic disk.* The only part of the central nervous system that can be seen, the optic disk contains no photoreceptors and thus constitutes the retina's blind spot.

The cones, which function best in bright light, provide detailed color vision. Cones are more numerous toward the *macula,* the center of the retina. The *fovea,* the center of the macula and the sharpest area of vision on the retina, is smaller than a pinhead and contains only specialized cones. The eye accomplishes its most detailed vision within this tiny area. In light too dim to stimulate cones, the fovea is blind.

The rods, which are most numerous in the periphery of the retina, provide vision in dim light. Their stimulation results in neutral, gray perceptions. As darkness increases, perception shifts from the cones to the rods. The rods

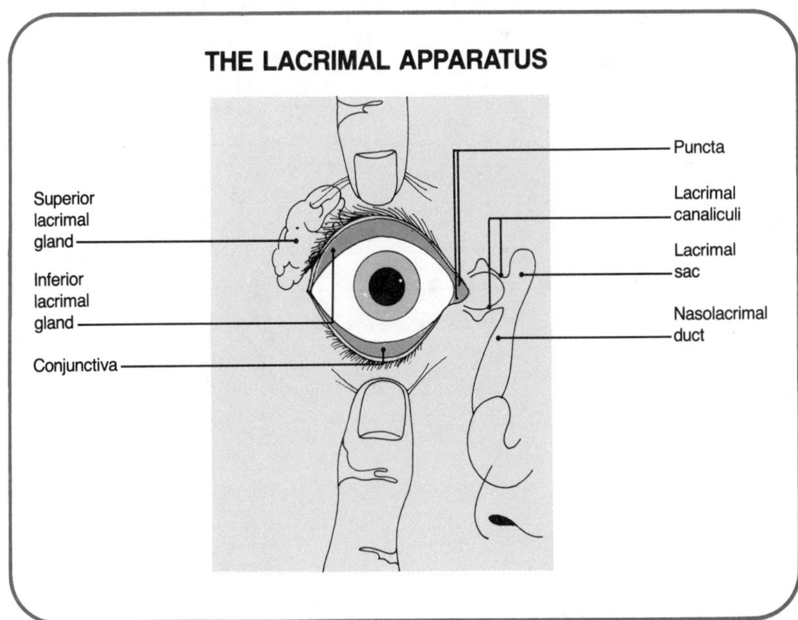

are also important in detecting movement of objects under lighted conditions.

251 Interior eye chambers

The eyeball's interior contains the anterior, the posterior, and the vitreous chambers. The *anterior chamber* and the *posterior chamber,* both filled with aqueous humor, form the *aqueous chamber,* which lies in front of the lens. The *vitreous chamber,* filled with vitreous humor, is a much larger compartment that lies behind the lens and occupies about four fifths of the eyeball.

Formed by the capillaries of the ciliary processes, *aqueous humor* is a clear, watery, slightly alkaline substance secreted continuously into the posterior chamber behind the iris. It circulates forward into the anterior chamber and then drains through the sinus venosus sclerae (Schlemm's canal). *Vitreous humor*—a transparent, gelatinous mass—fills the vitreous chamber. Its semisolid consistency prevents the eyeball from collapsing under extraocular pressure. Avascular, it receives nourishment from retinal blood vessels and the ciliary processes.

252 Refraction and accommodation

The *lens* is a transparent, encapsulated, biconvex structure held in place by the suspensory ligament. It has a firm central core and a soft outer rim. Posteriorly, it rests in a depression in the vitreous body; anteriorly, it contacts the free border of the iris.

The lens and the cornea are the principal structures of the eye that refract, or bend, light rays to focus them precisely on the retina so that (in a normal eye) a clear image may be seen. The shape of the cornea and of the lens, as well as the eyeball's length, determine where the light rays converge on the retina. To focus on objects closer than 20′ (6 m), the lens bulges and becomes more spherical—a process called *ac-*

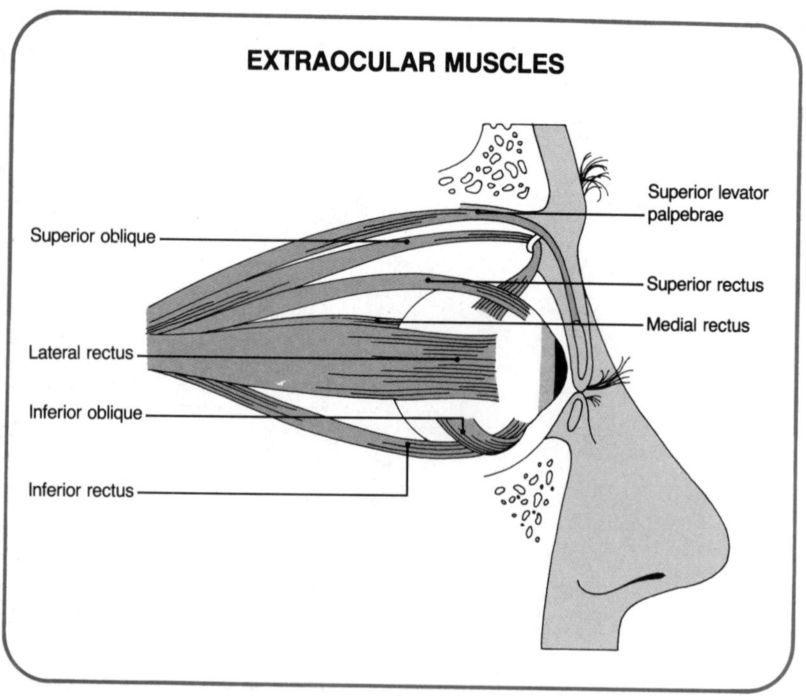

HOW THE EYEBALL MOVES

Six extraocular muscles control eyeball movement. To understand how they work, imagine three planes bisecting the eyeball.

- The *vertical* plane runs through the eyeball from top to bottom.
- The *transverse* plane runs through the eyeball from side to side.
- The *anteroposterior* plane runs through the eyeball from front to back.

Each of these planes contains an imaginary *axis* around which the eyeball rotates.

As you can see from these illustrations, each muscle has a main function and several additional functions. Which function it performs depends on which muscle group it's working with at a particular time. For example, the main function of the superior rectus is elevation, to rotate the eyeball upward on the transverse axis. It also performs these functions: adduction (to rotate the eyeball inward on the vertical axis) and intorsion (to rotate the eyeball to the right on the anteroposterior axis).

Remember that muscles of one eye work together, either supplementing or limiting one another's movements. Also, these muscles work together with the same muscles of the other eye to create simultaneous movement.

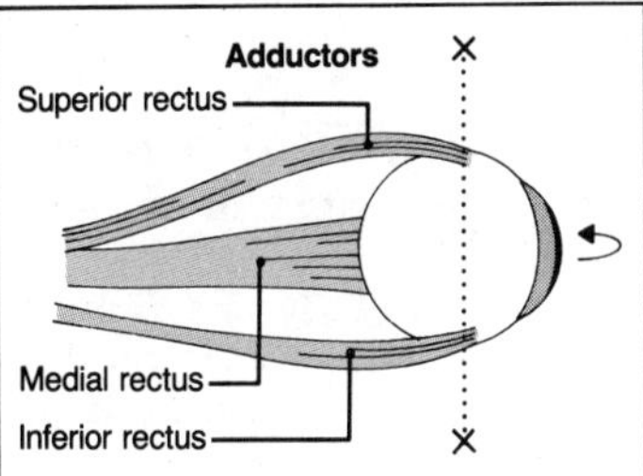

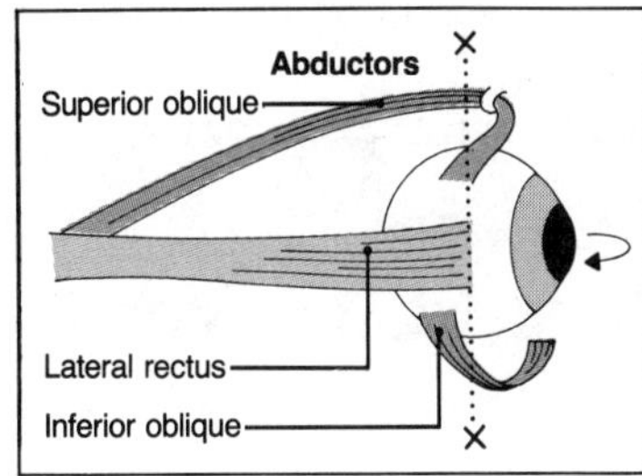

On the *vertical* axis, the *adductors* and *abductors* rotate the eyeball to the left and to the right.

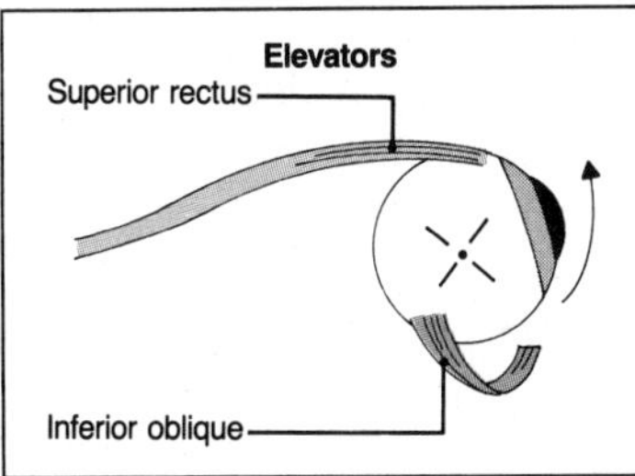

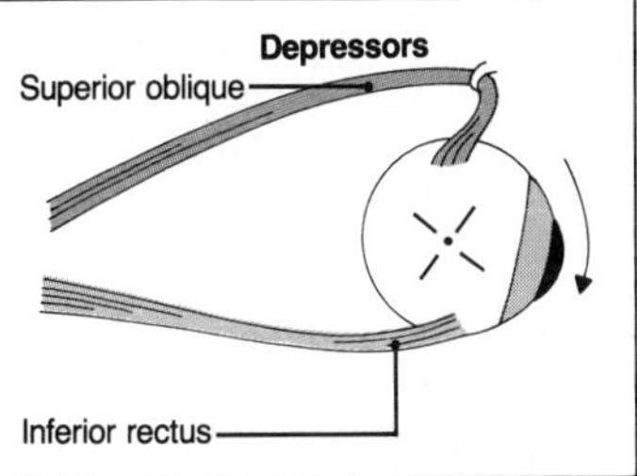

On the *transverse* axis, the *elevators* and *depressors* rotate the eyeball up and down.

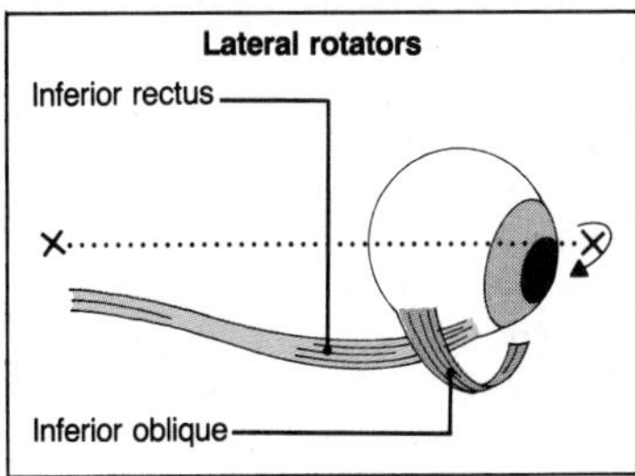

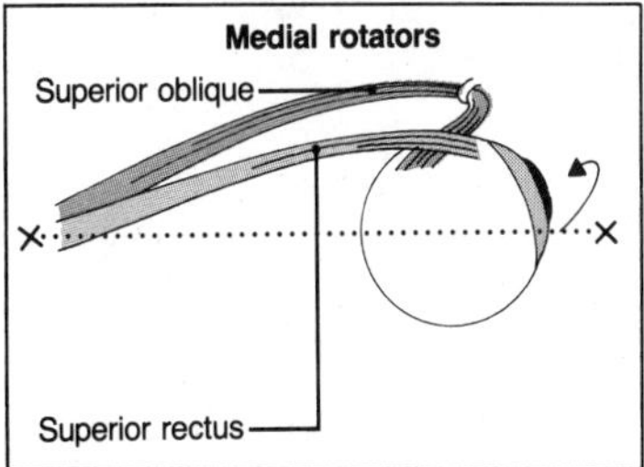

On the *anteroposterior* axis, the *medial* and *lateral* rotators rotate the eyeball in a circular fashion, either to the left (extorsion) or to the right (intorsion).

commodation. To do this, the ciliary muscle contracts, reducing tension on the suspensory ligament and allowing the lens to change shape. The lens becomes more spherical, because light rays must converge more sharply to focus on a close object than with a more distant object. The lens flattens when the muscle relaxes.

253 How the eyeball moves

Seven extraocular muscles control eyeball and upper eyelid movements. The *levator palpebrae superioris* raises the upper eyelid. The other six muscles move the eyeball within its socket. (See *How the Eyeball Moves,* page 211.)

The eyeball moves in relation to three axes (vertical, transverse, and anteroposterior) that pass through its center. These movements include abduction (direct lateral movement), adduction (direct medial movement), elevation, depression, and medial and lateral rotation. (These movements constitute the six cardinal fields of gaze.) Although each muscle has a specific mode of action, they all work together and reciprocally during most eye movements. (An exception is convergence—focusing on close objects.) Three cranial nerves innervate the extraocular muscles.

Collecting appropriate history data

254 Biographical data

Biographical data don't have particular significance in assessing patients with eye and vision disorders. Just obtain the information you need from your patient for identification purposes.

255 Chief complaint

Four groups of signs and symptoms constitute the most common chief complaints regarding the eyes and vision:
- pain/discomfort
- vision changes
- tearing/secretion
- appearance changes.

Vision changes include complaints about decreased or absent vision as well as blurred or double vision. Also in this category are reports of seeing distorted images, colors or lights, and floating particles. Complaints of pain and discomfort include tenderness or pressure. Changes in eye appearance include the presence of a lump or foreign body.

256 History of present illness

Using the PQRST mnemonic device, ask the patient to elaborate on his chief complaint. Then, depending on the complaint, explore the history of this present illness by asking the following types of questions:

- ***Decreased or absent vision.*** *Is your vision clearer in one eye than in the other?* Gradual visual loss usually indicates a chronic problem that may be correctable. Sudden visual loss is an ocular emergency that may indicate retinal artery or vein occlusion. *Do you see a blind spot? If so, does it move with eye movement? Is the problem in the center of your field of vision, or at the side? Does it occur only at night?* Visual loss in one specific area (scotoma) results from retinal or optic pathway damage. Reduced night vision can be from retinal degeneration.
- ***Blurred or double vision.*** *Does a shade, or curtain, seem to be covering your field of vision?* Find out whether the condition is constant or can be relieved by an action such as squinting. *Is it related to fatigue or eyestrain? Is it worse in the morning, or in the evening? In the dark, or in the light?*
- ***Distorted images, colors, or lights.*** *Does what you see look bent or warped?*

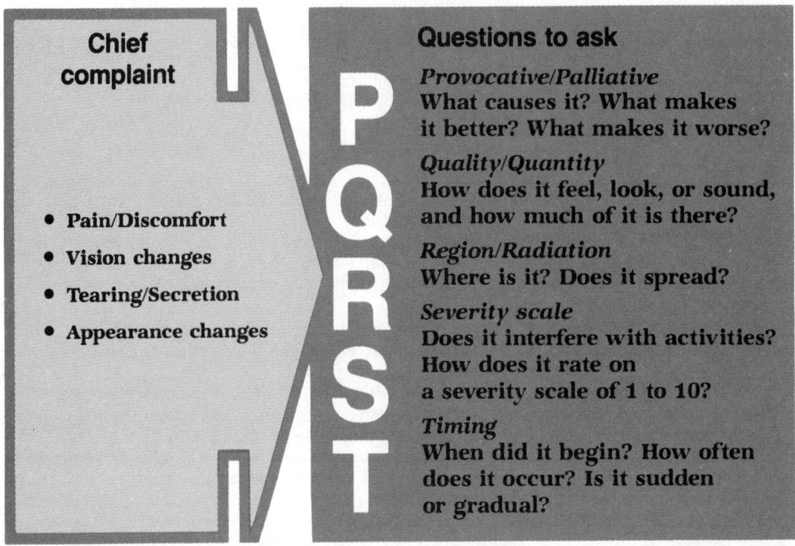

Is it difficult to differentiate colors, or do the colors blend together? Positive responses to these questions may indicate retinal disease. *Do you see lights or halos?* These symptoms may indicate acute glaucoma, cataracts, or corneal disease.

• ***Floating particles.*** *Do you see many particles, or only a few?* Seeing only a few spots is usually not significant. The sudden occurrence of many floaters, commonly described as *sooty vision,* may indicate vitreous detachment—a possible precursor of retinal detachment or intraocular inflammation.

• ***Pain and discomfort.*** *Is the pain on the eye, or does it seem to be in the eye? Is it worse at night?* Glaucoma and intraocular infections cause deep-seated pain that worsens at night. *Does it feel better when you keep your eyes closed? Does blinking make it better or worse?* Keeping the eyes closed relieves pain caused by infections, foreign bodies, or corneal injuries. Blinking makes it worse. *Does bright light cause pain in your eyes?* Photophobia may indicate an inflammation or injury involving the eye's external structures. *Do you sense pressure behind or around the eyes? Do your eyes feel as if they're bulging?* Brain tumors can cause pressure behind the eye, whereas diseases of the orbit can cause pressure around it. Thyroid disease can cause exophthalmos (bulging eyes), which may produce discomfort from conjunctival or corneal irritation.

• ***Lump or foreign body.*** *Does the lump or foreign body seem to be on the eyeball, or on the lid? Does it move with eye movement?* A stye (hordeolum) can feel like a lump or foreign body in one area of the eye or eyelid. A foreign body will move with blinking, unless it's imbedded in the cornea.

• ***Discharge.*** *What color is the discharge? Is it thick, or watery? Do you wake up with your eyelids stuck together?*

• ***Itching or redness.*** *Does the itching occur in a particular circumstance or environment? Do other parts of your body itch at the same time?* Itching is usually a symptom of allergy. *When did you first notice the redness—under what conditions? Did it seem to relate to a particular incident?* Redness may result from infection, trauma, or allergy.

• ***Excessive tearing or dryness.*** *Do your eyes tear a great deal?* Excessive

EMERGENCY

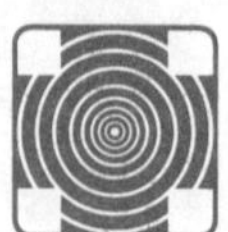

ASSESSING OCULAR TRAUMA

The patient with ocular trauma needs your immediate help. Notify the doctor, then quickly follow these emergency steps:

- Identify the nature and extent of the injury. Is it a blunt trauma—for example, from a cosmetic applicator; a penetrating injury—for example, from a BB gun pellet; or a chemical burn—for example, from lye in a drain cleaner? (Remember, he may also have other injuries that require immediate attention.)
- In a case of blunt trauma or a penetrating injury, have the patient lie down. Place a plastic or metal shield over the eye to prevent further injury until the doctor arrives. Then help the doctor treat and bandage the eye.

  In the case of a chemical burn, irrigate the eye with at least 1 qt (950 ml) of water. Be careful not to touch the eye with the irrigating catheter's tip. Also, never direct the irrigation flow toward the nasal cavity. To check the effectiveness of the irrigation, test the pH level of the inferior cul-de-sac by inserting litmus paper. Irrigate until the pH level returns to normal.
- Ask the patient about his past medical history. Especially note any allergies, current medications, and the date of his last tetanus shot.
- Following treatment, you'll want to test the patient's visual acuity. He'll need a complete eye examination, including a dilated fundus examination performed by an ophthalmologist.

tearing can result from chemical irritation, allergies, inflammation, or obstruction of the lacrimal drainage system. *Are your eyes excessively dry? How long have they felt dry?* Dryness occurs with aging and in several collagen disorders. Some people taking tranquilizers will report that their eyes feel dry.

257 Past history

Ask about the following health considerations and problems:

- ***Vision care.*** *Do you normally wear glasses or contact lenses? If so, who prescribed them, and how long ago? How many pairs do you have? What type of correction is involved? When did you have your last eye examination? Were you tested for glaucoma?* Visual symptoms, such as blurred vision, headaches, and eyestrain, can result from wearing improperly prescribed lenses.
- ***Allergies.*** *Has any allergy ever affected your eyes? Have you ever had a reaction to eye medications? If so, what happened, and what relieved it?* Both local allergies and systemic allergies can cause symptoms of eye disorders.
- ***Medications.*** *Do you use eye drops, ointments, or washes regularly? Why do you use them? How do your eyes react?* Repeated use of unprescribed eye medications sometimes can precipitate, rather than relieve, visual signs and symptoms. *What other medications are you using?* Note any regular use of systemic medications that can cause visual changes (see *Nurse's Guide to Some Drugs with Possible Ocular Side Effects*).
- ***Neurologic disorders.*** Visual changes may be seen in some neurologic disorders (see Entries 609 and 635).
- ***Endocrine disorders.*** Longstanding diabetes causes degenerative changes in the retinal vasculature that, if untreated, can lead to blindness. Thyroid disorders can also damage eye structures and affect eye function.
- ***Circulatory disorders.*** Damage to the retinal vasculature or the optic nerve can result from hypertension, hyperviscosity syndromes, or impaired circulation that decreases the oxygen and nutrient supply. Cerebrovascular accident may cause vision problems, such as diplopia.

DRUGS

NURSE'S GUIDE TO SOME DRUGS WITH POSSIBLE OCULAR SIDE EFFECTS

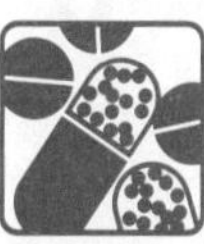

CLASSIFICATION	POSSIBLE SIDE EFFECTS
Antimalarials	
chloroquine (Aralen HCl)	• Corneal opacity, retinopathy, blurred vision, focusing difficulty
quinine sulfate (Coco-Quinine)	• Altered color vision, night blindness, photophobia, blurred vision, amblyopia
Antituberculars and antileprotics	
ethambutol (Myambutol*)	• Altered color vision, optic neuritis
isoniazid (Hyzyd)	• Optic neuritis, optic atrophy
streptomycin sulfate	• Nystagmus, blurred vision, extraocular muscle palsies
Cardiotonic glycosides	
digitalis leaf (Digifortis)	• Altered color vision, blurred vision, photophobia, diplopia
Corticosteroids	
prednisone (Meticorten)	• Cataracts, glaucoma
Diuretics	
hydrochlorothiazide (Hydro-Diuril*)	• Altered color vision, transient blurred vision
Nonnarcotic analgesics	
indomethacin (Indocin)	• Corneal opacity, blurred vision, retinal damage
phenylbutazone (Butazolidin*)	• Optic neuritis, blurred vision, retinal hemorrhage or detachment
Oral contraceptives	
estrogen with progestogen (Enovid)	• Worsening of myopia or astigmatism, intolerance to contact lenses
Phenothiazines	
chlorpromazine (Thorazine)	• Cataracts, retinopathy, visual impairment
Sedatives and hypnotics	
ethchlorvynol (Placidyl*)	• Optic neuritis, nystagmus, diplopia
Sulfonamides	
sulfisoxazole (Gantrisin)	• Periorbital edema, conjunctival and scleral injection
Vitamins	
vitamin D (Calciferol)	• Corneal and conjunctival calcifications

*Available in U.S. and Canada. All other products (no symbol) available in U.S. only.

• ***Hepatic and renal disorders.*** Disturbances of the liver's ability to detoxify chemicals (such as cirrhosis or liver failure) or of the kidney's ability to eliminate wastes (such as pyelonephritis or glomerulonephritis) can affect both neural and vascular eye structures.

258 Family history

Note any family history of *early vision loss, retinitis pigmentosa, strabismus, chronic glaucoma,* or *cataracts.* Also note if the patient's mother had an illness, such as *rubella,* during pregnancy.

259 Psychosocial history

Your patient's *occupation* is the main aspect of the psychosocial history. Ask whether he's routinely exposed to dust, smoke, chemical spraying, flying debris, or other irritants or hazards. If so, does he wear safety goggles or take any other precautions?

260 Activities of daily living

When you review your patient's activities of daily living, cover these areas:

• ***Smoking.*** *Do you smoke cigarettes? How many packs a day, and for how many years?* Nicotine causes arterial constrictions that can produce visual symptoms.

• ***Alcohol.*** *Do you drink alcoholic beverages? At what age did you first begin drinking? How much do you drink?* A type of amblyopia can result from heavy consumption of alcoholic beverages, especially in conjunction with heavy cigarette smoking. At times an alcoholic may suffer acute transient periods of blindness.

• ***Recreation.*** *Do you participate in sports that pose a hazard to your glasses or contact lenses, or that make you susceptible to eye injury?* Eye injuries are common in racquet sports. Swimming can cause eye infections.

• ***Cosmetics.*** *Do you regularly wear eye makeup?* Containers for eye makeup are excellent culture media for bacteria. Also ask if the patient uses lotions near the eyes.

• ***Self-care.*** *Do you sometimes burn yourself when cooking? Do you bump into things often?* A patient may be able to best describe his visual problem in terms of how it alters his activities.

261 Review of systems

Focus your questions on the following relevant areas:

• ***General.*** *Fever* that causes eye burning and tenderness can result from an infectious process.

• ***Skin.*** *Scabbing* and *crusting* result from infections and dermatoses.

• ***Cardiovascular.*** *Hypertension* and *arteriosclerosis* cause vascular changes in the eye.

• ***Gastrointestinal.*** *Nausea* and *vomiting* may occur with prolonged, elevated intraocular pressure.

• ***Nervous.*** *Motor disturbances from myasthenia gravis or multiple sclerosis can affect the eyes. Headache* can be caused by increased intraocular pressure, extraocular muscle imbalances, or space-occupying lesions (which may also cause visual disturbances).

• ***Musculoskeletal.*** *Muscle weakness, joint pain,* and *stiffness* may indicate a dystrophic or autoimmune disorder that can affect eye musculature.

• ***Hematopoietic and immune.*** *Anemias* can cause retinal changes.

Conducting the physical examination

262 Preparing for an eye examination

The best environment for an eye examination is a quiet room, free of distractions, in which you can control the lighting and make the patient comfortable. Be sure you have the following equipment on hand:

• Snellen or E chart (to test distance vision)

• Jaeger or Lebensohn card (to test near vision)

• hand light or penlight

• cover card or eye cover
• direct ophthalmoscope
• cotton-tipped applicator (to evert eyelids).

263 Testing distance vision

With most patients, use the Snellen chart to test distance vision (see *Using the Snellen Chart,* page 218). Make sure the chart is well-lighted and without glare.

Seat the patient 20′ (6 m) away from the chart. If he's wearing glasses or contact lenses, ask him to remove them so you can test his uncorrected vision first. Begin with the right eye. Have the patient occlude the left eye. Then, ask him to read the smallest line of letters he can see on the chart.

Visual acuity is recorded as a fraction: The numerator is the distance from the chart, and the denominator is the distance at which a normal eye can read this line. Record the fraction assigned to the smallest line your patient can read. A person who can read the 20/20 line on the Snellen chart is considered to have normal distance vision. If your patient's distance vision tests at less than 20/20, use a pinhole occluder and perform the test again; his tested vision may improve if it's a refractive error.

Now repeat the test for the patient's left eye, with the right eye occluded. If your patient wears glasses or contact lenses, use the same procedure to test his corrected vision.

If your patient can't read the largest letter on the Snellen chart from a distance of 20′, ask him to approach the chart until he *can* read it. Then record the distance between him and the chart. For example, if the patient can see the 20/200 line of the eye chart from a distance of 3′ (1 m), record the test result as *3′/200.*

Your patient's distance vision may be so poor that he can barely count the number of fingers you hold up in front of him. If he can count fingers (CF) at 2′ (61 cm), record his distance vision as *CF at 2′*. If the patient can't see your fingers, try hand movements (HM) at a distance of 2′. Move your hand up and down or from side to side, and ask him which way your hand is moving. If he responds correctly, record the result as *HM at 2′*. (Sometimes a patient may be able to see better if he turns his head slightly.)

A patient may have only light perception in his eyes from such disorders as trauma, dense cataracts, retinal degeneration, or hemorrhage. To test light perception (LP), first occlude the patient's left eye. Then darken the room, position an ophthalmoscope in front of the patient's right eye, and begin switching the instrument's light on and off. Ask the patient if he sees the light; if he does, ask when he first sees it and when he stops seeing it, and if he can tell you the direction from which the light is coming. Then vary the quadrants of the light. If he responds correctly, record the result as *LP with projection.* If he can't see the light at all, record *NLP* (no light perception).

If your patient is illiterate, you can use an E chart to test his distance vision. Ask him which way the legs of the E are pointing. Record the results as you would with the Snellen chart.

264 Near vision testing

If the patient wears glasses or bifocals, he should wear them throughout this test. Ask him to hold a well-lighted Jaeger or Lebensohn card at a comfortable distance—about 14″ [35 cm]—from his eyes. (If you don't have a near vision card, use a newspaper page with different type sizes on it.) Then ask him to cover his left eye and read the smallest paragraph he can see clearly on the card. After recording the results, have the patient cover his right eye and repeat the test.

265 Color vision testing

Using color plates, such as the Ishihara and the Hardy-Rand-Ritter plates, is

USING THE SNELLEN CHART

You'll use a Snellen chart like the one shown here to test your patient's distance vision.

P 6/30 20/100

T Z 6/21 20/70

E C F D 6/12 20/40

F C Z P 6/9 20/30

D E F P T E C 6/6 20/20

the preferred method for determining a patient's ability to distinguish reds, greens, and blues. You can also ask your patient to distinguish between the red and green lines on the Snellen chart.

266 How to inspect the external eye

Begin by standing directly in front of the patient. Inspect his eyes for symmetry in size, shape, contour, and movement of the eyes and surrounding structures. Observe their alignment: Do the eyes look alike? Normally, the upper quarter of the iris can't be seen on frontal view because the eyelid covers it. Are the eyes entirely exposed? Or, do the lids droop (ptosis)? Ask the patient to close his eyes gently; check for complete lid closure. Inadequate lid closure may expose the cornea during sleep and cause drying and ulceration.

Next, examine the patient's eyelids for edema, inflammation, or masses. A *stye* (hordeolum) is a staphylococcal infection of the eyelid glands characterized by a localized red, swollen, acutely tender area on the lid margin. Located deep in the eyelid, a *chalazion* is a sterile inflammation of the meibomian glands (or the glands of Zeis) that's swollen but, unlike a stye, is painless. The inflammation is chronic and doesn't subside spontaneously.

Yellow plaques on the skin of the lids *(xanthelasma)*—usually at the medial canthal area—indicate increased lipid deposits in the patient's blood. Note the turgor of the lids, and any extra skin folds. Do the lids appear to have lost elasticity? Are the changes bilateral?

Note whether the lid margins turn inward *(entropion),* causing the lashes to scrape against the eyeball, or outward *(ectropion),* at times preventing complete closure of the eye. Examine the lid margins closely for erythema and scales. Are the lashes clean and free of debris? (Note whether the patient wears eye makeup.)

Palpate both the preauricular and submandibular lymph nodes. Then, palpate each bony orbit for pain, edema, and masses, noting the eye's size and shape. The eyeballs shouldn't protrude excessively from their orbits *(exophthalmos)* or appear abnormally sunken *(enophthalmos).* Eye position should be the same bilaterally.

Inspect the skin around the patient's eyes for plaques, moles, discoloration, redness, and scaliness. Carefully observe any growths, such as moles, for color, shape, and contour.

Examine the inside of the patient's lower lid. You'll notice an initial blanching from this maneuver; the normal pink color should reappear promptly. (If the lid remains pale, your patient may be anemic.) Inspect also for foreign bodies, such as lashes or traces of eye makeup. Evert the upper lid to check for infection, swelling, or foreign bodies. To do this, have the patient look down, then gently pinch the lashes of the upper lid and bend the lid back over a cotton-tipped applicator.

Inspect the conjunctiva and sclera by separating the patient's eyelids widely, avoiding excessive pressure on the eyeball by holding the lids against the ridge of the bony orbit. Then, ask him to look right and left, then up and down.

The conjunctiva should be clear and transparent, free of cloudiness and redness.

The normal sclera is white and quiescent. Black patients may show scattered areas of brown pigment—a normal finding. Blue discoloration may indicate scleral thinning.

Note any change from normal in the sclera's color or vascular bed. Often such changes are among the first symptoms of a systemic disorder (for example, the yellow sclera of jaundice).

267 Assessing extraocular muscle function

Assessing extraocular muscle function involves three tests: the corneal reflex, the cover-uncover test, and checking the six cardinal fields of gaze. (See *How to Test Extraocular Muscle Function,* page 220.)

To test your patient's corneal light reflex, stand directly in front of him, and hold a penlight or small flashlight at his eye level and 12″ to 15″ (30 to 38 cm) away. Ask him to stare straight ahead. Then shine the light directly between his eyes. You'll see a dot of light on each cornea; the dots should be in the same spot on the cornea and equidistant from his nose. If they are, your patient's reflex is symmetrical. An asymmetrical reflex indicates a deviating eye—possibly from a muscle imbalance.

This finding is your cue to perform the cover-uncover test to see if the patient can maintain parallel gaze, necessary for binocular vision. To perform this test, have him fixate on a distant object. Cover his left eye, and watch the right eye to see if it moves to remain fixed on the distant object. Next, uncover the left eye: If it jerks into position to fix on the object the eye has drifted while resting, which indicates a muscle imbalance. Repeat this procedure, in reverse, covering the right eye.

You can test extraocular muscle function further by checking the fields of gaze. Hold a pencil or tongue depressor in front of your patient. Ask him to keep his head still and follow the object with his eyes as you move it clockwise, tracing the six cardinal fields of gaze. Stop at each field, and observe the patient's eyes. Note if they jerk *(nystagmus).* Minor nystagmus is normal only in the extreme lateral gaze. Consider all other nystagmus findings abnormal. Also note any *eye deviation.* If one of the patient's eyes deviates nasally, record the movement as *esotropic (ET).* Record temporal deviation as *exotropic (XT).* Record an upward deviation as *hypertropic (HT).*

268 Assessing peripheral vision

Confrontation visual field testing provides gross estimates of your patient's peripheral vision and also serves as a useful screening procedure for partial vision loss. (To perform this test, *you* must have normal peripheral vision.) Sit directly opposite the patient at a distance of about 2′ (60 cm). Have the patient cover his left eye while you cover your right eye. Then ask the patient to fixate on your nose or uncovered eye. Hold a brightly colored object, pencil, or penlight in your left hand, and extend your left arm to the side. Ask the patient to maintain his gaze while you slowly move the object into his line of vision, and to tell you when he first sees it. Use your own visual field as the normal for this test. Examine all quadrants of the patient's right eye (both directions horizontally, from above and from below); then examine his left eye in the same way.

If your patient's visual field is significantly constricted, more sophisti-

HOW TO TEST EXTRAOCULAR MUSCLE FUNCTION

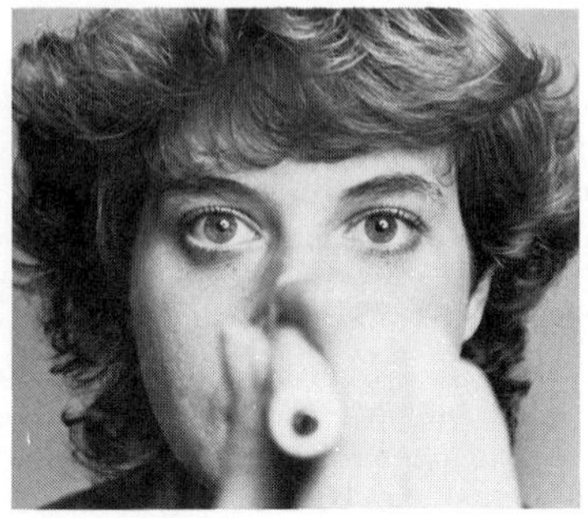

When performing the corneal light reflex test, watch the dots of light for symmetrical or asymmetrical positioning.

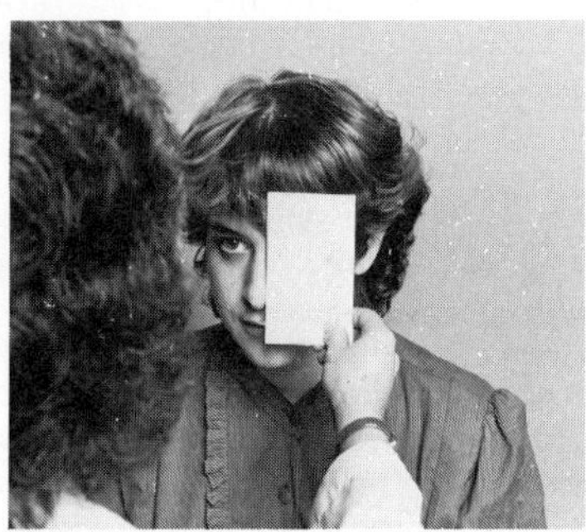

Use the cover-uncover test to evaluate your patient's eye muscles for weakness or imbalance.

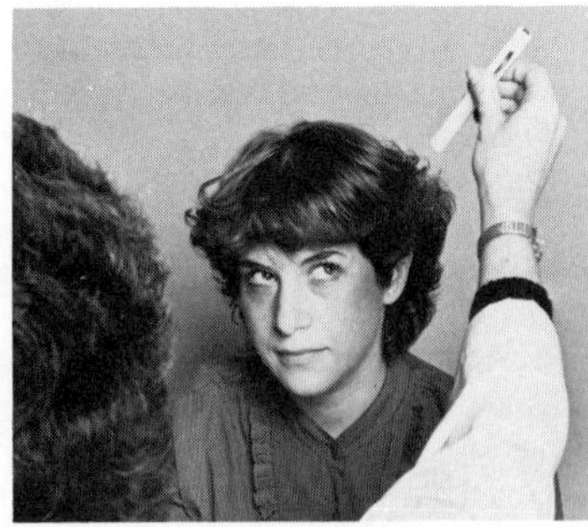

When testing the six cardinal fields of gaze, note normal and abnormal nystagmus.

cated testing (such as perimetry or a tangent screen examination) may be required to obtain further data.

269 How to measure intraocular pressure

Two kinds of tonometers are available: the indentation (Schiøtz) tonometer and the applanation (Goldmann) tonometer. As part of a general physical examination, the Schiøtz tonometer—which measures the depth of indentation produced on the cornea—is most commonly used.

For this test, have the patient lie on his back. Explain that he must keep both eyes open for this test and must fixate on a target (use a spot on the ceiling, positioned directly above his eyes). Reassure him that although you'll be touching his eye with an instrument, he won't feel any discomfort.

Then, instill a topical eye anesthetic, such as 0.5% tetracaine hydrochloride, and wait 15 to 20 seconds.

Now, gently retract the patient's upper and lower lids and, holding the tonometer vertically, rest the curved footplate gently on the center of the cornea. Don't put pressure on the eyeball. Note the position of the pointer on the scale. To determine the tension, refer to the table of measures that accompanies the tonometer (see *Applanation and Indentation Tonometers*). An average reading falls between 5 and 6 units on the tonometer scale and translates to a tension of between 12 and 20 mm Hg. Generally, the lower the reading on the tonometer scale, the higher the tension.

If the patient squeezes his eyelids together, it will falsely elevate the tension. Instruct him repeatedly to look at the fixation point with his other eye. This will distract him, relieve the tension in the eyelids, and enable him to be more cooperative. If the tonometer scale reads 3 units or less, use the 7.5 g weight or the 10 g weight and repeat the test.

After testing the right eye, repeat the procedure with the left eye.

APPLANATION AND INDENTATION TONOMETERS

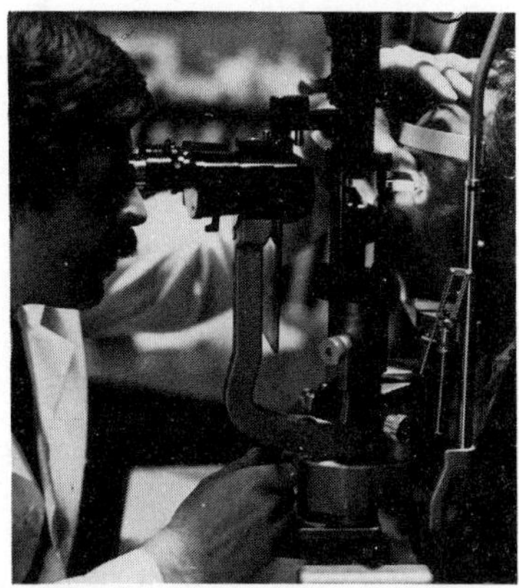

Applanation tonometry determines intraocular pressure by measuring the force required to flatten a small area of the central cornea. The Goldmann tonometer, shown here, is the most widely used applanation tonometer.

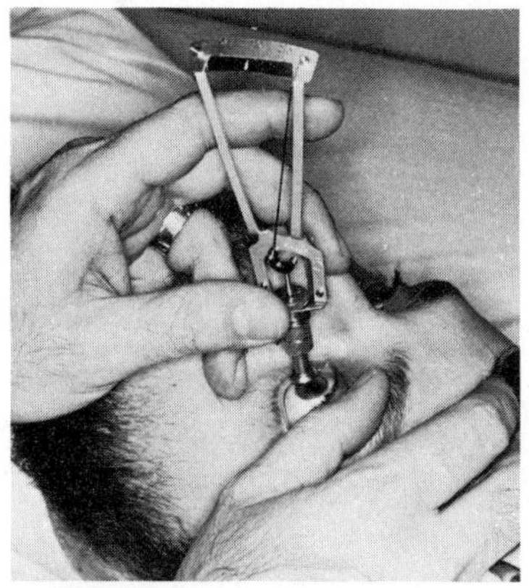

Indentation tonometry tests the resistance of the eyeball to extraocular pressure by measuring, on a calibrated scale, how deeply a known weight depresses the cornea. The Schiøtz tonometer, shown here, is the most widely used indentation tonometer.

270 Inspecting the cornea and anterior chamber

Inspect your patient's corneas for haziness, abnormal light reflex, and blood vessels. Direct a penlight beam slowly over all corneal areas. You should observe the light reflecting evenly across each cornea.

During corneal inspection, you can easily assess the anterior chamber—which should be clean, deep, shadow-free, and filled with clear aqueous humor.

If your patient's blink reflex is not obvious, test his corneal reflex (see *Testing the Corneal Reflex,* page 222).

271 Inspecting the iris and pupil

When inspecting the iris, note its color, size, shape, texture, and pattern. Look for evidence of previous surgery—such as sector iridectomy, which may appear as a wedge-shaped or roughly circular dark opening. Also inspect for evidence of trauma; for example, iris prolapse may be signaled by hyphema or a ragged, irregular pupil.

Your patient's pupils should be of equal size and roundness (although about 25% of the population have unequally sized pupils). Normal pupil size (which varies at different ages and from patient to patient) generally ranges from 3 to 4 mm. Note any change from round in the shape of the pupils.

To test the pupils, stand directly in front of the patient. Ask him to stare straight ahead as you shine a penlight into one of his eyes. (The light should come from the side, because direct light makes the pupil constrict before you can look at it.) The pupil should constrict quickly. Repeat this procedure on the patient's other eye. You should also notice a *consensual pupillary response:* The pupil of one eye constricts simultaneously when the opposite pupil is exposed to light. This response should occur even if the other eye is blind. (If only the blind eye is exposed to light, neither pupil will react.)

TESTING THE CORNEAL REFLEX

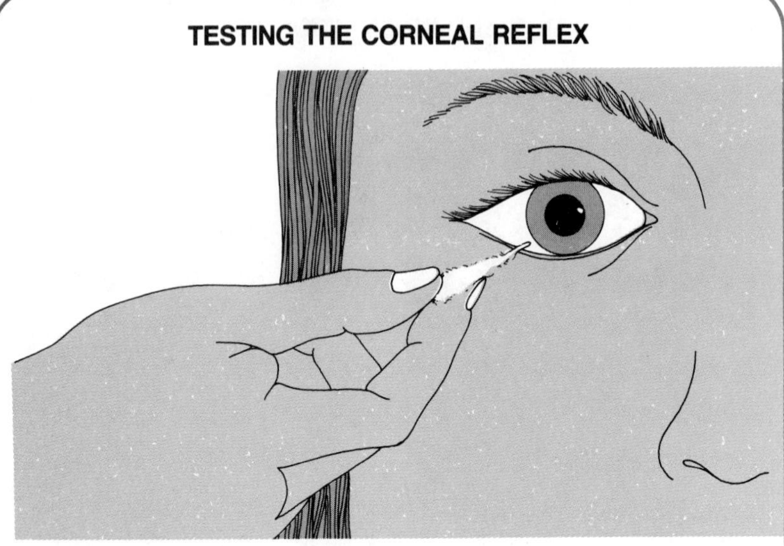

When testing your patient's corneal reflex, begin by asking her to look up. Approach the lateral side of her eye with a piece of cotton. Touch her cornea lightly, making sure you avoid her eyelashes. If her reflexes are normal, she should blink repeatedly. You can also perform this test on an unconscious patient.

HOW THE SLIT LAMP IS USED

The slit lamp is a combination light and microscope used to examine the anterior portion of the eyes, particularly the cornea. Ophthalmologists, and some nurse practitioners, use the slit lamp to detect:

- new blood vessels in the iris that are distributed erratically rather than radially. These may indicate diabetes mellitus.
- a shadow caused by bulging of the iris disk. This indicates shallowness of the anterior chamber.
- yellow pus in the anterior chamber. This may indicate inflammation.
- floating white blood cells in small quantities (recorded as *presence of cell)* or in large quantities (recorded as *presence of aqueous flare)*. These may also indicate inflammation.
- denuded areas. These are evident after instillation of a drop of 2% fluorescein and indicate corneal abrasion.
- opacities, seen in greater detail. These may indicate lens abnormalities, such as cataracts.

272 Using the direct ophthalmoscope

The direct ophthalmoscope lets you examine the interior of the patient's eyes. This hand-held instrument is equipped with a strong light source and various lenses that enable you to view the lens, the anterior chamber, and retinal structures and blood vessels. (See *Assembling the Ophthalmoscope.*)

You can regulate the amount of light you shine into your patient's eyes by using the aperture selection dial, located on the back of the ophthalmoscope head. You can select the lens you need (to focus the image you're looking at) using the lens selection wheel, which is located on the side of the ophthalmoscope head. To examine the patient's right eye, hold the ophthalmoscope up to your right eye with your right hand. Reverse the procedure to examine the left eye.

Flash the circle of light on the patient's pupil from a distance of about 1′ (30 cm) and also at a slight angle (about 25° to 30°), lateral to the patient's line of vision. You should notice a bright orange glow in the pupil—the *red reflex*. In some patients, an opacity may obscure your view of it. Keeping the red reflex in sight, instruct the patient to keep both eyes open and to maintain his gaze on a distant object. Then approach the patient slowly, until the ophthalmoscope is close to his pupil. This prevents eye rotation and encourages dilatation of the pupils.

Look next at the anterior chamber, which should be clear and free of particles. To do this, sit close to your patient, looking through his pupil with the ophthalmoscope, until some retinal structure, such as a blood vessel or the disk, comes into view. Focus the image. If the disk is not apparent, follow the vessels toward the midline until the optic disk comes into view. Focus the disk image.

To distinguish between arteries and veins in your patient's eye, remember that veins have a larger caliber and are dark red, with little or no light reflex. Arteries are small and bright red, with a bright light reflex. Note the normal light reflex present on the vessel. Vessels should appear regular in configuration and emanate from the optic disk into the vitreous.

Look for color differences in the blood vessels; copper or silver coloring can indicate arteriosclerosis. Also note the presence of any white blood vessels, called *ghost vessels*. These indicate previous vascular events. Note the general color, configuration, tortuosity, and course of the vessels. Are the veins beaded or sausage-shaped? Vascular irregularities may indicate systemic as well as ocular disorders.

Look at the background of the retina. Ask the patient to gaze upward, downward, and to each side. Its color may vary according to your patient's race and skin pigmentation, but normally you won't see areas of hemorrhage or small red dots (microaneurysms).

ASSEMBLING THE OPHTHALMOSCOPE

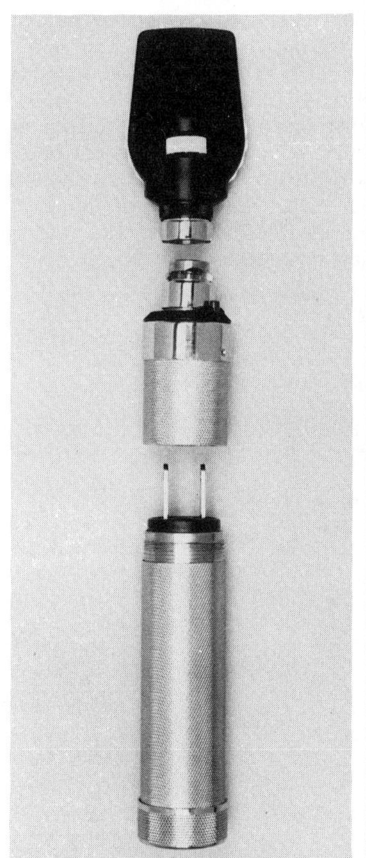

An ophthalmoscope consists of three parts: the handle, the battery housing, and the head. Note that the ophthalmoscope head has two dials on it: one on the back for aperture regulation and one on the side for lens selection. The ophthalmoscope shown here is a Welch Allyn ophthalmoscope. Your ophthalmoscope may come with an interchangeable otoscope, throat illuminator head, or nasal illuminator head, but it's basically similar to the one shown here.

To assemble the ophthalmoscope, screw the handle onto the battery housing. Next, align the base of the head with the lugs on the top of the handle, push down, and rotate the head until you hear it click into place.

Next, observe the optic disk directly. Note its size and shape, as well as how distinct its margins are. The nasal edge of the disk is normally not as distinct as the temporal edge, especially when the patient is myopic. The overall color of the optic disk is also important. It should be pink. Next, note the shape of the *physiologic cup*—the depressed central area of the disk—which is normally yellow-white. It should occupy one third of the optic disk diameter. If it's larger than this, or asymmetrical, consider the possibility that your patient has glaucoma.

Finally, examine the macula. Because this is the center of most acute vision, avoid directing the ophthalmoscope's light on it for long periods; the light can be uncomfortable for the patient. Instead, to find the macula, locate the disk and look temporally about two disk diameters away. The macula should appear darker than the rest of the retina, with a bright spot of light reflected from its center—the fovea. If you can't find it this way, ask the patient to look directly at the light. The macula is light reflective and should come into view.

NURSE'S GUIDE TO EYE DISORDERS

	CHIEF COMPLAINT
EYE INTEGRITY DISORDERS	
Blepharitis	• *Pain/Discomfort:* itching; burning; foreign-body sensation • *Vision changes:* none • *Tearing/Secretion:* crusted lids after awakening • *Appearance changes:* red-rimmed lids from unconscious rubbing; with seborrheic blepharitis, greasy scales on lashes; with ulcerative blepharitis, flaky scales on lashes, ulcerated areas on lid margins, loss of lashes
Chalazion	• *Pain/Discomfort:* none • *Vision changes:* astigmatism or distorted vision, depending on size of chalazion • *Tearing/Secretion:* none • *Appearance changes:* localized swelling of affected lid
Hordeolum (stye)	• *Pain/Discomfort:* acute pain and tenderness, depending on extent of swelling • *Vision changes:* none • *Tearing/Secretion:* pus formation within lumen of affected gland • *Appearance changes:* red and swollen lid gland
Orbital cellulitis	• *Pain/Discomfort:* dull to extreme pain • *Vision changes:* eye may be closed; visual loss from optic nerve compression or double vision from ocular muscle involvement • *Tearing/Secretion:* possibly purulent discharge from affected area • *Appearance changes:* unilateral lid edema, chemosis (swelling of conjunctiva at cornea), reddened eyeball, matted lashes, hyperemia of orbital tissues, impaired eye movement

Formulating a diagnostic impression

273 Classifying eye disorders

Proper eye function depends on the following conditions: eyeball integrity; light transmission into internal structures; image reception and transmission to the visual cortex of the brain.

Thus, eye disorders can be grouped by the function they primarily affect (see *Nurse's Guide to Eye Disorders*):
• disorders that interfere with the integrity of the eyeball by altering its protective structures, such as the eyelids and conjunctiva.
• disorders that inhibit proper refraction for image formation by interfering with the transmission of light rays
• disorders that prevent image reception by the retina, optic disk, and optic nerve.

	HISTORY	PHYSICAL EXAMINATION AND DIAGNOSTIC STUDIES
	• Seborrhea of scalp, eyebrows, or ears; recent *Staphylococcus aureus* infection; conjunctivitis; superficial keratitis on lower third of cornea; chronic meibomianitis in early morning	• Inspection reveals red-rimmed lids; scales, ulcers, or nits on lashes. • Loss of lashes possible. • Further diagnostic studies include culture of ulcerated lid.
	• Inflammation developed over a period of weeks	• Inspection reveals lump on upper or lower lid, pointing toward conjunctival side of lid; red-yellow raised arch inside lid. • Palpation reveals small lump on lid. • Further diagnostic studies include biopsy if chalazion recurs persistently.
	• Gradual onset of pain and swelling	• Inspection reveals red and swollen lid gland; outward-pointing lash possible. • With internal hordeolum, swollen lid gland points into conjunctival side of lid. • With external hordeolum, swollen lid gland points to skin side of lid margin. • Further diagnostic studies include culture and sensitivity tests of purulent matter.
	• Sudden onset of symptoms; recent streptococcal, staphylococcal, or pneumococcal infection of surrounding areas; recent orbital trauma, such as insect bite; recent history of sinusitis	• Inspection reveals lid edema, reddened eyeball, matted lashes, purulent discharge from affected areas. • Range-of-motion exercises reveal limited movement. • Further diagnostic studies include culture and sensitivity tests. *(continued)*

NURSE'S GUIDE TO EYE DISORDERS *(continued)*

	CHIEF COMPLAINT	
Dacryocystitis	• *Pain/Discomfort:* in acute form, pain, tenderness over nasolacrimal sac; in chronic form, discomfort from tearing • *Vision changes:* none • *Tearing/Secretion:* constant tearing; in acute form, purulent discharge from punctum, with pressure over nasolacrimal sac; in chronic form, mucoid discharge, with pressure over nasolacrimal sac • *Appearance changes:* in acute form, inflammation over nasolacrimal sac; in chronic form, none	
Keratoconjunctivitis	• *Pain/Discomfort:* burning, scratching, or sandy sensation • *Vision changes:* photophobia • *Tearing/Secretion:* diminished tear production, excess mucus secretion • *Appearance changes:* none	
Conjunctivitis	• *Pain/Discomfort:* varying degrees of pain and discomfort; itching; foreign-body sensation • *Vision changes:* photophobia when cornea affected • *Tearing/Secretion:* increased tearing; discharge (may be purulent) • *Appearance changes:* reddened cornea and conjunctiva; lids may be crusty or have sticky mucopurulent discharge; pseudoptosis, especially apparent in early morning	
Trachoma	• *Pain/Discomfort:* pain • *Vision changes:* photophobia, decreased acuity (if untreated, blindness may occur) • *Tearing/Secretion:* increased tearing during early infection; dry eyes if lacrimal ducts become obstructed; exudate • *Appearance changes:* early in disease, lids appear red and edematous, conjunctival follicles visible; 4 to 6 weeks after onset—hard, densely packed conjunctival papillae are beefy-red; later turn yellow or gray; late in disease, lids appear deformed and shortened, and conjunctival and corneal scarring occur.	
Corneal abrasion	• *Pain/Discomfort:* severe pain, despite size of injury; foreign-body sensation • *Vision changes:* decreased acuity, depending on size and location of injury • *Tearing/Secretion:* increased tearing • *Appearance changes:* reddened conjunctiva	
Keratitis	• *Pain/Discomfort:* irritation or mild pain • *Vision changes:* photophobia; blurred vision if infection occurs in center of cornea • *Tearing/Secretion:* increased tearing • *Appearance changes:* reddened cornea and conjunctiva; decreased corneal luster	

HISTORY	PHYSICAL EXAMINATION AND DIAGNOSTIC STUDIES
• Severe trauma to midface or nasal disease	• Inspection reveals evident tearing; in acute form, inflammation over affected lacrimal sac. • Palpation reveals lump over area; discharge, with pressure over affected area. • Further diagnostic studies include conjunctival smear.
• Sjögren's syndrome, rheumatoid arthritis, or other autoimmune diseases characterized by hypofunctioning lacrimal glands, excessive evaporation of tears, or a mucin deficiency	• Slit-lamp examination reveals interrupted or absent tear meniscus at lower lid margin; tenacious, yellow mucous strands in conjunctival fornix; thickened, edematous, and hyperemic bulbar conjunctiva; diminished luster. • Further diagnostic studies include Schirmer tearing test, tear film breakup time to test mucin deficiency, conjunctiva and corneal stain with rose bengal.
• Allergic reactions; infection; recent onset; in children, recent fever or sore throat	• Inspection may reveal enlarged regional nodes; reddened conjunctiva; sticky, crusty lids, with mucopurulent discharge; increased tearing. • Vision acuity tests reveal photophobia, with corneal involvement. • Further diagnostic studies include culture and sensitivity tests and stained smears of conjunctival scrapings.
• Poor hygiene; lack of water, especially in desert areas or poverty settings; patient may live (or recently have lived) in Africa, Asia, or Latin America, or among Southwest American Indians	• Inspection reveals excessive tearing; red and edematous lids; conjunctival follicles visible, possibly red, gray, or yellow, depending on stage of disease; exudates; conjunctival scarring and lid deformities late in disease. • Visual acuity tests reveal photophobia; possibly decreased acuity. • Further diagnostic studies include Giemsa-stained smears of conjunctival epithelial scrapings.
• Sudden onset of symptoms after eye trauma—such as from a piece of dust, metal, dirt, or grit embedded under the eyelid—or prolonged contact lens wear	• Inspection reveals reddened cornea and conjunctiva; foreign body (possibly visible with light); green affected area, after instilling 2% fluorescein. • Slit-lamp examination reveals depth of abrasion. • Vision acuity tests reveal decreased acuity.
• Exposed cornea; bacterial conjunctivitis; with dendritic keratitis, recent upper respiratory tract infection with herpes virus cold sores; with interstitial keratitis, congenital syphilis • Allergies to pollens, dusts, and some foods	• Inspection reveals reddened conjunctiva and decreased corneal luster. • Slit-lamp examination with fluorescein staining reveals one or more small dendritic lesions, ciliary injection, and reduced corneal sensation. • Visual acuity slightly decreased.

(continued)

NURSE'S GUIDE TO EYE DISORDERS *(continued)*

	CHIEF COMPLAINT
Corneal ulcers	• *Pain/Discomfort:* pain aggravated by blinking • *Vision changes:* blurred vision, especially in central corneal ulceration • *Tearing/Secretion:* increased tearing; purulent discharge if bacterial infection present • *Appearance changes:* injected cornea
Keratoconus	• *Pain/Discomfort:* none • *Vision changes:* blurred vision; acuity decreases as disorder progresses • *Tearing/Secretion:* none • *Appearance changes:* indentation of lower lid by cornea when patient looks down (Munson's sign); corneal hydrops may occur
Chronic open-angle glaucoma	• *Pain/Discomfort:* mild aching or dull headache; usually no pain • *Vision changes:* gradual, bilateral loss of peripheral vision; halos around lights; decreased acuity, especially at night • *Tearing/Secretion:* none • *Appearance changes:* none
Acute closed-angle glaucoma	• *Pain/Discomfort:* sudden onset of severe unilateral inflammation, pain, and pressure • *Vision changes:* sudden onset of blurring; decreased acuity; halos around lights; photophobia; if untreated, can produce blindness in 3 to 5 days • *Tearing/Secretion:* none • *Appearance changes:* cornea may appear hazy
Chronic closed-angle glaucoma	• *Pain/Discomfort:* none, unless left untreated until final stage • *Vision changes:* transient blurred vision; halos around lights • *Tearing/Secretion:* none • *Appearance changes:* none
LIGHT TRANSMISSION DISORDERS	
Uveitis	• *Pain/Discomfort:* moderate-to-severe pain • *Vision changes:* photophobia; blurred vision; with granulomatous uveitis, floating spots and loss of vision • *Tearing/Secretion:* none • *Appearance changes:* with nongranulomatous uveitis, none; with granulomatous uveitis, affected eye becomes diffusely red with circumcorneal flush

	HISTORY	PHYSICAL EXAMINATION AND DIAGNOSTIC STUDIES
	• Trauma • Contact lens wear	• Inspection reveals possibly injected cornea; irregular corneal surface apparent with light; outline of ulcer apparent with fluorescein dye instilled. • Vision acuity tests reveal decreased acuity in varying degrees. • Further diagnostic studies include culture and sensitivity tests.
	• Progressively decreased vision; uncorrectable (mostly affects females entering puberty)	• Inspection reveals cone-shaped cornea in later stages. • Placido's disk examination reveals distorted corneal reflection; unclear fundus. • Keratometer reveals abnormal readings. • Ophthalmoscopic examination with high plus lens reveals round, shadowlike reflex in central cornea. • Visual acuity tests reveal decreased acuity that worsens as disorder progresses.
	• Familial; genetically determined • Changes in the lens or uveal tract from systemic disorders • Family history of glaucoma	• Ophthalmoscopic examination reveals cupping and atrophy of optic disk. • Vision field tests reveal loss of peripheral vision. • Tonometer examination reveals increased intraocular pressure.
	• Sudden increase in volume of posterior chamber from hemorrhage, congestion or edema of uveal tract • Use of mydriatics	• Inspection reveals shallow or absent anterior chamber; corneal edema; hazy, fixed, and moderately dilated pupil; ciliary injection. • Ophthalmoscopic examination reveals pale optic disk. • Palpation reveals one eye harder than other.
	• Family history • Increase in volume of posterior chamber from hemorrhage, congestion, or edema of uveal tact • Gradual narrowing of angle	• Ophthalmoscopic examination reveals cupping and atrophy of optic disk late in disease. • Vision acuity tests reveal loss of peripheral vision.
	• May have history of tuberculosis, arthritis, exposure to toxoplasmosis, histoplasmosis, syphilis, arthritis, or genitourinary infection • With nongranulomatous uveitis, acute onset • With granulomatous uveitis, gradual onset	• *Nongranulomatous uveitis:* Inspection reveals small nonreactive pupils, severe injection, and sluggish pupil response to light. *Granulomatous uveitis:* Inspection reveals redness and distorted pupils. • Opthalmoscopic examination reveals active choroid and retina lesions appearing yellow-white through a cloudy vitreous. • Slit-lamp examination reveals keratitic precipitates; Koeppe nodules (cluswhite cells) in iris.

(continued)

NURSE'S GUIDE TO EYE DISORDERS *(continued)*

	CHIEF COMPLAINT
Uveitis *(continued)*	
Vitreous hemorrhage	• *Pain/Discomfort:* none • *Vision changes:* sudden unilateral, loss of vision; may see floaters or dark streaks • *Tearing/Secretion:* none • *Appearance changes:* none
Eyeball trauma resulting in hyphema	• *Pain/Discomfort:* varying degree of pain and discomfort • *Vision changes:* may have loss of vision (if injury caused retinal damage) • *Tearing/Secretion:* none • *Appearance changes:* blood obscuring iris; may have associated swelling of eyelid, ecchymosis (black eye)
Cataract	• *Pain/Discomfort:* none • *Vision changes:* photophobia; gradual blurring and loss of vision; misty vision; changes in color value (particularly loss of blue and yellow); halos around lights; difficulty with night driving from scattering of light • *Tearing/Secretion:* none • *Appearance changes:* none
IMAGE RECEPTION DISORDERS	
Optic atrophy	• *Pain/Discomfort:* none • *Vision changes:* decreased acuity; visual fields altered • *Tearing/Secretion:* none • *Appearance changes:* none
Extraocular motor nerve palsies	• *Pain/Discomfort:* may have pain, depending on cause of palsy • *Vision changes:* diplopia, depending on muscles innervated • *Tearing/Secretion:* none • *Appearance changes:* none

	HISTORY	PHYSICAL EXAMINATION AND DIAGNOSTIC STUDIES
		• Vision acuity tests reveal decreased acuity and photophobia. • Further diagnostic studies include skin tests for tuberculosis and histoplasmosis, and chest X-ray.
	• Diabetes, contusion, concussion, sickle cell anemia	• Slit-lamp examination reveals blood in vitreous chamber and retinal neovascularization. • Ophthalmoscopic examination reveals loss of fundus detail and floating red debris. • Vision acuity tests reveal decreased acuity. • Further diagnostic studies include ultrasonography.
	• Recent injury, such as being struck by a ball or fist	• Slit-lamp examination reveals blood in anterior chamber, obscuring the iris. • Tonometer examination reveals increased intraocular pressure. • Dilated fundus examination reveals retinal damage possibly. • Vision acuity tests reveal decreased acuity, depending on extent of injury.
	• Mostly affects older persons; also result of lens trauma from foreign body, or intraocular diseases; exposure to cataractogenic drugs, such as ergot, dinitrophenol, naphthalene • Diabetes	• Inspection with penlight reveals visible white area behind pupil. • Ophthalmoscopic examination reveals lens opacification. • Slit-lamp examination shows dark area or shadow in otherwise homogenous red reflex. • Vision acuity tests reveal decreased acuity often proportionate to density of cataract.
	• Central nervous system disorder, such as multiple sclerosis, intraorbital or intracranial tumors; other intraocular disorders • Ingested methanol • Arteriosclerotic changes; systemic degenerative diseases (such as multiple sclerosis); papilledema; metabolic diseases • Syphilis	• Ophthalmoscopic examination reveals nerve head pallor. • Slit-lamp examination reveals optic disk pallor and loss of pupillary reaction. • Vision acuity tests reveal decreased acuity, visual field changes (scotoma possible). • Further diagnostic studies include serology.
	• Tumors, diabetes, or recent sixth cranial nerve infection • Trauma • Aneurysm • Meningitis	• Inspection reveals, with third nerve palsy, ptosis, exotropia, dilated and unresponsive pupil, no eye movement, no accommodation; with fourth nerve palsy, head tilted to opposite shoulder to compensate for vertical diplopia (ocular torticollis); with sixth nerve palsy, eye unable to abduct beyond midline, esotropia. • Skull X-rays and scan performed to diagnose tumors; culture and sensitivity tests performed if caused by infection. *(continued)*

NURSE'S GUIDE TO EYE DISORDERS *(continued)*

	CHIEF COMPLAINT
Strabismus	• *Pain/Discomfort:* none • *Vision changes:* with binocular strabismus, diplopia; with monocular strabismus, amblyopia in deviated eye • *Tearing/Secretion:* none • *Appearance changes:* eyes crossed or deviated
Retinal artery occlusion	• *Pain/Discomfort:* none • *Vision changes:* sudden unilateral loss of vision, partial or complete • *Tearing/Secretion:* none • *Appearance changes:* none
Retinal detachment	• *Pain/Discomfort:* none • *Vision changes:* shade or curtain spreads across visual fields; floating spots or recurrent flashes of light; gradual loss of vision as detachment progresses • *Tearing/Secretion:* none • *Appearance changes:* none
Retinitis pigmentosa	• *Pain/Discomfort:* none • *Vision changes:* night blindness first symptom—usually occurs in adolescence; progressively decreased peripheral vision (gun-barrel vision leading to eventual blindness) • *Tearing/Secretion:* none • *Appearance changes:* none
Diabetic retinopathy	• *Pain/Discomfort:* none • *Vision changes:* glaring of vision; decreased acuity in later stages; dark spots, floaters • *Tearing/Secretion:* none • *Appearance changes:* none
Hypertensive retinopathy	• *Pain/Discomfort:* none • *Vision changes:* mild-to-severe decreased acuity • *Tearing/Secretion:* none • *Appearance changes:* none

HISTORY	PHYSICAL EXAMINATION AND DIAGNOSTIC STUDIES
• Family history indicates strabismus; amblyopia at early age; severe central nervous system disorders, such as Down's syndrome, cerebral palsy, or mental retardation	• Inspection reveals deviated, uncoordinated eye movements; ptosis; abnormal head position. • Vision acuity tests reveal decreased acuity and eccentric fixation.
• Unilateral loss of vision lasting several seconds to a few minutes; mostly affects older persons	• Ophthalmoscopic examination shows emptying of retinal arteries through transient attack; visible segmentation of blood column within 2 hours of occlusion; pale, opaque posterior retina; choroid seen as cherry-red spot; absent direct pupillary response. • Vision acuity tests show decreased acuity or complete loss of vision in affected eye. • Further diagnostic studies include carotid angiography and ultrasonography, to test condition of blood vessels.
• Gradual loss of vision; vitreous detachment	• Ophthalmoscopic examination shows—with dilation—gray, opaque retina, with an indefinite margin; in severe detachment, inward-bulging, gently rippled or folded retina; almost black arteriole and venules; one or more retinal holes possible • Vision acuity tests reveal decreased acuity corresponding to portion of retina detached
• Hereditary disorder	• Ophthalmoscopic examination shows, with early stage, degenerated retinal pigment epithelium, attenuated retinal arteries, gray or yellow atrophied disk; with final stage, posterior subcapsular cataracts, choroidal sclerosis, macular degeneration. • Vision acuity tests reveal decreased acuity, narrowing visual field. • Further diagnostic studies include electroretinography and electro-oculography.
• Adult or juvenile diabetes	• Slit-lamp examination reveals thickened retinal capillary walls. • Indirect ophthalmoscopic examination shows retinal changes, such as venous dilation and twisting, exudates, microaneurysms, hemorrhages, or edema. • Further diagnostic studies include fluorescein angiography to differentiate between microaneurysms and true hemorrhages, and BUN and serum creatinine for renal function.
• High blood pressure	• Ophthalmoscopic examination reveals hard, shiny deposits (in early stages); tiny hemorrhages; elevated arterial blood pressure; cotton-wool patches (in late stages); exudates; retinal edema; papilledema; hemorrhages and microaneurysms. • Vision acuity tests reveal decreased acuity.

CASE HISTORIES: NURSING DIAGNOSIS FLOWCHART

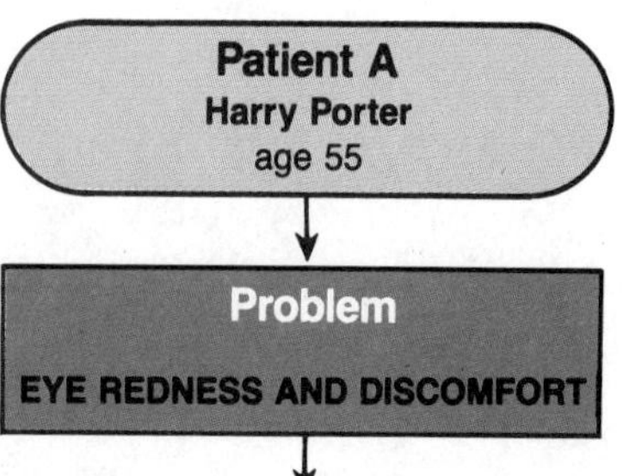

Subjective data

- Complains of moderate discomfort and irritation of left eye
- Noticed increased tearing over past several days
- Noticed difficulty seeing in sunlight without wearing dark sunglasses
- Noticed slightly blurred vision in past 24 hours
- Recorded history of cold sores—most recently, last week during an upper respiratory tract infection

Objective data

- Constantly blinking and rubbing left eye
- Eye reddened and irritated, with a moderate amount of tearing apparent
- Temperature: 98.6° F. (37° C.) orally
- Sclera white, corneal luster decreased, and ciliary injection present
- Pupils normal size and shape; equal, round, reactive to light and accommodation
- Visual acuity slightly decreased; tonometry reading, right eye, 15 mm Hg Schiøtz (5.5 g)
- Corneal lesion apparent after staining with fluorescein dentritic
- Ophthalmoscopic examination normal

Nursing diagnoses

- Alteration in comfort related to eye irritation and constant tearing
- Sensory perceptual alterations related to blurred vision
- When in bright light, alteration of comfort due to photophobia
- Potential for injury related to blurring of vision

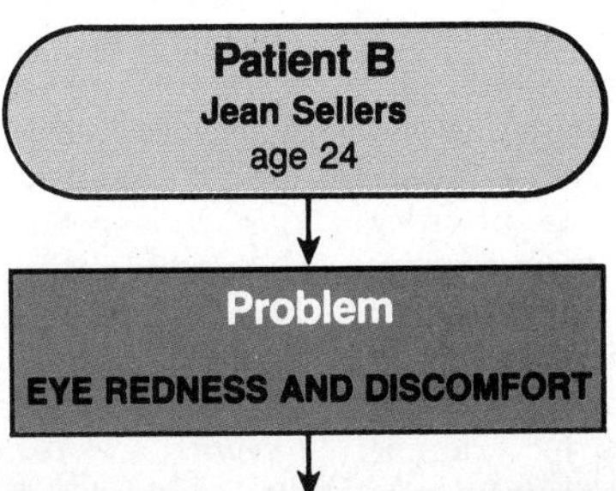

Subjective data

- Complains of right eye redness and discomfort
- Has foreign-body sensation in right eye
- Felt itching approximately 24 hours before clinic visit
- Reports purulent discharge in past 16 to 24 hours
- Noticed increased tearing
- Worries about permanent damage and states her eye "looks terrible"
- Says she missed 2 days of work last week because of a severe cold

Objective data

- Constantly blinking and rubbing right eye
- Purulent discharge from right eye
- Temperature: 99.6° F. (37.6° C.) orally
- Red and inflamed conjunctiva, with obvious conjunctival injection
- Sclera white; cornea clear
- Pupils normal size and shape; equal, round, reactive to light and accommodation
- Visual acuity 20/20 with Snellen chart; visual fields normal; tonometry reading, right eye, 14 mmHg Schiøtz (5.5 g)
- Ophthalmoscopic examination normal

Nursing diagnoses

- Alteration in comfort related to right eye itch, foreign-body sensation, and discharge
- Anxiety related to fear of permanent eye damage
- Alteration in body image related to severe redness of right eye and constant purulent discharge

• disorders that prevent the image from being received by the retina, optic disk, and optic nerve.

274 Making appropriate nursing diagnoses

Pain or discomfort—usually in the form of headaches, acute throbbing or boring pain, eyeaches, or burning—is most commonly associated with disorders of eye integrity. The concentration and distribution of nerve endings within each structure determine how much discomfort the patient experiences. The cornea and conjunctiva, for example, are extremely sensitive to painful stimuli, such as foreign bodies, increased intraocular pressure, and inflammation.

Nursing diagnoses for a patient with eye pain or discomfort include *alterations in comfort level* and possibly *alterations in level of cognitive functioning due to distractibility.*

Vision changes can result from disorders of any of the eye's structures, causing blindness in some patients. Spots before the eyes, or floaters, are usually caused by small opacities in the vitreous body, which affect the eye's ability to transmit light and thus inhibit correct image formation. Retinal disorders that affect image reception because of decreased innervation, altered contours of photoreceptors, or degeneration can cause visual field defects. The defects manifest as curtains or shadows across the visual field, distortions in which the edges of flat objects appear curved, and flashes of light. Sudden loss of vision in one eye generally results from circulatory changes caused by arteriosclerosis, emboli, or decreased blood supply. Diplopia is usually a result of extraocular muscle disorders that cause the retinas to be stimulated at different points, creating images that don't correspond.

Nursing diagnoses for patients who have experienced vision changes include *impaired physical mobility, anxiety, sensory perceptual alterations (visual),* and *potential for injury due to decreased vision.* Severe vision disturbances might require the additional nursing diagnosis of *fear of going blind.*

Tearing or secretion usually occurs in disorders of eye integrity. Inflammation can alter the protective structures, such as the conjunctiva, causing tearing and discharge. Tearing that occurs without discharge may result from excessive lacrimal fluid or an inability of the normal tear to pass into the lacrimal canaliculi. An appropriate nursing diagnosis for such a patient might be *potential impairment of skin integrity due to eye secretions.*

Eye appearance changes (redness, edema, lumps, or ptosis) may be diagnosed as *alterations in body image* or *alterations in psychological comfort level.* This can be due to the anxiety the patient may feel from the difficulty in conceding these changes.

Assessing pediatric patients

275 The child's health history

When taking a child's history, be alert for clues to familial eye disorders, such as refractive errors or retinoblastoma. A child whose family history includes relatives with glaucoma should be referred to an ophthalmologist, even if he has no obvious symptoms.

Ask if the child has been hurt during play. Children may suffer blows to the eye or head during play that can cause ocular trauma, such as hyphema. (Although you may detect the hemorrhage on external examination, it may not be readily visible to the parents, and the child may not complain of pain or discomfort.) If the child's history indicates he may have been hurt during play, ask

THE INFANT'S AND CHILD'S EYE: NORMAL ANATOMIC SITES

When examining an infant's eye, you'll notice that it differs in several ways from an adult's eye. The infant's eyes develop throughout his early years. You'll notice the infant's eye structure is larger in relation to the body than the adult's eye structure.

- The cornea is thinner and has a greater curvature.
- The cornea's exaggerated curve causes the lens to be more refractive, compensating for the eye's shortness.
- Initially, the iris appears blue. However, the blue coloring is actually from the posterior pigment layer, showing through a light or transparent anterior layer. Pigment, deposited in the anterior layer within the first 2 years, determines the adult iris color. Small deposits of pigment make the iris appear blue or green. Large deposits make the iris appear brown.
- The pupil, situated slightly on the nasal side of the cornea, appears larger on examination because of the high refractive power of the cornea. Despite this, the pupils are hard to dilate and small, widening at age 1 and reaching the greatest diameter during adolescence.
- For the first 3 or 4 months, foveal light reflection is not present; instead, the macula appears bright white and elevated and the peripheral fundus, gray. The fundus may also have a mottled appearance, which is normal in the infant.
- The sclera has a blue tinge because of its thinness and translucence. It turns white as it thickens and becomes hydrated.

the parents if the child has been unusually lethargic or drowsy. And because nausea and vomiting usually occur with hyphema, question the parents about these signs. Refer the child to an ophthalmologist if you suspect ocular trauma.

Often a school nurse or teacher will be the first to notice a child's vision problems and refer him for further evaluation. Behavior problems in school are often related to a child's having trouble seeing the chalkboard.

276 Testing a child's visual acuity

Because 20/20 visual acuity and depth perception are fully developed by age 7, you can test vision in school-age children as you would for adults. To test toddlers and preschoolers, you'll need to use different techniques. No accurate method is available to test visual acuity in children under age 3, but testing with Allen cards may give you some useful data. The Allen cards can make the eye examination seem like play and help reduce the child's anxiety.

Each Allen card is illustrated with a familiar object, such as a Christmas tree, birthday cake, or horse. Show the child the cards, and give him time to become familiar with them. Ask if he can identify the objects. Then test his right eye first (cover his left eye). As you flash the cards one by one, ask the child to identify each picture. Next, gradually back away from the child, and record the maximum distance at which he identifies at least three pictures. Record this distance as the numerator of the measure of visual acuity. (The denominator of 30′ (9 m) represents the maximum distance at which a child with normal vision can differentiate the cards; it's the standard for measuring children in this age-group.) For example, if the child identifies three pictures at a maximum of 15′ (4.5 m), you would record his visual acuity as *15/30*.

Normal visual acuity for children ages 2 to 3 ranges from 12/30 to 15/30. Children ages 3 to 4 normally have a visual acuity ranging from 15/30 to 20/30.

Test a child age 4 with the E chart, which is composed entirely of capital Es, their legs variously pointing up, down, right, or left. The child identifies what he sees by indicating with his hands or fingers the position of each E.

277 Testing a child's visual fields

Seat the child on his parent's lap, and have the parent hold the child's head straight forward (or ask the child to look at your nose) while you move an object, such as a small toy, into the child's visual field, following the same procedure you'd use for an adult.

Another way to perform this test is to have a co-worker or parent stand in front of the child and serve as the object for the child to fixate on; you stand behind the child and move the toy.

278 Testing a child's color vision

Color blindness is uncommon in girls, so you'll generally assess only boys' color vision. If a child can identify colors and is over age 4, perform color screening by asking the child to distinguish colored wools or to trace numbers on color-vision charts with his fingers.

279 Inspecting a child for strabismus

For a child to develop normal vision, both his eyes must work in unison. One of the most commonly seen abnormalities in preschool-age children is *strabismus,* caused by the misalignment of each eye's optic axis. As a result, one or both of the child's eyes turn in (crossed eyes), up, down, or out. Irreversible vision loss may occur if this condition is not detected early.

A child with a deviating eye usually develops double vision (*diplopia*) first, and then his brain compensates for the double vision by suppressing one image. Continued disuse of the deviating eye leads to *amblyopia*—an irreversible loss of visual acuity in the suppressed eye.

If the infant or toddler appears to have a deviating eye, refer him to an ophthalmologist for further evaluation. In older children, you can perform the *cover-uncover test.* Ask the child to fix-

INSTILLING EYE DROPS IN AN INFANT

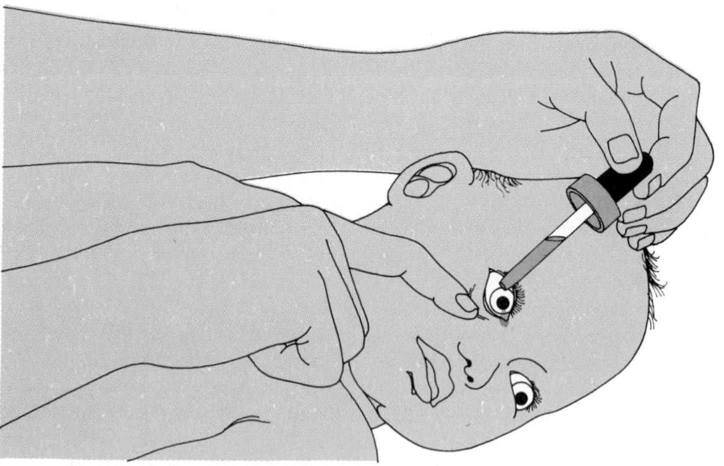

To instill eye drops in an infant, position him as the nurse is doing here. Note how she holds the dropper in one hand and uses her other hand to pull down the infant's lower lid.

ate on an attractive distant target, such as a stuffed animal, a lollipop, or a cartoon figure. Cover his left eye with an occluder (but don't touch it), and observe his right eye. It shouldn't move or change position to view the object. And when the occluder is removed, the other eye shouldn't jerk back into position. If you don't see any movement, the eye is straight. Cover the right eye and repeat the test. To detect more subtle deviations, repeat the test in all fields of gaze. Have the patient look up, down, right, and left.

The *light reflection test* (Hirschberg's test) also helps to detect strabismus. Shine a penlight into the child's eyes. The light reflection should appear in the same position on each pupil. A slight variation indicates strabismus.

280 Dilating a child's pupils

A complete ophthalmoscopic examination of a child, like that for an adult, frequently necessitates pupillary dilatation (mydriasis). Dilating drops sting, and you may have difficulty maintaining the child's cooperation. Some health-care professionals advocate instilling a topical anesthetic before the dilating drops, but anesthetic drops also sting. Generally, you'll need to use gentle force and perhaps enlist assistance from the parents or co-workers. (See *Instilling Eye Drops in an Infant.*)

Assessing geriatric patients

281 Eye and vision changes in the elderly

When you examine an elderly patient's eyes, keep in mind that ocular manifestations of aging can affect the entire eye. As you begin your inspection, you may note that his eyes sit deeper in the bony orbits. This normal finding results from fatty-tissue loss, which occurs with age.

Your patient's *eyelids* probably also show evidence of aging. Look for excess skin on the upper lid that results from normal loss of tissue elasticity. Entropion and ectropion are common in elderly persons. You may note drooping of the upper eyelids (blepharochalasis). When it results from normal aging changes, blepharochalasis usually occurs gradually and bilaterally. It may be so severe that it obscures vision. If sudden or unilateral, it may indicate a more serious problem.

When you inspect the *conjunctiva,* be aware that its luster may appear dimmed, and it may be drier and thinner than in younger patients. This dryness may trigger frequent episodes of conjunctivitis.

Aging can also affect the *lacrimal apparatus.* For example, the delicate *canaliculi* and *nasolacrimal ducts* may become plugged or kinked, resulting in constantly watering eyes. Such a blockage can also decrease tear production, causing dryness of an elderly person's eyes.

When you inspect the patient's *corneas,* you may note lipid deposits on the periphery, known as *arcus senilis.* In persons who are at least age 50, these deposits usually have no pathologic effect. The cornea also flattens with age, sometimes causing astigmatism.

You may see bilateral irregular *iris* pigmentation, with the normal pigment replaced by a pale brown color. If your patient had an iridectomy to treat glaucoma, the iris may have an irregular shape.

An elderly patient's *pupils* may be unusually small if he's taking medication to treat glaucoma. If an intraocular lens was implanted in the pupillary space after cataract removal, the pupil may be irregularly shaped.

Finally, when you examine an elderly patient's *macula* with an ophthalmoscope, you may note that the

THE ELDERLY PATIENT'S EYE: NORMAL ANATOMIC CHANGES

When examining the elderly patient's eyes, keep in mind that the eyes' structures and acuity change with age. For instance, the eyes sit deeper in the bony orbits. Other changes are detailed here.

- The eyelids lose elasticity and become wrinkled and baggy.
- The conjunctiva becomes thinner and yellow. Pingueculas—fat pads that form under the conjunctiva—may develop.
- The lacrimal apparatus loses fatty tissue. The quantity of tears decreases, and they tend to evaporate more quickly.
- The cornea loses luster and flattens. Arcus senilis, lipid deposits on the periphery, may develop.
- The iris fades or develops irregular pigmentation, turning pale. Increased connective tissue may cause sclerosis of the sphincter muscles.
- The pupil becomes smaller.
- The sclera becomes thick and rigid. Fat deposits cause yellowing. Senile hyaline plaques may develop.
- The vitreous can degenerate, revealing opacities and floating vitreous on examination.
- The vitreous can detach from the retina, appearing as an empty space on examination. Through the ophthalmoscope, the vitreous, detached from the area of the optic disk, looks like a dark ring in front of the disk.
- The lens enlarges and loses transparency. Accommodation decreases.

foveal light reflex is not as bright as in younger patients. This is a normal finding.

282 Effects of medications on the eyes

Because an elderly patient is likely to be taking medications for a systemic disease, remember that certain drugs used to treat such conditions as hypertension and congestive heart failure may have ocular sequelae. Make sure you've questioned your patient thoroughly about such medications in the history interview.

Certain ocular medications can cause systemic side effects that affect elderly patients more often than the general population. One example of this is scopolamine hydrobromide eye drops—a cycloplegic used in the treatment of uveitis and postoperatively in patients who have had cataract surgery. It may cause dizziness and disorientation.

283 Presbyopia

Gradual loss of accommodation because of decreased lens elasticity is an early indication of aging known as *presbyopia.* This condition usually begins during the fourth decade of life. The patient complains of near-vision blurring and fatigue from close work. Characteristically, he holds reading material farther and farther away, as presbyopia advances, in an attempt to focus clearly. Presbyopia is easily corrected with reading glasses or bifocals.

284 Cataracts

Cataracts, common in elderly patients, are lens opacities that arise from changes in the physical and chemical state of the lens. These changes occur very slowly and can cause painless vision loss.

Cataracts occur in different forms. They may occur on the lens peripherally—similar in appearance to the spokes of a wheel—or centrally. A cataract may be dense, occluding the lens, or appear as crystals in the lens, causing little (or no) vision loss. A dense, mature cataract (totally opaque and white) gives the pupil an obvious light-colored or white appearance. If your patient's cataract causes severe visual impairment, the lens can be surgically removed and replaced with an intraocular lens implant or contact lens.

285 Other geriatric vision disorders

Retinal detachment, in which the sensory portion of the retina separates from the pigment layer, most commonly affects persons over age 45—about 65% of them men. Many of these patients report recent eye trauma or have a history of nearsightedness. Patients with retinal detachment complain of vision loss (sometimes a cloud over part of the visual field) and the sudden appearance of *floaters*—spots flashing in their field of vision. If untreated, blindness may result.

Glaucoma, a slowly progressive disease characterized by abnormally increased intraocular pressure, may begin in a patient's early years, but its long-term effects are more readily seen in an elderly patient. Caused by overproduction of aqueous humor or obstruction of its outflow, glaucoma may produce pain, blurred vision, and eventual optic nerve damage, or it can progress to blindness with *no* discomfort.

Senile macular degeneration, a bilateral condition of unknown etiology, frequently occurs in persons age 60 and older. This condition—for which no treatment has yet been found—is a leading cause of blindness in the United States and is characterized by the presence of *drusen,* small, yellow defects in the retinal epithelium. Drusen result from breaks in the integrity of the retinal pigment. They may be scattered throughout the retina, causing no vision impairment, or may coalesce in the macular area, causing significant central vision loss.

Pterygium (an encroachment of a fold of conjunctiva onto the cornea) is a degenerative and hyperplastic process that progresses slowly and may eventually cover the cornea. The patient may complain of irritation or even vision loss.

Selected References

Alexander, Mary M., and Brown, Marie Scott. *Pediatric History Taking and Physical Diagnosis for Nurses,* 2nd ed. New York: McGraw-Hill Book Co., 1979.

Bates, Barbara. *A Guide to Physical Examination,* 2nd ed. Philadelphia: J.B. Lippincott Co., 1979.

Carotenuto, R., and Bullock, J. *Physical Assessment of the Gerontologic Client.* Philadelphia: F.A. Davis Co., 1981.

Hillman, Robert S., et al. *Clinical Skills: Interviewing, History Taking, and Physical Diagnosis.* New York: McGraw-Hill Book Co., 1981.

Luckmann, Joan, and Sorenson, Karen C. *Medical-Surgical Nursing: A Psychophysiologic Approach,* 2nd ed. Philadelphia: W.B. Saunders Co., 1980.

Malasanos, Lois, et. al. *Health Assessment,* 2nd ed. St. Louis: C.V. Mosby Co., 1981.

Miller, D. *Ophthalmology, The Essentials.* Boston: Houghton Mifflin Professional Publishers., 1979.

Moses, R., ed. *Adler's Physiology of the Eye: Clinical Application,* 6th ed. St. Louis: C.V. Mosby Co., 1975.

"Ophthalmic Nursing," *The Nursing Clinics of North America,* vol. 16, no. 3, September 1981.

Scheie, H., and Scheie, Albert D. *Textbook of Ophthalmology,* 9th ed. Philadelphia: W.B. Saunders Co., 1977.

Seedor, Marie M. *The Physical Assessment: A Programed Unit of Study for Nurses,* 2nd ed. New York: Teachers College Press, 1981.

Smith, J., and Nachazel, D. *Ophthalmologic Nursing.* Boston: Little, Brown & Co., 1980.

Vaughan, D., and Asbury T. *General Ophthalmology,* 8th ed. Los Altos, Calif.: Lange Medical Publications, 1977.

Walker, H. Kenneth, et al. *Clinical Methods: The History, Physical and Laboratory Examinations,* 2 vols. Woburn, Mass.: Butterworths Publishing Inc., 1976.

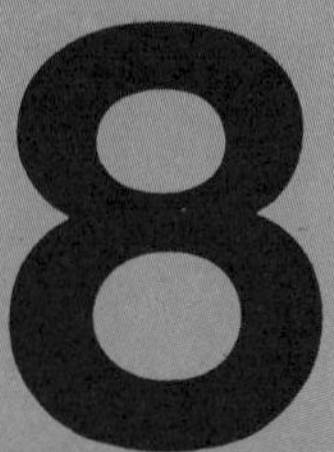

KEY POINTS IN THIS CHAPTER

KEY CHARTS IN THIS CHAPTER

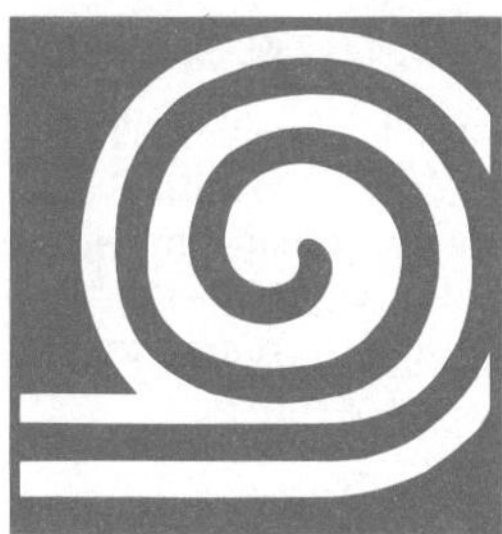

Ears and Hearing

Introduction

286 Importance of the sense of hearing

Hearing's importance derives from the basic human need to communicate, which colors every aspect of personal growth and development. Unimpaired hearing helps a person communicate with others by enabling him to receive oral messages accurately and hear himself speak. Language retardation in children is commonly caused by undetected deafness—proof of the causal relationship between auditory system functioning and development of language skills.

287 Assessing the ears and hearing

Assess your patient's ears thoroughly and methodically, keeping in mind the vital role the auditory system plays in his daily life. A thorough health history is especially important in assessing the auditory system, because many symptoms of ear disorders, such as dizziness and tinnitus, are subjective. After taking the health history, examine your patient physically (using the skills of inspection and palpation) to collect objective data that support or invalidate suspicions raised during the health history interview.

As part of the routine physical assessment, you'll perform several examination procedures, involving all three parts of the ear, including:

- inspecting the auricle
- palpating the pinna and tragus
- examining the external ear canal and eardrum, using an otoscope
- testing hearing with voice, watch, or a tuning fork.

288 Ear disorders: Etiology and testing

The causes of ear disorders are numerous, but the most common are fluid behind the eardrum, bacterial or viral infections, trauma, excessive wax buildup or a foreign body in the ear canal, and neurologic dysfunction. Tests of hearing acuity include your initial observation of the patient during conversation, his response to simple tests for hearing, and testing with a tuning fork when you conduct the Weber, Rinne, and Schwabach tests. (Additional tests that provide more precise information about a patient's hearing disorder, such as pure tone audiometry, must be performed by a specialist.) Remember that although hearing loss is irreversible in some patients, early recognition and intervention are still important. For persons in certain age or occupation categories—for example, schoolchildren and persons routinely exposed to industrial noise—hearing testing should be a regular part of any physical examination.

Reviewing anatomy and physiology

289 The ear's structure and function

The ear serves as both hearing organ and equilibrium sensor. It comprises three parts: the external ear, the middle ear, and the inner ear. The *external ear,* made up of the auricle and the ear canal, receives and funnels sound waves to the *middle ear,* an air-filled chamber that includes the eardrum (tympanic membrane) and contains the auditory ossicles. The middle ear transmits to the inner ear the vibrations caused by sound waves on the eardrum. The actual sensory structures within the *inner ear*—the semicircular canals, the vestibule, and the cochlea—enable a person to hear and to maintain balance.

290 External ear

The external ear consists of an auricle (or *pinna*) and an external ear canal (or *meatus*). Although the auricle's size and shape vary, these characteristics have no clinical significance. Made mostly of elastic cartilage, the auricle is soft and pliable in a child but less so in an adult. The only part of the auricle that doesn't contain cartilage

ANATOMY OF THE EAR

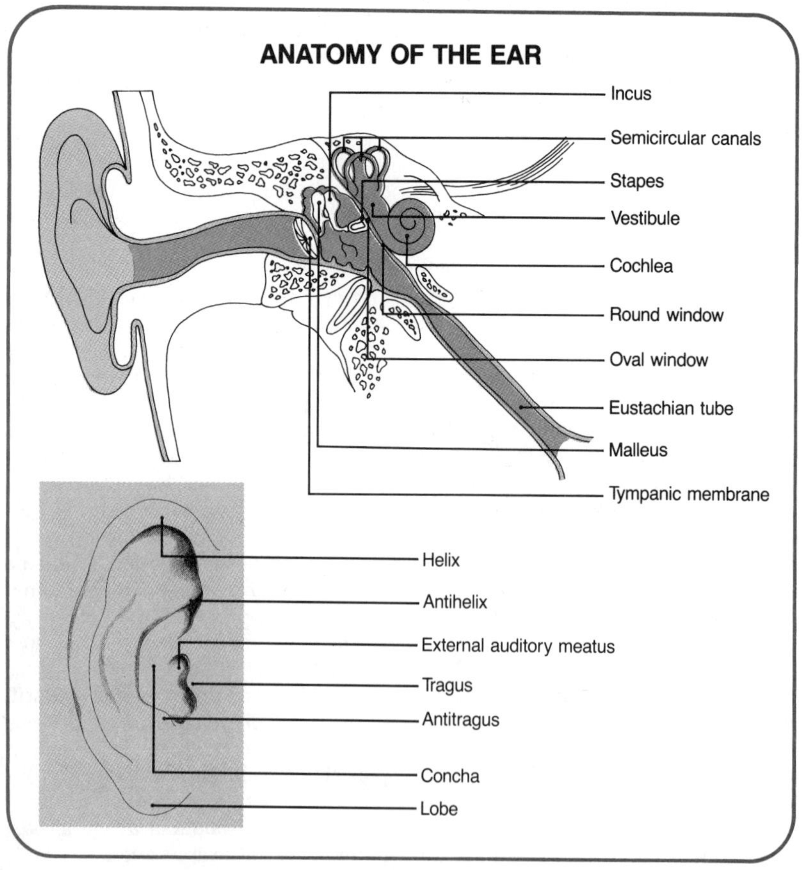

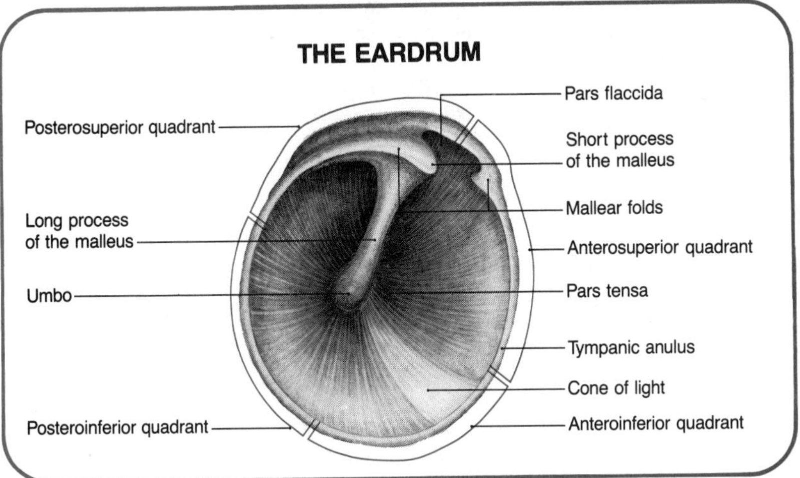

is the *earlobe,* which consequently is soft and fleshy.

The skin covering the entire auricle is thin, with little or no fat. Thus the auricle can easily become cold or even frostbitten when exposed to low temperatures. Fine hairs grow on the auricle; in elderly men, these hairs may be coarse and conspicuous, particularly on the *tragus,* the flap of cartilage in front of the ear canal's opening.

Cartilage forms the outer one third of the ear canal, whereas bone forms the inner two thirds. The canal is slightly S-shaped in an adult, but in a child, it's shorter, straighter, and almost flat. Thin, taut, extremely sensitive skin lining the canal contains guard hairs and ceruminous glands, which secrete wax.

In front of the external ear canal lies the temporomandibular joint. When a person opens his mouth, this joint moves forward, widening the ear canal's diameter slightly. This may explain why some people with hearing deficits listen intently with their mouths open.

291 Eardrum

The eardrum (tympanic membrane) separates the ear canal from the middle ear. Pearl gray and concave, the eardrum faces down and forward, as if to pick up sound waves bouncing off the ground in front of and slightly to the side of the body. When viewed through an otoscope, the eardrum's center reflects a shape that looks like a cone of light, called the *light reflex.*

Although the top of the eardrum—known as the *pars flaccida,* or Shrapnell's membrane—lacks support, the rest of the membrane—the *pars tensa*—is taut. The center, which corresponds to the tip of the long process of the malleus on the other side of the eardrum, is called the *umbo.*

292 Middle ear ossicles

The middle ear is a small, irregular, air-filled space, with a diameter of about 5 mm. Its small size is caused by the convex inner surface of the eardrum and a bulge in the medial wall. The middle ear contains three delicate bones (or auditory ossicles), linked in a kind of chain, which play a critical intermediate role in the transmission of sound. Their correct anatomic names are *malleus, incus,* and *stapes*, but they're more familiarly known as hammer, anvil, and stirrup, respectively (see *Anatomy of the Ear).*

The bones of the middle ear are an engineering marvel in miniature. The long process of the malleus is attached to the inner surface of the eardrum; the rounded head of the malleus fits into the incus to form a true joint. The incus, which resembles a bicuspid tooth as much as an anvil, is attached to the middle ear's posterior wall and moves as a unit with the malleus. The longer of the two processes beneath the incus connects to the stapes at the incudo-stapedial joint (the smallest joint in the body). Its diminutive footplate fits snugly into the oval window (fenestra vestibuli) in the medial wall.

Tiny muscles control the movements of two of the auditory ossicles. The *tensor tympani* muscle draws the long process of the malleus inward, maintaining the eardrum tension necessary for sound transmission. Another muscle, the *stapedius,* draws the stapes slightly away from the oval window, permitting sound wave transmission to the perilymph in the vestibule. Both these muscles may also help prevent the bones of the middle ear from oscillating uncontrollably when subjected to loud sound.

When sound waves strike the eardrum, the resulting vibrations—with help from the tensor tympani and stapedius—set the malleus, incus, and stapes in motion. This remarkable sequence of events culminates in the pistonlike action of the stapes as it moves rapidly in and out of the oval window, transmitting sound waves to the fluid of the inner ear.

293 Middle ear openings

Besides the oval window, the middle ear has three other important openings. The *round window* (fenestra cochlea), with its covering membrane, is an opening in the medial wall, below the oval window. In the middle ear's anterior wall is the *eustachian tube* opening, which leads to the upper (nasal) part of the pharynx. Tissue folds and muscles keep it closed, except during swallowing and yawning.

The posterior wall of the middle ear has an opening called the *aditus ad antrum,* which communicates with the mastoid antrum. This opening and the opening to the eustachian tube are so aligned that infectious organisms can travel easily from the pharynx, through the eustachian tube, across the middle ear, and into the area surrounding the mastoid process. Abundant mucous membrane contributes to the middle ear's warm, dark, moist environment.

THE COCHLEA

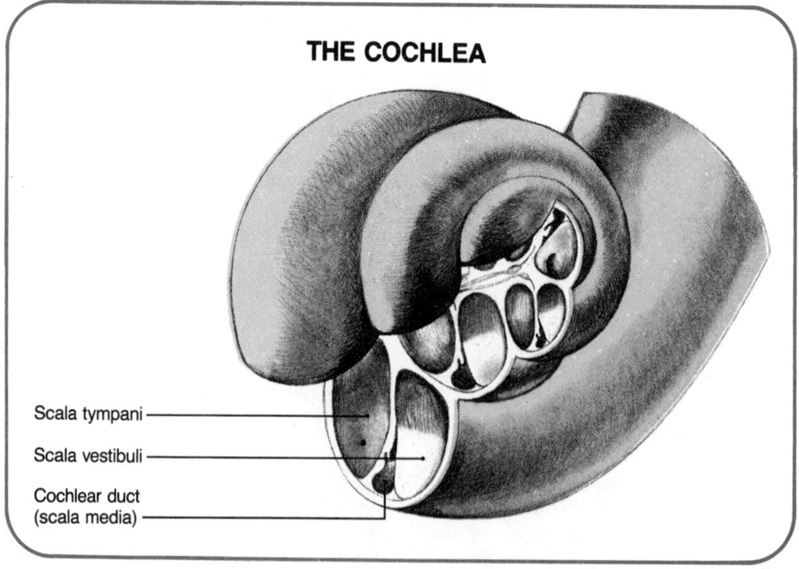

HOW THE BODY MAINTAINS BALANCE

Two structures within the inner ear—the semicircular canals and the vestibule, which contains the utricle and saccule—work together to help a person maintain his balance, or equilibrium. Components of the semicircular canals alert the brain to rotational movement, and components of the vestibule alert the brain to gravitational movement. Here's how:

The semicircular canals contain fluid (endolymph) that surrounds receptors (cristae). The instant the motion of rotation occurs, the endolymph moves, stimulating the cristae. The hair cells within the cristae bend. This releases nerve impulses that travel over the fibers of the vestibular nerve to the brain. The brain then properly orients the person to the motion.

On the walls of both the utricle and saccule are the maculae. Within the maculae lie otoliths and hair cells with cilia. When a person moves his head, the otoliths are pulled, coming to rest on the cilia. Their weight bends the cilia, causing the hair cells to send nerve impulses to the brain, by way of the vestibular portion of the eighth cranial nerve. The brain then properly orients the person to the forces of gravity.

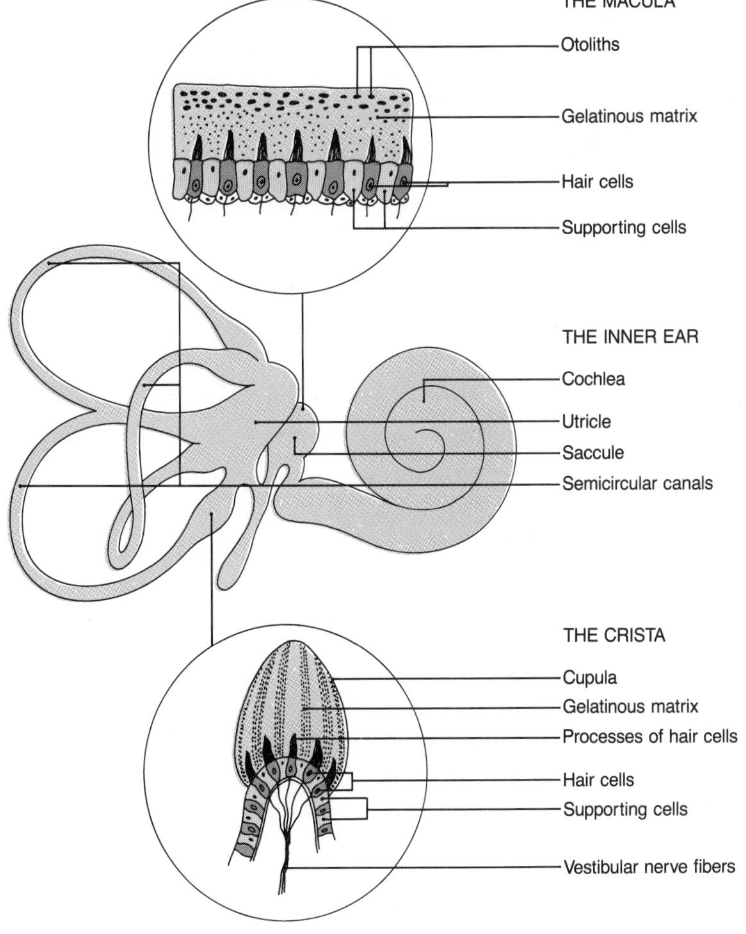

Adapted from J. Robert McClintic, *Physiology of the Human Body*, 2nd ed. (New York: John Wiley & Sons, 1978) with permission of the publisher.

294 Inner ear structures

The inner ear is a closed, fluid-filled space within the petrous portion of the temporal bone. It contains a bony labyrinth that, in turn, contains a membranous labyrinth. The *bony labyrinth* is made up of the osseous shells of three connected structures: the *vestibule,* the *semicircular canals,* and the *cochlea.* A fluid called *perilymph,* similar to cerebrospinal fluid but containing more protein, fills the space between the bony labyrinth and the membranous labyrinth. The membranous labyrinth is filled with a similar fluid, called *endolymph.* The *membranous labyrinth* consists of the sensitive inner portions of the same structures that make up the bony labyrinth, plus two membranous sacs in the vestibule—the *utricle* and the *saccule.*

The utricle, the saccule, and the semicircular canals help maintain equilibrium, whereas complex sensory receptors in the cochlea register sound waves and transmit them to the brain. Thus the inner ear is the most intricate of the three parts of the ear and the true center of hearing.

295 Vestibule and semicircular canals

The *vestibule* is the pear-shaped central cavity of the bony labyrinth, lying between the semicircular canals and the cochlea. It communicates with the oval window of the middle ear; perilymph that fills the vestibule transmits to the cochlea sound waves that have been generated by the stapes. Most of the vestibule is occupied by the utricle and the saccule, two membranous sacs containing maculae—oval areas of special columnar cells with hairlike processes that bend with the movement of endolymph, responding to the position of the head in relation to gravity. Impulses then travel to the brain through the vestibular nerve, to help maintain balance.

Above and to the side of the vestibule

UNDERSTANDING HEARING PATHWAYS

Sound waves are conveyed through the ear by two pathways—air conduction and bone conduction.

The air conduction pathway operates by transmitting sound waves in the *air* through the external and middle ear to the inner ear. The bone conduction pathway operates by transmitting sound waves through *bone* to the inner ear.

Both bone- and air-transmitted vibrations stimulate nerve impulses in the inner ear. The cochlear branch of the auditory nerve (eighth cranial nerve) transmits these vibrations to the brain so that sound can be heard.

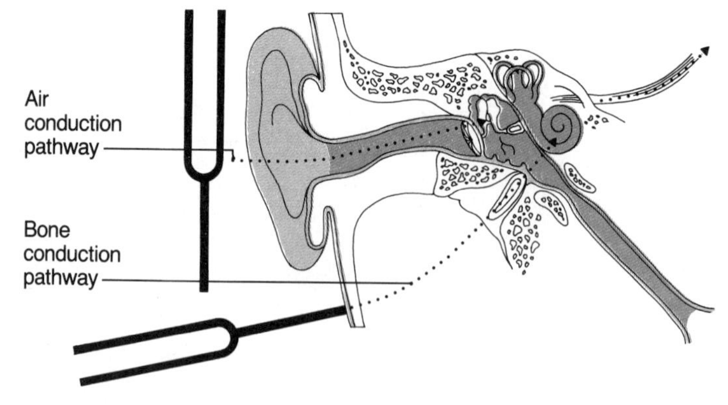

are three *semicircular canals,* positioned at right angles to one another. This arrangement ensures that any rotation of the body that affects balance will register in at least one of the canals—the *lateral, superior,* or *posterior.* The saclike dilatations (or *ampullae*) of the canals, which open into the utricle, contain hairlike processes called *cristae.* These respond to body movements and transmit impulses to the brain through the acoustic nerve's vestibular branch.

296 Cochlea

Situated in front of the vestibule, the cochlea is a spiral chamber that looks remarkably like a snail shell. It has three compartments: the *scala vestibuli,* the *scala tympani,* and the *scala media* (cochlear duct). The first two contain perilymph; the third contains endolymph. Sound waves, transmitted by air, pass through the auditory canal, vibrate the eardrum and the three ossicles of the middle ear, and enter the scala vestibuli through the oval window, causing the perilymph and the endolymph to vibrate. This process displaces or disturbs the hair cells of the organ of Corti. Associated nerve fibers transmit impulses through the cochlear branch of the auditory nerve to the brain. This is the process that enables us to hear.

Collecting appropriate history data

297 Biographical data

Acute ear disorders, conductive hearing loss, and reversible hearing loss occur most commonly in children. Otosclerosis most commonly affects females in their late teens and early 20s. The incidence of presbycusis increases with age.

298 Chief complaint

The most common chief complaints associated with ear or hearing disorders are *pain, discharge, hearing loss, tinnitus,* and *dizziness/vertigo.*

299 History of present illness

Using the PQRST mnemonic device (see page 250), ask your patient to elaborate on his chief complaint. Then, depending on the complaint, explore the history of his present illness by asking him the following types of questions:

- ***Pain.*** *Does the pain occur only when the ear is touched or pulled?* Ear pain that occurs with manipulation usually indicates an external ear problem. *Is the pain deep and throbbing?* Such pain may indicate an acute middle ear disorder. *Does the ear feel blocked?* If your patient's external ear is severely inflamed, the canal may be swollen or completely blocked. Sensations of pressure or blockage may be from eustachian tube dysfunction, which creates negative pressure in the middle ear, or from muscle spasm or temporomandibular joint arthralgia. *Did other health problems precede the ear pain?* Ear pain can be referred from adjacent areas of your patient's body, such as the nose, mouth, paranasal sinuses, and hypopharynx (see *Understanding Referred Ear Pain,* page 251).
- **Discharge.** *Was there a feeling of fullness, followed by a popping sound, before the discharge?* Discharge from your patient's ear can indicate an infection of the external canal or the middle ear. A feeling of fullness may indicate pus or fluid accumulation behind the eardrum. Discharge after a popping sound usually indicates a perforated eardrum caused by a middle ear disorder. *What color is the drain-*

age? If the drainage is a mixture of blood and pus, the patient's eardrum may have ruptured from a middle ear infection.

• ***Hearing loss.*** *Do you sometimes shout during a conversation, or ask others to repeat what they've said? Do you often have to turn up the television or radio volume? Is loss of hearing present to some degree in both ears?* Hearing loss resulting from an immobile stapes usually affects both ears. It typically begins to develop—most often in females—when the patient is in her late teens or early 20s. *Do voices sound as though your head is in a bucket?* This is a common complaint of patients with a blocked eustachian tube.

• ***Tinnitus.*** *Is the noise unilateral or bilateral? Does it seem to pulse?* Pulsations usually accompany middle ear inflammation. *Have you noticed that your own voice sounds hollow and other sounds are muffled?* Tinnitus may result from wax buildup in the ear canal, eardrum perforation, or fluid in the middle ear. *Is the tinnitus high-pitched and ringing?* Such tinnitus usually accompanies acoustic trauma and use of such medications as aspirin and quinine.

• ***Dizziness/vertigo.*** *Do you feel the room is turning when your eyes are open, and that you are moving when your eyes are closed?* These are the classic symptoms of vertigo. If your patient feels light-headed and unsteady, and *doesn't* have a sensation of turning, he's probably experiencing dizziness. *Does the vertigo come and go, or is it continuous?* Each of these types of vertigo is characteristic of specific diseases. Negative middle ear pressure may produce either set of symptoms. *Does the dizziness/vertigo cause nausea and vomiting?* Labyrinthine disease is the most common cause of severe vertigo or dizziness in a patient who doesn't have central nervous system disease. Dizziness that is less severe and doesn't follow a pattern may be caused by a disease or disorder anywhere in the body. *When did the vertigo begin? Is it associated with other symptoms?* Vertigo of several months' duration, accompanied by ringing tinnitus and hearing loss in one or both ears, is characteristic of edema of the membranous labyrinth in the inner ear. To help identify vertigo, you may also ask: *Does the condition force you to lie down or has it made you fall?*

Chief complaint

- **Pain**
- **Discharge**
- **Hearing loss**
- **Tinnitus**
- **Dizziness/Vertigo**

PQRST

Questions to ask

Provocative/Palliative
What causes it? What makes it better? What makes it worse?

Quality/Quantity
How does it feel, look, or sound, and how much of it is there?

Region/Radiation
Where is it? Does it spread?

Severity scale
Does it interfere with activities? How does it rate on a severity scale of 1 to 10?

Timing
When did it begin? How often does it occur? Is it sudden or gradual?

300 Past history

Focus on the following health problems and related matters when reviewing your patient's past history:

• ***Allergies.*** Allergic reactions to cosmetic preparations, such as hair dyes and sprays, can cause chronic dermatitis. Acute serous otitis media may also follow an allergic episode.

• ***Chronic ear discharge.*** Recurrent ear infections with persistent discharge can become chronic. If untreated, they may cause permanent perforation of the eardrum and eventual hearing loss.

• ***Upper respiratory tract infections.*** Complications of a common cold, such as sinusitis or bronchitis (usually with fever), can lead to infection of the middle ear through the eustachian tube.

• ***Endocrine disorders.*** Because patients with diabetes generally don't respond quickly to treatment of infections, ear disorders must be diagnosed and treated promptly to prevent complications. Hypothyroidism can cause hearing loss, usually reversible. Dizziness caused by endocrine dysfunction may occur during menstruation or pregnancy, or hormone (particularly estrogen) treatment.

• ***Hypertension.*** Hypertension, or a condition in which hypertension occurs (such as arteriosclerosis), causes a high-pitched tinnitus from vascular changes in the patient's central nervous system. Tinnitus fluctuates with blood pressure rise and fall.

• ***Drugs.*** Many drugs produce cochlear and vestibular toxicity (see *Nurse's Guide to Some Ototoxic Drugs,* page 252), resulting in related inner ear signs and symptoms, such as dizziness, gait disturbances, or hearing loss.

• ***Recent head trauma or injury.*** Head injuries can cause tinnitus, vertigo, or hearing loss. A cupping blow to the external ear may rupture the eardrum. A sudden loud noise, such as an explosive blast, can cause acoustic trauma.

• ***Previous hearing tests.*** The results of previous hearing tests give you baseline information about the progress of your patient's hearing loss.

• ***Recent head, facial, or dental surgery.*** Because your patient's ear pain may be referred from adjacent body areas, note evidence of any recent surgery involving these regions. For example, tonsillectomy commonly causes referred ear pain within 24 to 48 hours after surgery. Infected tonsils can also cause this type of pain.

301 Family history

Congenital syphilis can cause hearing loss. *Waardenburg's syndrome* may also cause deafness that's familial in origin but sometimes not until several generations have passed. Individuals born in intervening generations, although not deaf, may exhibit other characteristics of Waardenburg's syndrome, such as heterochromia, widely spaced eyes, or an epicanthal fold.

302 Psychosocial history

Your patient's occupation may cause, or contribute to, an ear or hearing disorder. Therefore, when you take his

UNDERSTANDING REFERRED EAR PAIN

When you interview your patient about an ear problem, remember that ear pain may be referred pain. Any of the sensory nerve pathways to the auricle—the great auricular nerve (the auricular branch of the vagus nerve), the lesser occipital nerve, Arnold's nerve, and the auriculotemporal nerve—may transmit pain from the nose and paranasal sinuses, mouth, teeth, esophagus, tonsils, or neck. Also, the temporomandibular joint is connected to the squamous portion of the temporal bone by the processus zygomaticus, which passes just above the ear canal. Consequently, disorders within this joint may cause ear pain. Review your patient's past medical history for surgery or illnesses affecting his mouth, throat, or nose—possible clues to the source of his pain.

DRUGS

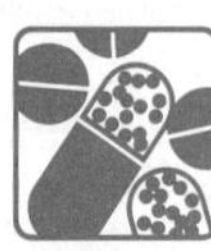

NURSE'S GUIDE TO SOME OTOTOXIC DRUGS

When recording your patient's medical history, note the drugs he's currently taking. Certain drugs, such as those listed below, may cause damage to the cochlea and vestibule. (Signs of such damage include tinnitus, vertigo, and hearing loss.) Other drugs also listed below may cause dizziness, but don't mistake this for an ototoxic reaction: These drugs may produce nervous system reactions, but *they will not damage the inner ear.*

DRUGS TOXIC TO THE COCHLEA AND VESTIBULE

Alkylating agents
cisplatin (Platinol)

Aminoglycosides
amikacin sulfate (Amikin*)
gentamicin sulfate (Garamycin*)
kanamycin sulfate (Kantrex*)
neomycin sulfate (Mycifradin Sulfate*)
streptomycin sulfate
tobramycin sulfate (Nebcin*)

Antiarrhythmics
quinidine bisulfate (Biquin Durules**)

Miscellaneous anti-infectives
vancomycin hydrochloride (Vancocin*)

Antimalarials
chloroquine hydrochloride (Aralen HCl)
quinine sulfate (Coco-Quinine)

Diuretics
ethacrynic acid (Edecrin*)

Nonnarcotic analgesics and antipyretics
sodium salicylate (Uracel)

DRUGS THAT CAUSE DIZZINESS

Antihypertensives
Barbiturates
Estrogens
Oral contraceptives
Phenothiazines

*Available in U.S. and Canada. **Available in Canada only. All other products (no symbol) available in U.S. only.

psychosocial history, ask if he works in a factory, an airport, or a place where he's frequently exposed to loud noise (for example, from motorcycles, trucks, loud music, or heavy industry). Exposure to loud noise may produce hearing loss that can become permanent if exposure continues.

303 Activities of daily living

Review of your patient's activities of daily living should include questions about the following:

• ***Cosmetics.*** Use of cosmetics, hair spray or other hair products, or earrings can irritate the earlobe or the ear canal. Ear piercing, if not done under sterile conditions, can cause an infection in the lobe.

• ***Recreation.*** Swimming in contaminated water can result in an ear infection, partly because the wax in the patient's ear can cause harmful microorganisms in the water to be retained in the ear canal. If your patient scuba dives or flies frequently, remember that failure to equalize pressures between the environment and the middle ear can cause barotrauma. Ask about hobbies—such as frequently listening to excessively loud music or taking part in skeet shooting—that may expose the patient to loud noises.

• ***Self-care.*** Using cotton-tipped applicators or bobby pins to clean the ears can irritate your patient's ear canal, introduce infectious organisms, or rupture his eardrum. Regular use of earplugs, earphones, or earmuffs can trap moisture in the ear canal, creating a favorable culture medium for bacteria.

304 Review of systems

Disorders of the labyrinthine apparatus in your patient's inner ear, such as Méniere's disease, may cause nausea and vomiting. Except for complications resulting from the spread of ear infections, no other body system is significantly affected by ear or hearing disorders.

Conducting the physical examination

305 Preparing to examine the ears

When examining a patient with an ear or hearing disorder, you inspect and palpate the auricles and surrounding tissues, use an otoscope to inspect the external ear canal and eardrum, and perform appropriate hearing and equilibrium tests. You'll need an otoscope with various-sized specula, cotton-tipped applicators to clear away soft wax, a wristwatch with an audible second hand, and a tuning fork of 512 or 1,024 cycles/second. You may also need a curette or cerumen spoon to remove dry wax or debris from your patient's ear canal.

Before you begin, make sure the examining room is well lighted and quiet. Seat the patient on an examining table or chair, depending on his size, so his head is level with or slightly below yours.

306 Examining the auricles

Begin examining your patient's ears by inspecting the auricles for bilateral symmetry, angle of attachment (a deviation of more than 10° from the vertical is abnormal), and size in proportion to the patient's head. Normally, the top of each auricle aligns with the canthi of the eye on the same side. Ears vary considerably in size and shape, however; so ignore any minor variations you see and note only striking deformities or deviations (see *Observing the External Ear: Abnormal Findings,* page 254).

Next inspect the auricles for appearance. The taut skin of a healthy auricle is intact and unblemished. Note any discolorations or lesions. (Of course, the color of the auricle depends on your patient's skin color.) If discharge is present in the auricle, note its color, consistency, and odor, and obtain a specimen for culturing.

Palpate all surfaces of each auricle for warmth and tenderness, as well as for swelling, deformities, nodules, skin lesions, or cysts. Press lightly on the tragus, then gently pull the auricle backward, observing the patient for any sign of discomfort.

Next press firmly on the mastoid area behind each auricle, noting any swelling or tenderness. Then, as your patient opens and closes his mouth, palpate the temporomandibular joint in front of the tragus. Note any crepitation or malalignment, because ear pain can be referred from temporomandibular joint pain. Another way to perform this test is to place the tips of your index fingers in your patient's ear openings while he opens and closes his mouth.

307 Using the otoscope

After inspecting and palpating the auricles and surrounding tissues, use the otoscope to inspect your patient's ear canal and eardrum. Before beginning, make sure the otoscope is in working order (see *Assembling and Operating the Otoscope,* page 256). Inspect the entrance to the ear canal to rule out obstruction by a foreign body. Note any irritation or discharge. With a cotton-tipped applicator or suction device, carefully remove any secretions near the ear canal entrance.

Select the largest speculum that will fit comfortably into your patient's ear canal without hurting him. To insert the speculum easily, stand to the adult patient's side and tilt his head away from you. Then gently pull his auricle up, back, and slightly out, to better align the S-shaped ear canal with his eardrum.

Before inserting the speculum into your patient's ear canal, brace the hand holding the otoscope against his head (see illustration on page 256) to avoid direct pressure on the canal. Then,

OBSERVING THE EXTERNAL EAR: ABNORMAL FINDINGS

When you examine a patient's external ear, be sure to document your findings. Because many of the nodules you find may look the same, you must note the specifics—especially, *where* a nodule occurs. If you observe any redness, swelling, lesions, or scales in the ear canal, note them as well.

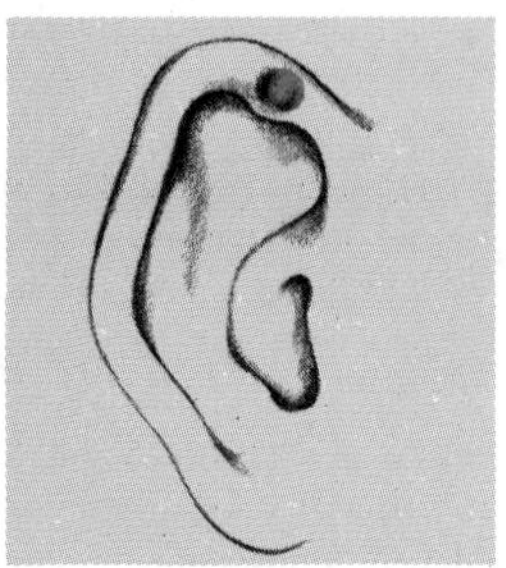

Chondrodermatitis helicis

External findings: small nodule in helix, most commonly occurring on superior rim of auricle

Characteristics: chronic, usually tender and painful; cause unknown; usually affects males

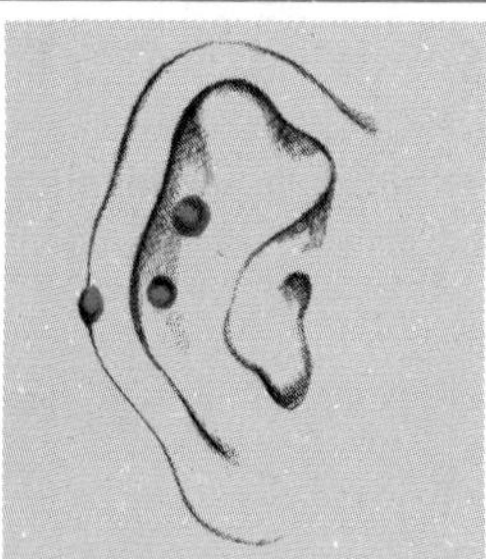

Tophi

External findings: hard nodule in helix or antihelix; varying size, orange color

Characteristics: may exude white, chalky crystalline discharge (monosodium waste crystals characteristic of gout); resembles squamous cell carcinoma

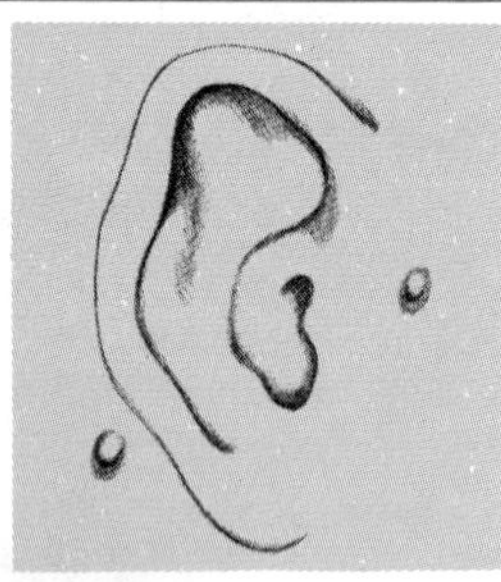

Lymph nodes

External findings: nodule anterior to tragus or overlying mastoid process

Characteristics: common; not always visible—best detected by palpation; may be caused by infection or malignancy

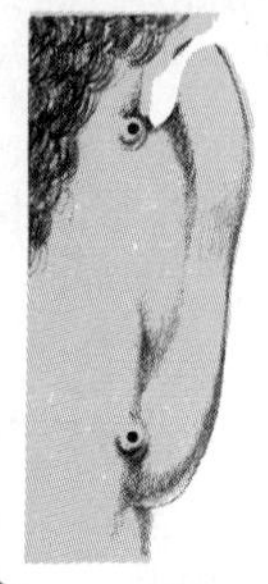

Sebaceous cysts

External findings: cyst behind ear, especially near lobule or in meatus, within skin

Characteristics: punctum (black dot in center of cyst) often visible; contents cheeselike, with rancid odor

while continuing to hold the auricle, carefully insert the speculum into the canal, moving it first downward, then forward. Remember that Arnold's nerve, the auricular branch of the vagus nerve, lies near the entrance to the ear canal. If you stimulate this nerve, you may cause your patient to cough or feel nauseated.

As you insert the speculum, observe the ear canal through the eyepiece, being careful not to insert the speculum too far. (If excessive hair in the ear canal is blocking your view, moisten the speculum with water or a water-soluble lubricant.) Note the width of the canal, as well as any swelling, redness, or obstructions. If you see wax in the canal, note its color. In a light-skinned patient, fresh wax is usually yellow or pink except when dry or impacted, when it's usually yellow brown. Normally, in a dark-skinned patient, earwax may be black or brown. If so

HOW TO REMOVE CERUMEN

To remove cerumen (earwax), position a speculum so you can view the ear canal and work on it at the same time. Insert a cerumen spoon into the canal, passing over the wax particle, as shown in the illustration. Then, lower the spoon into the wax and *carefully* withdraw it. The wax particle should come out.

Do not remove abnormally colored cerumen, impacted cerumen, or large wax plugs that completely block your view. Instead, notify the doctor.

Note: Don't perform this procedure unless you're a skilled practitioner. Sensitive epithelium on the inner aspect of the ear canal can be damaged easily, causing bleeding and pain.

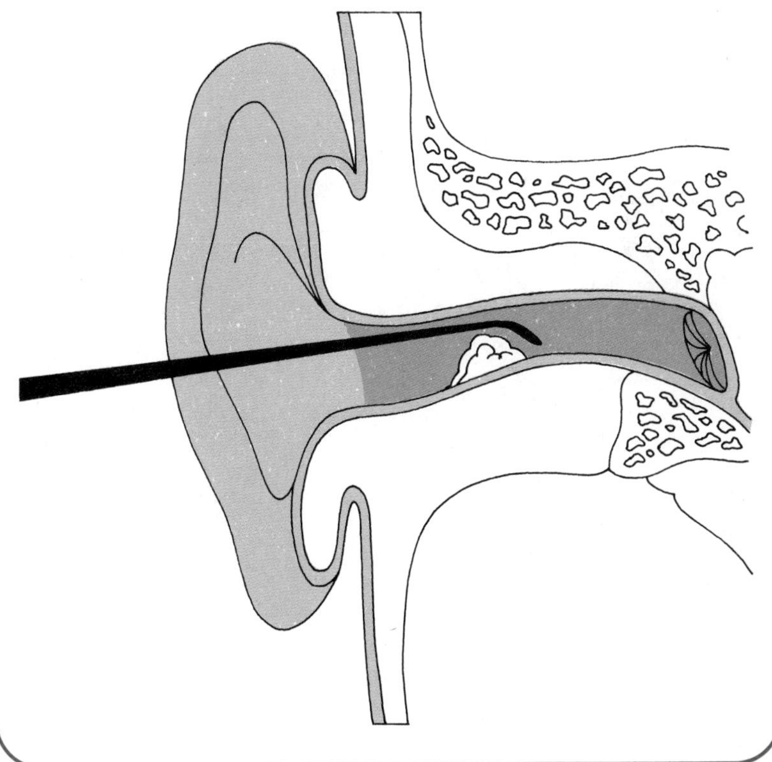

ASSEMBLING AND OPERATING THE OTOSCOPE

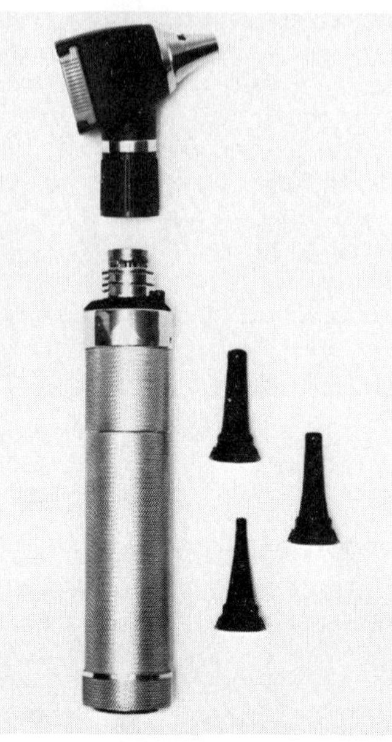

1 Shown here are the basic parts of the otoscope: the battery housing and handle (also used with ophthalmoscope attachments), a light source and magnifying lens, and various-sized specula.

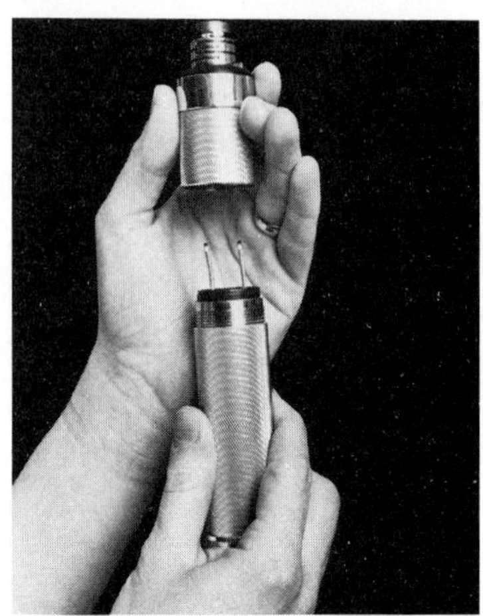

2 Here's how to assemble the parts: Screw the battery housing to the handle, as shown here. Attach the otoscope head to the handle by aligning the lugs on the head with the notches on the handle. Push down firmly, and twist the head clockwise until it clicks into place.

Attach an ear speculum—the largest one comfortable for your patient—by aligning the notch inside the speculum with the notch on the otoscope head. Gently snap the speculum into place.

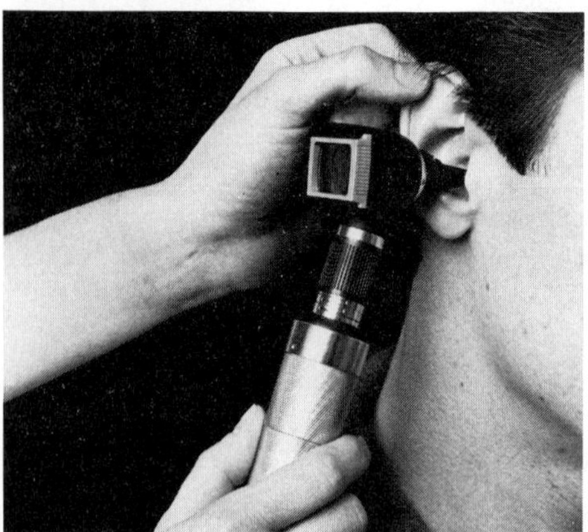

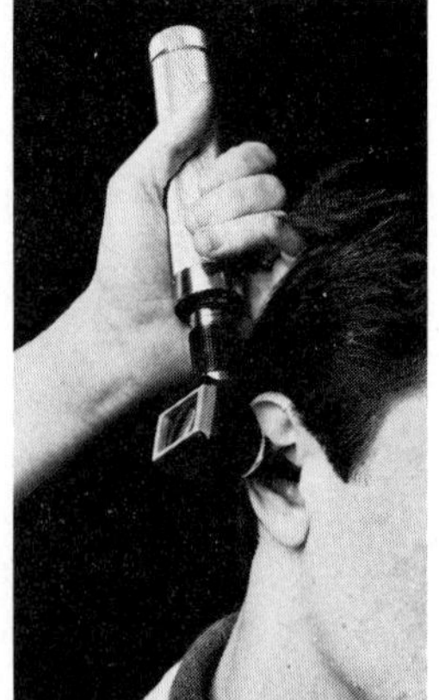

3 Hold the otoscope so the speculum's at the top. Insert the speculum into your patient's ear. Extend the third and fourth fingers of the hand holding the otoscope so that they rest against your patient's head. This will help you brace the otoscope and prevent any damage to your patient's ear. If your patient's uncooperative, try holding the otoscope so the speculum's at the bottom and the entire side of your hand rests against your patient's head, as shown on the right.

much wax has accumulated in the ear canal that you can't see the eardrum, you can remove the wax. To learn how to do this, see *How to Remove Cerumen* on page 255.

308 Examining the eardrum

Looking at your patient's eardrum through the otoscope requires that you manipulate the instrument skillfully, usually with some turning of the patient's head and a gentle tug on the auricle. With this technique, you should be able to see all the eardrum except the anterior inferior quadrant, which normally remains hidden from view because of the membrane's unique angle and the curvature of the anterior canal wall. Record the approximate percentage of the eardrum that you can see.

VIEWING THE EARDRUM

When you view a normal eardrum (tympanic membrane) through the otoscope, you'll see a shiny pearl gray or pale pink slanted disk that's slightly coned inward and toward you.

Behind the eardrum is the malleus handle, which extends downward in the center of the eardrum, as illustrated here. At the end of the malleus you'll see the umbo, which is where the malleus attaches to the eardrum.

If the eardrum's properly positioned, you'll also see a cone of light at approximately the 5-o'clock position in the right ear, and the 7-o'clock position in the left ear.

If the cone of light is displaced or absent, your patient's eardrum may be bulging, retracted, or inflamed. For more information on abnormalities of the eardrum, see pages 258 to 259.

Be sure to document your findings precisely.

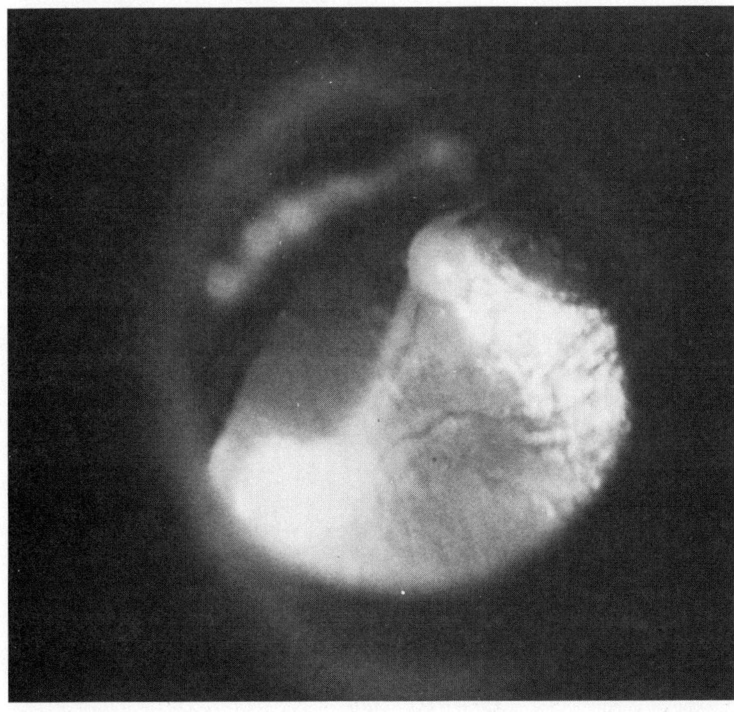

Once you have the eardrum in view, observe its color. A healthy eardrum is pearl gray, with a distinctive luster or translucence to its concave surface. The cone of light should stand out clearly between 4 o'clock and 6 o'clock in the right ear, and between 6 o'clock and 8 o'clock in the left ear, assuming your patient is sitting upright. (If he's in any other position, allow for the corresponding rotation of the cone of light.) Now, look for the malleus, which is creamy white; you should locate it easily. Its short process separates the anterior and posterior mallear folds; you'll see the umbo, the tip of the long process, at the vertex of the cone of light. The manubrium (handle) of the malleus, the most prominent landmark, appears as an opaque, narrow band starting at the drum's center. If your patient has an ear disorder, any of these landmarks may be affected, as well as the eardrum's integrity, thickness, vascularity, and symmetry (see *Viewing the Eardrum,* page 257).

309 How to perform hearing loss tests

Once you've inspected your patient's ear canal and eardrum with the otoscope, you're ready to test his hearing. But remember: The screening tests described here are qualitative and can only suggest that your patient has a hearing disorder; they can't determine the exact type or degree of his hearing loss. Depending on test results, you may have to refer the patient for further evaluation, including audiometry.

Actually, your assessment of a patient's hearing should begin—informally, at least—during the health history interview. At this time, note how he responds. If he seems to watch your lips when you talk, suspect he's lipreading. Test this suspicion by walking behind him and asking him a question. Does

OBSERVING THE EARDRUM: NORMAL AND ABNORMAL FINDINGS

FINDING	COLOR	CONCAVITY/CONVEXITY
Normal	Shiny pearl gray to pale pink	Slightly conical
Inflammation (mild to severe)	Bright pink to bright red	Ranges from loss of conical shape to convex bulging
Bubble, pus, or serum behind tympanic membrane	Yellow to white	Convex bulging
Blood	Blue	Convex bulging
Perforation	Pearl gray, with dark areas	Varies; normal if perforation is small
Obstructed eustachian tube	Normal	Concave
Plaque formation	Pearl gray, with dense white plaques throughout	Conical

he reply inappropriately or fail to answer? Poor articulation may also indicate hearing loss, because speech is learned through hearing.

The *watch-tick* and *whispering* tests provide a gross measurement of your patient's hearing. If the findings are abnormal, he'll need further testing. While you're performing these tests, ask your patient to rapidly—but gently—move the tip of his index finger back and forth within the canal entrance of the ear not being tested. This creates a masking effect: The patient hears a different-frequency sound in this ear than he hears in the ear you're testing, so you can be sure he's responding only to what he hears in the tested ear. The same effect may be accomplished by having your patient fold the earlobe over the canal or simply cover his ear with his hand. If he can't do this properly, do it for him; then proceed with one or both of the following tests:

Hold a ticking watch close to the patient's ear. Then move it away from his ear until he says he can't hear the ticking anymore. Record this distance in your notes.

Another version of this test involves whispering, or speaking softly, at a distance of 1′ to 2′ (30 to 60 cm) from the patient's ear. Exhale fully (to minimize the intensity of your voice), then softly whisper common two-syllable words (such as *airplane, watchman,* or *blackboard*) or numbers (*14, 18, 30*)—or a series of monosyllabic numbers (*2, 5, 10*). Usually two or three words or numbers are enough. Then ask the patient to repeat what you said. When you test his other ear, use different words or numbers. If your patient can't understand a low whisper, increase the intensity of your voice to a loud whisper. If he still can't hear you, try soft, medium, and loud speech until he responds correctly. To prevent

After examining your patient's eardrum through the otoscope and speculum, carefully document your observations, especially if you notice any abnormalities. Use the normal eardrum described below as a comparison.

Remember, if your patient's ear is inflamed, perform the examination gently to avoid causing pain.

LIGHT REFLECTION	APPEARANCE OF LANDMARKS
Bright to dim	Well defined; umbo appears regressed
Dim to lacking	Indistinguishable to lacking definition
Lacking	Variable (depending on fluid, pus, or serum levels)
Lacking	*Umbo and anulus:* not visible; *malleus:* variable (depending on amount of blood in the affected area)
Present *unless* perforation involves the anteroinferior quadrant	Defined *unless* perforation involves specific landmark area
Bent or lacking	Defined but smaller
Present *unless* plaque formation involves the anteroinferior quadrant	Defined *unless* plaques involve specific landmark area

TESTING YOUR PATIENT'S HEARING: TUNING FORK POSITIONS

1 For the Weber test, place a vibrating tuning fork firmly midline on your patient's forehead (as the nurse is doing here) or midline on the top of his head.

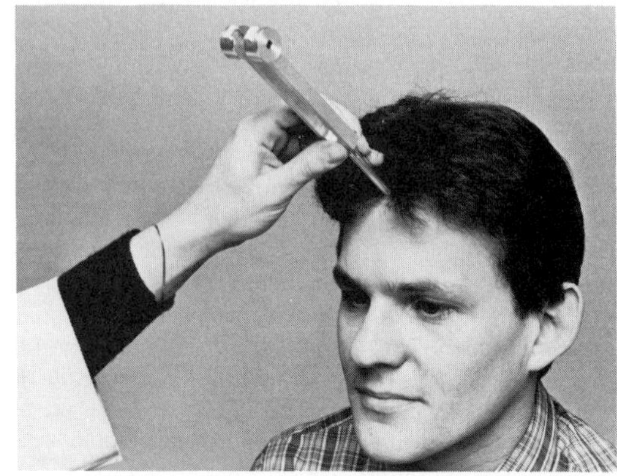

2 For the Rinne test, hold a vibrating tuning fork against the patient's mastoid process, as shown here, until the patient indicates he no longer hears the tone. This tests bone conduction. Then, quickly move the vibrating fork in front of his ear canal, as shown in the inset. This tests air conduction.

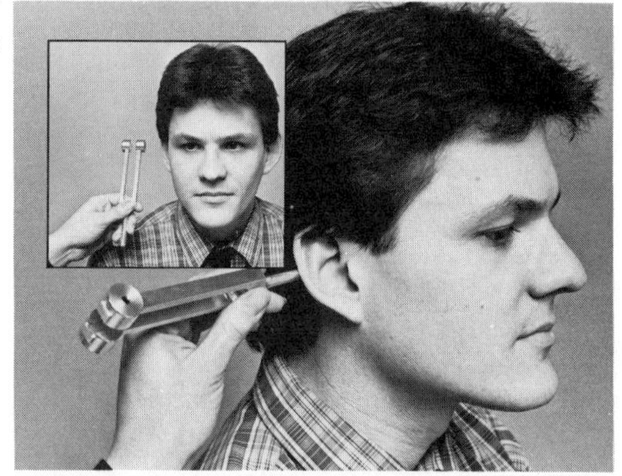

3 For the Schwabach test, position a vibrating tuning fork against the patient's mastoid process, as shown here. Then, place the tuning fork against *your* mastoid process, as shown in the inset. Alternate these positions until you or the patient no longer hears the tone. *Remember:* You must have normal hearing to conduct this test.

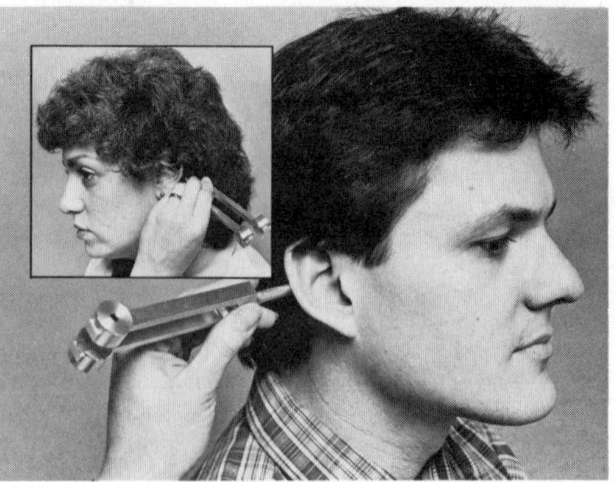

lipreading, ask him to cover his eyes (or do this for him) or simply mask your mouth with your hand.

310 Using the tuning fork

To perform the Weber, Rinne, and Schwabach tests, use a tuning fork with a frequency of 512 or 1,024 cycles/second, which corresponds to the frequency range of normal human speech (see *Testing Your Patient's Hearing: Tuning Fork Positions*). The results of these tests help differentiate *conductive, sensorineural* (perceptive), and *mixed* hearing loss, which is a combination of conductive and sensorineural hearing loss (see *Understanding Hearing Pathways,* page 248). Conductive hearing loss is caused by a blockage of sound conduction to the inner ear; sensorineural hearing loss results from disorders of the inner ear, auditory nerve, or brain.

Abnormal results of any of these tests require further quantitative testing.

311 How to perform the Weber test

To perform the Weber test, place the base of a vibrating tuning fork at the vertex of your patient's head or in the center of his forehead (see *Testing Your Patient's Hearing: Tuning Fork Positions*). As an alternate site, you may choose the bridge of his nose, his central incisors, or his mandibular symphysis. Ask him if he hears the tone equally well in both ears. (Don't bias his answer by asking which ear he hears it in.) If he does, record the results as *Weber negative,* a normal finding.

If the patient doesn't hear the tone equally well in both ears, ask him to point to the ear in which he hears the *louder* tone. Record the result as *Weber right* or *Weber left,* depending on which ear the patient points to. This is an abnormal finding, possibly indicating conductive hearing loss in this ear. The reason for this seemingly paradoxical conclusion is simple: The tone later-

INTERPRETING WEBER, RINNE, AND SCHWABACH TESTS

TEST	NORMAL HEARING	CONDUCTIVE HEARING LOSS	SENSORINEURAL (PERCEPTIVE) HEARING LOSS
Weber (bone)	• Patient hears same tone (intensity and volume) in both ears. Document result as *Weber negative: no lateralization.*	• Patient hears the tone louder in the affected ear. Document result as *Weber lateralizes to right* or *Weber lateralizes to left.*	• Weber test is inconclusive in this particular condition. However, you may expect the patient to hear the tone equally or louder in the ear you suspect is *unaffected.*
Rinne (air/bone)	• Patient hears an air-conducted tone twice as long as a bone-conducted tone. Document result as *+R* (Rinne positive): *AC>BC.*	• Patient hears a bone-conducted tone for as long or longer than he hears an air-conducted tone. Document result as *−R* (Rinne negative): *BC=AC* or *BC>AC.*	• Patient hears air-conducted tones longer than bone-conducted tones. Document result as *+R* (Rinne positive): *AC>BC.*
Schwabach (bone)	• Patient and nurse hear tone for equal amounts of time. Document result as *Time equal to examiner.*	• Patient hears tone longer than nurse. Document result as *Time more than examiner.*	• Patient hears tone shorter time than nurse. Document result as *Time less than examiner.*

alizes to the affected ear through bone conduction, while background noise prevents similar detection of the tone by the unaffected ear.

The Weber test isn't as specific for sensorineural hearing loss. But if one ear is normal and sensorineural loss exists in the other, the tuning fork is heard louder in the normal ear.

312 The Rinne test

The Rinne test compares your patient's responses, in both ears, to bone conduction and air conduction of sound. For this test, ask him to occlude the ear not being tested. Then strike the tuning fork and place it against his mastoid process (see *Testing Your Patient's Hearing: Tuning Fork Positions,* page 260). Hold it there until he no longer hears the tone. Note how many seconds this takes. Then quickly move the tuning fork, still vibrating, to a position in front of his ear canal, with the prongs parallel to the auricle's vertical axis. Hold the tuning fork in this position, without touching the auricle, until the patient no longer hears the tone. Again, note how long this takes. Then repeat the test on his other ear.

If your patient's hearing is normal, he'll hear the air-conducted tone twice as long as the bone-conducted tone (*Rinne positive*). If he hears the bone-conducted tone for as long as he hears the air-conducted tone or longer, it may indicate conductive hearing loss (*Rinne negative*). The Rinne test also produces a positive response in a patient with sensorineural hearing loss, because the inner ear's perception of sound waves by air *or* bone conduction is compromised.

313 The Schwabach test

The Schwabach test compares your perception of bone-conducted sound with the patient's. (If your hearing isn't normal, don't perform this test; the results will be inaccurate.) Begin by asking the patient to occlude the ear not being tested. Strike the tuning fork, then place it on the patient's mastoid process (see *Testing Your Patient's Hearing: Tuning Fork Positions,* page 260.) If he hears the tone, quickly place the tuning fork against *your* corresponding mastoid process. Listen for the tone, as you occlude your other ear. If you can hear the tone, place the tuning fork back against the patient's mastoid process. If he can still hear the tone, again place the tuning fork against your mastoid process to see if *you* can still hear it.

Repeat this back-and-forth procedure until neither of you can hear the tone. In most cases, the tone will become inaudible to both of you at the same time. If the patient continues to hear the tone after it's become inaudible to you, note for how many seconds he can still hear it. This abnormal finding indicates possible conductive hearing loss: The patient continues to hear the bone-conducted sound because he is less able to hear the air-conducted background noise that's made the bone-conducted tone inaudible to you. Conversely, the patient with sensorineural hearing loss won't hear the tone for as long as you do. Repeat this test on the other ear.

314 Testing your patient's equilibrium

Three common equilibrium tests that you should know how to conduct are the past-pointing test, the falling test, and Hallpike maneuvers. A fourth test—caloric testing—is only rarely done by nurses.

For the past-pointing test, sit across from the patient, and ask him to close his eyes, extend his arms in front of him, and point with his index fingers. Extend your arms in the same manner, placing your index fingers under and touching the patient's fingers. Ask the patient to raise his arms a few inches, then lower them so his fingers come down on top of yours. A patient with normal equilibrium can do this easily. If the patient misses your fingers (past-pointing), he may have a vestibular apparatus dysfunction.

To conduct the falling test, ask the patient to stand with his feet together, his eyes closed, and his arms at his sides. Normally, the patient remains erect or sways only slightly, but he shouldn't sway significantly—or fall (Romberg's sign). Make sure you stand close enough to the patient to stop him from falling if he does lose his balance.

Hallpike maneuvers evaluate (and also treat) benign paroxysmal positional vertigo. With the patient lying on his back, gently move his head to the right and hold it there for 1 minute. Positive signs (center and left nystagmus) usually occur within 5 to 10 seconds.

Formulating a diagnostic impression

315 Classifying ear disorders

Ear disorders are classified according to the primary function they mainly affect: disorders that interfere with the transmission of sound waves and disorders that cause an equilibrium disturbance (see *Nurse's Guide to Ear Disorders*, pages 264 to 269). *Normal hearing* depends on unobstructed transmission of sound waves through the ear to the organ of Corti in the cochlea and then to the auditory nerve for delivery to the auditory cortex—where sound waves are interpreted. *Equilibrium* depends on stimulation of the cristae of the semicircular canals and the maculae of the utricle and saccule by head movement and linear acceleration. Reflex responses result from this stimulation and help in the maintenance of orientation and balance.

316 Making appropriate nursing diagnoses

Ear disorders often cause pain or discomfort. These symptoms can range from a mild, uncomfortable feeling in the external ear canal to a severe, throbbing ache in the ear and head. Most pain receptors in the ear are located in the structures that transmit sound waves. Any type of tissue damage—inflammation, pressure, or irritation—stimulates the receptors in the ear to transmit impulses to the brain, where conscious perception of pain occurs. Nursing diagnoses for such conditions include *alteration in comfort* and possibly *altered cognition* if the pain is severe enough to interfere with concentration.

When inflammation or infection alters ear structures that serve as pathways for sound transmission, fluid or pus forms and is then emitted from the ear. Nursing diagnoses for disorders that cause ear discharge include *alteration in comfort* and *impaired skin integrity* (potential).

Another principal symptom of disorders that affect the transmission of sound waves is hearing loss. However, because no structural barriers exist between the cochlea and the labyrinth, hearing loss can also occur in equilibrium disturbances.

Conductive hearing loss results from an obstruction in the ear pathways that interferes with the transmission of sound waves to the cochlea. For example, occlusion of the external auditory canal blocks the transmission of sound waves to the eardrum. Damage to the eardrum, such as thickening, scarring, or perforation, decreases its vibrations—or prevents it from vibrating—and thus inhibits the transmission of sound waves to the middle ear.

The transmission of sound waves from the tympanic membrane to the oval window can be slowed or obstructed totally by the accumulation of pus, serum, or blood in the middle ear. Absent or decreased mobility of the

NURSE'S GUIDE TO EAR DISORDERS

	CHIEF COMPLAINT
EXTERNAL EAR DISORDERS	
Acute otitis externa	• *Pain/Discomfort:* mild-to-severe pain, which may be aggravated by jaw motion or pressure on the pinna or on the tragus; may be a throbbing ache over entire affected side of head • *Discharge:* usually yellow but may be serous, bloody, or cheesy; foul-smelling; tenacious • *Hearing loss:* may be mild, depending on degree of occlusion; conductive, low pitch • *Vertigo/Dizziness:* uncommon • *Tinnitus:* may be mild; low pitch
Chronic otitis externa	• *Pain/Discomfort:* severe itching of entire ear • *Discharge:* usually present • *Hearing loss:* none, unless discharge accumulates in the ear canal; then loss depends on the degree of occlusion; conductive • *Vertigo/Dizziness:* may be mild • *Tinnitus:* may be mild; low pitch
Otomycosis	• *Pain/Discomfort:* severe itching in canal often aggravated by scratching • *Discharge:* none except in severe cases; then foul-smelling, serous, or whitish secretion, with cheesy appearance • *Hearing loss:* may be mild, depending on degree of occlusion; conductive • *Vertigo/Dizziness:* may be mild • *Tinnitus:* may be mild; low pitch
Furunculosis	• *Pain/Discomfort:* severe; localized in outer cartilagenous half of ear canal • *Discharge:* after furuncle breaks, bloody or purulent for brief time • *Hearing loss:* may be moderate to severe, depending on degree of occlusion; conductive • *Vertigo/Dizziness:* may be mild • *Tinnitus:* may be mild; low pitch
MIDDLE EAR DISORDERS	
Acute serous otitis media	• *Pain/Discomfort:* little or none; pressure (as with nose-blowing, sneezing) • *Discharge:* none • *Hearing loss:* usually reversible; occasional sensation of canal blockage; conductive • *Vertigo/Dizziness:* occasional, slight dizziness, not true vertigo • *Tinnitus:* may be mild

	HISTORY	PHYSICAL EXAMINATION AND DIAGNOSTIC STUDIES
	• Summer swimming • Moist, hot climate • Cleaning ears with sharp object • Allergy to hair spray • Lymphadenopathy	• Tragus, acoustic meatus, and canal may be edematous. • May be unable to insert otoscope because of pain or occlusion • Possibly fever
	• Repeated episodes of dermatoses (psoriasis, dermatoses) • Allergy to hair spray and dyes, nail polish • Lymphadenopathy	• Eardrum normal • Auricle and canal red, thick, excoriated; often crusted • Canal and tympanic membrane insensitive
	• Often asymptomatic • Recent infection by candida, aspergillus, tinea organisms or actinomycosis • Moist, hot climate • No signs or symptoms unless ear tissues invaded by fungus	• Eardrum whitish gray with black dots; may be cottony • Canal edema and debris
	• Otitis media, with discharge	• Eardrum normal unless otitis media present • Furuncles visible in canal
	• Gradual onset; lasts several weeks or months • Recent upper respiratory tract infection, barotrauma; occasional fever, with upper respiratory tract infection present	• Eardrum retracted with prominent mallear folds • Yellow or blue fluid, or bubble line, behind tympanic membrane • Dark line lying horizontally across eardrum (sign of fluid level in eardrum) may be visible.

(continued)

NURSE'S GUIDE TO EAR DISORDERS *(continued)*

	CHIEF COMPLAINT
Acute suppurative otitis media	• *Pain/Discomfort:* severe, deep in head; throbbing; none with external ear motion • *Discharge:* purulent, if tympanic membrane is pierced • *Hearing loss:* conductive; moderate to severe • *Vertigo/Dizziness:* may be mild; accompanied by nausea • *Tinnitus:* may be present
Chronic suppurative otitis media	• *Pain/Discomfort:* little or none • *Discharge:* thick, purulent • *Hearing loss:* conductive; moderate to severe • *Vertigo/Dizziness:* none unless complications, such as irritation of labyrinth, occur • *Tinnitus:* none
Acute mastoiditis	• *Pain/Discomfort:* dull aching behind ear; deep, with pressure on mastoid process • *Discharge:* thick, foul-smelling, creamy, profuse • *Hearing loss:* none, unless complications occur • *Vertigo/Dizziness:* occasional • *Tinnitus:* may be mild
Otosclerosis	• *Pain/Discomfort:* none • *Discharge:* none • *Hearing loss:* conductive; progressive • *Vertigo/Dizziness:* little or none • *Tinnitus:* commonly present
Bullous myringitis (viral otitis media)	• *Pain/Discomfort:* severe in canal; fullness • *Discharge:* none • *Hearing loss:* conductive; mild • *Vertigo/Dizziness:* present • *Tinnitus:* present
Eustachian tube block	• *Pain/Discomfort:* intermittent; sensation of canal blockage • *Discharge:* none • *Hearing loss:* conductive • *Vertigo/Dizziness:* occasional • *Tinnitus:* may be present
INNER EAR DISORDERS	
Ménière's disease	• *Pain/Discomfort:* none • *Discharge:* none • *Hearing loss:* fluctuating low-frequency sensorineural loss; present usually in only one ear • *Vertigo/Dizziness:* sudden vertigo; lasts from minutes to hours; occurs weeks to months apart • *Tinnitus:* low buzz; fluctuates; present in one ear

	HISTORY	PHYSICAL EXAMINATION AND DIAGNOSTIC STUDIES
	• Progressive • Recent upper respiratory tract infection or measles, allergies, adenoid hypertrophy, barotrauma, fever, or chills • Sudden cessation of pain when tympanic membrane ruptures	• Eardrum hyperemic; minimal retraction, with dull red landmarks obscured • Perforation possible, accompanied by discharge • Canal normal or pus-filled
	• Untreated acute suppurative otitis media; occasional fever	• Eardrum perforated and covered with drainage
	• Previous acute suppurative otitis media (especially with adequate treatment) • Two weeks prior to onset of otitis media, fever, pinna displaced laterally or inferiorly	• Eardrum swollen, lusterless, dull, thick, edematous
	• Positive family history • Gradually worsening • Made worse with pregnancy • Monohybrid autosomal dominant inheritance (25% to 40% incidence)	• Eardrum normal • Schwartz's sign (faint pink blush seen behind eardrum) may be present. • Canal normal • Soft speaking despite hearing loss
	• Recent illness or exposure to virus • Recent upper respiratory tract infection	• Eardrum blood-filled, or blood in adjacent canal • Fine vascularity to diffuse hemorrhage • Numerous bubbles on tympanic membrane
	• Pressure change, such as during air travel	• Eardrum retracted; may be red • Air bubbles may be present in middle ear space.
	• Episodes recurrent • Asymptomatic between attacks • Altered activities of daily living • Audiography abnormal	• Sensorineural hearing loss in one ear • Fluctuating hearing loss

(continued)

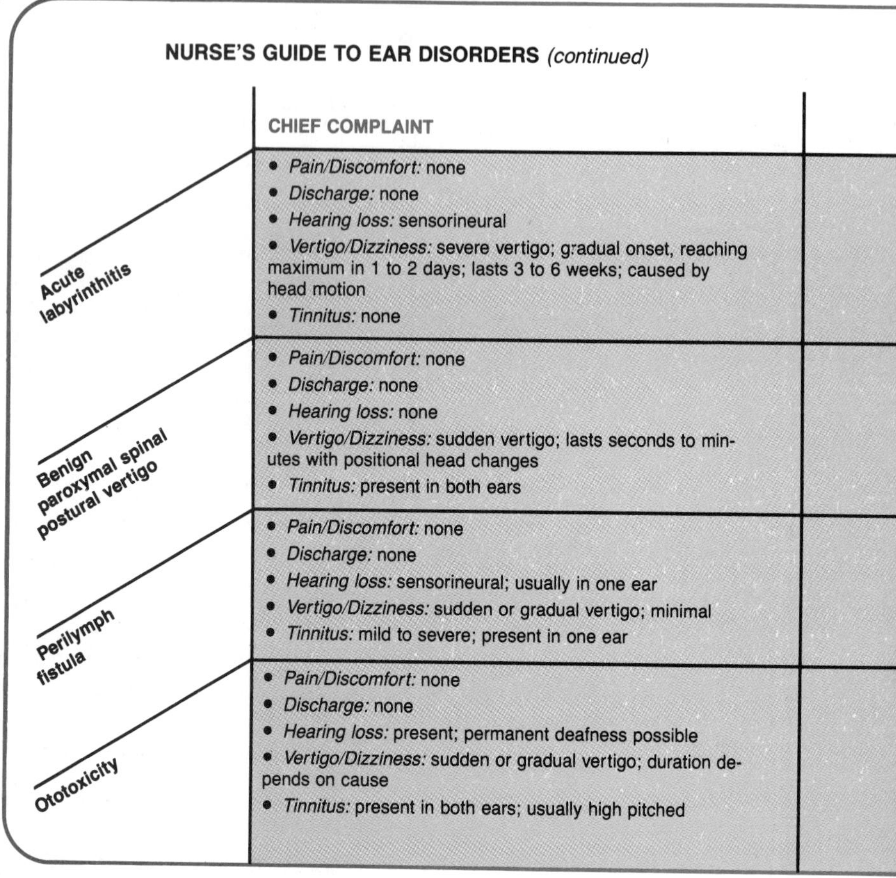

NURSE'S GUIDE TO EAR DISORDERS *(continued)*

	CHIEF COMPLAINT
Acute labyrinthitis	• *Pain/Discomfort:* none • *Discharge:* none • *Hearing loss:* sensorineural • *Vertigo/Dizziness:* severe vertigo; gradual onset, reaching maximum in 1 to 2 days; lasts 3 to 6 weeks; caused by head motion • *Tinnitus:* none
Benign paroxymal spinal postural vertigo	• *Pain/Discomfort:* none • *Discharge:* none • *Hearing loss:* none • *Vertigo/Dizziness:* sudden vertigo; lasts seconds to minutes with positional head changes • *Tinnitus:* present in both ears
Perilymph fistula	• *Pain/Discomfort:* none • *Discharge:* none • *Hearing loss:* sensorineural; usually in one ear • *Vertigo/Dizziness:* sudden or gradual vertigo; minimal • *Tinnitus:* mild to severe; present in one ear
Ototoxicity	• *Pain/Discomfort:* none • *Discharge:* none • *Hearing loss:* present; permanent deafness possible • *Vertigo/Dizziness:* sudden or gradual vertigo; duration depends on cause • *Tinnitus:* present in both ears; usually high pitched

middle ear bones or interruption in the normal bone placement can also interfere with transmission. Blockage of the eustachian tube can create a negative pressure in the middle ear that causes the tympanic membrane to retract, decreasing the membrane's vibration in response to sound waves.

Otosclerosis, which causes a progressive conductive hearing loss, results when spongy bone accumulates over the normal bone of the labyrinth. The overgrowth advances backward, immobilizing the foot of the stapes, which obstructs the oval window. As a result, hair cells of the organ of Corti don't bend as they should, preventing the transmission of sound waves.

Damage to the cochlea or to the acoustic nerve (CN VIII) can result from extensive exposure to loud noises, from infection, or from drug toxicity, and causes sensorineural hearing loss. Ear trauma that tears cochlear and vestibular tissue can impair hearing. Atrophy of ganglion cells in an elderly patient's cochlea causes presbycusis.

Appropriate nursing diagnoses for all disorders that impair hearing include *impaired communication, potential for injury, sensory perceptual alterations,* and *social isolation.*

A disturbance of the external auditory canal, tympanic membrane, cochlea, acoustic nerve, brain stem, or cerebral cortex can result in tinnitus. The cause of this symptom is unknown, but in most ear disorders it presents

	HISTORY	PHYSICAL EXAMINATION AND DIAGNOSTIC STUDIES
	• Recent acute febrile disease, drugs, alcohol, allergy, fatigue, upper respiratory tract infection, otitis media • Nausea and vomiting when severe • Fever, headache, nystagmus	• Otoscopy normal • Hearing tests indicate sensorineural loss • Nystagmus and past-pointing may be present.
	• Easily fatigued	• Otoscopy normal • Hearing tests normal • Nylen-Bárány maneuver positive for nystagmus
	• Stapedectomy • Pressure charge, such as during air travel • Round window rupture • Recent ear trauma	• Otoscopy normal unless trauma; then perforation of tympanic membrane and blood are seen.
	• Ototoxic medication use • Ataxia • Symptoms depend on drug	• Otoscopy normal • Hearing tests normal

as an intermittent or constant, high- or low-pitched noise (or ringing) in the ear. The patient may describe it as a tinkling, buzzing, or roaring. Tinnitus that occurs with acute inflammation of the middle ear usually results from irritation of the tympanic plexus. Blockage of the external ear canal diminishes external sounds, while sounds inside the head intensify and are often interpreted as tinnitus.

Appropriate nursing diagnoses for a patient with tinnitus include *alteration in comfort, impaired coping ability,* and possibly *lack of knowledge about tinnitus.*

Dizziness and vertigo, the principal symptoms of disorders that disturb equilibrium, can result from pressure on the eardrum from wax buildup, foreign bodies, or swelling in the external ear canal. Negative pressure in the middle ear from eustachian tube blockage can also cause these symptoms, as can irritation of the labyrinth or erosion of the labyrinth's bone. Any alteration in the normal physiology of the semicircular canals, saccule, utricle or vestibular branch of the acoustic nerve can cause dizziness or vertigo.

The unsteadiness that accompanies dizziness can cause the patient to misinterpret spatial relationships. Severe vertigo is normally accompanied by nausea and vomiting. Nursing diagnoses for these symptoms include *impaired physical mobility* and *self-care deficits.*

CASE HISTORIES: NURSING DIAGNOSIS FLOWCHART

Patient A
Mary Goldberg
age 42

Patient B
Billy Robertson
age 8

Problem
EARACHE

Patient A

Subjective data

- Severe pain in right ear on contact
- Mild, low-pitched ringing in ears
- No complaint of hearing loss or dizziness
- Slight itching of scalp and neck
- Dyes hair every 3 months; changed to new product 6 months ago

Objective data

- Right ear canal red, with yellow, foul-smelling discharge
- Only 50% tympanic membrane visible due to canal edema, but membrane appears normal
- Temperature: 99.6° F. (37.6° C.)
- Lymphadenopathy more marked than on left ear
- Hairline and scalp reddened
- Culture shows *Staphylococcus aureus*

Nursing diagnoses

- Alteration in comfort; pain due to swollen, excoriated ear
- Lack of knowledge concerning allergic potential of certain hair dyes
- Impaired skin integrity due to discharge

Patient B

Subjective data

- Deep throbbing pain on right side of head
- Seems not to hear at times
- Cries a lot, rubs right ear, and says he's chilly
- Nausea and vomiting since he started to feel hot 2 days ago
- Upper respiratory tract infection 2 weeks ago

Objective data

- Right ear canal appears normal
- Tympanic membrane red and bulging, landmarks unidentifiable
- Temperature: 104.6° F. (40.3° C.)
- Nasopharynx slightly inflamed
- Lymphadenopathy present
- Increased WBC count

Nursing diagnoses

- Fluid volume deficit due to loss through vomiting and fever
- Alteration in comfort; pain due to pressure in middle ear
- Alteration in sensory perception due to hearing loss

Assessing pediatric patients

317 Special history-taking considerations

A child may be having his ears examined and hearing tested because his parents have noticed that he seems less talkative or less responsive to sounds than usual. A school nurse may refer a child for further testing if he fails a hearing test in school or seems unusually restless or inattentive in class. Such situations are commonplace because of the high incidence of acute ear disorders among children.

When assessing a child with an ear or hearing disorder, remember that, as a rule, an infant can localize the direction of sound by age 6 months, and a child's hearing is fully developed by age 5. Interview one or both of the parents to obtain history data. Make it a point to investigate the child's speech development by listening to him carefully. Speech development reflects hearing acuity during childhood. By age 7, for example, most children can speak clearly enough to be understood by most adults. Also observe the child's nonverbal behavior for apparent signs of ear disorders. Does the child rub his ear as though it hurts? Does he tilt his head when listening?

318 Inquire about congenital disorders

If your patient's an infant or very young child, consider possible congenital causes of ear or hearing disorders. Obtain a detailed birth history, including precise information on the mother's health during pregnancy (see Entry 52). Prenatal causes of congenital hearing defects include maternal infection (especially rubella during the first trimester), maternal use of ototoxic drugs, and fetal exposure to X-rays. Events at birth that may cause hearing loss include hypoxia (or anoxia), jaundice, and trauma. If your patient has a con-

ANATOMIC VARIATIONS BASED ON AGE

You'll recognize three major differences between a young child's or infant's ear and an adult's ear.

In a child's, the tympanic membrane slants horizontally rather than vertically. Also, the entire external canal slants upward. These differences require that, during the otoscopic examination, you hold the child's pinna down and out—instead of up and back, as you would with an adult.

A child's eustachian tube also slants horizontally. This causes fluid to stagnate and act as a medium for bacteria. These anatomic differences make the infant and young child more susceptible to ear infection.

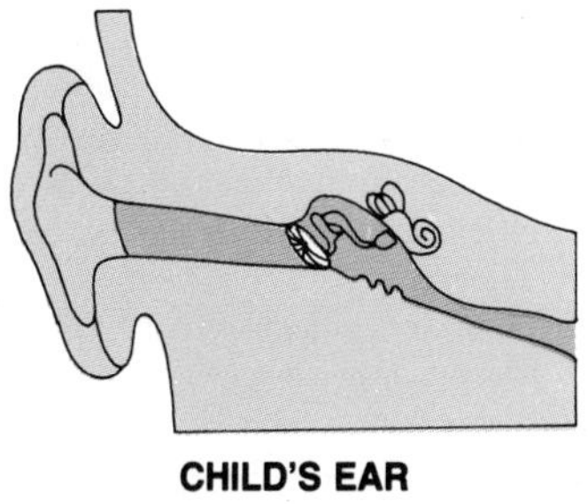

CHILD'S EAR

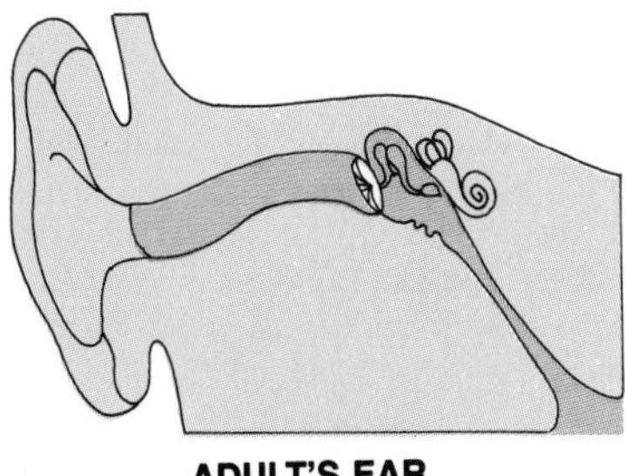

ADULT'S EAR

genital deformity, such as a cleft palate, he's more at risk for otitis media than normal children.

Also investigate the possibility of an inherited hearing disorder. Ask the parents of an infant or young child about inherited conditions, such as Waardenburg's syndrome, that predispose the patient to hearing loss.

319 Daily activities

Ask the mother of an infant with an ear or hearing disorder how she feeds him. If the infant drinks regularly from a bottle while lying down (especially on his back), the liquid may leak into his eustachian tubes when he coughs or cries. This happens because an infant's eustachian tube runs more horizontally from his pharynx to his middle ear, as opposed to its more vertical course in adults (see *Anatomic Variations Based on Age*, page 271). As a result, fluid entering the child's eustachian tube tends to stagnate, creating a perfect growth medium for the infectious organisms that cause otitis media.

Listen carefully to what the mother says. She may relate observations about her child that indicate possible hearing loss: for example, that he doesn't startle or wake up in response to a loud stimulus, or that (for a child who's old enough to understand commands) he has to be told several times to do something. In fact, any report of generally inattentive or unresponsive behavior should raise your suspicion of a hearing disorder. Remember that clues to hearing loss in children may be subtle, because the deficit may affect only one ear, and the child may compensate well with his good ear.

Always investigate external causes of hearing loss in children, such as ear damage from firecrackers, a cap pistol, or lead poisoning. Also ask if the child habitually puts things in his ears, because eardrum damage may result from foreign-body mechanical irritation in the ear canal.

320 Inspecting a child's auricles

Pay special attention to how a child's auricles are positioned (see *Recognizing Proper Auricle Alignment*). As in the adult, the top of the auricle should align with the inner and outer canthi of the eye. If a child's ears are low set, it may mean he has one or more birth defects, such as renal agenesis or anomalies.

Observe for other external ear deformities that may be associated with abnormalities. For example, in a child with Down's syndrome, you'll see hyperplasia of the superior crus of the antihelix, which causes the auricle to fold over. Microtia—an uncommon developmental anomaly in which the auricle is grossly undersized and the external ear canal is either blind or absent—can be associated with renal disease.

321 Using the otoscope to examine a child

Because inserting an otoscope may make a child uncomfortable, postpone this part of your assessment until the end of the physical examination, if possible. To help alleviate the child's fears, let him hold and look at the otoscope before the examination. You can also place the instrument at the opening of his ear canal (not *into* it), and then remove it, to show him that insertion doesn't hurt. When restraint is necessary, have the child sit or lie on his parent's lap. Instruct the parent to hold the child firmly.

To begin the examination, gently pull the child's auricle down, *but not back*, before inserting the otoscope. Remember that in an infant or young child the ear canal slants upward, and in an older child or adult the ear canal slants downward. Because the child's canal is also shorter, take care to insert the otoscope only about ¼" to ½" (6 to 13 mm). For maximum control of the otoscope, hold it upside down to insert it, with your hand braced against the child's head. This minimizes displacement of the otoscope if the child squirms or moves his head.

When you look through the otoscope, expect the cone of light on a normal child's eardrum to be indistinct, in contrast to its clear outline in a normal adult. Remember that a red eardrum in a crying child is often normal.

Pneumatic otoscopy—rarely performed by most nurses—can be used to evaluate a child's eardrum further.

322 Testing a child's hearing

You can't perform tuning fork tests on an infant or young child, but you can test his hearing with simpler procedures. For example, with an infant, make a sudden loud noise, such as clapping your hands or snapping your fingers, about 12″ (30 cm) from his ear. He should respond with the startle reflex or by blinking (see Entry 841). (If you clap your hands, be careful not to create an airstream that would cause the infant to blink.) Both these responses are normal, but they suggest only that the child did perceive the noise you made, not that he doesn't have some degree of hearing loss. Be sure to test both ears.

A 6-month-old infant normally reacts expectantly if he hears his mother's voice before she comes into view, so this is a good way to test hearing in such a young child. To evaluate hearing in a child between ages 2 and 5, use play techniques, such as asking him to put a peg in a board when he hears a sound transmitted through earphones. For an older child, try the whisper test, but be sure to use words he knows, and take care to prevent him from lipreading. The child should hear a whispered question or simple command at 8′ (2.5 m).

Recurrent otitis media, a major cause of hearing loss in young children, can block normal development of speech and socialization skills. For this reason, be sure to test the hearing of every child you examine who has a history of recurrent middle ear infections.

323 Common ear disorders in children

Acute otitis media is one of the most common childhood diseases, and many children have recurrent middle ear infections. A foreign body in the ear canal is another common problem in children.

RECOGNIZING PROPER AURICLE ALIGNMENT

As you inspect your pediatric patient's ears, look for proper auricle alignment. Normally, the top of the auricle lines up horizontally with the inner and outer canthi of the near eye, as shown in the first illustration. Abnormally high or low alignment, shown in the second and third illustrations, may indicate birth defects.

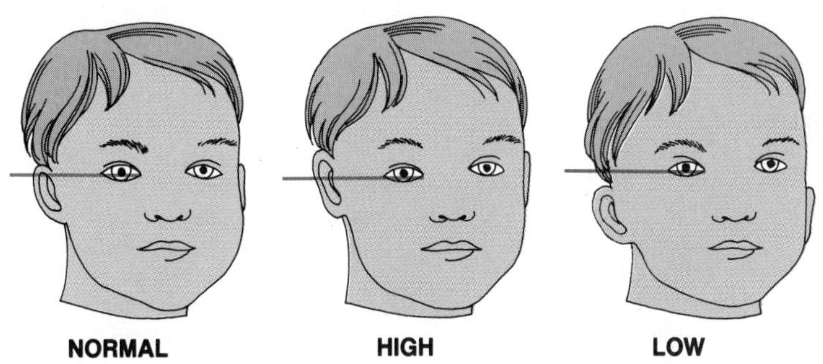

Eustachian tube malfunction is commonly associated with middle ear disease in children. Consider it whenever you see a child with recurrent ear infections, enlarged adenoids, a history of allergies, or a cleft palate.

A child who's had a myringotomy tube inserted may develop a middle ear infection, because the tube allows organisms normally present in the ear canal to enter the middle ear space. Usually the child experiences a significant discharge of pus and blood, but no pain.

Assessing geriatric patients

324 Hearing loss in elderly patients

Many elderly patients have some degree of hearing loss, most often caused by *presbycusis*, the slowly progressive deafness that often accompanies aging. Aging results in degenerative structural changes in the entire auditory system. The incidence of hearing loss in elderly persons is probably higher than statistics indicate. Often an older person isn't immediately aware of a hearing defect's onset or progression. He may recognize the problem but, accepting it as a natural aspect of aging, may not seek medical help.

Because hearing loss in an elderly patient may interfere significantly with his individual pursuits and social interactions, you must periodically assess each geriatric patient thoroughly to rule out conditions that can be treated by surgery or medication.

Interviewing an elderly patient who has a hearing defect requires patience, understanding, and the use of special techniques (see Entries 42 and 58). Be alert for signs that he's experiencing social isolation because of a hearing loss. Typical comments are, "I don't use the telephone anymore—it's too low," "I don't go to meetings—all the noise is too confusing," or "My family gets tired of talking to me."

Observe him, too, for behavioral patterns directly related to hearing loss. Insecurity and anxiety, perhaps coupled with disturbances in sleep patterns, may be manifestations of the feelings of loss and depression often experienced by an elderly person whose hearing is impaired. He may also be disorganized or unreasonable because of his inability to understand what is being said to him—and around him. Ask an elderly patient if he'd like to have a family member or a close friend remain with him during the health history interview and the physical examination.

325 Assessing for presbycusis

The most common cause of hearing loss in the elderly is presbycusis. Sometimes called *senile deafness*, presbycusis is irreversible, bilateral, sensorineural (perceptive) hearing loss that usually starts during middle age and slowly progresses. Four distinct forms of presbycusis are recognized. The most common form is *sensory presbycusis*, caused by atrophy of the organ of Corti and the auditory nerve.

Suspect presbycusis if your elderly patient complains of gradual hearing loss over many years but has no history of ear disorders or severe generalized disease. In most patients, the physical examination shows no abnormalities of the ear canal or eardrum. The Rinne test is positive—that is, the patient hears the air-conducted tone longer than the bone-conducted tone, with air conduction about equal in both ears. If your patient has a positive history of vertigo, ear pain, or nausea, suspect some pathology other than presbycusis. Any hearing or vestibular function abnormality requires immediate referral for audiometric testing.

326 Examining the elderly patient

During the physical examination, stand close to an elderly patient with a hearing disorder in case he experiences dizziness or vertigo. Try to make the examination as thorough as possible, without tiring him. If necessary, complete the examination later rather than accept inappropriate responses that may be prompted by fatigue.

As much as possible, combine interviewing techniques and examination procedures. For example, if your history interview elicits a particular complaint, ask the patient to elaborate on the symptom as you look for corresponding signs during the physical examination.

Inspection and palpation of the auricles and surrounding areas should yield the same findings as in the younger adult, with the exception of the normally hairy tragus in an older man. Examination with the otoscope yields similar results. Remember that the eardrum in some elderly patients may normally appear dull and retracted instead of pearl gray, but this can also be a clinically significant sign.

For early detection of hearing loss in an elderly patient, always perform tuning fork tests. Be particularly careful when you perform the Weber test, because the geriatric patient may become confused if he hears the tone better in his affected ear. As a result, he may falsely report that he hears the tone better in his other ear. Also evaluate the patient's ability to hear and understand speech (see Entry 56), in case you need to recommend rehabilitative therapy. Use the past-pointing and falling tests to evaluate patients who complain of vertigo, dizziness, or lightheadedness.

If your patient wears a hearing aid, inspect it carefully for proper functioning. Check how well the aid fits. Examine the earpiece, sound tube, and any connecting tubing for cracks and for the presence of dust, wax, or other sound-obstructing matter. Check that the batteries are installed correctly. Suspect that the aid isn't functioning properly if your patient reports that what he hears through it sounds fluttery or garbled.

Selected References

Bates, Barbara. *A Guide to Physical Examination,* 2nd ed. Philadelphia: J.B. Lippincott Co., 1979.

Bluestone, Charles D. "Otitis Media: Newer Aspects of Etiology, Pathogenesis, Diagnosis, and Treatment," *Consultant* 19:66, December 1979.

Davis, Hallowell, and Silverman, Richard S. *Hearing and Deafness,* 4th ed. New York: Holt, Rinehart & Winston, 1978.

De Gowin, Elmer L., and De Gowin, Richard L. *Bedside Diagnostic Examination,* 3rd ed. New York: Macmillan Publishing Co., 1976.

Guyton, Arthur C. *Textbook of Medical Physiology,* 6th ed. Philadelphia: W.B. Saunders Co., 1981.

Habel, D.W. "The E.N.T. Examination: Too Important to Overlook - Part I," *Consultant* 16:75, 1976.

Jaffe, B.F. *Hearing Loss in Children.* Baltimore: University Park Press, 1977.

Paparella, Michael M., and Shumrick, Donald, eds. *Otolaryngology: Ear,* vol. 2. Philadelphia: W.B. Saunders Co., 1973.

Senturia, Ben H., et al. *Diseases of the External Ear: An Otologic-Dermatologic Manual,* 2nd ed. New York: Grune & Stratton, 1980.

Smith, James D. "Evaluating Vertigo," *Emergency Medicine* 12(20):45, 1980.

Walker, H. K., et al. *Clinical Methods: The History, Physical, and Laboratory Examinations,* 2 vols. Woburn, Mass.: Butterworths Publishing, Inc., 1976.

West, Hugh H. "Pneumatoscopy," *Annals of Emergency Medicine* 9(12):634, 1980.

Wood, Raymond, and Northern, Jerry. *Manual of Otolaryngology: A Symptom-Oriented Text.* Baltimore: Williams & Wilkins Co., 1979.

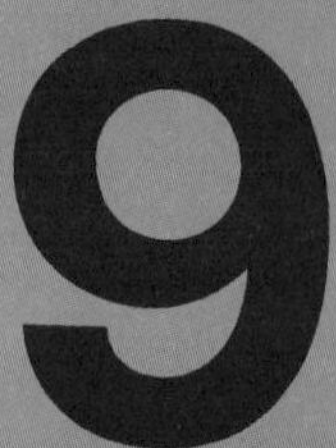

KEY POINTS IN THIS CHAPTER

KEY CHARTS IN THIS CHAPTER

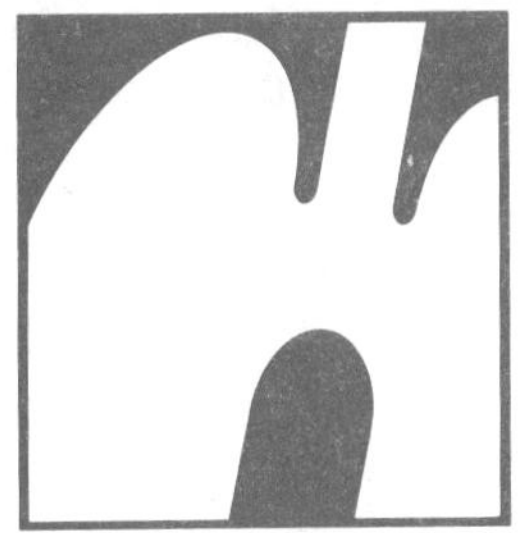

Respiratory System

Introduction

327 When to assess the respiratory system

Respiratory assessment is essential on hospital admission, at regular intervals during illness, and during routine health evaluation and screening. Perform respiratory assessment daily for ambulatory patients and more frequently for patients who are acutely ill or particularly susceptible to disease (pediatric and geriatric patients, for example) or those whose activities are limited by medication, surgery, or debilitating diseases. Your assessment can be deliberate and organized—as it would be for a newly admitted patient. Or it may be informal: For example, during your patient's bath, meals, and ambulation, you may observe for changes in his skin color and in the rate and depth of his respirations, for his use of accessory muscles, and for increased temperature. But whether your assessment is planned or informal, you'll probably be the first person your patient comes in contact with who can detect early changes in his pulmonary function, thus ensuring prompt treatment.

328 Acute changes demand quick detection

The two vital functions of the respiratory system are maintenance of oxygen and carbon dioxide exchange in the lungs and tissues, and regulation of acid-base balance. Any changes in this system affect all the other body systems. In chronic respiratory disease, pulmonary changes (such as hypoxia) occur slowly, and the person's body has time to adapt. But with acute pulmonary changes, such as those from pneumothorax or aspiration pneumonia, the patient's other body systems don't have time to adapt to sudden hypoxia, which can cause death.

Changes in other body systems may reduce the lungs' capability to provide oxygen. For example, a patient's poor cardiac function results in decreased tissue oxygenation, which causes his lungs to work harder to provide oxygen. In fact, any acute disease state increases the body's oxygen demands and the lungs' workload. Also, debilitation from acute disease makes a patient more susceptible to secondary infections, which may affect his lungs.

A patient with a less serious illness isn't immune from pulmonary complications. For instance, simple postanesthesia hypoventilation can develop into atelectasis that, if untreated, can cause a devastating pneumonia. Or, antibiotic therapy for a minor infection can alter the patient's normal lung flora and allow virulent pneumonia to develop. Regardless of their cause, changes in a patient's lung function can result in acid-base disturbances, tissue hypoxia, and even sudden death.

Using correct assessment techniques, you can detect changes in a patient's respiratory system early and intervene quickly, perhaps preventing serious complications.

Reviewing anatomy and physiology

329 Upper airways

The upper airways include the nose, the mouth, the nasopharynx, the oropharynx, the laryngopharynx, and the larynx. The *two portals for air* are the nose and the mouth. The nasal openings for air passage are the nares, or nostrils. Divided by the septum at the midline, the two separate nasal passages are formed anteriorly by cartilaginous walls and posteriorly by bony structures. The bony lateral walls of the two nasal cavities are called the *conchae* or *turbinates*. Covered with mucous membrane, they form additional surface areas over which air is humidified and warmed as it passes into the nasopharynx. Anteriorly, the nose hairs (vibrissae) trap dust and large particles; posteriorly, mucus traps finer particles, which the cilia carry to the pharynx to be swallowed. Posteriorly, the olfactory epithelium overlies the superior concha and upper portion of the septum. The superior portion of the hard palate forms the nasal floor.

The *paranasal sinuses* provide speech resonance. The maxillary and the frontal sinuses are large, paired, air-filled cavities. The sphenoidal and the ethmoidal sinuses, also covered with mucous membrane, consist of several small air spaces in the nasal cavity's bony posterior portion. All four sinuses drain through the meati, near the conchae.

The *nasopharynx* has lateral and posterior muscular walls. Air passes from the nasal cavity into the nasopharynx through the choanae, which are always open. The pharyngeal tonsils (adenoids) are located bilaterally near the choanae. In the lateral walls above the soft palate level are the eustachian tube openings. The eustachian tubes regulate middle ear pressure during swallowing or yawning.

The *oropharynx* is the posterior wall of the mouth that connects the nasopharynx with the laryngopharynx, the lowest pharyngeal region, which stretches down to the esophagus.

The *larynx,* which contains the vocal cords, is a cartilaginous and muscular organ connecting the pharynx and the trachea. Two of the nine principal cartilages—the large, shield-shaped thyroid cartilage (Adam's apple) and the cricoid cartilage inferior to it—can be palpated in the neck.

Formed by a flexible cartilage, the *epiglottis* bends reflexively on swallowing, closing off the larynx to swallowed substances. The inner laryngeal structures include the vestibule, the glottis, the vocal folds, and the infraglottic cavity. The vestibular folds (false vocal cords) are thick mucosal folds located just below the vestibule and superior to the true vocal cords. The opening between the folds is called the *glottis.* Located posteriorly, the small paired arytenoid cartilages act as a fulcrum for vocal cord muscles.

330 Lower airways

The lower airways begin at the top of the *trachea,* a tubular structure that extends about 5″ (12 cm) from the only complete tracheal ring, the cricoid cartilage, to the carina at the level of the sixth or seventh thoracic vertebra. C-shaped cartilage rings with posterior openings reinforce and protect the trachea, preventing its collapse. The isthmus of the thyroid covers the upper two or three rings. About half the trachea

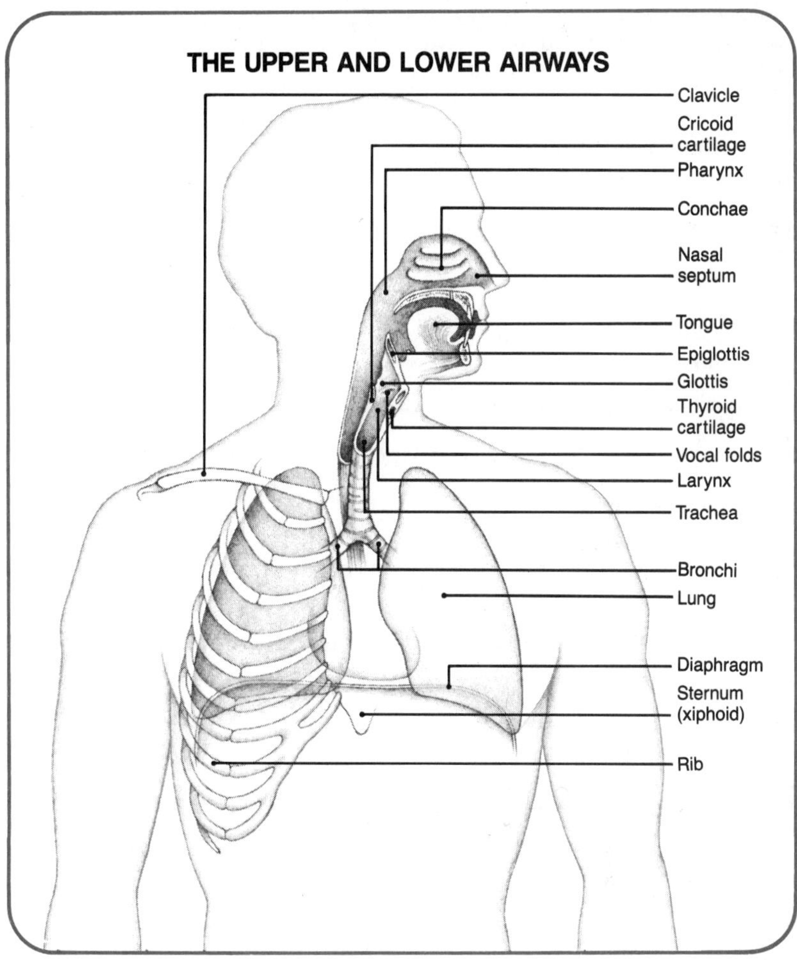

is in the neck and half is in the thorax; the right and the left primary bronchi (mainstem bronchi) begin at the carina, or tracheal bifurcation. Composed of tissue similar to that of the trachea, the walls of the primary bronchi are lined with epithelium containing cilia, goblet (mucus-producing) cells, and microvilli that increase surface area absorption. The right primary bronchus is shorter, wider, and more vertical than the left.

The *primary bronchi* divide into the secondary, or lobar, branches and—accompanied by blood vessels, nerves, and lymphatics—enter the lungs at the hilum. Each of the five secondary branches—right upper, middle, and lower, and left upper and lower—enters its own lung lobe. These branches further divide into the tertiary, or segmental, bronchi, which supply air to the 18 bronchopulmonary segments. From the tertiary bronchi, branching continues and airways become narrower, cartilage decreases, and smooth muscle increases.

The functional units of the lungs—the *lobules*—are supplied with air from the small airways (the terminal bronchioles), with an average diameter of 0.5 mm. The terminal bronchioles divide into two or more respiratory bronchioles, which are the entrances to the lobules. These passages continue to branch off, terminating in alveolar ducts, which lead to walled alveoli surrounded by a network of anastomosing capillaries. Alveolar cells are simple squamous epithelium as well as type II cells. Type II cells are capable of secreting surfactant, which reduces surface tension and enhances alveolar elasticity. Also, elastic fibers surround the alveoli and allow them to recoil to preinspiratory size.

331 Thoracic cage, lungs, and pleurae

The anterior boundary of the thoracic cage, which contains the lungs and pleurae, is the sternum. Its posterior boundary is formed by the thoracic vertebrae; the inferior boundary, by the costal margins, xiphoid process, and diaphragm.

The right lung has three lobes and is larger than the left—which has two. The medial inferior surface of the left lung curves slightly around and under the heart and forms a tonguelike struc-

LOCATING THORACIC LANDMARKS

Use the landmarks in these illustrations as guides when you assess your patient's respiratory status:

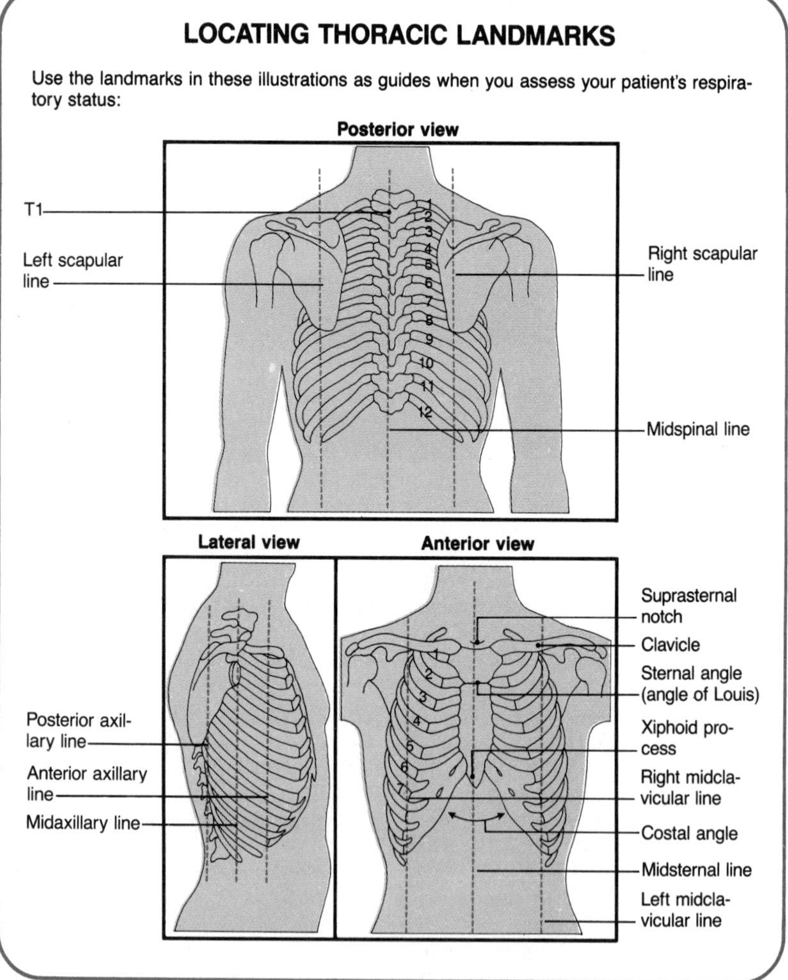

IDENTIFYING LUNG LOBES

Posterior view

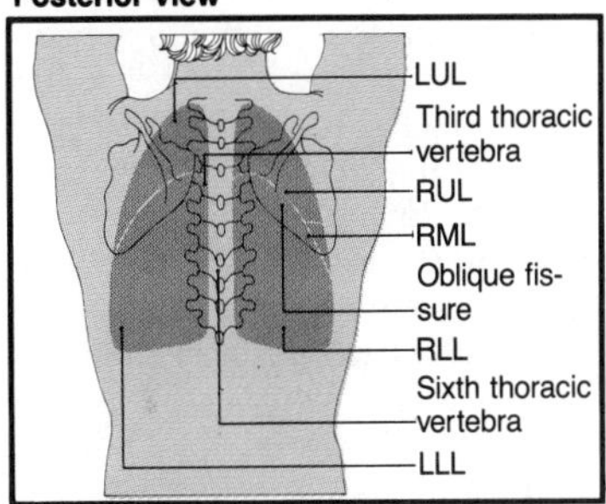

Left lateral view

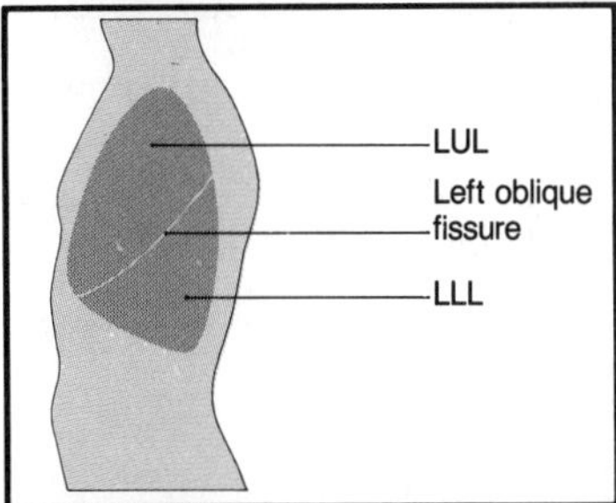

Right lateral view

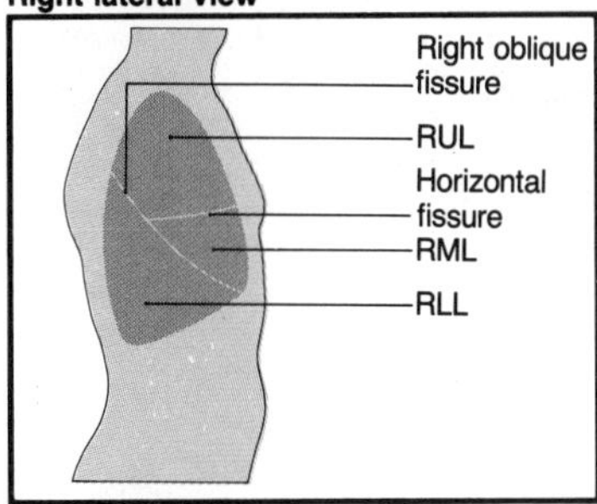

Anterior view

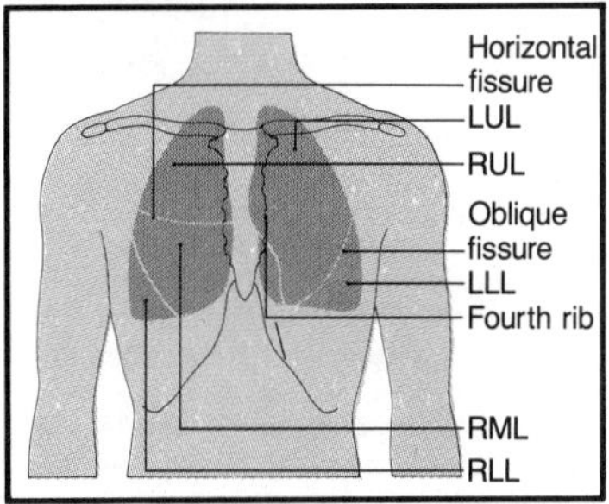

To locate lung lobes, you'll need to know the common chest wall landmarks shown in these illustrations.

In the posterior view, the oblique fissures divide the upper lobes from the lower lobes of both lungs. Externally, you can approximate the location of these fissures by imagining bilateral lines drawn laterally and inferiorly from the third thoracic spinous process to the inferior border of the scapula. You should remember that unlike the other views shown here, where all lobes can be identified, you can identify only two lobes in each lung in the posterior view.

In the left lateral view, the left oblique fissure divides the left upper lobe (LUL) from the left lower lobe (LLL). Externally, you can approximate the location of this fissure by imagining a line drawn anteriorly and inferiorly from the third thoracic spinous process to the sixth rib, midclavicular line.

In the right lateral view, you can determine the location of the right oblique fissure as you did for the left oblique fissure. But the right oblique fissure divides the upper *portion* of the lung (both upper and middle lobes) from the lower lobe (RLL). To approximate the division of the right upper lobe (RUL) and the right middle lobe (RML), imagine a line drawn medially from the fifth rib, midaxillary line, to the fourth rib, midclavicular line.

In the anterior view, you can locate the apices and the inferior borders of both lungs using external landmarks on the chest. The apices lie ¾" to 1½" (2 to 4 cm) above the inner portion of the clavicle. The inferior borders run from the sixth rib, midclavicular line, to the eighth rib, midaxillary line.

The horizontal fissure divides the right upper lobe from the right middle lobe. Externally, you can approximate the location of this fissure by imagining a line drawn anteriorly and superiorly from the fifth rib, midaxillary line, to the fourth rib, midclavicular line.

The right and left oblique fissures divide the lower lobe from the upper and middle lobes. Externally, you can approximate the location of these fissures by imagining bilateral lines drawn medially and inferiorly from the fifth rib, midaxillary line, to the sixth rib, midclavicular line.

Locating both chest wall landmarks and the imaginary lines noted above will help you perform a complete thoracic assessment of your patient.

ture called the *lingula pulmonis sinistri.* The inferior surfaces of both lower lobes are separated from the abdominal viscera by the diaphragm. The apices of the two upper lobes are slightly above the first rib, about 1″ (2.5 cm) above the clavicles. The lateral boundary of both lungs is the chest wall.

The *visceral pleura,* a serous membrane adhering closely to the lung parenchyma, envelops each lung and separates it from the mediastinal structures—the heart and its great vessels, the trachea, the esophagus, and the bronchi. The parietal pleura, which lines the thoracic cavity from the hilum, covers all areas that contact the lungs. The visceral pleura meets the parietal pleura at the hilum, forming a narrow fold called the *pulmonary ligament.* These membranes consist of connective and epithelial tissue and a single layer of secreting epithelium. As they rub together during respiration, secretions minimize friction. The area between the two membranes is only a potential space and can't be seen unless air or excess fluid occupies it. Normally, pleural fluid maintains the surface tension forces.

UNDERSTANDING THE PULMONARY BLOOD SUPPLY

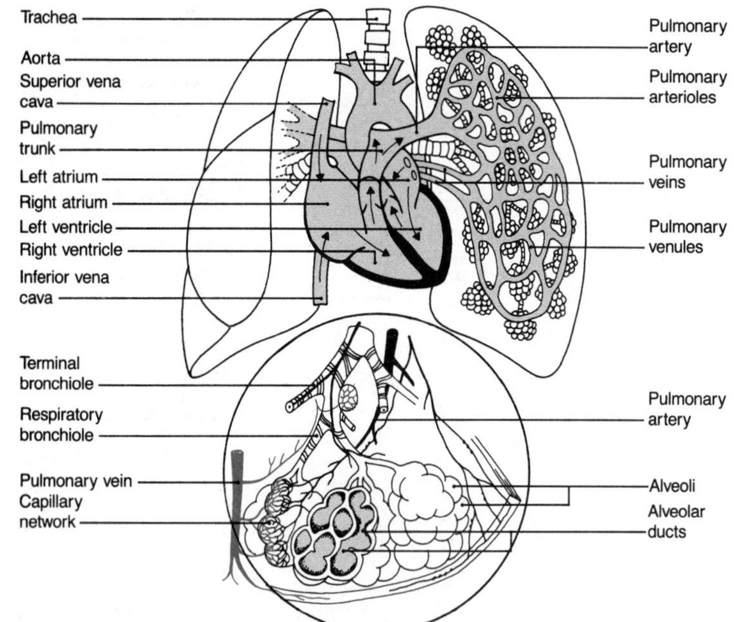

The respiratory and circulatory systems work closely together to transport gases to and from the lungs. To understand this relationship, follow the arrows in this illustration.

The right and left pulmonary arteries take deoxygenated blood from the right side of the heart to the lungs. These arteries divide into distal branches, called arterioles, that terminate as a concentrated capillary network in the alveoli and alveolar sacs. Here, gas exchange occurs. The pulmonary veins also divide into branches. The venules collect the oxygenated blood from the capillaries and pass it along to larger vessels, which carry it back to the heart. The pulmonary veins terminate at the left side of the heart, where they deliver oxygenated blood to be distributed throughout the body.

332 Pulmonary blood supply

Oxygen-deficient blood is pumped from the right ventricle of the heart to the pulmonary trunk. This trunk then branches laterally into the right and the left pulmonary arteries, which further divide into smaller arteries that closely follow the bronchial tree airways throughout the lungs. Eventually, pulmonary arterioles enter the lung lobules, where arterioles and venules form the capillary beds around the alveoli. This is where gas exchange occurs. The venous system then returns oxygenated blood to the left atrium of the heart to be pumped throughout the body. The tissues of the airways and pleura receive blood from the bronchial arteries, which arise from the aorta and its branches. (See *Understanding the Pulmonary Blood Supply.)*

333 Mechanics of respiration

Voluntary and intercostal muscles, working with the diaphragm, produce normal inspiratory and expiratory movement of the lungs and chest wall. The lungs' tendency to recoil inward, balanced by the chest wall's tendency to spring outward, creates a subatmospheric pressure in the closed pleural cavity. This pressure, which is about −5 mmHg below atmospheric pressure, makes lung ventilation (gas volume movement) possible (see *Understanding the Mechanics of Respiration*).

334 Neurologic control

Innervation of pulmonary structures varies according to their function. The phrenic nerves from the third to the fifth cervical vertebrae innervate the mediastinal and central diaphragmatic pleurae and the diaphragm. Intercostal nerves innervate the costal and peripheral diaphragmatic pleurae and the intercostal muscles. Vagus nerve branches innervate the larynx. Visceral sensation through these vagal fibers is

UNDERSTANDING THE MECHANICS OF RESPIRATION

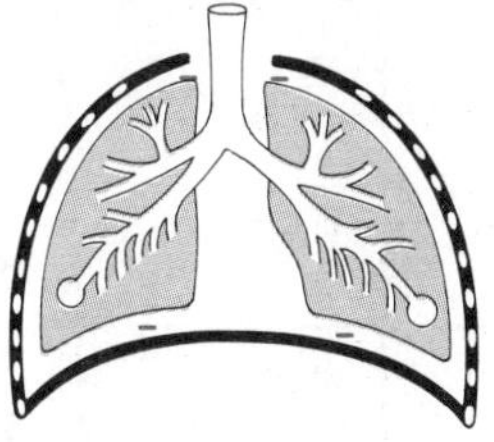

At rest
- Inspiratory muscles relax
- Atmospheric pressure present in tracheobronchial tree
- No air movement

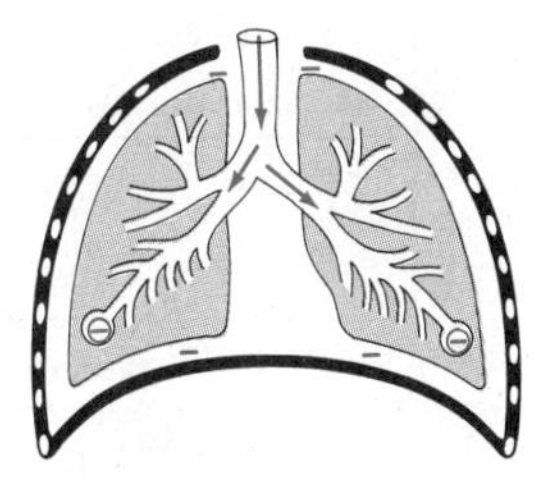

During inspiration
- Inspiratory muscles contract
- Chest expands
- Diaphragm descends
- Negative alveolar pressure present
- Air moves into lungs

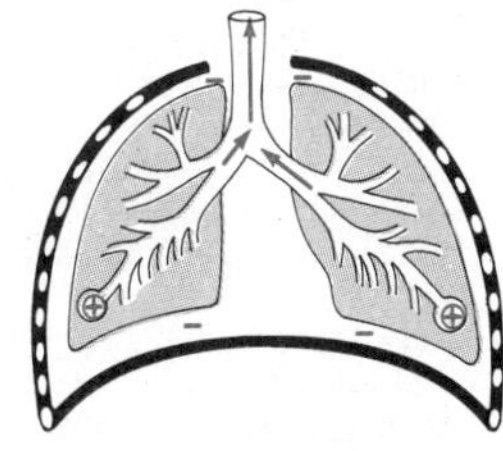

During expiration
- Inspiratory muscles relax, causing lung recoil
- Diaphragm ascends
- Positive alveolar pressure present
- Air moves out of lungs

KEY:
− = negative intrapleural pressure
⊖ = negative alveolar pressure
⊕ = positive alveolar pressure

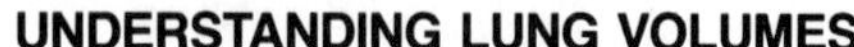

UNDERSTANDING LUNG VOLUMES

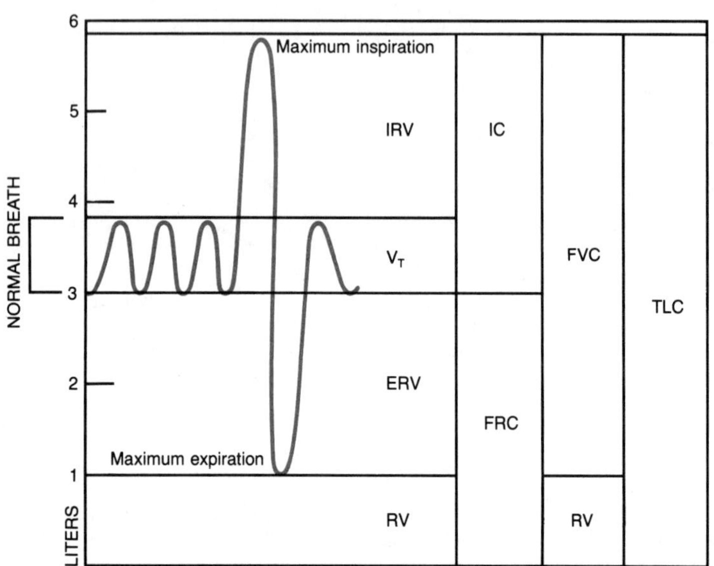

Basically, breathing is a rhythmic exchange of quantities of air. You can break down these quantities into specific lung volumes and capacities using a spirometer.

Lung volumes are measurements taken at various times during respiration. For example, *residual volume* (RV) is the amount of air in the lungs after your patient has expelled as much air as he can. The other volumes, identified in the above graph, include the following:

- *Tidal volume* (V_T): the amount of air that enters or leaves the lungs during normal breathing (inspiration and expiration)
- *Inspiratory reserve volume* (IRV): the amount of air inhaled, by forced maximum inspiration, above and beyond tidal volume
- *Expiratory reserve volume* (ERV): the amount of air forcibly exhaled beyond the tidal volume

If you added various lung volumes together in different combinations, you'd come up with several lung capacities. Here's how they're calculated:

- *Functional vital capacity* (FVC): the sum of tidal, inspiratory, and expiratory reserve volumes. It represents the total exchangeable air volume in the lungs.
- *Functional residual capacity* (FRC): the sum of the expiratory reserve volume and residual volume. This represents the amount of air remaining in the lungs after normal expiration.
- *Inspiratory capacity* (IC): the amount of air that can be inhaled after normal expiration
- *Total lung capacity* (TLC): the sum of vital capacity and residual volume. This represents the sum of all air in the lungs after the fullest possible inspiration.

Adapted from R.F. Wilson, ed., *Critical Care Manual: Principles and Techniques of Critical Care*, Vol. 1 (Kalamazoo, Mich.: Upjohn Co., 1976), with the permission of the publisher.

primarily limited to stretch, although some vagal (and sympathetic) fibers are motor fibers of the bronchial tree smooth muscle. In addition, other sympathetic fibers regulate vasoconstriction of the pulmonary arterioles.

The respiratory muscles respond to motor impulses from the respiratory center in the brain stem. The posterior medulla oblongata is functionally divided into inspiratory and expiratory centers. The apneustic center of the pons varolii constantly stimulates neurons in the inspiratory center. The expiratory center inhibits inspiration, thereby providing time for muscle relaxation. Impulses travel from the inspiratory center to the respiratory muscles (by way of the phrenic nerve) and to the pneumotaxic center of the pons. After a slight delay, impulses move from the pons to the expiratory center. Thus, the *pons* is the pacemaker that regulates the rhythm of respiration; the *medulla* regulates rate and depth.

The Hering-Breuer reflex also regulates respiratory excursion. Lung expansion stimulates stretch receptors that send impulses along the vagal afferent fibers to the expiratory center, thus inhibiting inspiration. When the lungs deflate, the stimulus stops, and inspiration again dominates.

Central chemoreceptors, located in the anterior medulla, respond to changes in pH, oxygen tension (PO_2), carbon dioxide tension (PCO_2), and peripheral chemoreceptors. These anterior neurons are particularly sensitive to pH changes in cerebrospinal fluid: A decrease quickly stimulates alveolar ventilation. The most active chemical stimulus is CO_2 tension of arterial blood: A small increase in inspired CO_2 (or hydrogen ion concentration) decreases the pH, causing quick medulla stimulation, which results in hyperventilation. The peripheral chemoreceptors (the aortic and carotid bodies) sense changes in oxygen tension and directly stimulate the central chemoreceptors. (Of course, respirations can also be partially controlled voluntarily.)

335 Gas exchange

Diffusion, also called *external respiration,* is the exchange of gases between the alveoli and the capillaries. In this process, oxygen diffuses across the alveolar epithelium, the epithelial basement membrane, the capillary basement membrane, and the capillary endothelial membrane. It then dissolves in the plasma and passes through the red blood cell membrane. Carbon dioxide diffuses in the opposite direction. Oxygen moves from the alveolus into the venous end of the capillary because oxygen pressure (PO_2) is greater in the alveolus; carbon dioxide diffuses from the venous end of the capillary, where carbon dioxide pressure (PCO_2) is greater, to the alveolus. Each gas acts independent of the other because of its distinctive partial pressure. A number of factors affect the rate of gas exchange, including drug use, geographic altitude, and the extent of the person's functional lung surface area.

Hemoglobin, which is normally about 98% oxygen-saturated, transports oxygen to the tissues for gas exchange between body cells and red blood cells. This exchange is called *internal respiration.* Because increased temperature and decreased pH trigger oxygen's release from hemoglobin, only tissues needing oxygen receive it. Blood also carries carbon dioxide to the lungs, primarily in the form of bicarbonate.

Collecting appropriate history data

336 Biographical data

When assessing a patient's respiratory system, remember that his age and sex can affect his thoracic configuration. When you note the area where a patient lives and what he does for a living, be alert to possible environmental or occupational hazards that can affect his lungs and breathing.

337 Chief complaint

The most common chief complaints for

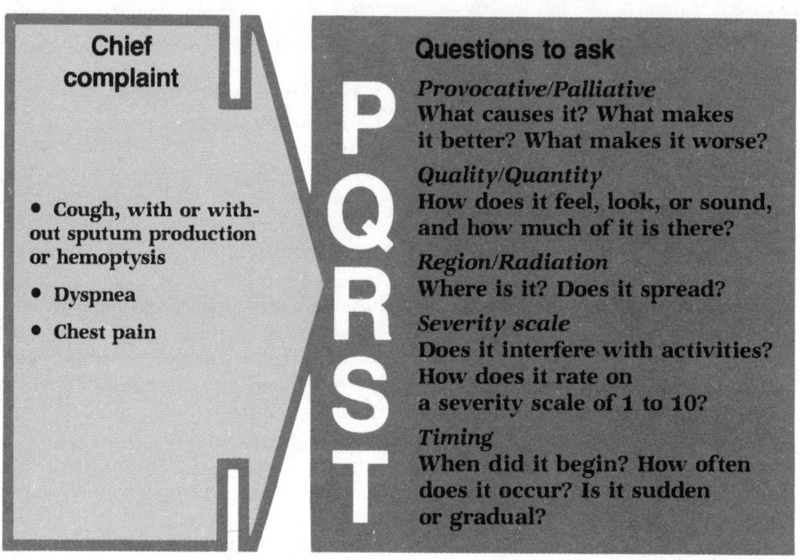

respiratory disorders are *cough*—with or without sputum production or hemoptysis—*dyspnea,* and *chest pain.*

338 History of present illness

Using the PQRST mnemonic device, ask your patient to elaborate on his chief complaint. Then, depending on the complaint, explore the history of his present illness by asking the following types of questions:

• ***Cough.*** *Does your cough usually occur at a specific time of day? How does it sound—dry, hacking, barking, congested?* (See *Analyzing Your Patient's Cough.*) Try to determine whether the patient's cough is related to cigarette smoking or irritants. (The most common causes of coughing are smoking and chronic bronchitis.) *Please describe any medication you're using or treatment you're receiving to clear the cough. How frequently do you take the medication or receive treatment? Have you recently been exposed to anyone with a similar cough? Was this person's cough caused by a cold or flu?*

• ***Sputum production.*** *How much sputum are you coughing up per day?* Remember, the tracheobronchial tree can produce up to 3 oz (90 ml) of sputum per day. *What time of day do you cough up the most sputum?* Smokers cough when they get up in the morning; nonsmokers generally don't. Coughing from an irritant occurs most often during exposure to it—for example, at work. *Is sputum production increasing?* This may result from external stimuli or from such internal causes as chronic bronchial infection or a lung abscess. Excess production of sputum that separates into layers may indicate bronchiectasis. *Does the sputum contain mucus, or look frothy? What color is it? Has the color changed? Does it smell bad?* Foul-smelling sputum may result from an anaerobic infection, such as an abscess. Blood-tinged or rust-colored sputum may result from trauma caused by coughing or from such underlying pathology as bronchitis, pulmonary infarction or infections, tuberculosis, and tumors. A color change from white to yellow or green indicates infection.

• ***Dyspnea.*** *Are you always short of breath or do you have attacks of breathlessness?* Onset of dyspnea may be slow or abrupt. For example, a patient with asthma may experience acute dyspnea intermittently. *What relieves the attacks—positioning, relaxation, medication? Do the attacks cause your lips and nail beds to turn blue? Does body position, time of day, or a certain type of activity affect your breathing?* Paroxysmal nocturnal dyspnea and orthopnea are commonly associated with chronic lung disease, but they may be related to cardiac dysfunction. *How many stairs can you climb or blocks can you walk before you begin to feel short of breath? Do such activities as taking a shower or shopping make you feel this way?* Dyspnea from activity suggests poor ventilation or perfusion, or inefficient breathing mechanisms. *Do you experience associated signs and symptoms, such as cough, diaphoresis, or chest discomfort? Does the breathlessness seem to be stable or getting worse? Is it accompanied by external sounds, such as wheezing or stridor?* Wheezing results from small-airway obstruction (for example, from an aspirated foreign body, from a tumor, from asthma, or from congestive heart failure). Stridor results from tracheal compression or laryngeal edema.

• ***Chest pain.*** *Is the pain localized? Is it constant or do you experience attacks? Have you ever had a chest injury? Does a specific activity (such as movement of the upper body, or exercise) produce pain?* Chest pain may be associated with cardiovascular disorders, but respiratory disorders usually cause musculoskeletal chest pain (the lungs have no pain-sensitive nerves). However, the parietal pleura and the tracheobronchial tree are sensitive to pain. *Is the pain accompanied by other signs and symptoms, such as coughing, sneezing, or shortness of breath? Does the pain occur when you breathe normally or only when you breathe deeply?* This distinction is important in determining whether your patient's pain is pleuritic. *Does splinting relieve the pain?* (See *Assessing Chest Pain,* pages 336 to 337.)

ANALYZING YOUR PATIENT'S COUGH

If you know how to interpret your patient's cough pattern, cough sound, and sputum, they can supply you with valuable information about his condition. This chart tells you how. Ask your patient these questions or, if possible, answer them yourself:

QUESTION	ANSWER	POSSIBLE CAUSE
When does he cough?	• Early morning	• Chronic inflammation of large airways in patients who smoke
	• Late afternoon	• Exposure to irritants during the workday
	• Evening	• Chronic postnasal drip or sinusitis, gastric reflux with nocturnal aspiration
What does the cough sound like?	• Dry	• Cardiac condition
	• Barking	• Croup or influenza
	• Hacking	• Atypical pneumonia or mycoplasmal pneumonia
	• Congested	• Cold, pneumonia, bronchitis
If he's coughing up sputum, what does it look like?	• Mucoid	• Tracheobronchitis, asthma
	• Yellow or green	• Some bacterial infections
	• Rust-colored	• Pneumococcal pneumonia, pulmonary infarction, tuberculosis
	• Pink and frothy	• Pulmonary edema

339 Past history

Focus on the following body systems, procedures, and conditions when reviewing your patient's past history:

• ***Respiratory system.*** Ask if your patient's ever had *pneumonia, pleurisy, asthma, bronchitis, emphysema,* or *tuberculosis.* Also ask him how often he gets colds.

• ***Cardiovascular system.*** Ask if your patient's ever had *high blood pressure, heart attack,* or *congestive heart failure.* A history of such a disorder is particularly significant, because of the close relationship between the cardiovascular system and the respiratory system.

• ***Chest surgery.*** Find out if the patient has had lung surgery or other chest surgery. Remember that physical examination findings differ for patients who've undergone such procedures as *thoracoplasty* or *pneumonectomy.*

• ***Invasive medical procedures.*** Ask the patient if he's undergone any chest- or lung-related procedures, such as *bronchoscopy* or *thoracocentesis.*

• ***Chest deformities.*** Note that *congenital* or *trauma-related deformities* may distort cardiac and pulmonary structures.

• ***Laboratory tests.*** Ask your patient for the dates and results of his last chest X-ray, pulmonary function test, electrocardiogram, arterial blood gas analysis, sputum culture, and skin test for tuberculosis.

• ***Allergies.*** Ask whether the patient reacts to such common allergens as medications, foods, pets, dust, or pollen. Also ask if he has any allergic signs and symptoms, such as coughing, sneezing, sinusitis, or dyspnea. Chronic allergies may predispose him to other respiratory disorders. Has he ever been treated for an allergy?

• ***Medications.*** Ask the patient if he takes any prescription or over-the-counter drugs for cough control, expectoration, nasal congestion, chest pain, or dyspnea. Also note any other medications the patient is taking (see *Nurse's Guide to Some Drugs That Affect the Respiratory System*).

• ***Vaccinations.*** Ask the patient if he's ever been vaccinated against pneumonia or flu.

340 Family history

When reviewing your patient's family history, ask if anyone in his family has ever had *asthma, cystic fibrosis,* or *emphysema,* all of which may be genetically transmitted. Other important disorders to ask about include *lung cancer* and *infectious diseases,* such as tuberculosis. Also inquire about *chronic allergies* in the family, *cardiovascular disorders* (such as hypertension, myocardial infarction, and congestive heart failure), and *respiratory disturbances* (such as frequent colds or episodes of flu, pneumonia, asthma, or emphysema). Disorders involving other body systems may be associated with pulmonary dysfunction, so ask about a family history of such conditions as *kyphosis, scoliosis, obesity,* and *neuromuscular dysfunction.*

341 Psychosocial history

Focus your questions about the patient's psychosocial history on the following aspects of his life:

• ***Home conditions.*** Persons living near a constant source of air pollution, such as a chemical factory, may develop respiratory disorders. Exposure to cigarette smoke in the home may aggravate respiratory symptoms. Crowded living conditions facilitate the transmission of communicable respiratory diseases.

• ***Work.*** Exposure on the job to cigarette smoke or to other substances that may be irritating to the respiratory system may be significant (see *Nurse's Guide to Occupational Lung Disorders,* page 291).

• ***Pets.*** Exposure to animals may precipitate allergic or asthmatic attacks.

• ***Hobbies.*** Seemingly innocent pastimes, such as building model air-

DRUGS

NURSE'S GUIDE TO SOME DRUGS THAT AFFECT THE RESPIRATORY SYSTEM

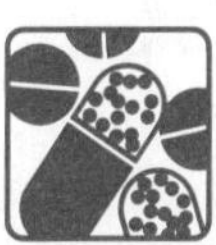

CLASSIFICATION	POSSIBLE SIDE EFFECTS
Adrenergics (sympathomimetics)	
epinephrine hydrochloride (Sus-Phrine)	• Pulmonary edema, dyspnea
isoproterenol hydrochloride (Isuprel*) isoproterenol sulfate (Medihaler-Iso*)	• Bronchial edema and inflammation
Adrenergic blockers (sympatholytics)	
methysergide maleate (Sansert*)	• Nasal congestion; pulmonary fibrosis causing dyspnea, tightness and pain in chest, pleural friction rubs and effusion
Alkylating agents	
busulfan (Myleran*)	• Irreversible pulmonary fibrosis, commonly known as busulfan lung
chlorambucil (Leukeran*)	• Allergic febrile reactions
cyclophosphamide (Cytoxan*)	• Pulmonary fibrosis with high doses
melphalan (Alkeran*)	• Pneumonitis
Aminoglycosides	
streptomycin sulfate	• Respiratory depression
Antibiotic antineoplastic agents	
bleomycin sulfate (Blenoxane*)	• Pulmonary fibrosis, fine rales, dyspnea
Antihypertensives	
guanethidine sulfate (Ismelin*)	• Nasal congestion
Anti-infectives	
polymyxin B sulfate (Aerosporin*)	• Respiratory paralysis
Antimetabolites	
methotrexate sodium (Mexate)	• Pulmonary interstitial infiltrates
Cephalosporins	
all types	• Dyspnea
Cholinergic blockers (parasympatholytics)	
atropine sulfate glycopyrrolate (Robinul)	• Bronchial plugging
Narcotic analgesics	
pentazocine hydrochloride pentazocine lactate (Talwin*)	• Respiratory depression
Nonsteroidal anti-inflammatory agents	
ibuprofen (Motrin*)	• Bronchospasm
indomethacin (Indocin)	• Respiratory distress

(*continued*)

NURSE'S GUIDE TO SOME DRUGS THAT AFFECT THE RESPIRATORY SYSTEM *(continued)*

CLASSIFICATION	POSSIBLE SIDE EFFECTS
Sedatives and hypnotics	
mephobarbital (Mebaral*)	• Respiratory depression, apnea
methotrimeprazine hydrochloride (Levoprome)	• Nasal congestion
paraldehyde (Paral)	• With I.V. administration, may cause pulmonary edema or hemorrhage, or respiratory depression
propiomazine hydrochloride (Largon)	• Respiratory depression
Urinary tract antiseptics	
nitrofurantoin (Furadantin) nitrofurantoin macrocrystals (Macrodantin*)	• Pulmonary sensitivity reactions, such as cough, chest pain, dyspnea

*Available in U.S. and Canada. All other products (no symbol) available in U.S. only.

planes or refinishing old furniture, may expose the patient to harsh chemical irritants.

• ***Stress.*** Some respiratory conditions, such as asthma and infection, can be aggravated by stress.

342 Activities of daily living

When reviewing your patient's activities of daily living, ask if he smokes cigarettes, cigars, pipe tobacco, or marijuana. If he smokes cigarettes, find out how many packs he smokes each day, and how long he's been smoking at this rate. If the patient doesn't smoke now, ask if he used to smoke, and how much. Learning about a patient's smoking habits is vital to completing a comprehensive respiratory history. Smoking can be associated with numerous and varied pathologies, such as lung cancer, chronic bronchitis, and emphysema.

The risk of lung disease is higher among smokers exposed to respiratory irritants either near their homes or on the job. So when asking your patient about his daily activities, be especially alert to a history of exposure to chemicals, noxious fumes, chromium, and dust containing nickel, uranium, or asbestos.

Your patient's daily routine is also important, because respiratory signs and symptoms can interfere with such activities as climbing stairs or traveling to work.

343 Review of systems

Complete your patient's health history by asking about the following signs and symptoms:

• ***General.*** *Fever, chills,* and *fatigue* may occur in association with respiratory symptoms.

• ***Skin.*** *Nocturnal diaphoresis* may be associated with tuberculosis.

• ***Blood-forming.*** *Anemia* decreases the blood's oxygen-carrying capacity; *polycythemia* may occur in response to chronic hypoxemia.

• ***Nose.*** *Nasal discharge, sinus pain or infection,* or *postnasal drip* may result from seasonal allergies or chronic sinus problems.

• ***Mouth and throat.*** *Halitosis* may result from a pulmonary infection, such as an abscess or bronchiectasis.

NURSE'S GUIDE TO OCCUPATIONAL LUNG DISORDERS

DISORDER	HIGH-RISK OCCUPATIONS	PATIENT HISTORY
Silicosis	Miners (lead, hard coal, copper, silver, and gold), foundry workers, potters, and sandstone and granite cutters	Exposure to free silica
Coal worker's pneumoconiosis (black lung disease)	Coal miners	Long-term exposure to coal dust in conjunction with excessive cigarette smoking
Berylliosis (beryllium disease, Wegener's granulomatosis)	Workers in chemical, military, ceramic, and aerospace industries who have contact with beryllium	Exposure to dust or fumes containing beryllium or its compounds, including sulfate and halide salts and beryllium oxide
Asbestosis	Workers involved in the mining, milling, manufacturing, or application of asbestos products, such as brake linings or insulation	Exposure to asbestos
Occupational asthma	Workers in cotton, leather, beer, wood, detergent, flax, and hemp industries (list is continually growing)	Exposure to irritants or allergenic particles or vapors
Acute exposure	Workers who handle chlorine, phosgene, sulfur dioxide, hydrogen sulfide, nitrogen dioxide, and ammonia gases	Excessive exposure to gas

- ***Cardiovascular.*** *Ankle edema, paroxysmal nocturnal dyspnea, orthopnea,* or *chest pain that worsens with exercise, eating, or stress* may reflect a cardiovascular disorder rather than a respiratory one.
- ***Gastrointestinal.*** *Weight loss* suggests possible deterioration from disease, such as from lung cancer.
- ***Nervous.*** *Confusion, syncope,* and *restlessness* may be associated with cerebral hypoxia.
- ***Musculoskeletal.*** Chronic hypoxia may cause *fatigue* and *weakness.*
- ***Psychological.*** Some respiratory signs and symptoms (for example, *wheezing* and *hyperventilation*) may be associated with emotional problems.

Conducting the physical examination

344 Environment and equipment

Before assessing your patient, be sure the examining area is quiet so you can auscultate his lungs accurately. Make sure the lighting is adequate to detect skin color variations. (If possible, use natural light, because fluorescent light doesn't show true skin color.)

You'll need a nasal speculum, a tongue depressor, a penlight, a cotton-tipped applicator or swabstick, and a stethoscope. You may also wish to use a marking pen and a centimeter stick to mark points of reference on the patient's body.

345 Patient preparation and positioning

Tell the patient to undress to the waist and to put on a loose-fitting examining gown. (If the patient's a woman and she's wearing a bra, ask her to remove it.) Be sure the patient is adequately draped for privacy and warmth.

Place the patient in a comfortable position that allows you access to his posterior and anterior chest. If he experiences shortness of breath, elevate his head. If the patient's condition permits, have him sit on the edge of a bed or examining table or in a chair, leaning slightly forward, with his arms folded across his chest. If this isn't possible, place him in the semi-Fowler's position for the anterior chest examination. Then ask him to lean forward slightly, using the side rails or mattress for support, so you can examine his posterior chest. If the patient can't lean forward for posterior chest examination, place him in a lateral position.

Assessment tip: Remember that when you use the lateral position to examine your patient's posterior chest, the bed mattress and the organ displacement involved distort sounds and lung expansion. To offset these effects, examine the uppermost side of your patient's chest first; then roll him on his other side and repeat the examination, for comparison.

When you assess the patient's thorax, keep in mind the three thoracic portions to be examined—posterior, anterior, and lateral. You can examine any of these areas first and perform the lateral examination during the posterior or anterior assessment. The most important point is to *proceed systematically,* always comparing one side of the patient's thorax with the other side. (In this way, the patient serves as his own control.) Remember to examine the apices during the posterior and the anterior examinations.

346 Quick observation of respiratory status

Before starting your detailed pulmonary assessment, quickly observe the patient for the following signs and symptoms of severe hypoxia or other acute respiratory difficulty:

- low level of consciousness
- shortness of breath when speaking
- rapid, very deep or very shallow, or depressed respirations
- use of accessory muscles when breathing
- intercostal and sternal retractions
- cyanosis
- external sounds (such as crowing, wheezing, or stridor)
- diaphoresis
- nasal flaring
- extreme apprehension or agitation.

A patient exhibiting most or all of these signs and symptoms requires immediate intervention. Position him appropriately to relieve distress, then notify the doctor.

347 Inspecting your patient's skin

Begin your detailed respiratory examination by inspecting your patient's skin color (see Entry 224). Look for central *cyanosis* in highly vascular areas: the lips, the nail beds, the tip of the nose, the ear helices, and the underside of the tongue. For a patient with dark brown or black skin, inspect those areas where cyanotic changes would be most apparent: the nose, the cheeks, and the mucosa inside the lips. Facial skin may be pale gray in a cyanotic dark-skinned patient.

Central cyanosis, which affects all body organs, results from prolonged hypoxia. Its presence helps you gauge the severity of a patient's illness. (Remember, though, that severely anemic patients with respiratory difficulty don't appear cyanotic.) Be sure you know how to distinguish central cyanosis from *peripheral cyanosis,* which is

RECOGNIZING RESPIRATORY PATTERNS

To determine the rate, rhythm, and depth of your patient's respirations, observe him at rest. Make sure he's unaware that you're counting his respirations. Why? A person conscious of his respirations may alter his natural pattern.

Always count respirations for at least 1 minute. If you count for only a fraction of a minute and then multiply, your count may be off by as much as four respirations per minute. Your patient's respiratory rhythm should be even, except for an occasional deep breath. Use this chart as a guide for noting differences in respiratory rates, rhythms, and depths.

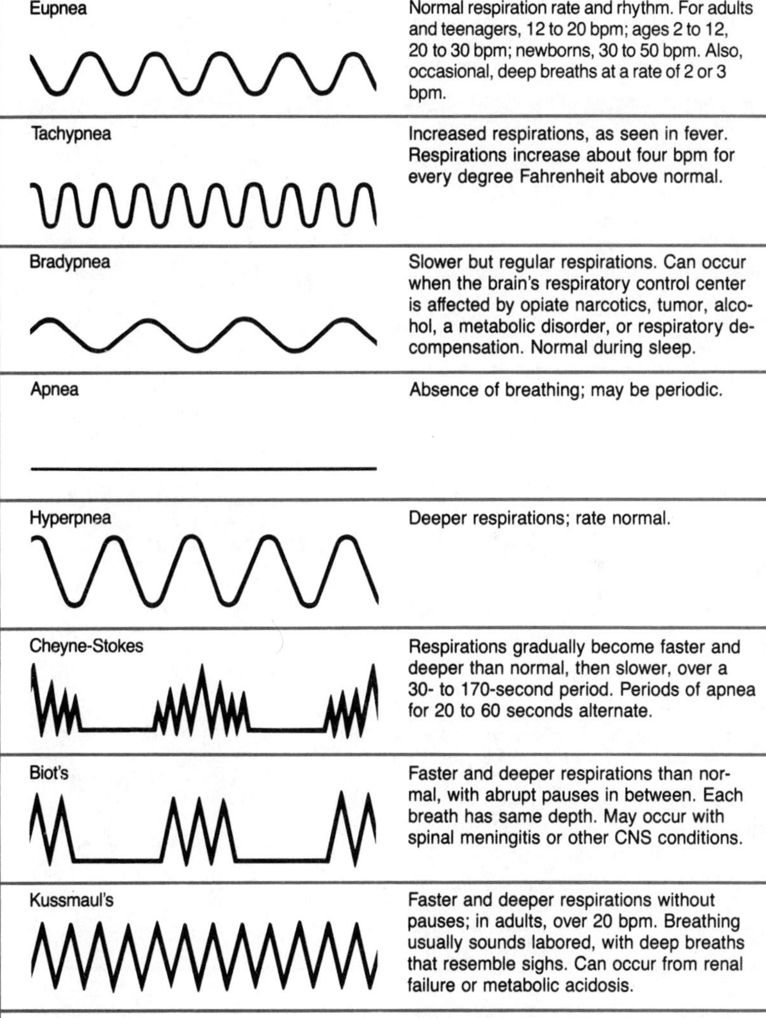

Pattern	Description
Eupnea	Normal respiration rate and rhythm. For adults and teenagers, 12 to 20 bpm; ages 2 to 12, 20 to 30 bpm; newborns, 30 to 50 bpm. Also, occasional, deep breaths at a rate of 2 or 3 bpm.
Tachypnea	Increased respirations, as seen in fever. Respirations increase about four bpm for every degree Fahrenheit above normal.
Bradypnea	Slower but regular respirations. Can occur when the brain's respiratory control center is affected by opiate narcotics, tumor, alcohol, a metabolic disorder, or respiratory decompensation. Normal during sleep.
Apnea	Absence of breathing; may be periodic.
Hyperpnea	Deeper respirations; rate normal.
Cheyne-Stokes	Respirations gradually become faster and deeper than normal, then slower, over a 30- to 170-second period. Periods of apnea for 20 to 60 seconds alternate.
Biot's	Faster and deeper respirations than normal, with abrupt pauses in between. Each breath has same depth. May occur with spinal meningitis or other CNS conditions.
Kussmaul's	Faster and deeper respirations without pauses; in adults, over 20 bpm. Breathing usually sounds labored, with deep breaths that resemble sighs. Can occur from renal failure or metabolic acidosis.
Apneustic	Prolonged gasping inspiration, followed by extremely short, inefficient expiration. Can occur from lesions in the brain's respiratory center.

EMERGENCY

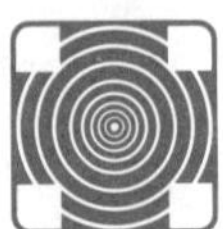

ASSESSING EMERGENCY RESPIRATORY SITUATIONS

Respiratory assessment of the emergency patient is critical because life-threatening problems may impair oxygen delivery to tissues.

Begin your assessment by simultaneously checking airway patency and adequate ventilation.

- Observe the chest for rise and fall.
- Listen to the sound of air movement near your patient's mouth and nose.
- Feel for air movement over his mouth and nose.

Use this chart to assess the emergency situation properly.

CONDITION	NURSING ASSESSMENT	NURSING INTERVENTION
Acute respiratory arrest	• No respiratory movement • No air felt over mouth and nose	• Position airway, using the head-tilt or jaw-thrust method. • Start mouth-to-mouth resuscitation immediately. • Once you've accomplished ventilation, continue until no longer needed. • Use endotracheal intubation and manual (or mechanical) ventilation, as ordered, for long-term support.
Complete airway obstruction	• No respiratory movement • No air felt over mouth and nose • If conscious, patient attempts to speak but fails, and typically reaches for his throat	• Administer four rapid blows between the scapulae, followed by the abdominal thrust or compression of the midchest, as is done in external cardiac massage. • If airway remains obstructed, manual clearing may locate and remove obstruction. • Anticipate cricothyrotomy or tracheotomy if other attempts fail. Perform cricothyrotomy only in life-threatening emergency when a doctor is unavailable. Usually a doctor performs a tracheotomy in the operating room.
Partial airway obstruction	• Increased respiratory effort (orthopnea in conscious patients) • Noisy respirations (whistling, wheezing, crowing) • Use of accessory muscles, including abdominals, sternocleidomastoid, and internal intercostals, to try to breathe • Possible intercostal retractions along with nasal flaring	• Administer back blows in succession. (This condition is unlikely to be relieved by an abdominal thrust or by chest compression.) • Administer oxygen until direct laryngoscopy becomes available.

caused by local vasoconstriction and is only apparent in the nail beds and sometimes the lips.

For all patients, examine the skin for dryness—a possible sign of dehydration—or for diaphoresis, which may be associated with fever and infection (see Entry 225). Bright cherry-red mucous membranes may result from carbon monoxide poisoning. While inspecting the skin, observe the fingers for clubbing, a sign of chronic respiratory dysfunction as well as certain cardiovascular and gastrointestinal disorders.

348 Examining the nose, mouth, and trachea

Inspect your patient's facial structures, observing for symmetry, deformities, and inflammation. Check his nasal septum for deviation and perforations. Using a nasal speculum, examine his nostrils for discharge, for the condition and color of their mucosa (it should be slightly redder than oral mucosa), for swelling and bleeding, and for any obstructions.

Next, palpate his nose to detect any swelling, pain, or fractures. Palpate the maxillary sinuses for tenderness and swelling by pressing the patient's cheeks over the maxillary areas. Palpate his frontal sinuses by placing your thumbs just below the patient's eyebrows and pressing upward. While observing and palpating these facial structures, listen for external sounds of moisture or mucus, and for stridor or wheezing.

If the patient wears dentures, ask him to remove them. Then, using a tongue depressor, a cotton-tipped applicator (or swabstick), and a penlight, examine his oropharynx for color changes, inflammation, white patches, ulcerations, bleeding, exudate, and lesions. Be sure to check his soft palate, anterior and posterior pillars of fauces, uvula, tonsils, posterior pharynx, teeth, gums, tongue, mouth floor, mucous membranes, and lips (see Entries 433 to 438). Remember that a dark-skinned patient has dark patches on his mucous membranes.

Using a tongue depressor, bring the patient's pharynx into view and ask him to say "eh." Observe for symmetrical rise and fall of the soft palate. Next, touch both sides of his posterior pharynx with the applicator to check his gag reflex. (This test is particularly helpful when you're assessing an older patient with decreased sensitivity to touch, or one who has suffered a cerebrovascular accident [CVA]; it helps you determine such a patient's ability to swallow oral secretions and food.) To determine the patient's ability to clear his respiratory tract of accumulated secretions, ask him to cough. If your patient is debilitated by CVA or other cerebral trauma or by drug or alcohol ingestion, elicit a cough by gently touching his posterior oropharynx with a swabstick.

Inspect the patient's trachea for midline position, and observe again for any use of accessory neck muscles in breathing. If you can't see his trachea, palpate for it at the midline position, using the fingertips of one hand. Starting at the middle base of the patient's lower jaw, gently slide your fingertips down the center of his neck. After locating his larynx, you should be able to feel his trachea in the area of the sternal notch. Any deviation of the trachea to either side indicates deformity and necessitates further investigation. Also, observe and palpate the patient's neck over the trachea for swelling, bruises, tenderness, and masses that might obstruct breathing.

349 Inspecting the posterior chest

Instruct the patient to sit and lean forward, with his shoulders rounded and his arms crossed on his chest. (Always note the patient's tolerance of position changes.) After checking his posterior chest for wounds, lesions, masses, or scars, observe the rate, rhythm, and depth of his respirations. The normal respiratory rate for an adult is 12 to 20 breaths/minute. Respirations should be regular and inaudible, with the sides of the chest expanding equally. Normal respirations consist of inspiration, a slight pause, and a slightly longer expiration. Prolonged expiratory time suggests air outflow impedance.

Next, observe the patient's chest for local lag or impaired movement. Normally, the chest moves upward and outward symmetrically on inspiration.

FOLLOWING THE PALPATION SEQUENCE

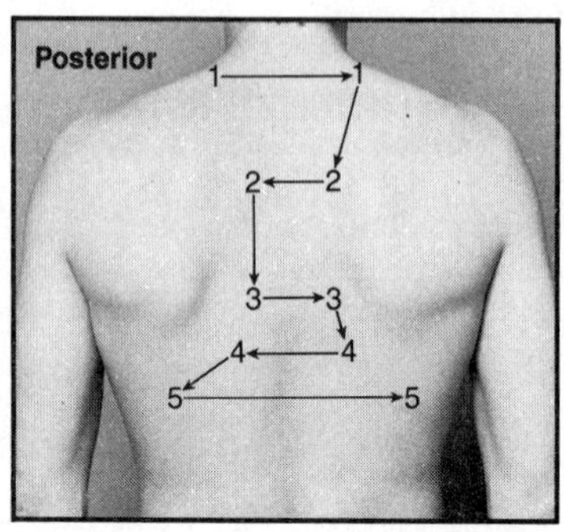

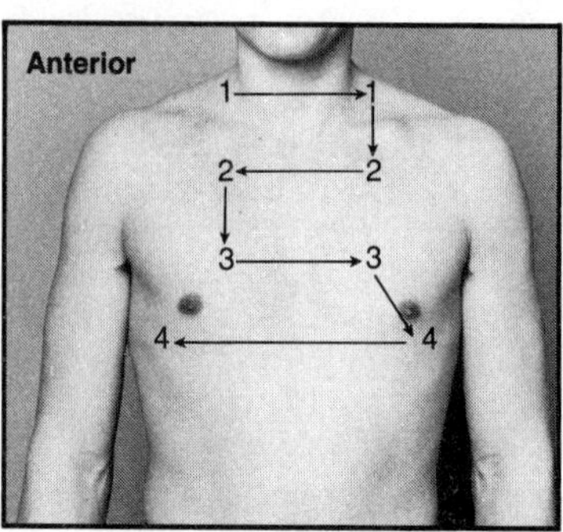

Use the palpation sequence illustrated here to palpate the posterior and anterior chest. It will help you detect any areas of increased or decreased fremitus.

When following the sequence, use the top portion of your palm to palpate. You'll also find using only *one* hand is best. Remember to avoid bony areas.

Impairment may result from pain, exertion from poor positioning, or obstruction from abdominal distention. Paradoxical movement of the chest wall may result from fractured ribs or flail chest.

Note the slope of the patient's ribs. Check for retraction of intercostal spaces during inspiration and for abnormal bulging of intercostal spaces during expiration. Then observe for such spinal deformities as lordosis, kyphosis, and scoliosis (see Entry 685).

350 Palpating the posterior chest

Palpate the patient's posterior chest to assess his thorax, to identify thoracic structures, and to check chest expansion and vocal or tactile fremitus (see Entry 86). Begin by feeling for muscle mass with your fingers and palms (use a grasping action of the fingers to assess position and consistency). Normally, it feels firm, smooth, and symmetrical. As you palpate muscle mass, also check skin temperature and turgor (see Entry 227). Be sure to note the presence of crepitus (especially around a wound site). Then palpate the thoracic spine, noting tenderness, swelling, or such deformities as lordosis, kyphosis, and scoliosis (see Entry 685).

Next, using your metacarpophalangeal joints and fingerpads, gently palpate the patient's intercostal spaces and ribs for abnormal retractions, bulging, and tenderness. Normally, the intercostal spaces delineate a downward sloping of the ribs. In a patient with an increased anteroposterior diameter caused by obstructive lung disease, you'll feel ribs that are abnormally horizontal.

Now palpate the thoracic landmarks to identify underlying lobe structures (see *Locating Thoracic Landmarks,* page 280). To help you identify the division between the patient's upper and lower lobes, instruct him to raise his arms above his head; then palpate the borders of his scapulae. The inner edges of the scapulae should line up with the divisions between the upper and lower lobes.

The inferior border of the lower lobes is usually located at the 10th thoracic spinous process and may descend, on full inspiration, to the 12th thoracic spinous process.

Assessment tip: To locate the lower lung borders in a patient lying laterally, palpate the visible free-floating ribs or costal margins; then count four intercostal spaces upward for the general location of the lower lung fields.

Palpate for symmetrical expansion of the patient's thorax (respiratory excursion) by placing your palms—fingers together and thumbs abducted toward the spine—flat on the bilateral sections of his lower posterior chest wall. Position your thumbs at the 10th-rib level, and grasp the lateral rib cage with your hands. As the patient inhales, his posterior chest should move upward and outward, and your thumbs should move apart; when he exhales, your thumbs should return to midline and touch each other again. Repeat this technique on his upper posterior chest.

Palpate for vocal or tactile fremitus by using the top portion of each palm and following the palpation sequence illustrated on the opposite page. To check for vocal fremitus, ask your patient to repeat "99" as you proceed. Palpable vibrations will be transmitted from his bronchopulmonary system, along the solid surfaces of his chest wall, to your palms and fingers.

Note the symmetry of the vibrations and the areas of enhanced, diminished, or absent fremitus. (Remember, fremitus should be most pronounced in the patient's upper chest where the trachea branches into the right and the left mainstem bronchi, and less noticeable in the lower regions of the thorax.)

You can estimate the level of your patient's diaphragm on both sides of his posterior chest by placing the ulnar side of your extended hand parallel to the anticipated diaphragm level. Instruct the patient to repeat "99" as you move your hand downward. The level where you no longer feel fremitus corresponds approximately to the diaphragm level.

351 Percussing the posterior chest

To learn the density and location of such anatomic structures as the patient's lungs and diaphragm, you must identify five percussion sounds: flat, dull, resonant, hyperresonant, and tympanic (see Entry 94 and *Identifying Percussion Sounds).* Start by percussing across the top of each shoulder. The area overlying the lung apices—approximately 2″ (5 cm)—should be resonant. Then percuss downward toward the patient's diaphragm, at 2″ intervals,

IDENTIFYING PERCUSSION SOUNDS

Use this chart to help you identify the sounds you may hear when you percuss your patient's chest. Be sure to document your findings.

SOUND	PITCH	INTENSITY	QUALITY	INDICATION
Flatness	High	Soft	Extreme dullness	*Normal:* sternum; *abnormal:* atelectatic lung
Dullness	Medium	Medium	Thudlike	*Normal:* liver area, cardiac area, diaphragm; *abnormal:* pleural effusion
Resonance	Low	Moderate to loud	Hollow	*Normal:* lung
Hyper-resonance	Lower than resonance	Very loud	Booming	*Abnormal:* emphysematous lung or pneumothorax
Tympany	High	Loud	Musical, drumlike	*Normal:* stomach area; *abnormal:* air-distended abdomen

USING THE PERCUSSION AND AUSCULTATION SEQUENCES

Posterior

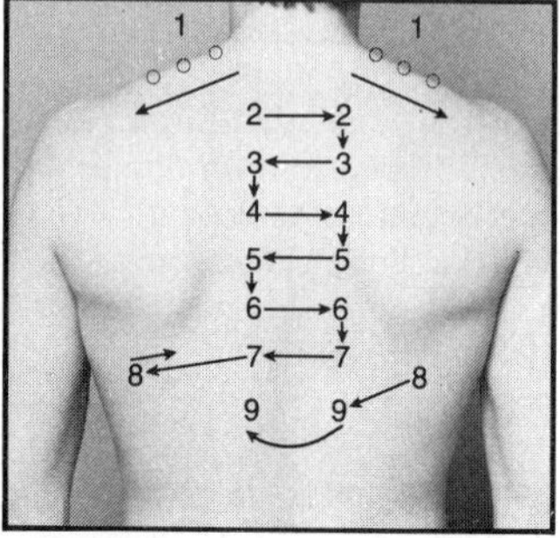

Anterior

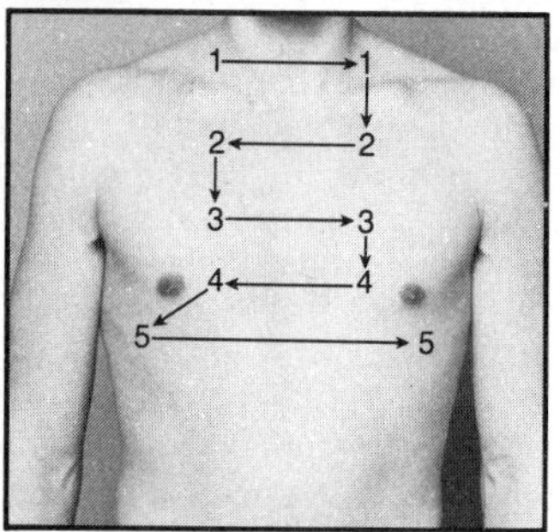

Left lateral

Right lateral

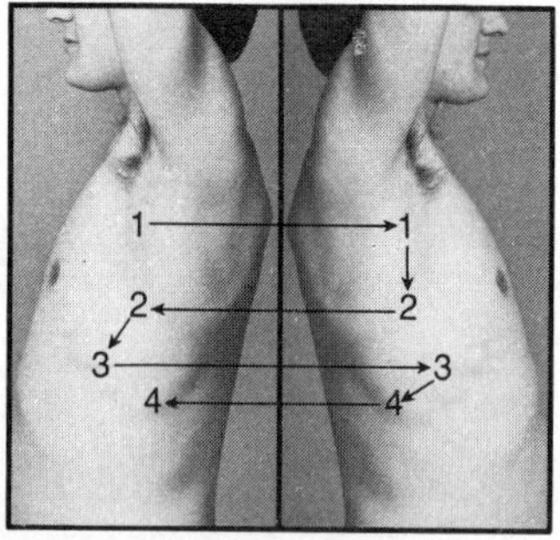

Follow the percussion and auscultation sequences shown here to help you identify abnormalities in your patient's lungs.

Remember to compare sound variations from one side to the other as you proceed. Document any abnormal sounds you hear and describe them carefully, including their location.

comparing right and left sides as you proceed (see *Using the Percussion and Auscultation Sequences*). Remember to avoid his scapulae and other bony areas. The thoracic area (except over the scapulae) should produce resonance when you percuss. At the level of his diaphragm, resonance should change to dullness. A dull sound over the lungs indicates fluid or solid tissue. Hyperresonance or tympany over a patient's lung suggests pneumothorax, massive atelectasis, or large emphysematous blebs. A marked difference in diaphragm level from one side to the other is an abnormal finding.

Next, measure diaphragmatic excursion. Instruct the patient to take a deep breath and hold it while you percuss downward until dullness identifies the lower border of the lung field. Mark this point. Now ask the patient to exhale and again hold his breath, as you percuss upward to the area of dullness. Mark this point, too. Repeat this entire procedure on the opposite side of the patient's chest. Now measure the distances between the two marks on each side. Normal diaphragmatic excursion measures about 1¼" to 2¼" (3 to 6 cm). (A person's diaphragm is usually slightly higher on his right side.)

352 Auscultating the posterior chest

To assess the flow of air through the patient's respiratory system, auscultate his lungs and identify normal and abnormal (adventitious) breath sounds (see *Assessing Normal and Abnormal Breath Sounds*). Lung auscultation helps detect abnormal fluid or mucus, as well as obstructed passages. You can also determine the condition of the alveoli and surrounding pleura.

Before auscultating the posterior chest, remove clothing and bed linen from the body area to be examined.

Assessment tip: If the patient has a lot of hair on his posterior chest, wet and mat it with a damp washcloth to prevent it from causing rubbing sounds

ASSESSING NORMAL AND ABNORMAL BREATH SOUNDS

Breath sounds are produced by air moving through the tracheobronchoalveolar system. Normal breath sounds are labeled *bronchial, bronchovesicular,* and *vesicular.* They're described according to location, ratio of inspiration to expiration, intensity, and pitch.

Abnormal (adventitious) breath sounds occur when air passes either through narrowed airways or through moisture, or when the membranes lining the chest cavity and the lungs become inflamed. These sounds include *rales, rhonchi, wheezes,* and *pleural friction rub.* You may hear them superimposed over normal breath sounds.

Use this chart as a guide to assess both normal and abnormal breath sounds. Document your findings.

NORMAL BREATH SOUNDS

TYPE	LOCATION	RATIO	DESCRIPTION
Bronchial	Over trachea	I 2:3 E	Loud, high pitched, and hollow, harsh, or coarse
Broncho-vesicular	Anteriorly, near the mainstem bronchi in the first and second intercostal spaces; posteriorly, between the scapulae	I 1:1 E	Soft, breezy, and pitched about two notes lower than bronchial sounds
Vesicular	In most of the lungs' peripheral parts (cannot be heard over the presternum or the scapulae)	I 3:1 E	Soft, swishy, breezy, and about two notes lower than broncho-vesicular sounds

ABNORMAL BREATH SOUNDS

TYPE	LOCATION	CAUSE	DESCRIPTION
Rales	Anywhere. Heard in lung bases first with pulmonary edema, usually during inspiratory phase	Air passing through moisture, especially in the small airways and alveoli	Light crackling, popping, nonmusical; can be further classified by pitch: high, medium, or low
Rhonchi	In larger airways, usually during expiratory phase	Fluid or secretions in the large airways or narrowing of large airways	Coarse rattling, usually louder and lower pitched than rales; can be described as sonorous, bubbling, moaning, musical, sibilant, and rumbly
Wheezes	May occur during inspiration or expiration	Narrowed airways	Creaking, groaning; always high-pitched, musical squeaks
Pleural friction rub	Anterolateral lung field, on both inspiration and expiration (with the patient in an upright position)	Inflamed parietal and visceral pleural linings rubbing together	Superficial squeaking or grating

IDENTIFYING CHEST DEFORMITIES

As you inspect your patient's anterior chest, you may notice deviations in size or shape. The illustrations below demonstrate three such deformities. Note the physical characteristics, signs, and associated conditions typical of each.

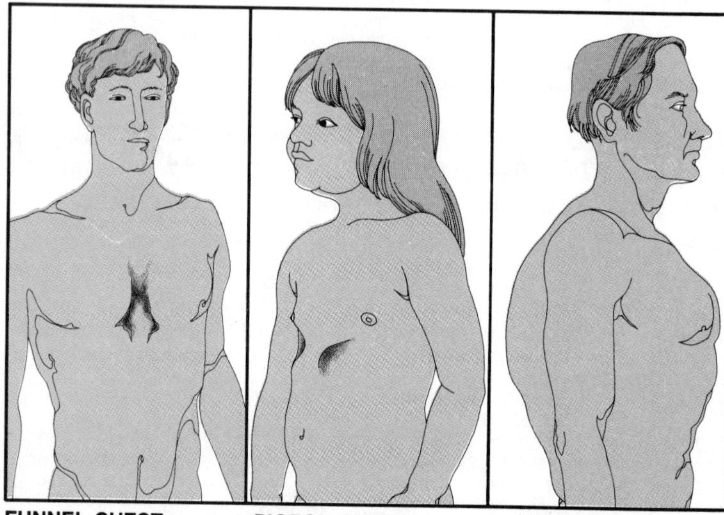

FUNNEL CHEST

Physical characteristics
- Sinking or funnel-shaped depression of lower sternum
- Diminished anteroposterior chest diameter

Signs and associated conditions
- Postural disorders, such as forward displacement of neck and shoulders
- Upper thoracic kyphosis
- Protuberant abdomen
- Functional heart murmur

PIGEON CHEST

Physical characteristics
- Projection of sternum beyond abdomen's frontal plane. Evident in two variations: projection greatest at xiphoid process; projection greatest at or near center of sternum

Signs and associated conditions
- Functional cardiovascular or respiratory disorders

BARREL CHEST

Physical characteristics
- Enlarged anteroposterior and transverse chest dimensions; chest appears barrel-shaped
- Prominent accessory muscles

Signs and associated conditions
- Chronic respiratory disorders
- Increasing shortness of breath
- Chronic cough
- Wheezing

that can be confused with rales.

When auscultating the patient's chest, instruct him to take full, slow breaths through his mouth. (Nose breathing changes the pitch of the lung sounds.) Listen for one full inspiration and expiration before moving the stethoscope. Remember, a patient may try to accommodate you by breathing quickly and deeply with every movement of the stethoscope—which can cause hyperventilation. If your patient becomes light-headed or dizzy, stop auscultating and allow him to breathe normally for a few minutes.

Using the diaphragm of the stethoscope, begin auscultating above the patient's scapulae. Move to the area between the scapulae and the vertebral column. Then move laterally beneath the scapulae, to the right and left lower lobes. Move the stethoscope's diaphragm methodically, and compare the sounds you hear on both sides of the chest before moving to the next area (see Entry 96).

Normally, you'll hear vesicular breath sounds—soft, low-pitched sounds lasting longer during inspiration—at the lung bases. Bronchovesicular breath sounds—medium-pitched sounds that are equal in duration on inspiration and expiration—can be heard between the scapulae. Decreased or absent breath sounds may result from bronchial obstruction, muscle weakness, obesity, or pleural disease.

If you hear an adventitious breath sound, note its location and at which point during the respiratory process it occurs—during inspiration, for example. Then continue auscultating the patient's posterior chest.

After auscultating, instruct the patient to cough and breathe deeply. Let him rest, and listen again to the area where you heard the adventitious sound or sounds. Note any changes. Sometimes rales and rhonchi can be cleared by coughing; wheezes and friction rubs can't be cleared this way.

If you've detected any respiratory abnormality during palpation, percussion, and auscultation, assess your patient's voice sounds for vocal resonance. The significance of vocal resonance is based on the principle that sound carries best through a solid, not as well through fluid, and poorly through air. Normally, you should hear vocal resonance as muffled, unclear sounds, loudest medially and less intense at the lung periphery. Voice sounds that become louder and more distinct signal *bronchophony,* an abnormal finding except over the trachea and posteriorly over the upper right lobe. To elicit bronchophony, ask your patient to say "99" or "one, two, three" while you auscultate his thorax in the systematic way described above.

Whispered pectoriloquy reveals the presence of an exaggerated bronchophony. Ask your patient to whisper a simple phrase like "one, two, three." Hearing the words clearly through the stethoscope is an abnormal finding.

Egophony is another form of abnormal vocal resonance. Ask your patient to say "ee-ee-ee." Transmission of the sound through the stethoscope as "ay, ay, ay" is an abnormal finding possibly indicating compressed lung tissue, as in a pleural effusion.

You may hear increased vocal resonance, whispered pectoriloquy, and egophony in any patient with consolidated lungs.

353 Inspecting the anterior chest

To inspect your patient's anterior chest, place him in semi-Fowler's position. Begin by inspecting the anterior chest for draining, open wounds, bruises, abrasions, scars, cuts, and punctures, as well as for rib deformities, fractures, lesions, or masses. Then inspect the rate, rhythm, and depth of respirations. Remember that men, infants, and children are normally diaphragmatic (abdominal) breathers, as are athletes, singers, and persons who practice yoga. Women are usually intercostal (chest) breathers.

Your patient's face should look relaxed when he breathes. Abnormal findings include nasal flaring, pursed-lip breathing, use of neck or abdominal muscles on expiration, and intercostal or sternal retractions. Inspect for local lag and impaired chest wall movement. Observe for thoracic deformities, such as pectus excavatum (funnel chest) and pectus carinatum (pigeon chest) (see *Identifying Chest Deformities*). Check the patient for barrel chest by noting the ratio between the anteroposterior diameter of his chest and its lateral diameter; the normal ratio ranges from 1:2 to 5:7.

354 Palpating the anterior chest

Begin palpating your patient's anterior chest, using your fingers and palms (see Entry 86). Feel for areas of tenderness, muscle mass, and skin turgor

UNDERSTANDING DIAGNOSTIC TESTS

Here are several essential diagnostic tests that help you assess pulmonary function:

• *Arterial blood gas analysis* helps detect ventilation and perfusion abnormalities by measuring oxygenation (Pao_2), arterial carbon dioxide pressure ($Paco_2$), and pH.

• *Hemoglobin* measurement can help support clinical findings. As you know, hemoglobin's the primary carrier of oxygen and carbon dioxide. Long-standing hypoxia causes hemoglobin to *rise. Low* hemoglobin (caused by anemia or primary bleeding) may produce such symptoms of hypoxemia as fatigue, tachycardia, and shortness of breath.

• *Hematocrit* measurement determines red blood cell (RBC) concentration. A decrease in RBC concentration causes a decrease in hemoglobin, because hemoglobin is the principal protein in the cytoplasm of circulating RBC.

• *Chest X-rays* help to further differentiate significant clinical findings. However, pulmonary changes aren't always apparent on X-ray films. Don't distrust clinical findings just because they're not immediately proven or disproven by X-ray.

• *Spirometry* is another reliable measure of pulmonary function. It helps determine maximum breathing capacity, forced vital capacity, and inspiratory and expiratory reserve volume. Changes in these sensitive indicators suggest the degree of dysfunction and your patient's capacity for normal activities.

and elasticity. Note any crepitus during your palpation, especially around wound sites, subclavian catheters, and chest tubes.

Palpate his sternum and costal cartilages for tenderness and deformities and then, using your metacarpophalangeal joints and fingerpads, palpate his intercostal spaces and ribs for abnormal retractions, bulging, and tenderness. Remember to proceed to the lateral aspects of the thorax.

Next, palpate the thoracic landmarks used to identify underlying structures (see *Locating Thoracic Landmarks*, page 280).

To assess for symmetrical respiratory expansion, place your thumbs along each costal margin, pointing toward the xiphoid process, with your hands along the lateral rib cage. Ask the patient to inhale deeply, and observe for symmetrical thoracic expansion.

Now palpate for vocal or tactile fremitus, remembering to examine the lateral surfaces and to compare symmetrical areas of the patient's lungs (see *Following the Palpation Sequence*, page 296). (If your patient is a woman, you may have to displace her breasts to examine her anterior chest.) Remember that fremitus will usually be decreased or absent over the patient's precordium.

355 Percussing the anterior chest

Percussing the patient's anterior chest allows you to determine the location and density of his heart, lungs, liver, and diaphragm. Begin by percussing the lung apices (the supraclavicular areas), comparing right and left sides. Then percuss downward in 1¼" to 2" (3- to 5-cm) intervals. You should hear resonant tones until you reach the third or fourth intercostal space (ICS), to the left of the sternum, where you'll hear a dull sound produced by the heart. This sound should continue as you percuss down toward the fifth ICS and laterally toward the midclavicular line. At the sixth ICS, at the left midclavicular line, you'll hear resonance again. As you percuss down toward the rib cage, you'll hear tympany over the stomach. On the right side, you should hear resonance, indicating normal lung tissue. Near the fifth to seventh ICS you'll hear dullness, marking the superior border of the liver.

To percuss his lateral chest, instruct the patient to raise his arms over his head. Percuss laterally, comparing right and left sides as you proceed. These areas should also be resonant.

356 Auscultating the anterior chest

In the same way you auscultated the

patient's posterior chest, auscultate his anterior and lateral chest, comparing sounds on both sides before moving to the next area. (See *Using the Percussion and Auscultation Sequences,* page 298.)

Begin auscultating the anterior chest at the trachea, where you should hear bronchial (or tubular) breath sounds (see *Assessing Normal and Abnormal Breath Sounds,* page 299).

Next, listen for bronchovesicular breath sounds where the mainstem bronchi branch from the trachea (near the second intercostal space, ¾″ to 1¼″ or 2 to 3 cm to either side of the sternum). Bronchial and bronchovesicular sounds are abnormal when heard over peripheral lung areas.

Now, using the standard chest landmarks, listen over the patient's peripheral lung fields for vesicular sounds. Be sure to auscultate his lateral chest walls, comparing right and left sides as you proceed. On the left side, heart sounds diminish breath sounds; on the right side, the liver diminishes them.

If you hear adventitious breath sounds, describe them and note their location and timing. After you've listened to several respirations in the area of the adventitious sound, instruct the patient to cough and breathe deeply. Then, using the technique described in Entry 352 for the posterior chest, auscultate the area producing the abnormal sound and, if necessary, auscultate for bronchophony, whispered pectoriloquy, and egophony.

Formulating a diagnostic impression

357 Classifying respiratory disorders

Gas exchange, the main function of the respiratory system, depends on three simultaneous processes:

- *Ventilation:* the process of air exchange between the lungs and environment, and air distribution to the alveoli
- *Diffusion:* the movement of oxygen and carbon dioxide across the blood-gas barrier (the alveolar-capillary membrane)
- *Perfusion:* the movement of blood to and from the alveolar capillary bed—the volume of blood flowing through the lungs.

Normally, major respiratory disorders are classified according to the body process or combination of these processes (ventilation-diffusion and ventilation-perfusion) that they affect. Disorders of ventilation, diffusion, and ventilation-diffusion are primarily respiratory in origin and are discussed in this chapter. Perfusion and ventilation-perfusion disorders are mainly extrapulmonary and are treated as primarily cardiovascular disorders (see Chapter 10, CARDIOVASCULAR SYSTEM).

The three cardinal symptoms of respiratory disorders—cough (with or without sputum production or hemoptysis), dyspnea, and chest pain—may occur in some disorders in each of the five categories. (See *Nurse's Guide to Respiratory Disorders,* pages 304 to 311.)

358 Making appropriate nursing diagnoses

A major effect of all respiratory disturbances is hypoxia—inadequate oxygen supply, which disrupts many body functions. Blood pressure, heart rate, and cardiac output increase (the initial response to hypoxia); later, hypotension and cyanosis occur. Cardiac arrhythmias may also develop, further compromising cardiac output. The patient becomes acidotic, less responsive to stimuli, drowsy, and confused. Acidosis affects tissue metabolism at the cellular level, thus increasing level of

NURSE'S GUIDE TO RESPIRATORY DISORDERS

	CHIEF COMPLAINT
VENTILATION DISORDERS	
Chest wall deformities (including pectus excavatum, kyphoscoliosis, thoracoplasty, and trauma)	• *Cough:* absent or productive, depending on severity or tendency toward infection • *Dyspnea:* present only in severe deformity • *Chest pain:* absent
Obesity, pickwickian syndrome	• *Cough:* absent or productive, depending on severity or tendency toward infection • *Dyspnea:* absent, or present only on exertion • *Chest pain:* absent
Pneumonectomy	• *Cough:* absent • *Dyspnea:* absent, unless remaining portion of lung is unable to compensate • *Chest pain:* absent
Tumor	• *Cough:* present; cardinal symptom of bronchial tumor or of tumor compressing bronchus • *Dyspnea:* usually present if tumor is large • *Chest pain:* possibly pleuritic or dull
Pleural effusion (small, acute)	• *Cough:* absent • *Dyspnea:* possible • *Chest pain:* possibly pleuritic or dull
Pleural effusion (large, chronic)	• *Cough:* absent • *Dyspnea:* usually present • *Chest pain:* possibly pleuritic or dull
Neuromuscular disorders	• *Cough:* absent • *Dyspnea:* possible • *Chest pain:* absent

	HISTORY	PHYSICAL EXAMINATION AND DIAGNOSTIC STUDIES
	• Possibly asymptomatic; signs and symptoms occur gradually; past history of chest trauma or congenital deformity	• Physical deformities; accessory muscle changes; lung distortion, making interpretation of findings difficult; flail chest (paradoxical movement of region of wall and local bulging during expiration, and retraction during inspiration); consolidation may be present; no adventitious sounds • Chest X-ray and pulmonary function test normal or abnormal, depending on severity of deformity; chronic deformity may cause increase in hematocrit and hemoglobin (polycythemia)
	• Possibly asymptomatic; history of weight gain; daytime somnolence	• Distant breath sounds; reduced respiratory excursion • Possible abnormal pulmonary function test
	• Possibly asymptomatic; history of lung surgery; fatigue	• Breath sounds absent; in partial pneumonectomy, remaining portion of lung may overexpand, causing hyperresonance; in total pneumonectomy, decreased respiratory excursion occurs on affected side • Chest X-ray and pulmonary function test normal or abnormal, depending on severity of deformity
	• Presence of signs and symptoms depends on tumor's size and location	• In large tumor, physical findings same as those of chronic pleural effusion • Chest X-ray abnormal
	• Possibly asymptomatic; history of neoplasms, congestive heart failure, rheumatoid arthritis, subphrenic abscess, pancreatitis	• Limited respiratory excursion may be present; tactile fremitus decreased or absent; dull percussion; decreased breath and voice sounds; adventitious sounds caused by underlying pathology • Chest X-ray abnormal
	• Possibly symptomatic; same history as small, acute pleural effusion	• Trachea deviates toward normal side; tactile fremitus absent; dull or flat percussion; voice sounds absent or decreased; breath sounds absent; adventitious sounds caused by underlying pathology and lung consolidation • Chest X-ray abnormal
	• *Neuromuscular disorders:* medulla or spinal cord dysfunction, bulbar poliomyelitis, cervical cord trauma, Guillain-Barré syndrome, muscular dystrophy, myasthenia gravis • *Respiratory center depression:* brain tumor, sedation, industrial or carbon monoxide poisoning, polymyxin or other antibiotic therapy, encephalopathy, high-flow uncontrolled oxygen therapy	• Shallow or absent respiration, requiring artificial ventilation; distant breath sounds; symptoms of neuromuscular disease; respiratory muscle atrophy; adventitious sounds caused by underlying pathology • Pulmonary function test abnormal; arterial blood gas analysis may be abnormal *(continued)*

NURSE'S GUIDE TO RESPIRATORY DISORDERS *(continued)*

	CHIEF COMPLAINT
Closed pneumothorax	• *Cough:* absent • *Dyspnea:* moderate • *Chest pain:* pleuritic; may be sudden and sharp
Open pneumothorax	• *Cough:* absent • *Dyspnea:* severe • *Chest pain:* severe, pleuritic; sudden and sharp
Tension pneumothorax	• *Cough:* absent • *Dyspnea:* severe • *Chest pain:* severe, pleuritic; sudden and sharp
Asthmatic attack	• *Cough:* dry and minimal; progresses to thick and productive • *Dyspnea:* severe, with audible wheezing • *Chest pain:* absent
Chronic obstructive pulmonary disease (COPD) Type A (pink puffer)	• *Cough:* present, with scant mucoid production • *Dyspnea:* insidious onset; slowly progresses to severe dyspnea on exertion • *Chest pain:* absent
Chronic obstructive pulmonary disease (COPD) Type B (blue bloater)	• *Cough:* chronic and productive cough occurring most often in the morning, for at least 3 months of the year for 2 consecutive years; possibly hemoptysis • *Dyspnea:* first occurs only during chest infections; less severe than Type A • *Chest pain:* absent, except in second-degree chronic cough

	HISTORY	PHYSICAL EXAMINATION AND DIAGNOSTIC STUDIES
	• Dizziness, emphysema, tuberculosis	• Crepitus; if small, no trachea deviation; *on affected side:* limited respiratory excursion; tactile fremitus absent; resonant or hyperresonant percussion; breath and voice sounds absent or decreased; no adventitious sounds • Chest X-ray abnormal
	• Dizziness	• Crepitus; trachea deviates to normal side; *on affected side:* limited respiratory excursion; tactile fremitus absent; hyperresonant or tympanic percussion; breath and voice sounds absent or decreased; no adventitious sounds; cyanosis • Chest X-ray abnormal
	• Acute symptoms	• Cyanosis; shock; possible tympanic percussion; other physical findings same as those of open pneumothorax • Chest X-ray abnormal
	• *Allergic asthma:* history of taking aspirin or other nonsteroidal anti-inflammatory agents; exposure to feathers, dander, molds, or certain foods; family history of allergies • *Idiosyncratic asthma:* attacks common following respiratory infection; no family history of allergies • *Precipitating or exacerbating asthma:* environment, stress, occupation, exercise, respiratory infection	• Tachycardia; pale and slightly cyanotic appearance; tendency to sit or lean forward; difficult speech; diaphoresis; nasal flaring on expiration; bulging neck veins; use of accessory muscles in retraction of intercostal, supraclavicular, and suprasternal spaces; markedly distended and fixed chest in inspiratory position; tactile fremitus decreased; hyperresonant percussion; diaphragm low on percussion; voice sounds decreased; breath sounds distant; expiration greater than inspiration; sibilant rhonchi (wheezing) throughout lung fields on expiration • Chest X-ray normal; arterial blood gas analysis abnormal during attack • Hyperinflation may be present.
	• Genetic predisposition; cigarette smoking; acute recurring respiratory illness (more common in Type B); exposure to environmental hazards; under age 60	• Reddish complexion; weight loss; neck veins distended on expiration, collapsed on inspiration; increased anteroposterior diameter; use of accessory muscles; decreased respiratory excursion bilaterally; decreased tactile fremitus; hyperresonant percussion; decreased diaphragmatic excursion; breath sounds distant with prolonged expiration; pursed lips when breathing; decreased voice sounds; adventitious sounds; occasionally sonorous or wheezing • Chest X-ray abnormal; pulmonary function test abnormal; arterial blood gas analysis abnormal; hematocrit abnormal
	• Exposure to air pollution, inorganic and/or organic dusts, or noxious gases; cigarette smoking; genetic predisposition; increased frequency of respiratory infections	• Red or blue complexion; cyanosis; overweight; increased anteroposterior chest diameter (barrel chest); hyperresonance on percussion; prolonged expiratory phase; sibilant and sonorous rhonchi and rales may be present; cor pulmonale may occur as complication • Chest X-ray normal or abnormal (may show evidence of past inflammatory disease); pulmonary function test abnormal; arterial blood gas analysis abnormal; hematocrit abnormal *(continued)*

NURSE'S GUIDE TO RESPIRATORY DISORDERS *(continued)*

	CHIEF COMPLAINT
Advanced bronchiectasis	• *Cough:* chronic, with copious, foul, purulent sputum; hemoptysis • *Dyspnea:* present in severe and extensive disease • *Chest pain:* absent, except in pneumonia or second-degree chronic cough
DIFFUSION DISORDERS	
Bacterial pneumonia	• *Cough:* present, productive, with mucoid, purulent sputum; hemoptysis • *Dyspnea:* present on exertion • *Chest pain:* present, pleuritic
Mycoplasmal pneumonia (atypical pneumonia)	• *Cough:* prolonged history of dry, hacking, possibly persistent cough; no hemoptysis • *Dyspnea:* absent • *Chest pain:* present, possibly from secondary musculoskeletal cough
Lung abscess	• *Cough:* present, productive with large amounts of bloody, purulent sputum • *Dyspnea:* present, frequent • *Chest pain:* present, pleuritic
Lung tuberculosis	• *Cough:* present, productive, purulent; hemoptysis • *Dyspnea:* present only in advanced disease • *Chest pain:* present, occasionally pleuritic
Pulmonary fibrosis, nonchemical (dust, industrial irritants, allergens)	• *Cough:* present, dry, irritable, progressing to productive hemoptysis • *Dyspnea:* present, progressive, exertional; wheezing; tachypnea • *Chest pain:* present

HISTORY	PHYSICAL EXAMINATION AND DIAGNOSTIC STUDIES
• Recurring pneumonia or sinusitis; congenital defects in bronchial system; hereditary predisposition; deficient immunities; local bronchial obstruction; general weakness and fatigue	• Cyanosis; clubbing; fever; night sweats; weight loss; sibilant or sonorous rhonchi and rales over lower lobes; in progressive advanced bronchiectasis, lung findings similar to Type A chronic obstructive pulmonary disease • Chest X-ray abnormal; bronchography abnormal; pulmonary function test normal or abnormal; arterial blood gas analysis abnormal
• Predisposing conditions include depressed cough and glottis reflexes; altered consciousness from alcoholism, drug abuse, seizure, head trauma, general anesthetic, cerebrovascular disease, old age; painful breathing; muscle weakness; neuromuscular diseases; obstructive diseases; impaired mucus transport; possibly aspiration of vomitus or oil; respiration or immunosuppressive drug therapy	• Fever, chills, tachycardia, tachypnea, cyanosis, hypotension, guarding and decreased excursion on affected side • *With adventitious sounds:* crepitant inspiratory rales, pleural friction rub with pleural involvement • *With consolidation:* tactile fremitus increased; percussion dull or flat; breath sounds tubular or bronchial; voice sounds increased, including bronchophony, egophony, and whispered pectoriloquy • *With bronchial plug and consolidation:* tactile fremitus absent; percussion dull; voice, breath sounds decreased or absent • Increased white blood cell count; chest X-ray abnormal; sputum examination abnormal
• Between ages 5 and 20; family history of disease; onset of signs and symptoms resembles that of viral respiratory tract infection (malaise, myalgia, sore throat, headache, mild cough, earache)	• Fever during first 2 weeks; in about 15% of cases, inflamed tympanic membrane, with bullae; fine crepitant rales at end of inspiratory cycle possible; dullness on percussion; rhonchi; coarse or musical wheezes; normal chest findings possible • Chest X-ray abnormal; complement fixation test shows level of specific antibody to *Mycoplasma;* no leukocytosis
• Recurrent dental infections; history similar to that of bacterial pneumonia but more insidious; history of altered mental status	• Fever, weight loss, fetid breath, poor dentition; respiratory findings may appear normal or similar to consolidation in bacterial pneumonia • Chest X-ray normal or abnormal; sputum culture should identify organism; increased white blood cell count (leukocytosis)
• Possibly asymptomatic; malaise, irritability at end of day; night sweats; exposure to active pulmonary tuberculosis; associated with uncontrolled diabetes, alcoholism, undernutrition, institutionalization, long-term treatment with corticosteroids	• Fever; weight loss; decreased respiratory excursion; in early stages, respiratory findings may appear normal; extensive fibrosis may cause consolidation: apical dullness, bronchial breath sounds, coarse rales • Chest X-ray abnormal; sputum culture positive for tubercle bacillus; positive tuberculin test
• Inhalation of dust, industrial irritants, or allergens; malaise; weight loss; anorexia	• Cyanosis on exertion; fine metallic crepitant basilar rales; decreased chest excursion in advanced disease • Chest X-ray abnormal; pulmonary function test abnormal

(continued)

NURSE'S GUIDE TO RESPIRATORY DISORDERS *(continued)*

	CHIEF COMPLAINT
Pulmonary fibrosis, chemical (irritant gases, chemicals)	• *Cough:* present, hemoptysis • *Dyspnea:* present, wheezing • *Chest pain:* present
VENTILATION/DIFFUSION DISORDERS	
Pulmonary edema	• *Cough:* dry at first, progressing to productive, with pink, frothy sputum • *Dyspnea:* in acute form: wheezing; in chronic form: paroxysmal nocturnal dyspnea; orthopnea • *Chest pain:* absent
Connective tissue disease affecting the lungs (such as systemic lupus erythematosus)	• *Cough:* may be present, with or without production • *Dyspnea:* present • *Chest pain:* pleuritic or dull sensation, with pleural effusion
Pulmonary embolism	• *Cough:* hemoptysis • *Dyspnea:* sudden, unexplained tachypnea • *Chest pain:* pleuritic, but only if infarction occurs
Lung tumor	• *Cough:* absent, mild, or change in pattern of chronic cough • *Dyspnea:* absent or on exertion • *Chest pain:* absent
Adult respiratory distress syndrome (ARDS)	• *Cough:* dry, progressing to rusty and frothy to burgundy red • *Dyspnea:* tachypnea, progressing to dyspnea • *Chest pain:* absent
Atelectasis	• *Cough:* present • *Dyspnea:* sudden; wheezing • *Chest pain:* absent or pleuritic

HISTORY	PHYSICAL EXAMINATION AND DIAGNOSTIC STUDIES
• Exposure to irritant gases or chemicals	• Burning and irritation of eyes, nose, throat, trachea; nausea and vomiting; cyanosis on exertion; fine metallic crepitant basilar rales; decreased chest excursion in advanced disease • Chest X-ray abnormal; pulmonary function test abnormal
• May be sudden or chronic; history of heart disease	• *Acute:* must sit up and lean forward to breathe; cyanosis; resonant percussion; normal voice sounds; breath sounds reveal prolonged expiratory phase; adventitious sounds reveal dry, fine rales usually at base, progressing to moist, bubbling rales throughout chest; sibilant rhonchi; rattle sound • *Chronic:* enlarged heart, peripheral edema, hepatomegaly, bilateral diffuse butterfly density from hilum • Chest X-ray abnormal
• Past history of connective tissue disease	• Signs of specific suspected disease; fibrosis; clubbing; decreased respiratory excursion; trachea deviates toward more affected side; resonant to dull percussion; decreased breath and voice sounds, especially in diffuse fibrosis; rales audible on inspiration and expiration; pleural friction rub • Chest X-ray abnormal; pulmonary function tests abnormal; specific tests to identify disease include antinuclear antibody and Rh factor
• Previous thromboemboli, recent surgery, dehydration, pregnancy, congestive heart failure, chronic pulmonary disease, use of oral contraceptives, leg fracture, deep venous insufficiency, extended inactivity, such as bed rest or prolonged air travel	• Tachycardia; may be normal except for rales and localized wheezing; pleural effusion and pleural friction rub possible if infarction occurs; atelectasis and pneumonia may occur as complications • Chest X-ray inconclusive; arterial blood gas analysis abnormal; pulmonary angiography abnormal. Ventilation/perfusion lung scan abnormal
• May be asymptomatic; cigarette smoking; possibly anorexia, weight loss, nausea, vomiting, weakness	• Possibly weight loss, consolidation, or atelectasis • Possibly abnormal chest X-ray, sputum cytology, bronchoscopy, and fiberoscopy
• Shock (septic, hemorrhagic, cardiogenic, anaphalactoid), direct chest trauma, aspiration, fat emboli, massive viral pneumonia	• Tachycardia; cyanosis; diffuse scattered rales, progressing to poor respiratory excursion; normal fremitus; normal percussion; normal breath and voice sounds • Chest X-ray abnormal; arterial blood gas analysis abnormal
• *Mild or chronic:* no signs or symptoms • *Acute:* sudden signs or symptoms; recent surgery	• Tachycardia; tracheal shift to affected side; respiratory excursion limited on affected side; tactile fremitus decreased or absent; dull to flat percussion over collapsed lung; hyperresonance over remaining portion of affected lung; decreased or absent breath and voice sounds; adventitious sounds high pitched with rales, especially on inspiration • Abnormal chest X-ray possible

CASE HISTORIES: NURSING DIAGNOSIS FLOWCHART

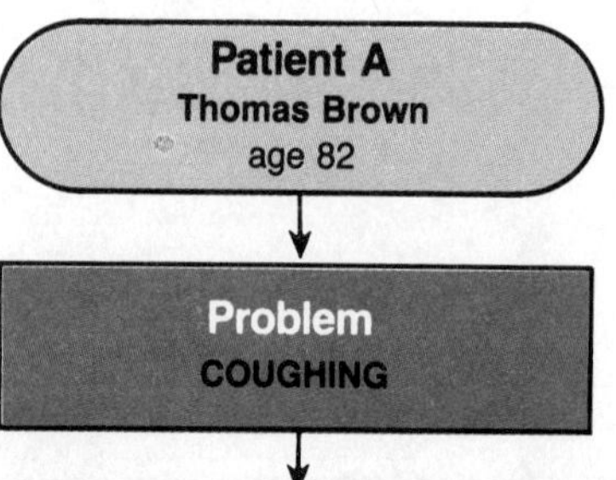

Subjective data

- Productive coughing, with large amounts of yellow-green sputum for 2 days
- No chills, no temperature taken
- Weakness, confusion, shortness of breath when he walked to bathroom
- History: Smoking one pack/day for 50 years
- Medications: Administered Tylenol with codeine #3, two tablets three times yesterday

Objective data

- *Inspection:* Restless; oriented to person but not to place and time; respirations shallow; 28 breaths/minute; less movement of chest seen on right side; shortness of breath noted on motion; cough weak, with small amounts of green production; temperature, 100.4° F. orally; pulse, 96; color, pale
- *Palpation:* Limited palpable expansion on right anterior and posterior thorax; increased vocal fremitus anterior right thorax, fourth to sixth intercostal spaces
- *Percussion:* Dullness over fourth to sixth intercostal spaces, right anterior and lateral thorax
- *Auscultation:* Increased bronchophony between fourth and sixth intercostal spaces, right anterior thorax; bronchial breath sounds, with coarse rales at fourth to sixth intercostal spaces; rhonchi in right base; no audible friction rub
- *Laboratory:* Chest X-ray shows right middle lobe infiltrated; white blood cell count elevated; Gram's stain sputum—gram-positive diplococci

Nursing diagnoses

- Ineffective breathing patterns
- Impaired gas exchange
- Impaired physical mobility
- Alteration in comfort

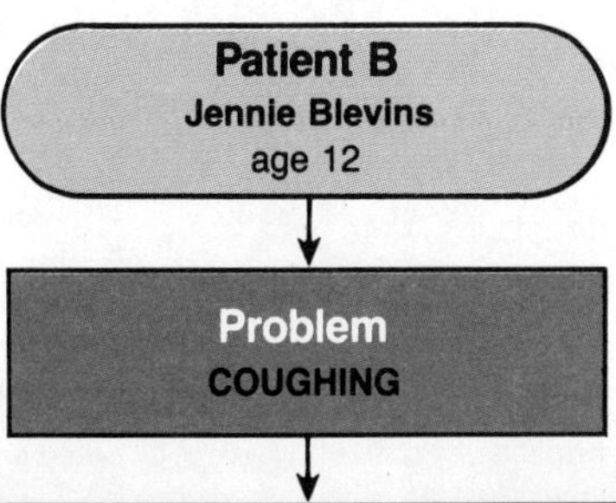

Subjective data

- Alteration in level of consciousness; ineffective airway clearance
- (Mother contributed to history) Had symptoms of common cold 4 weeks ago, with fever; cold symptoms disappeared, but dry, hacking cough persisted (no hemoptysis)
- No sharp stabbing pain in chest, but patient complains of chest discomfort when moving trunk
- No sore throat; no nasal congestion; no headache
- Mother concerned because patient is awake coughing all night, eating less, and missing school

Objective data

- *Inspection:* Appears tired but not in acute distress; temperature, 98.6° F. orally; pulse, 80; respirations, 16/minute; no nasal congestion; oropharynx normal; in ears, both eardrums visualized, with no hyperemia or bullae
- *Palpation:* No neck lymphadenopathy; tenderness on right lower posterior thorax
- *Percussion:* Normal
- *Auscultation:* Lungs clear
- *Laboratory:* White blood cell count within normal limits; chest X-ray shows right lower lobe infiltrated

Nursing diagnoses

- Alteration in comfort
- Alteration in sleep pattern
- Alteration in nutrition

FORMING SAMPLE NURSING DIAGNOSES

CHIEF COMPLAINT	EFFECT OF SIGN OR SYMPTOM	NURSING DIAGNOSIS
Dyspnea	*Acute:* • Diaphoresis; restlessness	• Alterations in comfort
	Chronic: • Barrel chest; accessory muscle change	• Ineffective breathing pattern
	Acute and chronic: • Fatigue, exhaustion • Emotional distress • Hypoventilation/hyperventilation (may lead to respiratory acidosis/alkalosis)	• Fear of breathlessness, ineffective breathing pattern, impaired gas exchange, impaired physical mobility
Chest pain	• Decreased ventilation (may lead to infection or pneumonia) • Increased CO_2 retention and respiratory acidosis	• Impaired gas exchange, ineffective breathing pattern
	• Discomfort • Pain	• Fear of chest pain, alterations in comfort
Cough	*Chronic and short term (less than 1 month):* • Hazardous elevation in intrathoracic pressure, intracranial pressure, and blood pressure (may lead to congestive heart failure, ruptured aneurysm) • Cough syncope	• Alteration in CO_2
	• Musculoskeletal pain • Fractured ribs	• Alterations in comfort
	Chronic and long term (more than 1 month): • Fatigue • Weight loss, anorexia	• Alteration in nutrition (less than body requirements)
	Forced cough: • Collapsed airways (atelectasis) • Rupture of thin-walled alveoli (may lead to pneumothorax)	• Impaired gas exchange
	• Hemoptysis, second-degree irritation of tracheobronchial tree	• Fear of seeing blood
Increased and abnormal secretions	*Increased sputum:* • Mucous plugs (may lead to airway obstruction, atelectasis, prevention of alveoli gas exchange, hypoxia, respiratory acidosis) • Increased secretions and/or abnormal fluids retained in lung (may lead to infection, tracheobronchitis, bronchopneumonia)	• Ineffective airway clearance, impaired gas exchange
	Hemoptysis: • Obstruction with blood (may lead to asphyxiation, atelectasis, pneumonia)	• Ineffective airway clearance, impaired gas exchange, alterations in tissue perfusion
	• Blood-streaked sputum; severe blood loss may lead to shock	• Fear of seeing blood

ventilation and possibly respiratory rate, aggravating arrhythmias, and further depressing the cardiovascular and central nervous systems.

Because hypoxia occurs to some degree in all respiratory conditions, always consider a nursing diagnosis of *inadequate oxygen available for body needs,* whether your patient's chief complaint is a cough, dyspnea, or chest pain. A cough's explosive force can cause musculoskeletal pain and even fractured ribs. Your nursing diagnosis for these conditions is *alterations in comfort.* A severe cough can collapse airways (atelectasis), rupture alveoli or blebs (which can lead to pneumothorax), and irritate the tracheobronchial tree, causing hemoptysis. Possible nursing diagnoses for airway collapse or for ruptured alveoli or blebs are *impaired gas exchange* and *ineffective breathing patterns.* Even mild hemoptysis may cause a patient to fear the worst—perhaps because of the historical description of consumption (tuberculosis) or the current emphasis on lung cancer. *Fear: incomplete understanding of disease* may be an appropriate nursing diagnosis in this situation.

A chronic cough (lasting more than a month) can drain your patient's energy. It may also reduce his appetite, especially when the cough is accompanied by sputum production. If your patient exhibits fatigue, anorexia, or weight loss, consider a nursing diagnosis of *altered nutritional intake: less than body requirements.*

Abnormally thick secretions may result in mucous plug formation. These plugs can obstruct airways and lead to atelectasis and respiratory acidosis. Possible nursing diagnoses for a patient with mucous plugs are *ineffective airway clearance* and *impaired gas exchange.* Increased secretions, abnormal fluids, or aspirates in the lungs can result in respiratory tract infections, such as pneumonia and possibly respiratory failure. Again, your nursing diagnosis would be *impaired gas exchange* and *altered comfort,* if pain during respiration exists.

Gross hemoptysis may result in *ineffective airway clearance* and *impaired gas exchange* by obstructing airways and causing asphyxiation and atelectasis.

Dyspnea is usually accompanied by hypoventilation (decreased carbon dioxide exchange) or hyperventilation (increased carbon dioxide exchange). Hypoventilation can lead to respiratory acidosis (elevated carbon dioxide and low pH); hyperventilation (usually less dangerous than hypoventilation) can lead to respiratory alkalosis (reduced carbon dioxide and increased pH). Nursing diagnoses would be *ineffective breathing pattern* or *impaired gas exchange,* or both.

When acute dyspnea causes diaphoresis and restlessness, *alterations in comfort* would be an appropriate nursing diagnosis. Both acute and chronic dyspneic patients may exhibit fatigue and exhaustion, resulting in *impaired physical mobility, deficits in self-care,* and *ineffective breathing pattern.* Emotional distress caused by straining for every breath or never knowing when an attack of dyspnea will come suggests a nursing diagnosis of *fear of breathlessness.*

Chest pain, of course, always requires a nursing diagnosis of *alterations in comfort.* Chest pain caused by pleuritic or musculoskeletal conditions results in decreased ventilation, which may lead to infection and respiratory acidosis. Appropriate nursing diagnoses are *impaired gas exchange* and *ineffective breathing pattern.* Because patients with chest pain commonly assume that this means they have cardiovascular disorders, consider a nursing diagnosis of *fear: incomplete understanding of disease.* All three cardinal symptoms, cough, dyspnea, and chest pain, may cause alterations in the patient's rest-activity patterns, as well as interfere with other activities of daily living (see *Forming Sample Nursing Diagnoses*).

Assessing pediatric patients

359 Anatomic and physiologic variations

A child's developing pulmonary system makes him more susceptible than an adult to certain respiratory diseases. For instance, upper respiratory tract infections commonly occur in children because a child's respiratory tract is immature, and the mucous membranes often can't produce enough mucus to warm and humidify inhaled air. Also, a child's developing immune system can't fight bacteria and viruses as well as an adult's can.

Kiesselbach's triangle, the cricoid cartilage, and the sinuses are important anatomic structures in a child's upper respiratory tract. *Kiesselbach's triangle*—also present in adults—is a fine network of small blood vessels near the tip of the nose and is especially significant in children as the most common site of nosebleeds. The *cricoid cartilage,* located just below the epiglottis, is the narrowest cartilage ring in the developing larynx; thus, swelling or small amounts of mucus easily occlude the narrow lumen. At birth, the *ethmoidal* and *maxillary sinuses* are present, the *sphenoidal* sinuses are very small, and the *frontal* sinuses are absent. The sphenoidal sinuses develop fully after puberty; the frontal, at age 7 or 8.

Because the lower respiratory tract is small in infants and children, breath sounds are louder and more bronchial, expiration is longer, and vesicular sounds are harsher. The infant's *thorax* is round, with equal anteroposterior transverse diameters. The lateral diameter increases rapidly with growth, resulting in characteristic adult proportions by age 6. (The thin chest wall and lack of muscle allow palpation of the floating ribs in young children.)

Infants are obligate nose breathers, which is one reason why colds are more serious for them. A child's breathing should be primarily abdominal until age 6 or 7 (longer if the patient has done breathing exercises for singing or athletics). Abdominal breathing beyond this age may indicate pain or splinting of the chest walls, as in pleuritis; respiratory movements before this age suggest pain or splinting of the abdomen, as in peritonitis.

A child's respiratory rate may double in response to exercise, illness, or emotion. Normally, the rate for newborns is 30 to 80 breaths/minute; for toddlers, 20 to 40; and for children of school age and older, 15 to 25. Children usually reach the adult rate (12 to 20) at about age 15.

360 Special pediatric history considerations

Ask the parents how often the child has had upper respiratory tract infections. Remember that a history of more than six nose or throat infections a year necessitates further evaluation of the child, because colds in preschool children are often a sign of streptococcal infection. Find out if the child has had other respiratory signs and symptoms, such as dyspnea, wheezing, rhinorrhea, or a stuffy nose. Ask if these appear related to the child's activities or to seasonal changes.

Also, ask if the child has had a cough that interrupts his sleep or causes vomiting. If so, does it produce sputum? Is the sputum blood-tinged? Ask if anyone in the family has ever had cystic fibrosis or other major respiratory diseases, such as asthma.

361 Examining a child's respiratory system

Positioning a child for a respiratory examination depends, of course, on his age, condition, and disposition. The sitting position offers you easiest access to his thorax, and usually a parent can help by holding the child in his lap. You and the parent can also form a mock examining table by sitting opposite each other, placing your knees together, and allowing the child to sit on the parent's lap.

If the child is quiet, auscultate his lungs first. If you hear fluid, place the stethoscope's diaphragm over his nose to determine if the fluid is in the nose or upper respiratory tract. This is important in children, because the sound of fluid in the nose can be transmitted through the short distance between nose and lungs.

To examine the child's nostrils for patency, occlude one, put the stethoscope's diaphragm over the other, and listen and watch for condensation on the diaphragm. With infants and young children, perform this procedure (which may provoke crying) after auscultating the lungs, because crying can cause an unnatural respiration rate and interfere with breath sound auscultation. Also, crying usually elicits mouth breathing, which can make determining the nostrils' patency difficult. To quiet a crying child and relax his breathing, hand him a plastic windmill and ask him to blow on it, or have him pretend to blow out a candle.

The procedure you should use for inspecting the child's mouth and throat also depends on his age and disposition. Position the *infant* on his back and ask the parent to hold him still. If the patient's a *young child,* have the parent hold the child on his lap, restraining the child's head with one arm and his arms with the other. Or, the parent can raise and hold the child's arms over his head, immobilizing the head between the arms. A child age *6 or older* will probably sit on the examining table without restraint. (To ease his anxiety, you might allow him to handle the equipment.)

Use a flashlight and tongue depressor to examine the child's mouth and throat. You can also use the tongue depressor to elicit the gag reflex in infants, but *remember, you should never test this reflex or examine the pharynx in a child suspected of having epiglottitis,* because these procedures can cause complete laryngeal obstruction, which could be fatal.

ABNORMAL PEDIATRIC CHEST ANATOMY

While you're examining the child, note any structural abnormalities of his chest. Chest abnormalities in children, and their significance, include the following:

- An unusually wide space between the nipples may indicate Turner's syndrome (the distance between the outside areolar edges shouldn't be more than one quarter of the patient's chest circumference).
- Rachitic beads (bumps at the costocondral junction of the ribs) may indicate rickets.
- Pigeon chest may be a sign of Marfan's or Morquio's syndrome or any chronic upper respiratory tract obstruction; funnel chest may indicate rickets or Marfan's syndrome; barrel chest may indicate chronic respiratory disease, such as cystic fibrosis or asthma.
- Localized bulges may suggest underlying pressures, such as cardiac enlargement or aneurysm.
- Multiple (more than five) café-au-lait spots may be associated with neurofibromatosis.

While examining the posterior thorax of the older child, be sure to check for scoliosis. If you observe an abnormality, refer him for treatment (see Entry 697). Also, remember that Harrison's groove (a horizontal ridge at the diaphragm level, accompanied by some flaring of the ribs below the groove, as by rickets or congenital syphilis) is considered normal in infants and young, thin children—if other pathologic signs aren't present (see *Abnormal Pediatric Chest Anatomy*).

362 Diagnosing childhood respiratory disorders

You may see laryngotracheobronchitis (croup)—the most common cause of respiratory distress in children over age 3—in a child with a history of upper respiratory tract infections, a hacking cough, fever, stridor, and diminished breath sounds with rhonchi. Signs and

RESPIRATORY DISTRESS IN CHILDREN

AGES 0 to 2

Common

Acute lower respiratory tract infections (bronchitis, bronchopneumonia)
Bronchiolitis
Aspiration pneumonia

Uncommon

Congenital laryngeal web
Laryngeal cyst
Subglottic stenosis
Congenital heart disease
Laryngomalacia

AGES 3 to 18

Common

Laryngotracheobronchitis (croup)
Acute pneumonia
Atelectasis
Foreign body (choking)
Asthma
Acute epiglottitis

Uncommon

Pneumothorax
Congenital heart disease
Neoplasms of laryngeal structure

symptoms of this usually benign disease are similar to those for epiglottitis. Usually, a chest X-ray determines the cause of respiratory distress in children.

Epiglottitis, a bacterial infection preceded by a minor respiratory illness, sometimes may be present in a child with sudden respiratory distress and a high fever, so-called seal bark, hoarseness, and anoxia. *Remember: Excitement or stress that causes the child to cry can produce immediate airway obstruction.* Epiglottitis is more common in children between ages 3 and 8; croup, which has similar signs and symptoms, is more common in children between ages 2 and 5. (See *Respiratory Distress in Children.*)

Intracostal, subcostal, and suprasternal retractions and expiratory grunts are always serious signs in children. Refer an infant or child with any of these signs for treatment immediately. He may have pneumonia, respiratory distress syndrome, or left-sided heart failure. An infant with untreated pneumonia can die within hours.

When a child's symptoms and signs include retractions, nasal flaring, cyanosis, restlessness, and apprehension—primarily on inspiration—the trachea or mainstem bronchi may be obstructed. If these signs and symptoms occur on expiration, his bronchioles may be obstructed, as seen with asthma or bronchitis. Foreign body aspiration is another major cause of respiratory distress in children. These signs and symptoms indicate serious respiratory distress.

Assessing geriatric patients

363 How aging affects the respiratory system

Age-related anatomic changes in the upper airways include nose enlargement from continued cartilage growth, general atrophy of the tonsils, and tracheal deviations from changes in the aging spine. Possible thoracic changes include increased anteroposterior chest diameter as a result of altered calcium metabolism and calcification of costal cartilages, reducing mobility of the chest wall. Also, because of such factors as osteoporosis and vertebral collapse, kyphosis advances with age (see Entry 700).

Pulmonary function also decreases in the elderly because of respiratory muscle degeneration or atrophy. Ventilatory capacity diminishes for several reasons. First, the lungs' diffusing capacity declines. Second, lung tissue degeneration causes a decrease in the lungs' elastic recoil capability, which results in an elevated residual volume. (The aging process alone can cause emphysema.) Last, the closing of some airways produces poor ventilation of the basal areas, resulting in both a decreased surface area for gas exchange and reduced Po_2. Thus, maximum breathing capacity, forced vital capacity, vital capacity, and inspiratory reserve volume diminish with age, leaving the elderly patient with lowered tolerance for oxygen debt.

364 Special health history concerns

During the health history interview, remember that the elderly patient may be confused or his mental function may be slow, especially if he has hypoventilation and hypoperfusion from respiratory disease. Also, keep in mind that because an elderly patient has reduced sensations, he may describe his chest pain as heavy or dull, whereas a younger patient would describe the same pain as sharp. When recording a retired patient's psychosocial history, be sure you ask about his former occupation, because it may have caused exposure to harmful substances.

365 Examining the elderly patient

As you inspect an elderly patient's thorax, be especially alert for degenerative skeletal changes, such as kyphosis (see Entry 700). Palpating for diaphragmatic excursion may be more difficult in the elderly patient because of loose skin covering his chest. Therefore, when you position your hands, slide them toward his spine, raising loose skin folds between your thumbs and the spine.

When you percuss his chest, remember that loss of elastic recoil capability in an elderly person stretches the alveoli and bronchioles, producing hyperresonance. During auscultation, carefully observe how well your patient tolerates the examination. He may tire easily because of low tolerance to oxygen debt. Also, taking deep breaths during auscultation may produce lightheadedness or syncope faster than in a younger patient. You may hear diminished sounds at the lung bases because some of his airways are closed.

366 Increased risk and incidence of illness

Elderly persons are subject to the same respiratory disorders and diseases as younger adults. However, in cold, damp weather, the incidence of chronic respiratory disease, colds, and flu rises more steeply among the elderly. Also, geriatric patients run a greater risk of developing pneumonia because their weakened chest musculature reduces their ability to clear secretions.

Selected References

Bates, Barbara. *Guide to Physical Examination,* 2nd ed. Philadelphia: J.B. Lippincott Co., 1979.

Blackburn, Nancy A., and Cebenka, Deborah L. "Honing Your Respiratory Assessment Technique," *RN* 43(5):28, 1980.

Brannin, P.K. "Physical Assessment of Acute Respiratory Failure," *Critical Care Quarterly* 1:27, March 1979.

Brown, Marie Scott, and Alexander, Mary M. "Physical Examination: Part 9, Examining the Nose," *Nursing74* 4(7):35, 1974.

Delaney, M. "Examining the Chest: Part 1, The Lungs," *Nursing75* 5(8):12, 1975.

Fuhs, Margaret F., and Stein, Alice M. "Better Ways to Cope with COPD," *Nursing76* 6(2):28, 1976.

Guyton, Arthur C. *Textbook of Medical Physiology,* 6th ed. Philadelphia: W.B. Saunders Co., 1981.

Hillman, Robert S., et al. *Clinical Skills: Interviewing, History Taking, and Physical Diagnosis.* New York: McGraw-Hill Book Co., 1981.

Jarvis, Carolyn Mueller. "Perfecting Physical Assessment: Part 2," *Nursing77* 7(6):38, 1977.

Thompson, June M., and Bowers, Arden C. *Clinical Manual of Health Assessment.* St. Louis: C.V. Mosby Co., 1980.

10

KEY POINTS IN THIS CHAPTER

KEY CHARTS IN THIS CHAPTER

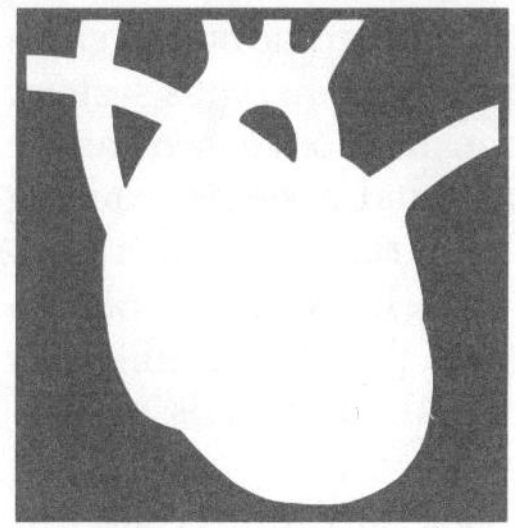

Cardiovascular System

Introduction

367 Importance of cardiovascular assessment

The phenomenally high incidence of heart disease and the seriousness of its complications continually reaffirm your need to know how to assess the complex cardiovascular system. As a nurse, you're already aware of the nationwide dimensions of this problem. In fact, the importance of cardiovascular assessment can be explained in terms of sheer numbers alone. Consider the following findings, released by the American Heart Association:

• Cardiovascular disease remains the *most common cause of death* in the United States. Overt coronary artery disease alone accounts for more than 600,000 deaths annually. More than one third of these deaths occur suddenly. (This last figure doesn't include deaths attributed to hypertension, cerebrovascular accident, and renal disease, which may result from underlying cardiovascular disease.)

• Increasingly large numbers of patients enter hospitals in the United States with a primary or secondary medical diagnosis related to cardiovascular dysfunction.

• The majority of serious complications in hospitalized patients involve cardiovascular dysfunction. These complications include pulmonary embolism, thrombophlebitis, congestive heart failure, stress response, shock, and cardiac arrhythmias.

No body system wears out, breaks down, or otherwise malfunctions so often, in so many people, as the cardiovascular system. Remember, heart disease affects people of all ages and takes many forms. It can be congenital or acquired, and it can develop suddenly or insidiously. (Atherosclerosis, for example, can be far advanced or even life-threatening before signs and symptoms appear.) Mastering cardiovascular assessment skills is therefore essential to your development as a member of the professional health-care team.

368 Assessment prerequisites

You perform some cardiovascular assessment techniques, such as recording pulse rates and blood pressures, routinely and easily. But complete assessment of the cardiovascular system, including evaluation of the heart and peripheral vascular system, is complex and requires special skills and knowledge. For instance, you must be adept at inspecting neck veins, palpating the precordium, and auscultating heart sounds and murmurs—advanced skills requiring many hours of practice.

You must also understand the complex relationships between the cardiovascular system and other body systems. For example, pathology of the nervous system resulting in increased intracranial pressure causes increased systemic vasoconstriction, hypertension, and decreased heart rate. This is the Cushing reflex. This cardiovascular response attempts to assure adequate perfusion of brain tissue. Pathology of the cardiovascular system, on the other hand, can stimulate a compensatory response in other body systems. For example, a drop in cardiac output stimulates the sympathetic nervous system, causing vasoconstriction, as well as the endocrine and renal systems, causing sodium and water retention (the renin-angiotensin cycle). These events attempt to increase the heart's efficiency as a pump in maintaining tissue perfusion.

Make sure you fully appreciate this delicate balance between the heart and other body functions before you assess your patient's cardiovascular system.

Reviewing anatomy and physiology

369 Basic functions of the cardiovascular system

The two basic functions of the cardiovascular system are to deliver oxygenated blood to the body tissues and to remove waste substances through the action of the heart. Specialized pacemaker cells and conduction fibers innervate the heart and initiate and propagate its beat. The average person's heart beats 60 to 100 times/minute, pumping 4 to 6 qt (4 to 6 liters) of blood in this time—and on the average, it does this for more than 70 years.

Controlled by the autonomic nervous system, the heart pumps blood through the entire body. The vascular network that carries blood through all body systems consists of high-pressure arteries, which deliver the blood, and low-pressure veins, which return it to the heart. This complex network keeps the pumping heart filled with blood and maintains blood pressure.

370 Pericardium

The pericardium is a closed, invaginated, serous sac that surrounds the heart and the roots of the great vessels. It has two contiguous layers: an inner (visceral) layer that forms the epicardium and an outer (parietal) layer that is continuous with the covering of the great vessels. The pericardial space or cavity, which contains 10 to 50 ml of serous fluid, lies between the two layers. Fibrous connective tissue (fibrous pericardium) strengthens the parietal layer, anchoring the sac to the diaphragm, the sternum, and the great vessels. The pericardium's posterior surface contacts the esophagus, thoracic aorta, and bronchi. Its lateral surfaces lie against the mediastinal pleurae, with only the phrenic nerves and blood vessels intervening.

371 The heart: Location and form

The heart is a hollow, muscular, four-chambered organ, enveloped by the pericardium. Roughly cone-shaped, the heart lies obliquely in the chest, with two thirds of it located to the left of the midline. An average man's heart weighs about 10.5 oz (300 g).

The heart varies in shape and position, depending on the person's age, body build, and the changing position of his body. Its axis is more vertical in a tall, slender person and more transverse in a person who is broad and stocky. Respiration also alters the position of the heart's axis. During inspiration, the axis becomes more vertical as the diaphragm descends; during expiration, as the diaphragm rises, it becomes more transverse.

THE CARDIOVASCULAR SYSTEM

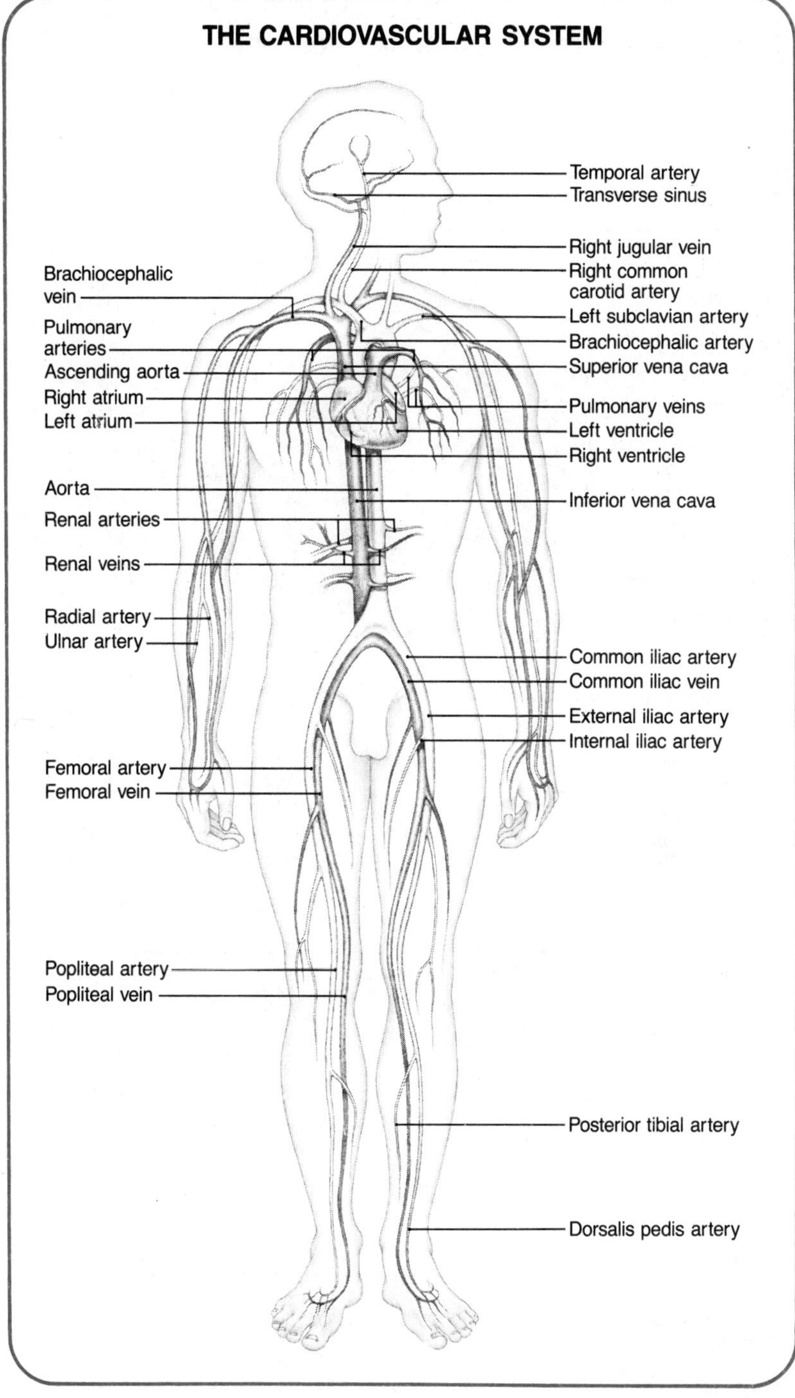

THE HEART: ANTERIOR AND POSTERIOR VIEWS

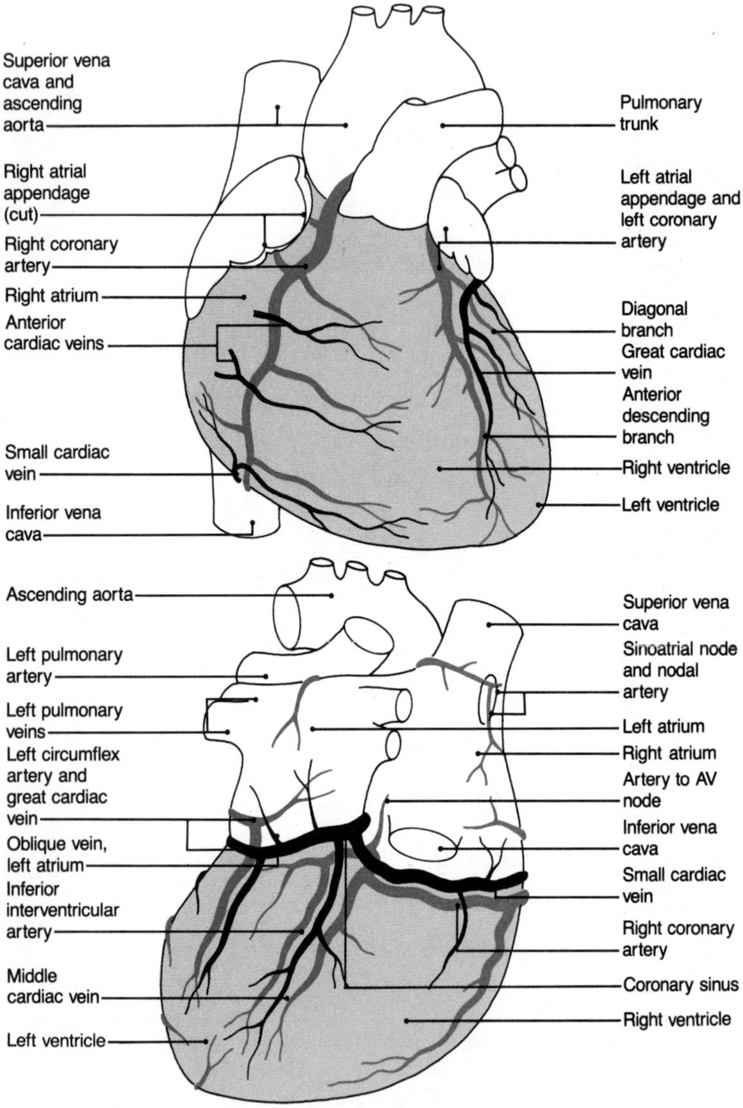

Superior vena cava and ascending aorta
Right atrial appendage (cut)
Right coronary artery
Right atrium
Anterior cardiac veins
Small cardiac vein
Inferior vena cava
Pulmonary trunk
Left atrial appendage and left coronary artery
Diagonal branch
Great cardiac vein
Anterior descending branch
Right ventricle
Left ventricle

Ascending aorta
Left pulmonary artery
Left pulmonary veins
Left circumflex artery and great cardiac vein
Oblique vein, left atrium
Inferior interventricular artery
Middle cardiac vein
Left ventricle
Superior vena cava
Sinoatrial node and nodal artery
Left atrium
Right atrium
Artery to AV node
Inferior vena cava
Small cardiac vein
Right coronary artery
Coronary sinus
Right ventricle

These illustrations show the arterial and venous blood supply of the heart, in addition to the position of its four chambers. The heart rests in the mediastinum, the space between the lungs. It slants forward, with its narrowest part, the apex, being forwardmost. As you know, the heart is not precisely centered in the thoracic cavity. About two thirds of it lies to the left of the midsternal line.

IDENTIFYING CARDIAC LANDMARKS

To perform an accurate cardiovascular assessment, familiarize yourself with the landmarks illustrated here.

The heart's base (the superior portion, where the ascending aorta and pulmonary trunk emerge and the superior vena cava enters) corresponds to a horizontal line at the third costal cartilages. This line begins about 1 cm from the right sternal margin and ends about 2 cm from the left sternal margin.

The heart's apex (the inferior portion that points down and to the left) is normally located at the fifth left intercostal space, about 8 to 9 cm to the left of the midsternal line. The right end of the inferior surface lies under the sixth or seventh chondrosternal junction.

You can determine the approximate size and shape of your patient's heart by identifying these points, marking them on his chest with a felt-tip pen, and connecting them with slightly convex lines.

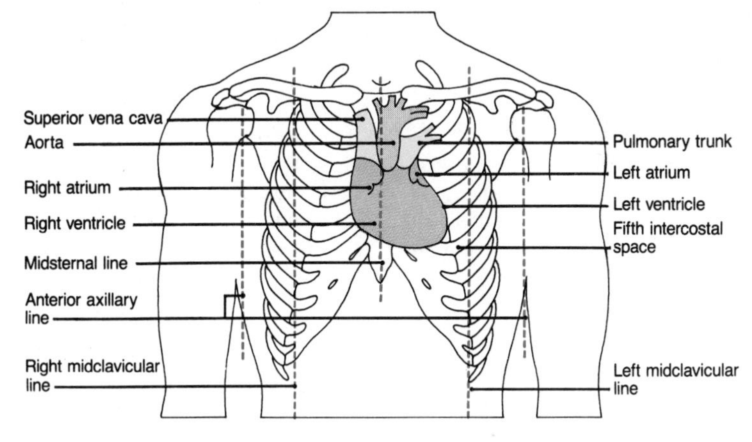

372 The heart's internal structure

The *endocardium,* an endothelial layer continuous with the lining of the vascular system, forms the smooth inner layer of the heart. The cardiac muscle (called the *myocardium*) makes up the bulk of the heart wall. Externally, the visceral layer of the pericardium comprises the *epicardium.* The interior heart has four chambers (two atria and two ventricles), eleven openings, and four valves.

The right atrium receives venous blood from the superior and the inferior venae cavae; the blood then passes through the tricuspid valve into the right ventricle. The right ventricular myocardium is thicker than that of either atrium but only one third as thick as that of the left ventricle. The right ventricle receives blood from the right atrium and expels it through the pulmonic valve into the pulmonary artery.

Smaller than the right atrium but with slightly thicker walls, the left atrium receives blood from the four pulmonary veins and delivers it to the left ventricle through the mitral valve. The posterior surface of the left atrium constitutes most of the heart's base.

Longer and more conical than the right ventricle, the left ventricle forms the heart's apex and most of its left border and diaphragmatic surface. A thick, muscular septum separates the two ventricles. The left ventricular myocardium is about three times as thick as the right ventricle's and produces about three times the pressure. The left ventricle receives blood from the left atrium and expels it through the aortic valve into the ascending aorta.

Functional valves guard four openings in the heart. The cusps of the two atrioventricular valves (the tricuspid, which normally has three leaflets, and the mitral, which normally has two) are connected to fibrous rings around the openings, part of the skeleton of the heart. Their free margins are attached by the thin but strong chordae tendineae to the ventricular papillary muscles. When blood passes through the opening, it pushes the cusps aside. During ventricular contraction, the papillary muscles contract, pulling on the cords and preventing the cusps from prolapsing into the atria.

The two semilunar valves guard the orifices of the pulmonary artery and the aorta. Each contains three crescent-shaped cusps (right, left, and anterior for the pulmonic valve and right, left, and posterior for the aortic valve) that appear concave when viewed from above. The aortic valve cusps are thicker, larger, and stronger than the pulmonic valve cusps. Blood expelled from the ventricles pushes the cusps into the orifices of the vessels. On ventricular relaxation, arterial pressure forces the blood back toward the heart and the cusps meet, closing the orifices and preventing backflow into the ventricles.

373 Blood supply to the heart

Two arteries supply blood to the heart; seven major veins drain blood from it. The two main coronary arteries encircle the heart like crowns. During left ventricular contraction, blood is ejected into the aorta, and the coronary ostia fill. During diastole, the ventricular muscle relaxes, allowing the coronary arteries to open and passively fill.

Ordinarily, the right coronary artery supplies all the right atrium (including the sinoatrial and atrioventricular nodes of the conduction system), part of the

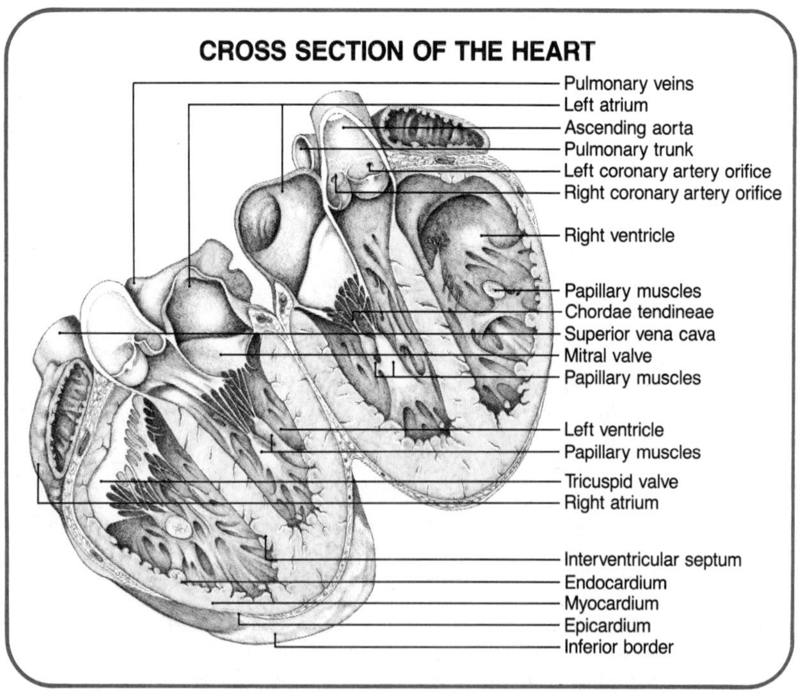

THE GREAT VESSELS

The three great vessels (the ascending aorta, the pulmonary trunk, and the superior vena cava) all appear at the heart's base, as illustrated here.

The ascending aorta eventually gives rise to the right and left coronary arteries.

The pulmonary trunk eventually branches into the right and left pulmonary arteries under the aortic arch.

The superior vena cava is formed by the junction of the right and left brachiocephalic veins.

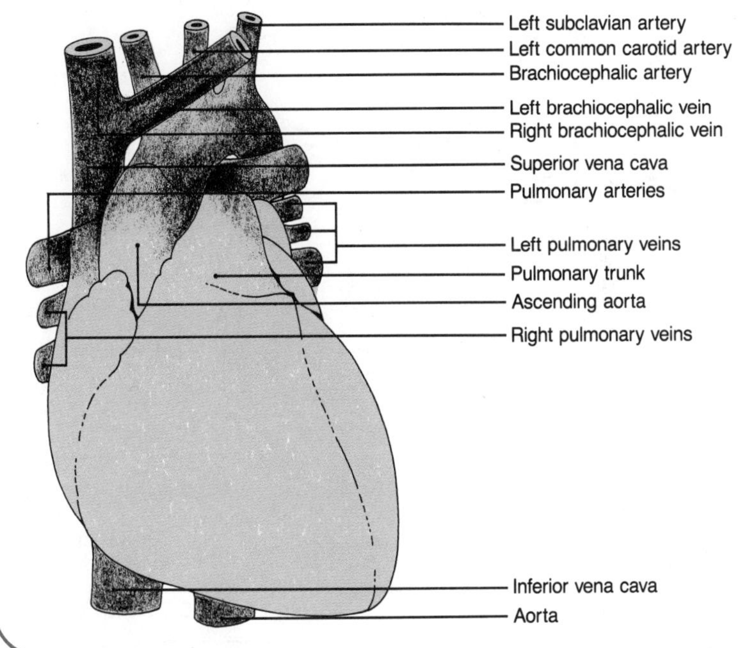

left atrium, and most of the right ventricle (including the atrioventricular bundle). The left coronary artery, which splits into the left anterior descending (interventricular) and circumflex arteries, usually supplies the left atrium, most of the left ventricle, and a large part of the ventricular septum.

Although anastomoses between the two coronary arteries are small or absent at birth, multiple anastamoses between *arterioles* develop with age. Despite this, however, sudden occlusion of a major branch usually leads to necrosis of the affected cardiac muscle region, with subsequent infarction and scar tissue replacement.

The major veins, which lie superficial to the arteries, drain venous blood from the myocardium. Except for the coronary sinus, these veins don't encircle the heart as the arteries do. They're called *cardiac* rather than *coronary* veins. The largest vein, the coronary sinus, lies in the posterior part of the coronary sulcus and opens into the right atrium. The coronary sinus is the terminus for most of the major cardiac veins except for the two or three anterior cardiac veins, which empty directly into the right atrium.

374 Cardiac innervation

The *intrinsic nerve supply* or *conduction system* for the heart includes the

THE CIRCULATORY SYSTEM

As you know, and can see in this schematic representation, arteries transport blood from the heart and distribute it throughout the body. Then, veins transport blood back to the heart. Note the pattern of distribution here, to better understand how blood circulation works.

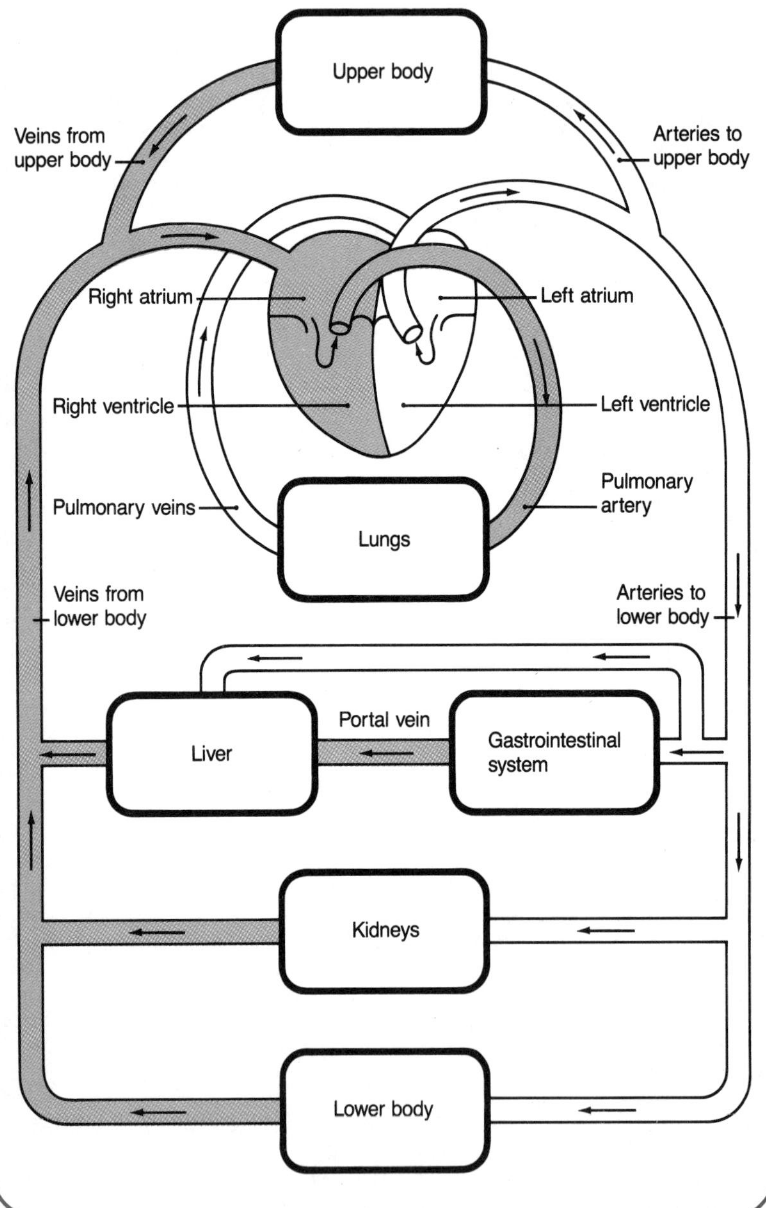

sinoatrial (SA) and atrioventricular (AV) nodes, the atrioventricular bundle of His and its branches, and the Purkinje system. Specialized cardiac muscle fibers initiate the heartbeat and coordinate chamber contraction. All these specialized fibers can initiate the contraction, but the SA node usually paces the heart because it has the fastest intrinsic rate.

The *extrinsic nerve supply* consists of cardiac nerves of the autonomic nervous system that control the conduction system and the heart's contractility. Thus the heart can respond to the body's changing physiologic needs by altering the rate and force of its contractions.

Stimulation of the sympathetic fibers that supply the SA and AV nodes and all four chambers increases the heart rate and contractility. Stimulation of the vagal (parasympathetic) fibers that supply the SA node and the atria decreases the rate. Dilatation of the coronary arteries results from stimulation of sympathetic fibers that supply the coronary arteries.

Visceral afferent pain fibers from the coronary arteries enter the first and second thoracic spinal cord segments. These segments also receive afferent pain fibers from the arm's ulnar aspect, which is the reason why angina pectoris attacks may cause referred pain in this area.

THE HEART'S CONDUCTION SYSTEM

The heart's conduction system works this way: Each electrical impulse travels from the sinoatrial node to the cardiac muscle cells of the atria, producing atrial contraction. The impulse slows momentarily as it passes through the atrioventricular node to the atrioventricular bundle (bundle of His). Then, the left and right bundle branches descend on both sides of the septum, immediately under the endocardium. Next, Purkinje fibers stimulate the ventricular contraction impulse, which spreads from the apex back toward the upper and outer parts of the ventricle.

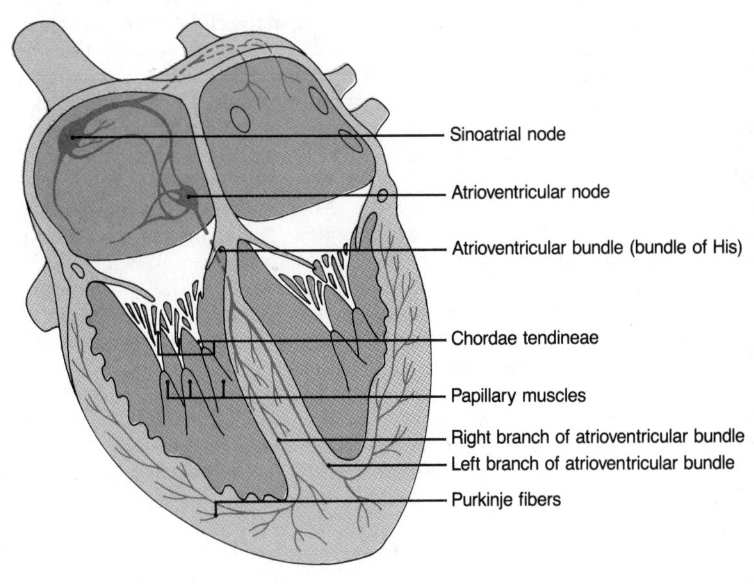

375 Blood vessels and peripheral pulses

Arteries are thick-walled vessels that carry blood from the heart and distribute it through the systemic and pulmonary circuits to all parts of the body. They serve both as low-resistance lines, conducting blood to the organs, and as a pressure reservoir, sending blood through the tissues.

The largest artery, the *aorta,* is the systemic circuit's trunk. The aorta and its branches are *elastic arteries*—so called because their middle layers contain many elastic fibers. The distributing arteries, which carry blood to the organs, have more smooth muscle in their middle layers and are called *muscular arteries.* The pulmonary artery and its branches constitute a low-pressure system that transports blood to the lungs for reoxygenation.

Veins, which have thinner walls but larger diameters than their companion arteries, return blood to the heart through the superior and inferior venae cavae and the pulmonary veins. The venous system consists of *deep veins,* which accompany companion arteries, and *superficial veins,* which lie in the superficial fascia under the skin. The veins are low-resistance lines that carry blood from the tissues to the heart and can adjust their own capacity to compensate for blood volume variations.

Capillaries are high-resistance thin-walled tubes composed of one endothelial layer. They connect the smallest arteries (arterioles) with the smallest veins (venules). About 5% of the total circulating blood is always flowing through the capillary beds. The capillaries' work is the ultimate function of the entire cardiovascular system: to exchange nutrients and metabolic end products. In effect, the rest of the system—the heart and vessels—functions solely to bring blood into and out of the body's several thousand miles of capillaries.

Maximum blood pressure (systolic pressure) occurs during peak ventricular ejection; minimum pressure (diastolic pressure) occurs just before ventricular contraction. The pulse that can be felt in any artery results from the difference between systolic and diastolic pressures (called *pulse pressure*). The easiest arteries to palpate are the radial, carotid, femoral, popliteal, posterior tibial, dorsalis pedis, ulnar, and superficial temporal.

376 Cardiac cycle

The cardiac cycle (one complete heartbeat) consists of two phases: contraction (systole) and relaxation (diastole). When the heart rate is 72 beats/minute, one cardiac cycle occurs every 0.8 second—0.3 second for ventricular systole and 0.5 second for ventricular diastole. Remember, the duration of the cardiac cycle varies with the heart rate. As the rate increases, systolic and diastolic phases shorten.

As ventricular systole begins, pressure builds in the ventricles, closing the atrioventricular valves and preventing the backflow of blood into the atria. When the ventricle contracts, ventricular pressure rises sharply—to about 120 mmHg in the left ventricle and 26 mmHg in the right ventricle. When this pressure becomes greater than aortic and pulmonary arterial pressures, the semilunar valves open. Blood is then ejected into the aorta and pulmonary artery—most of it during the first third of ventricular systole.

After ejection, ventricular diastole begins. The ventricles relax and pressure begins to drop. When it falls below the pressures in the aorta and pulmonary artery, the semilunar valves snap shut, preventing backflow into the ventricles.

Meanwhile, the pulmonary veins and venae cavae have filled the atria with blood, and atrial pressure starts to rise toward the end of ventricular systole. As ventricular pressure drops below atrial pressure, the atrioventricular valves open and the ventricles rapidly fill with blood. Atrial systole then completes ventricular filling.

377 Heart sounds

Heart sounds are thought to result from *vibrations* associated with the sudden closure of heart valves and the acceleration and deceleration of adjacent blood flow. These vibrations are transmitted to the body surface and are heard as heart sounds. The contribution of atrial and ventricular muscle contractions to audible heart sounds is uncertain.

Usually heard at the apex, the first heart sound (S_1) is associated with tricuspid and mitral valve closures. Because the mitral valve usually closes before the tricuspid, the sound splits into two components.

The second heart sound (S_2) is associated with aortic and pulmonic valve closures. Physiologic splitting of S_2 results when the pulmonic valve closes later than the aortic during inspiration. Two events cause this split. First, during inspiration, blood rushes into the thorax through large veins and increases venous return to the right heart, prolonging right ventricular filling and ejection and delaying pulmonic valve closure. Second, during inspiration, increased pulmonary capacity slightly reduces left ventricular blood volume, and the aortic valve closes slightly earlier than the pulmonic valve.

Although frequently heard in children, the physiologic third heart sound (S_3) isn't normally audible in adults. A low-pitched sound that occurs during rapid ventricular inflow, shortly after S_2 in early diastole, S_3 probably results from vibrations caused by abrupt ventricular distention or increased compliance.

The fourth sound (S_4) results from vibrations caused by the sudden forceful ejection of blood into a noncompliant ventricle (one that has lost its distensibility) during atrial systole. Murmurs are sounds resulting from turbulent blood flow in the heart.

Collecting appropriate history data

378 Biographical data

Age, sex, and race are all essential considerations in identifying patients with cardiovascular disorders. For example, coronary artery disease most commonly affects white men between ages 40 and 60; hypertension occurs most often in blacks.

379 Chief complaint

The most common chief complaints in cardiovascular disorders are the following: *chest pain* or *discomfort, dyspnea* (particularly paroxysmal nocturnal dyspnea and orthopnea), *fatigue* and *weakness, irregular heartbeat,* and *peripheral changes* (especially weight change with edema, dry skin, and extremity pain).

380 History of present illness

Using the PQRST mnemonic device on page 332, ask the patient to elaborate on his chief complaint. Then, depending on the complaint, explore the history of his present illness by asking the following types of questions:

• ***Chest pain.*** *How would you characterize the pain? For example, does it burn or produce a squeezing sensation? Where in your chest do you feel the pain? Can you point to the area? Does it radiate?* Ischemic pain usually affects a large chest area, and the patient has difficulty localizing it. If he can circumscribe the painful area, the pain probably isn't ischemic. *How long have you been having this chest pain? How long does an attack last?* The patient's answers will help you identify

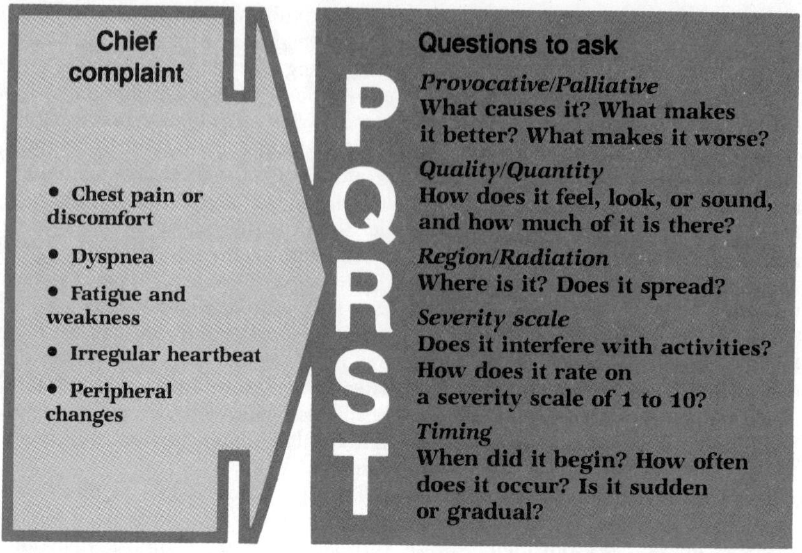

Chief complaint		Questions to ask
• Chest pain or discomfort • Dyspnea • Fatigue and weakness • Irregular heartbeat • Peripheral changes	P	*Provocative/Palliative* What causes it? What makes it better? What makes it worse?
	Q	*Quality/Quantity* How does it feel, look, or sound, and how much of it is there?
	R	*Region/Radiation* Where is it? Does it spread?
	S	*Severity scale* Does it interfere with activities? How does it rate on a severity scale of 1 to 10?
	T	*Timing* When did it begin? How often does it occur? Is it sudden or gradual?

the origin and severity of his cardiovascular disorder.

• ***Dyspnea.*** *When do you experience the shortness of breath?* This symptom may indicate transient congestive heart failure or left ventricular failure. If the dyspnea occurs with exertion, ask specifically how much activity is required to cause it. Dyspnea at rest suggests advanced disease; increasing dyspnea with less exertion may indicate progressive pathology and failing compensatory mechanisms.

• ***Paroxysmal nocturnal dyspnea (PND).*** A classic symptom of left ventricular failure, PND occurs at night when the patient is sleeping. He awakens with a feeling of suffocation. Maneuvers that cause gravity to drain fluid from the lungs to the feet—for example, sitting on the edge of the bed or walking to the window for fresh air—relieve PND. The attack usually subsides in a few minutes.

• ***Orthopnea.*** *How many pillows do you use to make breathing easier? Do you use more now than you used to?* An increase in the number of pillows indicates developing orthopnea. The number of pillows the patient uses helps determine the degree of left ventricular failure. Record your patient's response as *two-pillow orthopnea, three-pillow orthopnea,* and so on.

• ***Unexplained weakness and fatigue.*** *Do you tire easily? What type of activity causes you to feel tired? How long can you perform this activity before becoming tired? When did you first notice the feeling of weakness and fatigue? Is it getting worse? Is the feeling relieved by rest?* Fatigue and weakness on mild exertion, especially if relieved by rest, may be a sign of heart disease. Such a patient's heart can't provide sufficient blood to meet the cells' slightly increased metabolic needs. These symptoms are often the hallmark of early progressive heart failure.

• ***Irregular heartbeat.*** *Does your heart pound or beat too fast?* Palpitations usually reflect arrhythmias, especially tachyarrhythmias. *Does your heart ever skip a beat or seem to jump?* Skipped beats often indicate premature ventricular contractions. *Do you ever experience dizziness or faint? When?* These symptoms may be related to transient arrhythmias, often caused by intake of certain beverages, such as coffee, tea, and cola.

• ***Weight change with edema.*** *Does*

your weight fluctuate or have you gained weight recently? Weight changes are common in cardiovascular disease, especially weight gain from sodium and water retention secondary to congestive heart failure and hypertension. *Are your ankles or feet swollen? Do your shoes feel tight or uncomfortable at the end of the day? Is the swelling relieved by elevating your feet or lying down?* Edema associated with cardiovascular disease is readily mobilized.

• ***Dry skin.*** *Have you noticed any skin dryness or scaliness, especially on your legs?* Dry skin may be associated with peripheral vascular disease.

• ***Extremity pain.*** *Have you experienced any pain or discomfort in your arms or legs?* Ischemia from peripheral vascular disease can cause aches or cramps when the patient moves the affected arm or leg. *Do you feel pain or cramps in your legs when you walk? Is the pain relieved by rest? Does elevating the leg cause pain that's relieved by dangling or lowering the leg?* Intermittent claudication results from advanced atherosclerosis of the femoral arteries. *How many stairs or city blocks can you walk before the symptoms begin? Is the pain associated with walking over any particular kind of terrain, in certain temperatures, or at a particular pace?* These factors affect the intensity of exertion (see *Leg Pain Alert,* page 339). *Does the pain increase with prolonged standing or sitting?* Pain that's most severe during prolonged standing or sitting indicates venous insufficiency. Venous pain located in the calf and lower leg, usually described as an aching, tired, or full feeling, is commonly accompanied by leg edema and obvious varicosities.

EMERGENCY

CARDIAC EMERGENCY ASSESSMENT

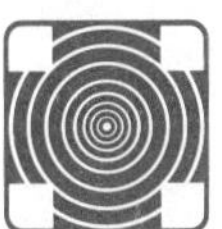

If your patient's in a state of cardiac emergency, you'll want to assess his condition quickly and accurately. If your patient's *unconscious,* check his respiration and pulse. If necessary, institute cardiopulmonary resuscitation. Assess the *conscious* cardiac emergency patient as follows:

Assess central pulse

• Assess the patient's central pulse by palpating his carotid or femoral arteries. Check his pulse for regularity and rate. *Note:* A weak, rapid pulse may precede cardiac arrest.

• Assess for chest pain. If present, note its location, duration, and severity.

Assess cardiac rhythm

• Assess his cardiac rhythm by instituting cardiac monitoring. Suspect impaired perfusion if the patient has tachyarrhythmias or bradyarrhythmias.

Assess perfusion status

• Assess his perfusion status by comparing central and peripheral pulses. Suspect impaired perfusion if the patient's peripheral pulse is weaker and/or slower than his central pulse.

• Measure his blood pressure. Remember, don't rule out shock just because hypotension's not evident.

• Determine his level of consciousness, and suspect shock if it's reduced.

• Check his skin; if it's cool and clammy, suspect impaired perfusion.

• Measure his urinary output. Consider shock confirmed if, along with the above findings, your patient's urinary output is severely decreased or absent.

381 Past history

Explore the following relevant areas when reviewing your patient's history:

• ***Hypertension.*** *Have you ever had your blood pressure taken? Can you recall what it was? Have you ever been told you had high blood pressure? Have you ever taken medication for blood pressure?* Pressure above 160/90 correlates positively with ischemic heart disease, renal failure, cerebrovascular accident, and an accelerated rate of coronary artery disease (CAD).

• ***Hyperlipoproteinemia.*** *Have you ever been told by your doctor that you have high cholesterol or triglyceride levels?* Elevated serum levels of cholesterol, triglycerides, and free fatty acids probably correlate directly with a higher incidence of CAD, although this relationship is still disputed. The two most

DRUGS

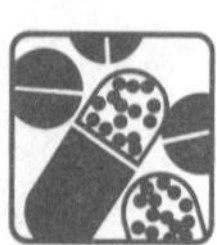

NURSE'S GUIDE TO SOME DRUGS THAT AFFECT THE CARDIOVASCULAR SYSTEM

CLASSIFICATION	POSSIBLE SIDE EFFECTS
Anticonvulsants	
diazepam (Valium*)	• Hypotension, bradycardia, cardiovascular collapse
phenytoin sodium (Dilantin*)	• Hypotension, ventricular fibrillation
Antidepressants	
amitriptyline hydrochloride (Elavil*) doxepin hydrochloride (Sinequan*)	• Orthostatic hypotension, tachycardia, EKG changes, hypertension
Antipsychotics	
chlorpromazine hydrochloride (Chlorprom**, Thorazine) thioridazine (Mellanil*)	• Orthostatic hypotension, tachycardia, arrhythmias
Cerebral stimulants	
amphetamine sulfate (Benzedrine*)	• Tachycardia, palpitations, hypertension, hypotension
caffeine (Nodoz, Vivarin)	• Tachycardia
Cholinergics (parasympathomimetics)	
bethanechol chloride (Urecholine*)	• Bradycardia, hypotension, cardiac arrest, tachycardia
Estrogens	
chlorotrianisene (Tace*) esterified estrogens (Amnestrogen, Climestrone**)	• Thrombophlebitis, thromboembolism, hypertension, edema, risk of cerebrovascular accident, pulmonary embolism, myocardial infarction
Nonnarcotic analgesics and antipyretics	
indomethacin (Indocid**, Indocin)	• Hypertension, edema
phenylbutazone (Butazolidin*)	• Hypertension, pericarditis, myocarditis, cardiac decompensation
Oral contraceptives	
estrogen with progestogen (Demulen*)	• Thromboembolism, thrombophlebitis, hypertension
Sedatives and hypnotics	
ethchlorvynol (Placidyl*)	• Hypotension
paraldehyde (Paral)	• By I.V. administration: pulmonary edema, hemorrhage, right-sided heart failure
Spasmolytics	
aminophylline (Aminophyllin)	• Sinus tachycardia, extrasystoles, flushing, hypotension

*Available in U.S. and Canada. **Available in Canada only. All other products (no symbol) available in U.S. only.

common hyperlipoproteinemia patterns in patients with premature atherosclerosis are Type II—elevated cholesterol with normal or slightly elevated triglycerides—and Type IV—elevated triglycerides with normal or slightly elevated cholesterol.

• ***Diabetes mellitus.*** *Have you ever been told you had sugar in your urine? Have you ever had a test for blood sugar? Was it normal?* The relationship between diabetes mellitus and CAD is still controversial, but patients with the most common types of hyperlipoproteinemia usually show abnormal carbohydrate metabolism. Patients with CAD also have a high incidence of diabetes mellitus, and patients with diabetes seem to have a tendency toward atheroma formation. Such atherosclerosis occurs not only in the coronary artery system, but also in the arteries of the systemic circulation, particularly in the aorta and in the femoral and carotid arteries.

• ***Rheumatic fever.*** *Did you ever have rheumatic fever? Were you ever told you had a heart murmur?* Many people have so-called innocent or functional heart murmurs unrelated to rheumatic fever or structural congenital heart disease. The effect of rheumatic fever or of repeated streptococcal infections, however, can be permanent damage to heart valves—especially the mitral and aortic—leaving them insufficient (unable to close) or stenosed (scarred, rigid, and unable to open fully). Knowing whether the patient has had these conditions will help you interpret heart murmurs common in patients with post–rheumatic fever heart disease.

• ***Medications.*** *Have you ever taken diuretics (water or fluid pills)? Do you know why the doctor prescribed the medication you took? Have you ever taken any drugs for your heart or circulation?* Knowledge of medications

IDENTIFYING THE TYPE A PERSONALITY

Cardiologists have identified a personality type that's especially vulnerable to myocardial infarction: the Type A personality. As you may know, the Type A person has a compulsion to achieve as much as possible in as little time as possible. Here's a list of specific characteristics:

CHARACTERISTIC	EXAMPLE
Chronically impatient; doesn't think there's enough time in each day	• Usually gives curt replies to questions; may answer with abrupt "Definitely!" or "Absolutely!" • Tries to rush conversations by interrupting with "Yes, yes," or "Right, right." • Annoyed by waiting in lines or being delayed in traffic • Walks quickly • May attempt to do several activities simultaneously, to save time
Fiercely competitive	• Hates to lose any type of contest • Doesn't like routine activities or hobbies that he feels have no worthwhile goals
Feels guilty for relaxing	• May duplicate his time-saving routine even at home—for example, reading the newspaper during a meal with the television set on
Thinks quickly and selectively	• Usually discusses only topics of personal interest; if forced to discuss a topic of no personal interest, he'll participate minimally, while attempting to think about something else

ASSESSING CHEST PAIN

CONDITION	LOCATION AND RADIATION	CHARACTER
Myocardial ischemia (angina pectoris)	• Substernal or retrosternal pain spreading across chest • May radiate to inside of either or both arms, the neck, or jaw	• Squeezing, heavy pressure, aching, or burning discomfort
Myocardial infarction	• Substernal or over precordium • May radiate throughout chest and arms to jaw	• Crushing, viselike, steady pain
Pericardial chest pain	• Substernal or left of sternum • May radiate to neck, arms, back, or epigastrium	• Sharp, intermittent pain (accentuated by swallowing, coughing, deep inspiration, or lying supine)
Pulmonary embolism	• Inferior portion of the pleura • May radiate to costal margins or upper abdomen	• Stabbing, knifelike pain (accentuated by respirations)
Spontaneous pneumothorax	• Lateral thorax • Does not radiate	• Tearing, pleuritic pain
Infectious or inflammatory processes (pleurisy)	• Pleural • May be widespread or only over affected area	• Moderate, sharp, raw, burning pain
Aortic (dissecting aortic aneurysm)	• Anterior chest • May radiate to thoracic portion of back	• Excruciating, knifelike pain
Esophageal pain	• Substernal • May radiate around chest to shoulders	• Burning, knotlike pain (simulating angina)
Chest wall pain	• Costochondral or sternocostal junctions • Does not radiate	• Aching pain or soreness

ONSET AND DURATION	PRECIPITATING EVENTS	ASSOCIATED FINDINGS
• Sudden onset • Usually subsides within 5 minutes	• Mental or physical exertion; intense emotion • Hot, humid weather • Heavy food intake; especially in extreme temperatures or high humidity	• Feeling of uneasiness or impending doom
• Sudden onset • More severe and prolonged than anginal pain	• Occurs spontaneously, with exertion, stress, or at rest	• Dyspnea • Profuse perspiration • Nausea and vomiting • Dizziness, weakness • Feeling of uneasiness or impending doom
• Severe, sudden onset • Usually relieved by bending forward • May occur intermittently over several days	• Upper respiratory tract infection • Myocardial infarction • Rheumatic fever • Pericarditis	• Distended neck veins • Tachycardia • Paradoxical pulse possible with constrictive pericarditis • Pericardial friction rub
• Sudden onset • May last a few days	• Anxiety (associated with coughing)	• Dyspnea; tachypnea • Tachycardia • Cough with hemoptysis
• Sudden onset • Relieved by aspiration of air	• Trauma • Ruptured emphysematous bleb • Anxiety	• Dyspnea; tachypnea • Mediastinal shift • Decreased or absent breath sounds over involved lung
• Occurs on inspiration • Relief usually occurs several days after effective treatment	• Underlying disease of lung, such as pneumonia	• Fever • Cough with sputum production
• Sudden onset • Unrelieved by medication or comfort measures • May last for hours	• Hypertension	• Lower blood pressure in one arm than in other • May have paralysis • May have murmur of aortic insufficiency or pulsus paradoxus • Hypotension and shock
• Sudden onset • Relieved by diet or position change, antacids or belching • Usually brief duration	• May occur spontaneously • Eating	• Regurgitation
• Often begins as dull ache, increasing in intensity over a few days • Usually long lasting	• Chest wall movement	• Symptoms and physical findings vary with specific musculoskeletal disorder

the patient is taking or has taken in the past can provide valuable information on past or present cardiovascular disorders (see *Nurse's Guide to Some Drugs That Affect the Cardiovascular System,* page 334).

382 Family history

Note any family history of the following conditions:

• ***Cardiovascular disease.*** Ask the patient specific questions about any family history of angina, acute myocardial infarction, hypertension, cerebrovascular accident, diabetes, or renal disease. The incidence of coronary artery disease (CAD) is higher in patients with a family history of advanced plaque disease or of one or more deaths from a CAD-related event.

• ***Acquired behavior.*** Genetic predisposition to cardiovascular disease may exist, but acquired behavior—including diet (high sodium intake, high lipid levels, obesity), personality (especially Type A personality), and a stressful life-style—is a significant contributing factor.

UNDERSTANDING AEROBIC EXERCISE

To be effective, aerobic exercise should elevate the heart rate to at least 120 beats per minute for at least 15 minutes. Most physiologists feel that such exercise performed at least three times a week results in a healthier heart. This is based on the overload principle: Repeatedly exercising a muscle set above its normal operating level for a sustained period will strengthen it.

During aerobic exercise, the heart beats faster than normal to pump additional oxygen-rich blood to the exercising muscles. The heart recuperates between exercise sessions and becomes stronger. The next time the muscles require more blood, the heart doesn't have to work as hard.

Examples of activities that provide aerobic exercise are running, swimming, and bicycling.

383 Psychosocial history

Explore the following areas in your patient's psychosocial history:

• ***Personality.*** How does the patient view himself? Your patient's personality is the most significant aspect of his psychosocial history.

• ***Personality traits and life-style.*** Although difficult to prove or define precisely, a positive correlation between the Type A personality and coronary artery disease seems to exist (see *Identifying the Type A Personality,* page 335).

• ***Occupation.*** The physical and emotional demands of a person's occupation can place him under a great deal of stress, a factor that may be important in the diagnosis of cardiovascular disease. Commuting long distances can also be stressful.

• ***Domestic problems.*** Problems at home can be more stressful than occupational problems and may also predispose a person to cardiovascular disease.

384 Activities of daily living

Examine the following aspects of your patient's daily life for patterns that may predispose him to cardiovascular problems:

• ***Physical activity.*** A healthy person should engage in aerobic activity at least three times a week (see *Understanding Aerobic Exercise*). Exercise is beneficial to general cardiovascular conditioning.

• ***Smoking.*** If your patient smokes cigarettes, determine the duration of his habit and the amount he smokes, and record this data as *pack years.* (Calculate pack years by multiplying the number of years by the number of packs per day.) Nicotine, a sympathetic nervous system stimulator, increases heart rate, stroke volume, cardiac output, cardiac work, and vasoconstriction. Smoking is a significant risk factor for peripheral vascular disease, and the mortality for patients with coronary artery disease is about 70% higher in middle-aged men who smoke one pack a day than in those who don't smoke. The percentage decreases for older men, and the correlation isn't as clear for women. Further, this risk doesn't apply to pipe and cigar smokers, probably because they generally don't inhale as much as cigarette smokers.

• ***Diet.*** A brief history of your patient's eating habits, particularly his intake of carbohydrates and fats, may help determine his potential for CAD. A high-sodium diet can aggravate the development of edema and may be one of the factors associated with the development of hypertension.

LEG PAIN ALERT

If you detect the following signs or symptoms in your patient, suspect a severe peripheral circulation problem, and notify the doctor immediately:

- sudden decrease in the distance the patient can walk without pain
- cold, mottled, or bluish legs
- cutaneous changes, such as reddened pressure areas, ulcers, or taut and shiny skin
- pain unrelieved by rest.

385 Review of systems

Ask the patient about the following signs and symptoms, which may indicate cardiovascular dysfunction (see *Cardiac Emergency Assessment,* page 333):

• ***Skin.*** Diaphoresis usually reflects strong sympathetic nervous system stimulation and is commonly associated with myocardial ischemia.

• ***Respiratory.*** Painful breathing may be pericardial or pleural in origin. Nocturnal or bloody coughing may indicate pulmonary edema, pulmonary embolism, pneumonia, or worsening congestive heart failure. Pain accompanying wheezing is most commonly associated with such bronchospastic obstructive diseases as asthma and bronchitis.

• ***Gastrointestinal.*** Nausea and vomiting are often associated with severe myocardial ischemia and myocardial infarction.

• ***Genitourinary.*** Nocturia can result when edema occurs during the day and renal perfusion increases at night, causing increased diuresis. In the absence of genitourinary disorders, nocturia is commonly associated with congestive heart failure.

• ***Nervous.*** Light-headedness, dizziness, or fainting may be related to hypotension, transient arrhythmias, or rapid heartbeat.

Conducting the physical examination

386 Positioning and equipment

After ensuring privacy, instruct your patient to change into a hospital gown that allows for thorough examination of his neck, chest, arms, and legs. Then ask him to assume the supine position, with his head and thorax comfortably supported at about a 45° angle. Make sure the bed or table height allows inspection of the patient in this and other positions—sitting forward, as well as in the left lateral recumbent position.

Make sure the lighting is adequate. Position the light source so the light *crosses* the areas you'll inspect—the neck and precordium—and doesn't shine directly on them. Also make sure the environment is quiet—particularly during your auscultation of cardiac sounds, which are usually subtle and low pitched.

Normally, the only equipment you'll need is a stethoscope, a blood pressure cuff, and a ruler. After inspecting the patient for overt signs of cardiac risk factors (such as xanthelasma) and recording his vital signs, you'll examine him from head to toe using inspection, palpation, and auscultation. (In cardiovascular assessment, percussion has limited value, because inspection, palpation, and chest X-rays more accurately determine heart size and borders as well as liver size.)

During the examination, stand on the patient's right side. This allows you to reach comfortably across the precordium for palpation and auscultation and to palpate the liver area on the right side correctly.

387 General inspection

During your general inspection, record your initial impressions of the patient's body type, posture, gait, and movements as well as his overall health and basic hygiene. Also note observable cardiac risk factors, such as cigarette smoking, obesity, and fatty skin deposits (xanthomas). Observe his facial expressions for signs of pain or anxiety. During conversation, assess his mental status, particularly the appropriateness of his responses and the clarity of his speech. Determine his apparent mood. Is he cooperative or withdrawn, fearful, or depressed?

Obtain some general information about the patient's cardiovascular system. Assess his skin color and condition and further assess his level of consciousness, if appropriate. Skin color, especially in the face, mouth, earlobes, and fingernails, helps determine the adequacy of cardiac output. Pallor or cyanosis may indicate poor cardiac output and tissue perfusion. (Remember, a dark-skinned patient with a cardiac disorder may appear gray. Inspect his lips and nail beds for cyanosis and his conjunctivas and mucous membranes for pallor, which may indicate anemia.)

Feel the patient's arm to assess its warmth and dryness. Dry, warm skin indicates adequate cardiac output and tissue perfusion. If the skin of the arm is perspiring and feels cool or cold, suspect peripheral vasoconstriction; this can be an early compensatory response in shock.

While assessing your patient's skin, you can also palpate his radial artery pulse to determine if the pulse rate, quality, and volume are within normal limits. Generally, the rate should be between 60 to 100 beats/minute; the quality should be strong and regular. This gross determination indicates whether your patient's cardiovascular system is stable or seriously compromised and requires immediate intervention. To complete your general inspection, record the patient's vital signs (see Entries 68 to 81).

388 Inspecting the venous pulse

Blood from the jugular veins flows directly into the superior vena cava and the right heart. Thus, you can assess the adequacy of your patient's circulating volume, right heart function, and venous pressure by examining external and internal jugular vein pulsations. External jugular veins, which lie superficially, are visible above the clavicle. Internal jugular veins are larger, lie deeper along the carotid arteries, and transmit their pulsations outward to the skin covering the neck.

Normally, a person's neck veins are visible when he lies down; they're flat when he stands up. The semi-Fowler's position is best for inspection, because at a 45° elevation, neck veins shouldn't be prominent if right heart function is normal. Position the patient properly, and turn his head slightly away from you. Use a small pillow to support the head, but don't flex the neck sharply. Remove clothing around the neck and thorax to prevent constriction. Arrange the lighting to cast small shadows along the neck.

You can learn about right heart dynamics by analyzing the venous waveform of your patient's right internal jugular vein. Use his carotid pulse or heart sounds to time the venous pul-

EXAMINING JUGULAR VENOUS PULSES

In your cardiovascular assessment, note how the patient's veins and arteries are distributed in the neck, as shown in this illustration.

You can observe internal jugular pulsations by shining a flashlight across your patient's neck. Doing so will create reflecting light waves that make his venous pulse visible.

Be sure to distinguish venous pulsations from arterial pulsations and to document your findings carefully.

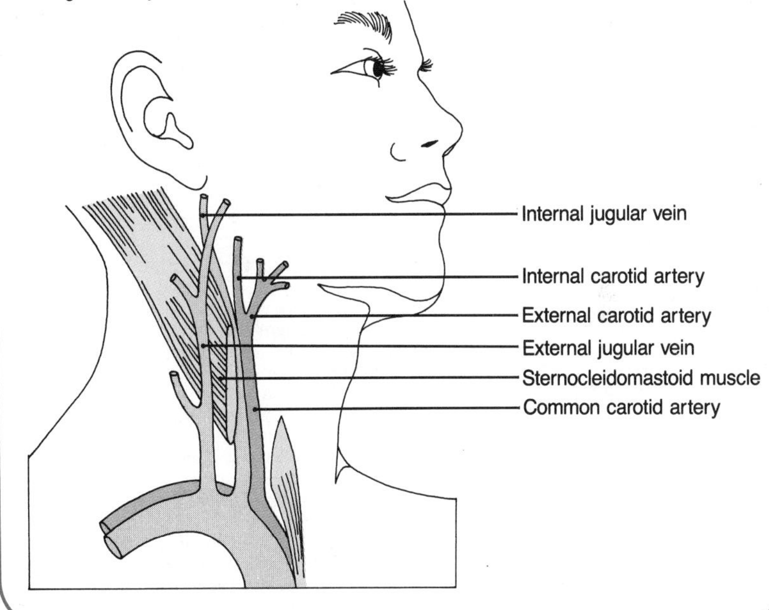

sations with the cardiac cycle.

The jugular venous pulse consists of five waves. The three ascending waves—*a, c,* and *v*—produce an undulating pulsation normally seen ⅜″ to ¾″ (1 to 2 cm) above the clavicle, just to the medial side of the sternocleidomastoid muscle, as follows:

• The *a wave* is the initial pulsation of the jugular vein, produced by right atrial contraction and retrograde transmission of the pressure pulse to the jugular veins. It occurs just before the first heart sound. You can time the atrial contraction by placing your index finger on the patient's opposite carotid, to feel the carotid pulse, or by listening for the first heart sound at the apex. The first jugular pulsation you see just before feeling the carotid pulse or hearing S_1 is the *a* wave. Remember that this wave won't appear in arrhythmias lacking atrial contraction, such as in atrial fibrillation, atrial flutter, and junctional rhythm. Also, the *a* wave may be exaggerated in chronic obstructive pulmonary disease, pulmonary embolism, and pulmonic or tricuspid stenosis—conditions causing elevated right atrial pressure. *Cannon wave* is a giant *a* wave occurring when the atrium contracts against a closed tricuspid valve during ventricular systole. This condition results from ectopic heartbeats, especially premature ventricular contractions, atrioventricular (AV) dissociation, or complete AV block.

• The *c wave* begins shortly after the first heart sound and may result from the carotid artery's impact on the adjacent jugular vein or pressure transmission from right ventricular contraction during ventricular systole. This wave may be hard to see.

• The *v wave* results from continued passive atrial filling during ventricular systole and peaks just after the second heart sound, when the tricuspid valve opens.

Two descending waves complete the jugular venous pulse:

• *x descent,* the descent of the *a* and *c* waves, results from right atrial diastole, as well as from the tricuspid valve's being pulled down during ventricular systole, reducing right atrial pressure.

• *y descent* is the fall in right atrial pressure from the peak of the *v* wave following tricuspid valve opening. It occurs during rapid atrial emptying into the ventricle in early diastole.

389 Measuring venous pressure

You can obtain more information about the right side of your patient's heart by determining his venous pressure level. (Venous pressure, the force exerted by the blood in the venous system, nor-

ESTIMATING CENTRAL VENOUS PRESSURE

This illustration shows how to indirectly measure your patient's central venous pressure. To begin, place the patient at a 45° angle, and identify his internal jugular vein. (Although you can use the external or the internal jugular vein, the internal jugular is more reliable.) Observe the internal jugular to determine the highest level of visible pulsation (meniscus).

Next, locate the angle of Louis, or sternal notch. To do this, palpate the clavicles where they join the sternum (the suprasternal notch). Place your first two fingers on the suprasternal notch, and then, without lifting them from the skin surface, slide them down the sternum until you feel a bony protuberance. This is the angle of Louis. The right atrium lies approximately 5 cm below the angle of Louis.

To estimate central venous pressure in centimeters, measure the vertical distance between the highest level of visible pulsation and the sternal notch. Normally, this distance is less than 3 cm. Add 5 cm to this figure to estimate the distance between the highest level of pulsation and the right atrium. If your estimate is more than 10 cm, consider your patient's central venous pressure elevated and suspect right heart failure.

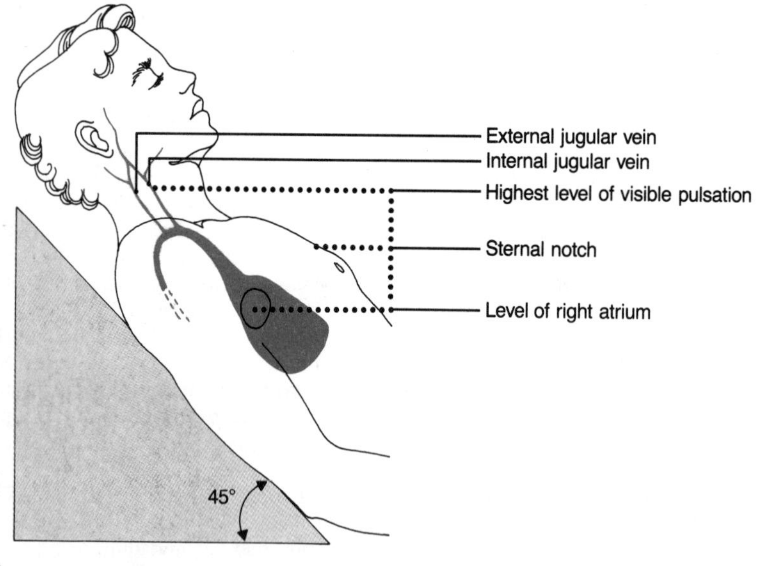

mally ranges from 6 to 8 cm of water.) Factors affecting venous pressure include circulating blood volume, vessel wall tone, vein patency, right heart function, respiratory function, pulmonary pressures, as well as the force of gravity.

Examples of alterations in venous pressure due to respiration include Kussmaul's sign and the hepatojugular reflux. *Kussmaul's sign,* a paradoxical rise in the height of jugular pressure during inspiration, may be seen in patients with chronic constrictive pericarditis. The *hepatojugular reflux* is increased venous pressure from abdominal compression during normal respirations. Although compressing the abdomen increases right heart volume, venous pressure shouldn't rise significantly. If it does (a positive hepatojugular reflux), the patient may have congestive heart failure.

You can describe jugular venous pressure by characterizing the neck veins as mildly, moderately, or severely distended and by measuring pressure levels in fingerbreadths of distention above the clavicle. Such a report might read: "The patient's neck veins are moderately distended to a level of three fingers above the clavicle, at a level of 45° from the horizontal." Generally, you should observe the veins bilaterally to confirm true venous distention. (Unilateral jugular venous distention may be caused by a local obstruction.)

390 How to examine the carotid pulse

Carefully inspect and palpate your patient's carotid arteries. This is essential, because the carotid pulse correlates with central aortic pressure and reflects cardiac function more accurately than peripheral vessels. During diminished cardiac output, a patient's peripheral pulses may be difficult or impossible to feel, but his carotid pulse should be easy to palpate.

Examine your patient's carotid pulse for rate, rhythm, equality, contour, and amplitude. Observe the carotid area for excessively large waves, indicating a hypervolemic or hyperkinetic state of the left ventricle, as in aortic regurgitation. With the patient in the semi-Fowler's position and his head turned toward you, use these techniques to palpate the carotid arteries:

- To prevent possible cerebral ischemia, palpate *only one* carotid artery at a time.
- Feel the trachea and roll your fingers laterally into the groove between it and the sternocleidomastoid muscle (below and medial to the angle of the jaw).
- Don't exert too much pressure or massage the area; this may induce excessive slowing of the heart rate.

The carotid pulse correlates with S_1. To gain information about heart rate and rhythm in a patient with a regular rhythm, palpate the pulse for 30 seconds. If the patient's rhythm is irregular, palpate for 1 to 2 minutes. Remember, you can't determine the pattern of irregularity or the presence of an apical-radial pulse deficit until you analyze the precordium and apical pulse.

Describe the amplitude of the carotid pulse as increased (hyperkinetic) or decreased (hypokinetic). Increased pulses are large and bounding, with wide pressures. You'll feel a rapid upstroke, a brief peak, and a fast downstroke. This is common during exercise and when a person feels anxious or afraid. Increased amplitude may also accompany hyperthyroidism, anemia, aortic regurgitation, complete heart block, extreme bradycardia, and hypertension. A bounding carotid pulse may indicate that the left ventricle is generating excessive pressures to accomplish adequate cardiac output.

Decreased amplitude is characterized by small, weak pulsations that demonstrate diminished pressure and a slow, gradual, or normal velocity of upstroke, a delayed systolic peak, and a prolonged downstroke. This type of pulse results from left heart failure, severe shock, constrictive pericarditis, or aortic stenosis.

DISTINGUISHING WAVE PULSATIONS

Because the carotid wave and internal jugular wave pulsations occur in the same part of the neck, you may have trouble differentiating between them. This listing will help.

CAROTID	INTERNAL JUGULAR
Number of positive waves: 1	*Number of positive waves:* 3
Characteristics: brisk, regular	*Characteristics:* wavelike
Position: no effect	*Position:* more prominent when supine
Respiration: no effect	*Respiration:* alters markedly—pulsation and distention decrease on inspiration; opposite occurs on expiration
Clavicular pressure: no effect	*Clavicular pressure:* pulsation eliminated
Abdominal pressure: no effect	*Abdominal pressure:* may increase prominence of pulsations

After palpating both carotid pulses, auscultate them in this fashion:

- Turn the patient's head slightly away from you to allow space for the stethoscope.
- Auscultate only one carotid artery at a time.
- Place the bell of the stethoscope on the skin overlying the carotid artery.
- Ask the patient to hold his breath. (Avoid Valsalva's maneuver—forced exhalation against a closed glottis—which may initiate arrhythmias in some patients.)

Blood flow through the arteries is silent except in a patient with occlusive arterial disease. Auscultation of the blood flow in such a patient usually produces a blowing sound called a *bruit.* Arteriovenous fistula and various high cardiac output conditions, such as anemia, hyperthyroidism, and pheochromocytoma, may also cause bruits. If you hear a bruit, gently repalpate the artery with the pads of your fingers to detect the *thrill* (a vibrating sensation similar to the one you perceive by feeling a purring cat's throat) that frequently accompanies it. A thrill results from turbulent blood flow caused by arterial obstruction.

391 Precordium inspection

Begin inspecting the patient's precordium by identifying anatomic landmarks. The critical landmarks for cardiovascular assessment are the suprasternal notch and the xiphoid process (see *Identifying Cardiac Landmarks,* page 325). Other important landmarks include the midsternal line, the midclavicular line (MCL), and the anterior axillary, midaxillary, and posterior axillary lines.

Place the patient in the supine position, and elevate his upper trunk 30° to 45°. Remember, you can examine the precordium best by standing to the right of the patient and using lighting that casts shadows across the chest area.

Inspect the patient's entire thorax for shape, size (including thickness), symmetry, obvious pulsations, and retractions. (Certain congenital heart diseases can cause (left-chest prominence.)

Next observe the apical impulse, which is normally located in the fifth intercostal space (ICS) at about the MCL. You can see this apical beat as a pulsation produced by the thrust of the contracting left ventricle against the chest wall during systole. This apical beat is evident in about half the normal adult population. Because it occurs almost simultaneously with the carotid pulse, simultaneous palpation of a carotid pulse helps you identify it.

The apical impulse reflects cardiac size, especially left ventricular size and location. In a patient with left ventricular hypertrophy, the impulse is sustained and forceful. In left ventricular distention, the impulse is laterally displaced. You'll see left ventricular hypertrophy in patients with hypertension, mitral regurgitation, aortic stenosis, and hypertrophic cardiomyopathy. A rocking motion at the apex is commonly associated with left ventricular hypertrophy.

Inspect the patient's right and left lower sternum for excessive pulsation and any bulging, lifting, heaving, or retraction. A slight retraction of the chest wall just medial to the MCL in the fourth ICS is a normal finding, but retraction of the rib is abnormal and may result from pericardial disease. When the work and force of the right ventricle increase markedly, a diffuse and lifting pulse can usually be seen or felt along the left sternal border. This impulse is called a *parasternal lift* and indicates right ventricular hypertrophy.

392 Precordium palpation

To palpate the patient's precordium, start at the apex and move methodically to the left sternal border and the base of the heart. (You may also palpate the epigastrium, the right sternal border, and the clavicular and left axillary areas.) Begin by placing your right palm over the apex area—the midclavicular line at the fifth intercostal space (ICS)—to locate the apical impulse (the point on the patient's anterior chest wall where the tip of the left ventricle hits during ventricular systole). Using light palpation, you should feel a tap with each heartbeat over an area the size of a nickel. The apical impulse correlates with the first heart sound and carotid pulsation. To be sure you're feeling it, you can use your left hand to palpate the patient's carotid artery. If you have difficulty palpating the apical impulse, turn the patient to the left lateral decubitus position, which brings the heart closer to the left chest wall.

The apical impulse may be abnormal in size, strength, and location. Generally, a weak apical impulse indicates poor stroke volume and a weakened contractile state, such as decompensated congestive heart failure from increased lung volume. Remember that the apical impulse may be imperceptible in a patient who's muscular or obese, or whose chest wall is enlarged (as in emphysema) or deformed. (Occasionally, in a patient with left ventricular hypertrophy, you may feel a lifting sensation under your examining hand in the apical impulse area.) An apical impulse that's sustained, forceful, and diffuse over a large area or that's displaced toward the axillary line usually indicates left ventricular enlargement. Generally, the degree of apical impulse displacement correlates with the degree of left ventricular enlargement. Displacement can indicate left ventricular dilatation. Conditions associated with volume overload, such as mitral and aortic regurgitation, left to right shunts (septal defects), and acute myocardial infarction, usually produce such dilatation and hypertrophy. Conditions that produce hypertrophy without dilatation include aortic stenosis, hypertrophic cardiomyopathy, and systemic hypertension. Hypertrophy without dilatation results in an apical impulse that's increased in force and duration but not necessarily displaced laterally.

After assessing the patient's apical impulse, palpate the apex for thrills resulting from turbulent blood flow (possibly due to mitral regurgitation and stenosis) in the following circumstances:

- across a damaged valve
- through a partially obstructed vessel
- through artificial changes between

CHEST AUSCULTATION: LISTENING FOR HEART SOUNDS

SOUNDS	TIMING	PHYSIOLOGY
S_1	Beginning of systole	Mitral and tricuspid valves close almost simultaneously, producing a single sound; S_1 corresponds to the carotid pulse.
Accentuated S_1	Beginning of systole	Mitral valve is still open wide at the beginning of systole, so the valve slams shut from an open position.
Diminished S_1	Beginning of systole	Mitral valve has time to float back into an almost closed position before ventricular contraction forces it shut, so it closes less forcefully. Softer closure may also be from an immobile, calcified valve.
Split S_1	Beginning of systole	Mitral valve closes slightly before the tricuspid valve.
S_2	End of systole	Pulmonic and aortic valves close almost simultaneously.
Physiologic split S_2 (split on inspiration but not on expiration)	End of systole	During inspiration, the pulmonic valve closes later than the aortic valve. (Pulmonic valve closure is normally delayed during inspiration, which causes decreased thoracic pressure and allows more blood into the right side of the heart, delaying pulmonic valve closure.)
Persistent wide split S_2 (split on both inspiration and expiration, but more widely split on inspiration)	End of systole	Pulmonic valve closes late or (less commonly) the aortic valve closes early.
Fixed split S_2 (equally split on inspiration and expiration)	End of systole	Pulmonic valve consistently closes later than aortic valve. Right side of heart is already ejecting a larger volume, so filling cannot be increased during inspiration. The sound remains fixed.
Paradoxical (reversed) S_2 split (widely split on expiration)	End of systole	On expiration, aortic valve closes after the pulmonic valve, from delayed or prolonged left ventricular systole. On inspiration, the normal delay of the pulmonic valve closure causes the two sounds to merge.
S_3 (ventricular gallop)	Early diastole	Ventricles fill early and rapidly, causing vibrations of the ventricular walls.
S_4 (atrial gallop)	Late diastole	Atrium makes an extra effort to fill against increased resistance.

When auscultating your patient's chest, listen carefully to each component of the cardiac cycle. This chart will also help you identify some abnormalities you may hear.

INDICATION	WHERE TO AUSCULTATE
• Normal	Apex
• During rapid heart rate • Mitral stenosis • After mitral valve disease, such as mitral prolapse	Apex
• First degree heart block • Mitral regurgitation • Severe mitral stenosis with calcified immobile valve	Apex
• Normal in most cases • Right bundle-branch heart block (wide splitting of S_1) • Pulmonary hypertension	Beginning at mitral area and moving toward tricuspid area
• Normal	Aortic and pulmonic areas (base); heard best at aortic area
• Normal; a physiologic S_2 split corresponds to the respiratory cycle.	Aortic and pulmonic areas; heard best at pulmonic area on inspiration
Late pulmonic valve closure: • Complete right bundle-branch heart block, which delays right ventricular contraction. As a result, the pulmonic valve closes later. • Pulmonary stenosis, which prolongs right ventricular ejection	Pulmonic area
• Severe right ventricular failure, which prolongs right ventricular systole • Atrial septal defect, which causes blood return to the right ventricle from lungs, prolonging the ejection	Pulmonic area
• Left bundle-branch heart block (most common cause) • Aortic stenosis • Patent ductus arteriosus • Severe hypertension • Left ventricular failure, disease, or ischemia	Aortic area
• Early congestive heart failure • Ventricular aneurysm • Common in children and young adults	Mitral area and right ventricular area, using stethoscope bell, with patient on his left side
• Hypertensive cardiovascular disease • Chronic coronary artery disease • Aortic stenosis • Hypertrophic cardiomyopathy • Pulmonary artery hypertension	Apex

LEARNING ABOUT HEART MURMURS

When you listen for heart sounds, you may hear more than the sounds identified as S_1 through S_4. You may hear a murmur, or audible vibration, when blood flow is obstructed or abnormal.

To help in identifying types of murmurs, carefully note the following indicators. Then, study the chart to learn about the different types of murmurs.

- *Timing:* Note the occurrence—is it in the systolic phase or the diastolic phase? A midsystolic murmur is also called an ejection murmur; a murmur heard throughout the systolic phase is called a pansystolic, or holosystolic, murmur.
- *Quality:* Describe the quality or sound of the murmur—is it blowing, harsh, musical, or rumbling?
- *Pitch:* Identify the pitch or frequency of the murmur—is it high, medium, or low?
- *Location:* Name the auscultation location where you hear the murmur best—is it aortic, pulmonic, tricuspid, or mitral?
- *Radiation:* List the bordering structures where the murmur is also heard.
- *Loudness:* Employ this rating system to describe the volume of the murmur: 1–barely heard; 2–faint but distinct;

TIMING	QUALITY	PITCH	LOCATION	RADIATION	CONDITION
Midsystolic (systolic ejection)	Harsh, rough	Medium to high	Pulmonic	Toward left shoulder and neck	Pulmonic stenosis
Midsystolic (systolic ejection)	Harsh, rough	Medium to high	Aortic and suprasternal notch	Toward carotid arteries or apex	Aortic stenosis
Holosystolic	Harsh	High	Tricuspid	Precordium	Ventricular septal defect
Holosystolic	Blowing	High	Mitral, lower left sternal border	Toward left axilla	Mitral insufficiency
Holosystolic	Blowing	High	Tricuspid	Toward apex	Tricuspid insufficiency
Early diastolic	Blowing	High	Midleft sternal edge (not aortic area)	Toward sternum	Aortic insufficiency
Early diastolic	Blowing	High	Pulmonic	Toward sternum	Pulmonic insufficiency
Mid- to late diastolic	Rumbling	Low	Apex	Usually none	Mitral stenosis
Mid- to late diastolic	Rumbling	Low	Tricuspid, lower sternal border	Usually none	Tricuspid stenosis

arteries and veins, such as atrioventricular shunts or fistulas

- through abnormal openings between heart chambers, such as ventricular or atrial septal defects
- because of high flow rates.

Next, place your right palm on the patient's left sternal border area. A diffuse, lifting systolic impulse indicates right ventricular hypertrophy, which occurs in fewer patients than left ventricular hypertrophy. It may be associated with a systolic retraction at the apex, resulting from posterior dis-

mia. Accurate interpretation of these abnormal variations will help you identify the cardiac abnormality.

Use the chart below to identify cardiac rates, rhythms, and sounds. Document your findings.

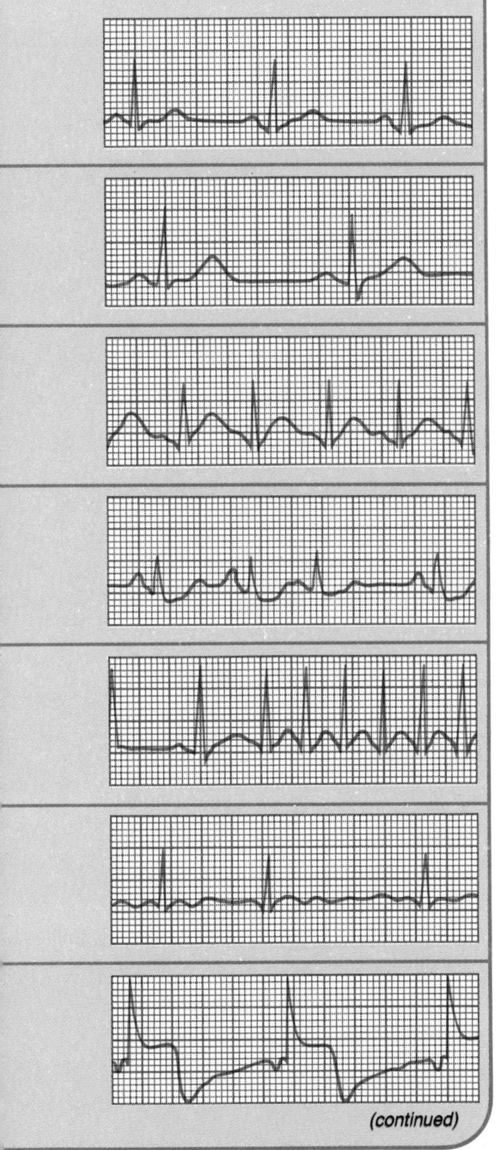

(continued)

First, using the stethoscope's diaphragm, listen to your patient's heart at the apex—the fifth intercostal space (ICS) at the midclavicular line—for the two normal heart sounds, S_1 and S_2. (S_1 is the *lub* and S_2 the *dub* of the *lub-dub* sound made by the normal heart.) You can hear S_1 best by listening as you palpate the carotid pulse, because the sound and the beat occur simultaneously. S_1 splitting is significant only if very pronounced.

S_2 immediately follows S_1. You'll hear it best at the heart's base (at the second ICS, right and left sternal borders). S_2 often splits into an aortic and a pulmonic component when the aortic valve closes slightly before the pulmonic valve, during inspiration. This physiologic split is most distinct at the second ICS, left sternal border. In systemic hypertension and dilatation of the ascending aorta, the aortic component is usually loud and sharp; in severe aortic stenosis, it may be diminished or absent. In pulmonary hypertension resulting from such conditions as mitral stenosis, left ventricular failure, pulmonary emboli, or pulmonary heart disease, the pulmonic component is louder; in severe pulmonic stenosis, it's diminished. Always identify S_1 and S_2 first, because you can only recognize abnormal sounds by their relationship to diastole and systole.

Now, use the stethoscope's bell to listen at the apex of your patient's heart for the abnormal S_3 and S_4 sounds. (Apply the bell lightly, because exerting pressure makes it work like a diaphragm.) S_3, a low-pitched sound immediately following S_2, is probably caused by abrupt limitation of left ventricular filling. Called *ventricular gallop* because of its triple sound, S_3 is an important early sign of heart failure and indicates more serious pathology than S_4. Learning to detect this extra sound takes practice and patience. But you should develop your skill, because S_3 often appears before other significant symptoms of congestive heart failure, such as rales, dyspnea, and elevated

IDENTIFYING CARDIAC RATE, RHYTHM, AND SOUND *(continued)*

CLASSIFICATION	RATE	RHYTHM	SOUND
Premature ventricular contraction (PVC)	*Atrial:* 60 to 100 *Ventricular:* 60 to 100 (Rates vary depending on the number of PVCs)	Irregular	Normal
Ventricular tachycardia	*Atrial:* variable *Ventricular:* 100 to 270	Fairly regular	S_1 intensity varies; abnormal S_2 splitting. If atria are captured retrogradely, may be constant.
Ventricular fibrillation	*Atrial:* cannot be determined *Ventricular:* 400 to 600	Irregular	Absent
First degree heart block	*Atrial:* 60 to 100 *Ventricular:* 60 to 100	Regular	Decreased S_1 intensity; normal S_2 splitting; S_4 heard with conduction delay
Type I second degree heart block	*Atrial:* 60 to 100 *Ventricular:* 30 to 100 (Atrial rate greater than ventricular)	Regular, although ventricular may be irregular, contraction not occurring with every atrial contraction.	S_1 intensity decreases cyclically, then increases after pause; normal S_2 splitting; S_4 heard with conduction delay
Type II second degree heart block	*Atrial:* 60 to 100 *Ventricular:* 30 to 100 (Atrial rate twice that of ventricular rate)	Regular, although ventricular may be irregular	Constant S_1 intensity; abnormal S_2 splitting
Complete atrioventricular block	*Atrial:* 60 to 100 *Ventricular:* less than 40	Regular	S_1 intensity varies; abnormal S_2 splitting

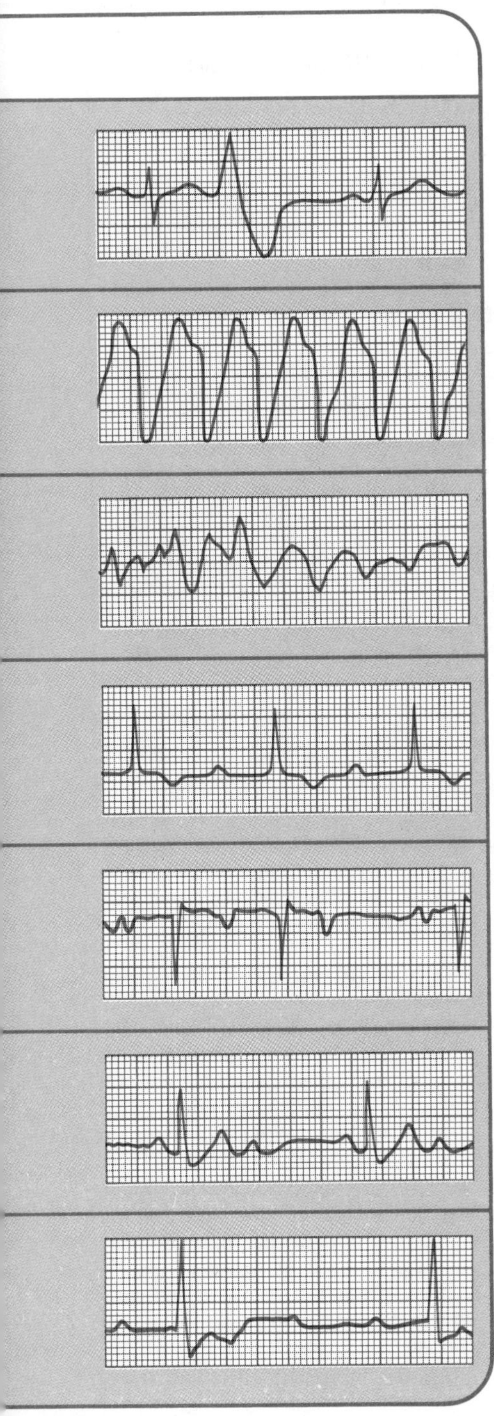

jugular venous pressure. This means that your skill in detecting it may contribute significantly to early identification of your patient's problems. In fact, S_3 is such an important indicator of congestive heart failure that many doctors begin drug therapy as soon as it's detected. (Remember: Effective treatment for heart failure makes this sound disappear.)

S_4 occurs just before S_1 and can be more difficult to hear than S_3. Called an *atrial gallop* because of its triple sound, S_4 results from atrial contraction during diastolic ventricular filling. Normally, atrial systole is silent, but when ventricular filling pressure is high and the ventricle is stiffer than normal (as in heart disease), the atria produce an extra sound as they contract against this greater ventricular resistance. (This explains why S_4 occurs just before S_1.) Although not as specific as S_3 for congestive heart failure, S_4 is a key sign for other forms of heart disease, including hypertension, cardiomyopathies, and aortic stenosis. In adults with severe myocardial disease and tachycardia, summation (a cumulative effect) of S_3 and S_4 may occur, producing a *summation gallop.*

Pericardial friction rub is an extra cardiac sound resembling squeaking leather or a grating, scratching, or rasping sound. You can hear it best between the apex and the sternum; it may be loud enough to mask other heart sounds. Inflammation of the pericardial sac causes the parietal and visceral surfaces to rub together.

Finally, listen carefully for *heart murmurs,* which result from turbulent blood flow produced by valvular or septal wall pathology. Murmur loudness is classified in six grades, with Grade 1 the softest audible murmur and Grade 6 the loudest—audible even when the stethoscope isn't touching the patient's chest. Murmurs can be classified as systolic or diastolic. Systolic murmurs occur during ventricular systole and may result from turbulent flow through a stenotic aortic or pulmonic

LEARNING CARDIAC AUSCULTATION LANDMARKS

To perform cardiac auscultation, you'll need to know the locations of the five areas shown here.

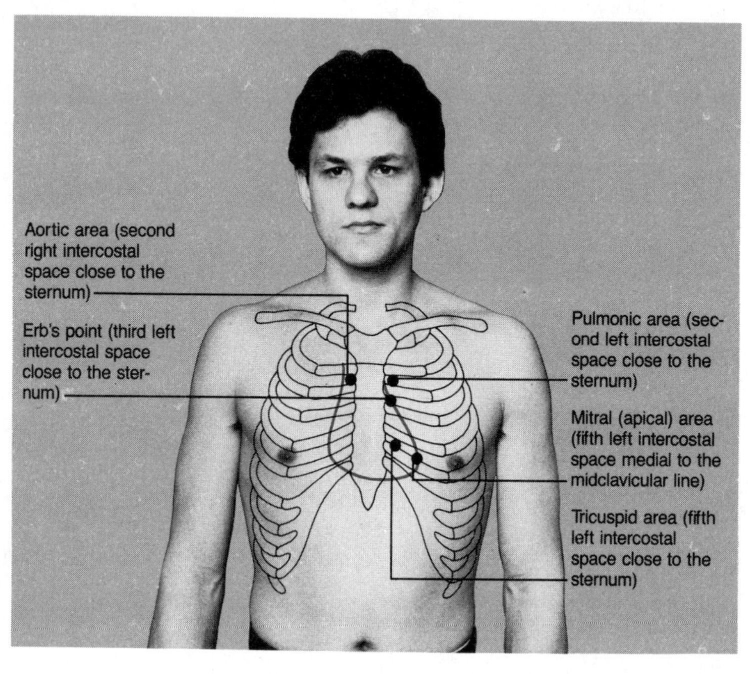

valve, regurgitant flow through an incompetent mitral or tricuspid valve, or flow through a ventricular septal defect. Diastolic murmurs occur during ventricular diastole and may result from turbulent flow through stenotic mitral or tricuspid valves or regurgitant flow through an incompetent aortic or pulmonic valve. Listen for a pansystolic murmur during the acute stage of myocardial infarction. A murmur of this type may indicate the presence of a ventricular septal defect. (The synonymous terms *pansystolic* and *holosystolic* indicate that the murmur occurs during the entire systolic cycle; you'll hear it as a whooshing sound between S_1 and S_2.)

Remember that identifying murmurs, like identifying heart sounds, is difficult. Developing this skill may take years of study and practice.

394 Auscultation sequence

Positioning your patient properly can help you hear heart sounds better. For the apex area, begin auscultation with the patient supine. Then turn him on his left side and listen with the bell to identify low-pitched filling sounds or murmurs (as in mitral stenosis). Finally, listen to the base with the patient sitting up. To hear high-pitched diastolic murmurs (as in aortic or pulmonic insufficiency), press the diaphragm firmly against the chest wall while the patient leans slightly forward.

Use the following auscultation sequence:

• With the patient in the supine or semi-Fowler's position, begin auscultating with the diaphragm at the *apex* to identify rate, rhythm, S_1 (the loudest sound at this location), and S_2. Then listen for extra sounds, such as murmurs, S_3, S_4, or pericardial friction rubs.
• Turn the patient on his *left side*, and listen with the bell to identify mitral valve murmurs and the filling sounds of S_3 and S_4.
• Position the patient on his back and inch the diaphragm up the *left sternal border* to the third intercostal space (ICS)—Erb's point. (Murmurs caused by tricuspid valve dysfunction and pulmonic valve disorders radiate to Erb's point.) Then proceed to the second ICS (pulmonic) area, where you can identify S_1 and S_2, and note the physiologic split of S_2 on inspiration. (S_2 is the more prominent sound in this base location.)
• Proceed to the second ICS at the right sternal border (aortic area), using the diaphragm. Note S_1 and S_2 (still the most prominent sound in this area). Then ask the patient to sit forward.

IDENTIFYING ARTERIAL PULSE ABNORMALITIES

You can identify heart problems, such as aortic insufficiency and cardiogenic shock, by properly interpreting pulse wave readings like the ones shown here.

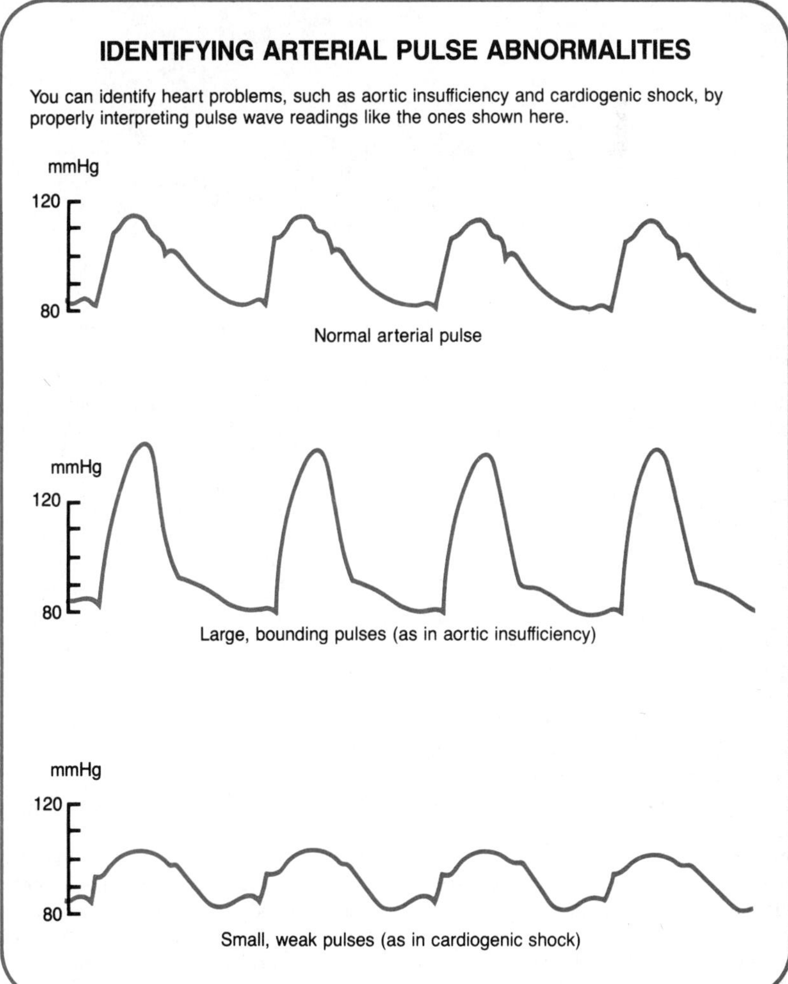

Normal arterial pulse

Large, bounding pulses (as in aortic insufficiency)

Small, weak pulses (as in cardiogenic shock)

PERFORMING THE ALLEN'S TEST

The Allen's test is used to check the patency of the ulnar and radial arteries. If you can't palpate a pulse in one or both of these arteries, follow these guidelines:

Instruct the patient to rest his right arm on a table. Support the wrist with a rolled washcloth, as shown here. Place your thumb over the radial artery and ask him to clench his fist tightly. Compress the artery firmly. Then ask him to relax his hand. Observe the color of his palms. If his hand flushes, the artery's patent. If it remains blanched, suspect ulnar artery occlusion. (Note, however, that slow blood return may also be caused by poor cardiac output or, in a patient in shock, poor capillary refill.) Continue the test, occluding the ulnar artery. Then, repeat the test on the patient's left arm and document your findings.

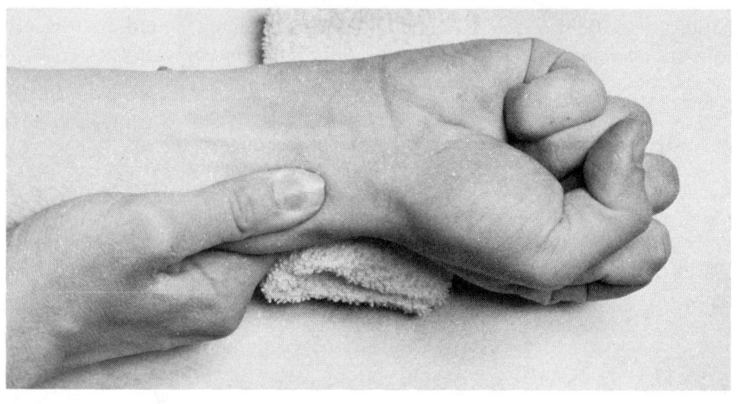

Press the diaphragm firmly against his chest wall and listen for the high-pitched murmurs of aortic regurgitation and, possibly, aortic stenosis.

395 Assessing the epigastric area

Assess your patient's upper abdominal area for evidence of cardiovascular disease. A normal patient may have visible or palpable pulsations in the epigastric area (upper central abdominal region). Abnormally large aortic pulsations may result from an aneurysm of the abdominal aorta or from aortic valvular regurgitation. To distinguish right ventricular hypertrophy—which can exaggerate epigastric pulsations—from an aortic pathology, place your palm on the epigastric area, and slide your fingers under the rib cage. You'll feel the aortic pulsations with your palm and the right ventricular impulses with your fingertips. Next, use the bell to auscultate the abdominal aorta from the epigastric area in the abdominal midline to the umbilicus, listening for bruits—which may indicate obstruction of the aorta by plaques.

Evaluating your patient's liver size by percussion or palpation can help determine the presence and extent of right-sided heart disease (for more information, see Entry 448). Remember to note whether liver percussion or palpation causes the patient discomfort, because tenderness is characteristic of right heart failure resulting from excessive venous congestion.

396 Palpating peripheral pulses

Your evaluation of the rate, rhythm, amplitude, and symmetry of peripheral pulsations, along with your auscultation of the femoral pulses for bruits, reveals important information about your patient's cardiac function and peripheral perfusion. Using your dominant hand, palpate his peripheral pulses lightly with the pads of your index, middle, and (when appropriate) ring fingers. Use three fingers where space permits and two fingers when the area you're palpating is small or angled (for example, the femoral pulses).

To determine *rate,* count all pulses for at least 30 seconds (60 seconds when recording vital signs). The normal rate is between 60 and 100 beats/minute. If you detect an irregular radial pulse, use the technique for apical-radial pulses.

To estimate the pulse's *volume* or *amplitude,* palpate the blood vessel during ventricular systole. Pulse amplitude reflects the adequacy of the circulating volume, the vessel tone, the strength of left ventricular contraction, and the elasticity and distensibility of the arterial walls. Normal arteries are soft and pliable. Sclerotic vessels are more resistant to occlusion by external pressure; when you palpate them, they feel beaded and cordlike. Characterize your patient's pulse volume using this scale:

- 3+: bounding, increased
- 2+: normal
- 1+: weak, thready, decreased
- 0: absent.

Palpate pulses on both sides of the patient's body simultaneously (except the carotid pulse) to determine *symmetry;* inequality is diagnostically significant. Always assess peripheral pulses methodically, moving from the patient's head (temporal, facial) to his arms (brachial, radial, ulnar) to his legs (femoral, popliteal, posterior tibial, pedal). For the *temporal pulse,* feel the ear immediately in front of the tragus, where the artery passes over the root of the temporal bone's zygomatic process. Then palpate the *facial pulse* where the artery passes over the mandible's lower border, at the anterior border of the masseter muscle.

Feel the patient's *brachial pulse* medial to the biceps tendon. Palpate the *radial pulses* on the palmar surface of the patient's relaxed, slightly flexed wrist, medial to the radial styloid process. (Remember, the radial pulse is the most frequently used indicator of pulsation rate and rhythm.) Feel the *ulnar artery* by pressing it against the ulna on the palmar surface of the patient's wrist. Be sure to note rate, amplitude, and symmetry for both of the patient's arms.

To assess the patient's *femoral pulses,* use the pads of your fingers to deep-palpate the area below the inguinal ligament, midway between the anterior superior iliac spine and the symphysis pubis. Then, auscultate the pulsation sites on both sides of the patient's body for bruits, which indicate arteriosclerotic changes.

To locate the patient's *popliteal* arteries, which are relatively deep in the soft tissues behind the knee, flex his knee slightly while he's supine or in the semi-Fowler's position. Use both hands to deep-palpate the pulsation. You may locate the pulse more easily by placing both thumbs on the patient's knee and palpating behind it with the first two fingers of both hands.

Assess the patient's *pedal pulses* by using the pads of your fingers to palpate the dorsum of the foot. To prevent excessive traction on the artery, dorsiflex the foot, preferably to 90°, and palpate where the vessel passes over the dorsum. To locate the pulsation, place your palm on the dorsum until you feel the dorsalis pedis pulse point. (Remember, the pedal pulse is a superficial pulse that can be obscured by heavy palpation.) Keeping the patient's foot in the dorsiflexed position, use the pads of your fingers to locate the posterior tibial pulsation on the posterior or inferior medial malleolus of the ankle.

Assessment tip: Always check the pedal pulse in patients with intermittent claudication or gangrene.

Remember that in some patients the dorsalis pedis may occupy a different position or be difficult to palpate; failure to find the pulse doesn't necessarily indicate arterial disease.

USING DIAGNOSTIC TESTS TO ASSESS CARDIOVASCULAR FUNCTION

The tests listed here may prove helpful when assessing the patient with a cardiac problem:

- *Blood gas tests:* determine acidity or alkalinity of the blood, partial pressure of oxygen, and carbon dioxide levels in the blood.
- *Cardiac enzyme and isoenzyme tests:* (CPK-MB, LDH_1 and LDH_2, HBD, SGOT): aid in identifying such cardiac disorders as myocardial infarction.
- *Electrolyte analysis:* may aid in identifying causes of some cardiac conduction disorders.
- *Electrocardiography:* records the conduction, magnitude, and duration of the electrical activity of the heart.
- *Chest X-rays:* permit visualization of the position, size, and contour of the heart and great vessels.
- *Fluoroscopy:* permits visualization of the pulsations of the heart and great vessels and helps detect and confirm malfunctions of prosthetic heart valves.
- *Ultrasonography* (echocardiography): helps evaluate cardiac structure and function and can reveal valve deformities.
- *Thallium imaging:* evaluates myocardial blood flow.
- *Technetium pyrophosphate scanning:* reveals damaged myocardial tissue as hot spots (areas where radioisotopes accumulate).
- *Cardiac catheterization:* permits visualization of cardiac contraction and cardiac structures, and measurement of intracardiac pressure and cardiac output.
- *Pulmonary artery catheterization:* permits measurement of pulmonary capillary wedge pressure (PCWP) and reflects both left atrial and left ventricular end-diastolic pressure.

Measurement of cardiac output (the amount of blood ejected from the right and left ventricles every 60 seconds) and estimation of the cardiac index (the cardiac output divided by the figure obtained from the patient's nomogram) are derived by using the four-lumen thermodilution catheter.

397 Assessing perfusion to arms and legs

Inspect the skin color of your patient's hands and feet. You can describe skin color as *normal, cyanotic, mottled,* or *excessively pale* (see Entry 224). Note if the patient has any petechial hemorrhages, evidence of Osler's nodes in his fingers or on his palms, or Janeway spots on his palms.

To assess arterial flow adequacy, have the patient lie down and raise his legs or arms 12″ (30 cm) above heart level; then ask him to move his feet or hands up and down briskly for 60 seconds. Next, tell the patient to sit up and dangle his legs or arms—which should show mild pallor, with the original color returning in about 10 seconds and the veins refilling in about 15 seconds. Significant arterial insufficiency may be present if one or both of the patient's feet or hands show marked pallor, delayed color return ending with a mottled appearance, or delayed venous filling—or if you note marked redness of his arms or legs.

Next, assess the adequacy of the patient's venous system by inspecting and palpating his legs for superficial veins. When the legs are in a dependent position, venous distention, nodular bulges at venous valves (bifurcations of veins), and collapsing veins are normal. Evidence of venous insufficiency (dilated, tortuous veins with poorly functioning valves) includes peripheral cyanosis, peripheral edema that pits with pressure, unusual ankle pigmentation, skin thickening, and ulceration—especially around the ankles.

To test capillary refill, squeeze a small area of the patient's foot or toe between your fingers to cause blanching, then release the pressure and observe how rapidly normal color returns. Immediate return indicates good arterial supply.

Test the patient's arms and legs for normal sensations to both light and deep palpation. Also note symmetry, areas of tenderness, and increased warmth or coolness.

Examine the patient's fingernails and toenails for quantitative changes, including decreased or increased thickness, and such qualitative changes as color, contour, consistency, and adherence to the nail bed (see Entry 231). Also check for clubbed nails, which are associated with lung and heart disease. In patients with long-standing heart disease, nail changes may result from hypoxemia. In these patients, you'll note chronic nail thickening and enlargement, as well as bulbous enlargement of the ends of fingers or toes. Inspection also reveals exaggerated curves in the nails, with obscuring of the obtuse angle between the distal portion of the finger or toe and the nail. The end root feels spongy or soft.

Now, inspect and palpate the patient's skin for texture and hair patterns. In a patient with chronic poor circulation, the skin appears thick, waxy, fragile, and shiny; normal body hair on the arms and legs is absent. These changes, characteristic of arterial insufficiency, also accompany long-standing diabetes mellitus. Also observe the patient for areas of unusual pigmentation that may indicate new skin lesions, rashes, or scarring from past injury or ulceration.

Inspect the patient's arms, hands, legs, feet, and ankles for edema caused by increased hydrostatic pressure and vascular fluid exudation into the tissue interspaces. (If the patient has been confined to bed, also check for edema in his buttocks and sacral areas, because edema occurs in the most dependent body parts.) Palpate for edema against a bony prominence and describe its characteristics:

- type (pitting or nonpitting)
- extent and location (ankle-foot area, foot-knee area, hands, or fingers)
- degree of pitting (described in terms of depth): 0″ to ¼″ is mild (1+); ¼″ to ½″, moderate (2+); and ½″ to 1″, severe (3+)
- symmetry (unilateral or symmetrical).

Inspect and palpate for evidence of deep vein inflammation or clot formation. Determine the presence of pain, tenderness, or a sense of fullness in the calf, which may be aggravated when your patient stands or walks. Next, assess for local redness, foot edema, or cyanosis of the foot, especially when it's dependent. Gently press the calf muscle with your palm; pain indicates possible thrombophlebitis. To test for Homans' sign, firmly and abruptly dorsiflex the patient's foot while supporting the entire leg, which must be extended or slightly bent (deep calf pain indicates thrombophlebitis); then palpate the foot. (For more information on general skin assessment, see Entries 223 to 228.)

Formulating a diagnostic impression

398 Classifying cardiovascular disorders

The cardiovascular system's primary tasks are delivering oxygenated blood to body tissues and carrying off metabolic wastes. For the system to accomplish these tasks successfully, four essential processes must take place: The myocardium must receive an adequate blood supply, the conduction system must properly innervate the heart, the heart must pump the blood it receives, and the peripheral vessels must provide adequate circulation.

Cardiovascular system disorders can thus be classified according to the functional process they interrupt (see *Nurse's Guide to Cardiovascular Conditions*, pages 360 to 371):

NURSE'S GUIDE TO CARDIOVASCULAR CONDITIONS

	CHIEF COMPLAINT	HISTORY
CONDITIONS OF REDUCED MYOCARDIAL PERFUSION		
Angina pectoris	• *Chest pain:* may be dull or burning, or described as pressure, tightness, heaviness; builds and fades gradually; may be in abdomen; may radiate to jaw, teeth, face, or left arm • *Dyspnea:* possible, with sense of constriction around larynx or upper trachea • *Fatigue:* absent • *Irregular heartbeat:* may be present; patient complains of palpitations or skipped beats • *Peripheral changes:* none	• Risk factors include family history of coronary artery disease, arteriosclerotic heart disease, cerebrovascular accident, diabetes, gout, hypertension, renal disease, obesity caused by excessive carbohydrate and saturated fat intake, smoking, lack of exercise, stress (Type A personality). • Higher incidence in men over age 40; lower incidence in women prior to menopause • Precipitating factors include exertion, stress, cold or hot weather, and emotional excitement.
Acute myocardial infarction	• *Chest pain:* sudden but not instantaneous onset of constricting, crushing, heavy weightlike chest pain occurring at any time—not relieved by nitroglycerin; located centrally and substernally, although not usually in left chest; may build rapidly or in waves to maximum intensity in a few minutes; may be accompanied by nausea and vomiting • *Dyspnea:* present; may be accompanied by orthopnea, cough, and wheezing • *Fatigue:* present; indicated by weakness and apprehension • *Irregular heartbeat:* may be present; patient complains of palpitations or skipped beats • *Peripheral changes:* peripheral cyanosis, with decreased perfusion	• Risk factors same as in angina pectoris. • Past medical history may include episodes of angina pectoris.
CONDITIONS AFFECTING PUMP ACTION		
Left ventricular failure	• *Chest pain:* usually absent • *Dyspnea:* present on exertion, accompanied by cough, orthopnea, paroxysmal nocturnal dyspnea; in advanced disease, present at rest	• Patient uses pillow to prop self up for sleep; wakes up gasping for breath; must sit or stand for relief. • History of present illness includes wheezing on inspiration

	PHYSICAL EXAMINATION	DIAGNOSTIC STUDIES
	• Inspection reveals patient anxiety and diaphoresis. • Palpation reveals tachycardia. • Auscultation reveals change in blood pressure, possibly hypertension, especially during anginal attack; transient rales associated with congestive heart failure; paradoxical splitting of S_2 possible.	• EKG may show depressed ST segments during ischemia attack but may be within normal limits; atrioventricular conduction defect. • Thallium stress imaging or stress EKG may show ischemic areas.
	• Fever after 24 hours • Inspection reveals anxiety, tenseness, sense of impending doom, nausea, vomiting, and possibly distended neck veins, sweating, pallor, cyanosis, and shock. • Palpation reveals tachycardia or bradycardia and weak pulse. • Auscultation reveals normal or decreased blood pressure (less than 80 mmHg), significant murmurs that may preexist or occur with ruptured septum or ruptured papillary muscle, diminished gallop rhythm, pericardial friction rub and rales. • In severe attack, shock, decreased urinary output, pulmonary edema.	• EKG at onset shows elevated ST segment, which then returns to baseline; T waves become symmetrically inverted; abnormal Q waves present; may also show arrhythmias. • WBC count shows leukocytosis on second day (lasts 1 week); erythrocyte sedimentation rate normal at first, rises on second or third day. • Enzyme testing shows elevated creatine phosphokinase (CPK) and CPK-MB initially; then increased SGOT.
	• Inspection reveals profuse sweating, pallor or cyanosis, frothy white or pink sputum, heaving apical impulse, hand veins that remain distended when patient puts hands above level of right atrium. • Palpation reveals enlarged, diffuse, and sustained left ventricular impulse at precordium,	• Pulmonary artery and pulmonary capillary wedge pressures elevated. • Central venous pressure elevated if condition has advanced to right ventricular failure, or hypervolemia from increased sodium and water retention.

(continued)

NURSE'S GUIDE TO CARDIOVASCULAR CONDITIONS *(continued)*

	CHIEF COMPLAINT	HISTORY
Left ventricular failure *(continued)*	• *Fatigue:* present on exertion, accompanied by weakness • *Irregular heartbeat:* may be present; patient may complain of rapid heart rate and skipped beats	and expiration (cardiac asthma), right upper abdominal pain or discomfort on exertion, daytime oliguria, nighttime polyuria, constipation (uncommon), anorexia, progressive weight gain, generalized edema, progressive weakness, fatigue, decreased mentation. • Past medical history includes severe chronic congestive heart failure.
Acute right ventricular failure	• *Chest pain:* usually absent • *Dyspnea:* respiratory distress secondary to pulmonary disease or advanced left ventricular failure • *Fatigue:* in severe cases, weakness and mental aberration • *Irregular heartbeat:* atrial arrhythmias common • *Peripheral changes:* dependent edema: begins in ankles but progresses to legs and genitalia; initially subsides at night, later does not; ascites; weight gain	• History of present illness includes anorexia, right upper abdominal pain or discomfort during exertion, nausea, and vomiting. • Past medical history includes left ventricular failure, mitral stenosis, pulmonic valve stenosis, tricuspid regurgitation, pulmonary hypertension, chronic obstructive pulmonary disease.
Cardiomyopathies	• *Dyspnea:* paroxysmal nocturnal, accompanied by orthopnea • *Fatigue:* present • *Irregular heartbeat:* palpitations; Stokes-Adams attacks with conduction defects • *Peripheral changes:* dry skin, extremity pain, edema and ascites with right-sided failure	• Past medical history includes viral illness, alcoholism, chronic debilitating illnesses.
Idiopathic hypertrophic subaortic stenosis (IHSS) or asymmetric septal hypertrophy	• *Chest pain:* present; similar to angina pectoris; but unrelieved by nitroglycerin • *Dyspnea:* present on exertion • *Fatigue:* present; accompanied by dizziness and syncope • *Irregular heartbeat:* may be present; patient may complain of palpitations or skipped beats • *Peripheral changes:* peripheral edema (uncommon)	• Symptoms may be induced by high temperatures, pregnancy, exercise, standing suddenly, Valsalva's maneuver.

	PHYSICAL EXAMINATION	DIAGNOSTIC STUDIES
	displaced to left; pulsus alternans at peripheral pulses. • Percussion reveals pleural fluid (indicated by dullness at lung bases) and decreased tactile fremitus. • Auscultation reveals S_3 and S_4 sounds, possibly mitral and tricuspid regurgitation murmurs, accentuated pulmonary component of second sound, decreased or absent breath sounds, rales (basilar) that don't clear on cough.	• EKG reflects heart strain or left ventricular enlargement, ischemia, and arrhythmias. • X-ray shows left atrial enlargement and pulmonary venous congestion.
	• Inspection reveals lower sternal or left parasternal heave independent of apical impulse. • Palpation and percussion reveal enlarged, tender, pulsating liver, with tricuspid regurgitation; abdomen fluid wave and shifting dullness; hepatojugular reflux, indicating jugular vein distention; tachycardia. • Auscultation reveals right ventricular S_3 sound; murmur of tricuspid regurgitation.	• Central venous pressure readings are elevated.
	• Fever • Signs of right and/or left heart failure • Palpation reveals displaced cardiac impulse to left; tachycardia. • Auscultation reveals systolic murmur, S_3 sound, and postural hypotension.	• EKG reveals nonspecific ST-T changes, decreased height of R wave; may show arrhythmias and conduction defects (especially atrial fibrillation). • Echocardiography and chest X-ray may help determine heart size.
	• Palpation reveals peripheral pulse with characteristic double impulse. • Auscultation reveals systolic ejection murmur. • In advanced stage, signs of mitral insufficiency (such as systolic murmur), congestive heart failure, and sudden death possible.	• EKG reveals left ventricular hypertrophy, ST segment, and T wave abnormalities. • Echocardiography shows increased thickness of the interventricular system and abnormal motion of the mitral valve. *(continued)*

NURSE'S GUIDE TO CARDIOVASCULAR CONDITIONS *(continued)*

	CHIEF COMPLAINT	HISTORY	
Pericarditis	• *Chest pain:* sudden onset; precordial or substernal, pleuritic, radiating to left neck, shoulder, back, or epigastrium; worsened by lying down or swallowing • *Dyspnea:* usually absent; breathing may cause pain • *Fatigue:* usually absent • *Irregular heartbeat:* absent • *Peripheral changes:* none	• Past medical history includes viral respiratory infection, recent pericardiotomy or myocardial infarction, disseminated lupus erythematosus, serum sickness, acute rheumatic fever, trauma, uremia, lymphoma, dissecting aorta. • Most common in men between ages 20 and 50	
Pericarditis with effusion	• *Chest pain:* may be present as dull, diffuse oppressive precordial or substernal distress; dysphagia • *Dyspnea:* present; associated with cough that causes patient to lean forward for relief • *Fatigue:* usually absent • *Irregular heartbeat:* absent • *Peripheral changes:* none	• Past medical history includes uremia, malignancy, connective tissue disorder, viral pericarditis.	
Subacute and acute bacterial endocarditis	• *Chest pain:* present; also in abdomen, and in flanks (uncommon) • *Dyspnea:* present in approximately 50% of cases; depends on severity of disease or valve involved • *Fatigue:* present, usually as malaise • *Irregular heartbeat:* absent • *Peripheral changes:* weight loss, redness or swelling, heart failure symptoms	• Present or recent history includes acute infection, surgery or instrumentation, dental work, drug abuse, abortion, transurethral prostatectomy. • Past medical history includes rheumatic, congenital, or artherosclerotic heart disease.	
Rheumatic fever (acute)	• *Chest pain:* absent • *Dyspnea:* may be present • *Fatigue:* malaise • *Irregular heartbeat:* absent • *Peripheral changes:* weight loss	• Recent history includes streptococcal infection of upper respiratory tract (in previous 4 weeks), anorexia. • Past medical history includes migratory, gradually beginning arthritis; recurrent epistaxis; "growing pains" in joints (arthralgia). • Increased clumsiness	

	PHYSICAL EXAMINATION	DIAGNOSTIC STUDIES
	• Fever: 100° to 103° F. (37.8° to 39.4° C.) • Palpation reveals tachycardia. • Auscultation reveals pericardial friction rub.	• EKG shows ST-T segment elevation in all leads; returns to baseline in a few days, with T wave inversion. • Possibly atrial fibrillation
	• Inspection reveals distended neck veins. • Palpation and percussion reveal tachycardia, enlarged area of cardiac dullness, apical beat that's within dullness border or not palpable. • Auscultation reveals abnormal blood pressure and possibly pericardial friction rub, and acute cardiac tamponade (inspiratory distention of neck veins, narrow pulse pressure, paradoxic pulse); may progress to shock.	• EKG shows T waves flat, low diphasic or inverted leads, QRS voltage uniformly low.
	• Daily fever • Inspection may reveal petechiae on conjunctivae and palate buccal mucosa; with longstanding endocarditis, clubbed fingers and toes; splinter hemorrhages beneath nails; tender red nodules on finger and toe pads (Osler nodes); pallor or yellow-brown tint to skin; oval, pale, retinal lesion around optic disk (seen with ophthalmoscope) • Palpation reveals splenomegaly. • Auscultation reveals sudden change in present heart murmur or development of new murmur and possibly signs of early heart failure or emboli.	• Blood cultures determine causative organism. • Echocardiography—particularly the two-dimensional (2-D) method—looks for vegetation.
	• Usually low-grade fever, with sinus tachycardia disproportional to fever level • Inspection reveals erythema marginatum (ring- or crescent-shaped macular rash), subcutaneous nodules (uncommon except in children), swollen joints (arthritis), Sydenham's chorea. • Palpation reveals enlarged heart. • Auscultation reveals mitral or aortic diastolic murmurs, varying heart sound quality, and possibly gallop rhythm arrhythmias and ectopic beats.	• Erythrocyte sedimentation rate and WBC count elevated. • Throat cultures positive for beta-hemolytic streptococci. • Antistreptolysin titer elevated. • Chest X-ray may show cardiac enlargement. • EKG shows PR greater than 0.2 seconds; may further define arrhythmias.

(continued)

NURSE'S GUIDE TO CARDIOVASCULAR CONDITIONS *(continued)*

	CHIEF COMPLAINT	HISTORY
CONDITIONS OF INCOMPETENT PERIPHERAL CIRCULATION		
Varicose veins	• *Chest pain:* absent • *Peripheral changes:* aching discomfort or pain in legs; pigmentation and ulceration of distal leg; possibly edema	• History of present illness includes leg cramps at night that may be relieved by leg elevation, itching in vein regions, leg fatigue caused by periods of standing. • Past medical history includes thrombophlebitis and family history of varicosities.
Thrombophlebitis	• *Chest pain:* present with pulmonary embolism • *Peripheral changes:* pain and swelling of affected extremity; if leg veins affected, pain may increase with walking	• Childbirth 4 to 14 days before onset • History of present illness includes fracture, trauma, deep vein surgery, cardiac disease, cerebrovascular accident, prolonged bed rest. • Past medical history includes malignancy, shock, dehydration, anemia, obesity, chronic infection, use of oral contraceptives. • In superficial vein thrombophlebitis, recent history includes superficial vein I.V. therapy with irritating solutions.
Dissecting thoracic aortic aneurysms	• *Chest pain:* present; sudden and severe, radiating to back, abdomen, and hips • *Peripheral changes:* paralysis of legs possible	• Recent history may include convulsions. • Past medical history includes hypertension, arteriosclerosis, congenital heart disease, Marfan's syndrome, pregnancy, trauma
Abdominal aortic aneurysm	• *Chest pain:* absent • *Peripheral changes:* absent	• Most common in men over age 50
Raynaud's disease and Raynaud's phenomenon	• *Chest pain:* absent • *Peripheral changes:* with Raynaud's disease: attacks of cyanosis, followed by pallor in fingers (rarely in thumbs or toes); redness, swelling, throbbing, and paresthesia during recovery, occurring when areas are warmed; numbness, stiffness, diminished sensation; with Raynaud's phenomenon: usually unilateral cyanosis, which may involve only one or two fingers	• Most common in females between puberty and age 40 • Precipitating factors include emotional upsets or a cold. • Past history includes immunologic abnormalities. • Family history of vasospastic diseases • Raynaud's phenomenon may accompany cervical rib, carpal tunnel syndrome, scleroderma, systemic lupus erythematosus, frostbite, ergot poisoning.

PHYSICAL EXAMINATION	DIAGNOSTIC STUDIES
• Inspection reveals dilated tortuous vessels in legs, visible when patient stands; brown pigmentation and thinning of skin above ankles; ulceration of distal leg; positive Trendelenburg's test.	• None usually performed.
• Slight fever • In deep vein involvement, inspection reveals, with severe venous obstruction, cyanotic skin in affected area; with reflex arterial spasm, pale and cool skin. • Palpation reveals warm affected leg, spasm and pain in calf muscles with dorsiflexion of foot (positive Homans' sign). • In superficial vein involvement, inspection reveals induration, redness, tenderness along course of vein; possibly no clinical manifestations.	• Ultrasound blood flow detector, thermography, and phlebography used to confirm diagnosis.
• Fever • Palpation reveals unequal or diminished peripheral pulses. • Auscultation reveals aortic diastolic murmur and murmurs over arteries.	• Aortography shows size and extent of aneurysm.
• Inspection reveals subcutaneous ecchymosis in flank or groin. • Palpation reveals pulsating midabdominal and upper abdominal mass.	• Aortography shows size of aneurysm. • EKG, urinalysis, BUN evaluate renal and cardiac function.
• Inspection reveals atrophy of terminal fat pads of fingers.	• None usually performed.

(continued)

NURSE'S GUIDE TO CARDIOVASCULAR CONDITIONS *(continued)*

	CHIEF COMPLAINT	HISTORY	
CONDITIONS AFFECTING VALVULAR FUNCTION			
Tricuspid stenosis	• *Chest pain:* usually absent • *Dyspnea:* present in varying degrees • *Fatigue:* present; often severe • *Irregular heartbeat:* usually absent • *Peripheral changes:* dependent peripheral edema	• Most common in women • Past medical history includes mitral valve disease.	
Tricuspid regurgitation (incompetence)	• *Chest pain:* absent • *Dyspnea:* present • *Fatigue:* present; tires easily • *Irregular heartbeat:* atrial fibrillation; usually not noticed by patient • *Peripheral changes:* none	• Past medical history includes right ventricular failure, rheumatic fever, trauma, endocarditis, pulmonary hypertension.	
Aortic stenosis	• *Chest pain:* present in severe stenosis • *Dyspnea:* present, with coughing, on exertion; paroxysmal nocturnal • *Fatigue:* usually present; syncope • *Irregular heartbeat:* present, as palpitations occasionally	• Most common in males • Usually asymptomatic unless severe	
Aortic regurgitation (incompetence)	• *Chest pain:* angina pectoris • *Dyspnea:* on exertion early in disease; paroxysmal nocturnal dyspnea; orthopnea and cough signal beginning of decompensation • *Fatigue:* present; weakness if left ventricular failure present • *Irregular heartbeat:* palpitations (signal beginning of decompensation) • *Peripheral changes:* none	• Past medical history includes Reiter's syndrome, rheumatoid arthritis, psoriasis, rheumatic fever, syphilis, subacute bacterial endocarditis.	
Mitral stenosis	• *Chest pain:* usually absent • *Dyspnea:* present; induced by exertion; may also occur during rest; orthopnea; paroxysmal nocturnal dyspnea; hemoptysis	• Most common in women under age 45 • Recent bronchitis or upper respiratory tract infection may worsen symptoms.	

	PHYSICAL EXAMINATION	DIAGNOSTIC STUDIES
	• Inspection may reveal olive skin. • Palpation may reveal presystolic liver pulsation if in sinus rhythm; middiastolic thrill between lower left sternal border and apical impulse. • Auscultation reveals diastolic rumbling murmur heard along lower left sternal border; slow y descent in jugular pulse; normal blood pressure.	• EKG shows wide, tall, peaked P waves; normal axis. • Echocardiography may permit stenosis recognition. • X-ray shows enlarged right atrium. • Cardiac catheterization may reveal site of stenosis.
	• Palpation reveals right ventricular pulsation, systolic liver pulsation, and possibly systolic thrill at lower left sternal edge. • Auscultation reveals blowing, coarse, or harsh systolic murmur heard along lower left sternal border; increases on inspiration.	• EKG usually shows atrial fibrillation.
	• Inspection reveals apical impulse localized and heaving, usually not laterally displaced. • Palpation reveals sustained localized forceful apical impulse; systolic thrill over aortic area and neck vessels; small, slowly rising plateau pulse, best appreciated in carotid pulse. • Auscultation reveals harsh, rough, systolic ejection murmur in aortic area, radiating to the neck and apex; possibly systolic ejection click at aortic area just before murmur; paradoxical splitting of second sound with significant stenosis; normal or high diastolic blood pressure.	• EKG shows criteria for left ventricular hypertrophy; possibly complete heart block. • X-rays and fluoroscopy may show calcified aortic valve, poststenotic dilatation of ascending aorta (hyperactivity evident with fluoroscopy), left ventricular hypertrophy. • Echocardiography may identify level of obstruction and a bicuspid aortic valve. • Cardiac catheterization indicates the severity and location of the obstruction as well as left ventricular function.
	• Inspection reveals generalized skin pallor; strong, abrupt carotid pulsations; forceful apical impulse to left of left midclavicular line and downward; capillary pulsations. • Palpation reveals sustained and forceful apical impulse, displaced to left and downward; rapidly rising and collapsing pulses. • Auscultation reveals normal heart sounds; soft, blowing, diastolic murmur (heard over aortic area and apex; usually loudest along left sternal border); in advanced aortic insufficiency, Austin Flint murmur that may be heard at apex; with diastolic pressure less than 60 mmHg, possibly wide pulse pressure.	• EKG shows evidence of left ventricular hypertrophy. • X-ray shows enlarged left ventricle. • Echocardiography helps establish aortic valve incompetence. • Cardiac catheterization and angiocardiography performed to exclude complicating lesions and to assess left ventricular function and magnitude of leak.
	• Inspection reveals malar flush; in young patients, precordial bulge and diffuse pulsation. • Palpation reveals tapping sensation over area of expected apical impulse, middiastolic and/or presystolic thrill at apex, small pulse,	• EKG shows notched and broad P waves in standard leads; inverted P in V_1 lead; atrial fibrillation common. • X-ray and fluoroscopy show left atrial enlargement.

(continued)

NURSE'S GUIDE TO CARDIOVASCULAR CONDITIONS *(continued)*

	CHIEF COMPLAINT	HISTORY
Mitral stenosis *(continued)*	• *Fatigue:* present; increased with decreased exercise tolerance • *Irregular heartbeat:* usually absent • *Peripheral changes:* extremity pain	• Past medical history includes rheumatic fever, congenital valve disorder, tumor (myxoma).
Mitral regurgitation (incompetence)	• *Chest pain:* absent • *Dyspnea:* present, progressive with exertion; orthopnea, paroxysmal dyspnea • *Fatigue:* present, progressive with exertion • *Irregular heartbeat:* present as palpitations • *Peripheral changes:* none	• Past medical history includes rheumatic fever, endocarditis, congenital mitral valve defect, papillary muscle dysfunction or rupture, chordae tendinae dysfunction or rupture, heart failure associated with left ventricular dilation, blunt injury to the chest.
Pulmonic stenosis	• *Chest pain:* usually not present • *Dyspnea:* present on exertion • *Fatigue:* present • *Irregular heartbeat:* absent • *Peripheral changes:* peripheral edema possible	• Congenital stenosis or rheumatic heart disease, associated with other congenital heart defects, such as tetralogy of Fallot
Pulmonic regurgitation (incompetence)	• *Chest pain:* absent • *Dyspnea:* present • *Fatigue:* present; patient tires easily; weakness • *Irregular heartbeat:* absent • *Peripheral changes:* peripheral edema	• Pulmonary hypertension • Congenital defect

• Some conditions reduce myocardial blood supply—for example, coronary vessel obstruction. Partial obstruction results in myocardial ischemia, causing angina pectoris; complete obstruction causes myocardial infarction.
• Conduction system problems, such as failure to form an impulse or to distribute it properly over the conduction system, may interfere with the heart's excitation and rhythmic contraction.
• Pump failure may result from such conditions as heart valve dysfunction, poor cardiac muscle contractility, or increased peripheral resistance.
• Poor peripheral circulation, from obstruction or incompetent valves in the vessels, may result in diminished systemic and pulmonary circulation. Peripheral artery disease may cause

	PHYSICAL EXAMINATION	DIAGNOSTIC STUDIES
	overactive right ventricle with elevated pulmonary pressure. • Auscultation reveals localized, delayed, rumbling, low-pitched, diastolic murmur at or near apex (duration of murmur varies depending on severity of stenosis; onset of murmur at opening snap early in diastole); possibly loud S_2 with elevated pulmonary pressure; normal blood pressure.	• Echocardiography helps assess severity of stenosis. • Cardiac catheterization and angiocardiography help determine amount of regurgitation that may also be present.
	• Inspection reveals forceful apical impulse to left of left midclavicular line. • Palpation reveals forceful, brisk apical impulse; systolic thrill over apical impulse; normal, small, or slightly collapsing pulse. • Auscultation reveals blowing, high-pitched, harsh, or musical pansystolic apical murmur maximal at apex and transmitted to axilla; abnormally wide splitting of S_2; possibly S_3 present; normal blood pressure.	• EKG shows P waves broad or notched in standard leads; with pulmonary hypertension, tall peaked P waves, right axis deviation, or right ventricular hypertrophy; possibly atrial fibrillation. • X-ray shows enlargement of left ventricle and moderate aneurysmal dilatation of left atrium. • Echocardiography shows dilated left ventricle and left atrium; pattern of contraction of left ventricle suggests diastolic overload. • Cardiac catheterization and ventriculography help determine amount of regurgitation and identify prolapsing cusps.
	• Inspection reveals jugular vein distention. • Palpation reveals hepatomegaly. • Auscultation reveals systolic murmur at left sternal border and split S_2 sound, with delayed or absent pulmonic component.	• EKG shows right ventricular hypertrophy, right axis deviation, right atrial hypertrophy.
	• Inspection reveals jugular vein distention. • Palpation reveals hepatomegaly. • Auscultation reveals diastolic murmur in pulmonic area.	• EKG shows right ventricular or right atrial enlargement.

decreased tissue perfusion. Venous insufficiency can cause some pooling of blood but usually does not cause significantly decreased venous return.

399 Making appropriate nursing diagnoses

Chest pain from myocardial ischemia and the buildup of metabolites in muscles results from a reduced blood supply to the heart. Any condition that decreases cardiac output, such as congestive heart failure, or that obstructs the coronary vessels (coronary artery disease, for example) may cause chest pain (angina). Exertion, anxiety, or extreme temperatures may exacerbate the pain. An appropriate nursing diagnosis for this symptom is *alteration in comfort due to myocardial ischemia.*

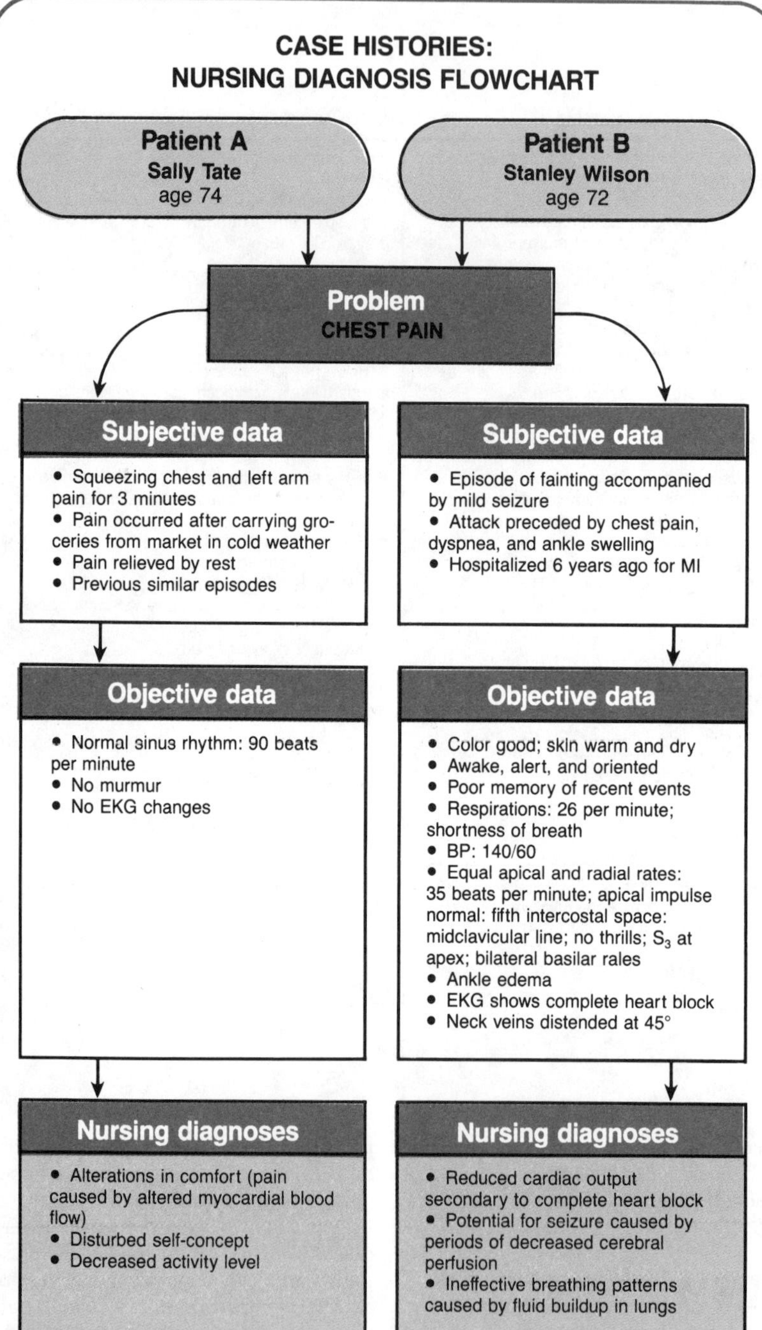
CASE HISTORIES:
NURSING DIAGNOSIS FLOWCHART
Patient A
Sally Tate
age 74
Patient B
Stanley Wilson
age 72
Problem
CHEST PAIN
Subjective data
• Squeezing chest and left arm pain for 3 minutes
• Pain occurred after carrying groceries from market in cold weather
• Pain relieved by rest
• Previous similar episodes
Subjective data
• Episode of fainting accompanied by mild seizure
• Attack preceded by chest pain, dyspnea, and ankle swelling
• Hospitalized 6 years ago for MI
Objective data
• Normal sinus rhythm: 90 beats per minute
• No murmur
• No EKG changes
Objective data
• Color good; skin warm and dry
• Awake, alert, and oriented
• Poor memory of recent events
• Respirations: 26 per minute; shortness of breath
• BP: 140/60
• Equal apical and radial rates: 35 beats per minute; apical impulse normal: fifth intercostal space: midclavicular line; no thrills; S_3 at apex; bilateral basilar rales
• Ankle edema
• EKG shows complete heart block
• Neck veins distended at 45°
Nursing diagnoses
• Alterations in comfort (pain caused by altered myocardial blood flow)
• Disturbed self-concept
• Decreased activity level
Nursing diagnoses
• Reduced cardiac output secondary to complete heart block
• Potential for seizure caused by periods of decreased cerebral perfusion
• Ineffective breathing patterns caused by fluid buildup in lungs

Dyspnea occurs in heart disease when left ventricular incompetence impedes the drainage of venous blood from the lungs (see Entry 358). An incompetent mitral or aortic valve, aortic stenosis, coronary artery disease, or cardiomyopathy may result in left ventricular failure. Nursing diagnoses may include *anxiety from inability to breathe; circulatory overload; real or potential decreased tissue perfusion, resulting in mental confusion, fatigue, and muscle weakness;* and *knowledge deficit related to need for rest and life-style change.*

Fatigue occurs when the heart can't meet the body's demand for oxygenated blood. Muscles become hypoxic and waste products build up. This symptom suggests a nursing diagnosis of *need to decrease energy demands on heart.*

Irregular heartbeat (arrhythmia) may result when physical damage to the conduction system accompanies myocardial damage. Other factors that can alter the heartbeat include anxiety, hyperthyroidism, medication, caffeine intake, and hypovolemia (which causes the heart to beat faster to compensate for the lack of tissue perfusion). Uncontrolled atrial fibrillation leads to reduced ventricular filling time and loss of atrial systole. This sequence of events reduces blood pressure and cardiac output, compromises perfusion of vital organs, and predisposes the patient to thrombus formation. Possible nursing diagnoses for irregular heartbeat include *potential for sudden death due to arrhythmias, possible syncope or confusion due to decreased cerebral perfusion, anxiety due to awareness of heartbeat,* and *anxiety due to uncertainty concerning medical condition.*

As for peripheral changes caused by cardiovascular disorders, weight change with edema and pain may result from the heart's inability to pump an adequate fluid volume. Edema reflects increased capillary hydrostatic pressure and sodium retention. This may result from the impaired pumping ability of the heart with arterial insufficiency or from obstructive vascular disease. The heart's inability to pump blood can result from a dysfunction in cardiac muscle, valves, or peripheral vessels. Extremity pain results from tissue and nerve damage caused by an inadequate supply of oxygenated blood, together with metabolic waste build-up.

These chief complaints lead to possible nursing diagnoses of *alterations in comfort due to ischemia or leg edema, anxiety due to worsening symptoms,* and (in patients who smoke) *knowledge deficit concerning the role of smoking in peripheral vascular diseases.*

Assessing pediatric patients

400 Developmental anatomy

The fetal heart has two extra openings: the *foramen ovale* (located between the two atria) and the *ductus arteriosus* (located between the aorta and the pulmonary artery). The foramen ovale, which normally fuses at birth, can function as an atrial septal defect. The ductus arteriosus, which normally closes soon after birth, may remain open for some time, resulting in a continuous murmur.

In children under age 8, the heart is proportionately smaller. The tip of the apex (and the apical pulse) is at the fourth, not the fifth, intercostal space. Located 2″ to 2½″ (5 to 6 cm) left of the sternum, the apex doesn't reach the midclavicular line.

401 Pediatric history questions

Ask if the child has frequent upper respiratory tract infections (see Entry

360). Then determine if he experiences shortness of breath. For an infant, ask the parents if their child has ever turned blue or had a bluish cast to his skin—especially on his face and around his mouth. Determine if the infant has trouble finishing a bottle without gasping or drinks only about 2 to 4 oz (60 to 120 ml) of milk at a time. Ask if other symptoms—such as increased breathing, rapid heartbeat, dyspnea, and diaphoresis—occur during feeding. Does the infant seem to tire easily and need rest? Also determine if the infant's breathing is greatly labored during bowel movements. Is loss of appetite, profuse sweating, or vomiting a problem?

Ask an older child if he can keep up physically with children his age. Next, determine if the child experiences cyanosis on exertion, dyspnea, or orthopnea. Ask the parents if he constantly assumes a squatting position or sleeps in the knee-chest position; either sign may indicate tetralogy of Fallot or other cyanotic heart disease. Finally, find out if he bleeds excessively when cut.

Check the family history for indications of possible congenital heart defects. If the child is old enough, talk with him to obtain a profile of his lifestyle and daily activities. What he tells you can provide important information about his symptoms, including whether they've affected his activities.

402 Inspecting the child

Examine the child for retarded growth or development. This condition may indicate significant chronic congestive heart failure or complex cyanotic heart disease. Then inspect his skin. Pallor can indicate a serious cardiac problem in an infant or anemia in an older child; in an infant or child, cyanosis may be an early sign of a cardiac condition. Cyanosis of the extremities (acrocyanosis) is a common and usually normal finding in neonates, but you should evaluate it when present. Acrocyanosis decreases when the infant is warm and active; cyanosis from decreased tissue oxygenation increases when the infant is crying and active.

Check for clubbed fingers, a sign of cardiac dysfunction. (Clubbing does not ordinarily occur before age 2.) Also, remember that dependent edema (a late sign of congestive heart failure in children) appears in the legs only if the child can walk; in infants, it appears in the eyelids. If the child is bedridden, also check his sacrum and buttocks.

Although it's difficult to do, you must measure blood pressure in children and infants, because it provides important diagnostic information—for instance, it can help confirm coarctation of the aorta. First, select an appropriate cuff size. It shouldn't be more than two thirds or less than one half of the upper arm length, and it should be about 20% wider than the arm's diameter. Pediatric cuff sizes are 2½", 5", 8", and 12". Remember, blood pressure may be inaudible in children under age 2. A Doppler stethoscope provides a more accurate measurement of blood pressure in children under age 2 than a regular stethoscope.

Before beginning, allow the child to handle the cuff and stethoscope to allay his fears. When you take his blood pressure, have him seated with his arm at heart level. Take an infant's blood pressure when he's supine. Also take an infant's thigh blood pressure, because lower diastolic readings in the legs than in the arms may indicate a coarctation of the aorta.

For children under age 1, the systolic thigh reading should equal the systolic arm reading; for older children, it may be 10 to 40 mmHg higher, but the diastolic thigh value should equal the diastolic arm value. If thigh readings are below normal, suspect coarctation.

Next, simultaneously palpate the child's radial and femoral pulses. If you feel the radial pulse before the femoral, suspect coarctation. (See *Nurse's Guide to Pediatric Pulse Rate and Blood Pressure.*)

NURSE'S GUIDE TO PEDIATRIC PULSE RATE AND BLOOD PRESSURE

AVERAGE RESTING PULSE RATE

Age	Normal Range		Average	
Newborn	70 to 170		120	
1 to 11 months	80 to 160		120	
2 years	80 to 130		110	
4 years	80 to 120		100	
6 years	75 to 115		100	
8 years	70 to 110		90	
10 years	70 to 110		90	
	Female	Male	Female	Male
12 years	70 to 110	65 to 105	90	85
14 years	65 to 105	60 to 100	85	80
16 years	60 to 100	55 to 95	80	75
18 years	55 to 95	50 to 90	75	70

AVERAGE RESTING BLOOD PRESSURE

Age	Female	Male
4 years	98/60	98/55
6 years	105/65	105/60
8 years	108/67	105/60
10 years	112/64	110/65
12 years	115/65	110/65
14 years	112/65	114/65

403 Palpation, percussion, and auscultation

In judging cardiac enlargement, remember that in children under age 8 the heart is proportionately smaller and the apical impulse is higher. Palpate or percuss the liver for enlargement, such as occurs in right ventricular failure, or for systolic pulsations, such as in tricuspid regurgitation (see Entries 447 and 448).

Before auscultating, try to obtain a young child's cooperation by letting him listen to his own heart.

Assessment tip: For infants, use a smaller bell on the stethoscope. If your stethoscope doesn't have interchangeable bells, remove the bell and use the base.

An S_3 sound is more common and more likely to be a normal finding in a child. Sinus arrhythmia (a variation in which the heart accelerates on inspiration and decelerates on expiration) is also more common and is normal in children. To confirm this variation in an older child, tell him to hold his breath; a true sinus arrhythmia will disappear.

Split sounds are significant in children. Carefully evaluate an S_2 split, which is easier to hear in a child than in an adult. Heard over the pulmonic area, this split occurs when the aortic valve closes slightly before the pulmonic valve. The difference in timing between the valve closures results in the S_2 split, which should increase during inspiration and decrease during expiration. A split that doesn't change

IDENTIFYING COMMON CONGENITAL HEART DEFECTS

Aortic stenosis
(narrowing of the aortic valve)

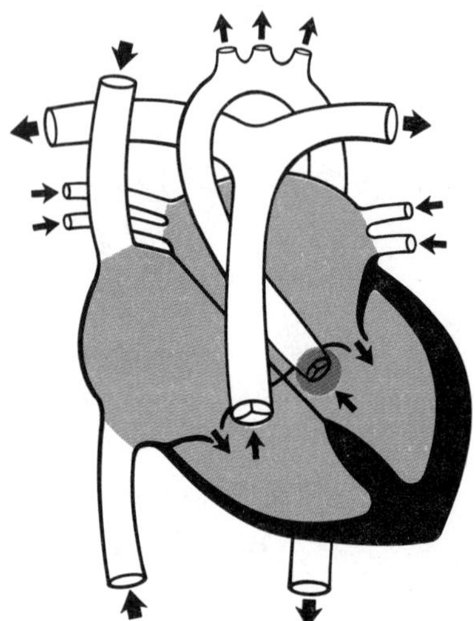

Circulatory effects
- To maintain aortic pressure, left ventricle pressure increases, causing left ventricular hypertrophy.

Clinical situation
- Systolic ejection murmur is atypical.
- With very severe condition, infant may have intractable congestive heart failure, dyspnea, hypotension, tachycardia, rales, and cyanosis.

Pulmonary stenosis
(narrowing of the pulmonic valve)

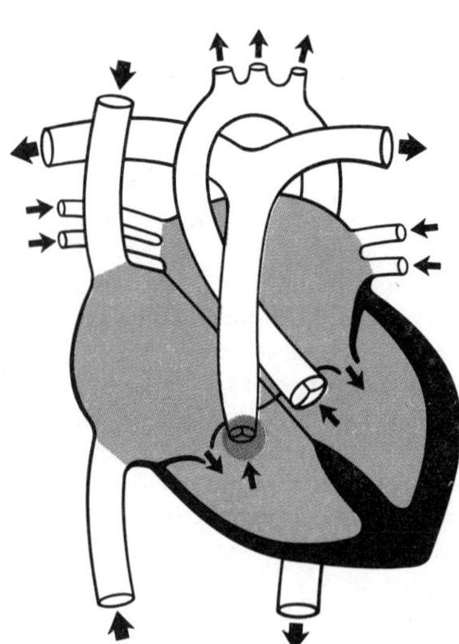

Circulatory effects
- To overcome obstruction, right ventricular pressure increases.

Clinical situation
- Midsystolic ejection murmur is prominent; thrill heard in second left intercostal space.
- Infant is normal in weight, growth, and development, unless defect is severe.
- Infant may also have narrowing of the pulmonary artery.
- Infant may experience dyspnea, fatigue, peripheral cyanosis, and cold extremities.

Transposition of great vessels
(aorta leaves right ventricle, pulmonary artery leaves left ventricle)

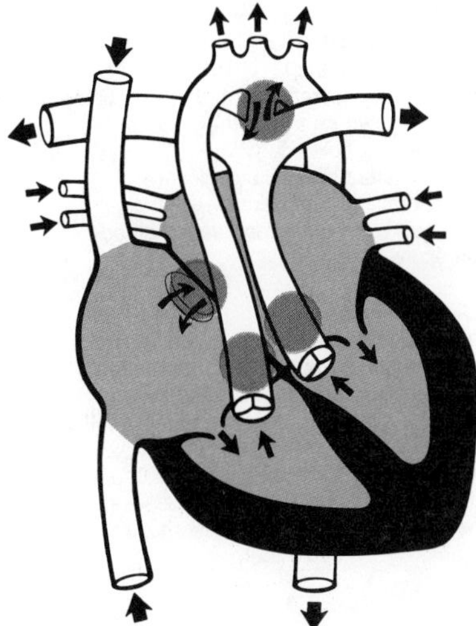

Circulatory effects
- Unoxygenated blood flows through right atrium and ventricle and out aorta to systemic circulation.
- Oxygenated blood flows from lungs to left atrium and ventricle and out pulmonary artery to lungs.

Clinical situation
- Systolic murmur heard if ventricular septal defect (VSD) is present.
- Infant may show signs of congestive heart failure, severe cyanosis, and extreme dyspnea shortly after birth.
- Infant exhibits poor sucking reflex.
- Condition associated with VSD or patent ductus arteriosus.
- Condition fatal if untreated.

Patent ductus arteriosus
(opening between the descending aorta and bifurcation of the pulmonary artery)

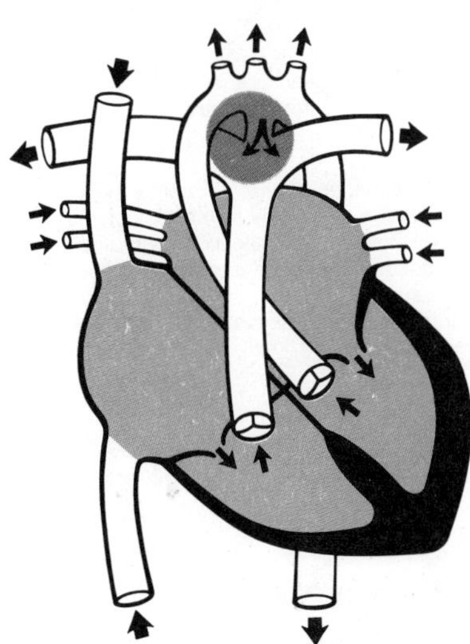

Circulatory effects
- Acyanotic defect
- Left to right shunt may cause pulmonary artery hypertension.
- Pulse pressure may be widened; pulses full or pounding.

Clinical situation
- Continuous murmur with machinelike sound may be only sign of defect. Murmur loudest at left upper sternal border and under clavicle.
- Bounding posterior tibial and dorsalis pedis pulses, dyspnea on exertion, and vigorous precordial movements
- Infant may show signs of congestive heart failure in severe defect.
- Incidence increases in premature infants.

(continued)

IDENTIFYING COMMON CONGENITAL HEART DEFECTS *(continued)*

Coarctation of the aorta
(constriction of descending aorta near the ductus arteriosus)

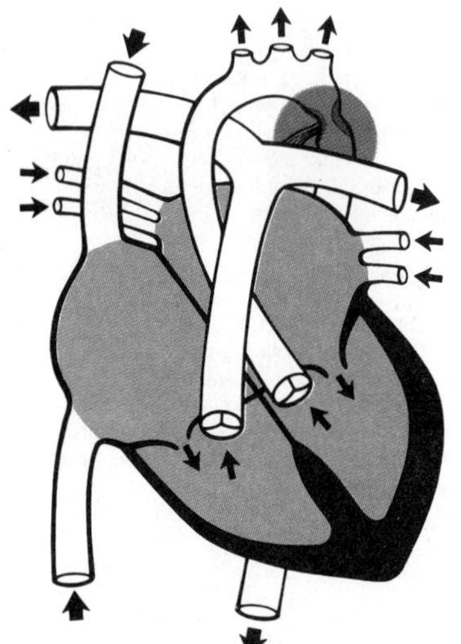

Circulatory effects
- Acyanotic defect
- Blood pressures elevated in ascending aorta, anywhere above the coarctation, and left ventricle.
- Insufficient mitral valve closure
- Pulmonary hypertension
- Aneurysms and/or increased blood pressure in arms

Clinical situation
- Murmur is systolic ejection click heard at base and apex of heart; associated with systolic or continuous murmur between scapulae; pulses in arms are full; pulses in legs are weak or absent.
- Pressure differences in child's upper and lower body may cause dizziness, headaches, fainting, nosebleeds, leg cramping, and cold feet.

Ventricular septal defect
(one or more openings between the ventricles)

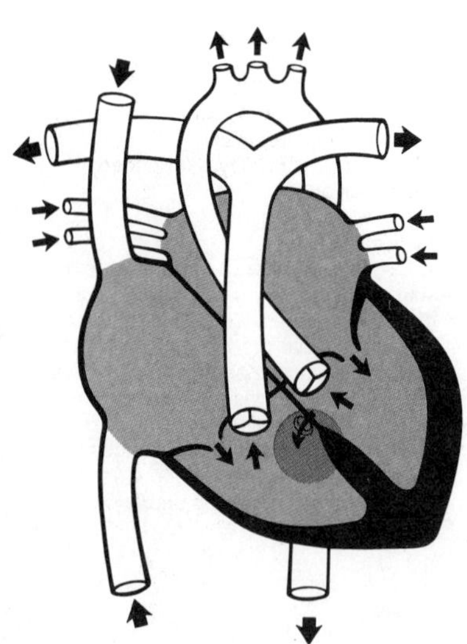

Circulatory effects
- Acyanotic defect
- Left to right shunt may cause pulmonary artery hypertension.

Clinical situation
- Murmur may be only sign of defect; soft pulmonic systolic ejection is greatest in second and third left intercostal spaces.
- Infant is usually acyanotic but may develop cyanosis.

Atrial septal defect
(one or more openings between the atria; includes ostium secondum, ostium primum, and sinus venosus)

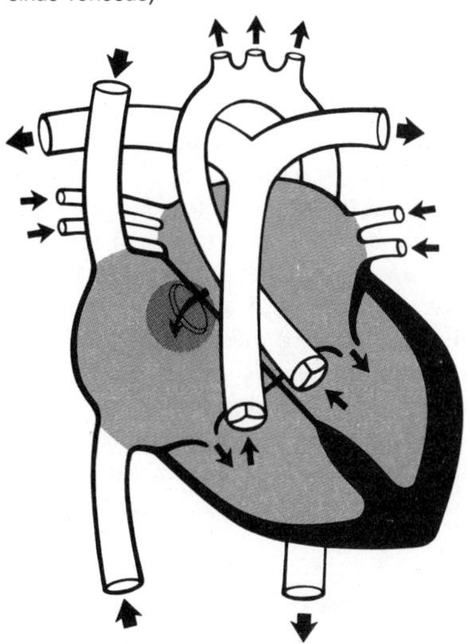

Circulatory effects
- Acyanotic defect
- Blood flows from area of higher pressure to area of lower pressure.
- With large defect, left to right shunt may cause pulmonary congestion and pulmonary artery hypertension over period of time.

Clinical situation
- Murmur may be only sign of defect; harsh, systolic sound heard in left lower sternal border, associated with palpable thrill.
- Infant may show signs of congestive heart failure in severe defect.

Tetralogy of Fallot
(four defects: ventricular septal defect, overriding aorta, pulmonic stenosis, and right ventricular hypertrophy)

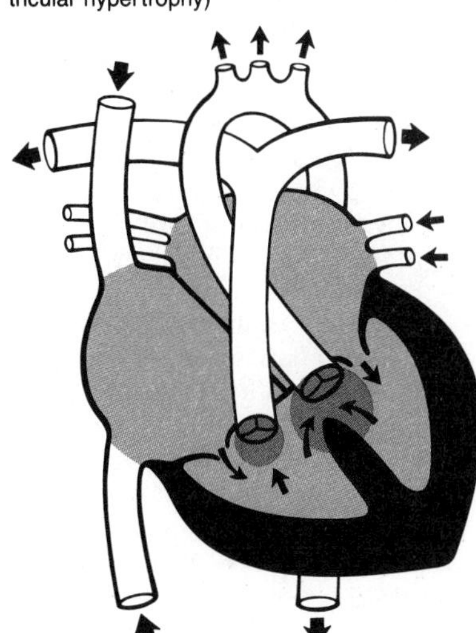

Circulatory effects
- Pulmonic stenosis restricts blood flow to lungs.
- Unoxygenated blood is shunted through the ventricular septal defect.
- Oxygenated and unoxygenated blood is mixed in the left ventricle and pumped out the aorta.

Clinical situation
- Single S_2 systolic murmur loudest in second and third intercostal spaces at left sternal border.
- Infant has intense cyanosis and severe dyspnea on exertion, and is limp.
- If untreated, may be fatal.

during respiration or that changes paradoxically is abnormal.

So-called innocent murmurs (functional murmurs) are those which don't reflect underlying pathology. Usually such a murmur is Grade I or Grade II early systolic, without transmission, and you'll hear it at the pulmonic area. Some organic murmurs have the same characteristics as innocent ones, so until you have considerable experience, refer every child with a murmur to a doctor for further evaluation.

404 Childhood heart problems

The two primary cardiac conditions of childhood are congenital heart problems and rheumatic fever (see *Identifying Common Congenital Heart Defects,* pages 376 to 379). Of every 1,000 full-term infants, 5 to 8 experience congenital heart problems, and this rate increases two to three times in premature infants. Neonates suffer the highest morbidity and mortality from congenital conditions—most deaths occur during the first week of life. Early detection and surgery could prevent at least 50% of these deaths.

The most common congenital cardiac conditions include atrial and ventricular septal defects, patent ductus arteriosus, tetralogy of Fallot, coarctation of the aorta, aortic stenosis, pulmonic stenosis, and transposition of the great vessels. Rheumatic fever (a complication of Group A streptococcal infection), unlike these conditions, most commonly strikes children between ages 5 and 15. Children in this age-group should always be given a thorough cardiac examination 2 weeks after a streptococcal infection.

Assessing geriatric patients

405 Cardiovascular changes in the elderly

As a person ages, his heart usually becomes smaller. Exceptions to this rule are persons suffering from hypertension or heart disease. By age 70, cardiac output at rest has decreased by about 35% in many persons. Fibrotic and sclerotic changes thicken heart valves and reduce their flexibility, sometimes causing a heart murmur. The elderly may also develop obstructive coronary disease and fibrosis of the cardiac skeleton. The heart's ability to respond to physical and emotional stress may decrease markedly with age. Usually, aging also contributes to arterial and venous insufficiency as the strength and elasticity of blood vessels decrease. All these factors contribute to elderly persons' increased incidence of cardiovascular disease; coronary disease is most common.

406 Geriatric history questions

As you begin the interview, assess your patient's *level of consciousness,* noting confusion or slowed mental status—occasionally, these are early signs of inadequate cardiac output. Remember that poor memory and generalized cerebral atherosclerosis may make it difficult for your patient to understand and respond to your questions.

Ask your elderly patient about *chest pain,* which could be interpreted as angina pectoris. Remember, however, that his chief complaint may be dyspnea or palpitations rather than chest pain, because although aging contributes to coronary artery plaque development, it also promotes collateral circulation to areas deprived of perfusion. Also keep in mind that these signs and symptoms in the elderly may indicate pathology in many systems other than cardiovascular, including the urinary, endocrine, musculoskeletal, and respiratory systems.

Ask your patient about his *activities of daily living,* any signs or symptoms

SELECTED CAUSES OF SECONDARY HYPERTENSION

BODY SYSTEM	DISORDERS
Urinary	
vascular	• Renal artery stenosis or occlusion
parenchymal	• Chronic glomerulonephritis, chronic interstitial nephritis, polycystic kidney disease
Endocrine	
adrenal	• Pheochromocytoma, Cushing's syndrome, hyperaldosteronism
pituitary	• Tumor, acromegaly
pancreas	• Uncontrolled diabetes mellitus
Cardio-vascular	• Coarctation of the aorta, increased intravascular volume
Miscellaneous	• Toxemia, oral contraceptives, hypercalcemia, increased intracranial pressure

associated with these activities, and his response to physical and emotional exertion. Reduced cardiac reserve limits the elderly patient's ability to respond to such conditions as infection, blood loss, hypoxia-induced arrhythmias, and electrolyte imbalance. Combine the information on your patient's daily activities with your assessment of his mental status, and try to correlate these signs and symptoms with any eating and sleeping difficulties he has.

Determine if the patient has a history of smoking, frequent coughing, wheezing, or dyspnea, which may indicate *chronic lung disease.* Pulmonary hypertension resulting from pulmonary disease is a chief cause of right-sided heart failure.

Ask, too, about *medication side effects.* Weakness, bradycardia, hypotension, and confusion may indicate elevated potassium levels; weakness, fatigue, muscle cramps, and palpitations may indicate inadequate levels of potassium. A patient's anorexia, nausea, vomiting, diarrhea, headache, rash, vision disturbances, and mental confusion may indicate an overdose of digitalis or antiarrhythmic medications.

407 Physical examination guidelines

In an elderly patient who may have *chronic lung disease,* check for evidence of cor pulmonale and advanced right-sided congestive heart failure: large, distended neck veins; hepatomegaly with tenderness; hepatojugular reflux; and peripheral dependent edema. Check, too, for evidence of chronic obstructive pulmonary disease (see *Nurse's Guide to Respiratory Disorders,* pages 304 to 311).

Carefully assess your elderly patient for signs and symptoms associated with *cerebral hypoperfusion*—such as dizziness, syncope, confusion or loss of consciousness, unilateral weakness or numbness, aphasia, and occasionally slight clonic, jerking movements. Cerebral hypoperfusion may result in transient ischemic attacks caused by cerebrovascular spasm, carotid stenosis, microembolic phenomena, or transient bradyarrhythmias resulting from degenerative disease of the heart's conduction system (Stokes-Adams attack). Check the carotid artery or femoral pulse when these signs and symptoms occur to help you differentiate between

HOW PROLONGED HYPERTENSION AFFECTS THE BODY

BODY SYSTEM	ASSOCIATED SIGN/SYMPTOMS	POSSIBLE CONDITIONS
Cardiorespiratory system	• Cough	• May be associated with early left heart failure
	• Chest pain	• May be associated with coronary artery insufficiency
	• Shortness of breath, paroxysmal nocturnal dyspnea, and orthopnea	• Left ventricular failure
	• Wheezing	• May be associated with congestive heart failure (CHF), asthma, and chronic obstructive pulmonary disease with bronchospasm
	• Edema	• May be associated with CHF, renal disease, or cirrhosis
Central nervous system	• Visual disturbances, numbness, tingling, and dizziness	• May be secondary to transient ischemia of cerebral tissue
	• Weakness, paralysis, and incontinence	• May be secondary to cerebrovascular accident
Genitourinary system	• Hematuria	• May be associated with renal involvement
	• Nocturia	• May be associated with edema, chronic renal insufficiency, or a partial obstruction; may also be an early sign of congestive heart failure

Adapted from Linda Pearson and M. Ernestine Kotthaff, *Geriatric Clinical Protocols* (New York: Lippincott/Harper & Row, 1979), with permission of the publisher.

transient ischemic attacks and Stokes-Adams attack. An extremely slow or absent pulse followed by rapid return of consciousness and a slightly increased or normal heart rate may indicate Stokes-Adams attack.

Record baseline blood pressures bilaterally and use them carefully to determine if pressures are consistently above 150 mmHg systolic. Because aging causes a person's arterial walls to thicken and lose elasticity, readings—especially systolic readings—may be higher than normal.

Measure the patient's heart rate for 60 seconds, apically and radially. (Remember that as a person ages, increased vagal tone slows the heartbeat.) If the apical rate is below 50 beats/minute in a hospitalized patient, monitor his vital signs frequently. Determine if the patient has palpitations or symptoms of inadequate cardiac output.

When palpating the carotid pulse, be alert for hyperkinetic pulses and bruits over the carotids, which are common in older patients with advanced arteriosclerosis.

Kyphosis and scoliosis, common in the elderly, distort the chest walls and may displace the heart slightly. Thus, your patient's apical impulse and heart sounds may be slightly displaced. According to some authorities, S_4 sound is common in the elderly population and results from decreased left ventricular compliance. Diastolic murmurs indicate pathology; soft, early systolic murmurs may be associated with normal aortic lengthening, tortuosity, or sclerotic changes and may not indicate serious pathology. Check for signs of peripheral arterial insufficiency (see *Nurse's Guide to Cardiovascular Conditions,* pages 360 to 371).

Selected References

Adler, Jack. "The Arterial Pulse," *American Journal of Nursing* 79:116, January 1979.

Alexander, Mary M., and Brown, Marie S. *Pediatric History Taking and Physical Diagnosis for Nurses,* 2nd ed. New York: McGraw-Hill Book Co., 1979.

Andreoli, Kathleen, et al. *Comprehensive Cardiac Care: A Text for Nurses, Physicians & Other Health Practitioners,* 4th ed. St. Louis: C.V. Mosby Co., 1979.

Bates, Barbara. "The Heart," in *A Guide to Physical Examination,* 2nd ed. Philadelphia: J.B. Lippincott Co., 1979.

Beeson, Paul B., et al. *Cecil Textbook of Medicine,* 2 vols., 15th ed. Philadelphia: W.B. Saunders Co., 1979.

Braunwald, Eugene. *Heart Disease: A Textbook of Cardiovascular Medicine.* Philadelphia: W.B. Saunders Co., 1980.

Burns, Kenneth R., and Johnson, Patricia J. *Health Assessment in Clinical Practice.* Englewood Cliffs, N.J.: Prentice-Hall, Inc., 1980.

Carotenuto, Rosine, and Bullock, John. *Physical Assessment of the Gerontologic Client.* Philadelphia: F.A. Davis Co., 1981.

Conover, Mary H. *Cardiac Arrhythmias: Exercises in Pattern Interpretation,* 2nd ed. St. Louis: C.V. Mosby Co., 1978.

Conover, Mary H. *Understanding Electrocardiography: Physiological and Interpretive Concepts,* 3rd ed. St. Louis: C.V. Mosby Co., 1980.

Daily, Elaine K., and Schroeder, John. *Techniques in Bedside Hemodynamic Monitoring,* 2nd ed. St. Louis: C.V. Mosby Co., 1980.

DeGowin, Elmer L., and DeGowin, Richard L. *Bedside Diagnostic Examination,* 3rd ed. New York: Macmillan Publishing Co., 1976.

Doyle, Jeanne. "If Your Legs Hurt the Reason May Be Arterial Insufficiency," *Nursing81* 11:74, April 1981.

Fowler, Noble O., ed. *Cardiac Diagnosis and Treatment,* 3rd ed. Philadelphia: Harper & Row, 1980.

Gillies, Dee A., and Alyn, Irene. *Patient Assessment and Management by the Nurse Practitioner.* Philadelphia: W.B. Saunders Co., 1976.

Harrison's Principles of Internal Medicine. New York: McGraw-Hill Book Co., 1980.

Humbrecht, Barbara, and Van Parys, Eileen. "From Assessment to Intervention: How to Use Heart and Breath Sounds as Part of Your Nursing Care Plan," *Nursing82* 12:34, April 1982.

Hurst, J.W., ed. *The Heart,* 4th ed. New York: McGraw-Hill Book Co., 1978.

Jackle, Mary, and Halligan, Marney. *Cardiovascular Problems: A Critical Care Nursing Focus.* Bowie, Md.: Robert J. Brady Co., 1980.

Jarvis, Carolyn Mueller. "Perfecting Physical Assessment: Part 2," *Nursing77* 7:38, June 1977.

Malasanos, Lois, et al. *Health Assessment,* 2nd ed. St. Louis: C.V. Mosby Co., 1981.

"Patient Assessment: Pulses-Section 1, The Arterial Pulse," *American Journal of Nursing* 79:115, January 1979.

Ritota, Michael. *Diagnostic Electrocardiography,* 2nd ed. Philadelphia: J.B. Lippincott Co., 1977.

Rogers, William J. "Current Concepts in Evaluation of Coronary Artery Disease," *Hospital Medicine,* March 1980.

Thompson, June M., and Bowers, Arden C. *Clinical Manual of Health Assessment.* St. Louis: C.V. Mosby Co., 1980.

Tilikian, Ara G., and Conover, Mary B. *Understanding Heart Sounds and Murmurs.* Philadelphia: W.B. Saunders Co., 1979.

Vandenhbelt, Ronald J., et al. "Cardiology—A Clinical Approach." Chicago: Year Book Medical Publishing, 1979.

Visich, Mary Ann. "Knowing What You Hear: A Guide to Assessing Breath and Heart Sounds," *Nursing81* 11:64, November 1981.

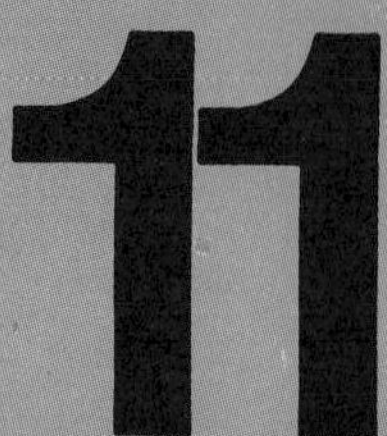

KEY POINTS IN THIS CHAPTER

KEY CHARTS IN THIS CHAPTER

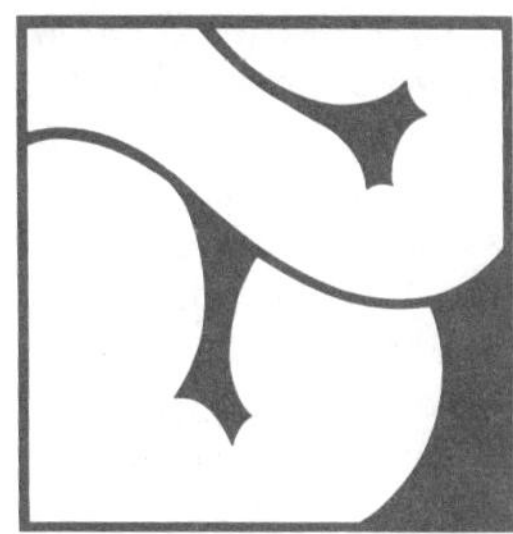

Gastrointestinal System

Introduction

408 Why assess the GI system?

The gastrointestinal (GI) system fuels the body, through the processes of ingestion, digestion, and absorption, and removes body wastes, through the process of elimination. Problems in the GI tract can have far-reaching metabolic implications for your patient. For example, dental caries or periodontal disease may affect a nutritionally deficient patient's ability to eat, exacerbating his nutritional problems and prolonging his recovery. Vomiting and diarrhea, if untreated, may cause acid-base imbalance. Bleeding from the GI tract may result in severe anemia.

The GI system often mirrors abnormal conditions in other systems. For example, gingival lesions that are infected and bleeding may accompany leukemia or uncontrolled diabetes. Projectile vomiting may result from a central nervous system disorder.

GI assessment may reveal a patient's need for preventive health teaching. You'll probably assess many patients who need to establish good bowel habits, others who need oral hygiene, and still others who need to eat a more nourishing diet.

GI assessment also lets you identify a patient's oral appliance, dentures, or bridges, so you can remove them before such procedures as intubation and suctioning—and prevent him from aspirating, choking on, or swallowing the appliance.

409 GI assessment: Three examinations

Comprehensive assessment of the gastrointestinal (GI) system requires that you perform oral, abdominal, and rectal examinations.

Perhaps because oral examination is a simple assessment procedure, it's often overlooked as part of a GI assessment. Yet, you may be the first to detect an oral lesion and refer the patient for early diagnosis and treatment.

Mastering abdominal assessment presents a real challenge. The abdomen contains most of the GI system: the lower end of the esophagus, the entire stomach, and the small and large intestines. It also contains parts of other body systems—the urinary, reproductive, cardiovascular, nervous, and blood-forming and immune systems, for example. In fact, only the respiratory system lies completely outside the abdomen—yet a distended abdomen certainly affects breathing. You can see, then, how you may encounter many abdominal signs and symptoms during assessment—and the myriad implications they might have. Differentiating among so many possible signs and symptoms is a nursing challenge.

You may complete your GI assessment with a rectal examination, which helps detect hemorrhoids, furnishes clues to possible rectal cancer, and allows you to evaluate adjacent reproductive organs for abnormalities. Because this part of the assessment is usually physically uncomfortable and emotionally distressing to the patient, you'll probably want to perform this examination last.

410 Your role in GI assessment

What do the following patients have in common?

- the elderly patient who has suffered a fractured hip and frequently becomes constipated
- the infant who's vomiting formula and losing weight
- the alcoholic who begins to vomit bright-red blood
- the hospitalized patient who's eating little or no food
- the patient who's experiencing severe nausea and vomiting during chemotherapy.

All these patients need gastrointestinal (GI) assessment. In fact, no matter which type of patient you care for, you'll use GI assessment frequently. Chief complaints related to the GI system are typically vague. Some patients with GI problems let seemingly innocuous symptoms go unattended; others report no symptoms at all. If you're a medical nurse, you've probably heard many patients dismiss their symptoms by saying, "Oh, it's only indigestion." Sometimes, though, the indigestion turns out to be a cardiac problem or has some other important medical significance. If you're a surgical nurse, you'll suspect that "I feel so full" may mean the patient has a distended bladder or bowel. Oral or rectal problems may be easier for you to recognize, although many patients neglect to report them because of fear, embarrassment, or lack of knowledge.

GI assessment helps you sort out abdominal complaints and sheds light on your patient's problem. Information gained through GI assessment can also help you monitor your patient's therapy, allowing you to identify any adverse developments, and providing a data base for your assessment of future patients.

Remember to reassess the patient with a GI complaint every time he experiences the problem. Don't assume his current abdominal pains are caused by previously diagnosed gallstones, for example. The nature and location of the pains may have changed, and they may signal a different problem.

Reviewing anatomy and physiology

411 Mouth: Structures and functions

The mouth is bounded anteriorly by the lips and posteriorly by the soft palate and base of the tongue. The superior plane is formed by the antral sinuses and floor of the nose, the inferior margin by the submandibular glands and the mylohyoid muscle.

The mouth's nonmovable upper jaw is called the *maxilla*. Its movable lower jaw, the *mandible*, attaches to the temporal bone, just anterior to the tragus of the ear at the temporomandibular joint. The muscles of mastication provide the motor activity for the temporomandibular joint and the jaws.

Normally, an adult has 32 permanent teeth, which begin forming during the first 6 months of neonatal life and start erupting at about age 6. *Teeth* consist of three types of mineralized tissue, surrounding an innervated and vascularized central pulp. The *alveolar bone* supports the teeth.

The *gingiva* (gums) are made up of stratified squamous mucosa. The gin-

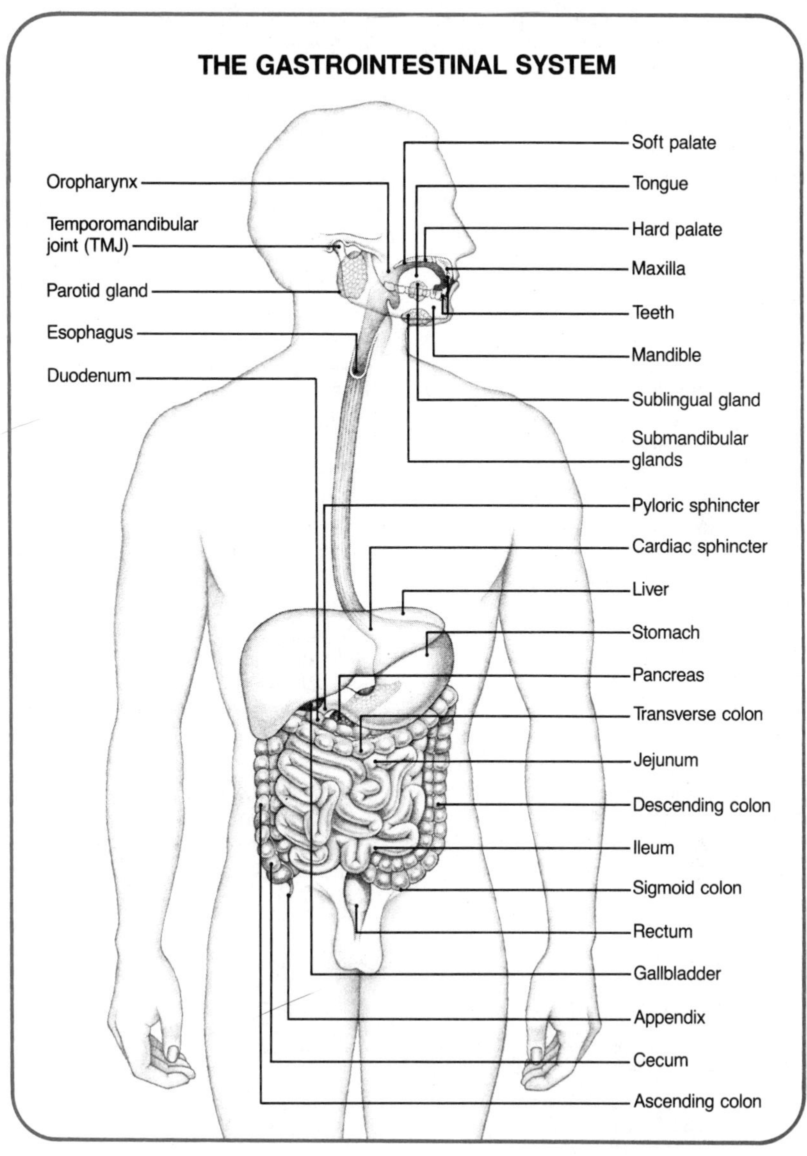

gival mucosa continues above the level of the bone and surrounds each tooth crown as free gingiva, supported by connective tissue. The *tongue* is a muscular organ coated on its dorsal surface by a keratinized, papilliferous mucosa. Smooth, flat, nonkeratinized pink mucosa covers its ventral aspect. All tongue mucosa contain minor salivary glands.

Many other areas of the mouth are covered with mucosa—the hard and soft palates, the floor of the mouth, the uvula, and the vestibular trough that attaches the labial and buccal mucosa to the alveolar mucosa.

The *oropharynx* comprises the soft palate, the uvula, the anterior pillars, and the tonsils and posterior pillars that make up the posterior pharynx.

In addition to minor salivary glands, three major pairs of salivary glands (the *parotid, submandibular,* and *sublingual glands*) provide more than half the volume of saliva—a colorless, hypotonic fluid.

The *lips* are muscular structures that are extremely sensitive because of innervation by many nerve fibers from the trigeminal nerve.

The mouth has many vital functions. The tongue, teeth, and lips modify sound for speech. The mouth also initiates the digestive process and salivary lubrication through mastication and hydrolysis of starches. It then delivers food to the digestive tract through swallowing. Its mucous membranes serve as a physical defense; its salivary secretions serve as an antimicrobial defense. Finally, the mouth is the medium for sensory response to taste.

412 Esophagus

The esophagus is a muscular tube that propels food from the pharynx to the stomach's cardiac sphincter. About 9″ (23 cm) long, the esophagus extends from the level of the sixth cervical vertebra to that of the eleventh thoracic vertebra.

413 Diaphragm

This domed musculotendinous sheet separates the thoracic and abdominal cavities. The phrenic nerve, which starts in the neck and courses through the thorax along the pericardium's lateral surfaces, supplies innervation. Because of the phrenic nerve's high origin, pain from the diaphragm is commonly referred to the posterior neck and shoulders.

414 Abdomen

The abdomen extends from the diaphragm superiorly to the inlet of the true pelvis inferiorly. Besides gastrointestinal organs, it contains the kidneys and ureters, the suprarenal glands, and the blood vessels, nerves, and lymphatics. The abdominal contents are partially protected superiorly by the lower ribs, posteriorly by the lumbar vertebrae, and laterally by the iliac bones. The rest of the anterior, anterolateral, and posterior abdominal walls consist largely of muscles and tendons.

415 Stomach

The stomach is roughly J-shaped. It lies under the diaphragm, to the left of and

THE SALIVARY GLANDS

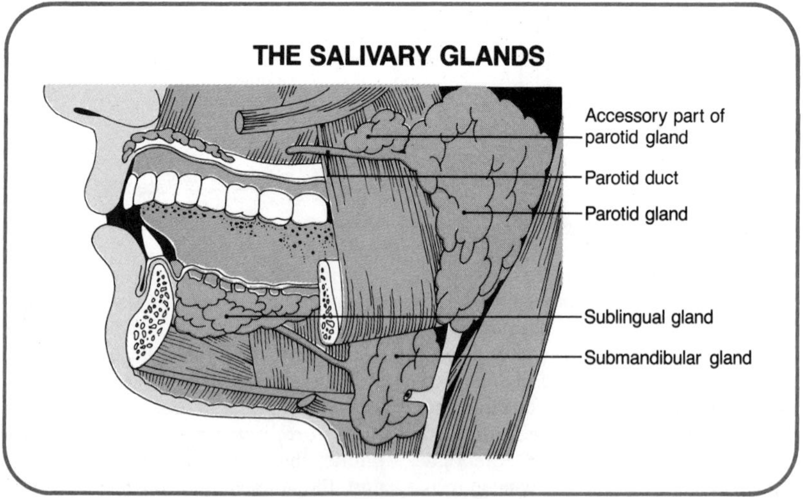

IDENTIFYING SURFACE LANDMARKS

To perform a thorough assessment of your patient, you'll need to know the surface abdominal landmarks illustrated here.

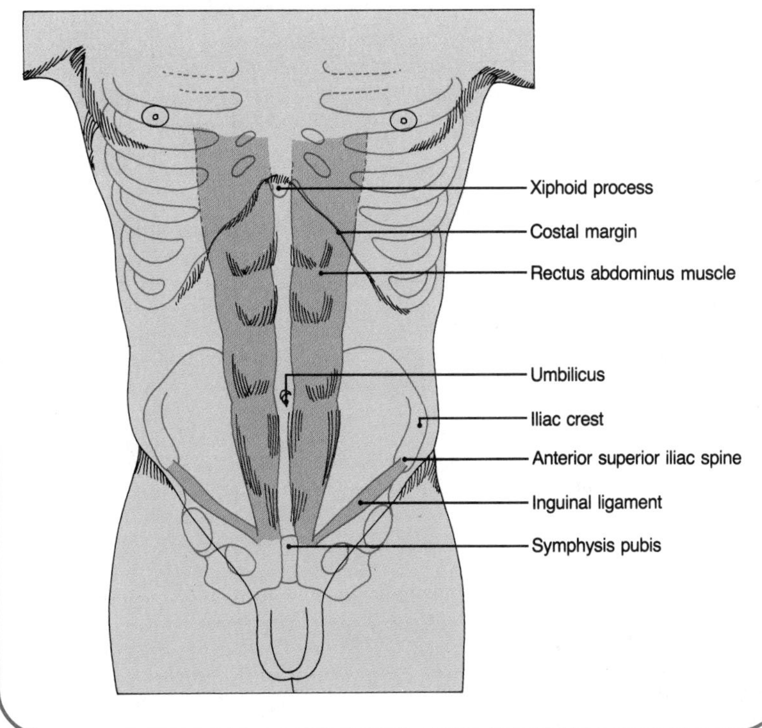

partially under the liver, to the right of the spleen, and in front of the pancreas. Mobile and easily displaced, when filled with food the stomach extends down to the second or third lumbar vertebra, slightly below the umbilicus. The cardiac sphincter opens at the esophageal entrance; the pyloric sphincter, at the duodenal entrance.

The stomach secretes gastric juices containing hydrochloric acid and enzymes. Together with the stomach's churning motion, these juices break food down into semisolid *chyme*. Serving as a reservoir, the stomach regulates the passage of chyme into the duodenum. (Hydrochloric acid kills most of the microbes in food.) The stomach's gastric mucosa can absorb small amounts of water, glucose, alcohol, and certain drugs.

416 Small intestine

The small intestine is about 21′ (6.4 m) long: the *duodenum* measures about 1′ (30.5 cm); the *jejunum*, about 8′ (2.4 m); and the *ileum*, the remaining 12′ (3.6 m). Highly mobile and quite active, the small intestine coils and loops through much of the abdominal cavity and part of the pelvic cavity.

The duodenum is a horseshoe-shaped organ, opening to the left. The pancreas lies in the concavity formed by the duodenum. Both the duodenum and pan-

LOCATING ABDOMINAL LANDMARKS: QUADRANT METHOD

As an aid to performing an abdominal assessment and recording your findings accurately, divide the patient's abdomen into quadrants, as shown in this illustration.

Memorize the shape, size, and location of all abdominal structures within each quadrant. Refer to these landmarks when you're performing your assessment.

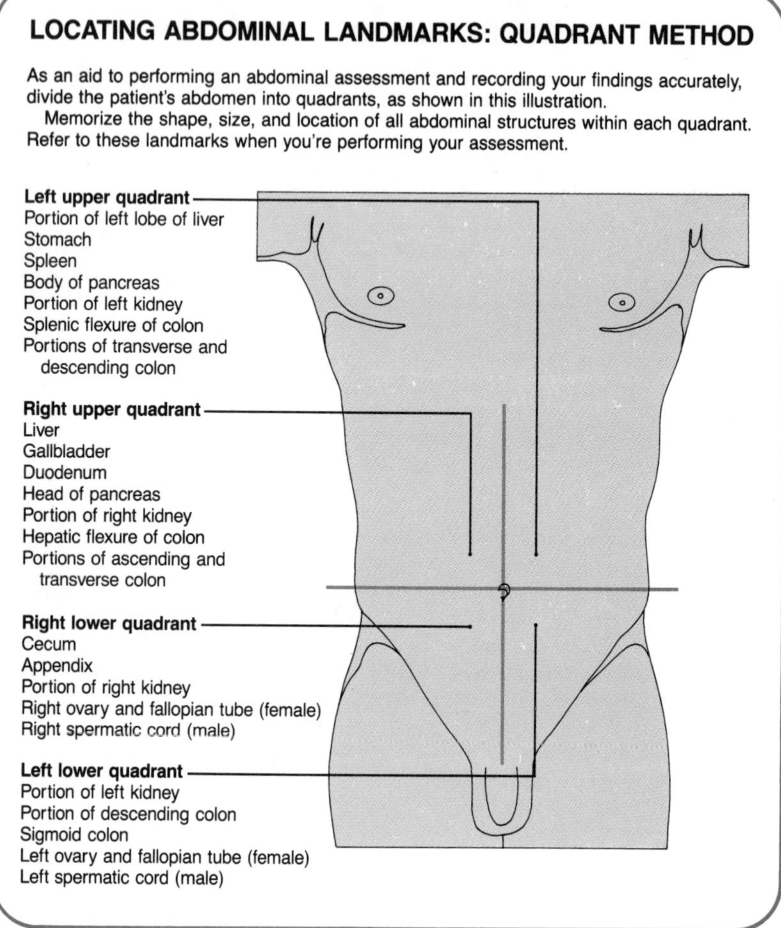

creas are located mainly behind the peritoneum. The duodenum enters the jejunum at the *duodenojejunal flexure,* in the left upper abdominal quadrant. Beyond this point, the mesentery's oblique attachment to the posterior abdominal wall forces the coils of the small intestine down and to the right. Most of the ileum, therefore, lies in the right lower quadrant.

The small intestine joins the large intestine at the *ileocecal valve,* near the right iliac fossa. Absorption and digestion take place mostly in the small intestine, where millions of villi increase the surface area. These villi control the absorption of carbohydrates, fat, and protein (see Entries 158 to 160).

417 Large intestine

The large intestine consists of the cecum; the ascending, transverse, descending, and sigmoid colons; and the rectum. Its primary functions are to absorb water and store feces. The rectum eventually excretes feces.

The *cecum,* a blind pouch, extends 3″ to 4″ (7.5 to 10 cm) below the ileocecal valve. The *appendix* opens into its inferomedian surface.

The *ascending colon* starts at the ileocecal valve and continues along the right side of the abdomen. It bends to the left at the *right colic flexure,* just in front of the right kidney.

The *transverse colon* runs obliquely across the abdominal cavity, usually paralleling the stomach's lower border. This portion of the colon is quite mobile, commonly occupying the lower quadrants of the abdominal cavity when the cavity is full. It meets the descending colon at the *left colic flexure.*

The *descending colon* starts just in front of the left kidney, approximately two vertebrae higher than the top of the ascending colon. It runs down the left side of the abdominal cavity to the *sigmoid colon,* which begins near the left iliac fossa. The sigmoid colon courses back in an S-shaped fashion near the pelvic brim and becomes the *rectum,* which descends and bends anteriorly along the back of the pelvic cavity, following the curve of the sacrum.

418 Peristalsis

Peristalsis is the involuntary process that propels food in waves through the esophagus, the stomach, and the intestines. Controlled mostly by vagus nerves, a peristaltic wave can travel the length of an organ or it can be a short, local reflex. The longitudinal layer of smooth muscle contracts first, followed by a brief contraction of the circular layer. Peristalsis can also result from the pressure of food or gas within the gastrointestinal (GI) tract.

Peristaltic waves in the stomach tend to mix its contents and move them into the duodenum. Waves occur at the rate of three per minute, and usually two or three waves are in progress at any

LOCATING ABDOMINAL LANDMARKS: NINE-REGIONS METHOD

This abdominal landmarks (nine-regions) method allows for more specific location identification than does the quadrant method.

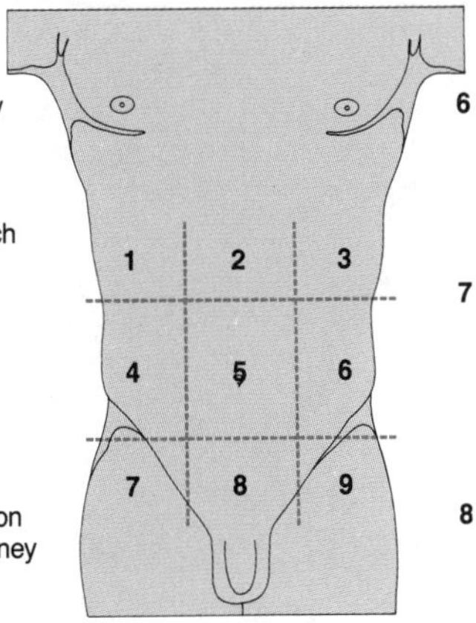

1 Right hypochondriac
- Right lobe of liver
- Gallbladder
- Portion of duodenum
- Hepatic flexure of colon
- Portion of right kidney
- Suprarenal gland

2 Epigastric
- Pyloric end of stomach
- Duodenum
- Pancreas
- Portion of liver

3 Left hypochondriac
- Stomach
- Spleen
- Tail of pancreas
- Splenic flexure of colon
- Upper pole of left kidney
- Suprarenal gland

4 Right lumbar
- Ascending colon
- Lower half of right kidney
- Portion of duodenum and jejunum

5 Umbilical
- Omentum
- Mesentery
- Lower part of duodenum
- Jejunum and ileum

6 Left lumbar
- Descending colon
- Lower half of left kidney
- Portions of jejunum and ileum

7 Right inguinal
- Cecum
- Appendix
- Lower end of ileum
- Right spermatic cord (male)
- Right ovary (female)

8 Hypogastric
- Ileum
- Bladder

9 Left inguinal
- Sigmoid colon
- Left spermatic cord (male)
- Left ovary (female)

one time throughout the GI tract. The waves in the small intestine are usually short and localized; they enhance absorption by bringing food into contact with the folded and villous mucosa, and they move food through the intestine. Peristaltic waves normally don't travel the extent of the small intestine.

In the large intestine, peristaltic waves do progress from one end to the other, propelling food and gas toward the rectum, usually at the rate of ½" to 1" (1 to 2 cm) per minute. Three or four times a day, much more powerful contractions move larger masses of waste material. Peristalsis also keeps bacteria moving along the walls of the large intestine, preventing the accumulation of harmful organisms. By moving gas toward the rectum, peristalsis helps prevent distention and pain.

419 Accessory organs

Accessory gastrointestinal (GI) organs (those that assist the digestive process but are not part of the GI tube) are the liver, gallbladder, and pancreas.

The *liver*, one of the largest organs in the body, lies under the thoracic cage, in the upper abdominal quadrants, covered superiorly by the diaphragm. About two thirds of the liver lies to the right of the midline. The liver is divided into large right and left lobes and smaller quadrate and caudate lobes.

The liver has many vital functions. It figures prominently in the metabolism of carbohydrates, producing and storing glycogen and metabolizing galactose. The liver also breaks down fat into glycerol and fatty acids and converts the fatty acids into small mole-

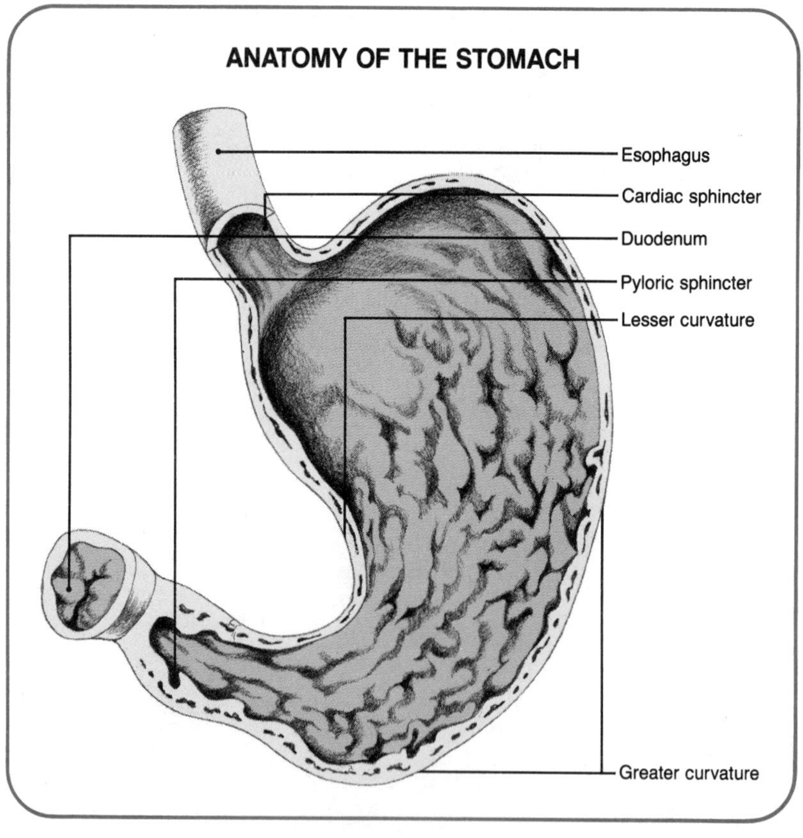

PERISTALSIS BEGINNINGS

Before peristalsis can begin, the neural pattern illustrated here must occur:

First, food pushed to the back of the mouth stimulates swallowing receptor areas that surround the pharyngeal opening. These receptor areas transmit impulses to the brain by way of the sensory portions of the trigeminal (V) and glossopharyngeal (IX) nerves. Then, the brain's swallowing center relays motor impulses to the esophagus by way of the trigeminal (V), glossopharyngeal (IX), vagus (X), and hypoglossal (XII) nerves, causing swallowing to occur.

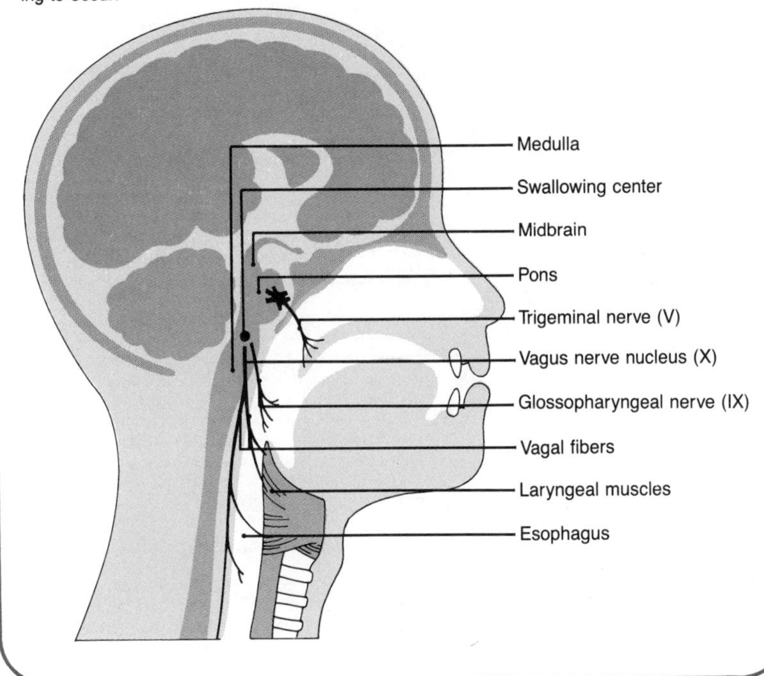

cules that can be oxidized. It deaminates amino acids and converts the resulting ammonia into urea. The liver also synthesizes plasma proteins—albumin, globulin, fibrinogen, and prothrombin—and nonessential amino acids. Lastly, the liver secretes bile, detoxifies harmful substances in plasma through the processes of inactivation and conjugation, forms vitamin A, and stores other essential nutrients (vitamins K, D, and B_{12} and iron).

The *gallbladder* lies just underneath the right lobe of the liver. About the size and shape of a small pear, the gallbladder stores bile until it's discharged into the biliary ductal system, which empties into the duodenum.

The *pancreas* lies horizontally behind the stomach. Its head is attached to the duodenum; its tail reaches the spleen. The pancreas serves as an exocrine gland, producing pancreatic juice that travels to the duodenum for use in digestion (see Entry 156). It also performs endocrine functions, releasing insulin and glycogen into circulation.

420 Autonomic nerves of the abdomen

The autonomic nerves of the abdomen consist of the *thoracic* and *lumbar splanchnic nerves* (sympathetic division) and the *vagus* and *pelvic splanch-*

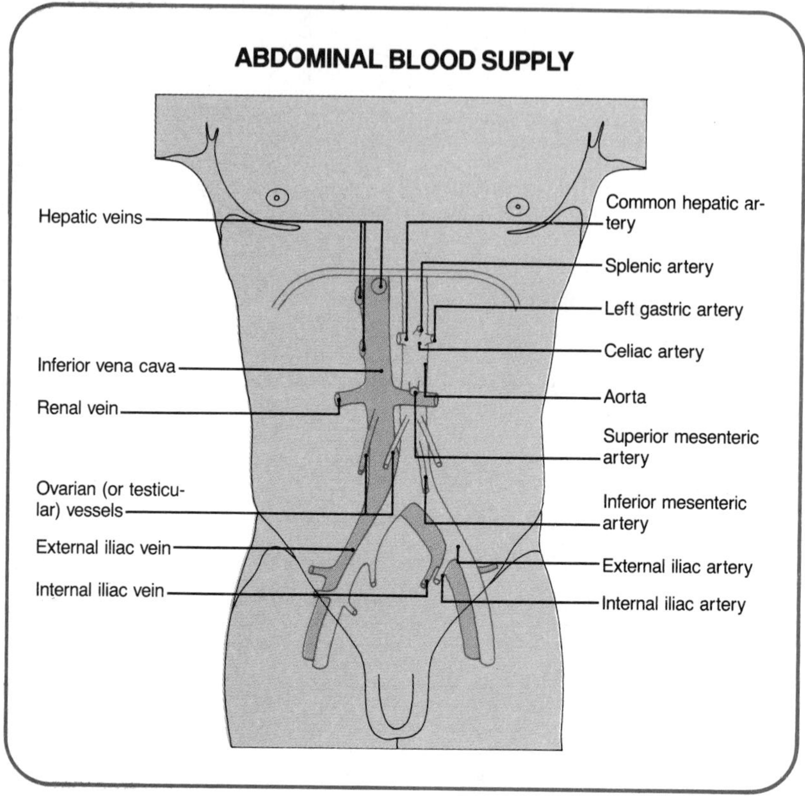

nic nerves (parasympathetic division). These form a number of plexuses that innervate the abdominal organs. Sympathetic impulses slow activity in the gastrointestinal (GI) tract, inhibit secretions, and contract sphincters. Parasympathetic impulses stimulate GI activity and secretions, and relax sphincters.

421 Abdominal vascularity

The *abdominal aorta* enters the abdomen at the level of the twelfth thoracic vertebra. After coursing slightly to the left of the vertebral column, it divides into the common iliac arteries at the fourth lumbar vertebra. In a thin person, the aorta may be palpable.

The *inferior vena cava* starts at the fourth or fifth lumbar vertebra and ascends in the abdomen, to the right of the aorta. The lumbar, renal, suprarenal, inferior phrenic, and hepatic veins empty into the vena cava, which leaves the abdomen through the diaphragm's central tendon, at the level of the eighth thoracic vertebra, and enters the heart's right atrium.

The union of the superior mesenteric veins and the splenic vein, joined by the inferior mesenteric in a variable fashion, forms the *portal vein.* The portal vein enters the liver and divides into sinusoids, which coalesce to eventually form the hepatic veins that enter the inferior vena cava.

422 Peritoneum

The peritoneum is a continuous serous membrane, lined with mesothelium. Its parietal layer lines the abdominal cavity; a visceral layer surrounds most of the abdominal organs. An organ surrounded by the peritoneum is called *intraperitoneal.* Such an organ is connected to the body wall or to other organs by double-walled layers of peritoneum known as *mesenteries* or *ligaments.* The mesenteries conduct blood vessels, nerves, and lymphatics to and from the viscera. An organ that lies behind the peritoneum and is covered only anteriorly, with no mesentery, is called *retroperitoneal.*

In men, the peritoneum forms a closed sac. In women, the fallopian tubes join the peritoneal cavity with the uterus. The peritoneum's slippery surface allows considerable mobility of certain organs, particularly the intestines.

423 Abdominal musculature

The anterolateral abdominal wall consists of three pairs of sheetlike muscles (*external* and *internal obliques* and the *transversis abdominis*) and a pair of bandlike muscles (*rectus abdominis*). In the posterior abdominal wall, the *psoas major* arises from the sides of the lumbar vertebrae and descends to meet the femur's lesser trochanter. The *iliacus,* which originates in the iliac fossa, joins the psoas major's lateral surface. The *psoas minor,* when present—only one out of two people has one—lies on the anterior surface of the psoas major. It probably assists in trunk flexion.

Collecting appropriate history data

424 Biographical data

Besides serving to identify your patient, biographical data—particularly age and sex—may indicate that your patient runs a greater risk of having certain gastrointestinal disorders. For example, more than 90% of oral cancer occurs in patients over age 45 (average age at onset is 60), and this disease affects twice as many men as women. Esophageal cancer occurs four times more frequently in men. Rectal cancer occurs most frequently in men between ages 50 and 60. Ulcerative colitis occurs primarily in young adult women. Diverticular disease is most prevalent in men over age 40.

425 Chief complaint

The most common chief complaints associated with gastrointestinal disorders are *pain, dysphagia, nausea, vomiting, diarrhea,* and *constipation.*

426 History of present illness

Using the PQRST mnemonic device (see *PQRST,* page 396), ask your patient to elaborate on his chief complaint. Then, depending on the complaint, explore the history of his present illness by asking the following types of questions:

• ***Pain.*** *What does the pain feel like? What symptoms accompany the pain?* Fever, malaise, nausea, vomiting, warmth, redness, and swelling (such as in the mouth) may indicate viral infection or inflammation of the gastrointestinal (GI) tract. If the patient has painful mouth ulcerations, ask if he notices any relation between exacerbation of symptoms and stress, food, change of seasons, or other factors. Aphthous ulcers are sometimes associated with these factors.

Do you have heartburn or dyspepsia? These conditions usually occur after eating certain spicy foods that produce excess acid in the stomach; dyspepsia may also occur with hiatal hernia or as a side effect of certain medications (such as salicylates), or it can reflect more serious GI disorders, such as cancer. If the patient has abdominal pain, ask about the relationship of the pain to meals. Peptic ulcer pain usually occurs about 2 hours after meals or whenever the stomach is empty; it may wake the patient at night. Arterial insufficiency to the bowel usually causes pain 15 to 30 minutes after meals and lasts up to 3 hours.

Have your bowel elimination patterns changed recently? When did you last have a bowel movement? Can you pass flatus? Does your abdomen feel distended? Your patient's answers may give clues to inflammatory or obstructive bowel disorders.

Do you have rectal discomfort? This type of pain can indicate local problems, such as pain from a large, hard stool that has torn the mucosa; inflammation from infections; and pain associated with hemorrhoids.

• ***Dysphagia.*** *When, during swallowing, do you feel discomfort? Does it occur between your mouth and esophagus? In the esophagus? Between the esophagus and stomach?* Asking the patient to point to the area of discomfort is important, because certain disorders affect specific points in the swallowing process. *Does the dysphagia result from ingesting solid food, or both solids and liquids? Did you have symptoms of reflux prior to the onset of dysphagia?* Dysphagia usually results from mechanical obstruction or loss of motor coordination. Because cancer is an important cause of mechanical obstruction, ask if the patient has experienced marked weight loss. Neurologic disease can cause loss of motor coordination, so ask about additional symptoms, such as dysarthria.

• ***Nausea and vomiting.*** *Do you feel nauseated before you vomit? Is the vomiting projectile?* Projectile vomiting often indicates central nervous system disorders. *Does the vomitus have an unusual odor?* A fecal odor, for example, usually indicates a small bowel obstruction. *Is the symptom related to a specific time period?* Pregnancy, metabolic disturbances, and excessive consumption of alcohol can cause early-morning vomiting. *Have you been emotionally upset recently? Have you vomited blood?* Hematemesis may reflect a GI disorder, such as severe esophagitis, or disorders outside the GI system, such as anticoagulant toxicity.

• ***Diarrhea.*** Ask about the frequency and consistency of the patient's bowel movements. *Have you been under emotional stress lately?* Psychogenic fac-

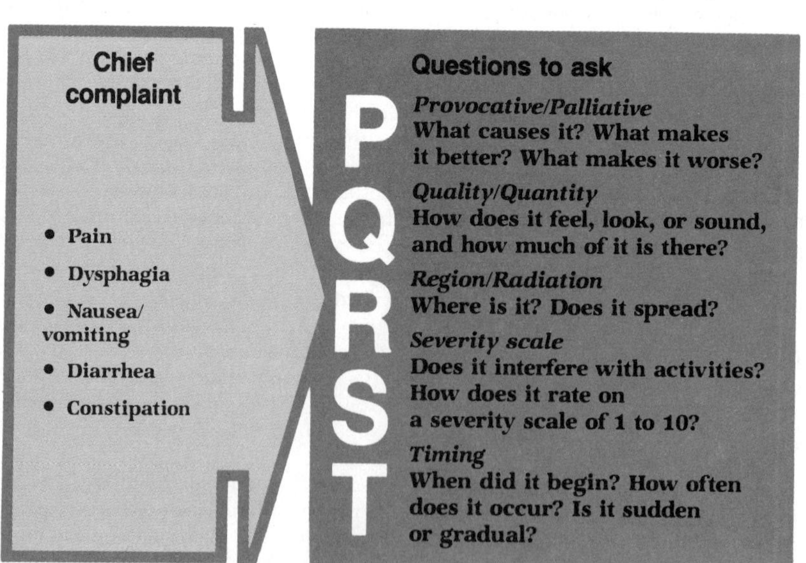

UNDERSTANDING REFERRED PAIN

Here's how referred pain occurs: Pain that's produced by an organ supplied with efferent nerves for pain from the same spinal cord segments supplying body walls and limbs is often felt on the surface. This pain may occur relatively near the affected organ or at some distance from it. Organ pain usually occurs more diffusely than surface pain. This chart identifies the areas to which organ pain is referred:

ORGAN	REFERRED PAIN AREA
Gallbladder	• Right upper quadrant • Right posterior infrascapular area
Diaphragm	• Posterior neck • Posterior shoulder area
Duodenum	• *Most commonly:* midline of the abdominal wall, just above the umbilicus
Appendix	• Umbilicus • Parietal peritoneal involvement, right lower quadrant
Ureter	• Inguinal region • Loin

tors may affect bowel motility. *What particular foods did you eat before the diarrhea's onset?* Food poisoning (such as from custard-filled pastries and processed meats contaminated by staphylococci) may cause diarrhea, usually accompanied by abdominal cramping and vomiting. Fever, tenesmus, and cramping pain associated with diarrhea usually indicate an infection, most commonly viral. *Is the stool bloody?* This may be from an inflammation or a neoplasm involving the bowel wall. *Is the stool foul-smelling, bulky, and greasy?* This suggests a fat malabsorption problem. Passage of mucus suggests irritable colon. *Do periods of diarrhea alternate with periods of constipation?* This combination may be associated with irritable colon, diverticulitis, or colorectal cancer.

• ***Constipation.*** *How would you describe the size, character, and frequency of your bowel movements?* Many patients mistakenly claim to have constipation, so always ask this type of question to determine if constipation exists. *What is your typical daily diet like?* The absence of fiber in the diet (or inadequate fluid intake) may lead to constipation. Laxative abuse, decreased physical activity, and emotional stress may also produce this symptom. *Do you experience cramping abdominal pain and distention related to the constipation?* These symptoms suggest mechanical obstruction, such as from stricture or tumor. Find out if the problem is acute—in which case it's more likely to have an organic cause—or chronic, which is commonly caused by a functional problem.

427 Past history

Explore the following relevant areas when taking your patient's past history:

• ***Gastrointestinal (GI) disorders.*** Long-term GI conditions, such as chronic ulcerative colitis or GI polyposis, may predispose a patient to colorectal cancer.

• ***Neurologic disorders.*** Such conditions as cerebrovascular accident, myasthenia gravis, amyotrophic lateral sclerosis, and peripheral nerve damage may cause GI disorders. For example, these conditions can impair movement of the tongue, the uvula, the larynx, or the pharynx, which can lead to drooling, dysarthria, and difficulty chewing or swallowing.

• ***Other major disorders.*** Gastrointestinal signs and symptoms may also result from pathologic conditions in other body systems. A patient with chronic obstructive pulmonary disease may be constipated from weakness of the diaphragm and decreased strength to defecate. Endocrine disorders, such as hypothyroidism and diabetes mellitus with neuromuscular dysfunction, may also predispose a patient to constipation. Diabetes mellitus may predispose the patient to oral candidal infections.

• ***Previous abdominal surgery or trauma.*** Intestinal adhesions may result from trauma, inflammation, or previous abdominal surgery. These adhesions may produce pain or intestinal obstruction. Even such a relatively simple procedure as oral surgery may cause infection or bleeding. A fractured jaw may result in malocclusion.

• ***Allergies.*** Allergic reactions to certain foods and medications can produce a variety of GI complaints, such as pain, nausea, and diarrhea. Check especially to see if the patient is hypersensitive to penicillin, sulfonamides, or local anesthetics (such as procaine or tetracaine), which can lead to severe allergic symptoms affecting GI mucous membranes. Also ask the patient about hypersensitivity to lipsticks, toothpastes, or mouthwashes, which may cause symptoms on contact.

• ***Chronic laxative use.*** Laxatives, including mineral oil and stool softeners, affect intestinal motility. Habitual use of laxatives may cause constipation (from insensitive defecatory reflexes).

• ***Medications.*** Anti-infectives, cytotoxic drugs, and many other drugs can produce various GI side effects, such as oral ulceration, nausea, vomiting, diarrhea, or constipation (see *Nurse's Guide to Some Drugs That Affect the Gastrointestinal System*).

428 Family history

Ask the patient if anyone in his family has ever had colorectal cancer or gastrointestinal (GI) polyposis. A family history of either disorder increases the patient's chances of developing colorectal cancer. GI symptoms may also result from diabetes mellitus, which can have a genetic basis.

429 Psychosocial history

To review your patient's psychosocial history, question him first about how his chief complaint is disturbing him. Then ask about his occupation. A sedentary occupation can contribute to constipation; a highly stressful job can lead to many gastrointestinal (GI) symptoms. An occupation that necessitates exposure to toxic substances can also cause GI disorders. For example, chronic lead or bismuth poisoning usually produces a blue-black or slate gray line next to the gingival crest.

Emotional problems can contribute significantly to GI symptoms—for example, pain, dyspepsia, nausea, anorexia, gluttony, or more idiosyncratic tendencies, such as cheek-biting.

Also pertinent in your patient's psychosocial history are financial problems, which may prevent him from seeking proper dental or medical care or from eating an adequate diet. In addition, financial worries contribute to stress-related GI symptoms. Odontophobia (an exaggerated fear of going to the dentist) may cause the patient to delay treatment for dental problems.

430 Activities of daily living

Explore the following aspects of your patient's daily life when investigating a gastrointestinal (GI) complaint:

• ***Oral hygiene.*** Ask your patient to describe his oral hygiene routine for a typical day. Note if he mentions using a toothbrush, dental floss, or gingival stimulants, but don't bias the patient's answers by naming these items in your

DRUGS

NURSE'S GUIDE TO SOME DRUGS THAT AFFECT THE GASTROINTESTINAL SYSTEM

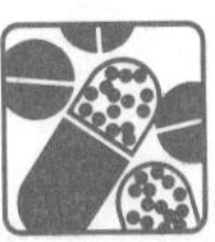

CLASSIFICATION	POSSIBLE SIDE EFFECTS
Analgesics	
aspirin	• Nausea, vomiting, GI distress, occult bleeding
indomethacin (Indocin)	• Nausea, vomiting, diarrhea, hemorrhage
phenazopyridine (Pyridium*)	• Nausea
phenylbutazone (Butazolidin*)	• Peptic ulceration or hemorrhage, nausea, vomiting
Antifungals	
griseofulvin (Fulvicin-U/F*, Fulvicin P/G)	• Nausea, vomiting, diarrhea, flatulence
Antidiabetics	
chlorpropamide (Diabinese*)	• Cholestatic jaundice, heartburn
Anti-infectives	
gentian violet	• Oral ulceration, nausea, vomiting
sulfonamides	• Nausea, vomiting, diarrhea, abdominal pain
tetracycline (Achromycin*)	• Tooth discoloration, nausea, vomiting, diarrhea, stomatitis
Antiarrhythmics	
isoproterenol (Isuprel*)	• Nausea, vomiting
phenytoin sodium (Dilantin*)	• Nausea, vomiting, gingival hyperplasia, constipation
Amebicides	
metronidazole (Flagyl*)	• Taste disturbances, abdominal cramping, diarrhea, vomiting
General anesthetics	
halothane	• Diffuse hepatocellular damage
Antihypertensives	
clonidine (Catapres*)	• Swelling of salivary glands, constipation
guanethidine sulfate (Ismelin*)	• Swelling of salivary glands, diarrhea
methyldopa (Aldomet*)	• Dry mouth, diarrhea, hepatic necrosis
reserpine (Serpasil*)	• Hyperacidity, nausea, vomiting
Hematinics	
ferrous sulfate (Fer-In-Sol*)	• Constipation, nausea, vomiting, black stools
Antineoplastics	
methotrexate	• Nausea, vomiting, diarrhea, stomatitis
vincristine	• Nausea, vomiting, stomatitis

(continued)

NURSE'S GUIDE TO SOME DRUGS THAT AFFECT THE GASTROINTESTINAL SYSTEM *(continued)*

CLASSIFICATION	POSSIBLE SIDE EFFECTS
Hypnotics	
secobarbital sodium (Seconal)	• Nausea, vomiting
Heavy metal antagonists	
dimercaprol (BAL in Oil)	• Halitosis, nausea, vomiting
Cardiotonic glycosides	
digitalis preparations	• Diarrhea, anorexia, nausea, vomiting
Uncategorized agents	
colchicine	• Diarrhea, nausea, vomiting, abdominal pain
levodopa (Levopa*)	• Nausea, vomiting, anorexia
Narcotics	
codeine phosphate, codeine sulfate	• Nausea, vomiting, constipation
meperidine hydrochloride (Demerol*) methadone hydrochloride (Dolophine) morphine sulfate	• Nausea, vomiting, dry mouth, constipation, biliary tract spasm

*Available in U.S. and Canada. All other products (no symbol) available in U.S. only.

questions. (Thus prompted, many patients who don't use these items will say they do.) If the patient wears a dental appliance, such as a bridge, note its type and location. Ask the patient with dentures if he wears them all the time. Ill-fitting dentures may cause gingival or palatal irritation. Ask the patient to describe how he cleans his dentures. Note how often he visits a dentist.

• ***Eating habits.*** Frequent between-meal snacking on sugar-rich foods may predispose a person to caries. Excessive consumption of very hot or very spicy foods may lead to stomatitis.

• ***Smoking.*** Remember, men between ages 45 and 64 who smoke cigarettes have a mortality ten times that of nonsmokers, and the effect of smoking on women's health is becoming increasingly significant. If your patient smokes cigarettes, note how much he smokes in *pack years* (number of packs of cigarettes smoked per day multiplied by the number of years the patient has been smoking at this rate). Cigarette smoking predisposes a person to oral cancer, and pipe smoking may cause stomatitis or lip cancer.

• ***Alcohol and caffeine consumption.*** Excessive alcohol consumption may be a factor in the development of oral cancer. A patient's stomach lining may be irritated by excess gastric secretions stimulated by the ingestion of large amounts of alcohol or caffeine.

431 Review of systems

Symptoms possibly related to gastrointestinal (GI) disorders may be revealed by assessment of your patient's other body systems.

• ***General.*** Ask your patient about recent *fever, weight loss, anorexia, fatigue,* or *weakness.*

• ***Skin.*** Generalized *jaundice* and *pru-*

ritus may result from hepatocellular damage or biliary obstruction. *Pruritus in the anal region* may be caused by local infections and lesions or by specific dermatologic disorders, such as psoriasis.

- ***Eye.*** Ask about *eye pain* and *photophobia. Uveitis* may accompany ulcerative colitis or Crohn's disease.
- ***Respiratory.*** *Dyspnea* may result from limited respiratory excursion caused by ascites.
- ***Urinary.*** *Uremia* may cause GI bleeding. Abdominal pain may be a symptom of urinary disorders.
- ***Musculoskeletal.*** *Arthritis* may occur with ulcerative colitis or Crohn's disease.
- ***Psychological.*** *Anxiety, depression* and *other emotional disturbances* commonly accompany GI disorders.
- ***Blood-forming and immune.*** *Swelling* of cervical, supraclavicular, or inguinal lymphatics may signal GI cancer.

Conducting the physical examination

432 Preparations for a GI examination

Physical assessment of a patient's gastrointestinal system usually consists of oral, abdominal, and rectal examinations. You'll assess his mouth by inspection and palpation; his abdomen by inspection, auscultation, percussion, and palpation; and his rectum by inspection and palpation.

For mouth assessment, you'll need a direct light source (such as a head lamp or penlight), a tongue depressor, an angled mouth mirror, 2″ × 2″ gauze pads, and rubber gloves or finger cots. For abdominal assessment, you'll need a stethoscope, a ruler, a skin-marking pencil, and a tape measure; for rectal assessment, rubber gloves or finger cots and a lubricant.

Before the examination, explain the procedure to the patient to reduce his anxiety. Tell him you'll be looking at and touching his mouth, abdomen, and rectum, and that you'll be listening to abdominal sounds with a stethoscope. Assure the patient that the examination is routine, and that you'll proceed carefully to avoid causing him any discomfort. Warn him that he'll feel some pressure during abdominal palpation. If the patient is experiencing abdominal pain, tell him that you'll assess the painful area last or not at all, as discussed in Entry 440. Inform him that the examination will take about 15 to 20 minutes.

If the patient is hospitalized, tell him and his family that some of the procedures you'll perform—possibly all of them—may be repeated frequently to monitor changes in his condition.

433 Initial assessment of the mouth

Unless your patient has an urgent abdominal complaint, begin your assessment of his gastrointestinal system by examining his mouth. After assisting the patient to a sitting position, inspect for asymmetry or swelling around the lips and jaws. Then inspect the temporomandibular joint, and palpate it bilaterally—just anterior to the ears—while the patient slowly opens and closes his mouth. Observe carefully for limited mobility and for tenderness and crepitus.

Next, tell the patient to close his mouth and clench his teeth. Retract his lips and check his bite. The teeth should meet, with the upper incisors and canines slightly outside the lower ones. Note any malocclusion.

434 Inspecting and palpating the lips

Be sure to ask a female patient wearing lipstick to remove it. Also ask the patient to remove any dental appliances, if necessary. Then, inspect your patient's lips for abnormal color or texture and for lesions. Next, put on a rubber glove or a finger cot to palpate the outer lips. Invert the lips and, using your light source, inspect and palpate the inner lips with the patient's jaw closed. Note any lesions, nodules, vesicles, or fissures, especially at the junction of the upper and lower lips.

435 Assessing the teeth and gums

With your patient's mouth open, use your light source to inspect his teeth. Normally, an adult has 32 teeth, 8 on each side of each jaw. Note obvious caries and any teeth that are missing, broken, stained, or displaced. Carefully palpate the teeth and note if any are loose.

Next, inspect and palpate your patient's gums (gingivae). They should be pink, moist, and smooth. Carefully check the gingival crest for recession, which may cause tooth loss. Also, note any redness, pallor, hypertrophy, ulcers, bleeding, or tenderness on palpation.

436 How to inspect and palpate the tongue

Ask your patient to stick out his tongue. Using your light source, inspect the tongue's superior surface. Normally, the lateral surfaces are pink and moist, with a slightly rough appearance because of the papillae. When the patient moves his tongue, note any deviation to one side, paralysis, or tremor. Also, note any abnormalities, such as redness, swelling, lesions, and any coating other than the tongue's normal thin white coating.

Next, grasp the tongue with a 2″ × 2″ gauze pad and palpate its superior surface and sides, paying special attention to its texture. Note any nodules or ulcerations. Ask the patient to touch the roof of his mouth with his tongue while you inspect and palpate the tongue's inferior surface and the floor of the mouth. Inspect carefully for ulcerations, which are especially prevalent in this area of the mouth and may be an early sign of oral cancer. Check, too, for leukoplakia (yellow-white leathery patches), which may be precancerous.

437 Assessing the buccal mucosa properly

With your patient's mouth open wide, your light source in position, and using your fingers as retractors, inspect and palpate the buccal mucosa on both sides. Record abnormalities, such as pallor, redness, excessive salivation or dryness, bleeding, swelling, ulcers or sores, and white patches or plaques. Be sure to move your fingers to various positions so you view the entire buccal mucosa area.

438 Assessing the hard and soft palates

Inspect and palpate the patient's hard and soft palates. Inspect the hard palate directly or, using a mouth mirror, indirectly. Normally, the hard palate is dome-shaped, pale, firm, and transversed irregularly by rugae. The soft palate is normally pink and soft (as its name implies). Note any redness, lesions, patches, petechiae, or pallor.

439 Inspecting your patient's pharynx

To examine your patient's pharynx, tilt his head back and depress his tongue with a tongue depressor (not too far back or you'll trigger the gag reflex). Ask the patient to say "Ah." His uvula and soft palate should rise. Inspect the anterior and the posterior pillars, the tonsils, and the posterior pharynx, which is normally pink and may be slightly vascular. Note abnormalities, such as uvular deviation; the absence, hypertrophy, or induration of the tonsils; and swelling of the tonsils or the posterior pharynx. Observe also for lesions, plaques, exudate, or a gray membrane. Finally, note any unusual mouth odor and describe it in your notes—for example, *sweet and fruity* or *fetid and musty*.

440 Contraindications to abdominal assessment

Before assessing your patient's abdomen, check for contraindications to palpation and percussion. Abdominal pain, for example, contraindicates repeated abdominal assessment. *Never* palpate the abdomen of a patient with suspected appendicitis or a dissecting abdominal aortic aneurysm, due to the possibility of rupture. Don't perform a physical examination on a patient with polycystic kidneys, because you might dislodge a cyst. The presence of transplanted kidneys or other organs in a patient also contraindicates percussion and palpation.

441 Abdominal examination sequence: IAPP

Assess your patient's abdomen according to the following sequence: inspection, auscultation, percussion, and palpation. Note that you'll perform auscultation—usually the last step in the assessment sequence—second. This is because percussing or palpating the abdomen *before* auscultating it can stimulate intestinal activity and produce misleading sounds.

When you auscultate your patient's abdomen, listen closely for bowel and vascular activity. Let the sounds you hear guide you in percussion, which helps outline major organs or masses. Your percussion findings then direct you in palpating for tenderness, size, mobility, consistency, and the location of masses or enlarged organs.

For assessment purposes, the abdomen is divided into four sections, as formed by a vertical line down the patient's midline and a horizontal line across his umbilicus. These sections are called the *left upper quadrant, right upper quadrant, left lower quadrant,* and *right lower quadrant.*

Your patient's history should tell you in which quadrant his symptoms are located. Examine all four quadrants, not just the symptomatic one, and examine the three asymptomatic quadrants first. Otherwise, any pain you elicit in the symptomatic quadrant will cause the muscles in the other quadrants to tighten and make your examination more difficult. The sequence you use to examine the three asymptomatic quadrants isn't significant, but you should develop a routine for performing an abdominal examination and do it the same way every time. Perform all four techniques in the modified sequence—IAPP—in each quadrant, concentrating on the organs underlying that section.

442 Abdominal assessment: Preparing the patient

Before you assess your patient's abdomen, instruct him to urinate. If he hasn't already removed all clothing from his abdomen, ask him to do so. Drape the pubic area for all patients—and the breasts, as well, for women. Position the patient comfortably on his back, with his knees bent and his arms at his sides, to prevent tensing of the abdominal muscles. Warm your hands and your stethoscope's diaphragm before beginning the examination.

443 Inspecting your patient's abdomen

Begin your abdominal assessment by inspecting the patient's entire abdomen. Position him so he's lying on his back, and stoop at his side to view his abdominal contour. A normal abdomen has a convex profile, even with the patient supine. A flat abdomen may be normal in an athlete or a muscular person. A hollow or scaphoid abdomen may indicate malnutrition. A distended or protuberant abdomen, usually having an everted umbilicus, could indicate excess air or fluid in the peritoneal cavity. Inspect the umbilicus for abnormalities besides eversion. For example, an umbilicus with a blue tinge may indicate intraabdominal bleeding.

Next, stand at the foot of the bed, and observe the patient's abdomen for symmetry of contour and for the presence of masses. An asymmetrical abdomen may result from previous abdominal trauma or surgery, an abnormal organ, or weak abdominal muscles.

Perform the rest of the examination from the patient's right side (if you're right-handed). Inspect the abdomen for movement from respiration, peristalsis, and arterial pulsations. Look for exaggerated abdominal movement during breathing that may indicate respiratory distress or severe anxiety. Normal peristaltic movement is rarely visible, even through a thin abdominal wall. If you can see strong contractions (peristaltic waves) crossing the patient's abdomen, report this finding to the doctor, because it may indicate impending bowel or pyloric obstruction.

The only arterial pulsations you may see are those of the abdominal aorta, which may be visible in the epigastric area. In a thin patient, you may see femoral arterial pulsations.

Inspect the abdominal skin thoroughly. Tense, glistening skin may indicate ascites or abdominal wall edema. Note any scars, lesions, ecchymoses, striae, rashes, or dilated veins. Also inspect for an abdominal hernia, which may become apparent when you ask the patient to cough. Draw a diagram of the abdomen's quadrants, and record the location, size, and color of such abnormalities.

Many skin and vascular findings relate to pressure caused by engorgement within the abdomen from obstruction of the vena cava or the portal vein. Malfunctioning organs, such as the liver or the spleen, may cause skin changes. For example, if your inspection reveals jaundice, it may result from liver disease or splenic hemolysis. Chronic uremia may cause abdominal pallor or frost. Although vascular lesions in the skin may result from various causes, always consider the possibility that your patient has a gastrointestinal system disorder.

444 Auscultating the abdomen systematically

After inspecting your patient's abdomen, auscultate it (see *Locating Abdominal Sounds*). Use the diaphragm of the stethoscope first. Exerting only light pressure, listen for bowel sounds in all quadrants. Normally, air and fluid movement through the bowel create irregular bubbling or soft, gurgling noises about every 5 to 15 seconds. If you don't hear bowel sounds immediately, listen for at least 5 minutes to confirm the absence of bowel sounds, which may indicate paralytic ileus or peritonitis. Report this finding. Conversely, rapid, high-pitched, tinkling bowel sounds or loud, gurgling noises with visible peristaltic waves commonly accompany diarrhea or gastroenteritis and indicate a hyperactive bowel. These findings may also signal an early intestinal obstruction.

Next, use the bell of the stethoscope to listen to vascular sounds. Place the bell lightly over the midline to check for *bruits,* blowing sounds that seem to elongate the pulsation normally heard over a vessel. Check also for bruits over the renal vessels, the result of dilatation or constriction. If you note any bruits in the abdominal aorta, assess arterial perfusion in the patient's legs. Absence of pulses indicates decreased blood flow to the legs: notify the doctor promptly. Meanwhile, keep your patient quiet and *don't* palpate his abdomen, because these symptoms may reflect a dissecting aneurysm, which is a surgical emergency. The same symptoms may indicate arteriosclerosis obliterans, a chronic condition, but a doctor must make the diagnosis.

You can also use the bell of the stethoscope to detect other abnormal abdominal sounds. If you hear a *venous hum*—a hum of medium tone created by blood flow in a large, engorged, vascular organ such as the liver or spleen—check for other signs of fluid overload. A *friction rub,* which sounds like two pieces of sandpaper being rubbed together, may originate in an inflamed spleen or a neoplastic liver.

While auscultating the patient's abdomen, assess the abdominal surface for edema by watching the imprint left by the bell of the stethoscope. If the circular imprint of a *lightly* placed stethoscope remains visible on the skin, fluid has probably accumulated within the abdominal wall. This often results from a nutritional deficiency, such as low circulating protein levels.

445 Abdominal percussion

Percussion is used mainly to check the size of abdominal organs and to detect excessive amounts of fluid or air in the abdomen. Percussion notes in each abdominal quadrant depend on the underlying structure. Keeping the positions of these underlying organs in mind, follow a pattern when you percuss (see *Percussing the Abdomen,* page 406). Abdominal percussion normally elicits tones ranging from dull or flat (over solids) to tympanic (over air). A sigmoid colon filled with stool produces dullness in the left lower quadrant. You'll usually hear high-pitched tympanic notes over a section of bowel filled with air (the degree of tympany reflects gaseous bowel distention). When ascites is present, you'll also detect dullness when you percuss the patient's flanks.

446 Fist percussion of the abdomen

Another percussion technique you can use during abdominal assessment of a patient is fist percussion (see Entry 91). Because this technique detects tender-

LOCATING ABDOMINAL SOUNDS

In abdominal auscultation, you'll find you can hear some sounds better in certain areas than in others. This illustration shows the best place to listen for each sound.

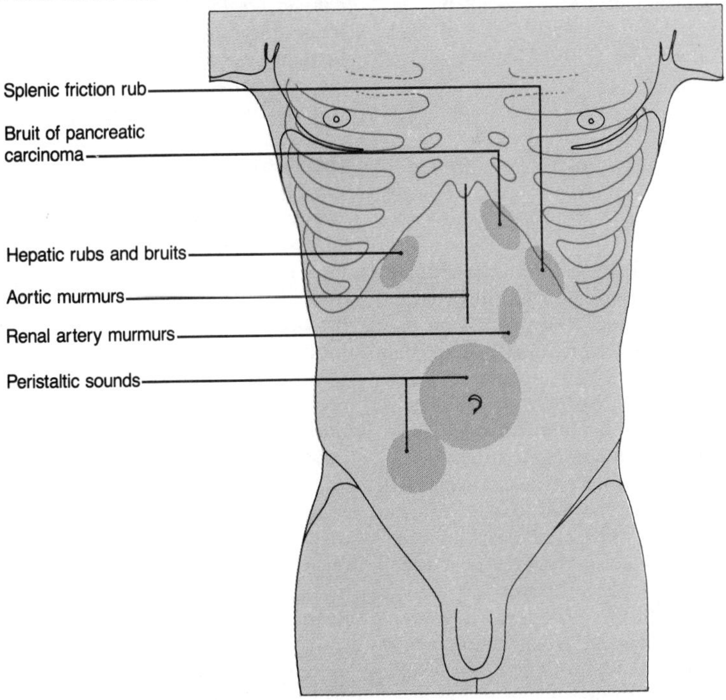

Splenic friction rub
Bruit of pancreatic carcinoma
Hepatic rubs and bruits
Aortic murmurs
Renal artery murmurs
Peristaltic sounds

PERCUSSING THE ABDOMEN

When percussing your patient's abdomen, move your hands clockwise, starting from the right upper quadrant unless your patient's experiencing pain. If he is, identify in which quadrant the pain's occurring and percuss that quadrant *last.* Remember, when tapping, to quickly move your right finger away so you don't damp vibrations.

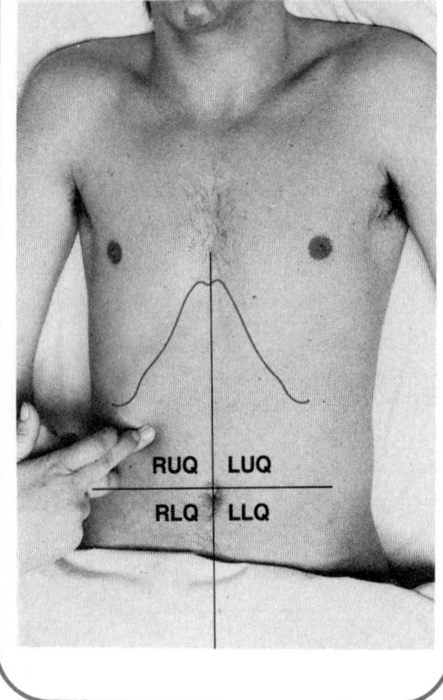

ness instead of producing percussion notes, don't perform it until the end of the examination. Fist percussion usually produces discomfort in a patient with deep-seated tenderness, organomegaly, or inflammation. It can also elicit signs of liver or gallbladder involvement. To use fist percussion for this purpose, place one hand parallel to and below the right costal margin and strike it with the fist of the other hand. You can also use fist percussion to test for tenderness over the kidneys (see Entry 501). *Don't* perform fist percussion routinely when pain or discomfort results, especially in the splenic area (the left upper quadrant and left upper midclavicular area).

447 Light and deep abdominal palpation

Techniques for abdominal palpation range from bimanual maneuvers to ballottement. The most frequently used are light palpation and deep palpation (see Entry 87). To perform *light palpation,* use your fingertips to depress the abdominal wall a little more than ½″ (1.3 cm), examining each quadrant systematically. Using light palpation you can determine skin temperature, detect large masses and tender areas, and elicit guarding. You can also assess the patient's abdominal vasculature through light palpation. For example, you can usually palpate the femoral pulse in the groin area. To palpate the aortic pulse, press the patient's upper abdomen slightly to the left of the midline. (Deeper palpation may be necessary to locate this pulse.)

Light palpation may not allow you to feel normal-sized abdominal organs, especially in a patient with a significant adipose layer. But if you place your index finger parallel to and slightly beneath the right costal margin and ask the patient to take a deep breath, you may be able to feel the liver's lower edge. The deep breath pushes the liver's lower edge farther under the costal margin. Normally, this edge stops just below the margin. It feels like a firm, sharp, even ridge, with a smooth surface. If the patient grimaces during this maneuver or tells you it's painful for him, report the tenderness to the doctor immediately.

With the patient in the right lateral decubitus position, use light palpation under the left costal margin to assess for splenic tenderness. If you suspect an enlarged spleen, use very light pressure and watch the patient for signs of discomfort. *Never* use deep palpation on a tender spleen. (For more information on assessing the spleen, see Entry 729).

To perform *deep palpation,* press the fingers of one hand in about 3″ (7.5 cm) with the aid of the other hand. With deep palpation you can determine the position of organs and detect abdominal masses. Never use deep palpation on a patient who's just had a kidney transplant, on a patient whose organs are tender, or on a patient with polycystic kidneys. Defer deep palpation of a known abdominal mass because of the danger that tumor cells may spread. Deep palpation may also evoke rebound tenderness when you suddenly withdraw your fingertips, a possible sign of peritoneal inflammation. This technique is often used to assess a patient for appendicitis, but it should not be used repeatedly on such a patient. *Don't palpate the abdomen at all after a diagnosis of appendicitis.*

Deep palpation can also be used to assess the inferior liver border. Standing at the right of the recumbent patient and facing his feet, hook the fingers of both your hands over the costal margin and ask the patient to take a deep breath. You should be able to feel the border of the liver's right lobe. Assess it for contour, mobility, consistency, and tenderness.

448 Percussing for liver size and position

You can estimate the size and position of your patient's liver through percussion (see *Estimating Liver Size*). Beginning at the right iliac crest, percuss up the right midclavicular line (MCL). The percussion note becomes dull when you reach the liver's inferior border, usually at the costal margin, although it may be lower with liver disease. Mark this point, then percuss down from the right clavicle, again along the right MCL. Place your pleximeter between the patient's ribs as you tap, to avoid confusing the dull note of the liver's superior border (usually between the fifth to seventh intercostal spaces) with the dull note that results from percussing bone. Mark the superior border. The distance between the two marked points represents the approximate size of the liver's right lobe, normally from 2⅜" to 4¾" (6 to 12 cm). A liver size of more than 4¾" in the MCL suggests hepatomegaly.

Assess the liver's left lobe similarly, percussing along the sternal midline. Again, mark the point where you hear dull percussion notes, and measure the size of the left lobe, normally 1½" to 3⅛" (4 to 8 cm).

Several structures and conditions—the sternum, ribs, breast tissue, pleural effusions, or gas in the colon—can obscure the dull percussion notes you're listening for. This situation may require you to use palpation and auscultation, along with percussion, to determine the patient's liver size and position.

The *scratch test* can locate the liver's inferior border if you can't find it through

ESTIMATING LIVER SIZE

To estimate the size of the liver, follow the percussion pattern shown here. First, percuss upward and then downward on the right midclavicular line. By noting in each sequence when dullness begins, you can approximate the lower and upper borders of the liver. Normally, the distance between these borders, or liver size, is 2⅜" to 4¾" (6 to 12 cm) at the midclavicular line.

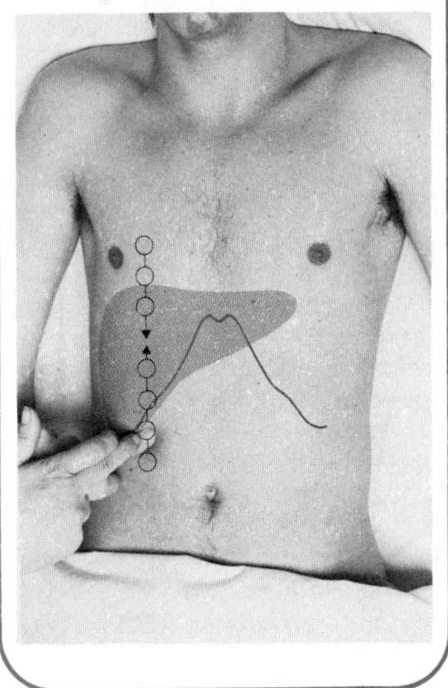

percussion. To perform this test, lightly place the stethoscope's diaphragm over the approximate location of the inferior border. Then auscultate while stroking the patient's abdomen lightly with your right index finger in the pattern you used for locating the liver's inferior border through percussion. Start your stroke along the MCL at the right iliac crest and move upward. Because the liver transmits sound waves better than the air-filled ascending colon, the scratching noise you hear through your stethoscope becomes louder over the solid liver.

449 Assessing abdominal masses carefully

If you detect an abdominal mass through palpation, note its location and the patient's position. (A mass in the splenic area, for example, may be palpable only when the patient is in the right lateral decubitus position.) Determine the size and shape of the mass. Describe its contour as *smooth, rough, nodular,* or *irregular.* Its consistency may be *soft, doughy, semisolid,* or *hard.* Percuss the mass to determine whether it's tympanic (filled with air) or dull (filled with fluid). Also assess the mass for tenderness, and ask the patient about changes in its location or size.

Determine the relation of the mass to other abdominal organs. Note whether it's attached to the abdominal wall. Evaluate its mobility. Does it seem to float in surrounding tissues, or does it adhere to underlying structures? Lastly, assess the mass for pulsations that may be caused by a highly vascular tumor, an anomalous vessel, or a mass located over an artery.

450 Assessing ascites

You can assess your patient for ascites through three techniques: testing for shifting dullness (see *Assessing Ascites: Shifting Dullness Test*), testing for fluid wave, and measuring the patient's girth. A dull percussion note may suggest fluid accumulation in the abdomen without visual signs of ascites. To confirm fluid accumulation, with the patient lying on his back, percuss his abdomen from the umbilicus toward each flank. On the patient's abdomen, draw a line between areas of dullness and tympany. Then, turn the patient to one side, causing ascitic fluid to shift, and repeat percussion from the umbilicus toward the flanks. Again draw a line between areas of dullness and tympany, and compare this line to the one you drew previously. The distance between these lines indicates the presence of fluid. Repeat the procedure with the patient lying on his other side.

The *shifting dullness* sign confirms ascites and also provides a baseline for daily comparison of the distance between the lines, which may indicate an increase or decrease in the accumulated fluid. However, the shifting dullness sign can produce a false finding, such as when an engorged loop of bowel—not free peritoneal or ascitic fluid—shifts and causes dull percussion tones. Adhesions from previous surgery or cancer may also prevent fluid from shifting freely in the patient's abdomen. Be sure to analyze all your findings carefully and consider possible false or misleading causes when performing this test.

Eliciting a *fluid wave* can help you distinguish between fluid retention and air retention in a patient with a slightly distended abdomen. You'll need someone to help you perform this technique—perhaps the patient himself, a family member, or a co-worker. Have the other person place the ulnar surface of his hand on the patient's abdominal midline and push down slightly, to dampen any movement of the abdominal wall. Then, place one of your palms on one of the patient's flanks and sharply tap the opposite flank. If a large amount of fluid is present, you'll feel a moving wave in the palm that's resting on the patient's flank.

You can also monitor abdominal dis-

ASSESSING ASCITES: SHIFTING DULLNESS TEST

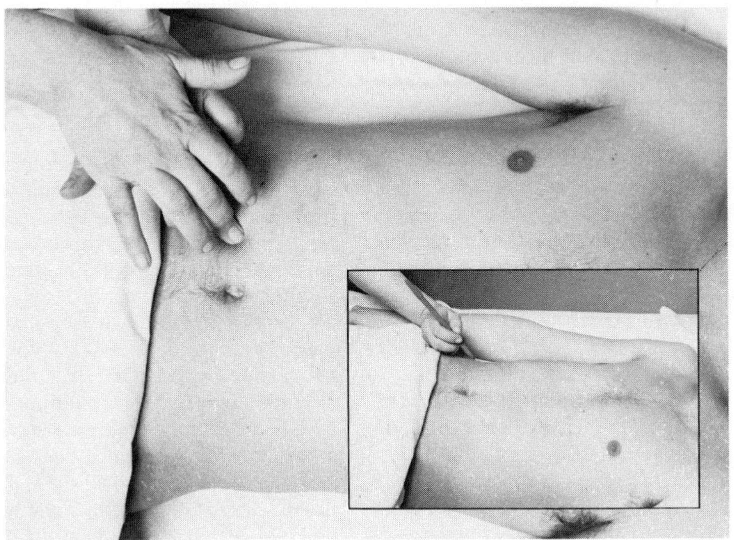

1 To assess for ascites, or fluid buildup, the nurse shown here is testing for shifting dullness. With the patient on his back, she percusses from the umbilicus to each flank. Next, she draws a line to demarcate dullness (fluid accumulation) from tympanic sounds (air-filled structures).

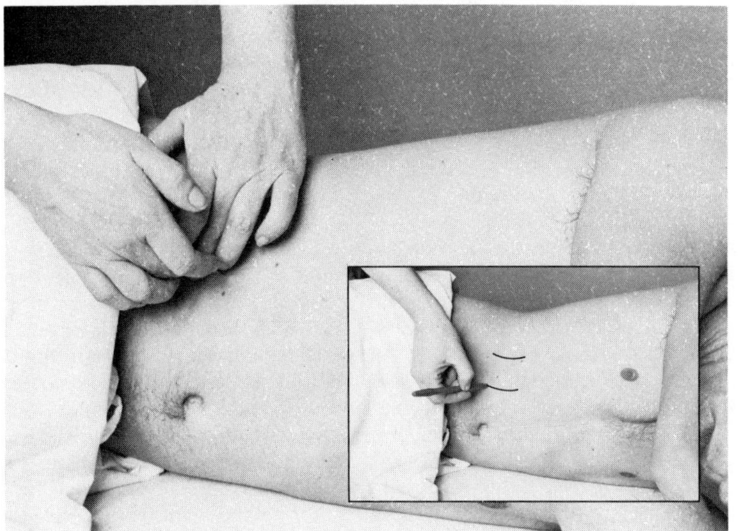

2 Then, she positions the patient on his side and repeats the percussion procedure, again marking the demarcation lines. Any change between the first set of lines and the second set of lines indicates the presence of fluid.

tention by measuring your patient's *girth* (probably the most reliable method). The patient must be lying down when you do this. Draw the tape firmly but not tightly around his abdomen, and then measure his girth during exhalation. Mark the patient's flanks to ensure the same area is measured each time.

451 Inspecting the rectum

Always examine the rectum last. Turn the patient on his left side, with his knees up and his buttocks close to the edge of the examining table. (If the patient is ambulatory, ask him to stand and bend over the examining table.) Spread his buttocks to expose the anus. Rectal skin is normally darker than the surrounding area. Inspect for inflammation, lesions, scars, outpouching, fissures, and external hemorrhoids. Check for hemorrhoids while the patient strains as though to defecate.

452 Palpating the rectum

For this technique, which follows inspection of the rectum, use a disposable glove and a lubricant. While the patient strains as though to defecate, use your index finger to palpate any weak anal outpouchings, nodules, or tenderness on movement. Then, explain to the patient that you'll insert your gloved finger a short distance into his rectum and that this pressure may make him feel as though he needs to move his bowels. Wait for the anal sphincter to relax, then insert your finger gently and rotate it to palpate as much of the rectal wall as possible. Palpate for any nodules, irregularities, or tenderness, and for fecal impaction. As you palpate the anterior rectal wall of the male patient, remember to assess the prostate's lateral lobes and median sulcus. Test any fecal matter adhering to the glove for occult blood, using the correct guaiac or Hematest procedure.

Formulating a diagnostic impression

453 Classifying GI disorders

Gastrointestinal disorders can be classified according to the physiologic processes of ingestion, digestion, and elimination (see *Nurse's Guide to Gastrointestinal Disorders,* pages 412 to 419). These processes include the absorbing and transferring of fluid, nutrients, electrolytes, and trace elements all along the alimentary canal. Disorders of ingestion affect the mouth and esophagus. Most disorders of digestion occur in the stomach, small intestine, liver, gallbladder, and pancreas. Elimination disorders are usually associated with exocrine gland malfunction or intestinal problems.

454 Your nursing diagnosis

Pain, a common complaint of patients with gastrointestinal (GI) disorders, may occur with problems of ingestion, digestion, or elimination. Oral pain commonly results from an acute benign inflammatory process. Heartburn, or substernal burning, results from an incompetent lower esophageal sphincter, which causes esophageal reflux. Abdominal pain has many possible causes. Acute pain may result from obstruction, as receptors in the bowel or biliary tract respond to increasing distention. Peritoneal irritation produces severe pain, because the parietal peritoneum has many sensitive nerve endings. Altered bowel motility from inflammatory or functional disturbances usually results in abdominal cramps. Abdominal wall pathology causes constant, aching pain that worsens when the patient moves. Mucosal ulceration produces burning, or gnawing discomfort, in the epigastrium.

Capsular inflammation or distention causes aching, unremitting pain, because the connective tissue covering the liver and spleen contains many nerves. Reduced arterial blood flow to the bowel may initially produce mild, then severe, discomfort from ischemic nerve endings. Metabolic disturbances and nerve injury may simulate intraabdominal causes of pain. Psychogenic pain varies in intensity and nature. Referred pain may occur from a process outside the abdomen that affects common nerve pathways.

Rectal pain may result from ulceration, edema, distention, or a late-stage tumor. Because of the extensive nerve supply to this area, pain may be severe.

Nursing diagnoses for all types of pain caused by GI disorders include *alterations in comfort* and possibly *fear of serious illness,* as well as *alterations in rest/activity patterns.*

Dysphagia affects ingestion and specifically involves the esophagus. This symptom can result from mechanical obstruction, such as a tumor or stricture, that interferes with the passage of solids. Achalasia is the most frequent cause of dysphagia, resulting from impaired motor activity. Diminished peristalsis, incomplete relaxation of the lower esophageal sphincter, and increased pressure in the same resting sphincter combine to produce the symptom. Neurologic disease may account for upper esophageal dysphagia.

Possible nursing diagnoses for dysphagia are *alterations in nutrition* (less than body requirements) and *fluid volume deficit.*

Nausea and vomiting always affect ingestion and digestion. These symptoms specifically involve the GI system. Decreased gastric motor activity, gastric mucosal pallor, and duodenal contraction usually accompany nausea. Many factors within and outside the GI tract may cause nausea and vomiting. For example, both parasympathetic (vagal) and sympathetic nerves in the pharynx, stomach, bile ducts, bowel, mesentery, and peritoneum (as well as in the heart) carry impulses to the brain's vomiting center. Therefore, pharyngeal, gastric, or peritoneal irritation, as well as distention of a hollow viscus and myocardial ischemia, may result in nausea and vomiting. Vestibular, neurologic, and metabolic disturbances that stimulate the brain's vomiting center do so by way of a chemoreceptor trigger zone, located in the fourth ventricle. Drugs and toxins may have this same effect.

Nursing diagnoses for patients with nausea and vomiting may include *fluid and electrolyte deficit, alterations in comfort,* and *alterations in nutrition* (less than body requirements) if vomiting is prolonged and/or severe.

Diarrhea affects elimination and specifically involves the small or large intestine and the rectum. Increased intestinal fluid secretion (possibly caused by toxins, hormones, or inflammation) raises the water content in stools and causes this symptom. Increased stool water content may also result from decreased intestinal absorption caused by malfunctioning bowel mucosa or loss of reabsorptive surface, as well as by increased intestinal motility.

Nursing diagnoses for patients with diarrhea include *alteration in bowel elimination, potential for impaired skin integrity,* and possibly *fluid volume deficit.*

Constipation also affects elimination and specifically involves the colon and rectum. Interference with rectal filling or with the defecation reflex can cause constipation. Physical inactivity and a low-fiber diet impede colonic transport and rectal filling. Mechanical obstruction, such as from stricture or tumor, also may interfere with stool passage. Neurogenic factors, voluntary suppression, and chronic laxative use can diminish the defecation reflex.

Possible nursing diagnoses for constipated patients include *alteration in bowel elimination, alterations in comfort,* and possibly *knowledge deficit related to proper bowel or nutritional habits.*

NURSE'S GUIDE TO GASTROINTESTINAL DISORDERS

	CHIEF COMPLAINT
INGESTIVE DISORDERS	
Zenker's diverticulum (pulsion-type diverticulum)	• *Pain:* scratchy throat • *Nausea/vomiting:* regurgitation of food partially digested or eaten the day before • *Dysphagia:* intermittent; progresses with continued eating
Esophagitis	• *Pain:* heartburn 1 hour after eating; aggravated by bending over, lying down, or straining; relieved by drinking or standing; pain may radiate to neck, arms, or jaws • *Nausea/vomiting:* possible nocturnal regurgitation into mouth • *Dysphagia:* intermittent
Achalasia (second-degree abnormal peristalsis or obstructed esophagogastric junction)	• *Pain:* usually absent • *Nausea/vomiting:* possible regurgitation of food eaten hours before, without acid taste • *Dysphagia:* progressive difficulty with both solids and liquids
Esophageal cancer	• *Pain:* may be present under sternum, or in back or neck; progresses with advancing disease • *Nausea/vomiting:* present in late stages • *Dysphagia:* difficulty with solids, progressive difficulty with liquids
Hiatal hernia	• *Pain:* usually absent; occasional heartburn (gastroesophageal reflux); severe pain if incarcerated • *Nausea/vomiting:* nocturnal regurgitation, aggravated by lying down, relieved by standing • *Dysphagia:* if hernia produces esophagitis, esophageal ulceration or stricture
Necrotizing ulcerative gingivostomatitis (Vincent's disease, trench mouth)	• *Pain:* may be severe enough to interfere with eating • *Nausea/vomiting:* absent • *Dysphagia:* may be severe
Gingivitis	• *Pain:* may be present • *Nausea/vomiting:* absent • *Dysphagia:* usually absent
Aphthous stomatitis	• *Pain:* may be severe • *Nausea/vomiting:* absent • *Dysphagia:* may be present

	HISTORY	PHYSICAL EXAMINATION	DIAGNOSTIC STUDIES
	• Nocturnal coughing, halitosis, and weight loss are related signs and symptoms.	• Protrusion on neck	• Barium swallow shows pouching in upper esophagus; esophagoscopy performed to rule out other problems.
	• Hematemesis, melena, frequent eructation, increasing salivation, and nocturnal coughing are related signs and symptoms, aggravated by lying down.	• Physical signs usually absent	• Esophagoscopy shows eroded or ulcerated mucosa; cineroentgenography of esophagus with barium swallow shows weak peristalsis and failure of sphincter to relax.
	• Weight loss, slowed eating, coughing, wheezing, and choking are related signs and symptoms, aggravated by emotional stress.	• Physical signs absent	• Barium swallow shows narrowed distal end of esophagus; proximal dilatation and fluid appear high in esophagus; biopsy and cytology done to exclude cancer.
	• Rapid weight loss and substernal burning after drinking hot fluids are related signs and symptoms.	• Cachexia, frequent coughing	• Cytology shows cancer cells; barium swallow outlines tumor obstruction with irregular lesion; esophagoscopy visualizes lesion.
	• Increased intraabdominal pressure, caused by straining, obesity, ascites, or coughing, is a predisposing factor; most common in elderly women.	• Physical signs absent	• Barium swallow shows pouching in lower esophagus.
	• Poor oral hygiene, lowered resistance, agranulocytosis, and leukemia are possible predisposing factors; headache and malaise are related symptoms; most common in men ages 20 to 25.	• Ulcerative erosion of gingival papillae, gray pseudomembrane oval covering, low-grade fever, regional lymphadenitis	• Culture may reveal fusiform bacillus or spirochete.
	• Local irritation, blood dyscrasias, little or no gingival stimulation, mouth breathing, and pregnancy are predisposing factors; most common during puberty.	• Gingival swelling, redness, bleeding, change in normal contour	• None pertinent
	• Stress, fatigue, anxiety, and menstruation are predisposing factors; common in young girls.	• Single or multiple shallow ulcers with white centers and red borders	• None pertinent

(continued)

NURSE'S GUIDE TO GASTROINTESTINAL DISORDERS *(continued)*

	CHIEF COMPLAINT
Glossitis	• *Pain:* usually present; may be severe • *Nausea/vomiting:* absent • *Dysphagia:* usually present
Periodontitis	• *Pain:* usually absent at first; later, slightly painful around teeth's supporting area; if abscess develops, severe local pain may occur • *Nausea/vomiting:* absent • *Dysphagia:* usually absent
Herpes simplex, primary (herpes simplex Type 1 virus)	• *Pain:* may be severe • *Nausea/vomiting:* absent • *Dysphagia:* may be present
Oral cancer	• *Pain:* usually absent; presence depends on location, degree of invasion, and pressure on surrounding tissue • *Nausea/vomiting:* absent • *Dysphagia:* usually present only in advanced stages
DIGESTIVE DISORDERS	
Upper gastrointestinal (GI) bleeding (secondary)	• *Pain:* present; in ulcer disease, usually relieved by bleeding • *Nausea/vomiting:* vomiting present; bright red from acute bleeding; dark red suggests past bleeding • *Constipation/diarrhea:* bloody diarrhea with acute GI hemorrhage; melena with chronic upper GI bleeding
Peptic ulcer	• *Pain:* gnawing, burning pain more than 1 hour after eating; described as a feeling of nausea or hunger; relieved by eating; gastric ulcers may cause pain immediately after eating
Gastritis (acute and chronic)	• *Pain:* epigastric pain slightly left of midline; indigestion • *Nausea/vomiting:* if both present, hematemesis may occur • *Constipation/diarrhea:* melena; diarrhea may occur

HISTORY	PHYSICAL EXAMINATION	DIAGNOSTIC STUDIES
• Irritation, injury, poorly fitting or improperly fitted dentures, alcoholism, tobacco smoking, diet of spicy foods, allergy to toothpastes and mouthwashes are predisposing factors; difficulty in speaking and chewing and changes in taste are related signs.	• Reddened, ulcerated, or swollen tongue; swelling may obstruct airway	• None pertinent
• Uncontrolled diabetes, blood dyscrasias, pregnancy, traumatic irritation, and poor oral hygiene are predisposing factors; most common in pubescent females.	• Gingival recession; periodontal pocket containing food, bacteria, calculi; tenderness on percussion; teeth mobility in advanced stage	• Dental X-ray shows destruction of supporting osseous tissues; biopsy provides differential diagnosis.
• Irritability, headache, and fever are related symptoms; most common in children.	• Multiple vesicles that ulcerate rapidly, forming yellow-white ulcers with red halos; lesions may appear on gingival, labial, or buccal mucosa	• Confirmation requires isolation of the virus from local lesions, histologic biopsy, and serologic tests.
• Smoking or chewing tobacco, overexposure to sunlight, and alcoholism are predisposing factors; most common in men over age 40.	• Early lesions are white with varying texture, or red, soft, and smooth; ulcerating cancer has raised, firm, and fixed margins; may bleed	• Biopsy provides differential diagnosis.
• Prior ulcer disease, alcoholism, and abuse of certain drugs, such as inflammatory agents, are predisposing factors.	• Weakness, fainting, orthostatic changes in blood pressure, tachycardia, diaphoresis	• Hemoglobin and hematocrit measured to evaluate extent and type (acute or chronic) of blood loss; prothrombin time measured to determine clotting problems.
• Emotional stress and drugs irritating to gastrointestinal (GI) tract are possible predisposing factors; signs and symptoms occur in clusters, then subside and later recur.	• Abdominal tenderness	• Upper GI series: crater easily visualized; endoscopy performed to confirm diagnosis; biopsy performed to rule out cancer; serum gastrin level elevated.
• Drug or chemical irritation, ingestion of irritating foods, alcoholism, pernicious anemia, severe stress, burns, surgery, trauma, and sepsis are predisposing factors.	• Abdominal tenderness	• Fiberoptic endoscopy; mild leukocytosis; biopsy performed to diagnose chronic condition.

(continued)

NURSE'S GUIDE TO GASTROINTESTINAL DISORDERS *(continued)*

	CHIEF COMPLAINT
Viral hepatitis, Type A and Type B	• *Pain:* mild, constant pain in right upper quadrant • *Nausea/vomiting:* nausea present; vomiting may be present • *Constipation/diarrhea:* clay-colored stool may be present
Cirrhosis	• *Pain:* mild right upper quadrant pain; increasing as disease progresses • *Nausea/vomiting:* both present • *Constipation/diarrhea:* both present
Pancreatitis (acute and chronic)	• *Pain:* constant epigastric pain; may radiate to back; pain worsened by lying down • *Nausea/vomiting:* both present with bilious vomiting • *Constipation/diarrhea:* absent
Cholecystitis	• *Pain:* severe, cramping pain in epigastrium or right upper quadrant; may be referred to back of right scapula; onset sudden, but subsides after about 1 hour; followed by dull ache • *Nausea/vomiting:* both present • *Constipation/diarrhea:* absent
Appendicitis	• *Pain:* sudden epigastric or periumbilical pain; later localizes in right lower quadrant at McBurney's point • *Nausea/vomiting:* both may be present following pain • *Constipation/diarrhea:* diarrhea or, later, constipation

	HISTORY	PHYSICAL EXAMINATION	DIAGNOSTIC STUDIES
	• *Type A:* Contaminated food or water and contact with infected person are predisposing factors; *Type B:* usually transmitted parenterally but also through contact with infected secretions; headache, cough, coryza, loss of appetite, aversion to smoking, fatigue, arthralgia, myalgia are related symptoms.	• Fever, chills, abdominal tenderness in right upper quadrant; in second stage: hepatomegaly, jaundice, and possibly splenomegaly and cervical adenopathy	• Serum glutamic-oxaloacetic transaminase (SGOT) and serum glutamic-pyruvic transaminase (SGPT) levels elevated; bilirubin level elevated; prolonged prothrombin time indicates impending hepatic failure; serum alkaline phosphatase level slightly elevated; serum albumin level low; serum globulin level elevated; antibody to hepatitis A virus (antiHAV) confirms hepatitis A; hepatitis B surface antigens (HB_sAg) and hepatitis B antibodies (antiHB) confirm hepatitis B.
	• Alcoholism, hepatitis, heart failure, and hemochromatosis are predisposing factors; malaise, fatigue, anorexia leading to weight loss, pruritus, dark urine, and bleeding tendencies are related symptoms.	• Palpable liver and possibly spleen, jaundice, spider angioma, peripheral edema; in progressive stages, ascites	• Liver biopsy provides definitive diagnosis; serum glutamic-oxaloacetic transaminase (SGOT), serum glutamic-pyruvic transaminase (SGPT), and lactate dehydrogenase (LDH) levels elevated; serum alkaline phosphatase and bilirubin levels elevated, reflecting liver damage; prothrombin time and partial thromboplastin times may be prolonged.
	• Alcoholism, previous cholelithiasis, peptic ulcer, and use of drugs, such as azathioprine, are predisposing factors; pain aggravated by food or alcohol ingestion and restlessness are related symptoms.	• Mild fever, tachycardia, hypotension, abdominal distention, decreased bowel sounds, abdominal tenderness, and, if severe, abdominal rigidity and rales at lung base	• Serum amylase level elevated; marked leukocytosis; serum calcium level decreased; hyperglycemia; X-rays show distortion or edema of duodenal loop or calcification of pancreas.
	• Fatty food intolerance, indigestion, flatulence, and belching are related signs and symptoms; most common in obese multiparous women over age 40	• Fever, abdominal tenderness in right upper quadrant, abdominal rigidity and guarding, palpable liver, palpable gallbladder, possibly jaundice, elevated pulse	• Cholecystography and ultrasound detect calculi; white blood cell count may be elevated; serum alkaline phosphatase and bilirubin levels may be elevated.
	• Sudden onset of symptoms	• Mild fever, pain increases with right thigh extension, abdominal rigidity in right lower quadrant, rebound tenderness	• White blood cell count elevated; X-ray may show local distention.

(continued)

NURSE'S GUIDE TO GASTROINTESTINAL DISORDERS *(continued)*

ELIMINATION DISORDERS	CHIEF COMPLAINT
Diverticular disease (diverticulitis)	• *Pain:* occasional lower left quadrant pain • *Nausea/vomiting:* mild nausea present, but vomiting usually absent • *Constipation/diarrhea:* constipation more common than diarrhea; occurs with onset of pain
Ulcerative colitis	• *Pain:* cramping abdominal pain • *Nausea/vomiting:* both present • *Constipation/diarrhea:* profuse, episodic, bloody diarrhea with mucus possible
Crohn's disease	• *Pain:* cramping lower right quadrant pain • *Nausea/vomiting:* nausea present, but vomiting usually absent • *Constipation/diarrhea:* mild, urgent diarrhea
Intestinal obstruction	• *Pain:* colicky abdominal pain in epigastric or periumbilical area; in distal colon obstruction, pain referred to lumbar spine area • *Nausea/vomiting:* in high obstruction, present; in large bowel obstruction, vomiting usually absent • *Constipation/diarrhea:* in complete obstruction: constipation; in partial obstruction (by tumor): pencil-thin stools; in obstruction caused by adhesions: diarrhea possible
Colorectal cancer	• *Pain:* abdominal cramping pain in later stages • *Nausea/vomiting:* absent • *Constipation/diarrhea:* blood-streaked stools occur as early sign; pencil-thin stools possible; constipation alternating with diarrhea
Peritonitis	• *Pain:* sudden, severe abdominal pain • *Nausea/vomiting:* both present • *Constipation/diarrhea:* inability to pass flatus or feces
Hemorrhoids	• *Pain:* occasional pain on defecation; sudden, severe pain, if thrombosed • *Nausea/vomiting:* absent • *Constipation/diarrhea:* absent

	HISTORY	PHYSICAL EXAMINATION	DIAGNOSTIC STUDIES
	• Long-term diet low in roughage and fiber is a predisposing factor.	• Low-grade fever; in severe disease, abdominal tenderness	• Leukocytosis; flat plate abdominal view shows free air with perforation; barium enema visualizes diverticula.
	• Family history of disease and emotional stress are predisposing factors; weight loss and anorexia are related signs.	• Low-grade fever; abdominal tenderness	• Leukocytosis; electrolyte imbalance; anemia; increased erythrocyte sedimentation rate; sigmoidoscopy shows increased friability and pus, mucus, and blood; barium enema shows extent of disease.
	• Family history of disease and emotional stress are predisposing factors; flatulence, weight loss, weakness, and malaise are related signs and symptoms	• Low-grade fever; abdominal tenderness; possible mass in right lower quadrant	• Leukocytosis; sigmoidoscopy usually negative; barium enema shows string sign (segments of stricture separated by normal bowel); biopsy confirms diagnosis.
	• Family history of cancer is a predisposing factor; weight loss and weakness are related signs and symptoms.	• Abdominal distention and tenderness; paralytic ileus with absent bowel sounds; low-grade fever; possible palpable mass	• Leukocytosis; X-ray shows distention; sigmoidoscopy and colonoscopy visualize obstruction; small intestine X-ray shows stepladder fluid and gas distribution.
	• Family history of cancer, polyposis, history of ulcerative colitis are predisposing factors; malaise and loss of appetite are related signs and symptoms.	• Weight loss; digital rectal examination may reveal palpable mass	• Sigmoidoscopy, colonoscopy, and barium enema visualize tumor; biopsy reveals cancer cells.
	• Abdominal distress, abdominal surgery, and traumatic abdominal injury are predisposing factors.	• Fever; abdominal rigidity; pallor; sweating; hypotension; thirst; tachycardia, shallow respirations; decreased bowel sounds; paralytic ileus causes resonance and tympany; rebound tenderness	• Leukocytosis; abdominal X-ray shows free gas and fluid in abdomen; paracentesis reveals cause.
	• Prolonged sitting and multiple pregnancies are predisposing factors.	• External hemorrhoids	• Proctoscopic examination visualizes internal hemorrhoids.

CASE HISTORIES: NURSING DIAGNOSIS FLOWCHART

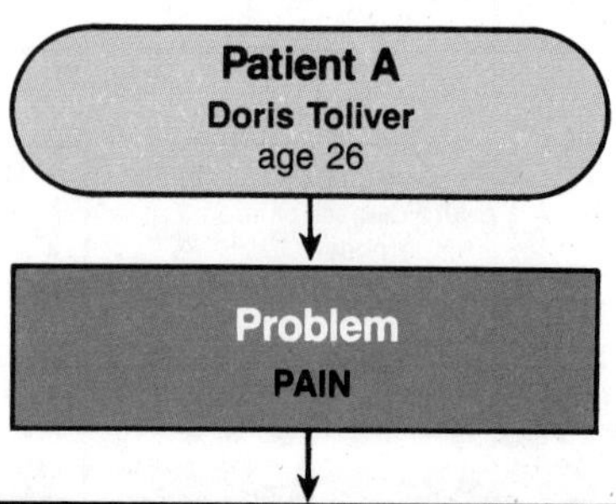

Subjective data

- Progressive abdominal cramping, relieved with bowel movement; duration 1 month
- Diarrhea: four to six stools daily, semisolid with mucus
- Weight loss: 7 lb (3.15 kg) in last month
- Lassitude and fatigue
- Anorexia

Objective data

- Inspection: pallor; dry, thickened tongue; sunken eyes with dark circles; cracked lips; abdomen slightly distended; rectal excoriation
- Auscultation: increased bowel sounds
- Percussion: increased tympany over bowel
- Palpation: abdominal tenderness, not increased during right thigh extension; detection of sausagelike mass in right lower quadrant
- Height: 5′6″ (167.6 cm)
- Weight: 110 lb (49.5 kg)
- Temperature: 100.8° F. (38.2° C.)
- Pulse: 104
- Blood pressure: 92/60
- Respiration: 26

Nursing diagnoses

- Alterations in comfort due to crampy abdominal pain
- Fluid volume deficit due to anorexia and diarrhea
- Alteration in bowel elimination: diarrhea
- Alterations in nutrition secondary to anorexia
- Difficulty maintaining home due to debilitating symptoms

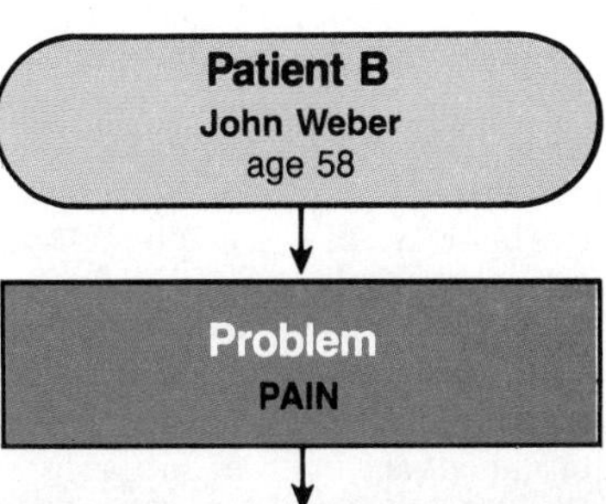

Subjective data

- Recurrent epigastric pain that began 2 years ago and varies in intensity
- Nausea, frequent vomiting, accompanying pain, anorexia
- Weight loss: 25 lb (11.25 kg) over 2 years
- Passage of frequent, frothy, foul-smelling stools over past 2 months
- Addiction to alcohol
- Unemployed
- No health insurance
- Recently divorced

Objective data

- Inspection: thin, pale, gaunt, unshaven appearance; icteric sclera; slight abdominal distention
- Auscultation: bowel sounds present
- Percussion: normal findings
- Palpation: moderate abdominal tenderness over epigastric region
- Height: 5′11″ (180 cm)
- Weight: 145 lb (65.3 kg)
- Temperature: 99.2° F. (37.3° C.)
- Pulse: 96
- Blood pressure: 110/84
- Respiration: 24

Nursing diagnoses

- Alterations in nutrition related to anorexia, vomiting, alcoholism, and steatorrhea
- Alterations in comfort related to abdominal pain
- Alteration in bowel elimination: frequent passage of fatty stools
- Self-care deficit (hygiene, grooming) related to alcoholism
- Ineffective individual coping with social, financial, and health problems

Assessing pediatric patients

455 Primary and permanent teeth

A child has 20 primary (baby) teeth (compared with the adult's 32). Each arch has 10 teeth: 4 incisors, 2 cuspids, and 4 molars. These teeth usually begin forming by the third month of fetal life, and when the infant's about age 6 months, they begin to erupt. By age 24 eruption is usually complete.

Permanent teeth begin to develop inside the gums during the first 6 months of neonatal life and start to replace the primary teeth by about age 6. Tooth replacement normally begins with the mandibular incisors and continues in orderly fashion until the final permanent teeth—the third molars (wisdom teeth)—erupt between ages 17 and 21 (see *Usual Sequence of Tooth Eruption*).

456 Abdominal differences

The *spleen* increases in weight from ½ oz (17 g) at birth to 6 oz (170 g) by age 20. In children under age 1, it may extend ⅜" to ¾" (1 to 2 cm) below the left costal margin. Thus, the spleen may be palpable in a thin child or in an infant who is only a few months old. A child's spleen is more likely to enlarge as the result of disease (such as blood dyscrasia) than an adult's. The function of the spleen changes as a child grows. During the first year of life, it helps produce red blood cells; after the first year, it helps destroy red blood cells and form hemoglobin (for more information on the spleen, see Entry 709).

A child's *liver* is proportionately larger than an adult's. During the first year of life it may extend ⅜" (1 cm) below the right costal margin. Like the spleen, a child's liver enlarges more quickly than an adult's in response to disease (especially cardiac disease). The *bladder* is much higher in a child than in an adult and lies between the symphysis pubis and the umbilicus; its accessibility is one reason for the prevalence of suprapubic punctures in children. (For more information on the pediatric urinary system, see Entry 507.)

457 Pediatric history

To assess a child's gastrointestinal system properly, you'll need to obtain a thorough nutritional history (see Entry 195). For example, if you note periods of decreased appetite in a young child, check to see if his growth and weight have been affected. Remember, decreased appetite may be normal for the child's age (for instance, for a toddler).

Because abdominal pain is a common childhood complaint, be sure to ask about it. Instead of asking the child directly about stomach pain, determine the pain's nature and severity through such indirect questions as *Did you eat your dinner last night? Did you sleep last night? What toys did you play with this morning?* Use indirect questions to obtain objective answers from anxious parents too.

Determine the characteristics of any nausea and vomiting (especially projectile vomiting) the child has experienced, as well as the frequency and consistency of his bowel movements. Does the child suffer from diarrhea or constipation? (When asking these questions, make sure the parents understand such terms as nausea, diarrhea, and constipation.) Remember, diarrhea can be serious in infants, because their extracellular fluid volume is proportionately larger than that of an older child or adult. Thus, diarrhea can quickly lead to dehydration, electrolyte imbalance, and possibly metabolic acidosis. Also determine if bowel symptoms occur during toilet training periods. (Ask at what age the child was

USUAL SEQUENCE OF TOOTH ERUPTION

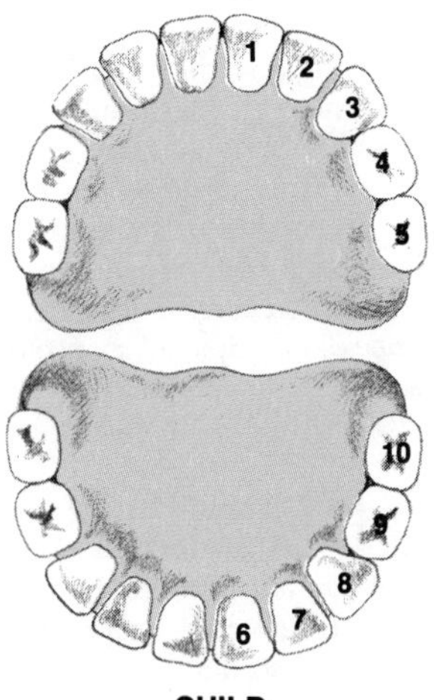

CHILD

PRIMARY DENTITION

Maxillary

1 Central incisor: 8 to 12 months
2 Lateral incisor: 10 to 12 months
3 Cuspid: 18 to 24 months
4 First molar: 12 to 15 months
5 Second molar: 24 to 30 months

Mandibular

6 Central incisor: 5 to 9 months
7 Lateral incisor: 12 to 15 months
8 Cuspid: 18 to 24 months
9 First molar: 12 to 15 months
10 Second molar: 24 to 30 months

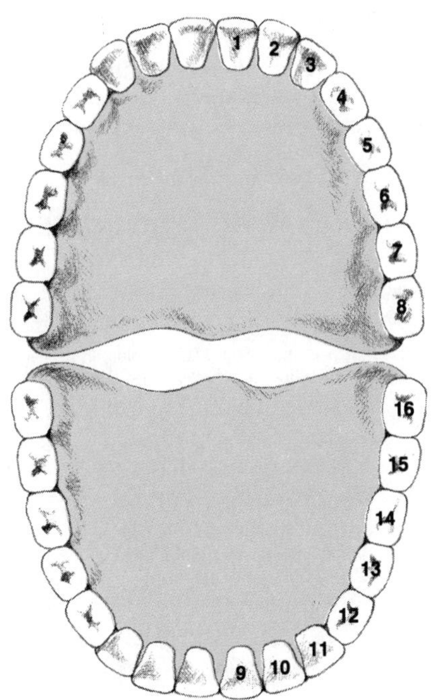

ADULT

PERMANENT DENTITION

Maxillary

1 Central incisor: age 7 to 8
2 Lateral incisor: age 8 to 9
3 Cuspid: age 11 to 12
4 First bicuspid: age 10 to 11
5 Second bicuspid: age 10 to 12
6 First molar: age 6 to 7
7 Second molar: age 12 to 13
8 Third molar: age 17 to 21

Mandibular

9 Central incisor: age 6 to 7
10 Lateral incisor: age 7 to 8
11 Cuspid: age 9 to 10
12 First bicuspid: age 10 to 12
13 Second bicuspid: age 11 to 12
14 First molar: age 6 to 7
15 Second molar: age 11 to 13
16 Third molar: age 17 to 21

toilet-trained.) Does the child ever eat dirt, grass, paint chips, or other nonfood materials?

Ask about any changes in life-style, such as a recent death in the family or a change in schools, that may be creating stress for the child.

Inquire if the child brushes his own teeth. Determine, too, if the parents leave a bottle of formula, milk, or juice in the crib with him at night, which may predispose the child to caries from nursing bottle syndrome. Ask about thumbsucking, which may cause malocclusion, especially if continued after age 4. Question the child's parents about family members who have malocclusion; this finding increases the child's risk of developing it.

Because abdominal symptoms may also indicate pathology outside the abdomen, ask if the child has other symptoms, such as a sore throat, a cough, or burning on urination.

458 Positioning the child

You'll usually assess a child's mouth while he's sitting. An uncooperative child will have to be restrained—an infant in the supine position and a toddler in the supine or sitting position, preferably in the parent's lap.

When examining a young child's abdomen, you may want to place your knees against the parent's knees to form an impromptu examining table. Or, if possible, have a parent hold the child. If this isn't possible, position the child so he can see his parent. Abdominal tenseness can impede your examination. To ease tenseness, flex an infant's knees and hips. Ask an older child to assume this position so you can examine him.

459 Inspecting the child's abdomen

The contour of a child's abdomen may be your first clue to a possible gastrointestinal disorder. In a child under age 4, you may see a mild potbelly (a normal finding) when the child stands or sits; from about age 4 to age 13, a mild potbelly is usually noticeable only when the child stands. An extreme potbelly may result from organomegaly, ascites, neoplasm, defects in the abdominal wall, or starvation; a depressed or concave abdomen may indicate a dia-

UNDERSTANDING ACUTE ABDOMINAL PAIN IN CHILDREN

DISORDER	DESCRIPTION
Hirschsprung's disease (congenital megacolon)	Developmental defect; absent ganglion cells in colon, impeding peristalsis; may result in intestinal obstruction
Intussusception	Telescoping of one intestinal segment into another (usually ileum into cecum), leading to acute intestinal obstruction
Incarcerated inguinal hernia	*Indirect:* weakness in fascial margin of internal inguinal ring *Direct:* weakness in fascial floor of inguinal canal; protrusion of sac (containing intestinal contents) at inguinal opening, with resultant bowel obstruction
Appendicitis	Obstruction of lumen of appendix, leading to inflammation and possibly perforation with peritonitis

phragmatic hernia. Look for an area of localized swelling.

Note any scars or abdominal vascularity. Superficial veins are readily visible in a normal infant (to a degree considered pathologic in an adult).

In children, respiratory movements are primarily abdominal; costal respiratory movements may indicate peritonitis, obstruction, or accumulation of ascitic fluid. The transition from abdominal to costal respirations is rather gradual.

To inspect an infant's abdomen, stand at the foot of the table and direct a light across his abdomen from his right side. Observe for peristaltic waves. (These waves normally progress unseen across an infant's abdomen from left to right during feeding.) Because peristaltic waves aren't normally visible in a full-term infant, their appearance probably indicates obstruction. Reverse peristalsis generally indicates pyloric stenosis; other possible causes include bowel malrotation, duodenal ulcer, gastrointestinal allergy, or duodenal stenosis.

Also observe a young child for diastasis recti abdominis (separation of the two abdominal recti muscles, with a protrusion between them). This benign condition is common, especially in black infants. A normal variation, it usually disappears during the preschool years. Inspect for umbilical hernia. The best time to perform this inspection is when the child cries. Also inspect the umbilicus for cleanliness and scar tissue.

460 Auscultating a child's abdomen

Auscultate a child's abdomen as you would an adult's. Significant findings (and their possible implications) include:

- *abdominal murmur:* coarctation of the aorta
- *high-pitched bowel sounds:* impending intestinal obstruction or gastroenteritis
- *venous hum:* portal hypertension
- *splenic or hepatic friction rubs:* inflammation
- *double sound,* or so-called *pistol shot,* in the femoral artery: aortic insufficiency
- *absence of bowel sounds:* paralytic ileus and peritonitis.

Acute abdominal pain (acute abdomen) occurs frequently in infancy and childhood. This chart details the most common causes of this problem.

HISTORY	PHYSICAL ASSESSMENT
Vomiting; abdominal distention; constipation possibly alternating with diarrhea	Palpable midline suprapubic mass, caused by feces-filled rectosigmoid
Colicky abdominal pain, with restlessness and intense crying; passage of bloody, mucoid "currant jelly" stools	Palpable sausage-shaped tender mass in right upper or lower quadrant
Cramping, abdominal pain; vomiting; abdominal distention; lump in inguinal area	Palpable, irreducible, tender swelling or lump in inguinal area
Vomiting common in children under age 8; midabdominal crampy pain, possibly progressing to right lower quadrant pain; slight fever	Request to cough will produce pain over site of peritoneal inflammation; bowel sounds may be depressed; rebound tenderness on palpation (performed by doctor)

461 Palpating the child's abdomen

Because of the child's underdeveloped abdominal wall, you should find palpation easier than in an adult. This part of an abdominal examination is very subjective; be sure to gain the child's cooperation so he'll report his symptoms truthfully. Because children tend to be more ticklish and tense than adults, you may need to distract a child while you're examining him—perhaps by starting a discussion or asking him to count or say the alphabet. Sometimes you can get a preschool child to cooperate by playing a game ("Let me feel what you had for breakfast.") and ensure his continued cooperation with amusing guesses ("A watermelon? A box of candy?"). To relax an infant's abdomen, have him suck a pacifier (not a bottle of milk, which may cause regurgitation).

Abdominal guarding is more common in children than in adults when pain is present (see *Understanding Acute Abdominal Pain in Children,* pages 424 to 425). Remember to palpate the painful quadrant last. To minimize ticklishness and let the child feel he has some control over the situation, you can palpate with the child's hand under your own, which can identify localized pain. This procedure isn't sufficiently sensitive, of course, to detect most palpable findings. Other clues to a child's pain include facial grimacing, sudden protective movement with an arm or leg, and a change in the pitch of the child's cry. Palpation in a quadrant other than the painful quadrant should reveal a soft, nontender abdomen. If it doesn't, the child is still tense. Try to relax him before proceeding or you're certain to evaluate inaccurately. A slightly tender descending colon may be caused by stool. Tenderness in the right lower quadrant may indicate an inflamed appendix. If your palpation consistently reveals generalized tenderness and rigidity in the affected quadrant, peritoneal irritation is probably present.

Next, ask the child to cough. A reduced or withheld cough may confirm peritoneal irritation, contraindicating checking for rebound tenderness—a potentially painful procedure for the child.

Check the child for a hernia as you would an adult. (To get a child to perform the Valsalva's maneuver, have him puff out his cheeks or blow up a balloon.)

Umbilical hernias are commonly present at birth. They usually increase in size until age 1 month and then gradually decrease until about age 1 year. An umbilical hernia may not always be visible. Here's a test: Press down on the infant's umbilicus. If you can insert one fingertip, the infant has a small hernia. Treatment usually consists of letting the hernia close by itself without surgery. Any hernia larger than ¾" (2 cm) or one that increases in size after age 1 month requires further assessment. (Black children have a higher incidence of all types of hernias.)

In most infants with pyloric stenosis, pyloric tumors are palpable. (Palpation is easiest immediately after the infant vomits.) Stand at the infant's left side and palpate with the middle finger flexed at a right angle. You'll find a tumor about the size and shape of an olive deep between the edges of the rectus muscle and the costal margin on the right side.

A child's potbelly with a plastic feel to the abdominal masses indicates megacolon.

462 Percussing a child's abdomen

Because a child swallows a lot of air when he eats and cries, you may hear louder tympanic tones when you percuss his abdomen, compared with those in an adult. Minimal tympany with abdominal distention may result from fluid accumulation or solid masses. To test for abdominal fluid, use the test for shifting dullness, instead of the test for a fluid wave.

In a neonate, ascites usually results from gastrointestinal or urinary perforation; in an older child, the cause may be heart failure, cirrhosis, or nephrosis.

463 Checking abdominal skin turgor

Tissue turgor is important in an infant, because dehydration—which may be fatal—proceeds so rapidly. Diarrhea accompanying gastroenteritis is a common cause of dehydration in infants. To test abdominal skin turgor, gently pull the child's skin and subcutaneous tissue up and then release it. Do the resulting creases disappear immediately after you let go of the skin? If not, consider the child dehydrated. If you suspect dehydration, assess the child's urinary output (see *Assessing Fluid Status*, page 444).

464 Assessing the mouth

Usually you'll examine a child's mouth as you would an adult's, but the patient's age may require you to modify your methods.

A toddler or preschool-age child may cooperate more easily if you examine his parent's mouth first. He'll probably want *his* mouth examined, too. Let the child handle the tongue depressor before you examine him to allay any fears he may have. You can also let the child place the depressor on his tongue as you guide his hand.

Inspecting an uncooperative child's mouth isn't easy or pleasant. One technique for bypassing clenched teeth is to ease a depressor along the lips, toward the back of the mouth, and then insert it between the posterior teeth in a downward motion, which triggers the gag reflex when you depress the posterior tongue. You then have a brief period to examine the child's mouth.

465 Avoiding the gag reflex

To avoid making a child gag when examining his mouth, try these tips:

- Tell the child to stick his tongue out and pant like a puppy while you examine his mouth.
- Avoid touching the patient's posterior tongue when using a tongue depressor except when viewing the posterior pharynx (or examining an uncooperative child).
- Use the tongue depressor on each side of his tongue and examine one half of his throat at a time.

466 Examining a child's teeth

If you can identify dental or mouth problems in a child, he may be able to receive treatment before costlier (or permanent) sequelae occur. First, observe the child for malocclusion. Don't ask him to *show* you his teeth, because reflex alignment may make his bite appear normal. Instead, ask him to bite down hard while his mouth is closed; then evert his lips and observe his bite.

Inspect the child's teeth carefully for dental caries and tooth eruption. Dental caries in primary teeth pose a special problem because of possible infection, loss of teeth, and loss of space for permanent tooth eruption. Also check for lack of tooth eruption by age 1 and for missing teeth in older children.

467 Inspecting for gingivitis

Inspect the child's gums carefully. Gingivitis, a common condition among children, usually results from a combination of such factors as:

- mouth breathing (often associated with nasal insufficiency from such problems as enlarged adenoids or allergies) in which constant passage of air dries out the gums and inflames the anterior labial gingiva
- tooth eruption (the presence of both primary and permanent teeth commonly causes abnormal gingival stimulation from chewing and from food impaction)
- puberty (hormonal stimulation, especially in girls, contributes to gingivitis).

Gingivitis may also result from a combination of poor hygiene, crooked teeth, retained primary roots, and poor diet. (*Note:* Gingivitis may also be the first clinical sign of leukemia.)

468 Tongue and buccal mucosa

When you inspect and palpate a child's tongue, check for abnormalities that are often seen in children. These include the strawberry (later raspberry) appearance that occurs during scarlet fever and the condition of being tongue-tied—unable to touch the tongue to the lips because of shortness of the frenulum.

In a child with a history of fever, chills, and coughing, be sure to check the buccal mucosa opposite the first and second molars for small white spots on erythematous bases (Koplik's spots), the prodromal hallmark of measles.

White, slightly raised patches on the buccal mucosa (or on the tongue and pharynx) that are indurated and tend to bleed when removed characterize *thrush,* an infection caused by *Candida albicans.* Thrush usually begins on the buccal mucosa or tongue and spreads to other areas of the mouth.

Inspect a young child's tongue for a dry, shriveled appearance, which may be a clue to dehydration. Absence of tongue papillae suggests avitaminosis.

469 Palate and lips

Abnormalities of a child's palate that you may encounter during inspection and palpation include bruising, which may result from forced feeding, and cleft palate, a congenital abnormality. Cleft palate may be partial or complete. It may affect only the soft palate, or it may extend through the hard and soft palate to the incisive foramen. Cleft palate commonly occurs with cleft lip, another congenital defect, which may be unilateral or bilateral. Cleft lip usually affects the alveolar ridge and varies in severity from a notch in the border of the lip to a complete cleft involving the floor of the nose. The nasal cartilage may also be deformed or displaced.

Assessing geriatric patients

470 Normal physiologic variations

When assessing an elderly patient's gastrointestinal (GI) system, pay particular attention to the physiologic changes that accompany aging. Fortunately, these are less debilitating in the GI system than in most other body systems. Normal changes include diminished mucosal elasticity and reduced GI secretions that, in turn, modify some processes—for example, digestion and absorption. GI tract motility, bowel wall and anal sphincter tone, and abdominal muscle strength may also decrease with age. Any of these changes may cause complaints in an elderly patient, ranging from loss of appetite to constipation.

Normal physiologic changes in the liver include decreased liver weight, reduced regenerative capacity, and decreased blood flow to the liver.

471 Assessment technique differences

Assessing an elderly patient's GI system is similar to examining the younger adult, with these differences: Abdominal palpation is usually easier and the results more accurate, because the elderly patient's abdominal wall is thinner (from muscle wasting and loss of fibroconnective tissue), and his muscle tone is usually more relaxed. A rigid abdomen, which in a younger patient may be from peritoneal inflammation, is less common in the elderly. Abdominal distention is more common.

472 Assessing the mouth

When assessing an elderly patient's mouth, inspect carefully for limited movement of the temporomandibular joint, and be alert for complaints of pain. These symptoms may indicate degenerative arthritis.

Pay particular attention to the elderly patient's teeth. Often you'll find loose teeth (from bone resorption that occurs in periodontal disease) or missing or replaced teeth (see *Identifying Dental Appliances*, page 430). Because many elderly patients don't replace lost teeth, common problems in this age-group include keratosis of the ridge, irritation, fibromas, and malocclusion. Mouth pathology is more common among the elderly for several reasons. For one, they are predisposed to mouth disorders by the normal physiology of the aging process. Other contributing factors include:

- physical disability (such as arthritis) that inhibits proper oral hygiene
- inadequate diet, resulting in nutritional deficiencies, which in elderly persons may initially produce gastrointestinal symptoms
- chronic systemic illnesses, especially diabetes mellitus
- chronic irritation from smoking or alcohol consumption
- inadequate dental care because of insufficient income.

Pathologic changes that are more common in the elderly include oral carcinoma, dysplasia, atrophic glossitis, xerostomia (dry mouth), and denture-related fibrous hyperplasia.

473 Esophageal disturbances

Esophageal peristalsis may decrease with age, leading to delayed emptying, irritation, and dilatation, and producing signs and symptoms of gastric reflux. Ask the elderly patient about any burning sensation after meals, because gastric reflux is the most common cause of heartburn. Chest pain, the other major symptom of gastric reflux, is usually substernal and varies from mild discomfort to a severe stabbing sensation. Pain is usually associated with food intake and may be accentuated when the patient stoops or lies down; antacids usually relieve it. The pain from gastric reflux is difficult to differentiate from cardiac or hiatal hernia pain, and necessitates medical consultation.

Because dysphagia is characteristic of esophageal cancer (and the incidence of this disease rises with age), refer any elderly patient with this symptom to a doctor.

In the elderly, hiatal hernia is the most common upper gastrointestinal tract problem, affecting about 70% of persons over age 70. This condition commonly results from weakened musculature around the diaphragmatic hiatus that allows herniation of the lower esophagus and cardiac sphincter into the thorax. Signs and symptoms, including substernal pain, usually appear after periods of intraabdominal pressure. Be sure to ask the patient if his problems seem to occur following bending or straining, or even vomiting or coughing. Also assess for ascites and obesity, which also can increase intraabdominal pressure (see Entry 185). Ask the patient if changing his body position relieves the symptoms, because many of these hernias are sliding hernias, which move into the thoracic cavity when the patient lies down and return to the abdominal cavity when he sits or stands up. Ask the patient how many pillows he uses when he sleeps. Patients with hiatal hernia or gastric reflux often use two or three pillows. (Remember that patients with chronic obstructive lung disease may also use several pillows.)

474 Stomach disturbances

Atrophic gastritis, a common stomach disorder among the elderly, is chronic inflammation of the stomach. It causes gradual mucosal degeneration, diminishing the number of parietal and chief

IDENTIFYING DENTAL APPLIANCES

Although patients of any age may require tooth replacement, this problem is most common in elderly persons. During your examination, you may encounter any of these dental appliances:

- *Fixed bridge:* a permanent artificial tooth or teeth designed to replace a missing tooth or teeth. Usually one tooth on either side is crowned (capped) to support the replacement teeth that are cemented to them. Because bridges are often made of gold and porcelain, take care handling them; they're brittle.
- *Removable partial denture:* a removable appliance designed to replace long spans of missing teeth or teeth missing on both sides of the mouth. In many cases, maxillary partial dentures cover the palate partially or fully; mandibular partial dentures cross the midline by way of a connector lingual to the mandible. Most partial dentures are attached mechanically, usually with clasps to supporting teeth. Partial dentures usually consist of porcelain or plastic teeth on an acrylic and metal framework. These appliances can be removed or dislodged; their clasps can be easily bent.
- *Complete denture:* upper and lower appliances usually made of porcelain and acrylic; can be easily broken. An upper denture usually covers the palate and is held in place by a partial vacuum. A lower denture fits on the mandibular ridge and is designed to permit movement of the tongue. The lower denture is easier to dislodge, to break, or to aspirate than the upper denture.

Note the type and location of any of these appliances, and check for deterioration. Pathologic lesions commonly associated with dental appliances include periodontitis, gingivitis, candidiasis, fibrous hyperplasia, and chronic irritative ulcers.

cells. As a result, the gastric acid content of the stomach also decreases (achlorhydria), which can lead to malabsorption of calcium and iron. Loss of parictal cells decreases production of the intrinsic factor necessary for the absorption of vitamin B_{12}; this can cause pernicious anemia.

About 15% of the U.S. population over age 60 suffers from peptic ulcers. The incidence of complications from peptic ulcers and of associated mortality is also higher in the elderly population. Testing the stool for occult blood is a good screening device to use for all elderly patients.

475 Problems of the small intestine

Decreased enzyme secretion, which begins at about age 40, can cause problems in elderly persons because of decreased nutrient absorption (chiefly carbohydrates) and delayed fat absorption (causing interference with absorption of fat-soluble vitamins). Diminished gastrointestinal tract motility and impaired blood flow to the small intestine can also impair nutrient absorption. Remember, however, that an inadequate diet commonly causes vitamin and other nutritional deficiencies.

476 Problems of the large intestine

Assess for *dehydration* in an elderly patient with inadequate water intake, excessive salt intake, or a gastrointestinal (GI) disorder that disturbs water absorption in the large intestine (such as inflammation, diarrhea, and vomiting).

Atherosclerosis narrows abdominal blood vessels, compromising circulation to the colon. This can lead to pathology ranging from irritation and diminished absorption to complete vascular occlusion and bowel obstruction.

Diverticulosis, which occurs often in the elderly, is the asymptomatic presence of diverticula—pouches that bulge through the weakened intestinal wall because of persistent high intraluminal pressure. Diverticulosis may progress to a symptomatic form *(diverticulitis),* in which inflamed diverticula produce pain (in the lower left or middle abdomen), changed bowel habits, flatulence, and possibly bowel obstruction.

The elderly population has the highest incidence of *colorectal cancer.* Although some signs and symptoms, such as rectal bleeding, usually receive prompt attention, others—such as constipation, diarrhea, and changes in bowel habits—are typically vague and may be minimized by the patient.

Rectal polyps usually affect elderly persons; normally, they're difficult to palpate, because they're soft.

Constipation is a common GI problem among the elderly. It may result from several factors, so be sure to ask the patient about the following points:

- overdependence on laxatives
- anorectal lesions
- low dietary fiber
- habitual disregard of the urge to defecate
- emotional upset or stress
- lack of exercise
- insufficient fluid intake
- use of drugs (such as some tranquilizers, antacids, and iron preparations).

Ask the patient if he has difficulty passing stool. (Some patients think constipation means a decrease in elimination frequency to a degree they consider abnormal.) Refer the patient to a doctor if his constipation continues after correction of the apparent cause.

Fecal incontinence occurs in many elderly patients and probably results from such age-related conditions as changes in intestinal motility, loss of internal sphincter muscle tone, or compromise of voluntary and involuntary brain centers controlling defecation. In your patient history, include questions about the patient's mobility (immobility may prevent him from reaching the bathroom in time). Also rule out fecal impaction and rectal anomalies, such as painful fissures, as causes of fecal incontinence.

477 Liver and biliary system

Always assess an elderly patient for jaundice, which may indicate such causes of obstruction of the common bile duct as cancer of the head of the pancreas or cholelithiasis. Patients with cholelithiasis (a condition that affects more than one third of all persons between ages 70 and 80) usually complain of midepigastric pain 3 to 6 hours after a heavy or fatty meal.

Selected References

Antoon, J.W., and Miller, R.L. "Aphthous Ulcers: A Review of the Literature on Etiology, Pathogenesis, Diagnosis and Treatment," *Journal of the American Dental Association* 101:803, 1980.

Brown, M.S., and Alexander, M.M. "Physical Examination: Part 10, Mouth and Throat," *Nursing74* 4:57, August 1974.

Daly, K.M. "Oral Cancer: Everyday Concerns," *American Journal of Nursing* 79:1415, August 1979.

Gannon, E.P., and Kadezabek, E. "Giving Your Patients Meticulous Mouth Care," *Nursing80* 10:70, March 1980.

Kirkis, E.J. "This Oral Technique Gets Results," *RN Magazine* 41:82, October 1978.

Kolb, L. *Modern Clinical Psychiatry*, 9th ed. Philadelphia: W.B. Saunders Co., 1977.

Meissner, J.E. "A Simple Guide for Assessing Oral Health," *Nursing80* 10:84, April 1980.

Miller, J.K., and Miller, R.L. "Identifying and Assessing Oral Ulcers," *Nursing81* 11:10, July 1981.

Ostchega, Y. "Preventing...and Treating...Cancer Chemotherapy's Oral Complications," *Nursing80* 10:47, August 1980.

Sutton, R.B.O. "Acute Periodontal Conditions," *Nursing Mirror* 139:67, July 5, 1974.

Zegarelli, Edward V., et al., eds. *Diagnosis of Diseases of the Mouth and Jaws*, 2nd ed. Philadelphia: Lea and Febiger, 1978.

12

KEY POINTS IN THIS CHAPTER

KEY CHARTS IN THIS CHAPTER

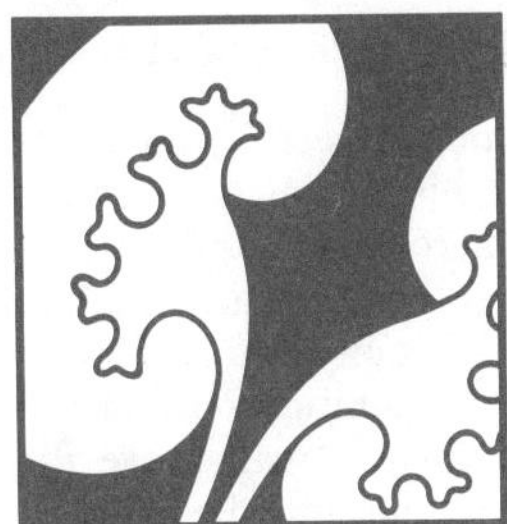

Urinary System

Introduction

478 Recognizing urinary system disorders

Knowing when to assess your patient's urinary system can be difficult, because patients with urinary disorders may exhibit a wide range of signs and symptoms. For instance, a patient with impending renal failure from Goodpasture's syndrome may exhibit only hemoptysis. Or consider the patient with severe chronic renal insufficiency (a 50% to 75% loss of normal function). He may have a brief history and few signs and symptoms; he may even look and feel well because his body has compensated as the disease has slowly progressed. Unfortunately, sometimes such a patient is treated only to relieve his signs and symptoms, while the underlying cause of his problem goes undetected.

When you assess any patient (regardless of his chief complaint), always look for subtle changes in his well-being, and explore further any signs and symptoms of possible urinary system disorders. (Remember, kidney failure may be insidious.) The investigation should include not only a detailed history and a thorough physical examination but also such basic laboratory tests as urinalysis, complete blood count, coagulation profile, and blood chemistries (especially blood urea nitrogen, creatinine, and electrolytes).

479 The kidneys' role in homeostasis

The body's systems depend on the kidneys to maintain homeostasis. In turn, the kidneys depend on other body systems for the same critical purpose. For example, the *cardiovascular system* must deliver blood to the kidneys at a pressure adequate for filtration. The kidneys reciprocate by regulating fluid balance, which maintains the circulating blood volume and electrolyte balance necessary for myocardial function. The kidneys also play an important role in the production of erythropoietin (a hormone regulating red blood cell production).

The kidneys are coordinated with the *nervous system,* which helps regulate blood pressure and control urination; with the *endocrine system,* which maintains sodium and water balance by producing aldosterone and antidiuretic hormone; and with the *musculoskeletal system,* which relies on the kidneys for vitamin D synthesis.

These are just a few examples of the kidneys' importance to a person's overall health and ability to function. Remember, you may uncover clues to possible problems in *any body system* when you assess a patient's renal system. So remain alert to the kidneys' vital homeostatic role every time you assess a patient.

Reviewing anatomy and physiology

480 Kidneys

The kidneys are smooth, bean-shaped organs, about 5″ (12.7 cm) long, 2½″ (6.5 cm) wide, and 1½″ (4 cm) thick. Located retroperitoneally, they lie primarily in the lumbar region, on both sides of the vertebrae. In a standing patient, the left kidney normally occupies the space between the first and fourth lumbar vertebrae, with the right kidney slightly lower because of the liver above it. In a supine patient, the kidneys are one vertebra higher. Because of their protective layers, the kidneys aren't usually palpable, except in very thin patients with weak abdominal muscles.

Internally, each kidney contains two distinct regions: the *cortex* (outer portion) and the *medulla* (inner portion). The *hilus* is the medial indentation where renal blood vessels, nerves, and the ureter enter and exit the kidney. The renal medulla contains the renal pyramids, triangular divisions containing most of the nephrons. The pyramids' papillae extend into the calices of the kidney, which then join to form the renal pelvis (upper end of the ureter). The cortex surrounds the base of the pyramids and projects between them.

Highly vascular organs, the kidneys regulate fluid and electrolyte balance through glomerular filtration and rid the body of waste products by passing urine. They receive almost one fourth of the total cardiac output. Blood enters the kidney through the two renal arteries at each hilus.

481 Ureters

Once formed, urine collects in the renal pelvis (upper end of the ureter). It exits the kidney through the hilus by way of the ureter, which descends along the posterior abdominal wall and enters the bladder anteromedially. Each ureter is about 1′ (30 cm) long, lying half in the abdominal cavity and half in the pelvic cavity. Peristaltic contractions of the smooth muscle wall move the urine down the ureter into the bladder.

482 Bladder

When the bladder is full, it lies under the peritoneal cavity; when empty, it's positioned behind the pubic bones. In women, the supporting urogenital diaphragm lies directly below the bladder; in men, it's below the prostate gland, which surrounds the upper portion of the urethra. Low in the bladder's posterior wall, the ureteral and urethral orifices form the *trigone,* a triangular structure. The urethral orifice is the lowest of the three openings.

The muscular bladder can hold as much as 1 qt (1 liter) of urine. The rugal folds of its inner tissues and its transitional epithelial lining account for its remarkable holding capacity. Parasympathetic stimulation of the bladder's smooth muscle layers precipitates micturition (urination) through the urethra.

483 Urethra

In women, the urethra is short—about 1½″ (4 cm)—and is located in the vagina's anterior wall. Muscle surrounds it as it extends from the bladder to the urethral meatus, between the clitoris and vaginal orifice. In men, the urethra is much longer—about 8″ (20 cm)—because it must pass through the penis (surrounded by erectile or cavernous tissue), connecting the urethral meatus distally and the prostate proximally.

484 Urine formation

Each kidney contains about 1.3 million nephrons—its functional units. The

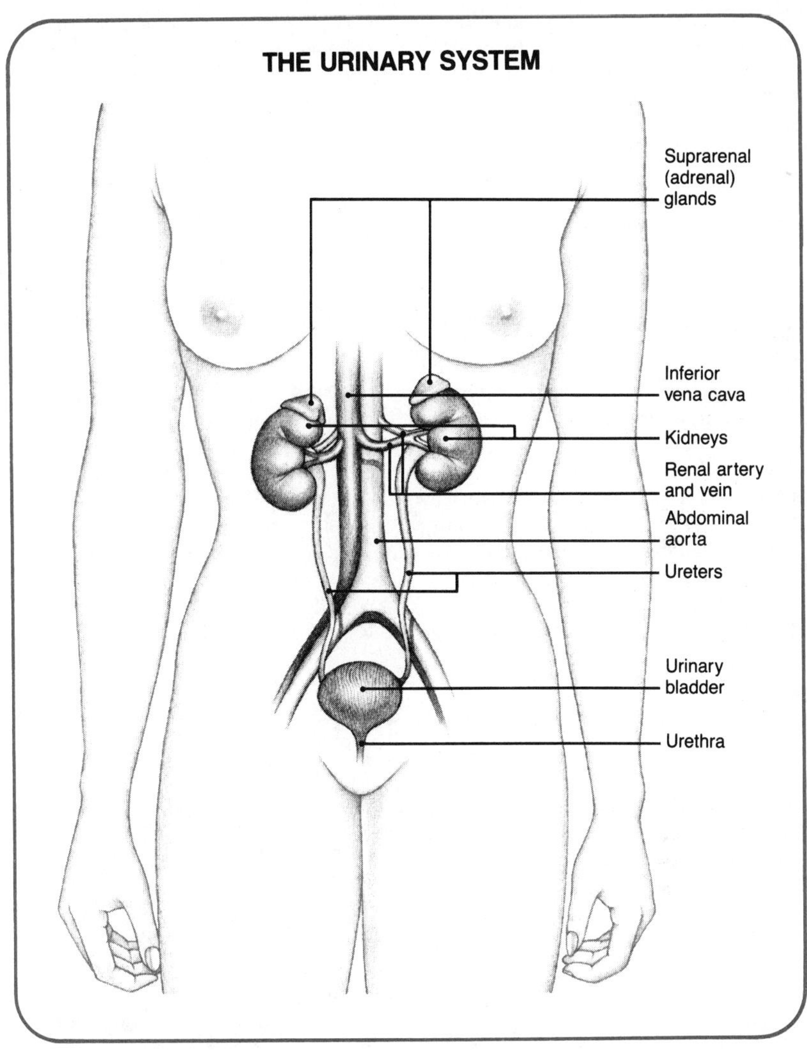

nephron includes the *renal corpuscle* and the *tubules.* Nephrons in the kidney's outer cortex, called *cortical nephrons,* may be too short to reach the medulla. But the *juxtamedullary nephrons* have long limbs and can enter the medullary pyramids, which contain the collecting tubules.

Nephrons receive blood from the *afferent arterioles,* subdivisions of the renal artery. An afferent arteriole enters the renal corpuscle and divides into the capillary network of the *glomerulus.* As blood passes through the glomerular capillaries to the efferent arterioles, pressure inside the glomerular capillaries causes fluid to filter through the capillary membranes into *Bowman's capsule,* which is made up of highly differentiated cells. A normal glomerulus produces an ultrafiltrate of plasma as blood passes from the afferent arteriole to the narrower *efferent arteriole.* The pressure within the glomerulus forces the filtrate through the visceral layer of Bowman's capsule into

Bowman's space. To enter the nephron's tubular system, the filtrate must then penetrate a parietal layer of epithelial cells surrounding Bowman's space.

Because glomerular capillaries are situated between two arterioles, their blood pressure is about twice that of other capillaries. Glomerular filtration depends on blood pressure, and the filtration rate is directly proportional to blood flow. (A drastic and prolonged blood pressure reduction can result in permanent kidney shutdown.) Assisted by capsular osmotic pressure, the blood hydrostatic pressure is the main force opposing blood osmotic pressure and capsular hydrostatic pressure. Thus water, polypeptides, sugars, electrolytes, urea, amino acids, and many other molecules push through the pores of the capillary endothelium, the basement membrane, and the visceral layer. However, the basement membrane repels many intermediate-sized plasma proteins, such as albumin, because of their negative charge. Therefore, they don't usually appear in normal urine. Because of their size, large proteins, red blood cells, and platelets don't usually pass through the endothelial pores. If they do, they're stopped by the basement membrane. All these barriers are permeable to water, allowing a 42½- to 48-gal (160- to 180-liter) daily volume of glomerular filtrate for an adult kidney.

485 Tubular reabsorption and secretion

After the filtrate leaves the renal corpuscle, 70% to 80% of it is selectively reabsorbed through the proximal tubule pores. The reabsorbed filtrate then passes back into the peritubular capillaries; the remainder of the filtrate enters the loop of Henle. As the filtrate passes along the tubules, substances

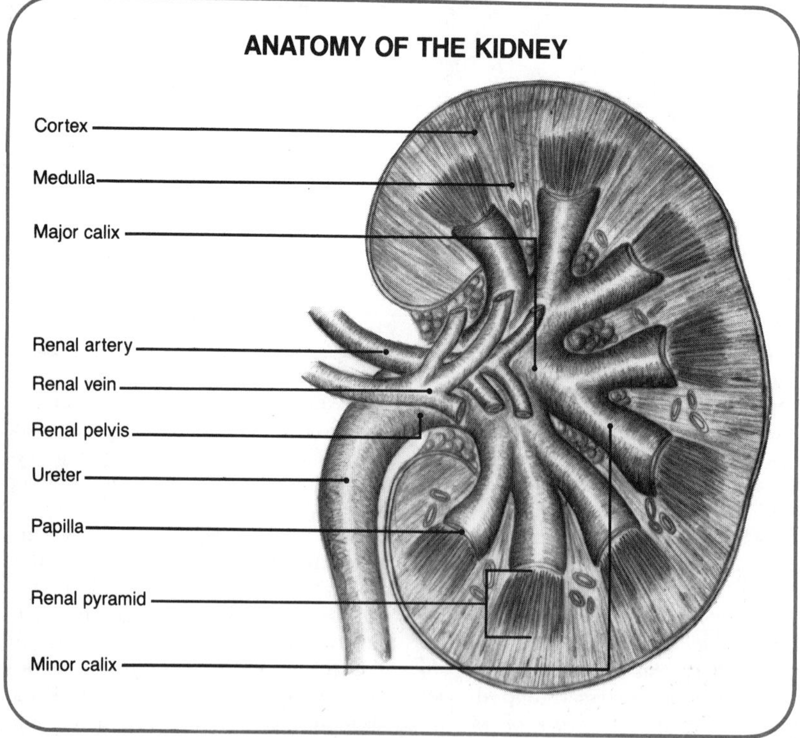

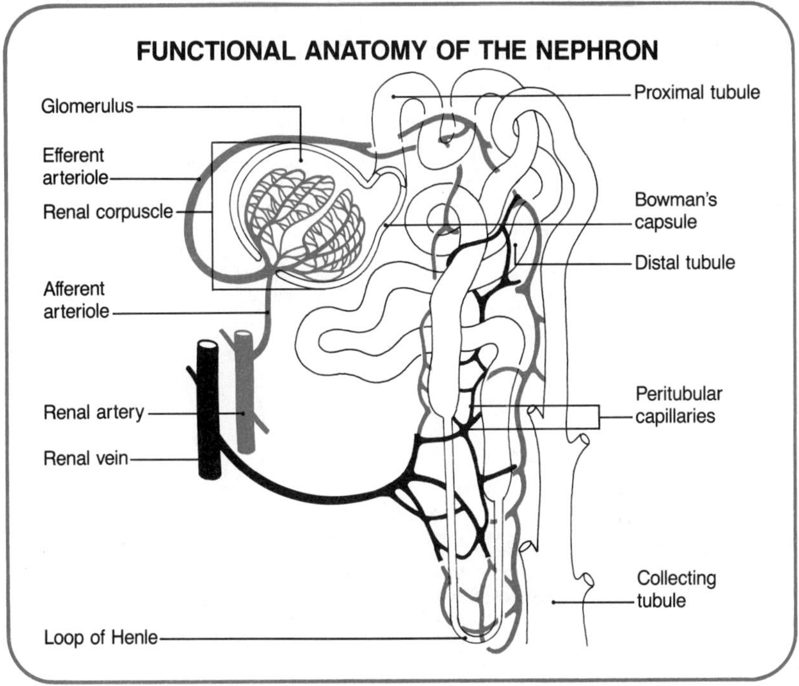

are selectively reabsorbed and secreted until the filtrate enters the renal pelvis as urine. Active and passive transport are the primary mechanisms of reabsorption and secretion. (In active transport, a substance moves against a gradient of electrical or chemical potential; in passive transport, or diffusion, a substance moves down a gradient and so expends no energy.) Electrical differences cause diffusion of ions through the tubules. For example, negatively charged chloride ions follow positively charged sodium ions out of the tubule to keep the electrical charge neutral. Specific substances (water, nutrients, and ions) are reabsorbed or secreted in different segments of the tubules. Water is reabsorbed by osmosis. (See *How Urine Is Formed*, page 438.) About 90% of bicarbonate is indirectly reabsorbed in the proximal tubule through sodium and hydrogen exchange. Bicarbonate is the principal buffer that contributes to maintaining blood pH within normal limits.

The distal tubule regulates final water and acid-base balance. The total solute concentration of body fluids remains constant, despite fluctuations in water and solute intake or excretion. On ingestion of a large volume of fluid, urine becomes dilute and excess water is rapidly excreted. During water deprivation or excessive solute intake, urine becomes highly concentrated, and water is retained to restore the body fluids' normal concentration.

Of the approximately 48 gal (180 liters) of fluid filtered by the glomeruli each day, the kidneys excrete only about 1 qt (1 liter). The rest is reabsorbed by the peritubular capillaries—one of two capillary beds supplying the nephron.

486 Hormonal regulation

Hormones regulate tubular reabsorption and secretion of solutes and water. *Antidiuretic hormone* (ADH) influences the distal and collecting tubules by stimulating urea and water diffu-

HOW URINE IS FORMED

The body excretes urine only after several processes take place within the convoluted tubules. These processes include selective tubular reabsorption of water and solutes as well as selective tubular secretion of solutes.

This chart and functional drawing help explain where most products are reabsorbed and/or secreted during the process of urine formation. Note that the collecting tubules may reabsorb *or* secrete sodium, potassium ions, hydrogen ions, ammonium ions, and urea, depending on the patient's physiologic needs.

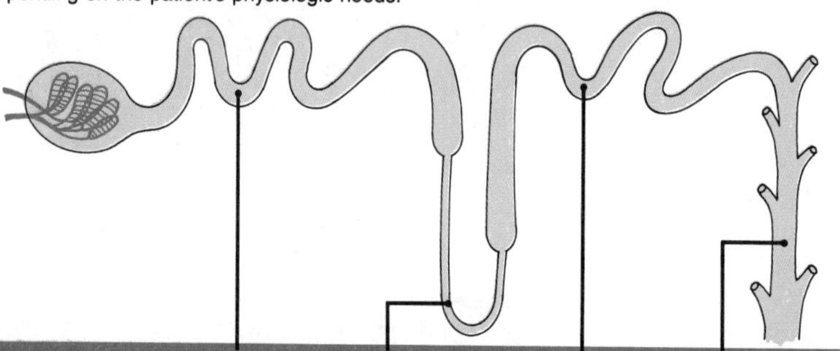

	PROXIMAL TUBULE	LOOP OF HENLE	DISTAL TUBULE	COLLECTING TUBULE
Products reabsorbed	- - Chloride ions — Glucose — Potassium ions — Amino acids — Bicarbonate ions — Phosphate ions - - Urea — Sodium ions - - Water — Uric acid — Magnesium ions — Calcium ions	- - Sodium ions — Chloride ions	- - Chloride ions — Sodium ions+ - - Water* — Bicarbonate ions	- - Water* — Sodium ions — Potassium ions — Hydrogen ions - - Ammonium ions - - Urea
Products secreted	— Hydrogen ions — Foreign substances — Creatinine	- - Sodium chloride	— Water — Potassium ions+ - - Urea — Hydrogen ions - - Ammonium ions — Uric acid	— Urea — Sodium ions — Potassium ions — Hydrogen ions - - Ammonium ions
Character of filtrate	Isotonic	Hypotonic	Isotonic or hypotonic	Concentrated

KEY - - passive transport
— active transport

* Antidiuretic hormone required for absorption to occur.
+ Stimulated by aldosterone, which is controlled by the renin-angiotensin system.

sion into the medullary interstitium and forming a concentrated urine. Thus, a lack of ADH results in a dilute urine.

Sodium concentration in the tubule stimulates secretion of the hormone *renin*. A proteolytic enzyme, renin converts the plasma protein angiotensinogen to angiotensin I, which is modified in the lungs to angiotensin II, a potent vasoconstrictor and a powerful stimulator of aldosterone from the adrenal cortex. Elevated aldosterone levels then stimulate sodium reabsorption from the distal tubules and collecting ducts. Water is passively attracted to sodium and will move with sodium to be reabsorbed into the blood, where it increases blood volume and pressure, ensuring adequate glomerular function.

The distal tubules regulate potassium excretion. The adrenal cortex responds to elevated serum potassium levels by increasing aldosterone secretion. Aldosterone influences the potassium-secreting capacity of the distal tubular cells, but the action isn't understood. Regardless of the mechanism, the kidneys—the site of sodium-potassium exchange—regulate serum potassium levels, because potassium and hydrogen ions compete for sodium's place in the tubular cells.

487 Urine characteristics

Urine, the final product of nephron and collecting tubule activity, is normally sterile, with a pH ranging from 4.5 to 8.0. Its constituents include sodium, chloride, potassium, calcium, magnesium, sulfates, phosphates, bicarbonates, uric acid, ammonium ions, enzymes, urea, modified hormones and drugs, creatinine, urobilinogen, epithelial cells, crystals, a few sperm or leukocytes, and as many as five red blood cells per high-power field. Urine volume varies with intake and climate, but 30 to 60 oz (1,000 to 2,000 ml) per 24 hours—which represents 1% or less of the original glomerular filtrate—is normal. Normal concentration, measured by specific gravity determination, ranges from 1.008 to 1.030.

Collecting appropriate history data

488 Biographical data

When you collect biographical data, pay particular attention to age and race. Age is significant because the signs and symptoms of some renal diseases are more common in certain age-groups. For instance, polycystic kidney disease, which can remain dormant for years, usually manifests its first signs and symptoms in persons between ages 40 and 60. Race is also related to the incidence of some renal diseases; for example, malignant hypertension, which can lead to nephrosclerosis and renal failure, is most prevalent in blacks.

489 Chief complaint

The most common chief complaints regarding urinary disorders are *output changes* (polyuria, oliguria, anuria), *voiding pattern changes* (frequency, urgency, nocturia), *urine color changes,* and *pain* (suprapubic pain, flank pain, dysuria).

490 History of present illness

Using the PQRST mnemonic device (see page 440), ask the patient to elaborate on his chief complaint. Then, depending on the complaint, explore the history of his present illness by asking the following types of questions:

• ***Output changes.*** *Have you noticed a change in the amount of urine excreted? How often do you have this problem? Does it occur only if you drink a lot of fluids?* Always compare

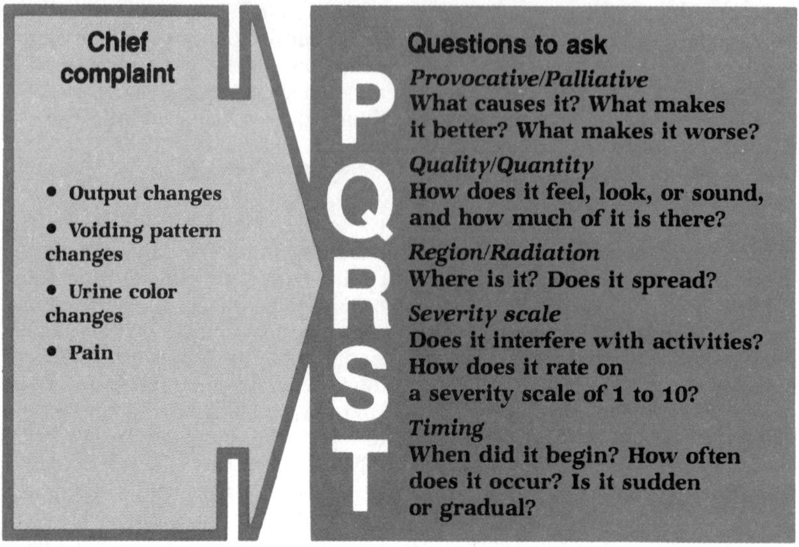

Chief complaint

- Output changes
- Voiding pattern changes
- Urine color changes
- Pain

Questions to ask

P *Provocative/Palliative*
What causes it? What makes it better? What makes it worse?

Q *Quality/Quantity*
How does it feel, look, or sound, and how much of it is there?

R *Region/Radiation*
Where is it? Does it spread?

S *Severity scale*
Does it interfere with activities? How does it rate on a severity scale of 1 to 10?

T *Timing*
When did it begin? How often does it occur? Is it sudden or gradual?

intake and output before considering a patient's output abnormal.

• ***Voiding pattern changes.*** *How many times a day do you usually urinate? Recently, how many times a day have you been urinating? Have you noticed a change in the size of your urine stream? Does your bladder still feel full after you've urinated? Do you urinate small amounts frequently? Do you wake up during the night to urinate? Are you unable to wait to urinate? Do you have a problem controlling your urine?* Most voiding pattern changes suggest bladder dysfunction or an infectious process. In an edematous patient on bed rest, nocturia may result from rapid fluid reabsorption.

• ***Urine color changes.*** *What color is your urine? How long has it been this color?* A dark amber color may indicate concentrated urine, usually associated with diminished volume. A clear, watery appearance may indicate dilute urine, associated with increased volume. Brown or bright-red urine may contain blood. Other color variations may result from taking certain medications.

• ***Pain.*** *Do you ever have pain when trying to urinate? Do you ever feel a burning sensation when urinating? How often?* Painful spasms during urination suggest calculi. Dysuria described as a burning sensation usually indicates a disorder of the lower urinary tract. *Do you have painful distention of your abdomen? Do you have pain over the pubic area or in your lower back? Is the pain dull or sharp? Does repositioning relieve suprapubic or flank pain?* Position changes don't relieve pain from renal colic, but lying down does reduce inflammatory pain.

491 Past history

Focus your past history questions on the following areas:

• ***Kidney or bladder problems.*** Kidney and bladder stones tend to recur.

• ***Systemic diseases.*** Signs and symptoms of diabetic nephropathy—hypertension, edema, and azotemia—may appear 10 to 15 years after onset of diabetes mellitus. Urinary symptoms of systemic lupus erythematosus (SLE), such as nephritis, may appear at onset or later. (SLE may also produce recurrent swelling that's characteristic of the nephrotic syndrome.) Tuberculosis may reach the urinary tract; disseminated intravascular coagulation can lead to severe renal perfusion problems; and hepatic disease can occur with renal failure.

- ***Nerve damage.*** In multiple sclerosis, demyelination can affect bladder musculature, causing urinary hesitancy and chronic urinary tract infections.
- ***Sexually transmitted disease.*** Gonorrhea causes urinary tract problems (discharge, dysuria, urgency, and frequency) that may be the first indications of the disease.
- ***Streptococcal infection.*** A recent episode of streptococcal infection increases a patient's risk of glomerulonephritis.
- ***Allergies.*** Some immune complex reactions (to foods, insects, drugs, or contrast media, for example) can cause tubular damage; severe anaphylactic reactions can produce temporary renal failure and permanent tubular necrosis.
- ***Medications.*** Many drugs can produce signs and symptoms of urinary disorders (see *Nurse's Guide to Urinary Disorders,* pages 452 to 455).
- ***Urinary tract surgery.*** Be sure to ask your patient whether he's ever had surgery for a urinary disorder. If so, ask how long ago it was performed.

492 Family history

Ask your patient if anyone in his family has ever had any of the following conditions:

- ***Noninherited renal disorders.*** Although they're not hereditary, such disorders as urinary tract infections, congenital anomalies, and urinary calculi recur in some families.
- ***Hereditary renal diseases.*** Polycystic kidney disease and all types of hereditary nephritis (such as Alport's syndrome) are genetically transmitted conditions that can progress to end-stage renal disease.
- ***Inheritable systemic diseases.*** Hypertension and diabetes mellitus can eventually cause nephropathies.

493 Psychosocial history

An occupation or activity may keep a person so busy he can't (or won't) take time to urinate when he feels the urge. This can predispose him to bladder or urinary tract infections.

494 Activities of daily living

When questioning your patient about his daily activities, concentrate on the following areas:

- ***Diet.*** Learning about your patient's diet may provide valuable information (see Entry 173). As the patient describes his usual diet, determine if he takes in an adequate amount of fluid, salt, and protein. Ask if he's on a special diet and, if so, whether a doctor prescribed it. (Prolonged reducing diets involving liquid protein are associated with kidney dysfunction.) Special diets for renal patients include sodium, potassium, protein, and fluid restrictions.
- ***Sleeping.*** Disturbed sleep from nocturnal muscle cramps of the calves and thighs is common in early renal failure. A reversal in sleep patterns (awake at night, asleep during the day) is also a symptom of renal failure.

495 Review of systems

Your review of systems should include questions about the following signs and symptoms:

- ***Skin.*** Itchy skin may indicate calcium or uremic deposits.
- ***Cardiovascular.*** Hypertension may result from renal disease or predispose a person to it. Shortness of breath, paroxysmal nocturnal dyspnea, orthopnea, and edema may indicate kidney disease. Sudden weight change may result from an altered water balance.
- ***Gastrointestinal.*** A metallic taste or urinous breath odor (uremic fetor) may indicate diminished renal function. Anorexia, nausea, and vomiting may accompany any stage of renal dysfunction.

DRUGS

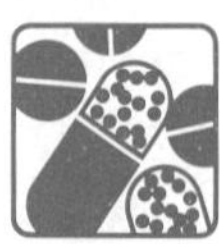

NURSE'S GUIDE TO SOME DRUGS THAT AFFECT THE URINARY SYSTEM

CLASSIFICATION	POSSIBLE SIDE EFFECTS
Adrenergic blocker (sympatholytic)	
methysergide maleate (Sansert*)	• Retroperitoneal fibrosis, causing urinary obstruction
Alkylating agents	
cisplatin (Platinol)	• Hemorrhagic cystitis, bladder fibrosis
cyclophosphamide (Cytoxan*)	• Nephrotoxicity
Aminoglycosides	
gentamicin sulfate (Garamycin*) tobramycin sulfate (Nebcin*)	• Nephrotoxicity
Narcotic analgesics	
meperidine hydrochloride (Demerol*) morphine sulfate*	• Urinary retention
Anti-inflammatory agents	
ibuprofen (Motrin*)	• Hematuria, acute interstitial nephritis
indomethacin (Indocin)	• Hematuria, acute renal failure, acute interstitial nephritis
phenacetin (APC)	• Papillary necrosis, chronic interstitial nephritis
Antiarrhythmics	
atropine sulfate disopyramide phosphate (Norpace*)	• Urinary retention, hesitancy
Anticoagulants and heparin antagonists	
dicumarol (Dufalone**)	• Hematuria
phenprocoumon (Liquamar)	• Nephropathy, hematuria
Antidepressants	
amitriptyline hydrochloride (Elavil*)	• Urinary retention, frequency, dilatation of urinary tract
desipramine hydrochloride (Norpramin*)	• Urinary frequency, retention, nocturia, dilatation of urinary tract, delayed micturition
Cephalosporins	
cephalexin monohydrate (Keflex*) cephaloridine (Loridine*) cephalothin sodium (Keflin Neutral*)	• Nephrotoxicity
Cholinergic blockers (parasympatholytics)	
benztropine mesylate (Cogentin*) scopolamine hydrobromide trihexyphenidyl hydrochloride (Artane*)	• Urinary hesitancy or retention

CLASSIFICATION	POSSIBLE SIDE EFFECTS
Diuretics	
acetazolamide (Diamox*) dichlorphenamide (Daranide*) ethoxzolamide (Cardase)	• Renal calculi
furosemide (Lasix*)	• Electrolyte imbalance, hyperuricemia, dehydration, interstitial nephritis
mannitol (Osmitrol*)	• Urinary retention
thiazides	• Interstitial nephritis
Gold salts	
gold sodium thiomalate (Myochrysine*)	• Nephritis, acute tubular necrosis, nephrotic syndrome
Penicillins	
methicillin sodium (Staphcillin*) oxacillin sodium (Prostaphilin*)	• Interstitial nephritis
Miscellaneous	
amantadine hydrochloride (Symmetrel*)	• Urinary retention
cimetadine (Tagamet) lead	• Interstitial nephritis
polymyxin B sulfate (Aerosporin*)	• Albuminuria, hematuria, cylinduria, nephrotoxicity
spectinomycin dihydrochloride (Trobicin*)	• Oliguria
Psychotherapeutics	
haloperidol (Haldol*)	• Urinary retention
lithium carbonate (Lithane*)	• Polyuria, glycosuria, renal toxicity, incontinence
Sulfonamides	
sulfacytine (Renoquid) sulfadiazine (Microsulfon) sulfamethoxazole (Gantanol*) sulfisoxazole (Gantrisin*)	• Acute toxic nephrosis, with oliguria and anuria; crystalluria; hematuria
Uricosuric	
probenecid (Benemid*) sulfinpyrazone (Anturane)	• Urinary frequency, hematuria
Vitamins	
ascorbic acid	• Acid urine, oxaluria, renal calculi
calciferol (vitamin D)	• Polyuria, albuminuria, hypercalciuria, nocturia, impaired renal function, renal calculi

*Available in U.S. and Canada. **Available in Canada only. All other products (no symbol) available in U.S. only.

• ***Musculoskeletal.*** Weakness and lethargy may indicate neuropathy or anemia caused by renal insufficiency.

• ***Neurologic.*** Progressive renal failure can cause increased intracranial pressure, headaches, fasciculations, asterixis (flapping tremor), seizures, or coma.

• ***Psychologic.*** Extreme behavior changes, such as agitated depression, delusions, and psychosis, can occur in a patient with renal failure.

Conducting the physical examination

496 General physical status

Begin the examination by weighing the patient and comparing the result with a baseline figure, if available. Significant weight gain or loss within 24 to 48 hours indicates a change in fluid status, not body mass. Weight monitoring is especially valuable during hospitalization of patients with urinary disorders (see *Assessing Fluid Status*).

Observe the patient's position and movements, noting any abnormalities. For example, a patient who can't lie flat in bed may be suffering from severe respiratory distress, as in acute pulmonary edema, which can coexist with primary renal failure. Such a patient may sit with his arms extended in front of him, perhaps resting them on his overbed table. The patient who keeps changing position, attempting to relieve severe stabbing flank pain, may have renal colic.

Monitor the patient's vital signs (see Entries 68 to 81). Measure blood pressure in both arms for comparison. Also take blood pressure readings with the patient lying down and sitting up. If blood pressure drops severely when the patient sits up, he may have volume depletion. Fever may suggest an acute urinary tract infection. Tachycardia with systolic hypotension is a sign of shock and demands immediate intervention. Mild tachycardia and normal or slightly elevated blood pressure suggest fluid overload. Pulse irregularities, such as bradycardia or other arrhythmias, may indicate potassium imbalance. The rate and character of respiration also may be altered by severe electrolyte imbalance. For example, Kussmaul's respiration suggests severe acidosis or right heart failure secondary to renal insufficiency. Severe hypotension (systolic pressure less than 90 mmHg) and severe hypertension (diastolic pressure greater than 120 mmHg) are ominous signs. Sustained severe hypotension (systolic pressure less than 70 mmHg) results in diminished renal blood flow and may produce acute renal failure.

Hypertension can cause renal insufficiency and can also result from vascular damage caused by a primary renal disorder.

ASSESSING FLUID STATUS

To assess your patient's fluid status, weigh him daily at the same time, using the same scale. He should wear the same type of clothing. If maintaining these constants isn't possible, document whatever's different about each weigh-in. Measure and compare intake and output daily, and report changes in output. Because of insensible loss from skin and lungs, output should equal only about two thirds of intake over 24 hours. The normal hourly output is 30 to 100 ml; normal 24-hour output, 720 to 2,400 ml. When measuring output, be sure to consider fluid loss from diarrhea, vomiting, fever, or wound drainage. Use daily intake-output records and weights to validate each other. One ml of water weighs 1 g, so if a patient's intake exceeds his output by 1,000 ml in 24 hours, his weight should increase by about 1 kg. If his output exceeds his intake, the negative fluid balance should produce weight loss.

497 The patient's mental status

Evaluate your patient's general appearance and behavior (see Entries 125 to 135). Then check his motor activity; orientation to person, place, and time; and memory of the immediate past. Renal dysfunction may cause an inability to concentrate and loss of recent memory. Chronic, progressive renal failure can lead to toxin accumulation and electrolyte imbalance, producing neurologic signs and symptoms, such as lethargy, confusion, disorientation, stupor, somnolence, coma, and convulsions.

498 Internal eye examination

Perform an internal eye examination, especially if your patient has malignant hypertension, because renal vascular changes parallel retinal arteriolar changes (see Entry 272). Hypertension may result from kidney disease or cause urinary symptoms by compromising renal microcirculation. Thickened retinal arteriolar walls with small areas of infarction or hemorrhage indicate damage to the intimal layer of the retinal vessels. An internal eye examination may also reveal papilledema; cottonwool patches from edema; and dilated, tortuous veins. Reddened conjunctivae due to calcium deposits may result from chronic renal failure.

499 Examining skin, hair, and nails

Inspect your patient's skin color for anemic pallor and for the yellow-tan coloration that results from retained urochrome pigment. Pallor results from a normocytic, normochromic anemia that gradually worsens as the kidneys fail. End-stage renal failure results in reduced erythropoietin production that in turn causes decreased red blood cell production. Also, uremic toxins shorten the life span of red blood cells.

Inspect the patient's skin for large bruises and for purpura, both characteristic of clotting abnormalities and decreased platelet adhesion from chronic renal failure. Check also for uremic frost (white or yellow urate crystals on the skin), which indicates a late stage of renal failure. Then note his skin integrity and observe for possible secondary infection, because a patient with chronic renal disease is more susceptible to infections.

Assess your patient's hydration by inspecting the mucous membranes in his mouth. A dry mucosa indicates mild dehydration; parched, cracked lips with a very dry mucosa and sunken eyes suggest severe dehydration. Then inspect the patient's skin for dryness and scratches, because renal failure causes sweat and oil glands to atrophy and results in subcutaneous calcium deposits. In a patient with long-standing renal failure, the scratches from itching may be severe. Next, evaluate his skin turgor (see Entry 227). If the skin doesn't return to its normal shape immediately—and your patient isn't old and hasn't recently lost weight—dehydration is advanced.

Inspect your patient's neck veins for distention. Dependent edema (ankle, sacral, and scrotal) or total body edema (periorbital, abdominal, and pulmonary), together with distended neck veins, indicate fluid overload (see *How to Test for Peripheral Edema,* page 448).

Examine your patient's hair for dryness and hair loss and his nails for thinness and brittleness. Then check for anemia by pressing two or more of the patient's fingernails; the normal pink color should return immediately after blanching. If capillary refill is delayed and the patient's skin is cool and clammy, he may have circulatory insufficiency and peripheral vasoconstriction from dehydration.

500 Assessing the chest and abdomen

When examining your patient's chest and abdomen for signs and symptoms of kidney disorders, use the same basic preparatory procedures used for cardio-

ASSESSING YOUR PATIENT'S KIDNEYS

1 To bimanually palpate your patient's kidneys, follow the technique shown here. If palpable, note each kidney's contour and size. Also, check for lumps and masses.

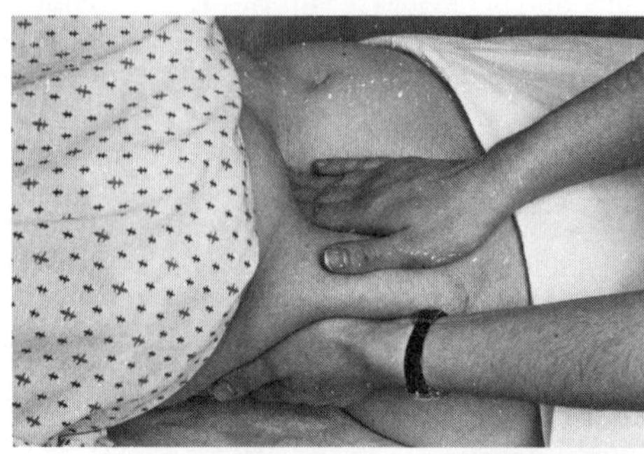

2 To check for kidney tenderness, use fist percussion, as shown here. Alert your patient before you percuss. Otherwise, you may startle him, causing a reaction similar to that associated with acute tenderness.

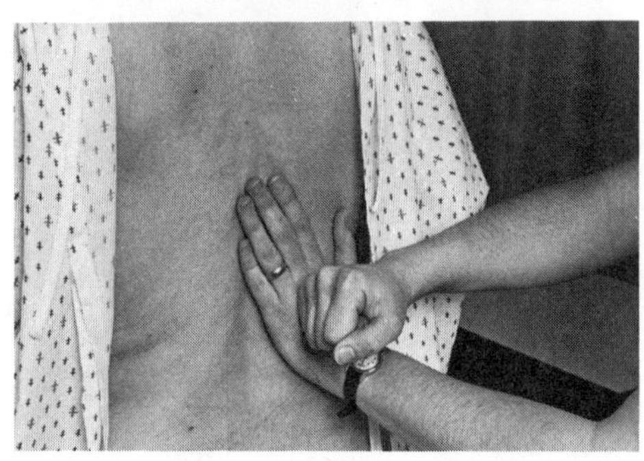

respiratory and GI assessment (see Entries 344, 345, 386, and 432).

Observe the patient's chest for symmetrical expansion and possible retractions. Auscultate all lung fields for rales and rhonchi, which suggest fluid overload. Then note the patient's cardiac rate and rhythm and the quality of his heart sounds (see Entries 393 and 394). (Remember that fluid overload may obscure normal heart and breath sounds.) Changes in heart rate and rhythm without underlying cardiac disease may indicate that the patient has severe fluid or electrolyte imbalance (especially of calcium or potassium). A gallop rhythm suggests fluid overload; a systolic murmur may indicate anemia from renal failure.

Examine the patient's abdomen for indications of fluid retention—distention, tight and glistening skin, and umbilical protrusion. Note any striae—a sign of rapid skin stretching. Note and inquire about any surgical scars not mentioned in your patient's history. If you suspect ascites, perform the fluid wave test (see Entry 450). If the patient has an ileal loop diversion or ureterostomy, remove the collection bag and inspect the site. Usually, you'll see immediate urine production and a cherry-red stoma. Note any irritation or excoriation of the surrounding skin—usually an indication of a poorly fitted appliance or inadequate care.

501 Examining your patient's kidneys

Palpate the patient's kidneys for size and tenderness. The kidneys lie behind other organs, protected by muscle—so unless they're enlarged, they may not be palpable. If the patient is very thin, you may feel the lower pole of the right one and, rarely, the tip of the left. Remember that excessive pressure on a kidney can cause your patient intense pain.

To perform bimanual deep palpation of the right kidney, stand at the patient's right side and elevate his right flank with your left hand (see *Assessing Your Patient's Kidneys*). Then place your right hand below the costal margin, with your fingers facing left. Ask your patient to breathe in deeply, so you can palpate the abdominal tissues. When he releases his breath, release the pressure and you may feel the right kidney's lower pole move back into place. To palpate the left kidney, reach across the patient's abdomen and repeat this technique, using your left hand to support the left flank and your right hand to palpate.

Next, use blunt percussion to evaluate kidney tenderness. Ask your patient to sit or—if he can't sit—to lie on his side. Then, place one palm over the costovertebral angle, between the spine and 12th rib, and strike lightly with your fist. The spleen's sound is dull; the kidney's is resonant.

Usually, you can help a patient localize mild or vague back pain by percussing bilaterally or pressing one finger into the soft tissue of the costovertebral angle. Be sure to ask if the pain radiates to the groin or labia (or scrotum). If percussion elicits tenderness, suspect kidney, liver, or gallbladder inflammation. Suprapubic or low back pain suggests simple cystitis.

Now, using the bell of your stethoscope, try to auscultate the renal arteries. This is especially important if the patient is hypertensive. Listen in

ASSESSING THE BLADDER

1 Percuss the area over the bladder, starting 2″ (5 cm) above the symphysis pubis. Continue percussion, moving downward. You'll hear a tympanic sound if the bladder is normal. If you hear a dull sound, the bladder may be retaining urine.

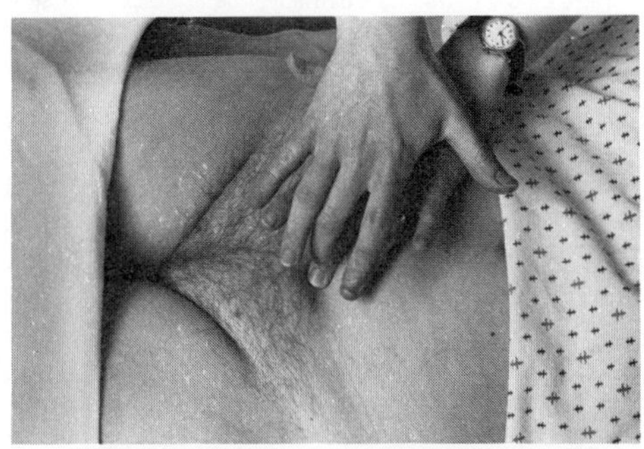

2 Palpate your patient's bladder bimanually, beginning midline about 1″ to 2″ (2.5 to 5 cm) above the symphysis pubis, as the nurse is doing here. Continue palpating until you locate the edge of the bladder, which normally is not accessible when empty.

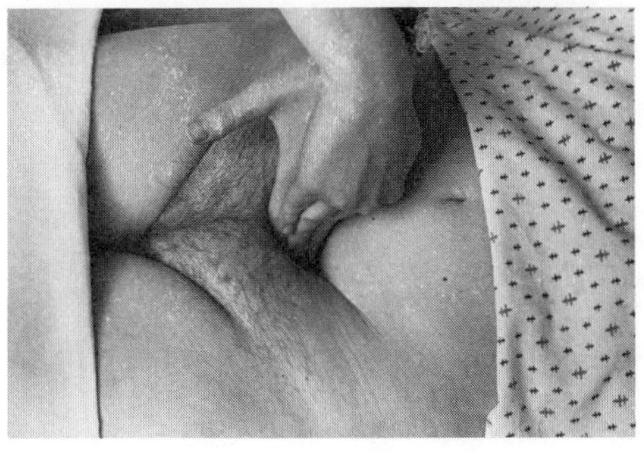

the periumbilical region for bruits, which are characteristic of renal artery stenosis.

502 Assessing the bladder and genitalia

Inspect the contour of your patient's lower abdomen for bladder distention. Then palpate and percuss the area, starting at the umbilicus and proceeding toward the symphysis (see *Assessing the Bladder*, page 447). If the bladder is normal, you won't feel it. A slightly dull percussion note above the symphysis indicates mild distention. On palpation, a smooth, rounded, fluctuant suprapubic mass suggests severe distention; a fluctuant mass extending to the umbilicus indicates extreme distention. (Remember that palpation and percussion usually stimulate the micturition reflex.)

Check the patient's genitalia for swelling from localized edema. Also observe for such signs and symptoms of obstruction as dribbling, frequency, or urgency. In a man, these problems indicate the need for examination for prostatic enlargement (see Entry 535).

503 Examining your patient's extremities

Examine the patient's legs and ankles for edema by pressing your fingers against his lower tibia (see *How to Test for Peripheral Edema*). Also check for arm and leg pain and limited range of motion (see Entry 679), because chronic

HOW TO TEST FOR PERIPHERAL EDEMA

When you're assessing your patient's urinary function, you'll want to test for edema—the buildup of excess sodium and water in interstitial spaces. Edema can be a sign of kidney malfunction. Suspect it in any swollen area, especially in the legs.

Here's how to test for edema: Press a finger against the suspected edematous area for 5 seconds. Then, remove your finger quickly and completely. If edema's present, the skin won't rebound to its original contour right away. Instead, you'll notice a small depression, or pit, in the skin. Measure the pit with a scale approved by your hospital. Here's how to use one widely accepted system, the four-point scale: Record a barely perceptible pit, like the one shown on the left, as *+1*. Record a deep pit like the one on the right, which takes over 30 seconds to rebound, as *+4*.

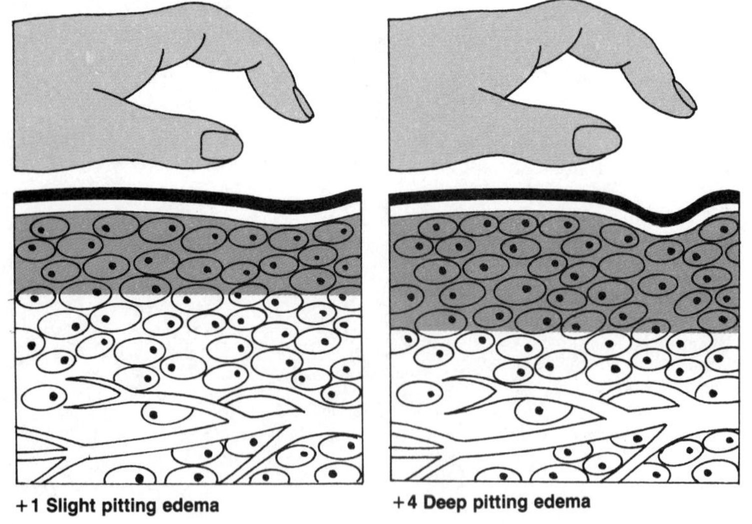

+1 Slight pitting edema

+4 Deep pitting edema

EVALUATING URINE COLOR

APPEARANCE	POSSIBLE CAUSES
Colorless or straw-colored (diluted urine)	• Excessive fluid intake, chronic renal disease, diabetes insipidus, nervous conditions
Dark yellow or amber (concentrated urine)	• Low fluid intake, acute febrile disease, vomiting, diarrhea
Cloudy	• Infection, purulence, blood, epithelial cells, fat, colloidal particles, urates, vegetarian diet, parasitic disease
Yellow to amber, with pink sediment	• Hyperuricemia, gout
Orange-red to orange-brown	• Urobilinuria, such drugs as phenazopyridine (Pyridium), obstructive jaundice (tea-colored)
Red or red-brown	• Porphyria, hemoglobin, erythrocytes, hemorrhage, such drugs as pyrvinium pamoate (Povan)
Green-brown	• Bile duct obstruction, phenol poisoning
Dark brown or black	• Acute glomerulonephritis, chorea, typhus, methylene blue medication
Smoky	• Prostatic fluid, fat droplets, blood, chyle, spermatozoa

renal insufficiency can lead to osteodystrophy as a result of hyperparathyroidism and changes in calcium metabolism.

504 Laboratory tests

Laboratory tests and radiography are regularly used to confirm the cause of a patient's renal problems (see *Nurse's Guide to Urinary Tract X-ray Studies*, page 450). The simplest (and perhaps most informative) laboratory test is routine urinalysis, which measures pH and specific gravity and also tests for protein, glucose, blood, and bacteria (see *Evaluating Urine Color*). The pH is a measure of the body's acid-base balance; when renal tubular absorption is impaired, pH is low (acidic). Specific gravity (or the solute-solvent ratio) indicates the kidneys' ability to dilute or concentrate urine.

Glycosuria, in the presence of normal serum glucose levels, indicates impaired proximal tubular reabsorption. This condition may appear with chronic renal insufficiency or primary tubular defect. Transient proteinuria may result from febrile illness or strenuous exercise, but persistent proteinuria suggests significant glomerular disease and indicates the need for quantitation of a 24-hour urine specimen. Urinalysis may also show gross or microscopic hematuria. Pyuria can appear with some nonbacterial inflammatory diseases, but a large number of white cells with bacteria probably indicates urinary tract infection (a culture is required for confirmation).

The most accurate and clinically practical laboratory measure of kidney function is the glomerular filtration rate, which represents the amount of blood filtered per minute (cc/minute).

NURSE'S GUIDE TO URINARY TRACT X-RAY STUDIES

Here's a list of common X-ray studies used to detect and evaluate urinary tract disorders. Although you won't perform these studies, which one the doctor selects for the patient can be influenced by *your* assessment findings.

Note that, except for ultrasonography, these studies are invasive and should not be performed on a pregnant patient. Also, check your patient's records to make sure he's not allergic to the contrast medium.

Computerized tomography (CT scan): uses contrast medium to produce a three-dimensional image from a series of X-rays taken at various angles. Helps evaluate renal pelvis size, parenchymal thickness, and structural abnormalities.

Renal scan: shows kidney function size, blood flow, and excretion, using ^{131}I or iodohippurate sodium (Hippuran). Helps detect renal artery stenosis and renal parenchymal disease.

Intravenous pyelography (IVP): shows renal parenchyma, ureters, and bladder, using contrast medium. Helps determine kidney size and shape and detect the presence of soft- or hard-tissue lesions.

Cystography: determines size and shape of a fluid-filled bladder, using contrast medium. Helps diagnose lower abdominal or pelvic trauma, disorders affecting the bladder wall, and some instances of pyuria or hematuria.

Ultrasonography: produces oscilloscopic, time-lapse image by transmitting high-frequency sound waves into the abdomen. Helps determine kidney size and shape, detects the presence of calculi, and differentiates between solid masses and fluid-filled cysts.

Renal angiography: shows renal vascular pathways, using contrast medium. Helps diagnose renal artery stenosis, renal vein thrombosis, or vascular damage from trauma; differentiates vascular tumors from avascular cysts.

Voiding cystourethrography: delineates the bladder while patient voids contrast medium. Helps diagnose urethral obstructions or lesions.

This test measures serum creatinine levels in a blood sample drawn during a timed urine collection (usually a period of 4 to 72 hours).

Additional laboratory tests include measurements of hemoglobin and hematocrit—which are usually low in chronic renal disease. Depending on the type and severity of the patient's disease, blood chemistries show changes in serum electrolytes (including potassium, sodium, chloride, and bicarbonate ions), blood urea nitrogen (BUN), creatinine, calcium, and phosphorus. BUN and creatinine are routinely measured to screen for kidney disease.

Formulating a diagnostic impression

505 Classifying urinary system disorders

The urinary system regulates blood volume and chemical composition by excreting metabolic end products and water. For the system to accomplish these essential functions, the following processes must occur: Unnecessary chemicals must be filtered from the plasma, necessary solutes and fluids must be returned to the blood, and urine must be collected and excreted. Urinary disorders, when classified according to the processes they interrupt, fall into two broad categories: those which affect filtration and reabsorption and those which affect urine collection and excretion (see *Nurse's Guide to Urinary Disorders,* pages 452 to 455).

506 Making appropriate nursing diagnoses

Output changes include polyuria, oliguria, and anuria. Polyuria may result from a failure of the nephrons' concentrating mechanism, which causes solute—but not water—reabsorption in the tubules and results in dilute urine (low specific gravity). Polyuria can also result from hypercalcemia, osmotic diuretic states (such as diabetes mellitus), intravenous pyelography, or excessive fluid intake. This symptom usually occurs with filtration and reabsorption disorders, although it can appear in collection and excretion problems. Your nursing diagnosis for polyuria is *fluid volume excess.*

The pathophysiology of oliguria and anuria isn't well understood. Their appearance in acute renal failure is most commonly explained as resulting from any of the following conditions:

- diminished renal blood flow from ischemia
- tubular collapse caused by changes in the interstitial-intratubular pressure gradient
- back diffusion of filtrate when damaged epithelial tissue causes tubule blockage.

Of course, oliguria may result from an obstruction that prevents urine excretion. But oliguria, like polyuria, usually occurs in disorders of filtration and reabsorption. Anuria is uncommon. Your nursing diagnosis for oliguria or anuria is *fluid volume deficit.*

Voiding pattern changes result from changes in the bladder's ability to collect urine. An inflammatory process, an innervation disturbance, a foreign body, or a thickened detrusor muscle wall may impair this ability, causing frequency, urgency, and nocturia. Of course, these symptoms appear in disorders of collection and excretion. Your nursing diagnoses for these symptoms are *alterations in urinary elimination patterns* and (for nocturia) *sleep disturbances.*

Urine color changes usually result from hematuria. The extent of hematuria—microscopic or gross—doesn't help determine the cause. However, the stage of urination at which the symptom occurs can provide diagnostic clues. Initial hematuria indicates a urethral disorder; terminal hematuria suggests dysfunction near the bladder neck or posterior urethra. Hematuria throughout urination indicates that the source of the problem is located above the

IDENTIFYING UREMIC SYNDROME

Any chronic renal disease that results in renal failure causes retention of nitrogenous wastes in its end stage. This life-threatening situation can affect the following major body systems, as indicated.

- *Urinary:* polyuria, leading to oliguria and anuria; nocturia; loss of diurnal pattern; changes in size of kidneys
- *Cardiovascular:* hypertension, congestive heart failure, pericarditis, cardiac arrhythmias
- *Respiratory:* Kussmaul breathing, dyspnea; pulmonary edema; pneumonia
- *Hematologic:* anemia (pallor, fatigue), bleeding tendencies, decreased ability to fight infections
- *Dermatologic:* uremic frost, pruritus, purpura, decreased perspiration, thin and brittle nails, dry hair that falls out
- *Gastrointestinal:* anorexia, nausea, vomiting, weight loss, uremic fetor (urinous breath), metallic taste, stomatitis, gastritis, gastrointestinal bleeding, diarrhea
- *Musculoskeletal:* muscle wasting, weakness, easy fatigability, renal osteodystrophy, pathologic fractures, bone pain
- *Neurologic:* changes in level of consciousness (confusion, stupor, coma), behavior changes (irritability, labile moods, psychosis), peripheral neuropathy (restless legs, footdrop), paresthesias, twitches, fasciculations, asterixis
- *Reproductive:* impotence, amenorrhea, decreased libido

Laboratory studies reveal decreased glomerular filtration rate—including increased BUN and creatinine levels, hyperkalemia, hypermagnesemia, metabolic acidosis, abnormal glucose tolerance test, EKG changes, decreased erythrocyte sedimentation rate, and increased bleeding time.

NURSE'S GUIDE TO URINARY DISORDERS

	CHIEF COMPLAINT
FILTRATION AND REABSORPTION DISORDERS	
Polycystic kidney disease	• *Output changes:* polyuria • *Voiding pattern changes:* nocturia possible • *Urine color changes:* hematuria, possibly gross • *Pain:* flank pain
Acute pyelonephritis	• *Output changes:* polyuria or none • *Voiding pattern changes:* frequency, urgency • *Urine color changes:* hematuria • *Pain:* tenderness over one or both kidneys
Chronic interstitial nephritis	• *Output changes:* polyuria • *Voiding pattern changes:* nocturia • *Urine color changes:* light color due to poor concentration • *Pain:* none
Hypernephroma	• *Output changes:* none • *Voiding pattern changes:* none • *Urine color changes:* hematuria, gross or microscopic • *Pain:* flank pain
Nephrolithiasis	• *Output changes:* none • *Voiding pattern changes:* frequency, urgency • *Urine color changes:* hematuria • *Pain:* severe, radiating pain
Acute glomerulonephritis	• *Output changes:* oliguria, possibly progressing to anuria • *Voiding pattern changes:* none • *Urine color changes:* hematuria, smoky or coffee-colored • *Pain:* none
Chronic glomerulonephritis	• *Output changes:* none • *Voiding pattern changes:* none • *Urine color changes:* none • *Pain:* none
Acute renal artery occlusion	• *Output changes:* oliguria possible • *Voiding pattern changes:* none • *Urine color changes:* none • *Pain:* sudden, sharp, constant pain over upper abdomen or flank

	HISTORY	PHYSICAL EXAMINATION AND DIAGNOSTIC STUDIES
	• Family history of polycystic disease • Symptoms start after age 40	• Enlarged, palpable kidneys • Hypertension • Urine analysis reveals proteinuria, bacteriuria, and calculi. • Further diagnostic studies include urography, ultrasonography, radioisotopic renal scan, renal computerized tomography.
	• Sudden onset	• Fever and chills • Nausea and vomiting • Kidneys tender on palpation • Urine analysis reveals pyuria and bacteriuria.
	• Urinary abnormality, such as obstruction or reflux • Early stages may have no specific symptoms.	• Hypertension • Blood analysis reveals elevated BUN. • Urine analysis reveals WBC casts. • Further diagnostic studies include intravenous pyelography and biopsy.
	• Allergies • Use of nephrotoxic drugs	• Palpable mass • Fever, hypertension, weight loss • Fatigue and malaise • Blood analysis reveals anemia or polycythemia. • Further diagnostic studies include intravenous pyelography, ultrasonography, angiography, renal computerized tomography.
	• Excessive dehydration and infection • Previous kidney stones • Hyperparathyroidism • Renal tubular acidosis	• Fever and chills • Nausea and vomiting • Blood analysis reveals leukocytosis. • Urine analysis reveals increased specific gravity, crystalluria, and leukocyturia. • Further diagnostic studies include retrograde intravenous pyelography.
	• Poststreptococcal infection of throat or skin • Systemic lupus erythematosus, Schönlein-Henoch purpura, pregnancy, vasculitis, or scleroderma	• Hypertension • Edema; starts in periorbital areas and progresses to dependent areas, ascites, and pleural effusion • Costovertebral tenderness • Urine analysis reveals proteinuria and RBC casts. • Further diagnostic studies include renal computerized tomography and biopsy.
	• May be asymptomatic until advanced stages	• Renal failure • Hypertension • Urine analysis reveals proteinuria. • Blood analysis reveals anemia. • Further diagnostic studies include biopsy.
	• Emboli from endocarditis or atherosclerosis	• Severe hypertension present • Further diagnostic studies include renal arteriography. *(continued)*

NURSE'S GUIDE TO URINARY DISORDERS *(continued)*

	CHIEF COMPLAINT
Chronic renal artery stenosis	• *Output changes:* none • *Voiding pattern changes:* none • *Urine color changes:* none • *Pain:* none
Renal vein thrombosis	• *Output changes:* oliguria possible if thrombosis is bilateral • *Voiding pattern changes:* none • *Urine color changes:* hematuria • *Pain:* severe lumbar pain
Acute tubular necrosis	• *Output changes:* oliguria dominates in early stages; leads to renal failure • *Voiding pattern changes:* none • *Urine color changes:* dark and smoky or clear • *Pain:* none
URINE COLLECTION AND EXCRETION DISORDERS	
Bladder neck obstruction	• *Output changes:* anuria with complete obstruction • *Voiding pattern changes:* frequency, urgency • *Urine color changes:* none • *Pain:* dysuria
Carcinoma of the bladder	• *Output changes:* oliguria possible, depending on mass size • *Voiding pattern changes:* frequency, urgency, nocturia • *Urine color changes:* hematuria, intermittent or constant • *Pain:* dysuria, flank pain
Cystitis	• *Output changes:* none • *Voiding pattern changes:* frequency, urgency, nocturia • *Urine color changes:* cloudy hematuria • *Pain:* dysuria, low back pain or flank pain
Urethral obstruction	• *Output changes:* polyuria • *Voiding pattern changes:* incontinence, hesitancy, urgency • *Urine color changes:* none • *Pain:* dysuria
Urethritis	• *Output changes:* polyuria may result from forced fluids • *Voiding pattern changes:* frequency, urgency • *Urine color changes:* hematuria • *Pain:* dysuria possible; burning at start of urination; urethral pain

HISTORY	PHYSICAL EXAMINATION AND DIAGNOSTIC STUDIES
• Fibromuscular dysplasia or atherosclerosis	• Hypertension that's difficult to control • Renal arteriography
• Metastatic disease, nephrotic syndrome, thrombophlebitis, periarteritis, abdominal injury, unexplained leg edema, or recurrent emboli	• Enlargement of affected kidney • Blood analysis reveals leukocytosis. • Urine analysis reveals proteinuria and RBC casts. • Further diagnostic studies include inferior vena cavography.
• Crush injury or illness associated with shock, such as burns or trauma • Muscle necrosis • Use of a nephrotoxic agent, such as lead, or intravenous pyelography dye	• Anorexia • Vomiting • Pulmonary edema, heart failure • Urine analysis reveals low specific gravity, granular casts, and hematuria. • Blood analysis reveals elevated BUN and creatinine levels. • Further diagnostic studies include spot urine sodium and urine creatinine analyses.

HISTORY	PHYSICAL EXAMINATION AND DIAGNOSTIC STUDIES
• May be acquired or hereditary	• Incontinence • Nausea and vomiting • Distended bladder • Diagnostic studies include cystoscopy and cystography.
• Exposure to analine dyes • Chronic infestation of schistosomes • Heavy cigarette smoking	• Fever • Flank tenderness, muscle weakness • Blood analysis reveals elevated WBC count and anemia. • Positive urine cytology • Further diagnostic studies include cystography, cystoscopy, and biopsy.
• Recurrent urinary tract infections • Recent chemotherapy, systemic antibiotic therapy • Recent vigorous sexual activity • Commonly affects women	• Suprapubic pain on palpation • Fever • Nausea and vomiting • Inflamed genital area • Urine analysis reveals bacteriuria (10^5/ml). • Urine culture and sensitivity tests repeated 2 weeks after therapy ends.
• Injury, infection, carcinoma, or congenital anomalies • Past history of calculi	• Enlarged kidney (to compensate for obstructed kidney) • Renal failure • Distended bladder • Urine analysis reveals proteinuria. • Further diagnostic studies include cystoscopy.
• Infections • Exposure to chemicals or bubble bath • Recent vigorous sexual activity	• Fever • Edema and redness around urinary meatus and vulva • Urethral and/or vaginal discharge

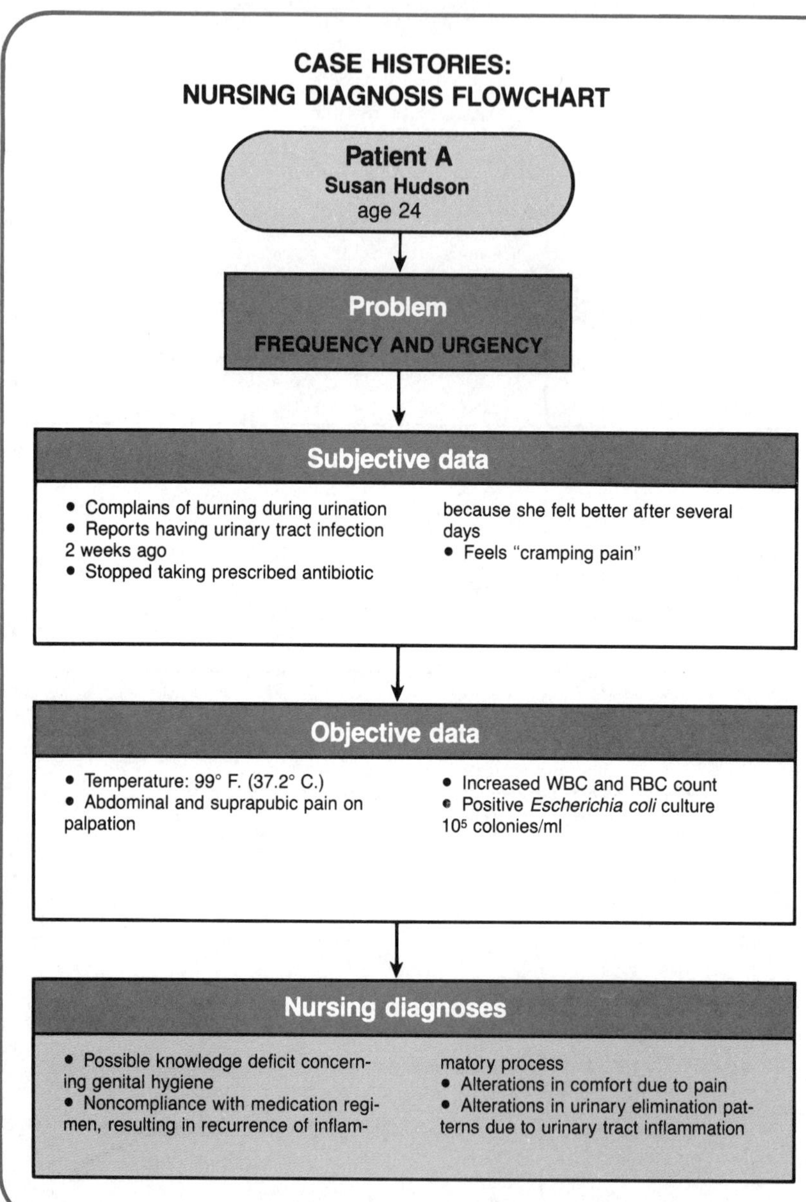

bladder neck, where blood has mixed with urine. Regardless of its timing, this symptom may result from sickle cell anemia, calculi, infections, tumors, or trauma. It may appear in disorders of filtration and reabsorption or in those of collection and excretion. Various foods, dyes, and medications may also cause urine color changes that mimic hematuria but don't indicate urinary system damage. A possible nursing diagnosis is *anxiety related to*

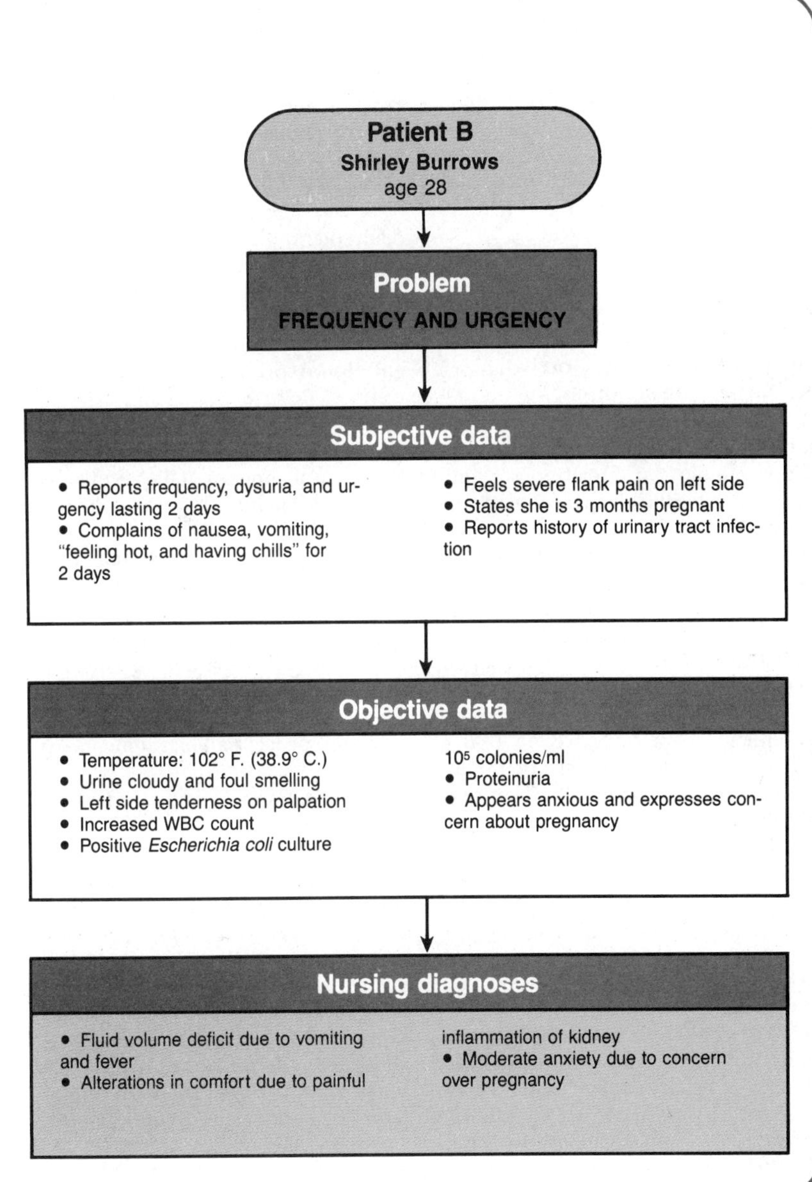

unknown cause of hematuria.

Pain is the urinary symptom that most often causes patients to seek treatment. Dysuria, described as a burning sensation in the urethra or an ache in the suprapubic area, usually results from an inflammatory process in the lower urinary tract. A calculus, a tumor, or a foreign body can also cause dysuria.

Mild to agonizingly severe flank pain results from distention. Colicky pain is caused by violent hyperperistalsis and paroxysmal spasms in the renal pelvis or ureter as it tries to expel the obstruction (calculus or clot). Such pain may also result from an inflammatory process or tumor.

Pain indicates disorders of collection and excretion. Your nursing diagnoses may include *alterations in comfort* and *alterations in cognitive function: distraction due to severe pain* (see *Nursing Diagnosis Flowchart,* pages 456 to 457).

Assessing pediatric patients

507 Anatomy and physiology

A newborn infant's kidneys are anatomically and functionally immature. Their glomerular filtration rate and ability to concentrate urine and excrete acid, as well as their tubular reabsorption of sodium, are less than those of adult kidneys. Generally, a child's kidneys become functionally mature between ages 6 months and 1 year, although creatinine clearance (dependent on lean muscle mass), normal serum creatinine, and urinary output per kilogram of body weight (.50 to .75 cc/kg of body weight/hour) are lower than in an adult. Lack of perirenal fat increases the immature kidneys' vulnerability to traumatic injury.

A normal child develops the physiologic ability to control urination between ages 2 and 3.

508 Pediatric history questions

Ask your patient's mother about problems during pregnancy and delivery that may be associated with urinary tract malformations. Inquire about congenital anomalies: low-set, malformed ears; chromosomal disorders, such as trisomy D and E; imperforate anus; or a single umbilical artery. A history of an imperforate anus associated with fistula development or spina bifida also makes a child more susceptible to infection because of impaired innervation.

Other history considerations include delayed growth and development, feeding problems, vomiting, unexplained fevers, colic associated with voiding, and persistent enuresis after age 5. Bladder or urethral irritation or an emotional problem can cause bedwetting.

Also ask the parent about the child's urinary stream—its color, odor, frequency, and amount. If the child is very young, ask if his diaper is soaked or barely wet, or blood-stained, when the parent changes it. Also ask how many times a day the child's diaper must be changed.

Finally, determine if the child has had pharyngitis or a skin infection, such as impetigo, in the past 3 weeks. These conditions can cause acute poststreptococcal glomerulonephritis.

509 Examining a child

Take the child's blood pressure using an appropriate-sized cuff. Inspect his skin for anemic pallor, which may indicate a congenital renal disorder, such as medullary cystic disease. Also inspect for anomalies associated with congenital urinary tract malformations: low-set or malformed ears, absence of abdominal musculature, undescended testes, and inguinal hernia.

Palpate the child's abdomen carefully for bladder distention and kidney enlargement. Remember, you'll probably be able to palpate and percuss an infant's bladder at the umbilical level. Bladder distention in an older child may indicate urethral dysfunction or a central nervous system defect. Unless a child has ascites, you'll be able to palpate his kidneys more easily than

RECOGNIZING CONGENITAL ANOMALIES OF THE URETER, BLADDER, AND URETHRA

When taking the child's history, ask the parent about any congenital anomalies the child may have that affect the ureter, the bladder, and the urethra. Remember, such congenital anomalies aren't always obvious at birth. Carefully evaluate the child's urinary system for possible undiscovered anomalies, such as those that follow:

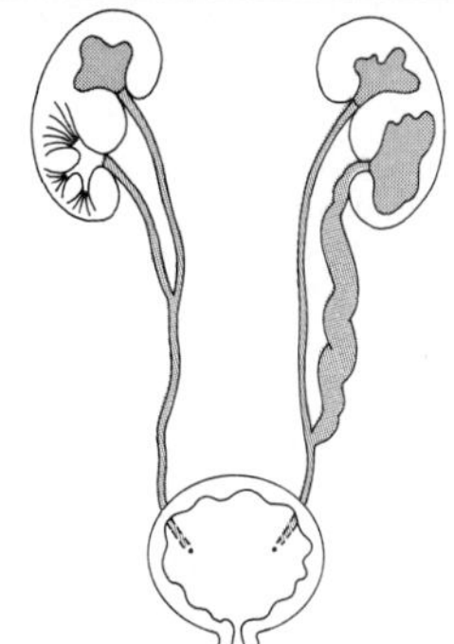

DUPLICATED URETER

- *Complete:* a double collecting system with two separate pelves, each with its own ureter and orifice
- *Incomplete* (y type): two separate ureters join before entering the bladder
- Most common ureteral anomaly

Signs and symptoms

- Persistent or recurrent infection
- Frequency, urgency, or burning on urination
- Diminished urinary output
- Flank pain, fever, and chills

Diagnostic tests

- Intravenous pyelography
- Voiding cystoscopy
- Cystoureterography
- Retrograde pyelography

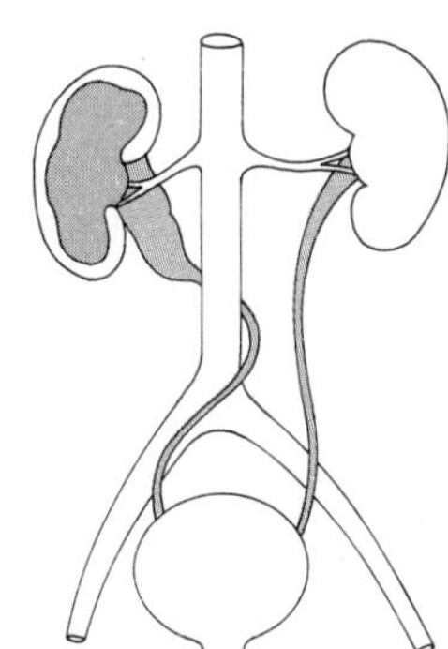

RETROCAVAL URETER (PREURETERAL VENA CAVA)

- Right ureter passes behind the inferior vena cava before entering the bladder. Compression of the ureter between the vena cava and the spine causes dilatation and elongation of the pelvis, hydroureter (urine-distended ureter), hydronephrosis, and ureteral fibrosis and stenosis in the compressed area.
- Relatively uncommon; higher incidence in males

Signs and symptoms

- Right flank pain
- Recurrent urinary tract infection
- Renal calculi
- Hematuria

Diagnostic tests

- Intravenous or retrograde pyelography demonstrates superior ureteral enlargement, with spiral appearance.

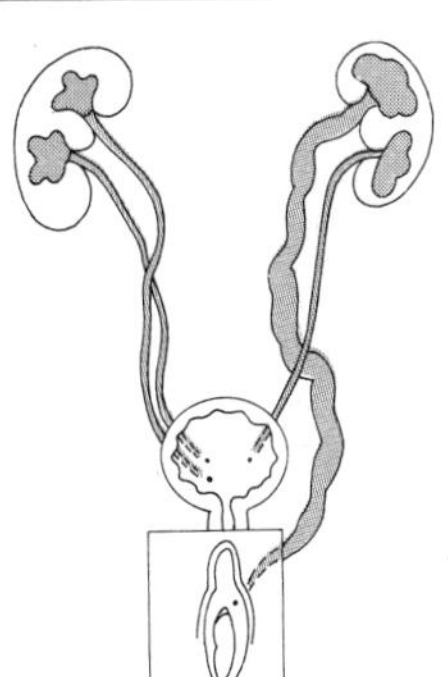

ECTOPIC ORIFICE OF URETER

- *In females:* ureteral orifice usually inserts in urethra or vaginal vestibule, beyond external urethral sphincter
- *In males:* ureteral orifice usually in prostatic urethra or in seminal vesicles or vas deferens

Signs and symptoms

- Symptoms rare when ureteral orifice opens between trigone and bladder neck.
- *In females:* obstruction, reflux, and incontinence (dribbling) possible
- *In males:* flank pain, frequency, urgency

Diagnostic tests

- Intravenous pyelography
- Urethroscopy, vaginoscopy
- Voiding cystourethrography

(*continued*)

RECOGNIZING CONGENITAL ANOMALIES OF THE URETER, BLADDER, AND URETHRA (*continued*)

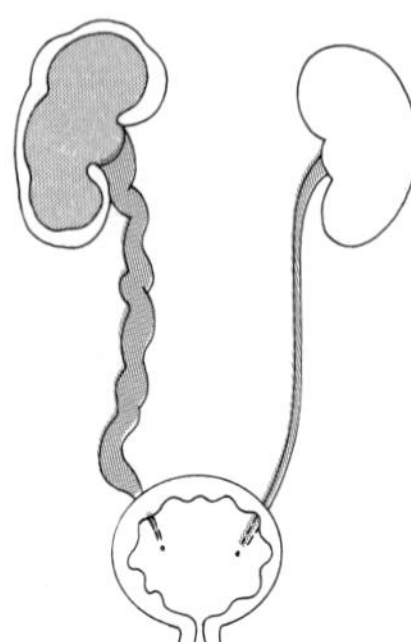

STRICTURE OR STENOSIS OF URETER

- Most common site, the distal ureter above ureterovesical junction; less common, ureteropelvic junction; rare, midureter
- Detected during infancy in 25% of patients; before puberty in most
- Most common in males

Signs and symptoms

- Megaloureter or hydroureter, with hydronephrosis when stenosis occurs in distal ureter
- Hydronephrosis alone when stenosis occurs at ureteropelvic junction

Diagnostic tests

- Ultrasound
- Intravenous and retrograde pyelography
- Voiding cystography

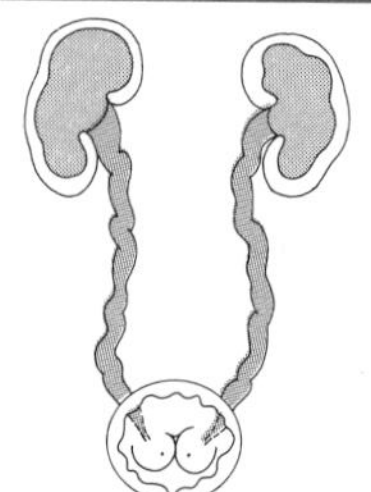

URETEROCELE

- Bulging of submucosal ureter into bladder, ranging from ⅜" (1 cm) to filling entire bladder
- Unilateral, bilateral, ectopic, with resulting hydroureter and hydronephrosis

Signs and symptoms

- Obstruction
- Persistent or recurrent infection

Diagnostic tests

- Voiding cystourethrography
- Intravenous pyelography and cystoscopy show thin, translucent mass

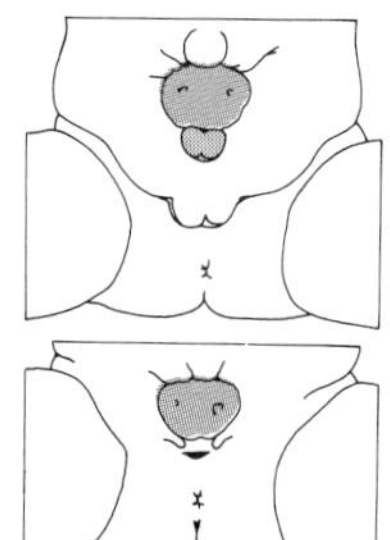

EXSTROPHY OF BLADDER

- Absence of anterior abdominal and bladder wall makes the bladder appear inside out
- *In males:* epispadias and undescended testes
- *In females:* cleft clitoris, separated labia, or absent vagina
- Skeletal or intestinal anomalies possible

Signs and symptoms

- Obvious at birth, with urine seeping onto abdominal wall from abnormal ureteral orifices
- Excoriated surrounding skin, ulcerated exposed bladder mucosa, associated anomalies and infection

Diagnostic tests

- Intravenous pyelography

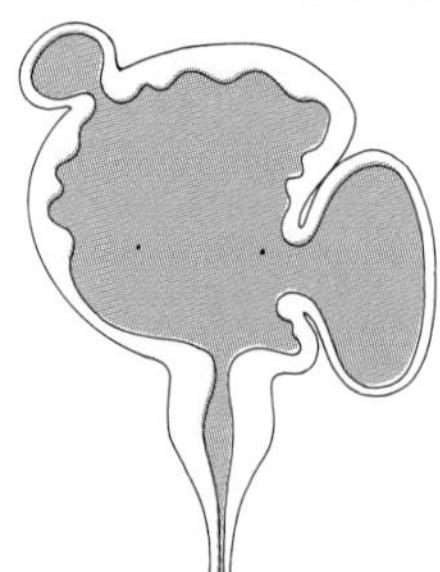

CONGENITAL BLADDER DIVERTICULUM

- Circumscribed sac (diverticulum) of bladder wall
- Can occur anywhere in bladder, usually lateral to ureteral orifice; large diverticulum at orifice can cause reflux

Signs and symptoms

- Fever, frequency, and painful urination
- Urinary tract infection
- Cystitis, particularly in males

Diagnostic tests

- Intravenous pyelography shows diverticulum.
- Retrograde cystography shows vesicoureteral reflux in ureter.

in an adult, so always try to feel the kidneys to detect enlargement. In a preschool-age child, a firm, smooth, and palpable mass adjacent to the vertebral column—but not crossing the midline—suggests Wilms' tumor. If you detect such a mass, avoid further deep palpation and refer the patient immediately for additional evaluation.

Next, inspect the patient's external genitalia closely for abnormalities associated with congenital anomalies of the urinary tract. A child may be bashful about allowing you to examine his or her genitalia, so take time to explain the procedures and their purpose. Be gentle but thorough, and complete your examination as quickly as possible. Note the location and size of a boy's urethral meatus, the size of his testes, and any local irritation, inflammation, or swelling. The meatus should be in the center of the shaft; you may note epispadias (urethral opening on the dorsum of the shaft) or hypospadias (urethral opening on the underside of the penis or on the perineum). Note the location of a girl's clitoris, urethral meatus, and vaginal orifice. So-called female epispadias, with the mons and clitoris divided along the midline, may indicate hermaphroditism. Also check for irritation, swelling, and abnormal discharge—possible signs of urethritis. Then palpate the meatus for urethral caruncles.

510 Detecting childhood disorders

After the respiratory tract, the urinary tract is the most commonly infected area in infants and children. In an infant, signs and symptoms of a urinary tract infection (UTI) may be nonspecific. Look for fever, irritability, feeding problems, vomiting, diarrhea, and jaundice. Usually the presenting sign is fever: When it occurs with such specific urinary tract signs as hematuria, odorous urine, and recurrent enuresis, obtain a urine culture of a clean-catch specimen.

In an infant or young child, a UTI (especially if recurrent) that's confirmed by urine culture suggests a congenital structural anomaly of the urinary tract, such as retrocaval ureter, ureterocele, bladder diverticulum, or vesicoureteral reflux (see *Recognizing Congenital Anomalies of the Ureter, Bladder, and Urethra*). The underlying cause of any UTI must be found and treated to prevent acute pyelonephritis and renal damage.

Acute glomerulonephritis is the most common form of nephritis in children. A group A beta-hemolytic streptococcal infection usually precedes the disease 7 to 14 days before the sudden onset of symptoms. Symptoms include urinary abnormalities (hematuria, proteinuria, and decreased urinary output), edema, and hypertension. The child is lethargic, pale, and anorexic. If only the urinary abnormalities appear, diagnosis is more difficult. A bacterial urine count should be used to rule out a UTI. If proteinuria persists for a week, postural proteinuria may be present.

Assessing geriatric patients

511 Anatomy and physiology

After age 40, a person's renal function may diminish; if he lives to age 90, it may have decreased by as much as 50%. This change is reflected in a decline in the glomerular filtration rate resulting from age-related changes in renal vasculature that disturb glomerular hemodynamics. Diminished renal blood flow from reduced cardiac output and from atherosclerotic changes also occurs with age. In addition, tubular reabsorption and renal concentrating ability decline in elderly persons,

WHAT YOU SHOULD KNOW ABOUT URINARY INCONTINENCE IN THE ELDERLY

This chart on urinary incontinence in the elderly distinguishes popular myth from actual fact. It will help you recognize the reasons for urinary incontinence in your elderly patients and assist you in proper management of the problem.

MYTH	FACT
All old people are incontinent.	About 86% to 90% of community-living elderly and 55% to 60% of nursing home residents have no trouble with urinary control.
Urinary incontinence is a normal development in old age.	Age changes may predispose to, but do not cause, incontinence.
There is nothing you can do for incontinent old people.	Many causes of urinary incontinence can be treated. Some of your patients may even be able to regain urinary control.

because the size and number of functioning nephrons decrease. As a person ages, his bladder muscles weaken; this may result in incomplete bladder emptying and chronic urine retention—predisposing the bladder to infection.

512 Geriatric history concerns

An older patient who has had scarlet fever or other streptococcal infections, especially before the introduction of sulfonamides and penicillin, is at risk to develop renal damage secondary to glomerulonephritis. Prolonged hypertension predisposes the patient to arteriolar nephrosclerosis, which can impair renal function. Atherosclerosis can reduce renal circulation.

513 Tests: Values and hazards

For geriatric patients, normal values for some laboratory tests are different from those established for younger adults, because of decreased renal function. An elderly patient's blood urea nitrogen level, for example, is normally higher by 5 mg/100 ml. Because an older person's kidneys have diminished concentrating ability, some diagnostic tests are more hazardous to him than to a younger patient. For instance, dehydration induced in preparation for radiologic studies, or resulting from the osmotic diuresis produced by contrast agents, may predispose an elderly patient to intravascular volume contraction and further renal function deterioration.

514 Common geriatric urinary disorders

Because of degenerative changes affecting body functions, elderly persons are more susceptible than younger adults to some renal disorders. Susceptibility to infection, for example, increases with age, and kidney infection from obstruction is a common cause of hospitalization among older patients. An immobilized elderly patient is especially vulnerable to infection from urinary stasis or poor personal hygiene.

An alteration in cardiac output (such as in congestive heart failure) lowers renal perfusion and may result in azotemia. The kidneys compensate by retaining sodium and increasing edema. Medications to improve a patient's myocardial contractility, and therapy with diuretics, may increase his renal function temporarily, but prerenal azotemia from depletion of intravascular volume often results.

Poor musculature from childbearing

and from aging may predispose elderly women to cystocele (see *Nurse's Guide to Female Reproductive System Disorders,* pages 520 to 529). This condition can result in frequent urination, urgency, incontinence, urine retention, and infection. Obstruction in an elderly woman may result from uterine prolapse or pelvic cancer.

Prostatic enlargement, common among elderly men, may contribute to obstruction (see Entry 544). Retrograde pressure from urine causes distention of the kidneys, pelvis, and calices, resulting in renal tissue damage. If untreated, prostatic enlargement may also result in hydronephrosis, infection, and uremia. Prostatic cancer, the most common type of cancer in men over age 50, may also lead to urinary tract obstruction.

The potential for cancer is higher in the elderly. Bladder cancer, common after age 50, is more prevalent in men than in women. Symptoms of bladder cancer include frequency, dysuria, and hematuria.

You may have difficulty identifying uremia as the cause of an elderly patient's confusion, because an altered level of consciousness in an elderly person can also arise from organic brain syndrome or environmental disorientation.

Selected References

Alexander, Mary M., and Brown, Marie Scott. *Pediatric Hisotry Taking and Physical Diagnosis for Nurses,* 2nd ed. New York: McGraw-Hill Book Co., 1979.

Beeson, Paul B., et al. *Cecil Textbook of Medicine,* 15th ed. Philadelphia: W.B. Saunders Co., 1979.

Brenner, Barry M., and Rector, Floyd C., eds. *The Kidney,* 2 vols. Philadelphia: W.B. Saunders Co., 1976.

Brundage, Dorothy J. *Nursing Management of Renal Problems,* 2nd ed. St. Louis: C.V. Mosby Co., 1980.

Burrell, Zeb, Jr., and Burrell, Lenette O. *Critical Care,* 3rd ed. St. Louis: C.V. Mosby Co., 1977.

Conn, Howard F., and Conn, Rex B., eds. *Current Diagnosis,* 6th ed. Philadelphia: W.B. Saunders Co., 1980.

DeGowin, Elmer L., and DeGowin, Richard L. *Bedside Diagnostic Examination,* 3rd ed. New York: Macmillan Publishing Co., 1976.

Gault, Patricia L. "How to Break the Kidney Stone Cycle," *Nursing78* 8:24, December 1978.

Ginsburg, A. David. *Clinical Reasoning in Patient Care.* Philadelphia: Harper & Row, 1980.

Guyton, Arthur F. *Textbook of Medical Physiology,* 6th ed. Philadelphia: W.B. Saunders Co., 1981.

Harrison, J., et al., eds. *Campbell's Urology,* 4th ed. Philadelphia: W.B. Saunders Co., 1978.

Hillman, Robert S., et al. *Clinical Skills: Interviewing, History Taking, and Physical Diagnosis.* New York: McGraw-Hill Book Co., 1981.

Isselbacher, Kurt H., et al. *Harrison's Principles of Internal Medicine,* 9th ed. New York: McGraw-Hill Book Co., 1980.

James, J. *Renal Disease in Childhood,* 3rd ed. St. Louis: C.V. Mosby Co., 1976.

Kagan, Lynn. *Renal Disease: A Manual of Patient Care.* New York: McGraw-Hill Book Co., 1979.

Kraytman, Maurice. *The Complete Patient History.* New York: McGraw-Hill Book Co., 1979.

Krupp, Marcus A., and Chatton, Milton J., eds. *Current Medical Diagnosis & Treatment,* rev. ed. Lange Medical Publications, 1980.

Lapides, Jack. *Fundamentals of Urology,* Philadelphia: W.B. Saunders Co., 1976.

Price, Sylvia, and Wilson, Lorraine. *Pathophysiology: Clinical Concepts of Disease Processes.* New York: McGraw-Hill Book Co., 1978.

Prior, John A., and Silberstein, Jack S. *Physical Diagnosis: The History & Examination of the Patient,* 5th ed. St. Louis: C.V. Mosby Co., 1977.

Roberts, S.L. "Renal Assessment: A Nursing Point of View," *Heart and Lung* 8:105, January/February 1979.

Warwick, Roger, and Williams, Peter L., eds. *Gray's Anatomy,* 35th ed. Philadelphia: W.B. Saunders Co., 1973.

13

KEY POINTS IN THIS CHAPTER

KEY CHARTS IN THIS CHAPTER

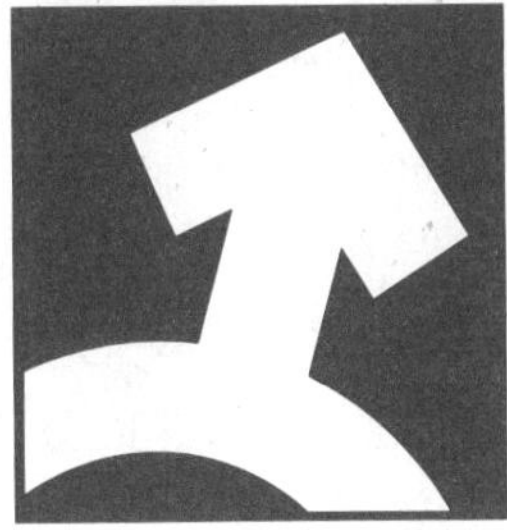

Male Reproductive System

Introduction

515 Why assess the male reproductive system?

You need keen assessment skills to understand and evaluate the male reproductive system. You know that many common disorders of this system have serious consequences. And disorders in this system, along with possibly altering other body systems, can also affect male sexuality. A patient with heart disease may fear he'll have more symptoms, or a heart attack, if he resumes sexual activities. Or, a patient with an ileostomy may be afraid of intimacy because a sexual partner might reject him. Such psychological maladjustments can lead to sexual dysfunction. If your assessment helps to uncover a male patient's potential sexual dysfunction, you'll have contributed not only to his health but also to the quality of his life.

Another important reason for this assessment is that many patients don't volunteer any information about their sexual dysfunction. They're either afraid or too uneasy to inquire about it—or they're unsure whether it can be treated.

Remember, too, that every nurse needs to be attuned to the signs and symptoms of sexually transmitted diseases (formerly referred to as *venereal diseases*), the most common communicable diseases in the United States. Only early detection and prompt treatment can prevent the potentially devastating secondary complications of these diseases.

516 Assessing male sexual disorders

When you must deal with a male patient's psychological reactions to a reproductive system disorder, your tact and skill are as critical in your assessment as identifying his chief complaint and examining him. For example, when assessing a patient with a disease that can be sexually transmitted, remember that he's probably anxious about his signs and symptoms. This may interfere with his recall of historical data vitally needed to limit the spread of the disease—not only in his body, but also in the community. An adolescent may complain of dysuria and discharge but not admit he's had a number of sexual partners until later in the examination. Or a married, middle-aged man may schedule a routine physical examination and never mention the small genital lesion that appeared recently.

Before you can help your patient talk comfortably about his sexual problems, you need to explore your own feelings about reproduction and sexuality and to feel at ease in discussing sexual dysfunctions. Each person's psychological and moral attitudes about sexual matters differ from everyone else's. Because of this, you need to be prepared for a variety of patient reactions when you introduce the subject of sex. By working to overcome any reluctance you may have about managing sexual situations, you enhance your professional skills and provide your patient with the care and attention he requires.

Reviewing anatomy and physiology

517 Testes and spermatogenesis

The testes are ovoid structures somewhat larger than the ovaries. The paired testes lie outside the abdominal cavity, in a pouchlike sac called the *scrotum.* Each testis measures about 2″ (5 cm) in length and 1″ (2.5 cm) in width, and weighs about ½ oz (15 g).

Spermatogenesis occurs in the seminiferous tubules within the testes (see *How Sperm Develop,* page 469). Two types of cells—those which produce sperm and those which nourish it during development—line the tubules so that sperm production occurs continually, throughout the entire length of each tubule.

Testosterone production occurs in specialized cells (Leydig's cells), which form large quantities of testosterone in the newborn and again in the pubescent male.

518 Transport ducts

A paired system of ducts conveys sperm from the testes to the ejaculatory ducts. Each system forms a continuous channel beginning with the *testis,* which holds the sperm discharged by the seminiferous tubules, and continuing with the *efferent ductules,* which convey the sperm into the *epididymis*—a convoluted, tubular reservoir for sperm maturation (during maturation, the sperm becomes fertile and motile). The storage site for mature sperm is the *vas deferens,* which enlarges into an ampulla within the pelvis. This duct travels from the epididymis through the inguinal canal, then alongside the bladder to the ejaculatory duct inside the prostate. The *spermatic cord* consists of a compact bundle of blood vessels, lymphatics, nerves, muscle bundles, and the vas deferens.

519 Glands

The *seminal vesicles* are paired, saclike glands lying below the ampulla and against the posterior bladder. They're lined with epithelium, which secretes a mucoid material. During ejaculation, each vesicle empties this fluid into the ejaculatory duct at the same time the vas deferens empties the sperm. The resulting mixture is thought to protect the ejaculated sperm until one of them reaches the ovum.

The *prostate* is a spherical gland, about 2″ (5 cm) in diameter, that surrounds the urethra just below the base of the bladder. Glandular tissue makes up about half the prostate; the other half is made up of fibromuscular tissue. The glandular tissue is arranged in two groups—an inner group that surrounds the urethra and a larger outer group that forms the bulk of the tissue. The prostate gland continuously secretes a thin, milky, alkaline fluid.

During ejaculation, the prostate's fibromuscular tissue contracts simultaneously with the vas deferens and seminal vesicles, thickening the seminal fluid (semen). Later, prostatic fluid greatly enhances the motility and possibly the fertility of the sperm by neutralizing the acidity of the urethra and of the woman's vagina.

520 The penis and the male sexual act

The penis consists of three cylinders of highly vascular erectile tissue: two *corpora cavernosa,* which form the major part of the penis, and the *corpus spongiosum,* which encases the urethra. The two corpora cavernosa are encased in a capsule of fibrous tissue, and all three cylinders are enveloped in a fascial sheath and loose skin.

Bulbourethral (Cowper's) *glands* are small paired glands, about 5 mm in diameter, located below the prostate gland within the pelvic floor's tissues. Before ejaculation, these glands secrete a mucoid material that empties into the posterior urethra to become part of the semen.

The stages of the male sexual act are erection, lubrication, and emission and ejaculation. The degree of erection is proportional to the degree of stimulation, whether the source is physical or psychological. When parasympathetic impulses received from the sacral portion of the spinal cord pass to the arteries and veins of the penis, blood fills the erectile tissues and causes the penis to elongate and become rigid. At the same time, the parasympathetic impulses cause the bulbourethral glands to secrete mucus, which flows through the urethra during intercourse to aid in lubrication. In addition, the scrotum thickens and the testes increase in size, rotate anteriorly, and elevate.

When the sexual stimulus reaches a critical intensity, the spinal cord reflex mechanisms emit rhythmic sympathetic impulses from the first and second lumbar vertebrae to the genital organs. Emission begins with contractions of the epididymis, the vas deferens, and ampulla, causing expulsion of sperm into the internal urethra. Con-

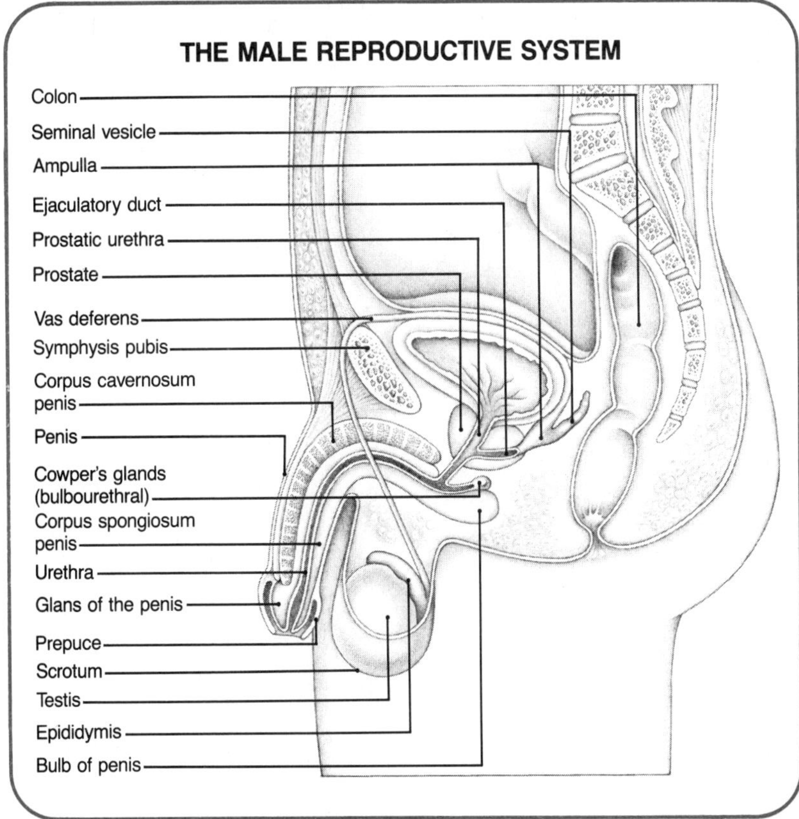

tractions in the seminal vesicles and prostate gland expel fluid and propel the sperm forward, where more mucus is added by the bulbourethral glands. In response to the filling of the internal urethra, more rhythmic impulses are sent, this time to the skeletal muscles. These encase the base of the erectile tissue and cause peristaltic pressure changes that forcefully expel the semen from the urethral meatus. This process is known as *ejaculation.* Its progress can be inhibited by adverse environmental conditions (for example, extremes of temperature), psychological disturbances, physical fatigue, illness, or recent orgasm.

521 Scrotum and spermatogenesis

A skin-covered sac composed of fibrous tissue and muscle fibers, the scrotum contains a pair of testes, the epididymides, and the proximal vasa deferentia. A vertical fibrous partition bisects the scrotum; each half contains a testis, an epididymis, and a proximal vas deferens.

The scrotum maintains the proper testicular temperature for spermatogenesis (which occurs at below normal body temperature) through contraction and relaxation. Sexual stimulation or cold causes the scrotal muscles to contract, which elevates the testes and draws them closer to the body's warmth. Heat causes the scrotum to relax, which moves the testes away from the body and lowers the intratesticular temperature.

522 Hormonal regulation

The pituitary gonadotropins that control ovarian function in women also regulate testicular function in men. *Follicle-stimulating hormone* (FSH) stimulates spermatogenesis, and *luteinizing hormone* (LH), also known as *interstitial cell-stimulating hor-*

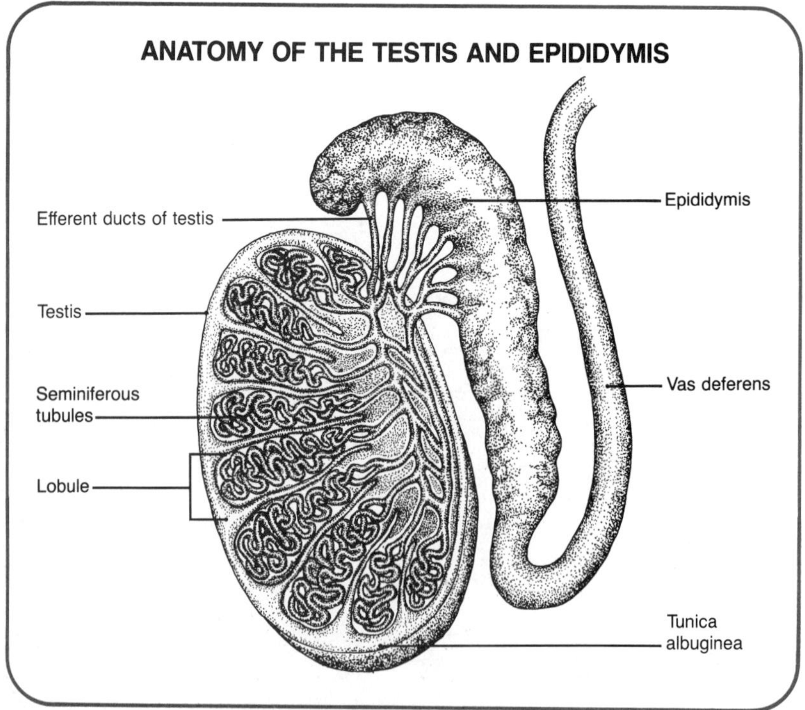

HOW SPERM DEVELOP

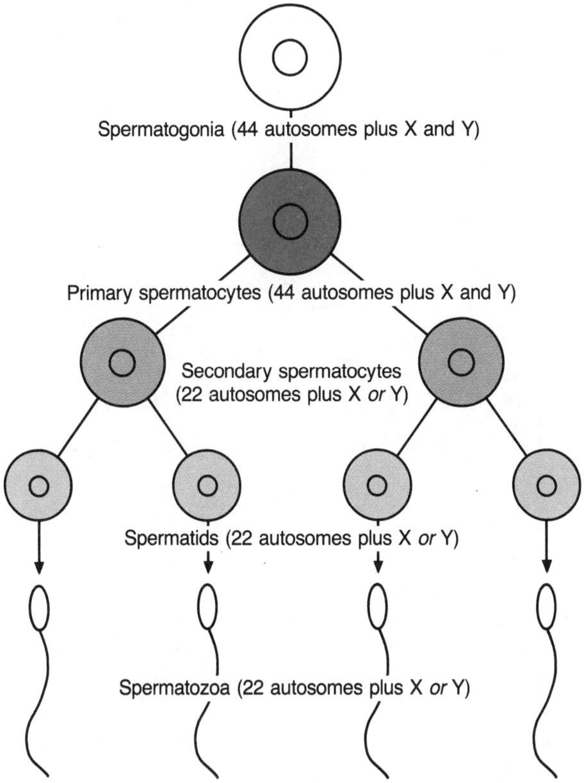

Spermatogonia (44 autosomes plus X and Y)

Primary spermatocytes (44 autosomes plus X and Y)

Secondary spermatocytes (22 autosomes plus X *or* Y)

Spermatids (22 autosomes plus X *or* Y)

Spermatozoa (22 autosomes plus X *or* Y)

Spermatogenesis, the formation of mature spermatozoa within the seminiferous tubules, occurs in several stages:

- As you can see in this illustration, spermatogonia, the primary germinal epithelial cells, grow and develop to become *primary spermatocytes.*

Both spermatogonia and primary spermatocytes contain 46 chromosomes. Forty-four of these are called *autosomes.* The other two are the sex chromosomes, X and Y.

- Primary spermatocytes divide meiotically to form *secondary spermatocytes.* No new chromosomes are formed in this stage—the pairs only divide. Each secondary spermatocyte contains a haploid number of chromosomes—one spermatocyte contains an X chromosome and the other contains a Y chromosome.
- Each secondary spermatocyte divides meiotically again to form *spermatids.*
- Finally, the spermatids undergo a series of structural changes that transform them into motile spermatozoa.

mone, stimulates testosterone secretion by the Leydig's cells, located between the testicular tubules.

Testosterone enlarges the primary sexual structures from puberty to about age 20, after which the penis, scrotum, and testes remain essentially the same until after about age 50.

Responding to releasing hormones liberated by the hypothalamus, FSH and LH are continually secreted in men by the pituitary gland. A feedback

REGULATING MALE SEXUAL HORMONAL FUNCTION

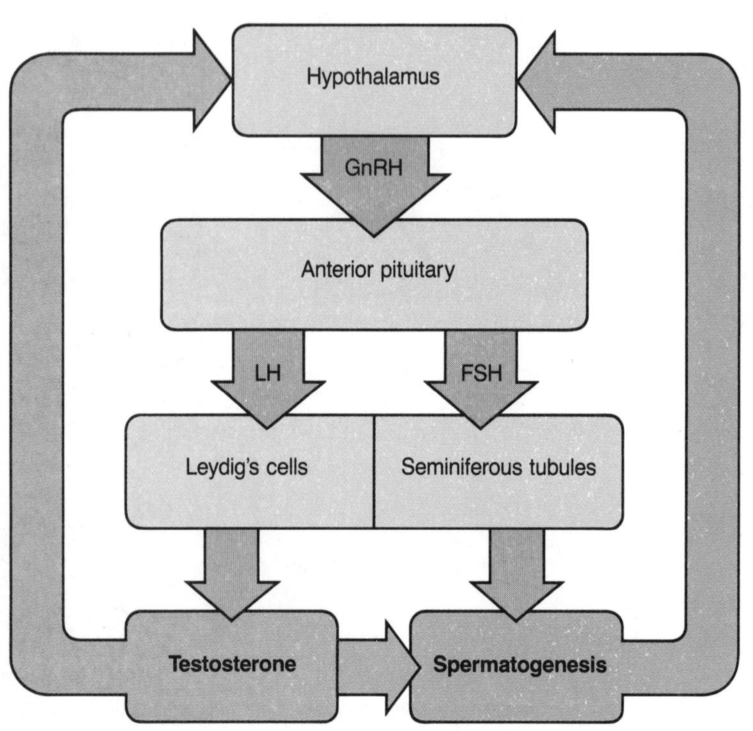

In all normal males, hormonal function is controlled by a negative feedback mechanism stimulating the hypothalamus. Here, the hypothalamus secretes substances, gonadotropin-releasing hormones (GnRH), that stimulate the anterior pituitary. Once stimulated, the anterior pituitary releases luteinizing hormone (LH) and follicle-stimulating hormone (FSH). Both LH and FSH are found in plasma and urine as gonadotropins.

LH acts on the Leydig's cells of the testis. LH causes these cells to mature and secrete testosterone—the hormone necessary for normal growth and development of male sex organs. Normal testosterone production develops and maintains the male secondary sex characteristics, such as thickening skin and increased growth of muscles and of body hair. Unlike the female hormonal cycle, male hormonal function is continuous and constant. When testosterone concentrations rise, the body sends negative feedback messages to the hypothalamus to keep testosterone levels stable.

FSH acts on the germinal epithelial cells of the seminiferous tubules. This promotes complete spermatogenesis.

mechanism, similar to the one regulating other pituitary tropic hormones, controls their release (see *Regulating Male Sexual Hormonal Function*).

Testosterone is also responsible for the development and maintenance of secondary sex characteristics and is required for spermatogenesis. Puberty marks the onset of male secondary sex characteristics: distinct body hair distribution; skin changes, such as increased sweat and sebaceous gland secretion; voice change, caused by laryngeal enlargement; increased musculoskeletal development; and intracellular and extracellular changes.

Collecting appropriate history data

523 Biographical data

Age is perhaps the primary consideration in assessing the male reproductive system. For example, gonorrhea is usually associated with young people and is most prevalent between ages 19 and 25. On the other hand, elderly men are more likely to develop prostate disorders, primarily benign prostatic hypertrophy and prostatic cancer. In fact, more than half of all men over age 50 have some degree of prostatic enlargement, and prostatic cancer is one of the most common malignant neoplasms in men over age 50. When it occurs, testicular cancer usually develops in men between ages 15 and 40, with the highest incidence occurring at age 32; in the United States, it's also the most common type of solid tumor in males.

Race is another significant biographical factor. For example, the highest incidence of prostatic cancer occurs in blacks and the lowest incidence occurs in Orientals.

524 Chief complaint

The most common chief complaints associated with the male reproductive system are *changes in voiding pattern, penile discharge, scrotal or inguinal mass, pain or tenderness, impotence,* and *infertility.*

525 History of present illness

Using the PQRST mnemonic device, ask the patient to elaborate on his chief complaint. Then, depending on the complaint, explore the history of the patient's present illness by asking him the following types of questions:

• ***Changes in voiding pattern.*** *Do you have to wait longer than a few seconds before urine flow begins? Do you strain to urinate? Do you have a feeling of urgency to urinate? Does the urinary stream seem smaller in caliber or less*

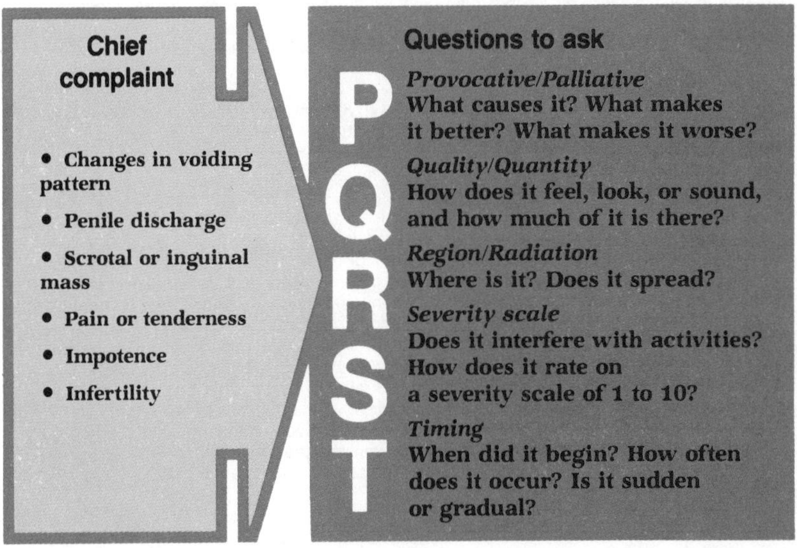

Chief complaint

- **Changes in voiding pattern**
- **Penile discharge**
- **Scrotal or inguinal mass**
- **Pain or tenderness**
- **Impotence**
- **Infertility**

Questions to ask

P — *Provocative/Palliative*
What causes it? What makes it better? What makes it worse?

Q — *Quality/Quantity*
How does it feel, look, or sound, and how much of it is there?

R — *Region/Radiation*
Where is it? Does it spread?

S — *Severity scale*
Does it interfere with activities? How does it rate on a severity scale of 1 to 10?

T — *Timing*
When did it begin? How often does it occur? Is it sudden or gradual?

forceful than usual? Have you been urinating more frequently, or do you wake up in the middle of the night to urinate? An obstructed or decreased urinary flow or an increase in urinary frequency (including nocturia) is commonly caused by an enlarged prostate gland. Also consider that the patient may have a urinary system disorder. (See *Nurse's Guide to Urinary Disorders,* pages 452 to 455.)

• ***Penile discharge.*** *How much discharge is there? Is the discharge present only during urination? What color is it? What consistency is it?* Large quantities of thick, creamy, yellow-green discharge usually indicate gonorrhea. A thin, watery discharge may suggest a nonspecific urethritis or a prostate infection. A bloody discharge may indicate an infection or cancer in the urinary or reproductive tract.

• ***Pain or tenderness.*** *Is urination painful for you?* This may suggest a nonspecific urinary tract infection or a sexually transmitted disease. *Is the painful passage of urine accompanied by spasms (strangury)?* This may result from bladder or prostate infection. *Does dull, aching scrotal pain worsen when you strain?* This could indicate an inguinal hernia. On the other hand, extreme scrotal pain that begins suddenly suggests testicular torsion. Gradual onset of acute pain, accompanied by warmth, heat, and swelling, usually indicates an infection. Flank pain suggests renal calculi.

• ***Scrotal or inguinal mass.*** *Does the mass disappear when you lie flat on your back?* Normally, this indicates an inguinal hernia. *Have you recently received an injury to your genitals?* This may cause a hematocele. *How long has the mass been present? Are there any associated symptoms, such as pain?*

DISCUSSING SEXUAL PROBLEMS

Knowing how to discuss your patient's sexual problems or concerns is important for two reasons. First, it helps you identify areas that require active treatment. Second, it shows the patient that you view sexual function as an integral part of his life-style, and that you're willing and able to discuss the subject. Here are some guidelines to help you:

• To begin, tell the patient that you need some information about his sexual functioning so you can provide appropriate care. Explain which areas of questioning you'll explore—such as his relationship with his partner, his sexual experiences, and his sexual preferences. Assure him that his answers will remain confidential.

• In your discussion, move from less sensitive to more sensitive areas. For example, discuss the patient's urinary problems before you bring up the subject of his sexual functioning.

• Integrate your questions with those dealing with his activities of daily living. This way you'll help him feel that discussing sexual functioning is acceptable. To encourage discussion, ask open-ended questions. Instead of asking, "Did you just notice this problem recently?", ask, "When did you first notice this problem?"

• Because medical terminology may be confusing to him, try using the sexual terms your patient understands. But be sure you're both talking about the same thing. Misunderstandings can easily occur if your patient uses slang (or accepted terms) incorrectly. To avoid confusion, you might begin by using several different words that mean the same thing, to clarify your point and get an idea of the type of terminology he uses. For example, you might ask: "Do you have any pain in your penis—your sexual organ?" Use his response to guide your use of terminology as the discussion continues.

• Introduce common or slang terms into the conversation selectively and cautiously. You'll do this more often with younger patients, because they tend to use more slang in general conversation. First make sure you've established rapport, so the patient doesn't feel uncomfortable with the familiarity that slang implies.

• Don't react to your patient's comments in ways that discourage conversation. If he senses your disapproval, he'll be less willing to continue the discussion.

• Be sure to end your discussion by asking the patient if he has additional questions or concerns that he wants to discuss.

Although benign conditions may be painless, testicular cancer must be considered.

• ***Sexual impotence.*** *Sexual impotence means different things to different people, so can you tell me what you mean by the term?* Clarifying the patient's understanding of impotence is important, because sexual terms are frequently misunderstood and misused. *What was your life-style like at the time the problem began? Did the problem begin suddenly or gradually?* Sudden impotence that occurs during a stressful time in the patient's life most likely originates psychogenically. (About 80% of all occurrences of sexual impotence are psychogenic.) *Do you have nocturnal or morning erections? Can you achieve an erection through fantasizing or masturbation?* Patients with psychogenic impotence usually retain these capabilities.

• ***Infertility.*** *How long have you and your sexual partner been trying to achieve pregnancy?* Suspect infertility only if the couple have engaged regularly in intercourse, without using birth control, for at least 1 year. *Do you have a low sex drive, premature ejaculation, or impotence? Was your sexual development normal? Have you had any infections or injuries to your testes?*

UNDERSTANDING YOUR PATIENT'S SEXUAL PROBLEM

If your patient complains of impotence, don't assume that's his primary problem. Impotence may be only a symptom of another condition. You'll want to find out the reason for his problem to help him deal with it. Consider these other possibilities:

- Loss of libido
- Lowered quality or quantity of sexual performance
- Ejaculatory incompetence
- Premature ejaculation
- Decreased volume or force of ejaculate
- Increased postcoital refractory period
- Disinterest in sexual partner
- Unwillingness or inability to meet sexual desires of actual or potential sexual partner
- Sexual exhaustion
- Normal aging changes
- Anxiety about penis size.

526 Past history

Focus on the following health problems when reviewing your patient's past history:

• ***Metabolic and endocrine disorders.*** *Diabetes mellitus* can cause irreversible, organic sexual impotence, probably from vascular impairment. (About half of all men with diabetes are impotent.) Diabetes mellitus can result in infertility, as can *panhypopituitarism* and, infrequently, *hypothyroidism* and *congenital adrenal hyperplasia.*

• ***Nervous disorders.*** Nerve damage occurring with *multiple sclerosis* may result in sexual impotence and infertility. *Spinal cord trauma* also can cause sexual impotence.

• ***Infections.*** About 25% of all postpubertal males who acquire *mumps* (viral parotitis) develop orchitis, which can cause extreme pain and tenderness. If bilateral degeneration of the seminiferous tubular epithelium accompanies the infection, infertility may result. Sexually transmitted diseases and other *genital infections* can cause infertility.

• ***Urinary disorders.*** *Chronic renal failure* can result in sexual impotence and infertility. Previous surgical procedures—such as cystectomy, radical prostatectomy, and bilateral orchiectomy—can also cause impotence.

• ***Drugs.*** Many drugs, as well as alcohol, can impair the function of the male reproductive system (see *Nurse's Guide to Some Drugs That Affect the Male Reproductive System,* page 474).

527 Family history

Klinefelter's syndrome, a chromosomal pattern marked by the presence of two

DRUGS

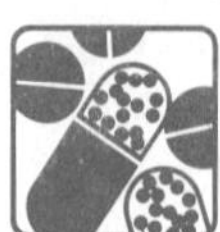

NURSE'S GUIDE TO SOME DRUGS THAT AFFECT THE MALE REPRODUCTIVE SYSTEM

CLASSIFICATION	POSSIBLE SIDE EFFECTS
Anticonvulsants	
carbamazepine (Tegretol*) primidone (Mysoline*)	• Impotence
Antidepressants	
doxepin hydrochloride (Sinequan*)	• Testicular swelling
imipramine hydrochloride (Tofranil*)	• Painful ejaculation, testicular swelling, erectile difficulty
tranylcypromine sulfate (Parnate*)	• Altered libido, impotence
Antihypertensives	
clonidine hydrochloride (Catapres*)	• Inhibited ejaculation, impotence
guanethidine sulfate (Ismelin*)	• Inhibited ejaculation
mecamylamine hydrochloride (Inversine)	• Decreased libido, impotence
methyldopa (Aldomet*) reserpine (Serpasil*)	• Impotence
Antipsychotics	
chlorpromazine hydrochloride (Chlorprom**, Thorazine) prochlorperazine maleate (Compazine, Stemetil**) thioridazine hydrochloride (Mellaril*)	• Diminished libido, inhibited ejaculation
Gastrointestinal anticholinergics	
atropine sulfate and other anticholinergics	• Impotence
Miscellaneous gastrointestinal drugs	
cimetidine (Tagamet*)	• Reduced sperm count, impotence
Tranquilizers	
diazepam (Valium*) oxazepam (Serax*)	• Changed libido

*Available in U.S. and Canada. **Available in Canada only.
All other products (no symbol) are available in the U.S. only.

or more X chromosomes with at least one Y, is a relatively common condition resulting in primary hypogonadism. This condition is characterized by gynecomastia, underdeveloped testes, sparse facial hair, and azoospermia (semen that doesn't contain spermatozoa). Many of these patients are tall as a result of delayed epiphyseal closure.

528 Psychosocial history

When appropriate, ask your patient about his *sexual practices and attitudes.* For example, does he have guilt feelings, fears, or other negative emotions about women? Inquire about his sexual relationships, including possible exposure to sexually transmitted diseases.

Because *stress* can interfere with sexual performance, ask your patient if he has any emotional conflicts at work or at home. Don't forget to question him about his work environment. A job that exposes him to harmful chemicals or radiation may cause infertility.

529 Activities of daily living

Ask your patient if he takes hot baths, rides a bicycle frequently, or wears tight underwear or an athletic supporter. These circumstances elevate scrotal temperature and may interfere with spermatogenesis, possibly producing temporary oligospermia. If your patient participates in sports, ask him how he protects himself from possible genital injuries. Also ask if he performs testicular self-examinations routinely.

530 Review of systems

Ask your patient if he has any of the following symptoms:

- ***Skin.*** *Pruritus* may accompany many infectious diseases of the reproductive system that cause an exudate.
- ***Gastrointestinal.*** Severe pain, such as the pain associated with testicular torsion, may cause *nausea* and *vomiting.*
- ***Psychological.*** Typical reactions to anxiety, such as *insomnia* and *restlessness,* may also accompany possible psychogenic sexual dysfunction.

Conducting the physical examination

531 Preparing to examine your patient

Before you begin examining a patient, be sure you have adequate lighting and the following equipment on hand: disposable gloves, lubricant, a flashlight (for transilluminating the scrotum), cotton swabs, culture tubes, and an agar plate (in case you notice a penile discharge during the examination).

Explain to the patient the procedures you're about to perform, to allay any fears he may have. Then conduct your general survey (see Entry 67). Determine whether the patient can stand or whether you'll have to position him supine on an examining table. If he has to lie on the examining table, drape him carefully, exposing only his genitalia and groin.

532 Inspecting and palpating the penis

Inspection and palpation are the two most important techniques used to examine the male genitalia. Begin by observing the amount and distribution of your patient's pubic hair. It should be thickest at the symphysis pubis and continue over the scrotum and inner thighs. Then, observe his penis. Inspect its anterior surface first; then lift it to inspect the posterior surface.

Normally, the penis appears pink and smooth. Note any swelling, erythema, nodules, or ulcers. Remember, the size of the penile shaft varies; evaluate it in terms of your patient's age and general development. Suspect an abnormality only if it appears extremely small and infantile.

Inspect the glans, noting whether the patient is circumcised. If he isn't, you'll have to retract the foreskin (see *Inspecting and Palpating the Penis,* page 477). You should be able to do this easily. (If you can't, the patient probably has *phimosis,* constriction of the foreskin over the glans, usually from a previous inflammation.) Normally, the glans is smooth. Note any lesions, erythema, discharge, or smegma. (A potential carcinogen, smegma may be responsible for the higher incidence of penile carcinoma in uncircumcised men.)

Next, inspect the urethral meatus.

HOW TO CULTURE A PENILE DISCHARGE

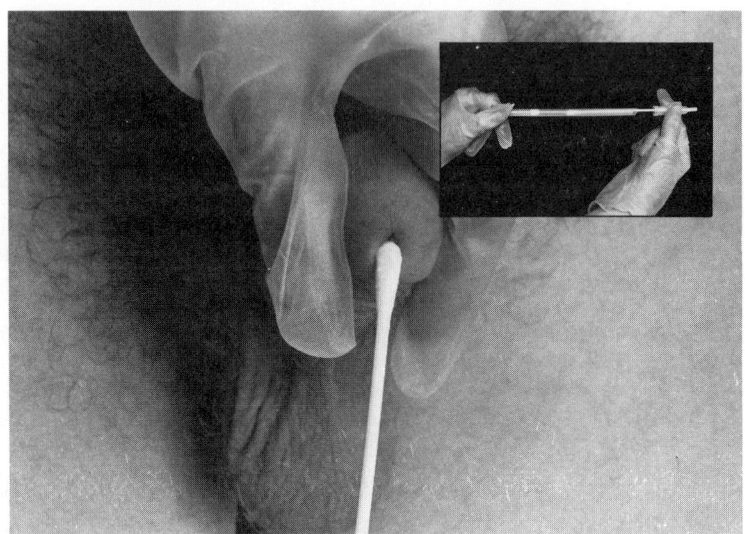

1 If you notice a discharge from your patient's penis, document its color, consistency, and odor. Then, to check for bacterial growth, take two separate specimens for cultures. To do this, first roll a sterile cotton swab in the discharge. Then, place the swab in a Culturette™ tube, as shown in the inset.

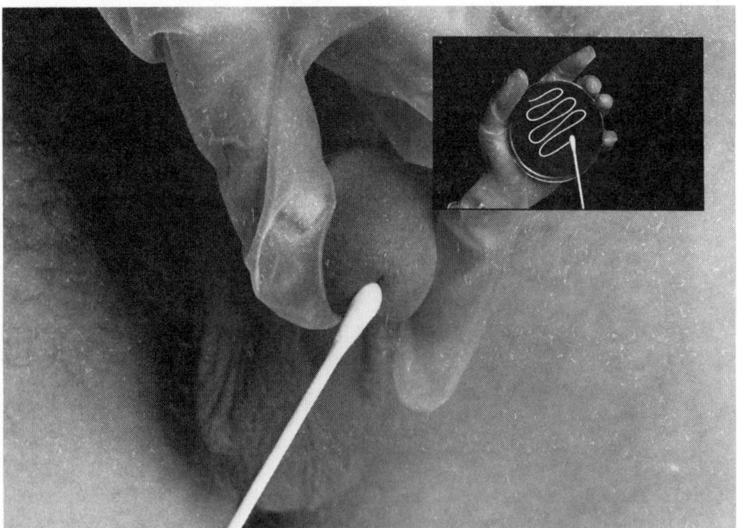

2 With a second sterile cotton swab, obtain another specimen for a gonorrheal culture. Roll the swab over a Thayer-Martin plate in a Z-pattern, as shown in the inset. Then immediately use the swab to cross-streak the plate, unless the laboratory performing the test handles cross-streaking. Finally, label both cultures, and send them to the laboratory for analysis.

Note any abnormalities, such as hypospadias or epispadias. Also note any discharge.

Finally, palpate the entire penile shaft between your thumb and first two fingers. In its nonerect state, the penis should feel soft. Note any indurations, nodules, or thickening.

INSPECTING AND PALPATING THE PENIS

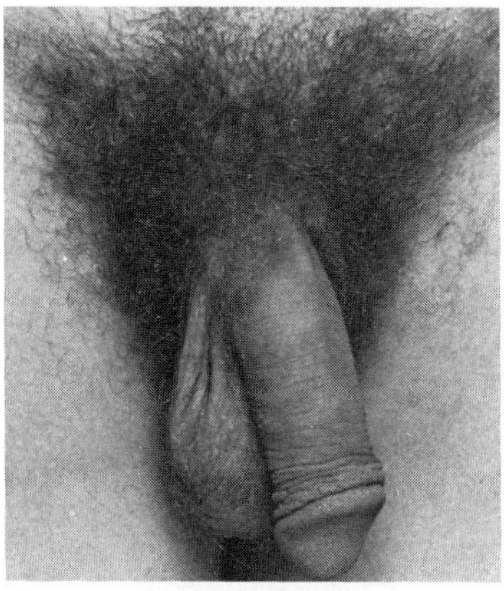

1 To inspect and palpate your patient's penis, begin by observing his pubic hair; it should be thickest at his symphysis pubis and extend over his inner thighs and scrotum.

Inspect the anterior surface of the penis first. Then lift the penis to check the posterior surface. Note any ulcers, swelling, scars, nodules, or skin discoloration.

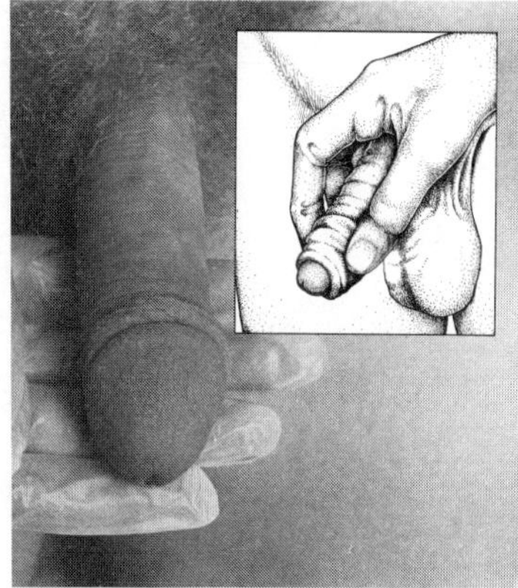

2 Inspect the glans to note any lesions, discharge, growths, swelling, or inflammation. If your patient's uncircumcised, retract his foreskin to see the glans. To do this, place your thumb and forefinger on either side of the glans and, using gentle pressure, draw the foreskin over the penile shaft, as shown in the inset. Note any abnormalities. After this examination, replace the foreskin.

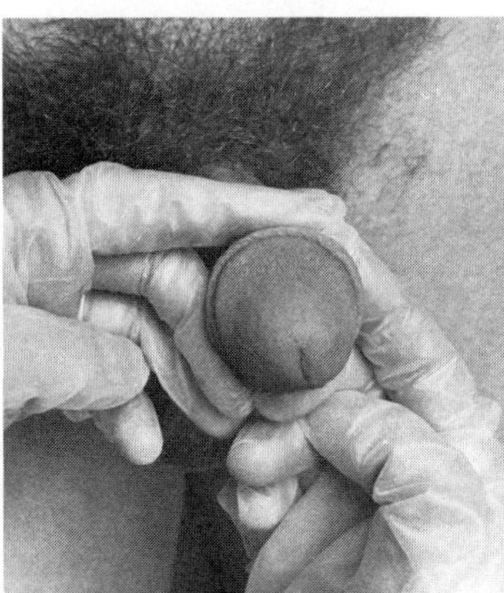

3 Inspect the urethral meatus by holding the glans between your index and middle fingers. Observe for lesions, discharge, and stenosis.

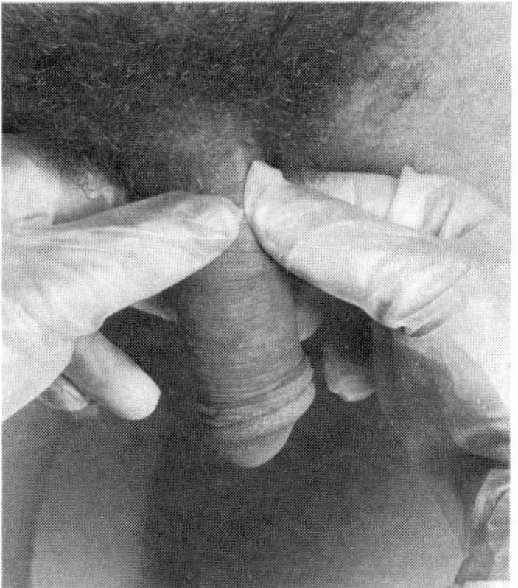

4 Finally, palpate the entire penile shaft between your thumb and first two fingers. Note any thickening, nodules, or hardness.

RECOGNIZING PENIS ABNORMALITIES

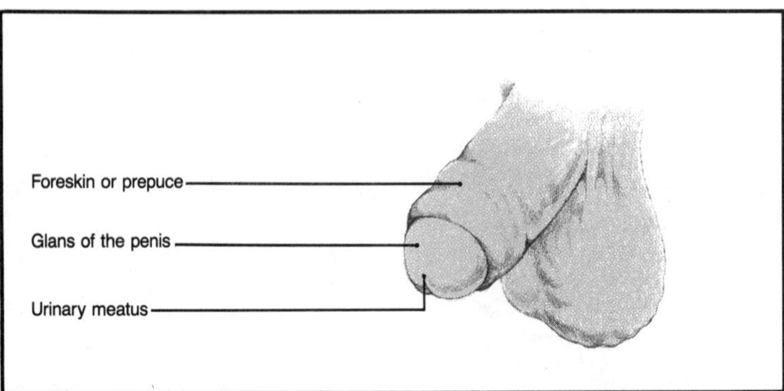

Normal: foreskin retracts easily from the glans and readily returns to its original position

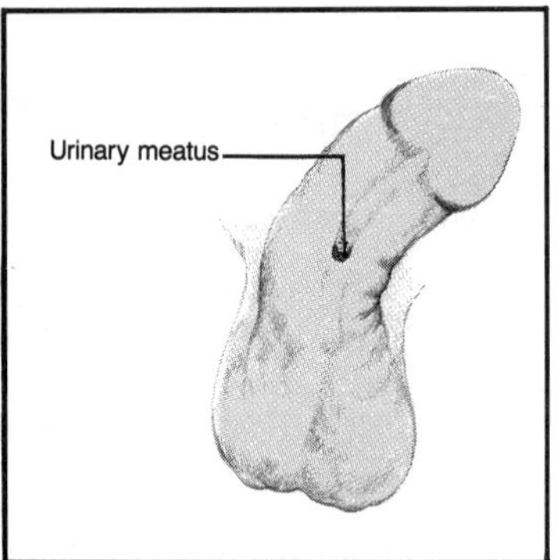

Hypospadias: urethral opening on posterior side of penis or on perineum

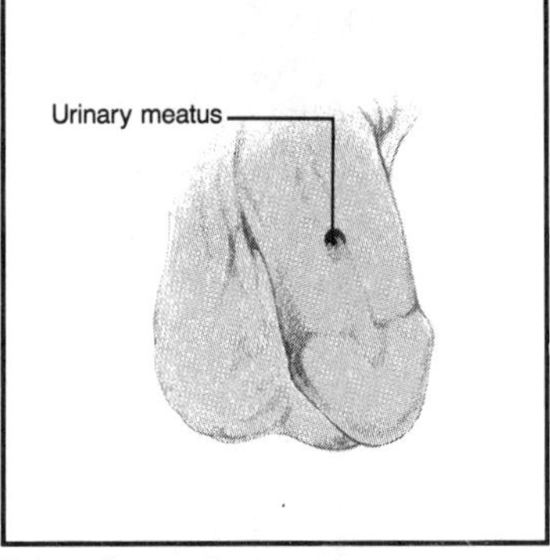

Epispadias: urethral opening on anterior side of penis

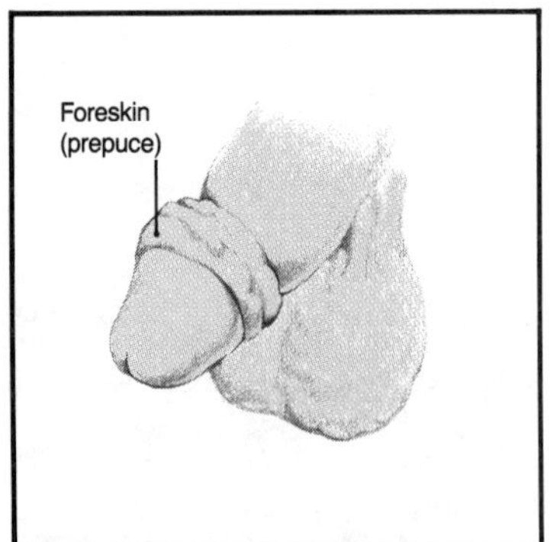

Paraphimosis: constricting foreskin behind glans, preventing its return to original position

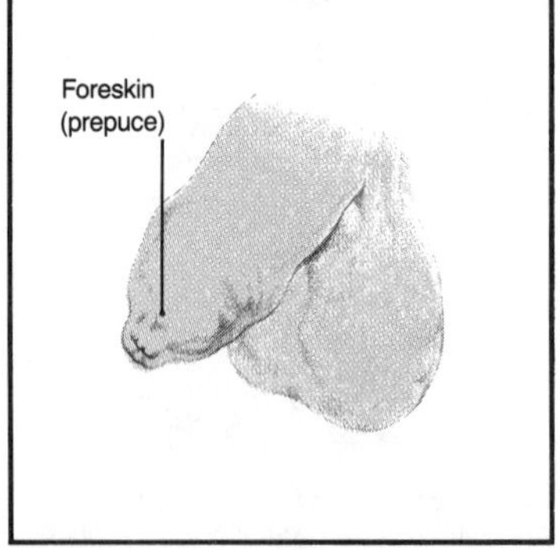

Phimosis: constricting foreskin covering the glans, preventing foreskin retraction

INSPECTING AND PALPATING THE SCROTUM

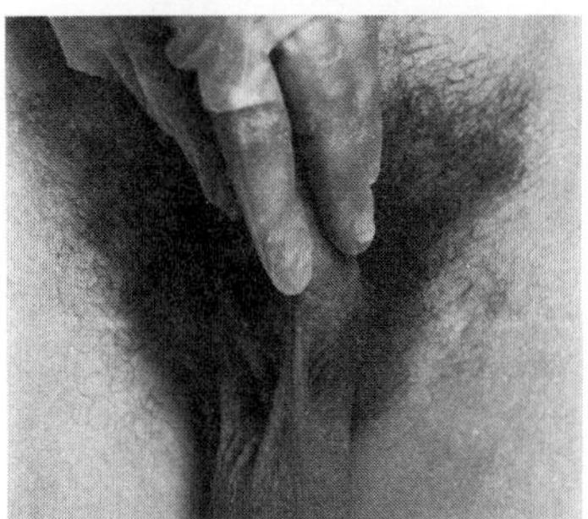

1 To inspect your patient's scrotum, support his penis against the symphysis pubis. Note that the left testis normally rests slightly lower than the right testis.

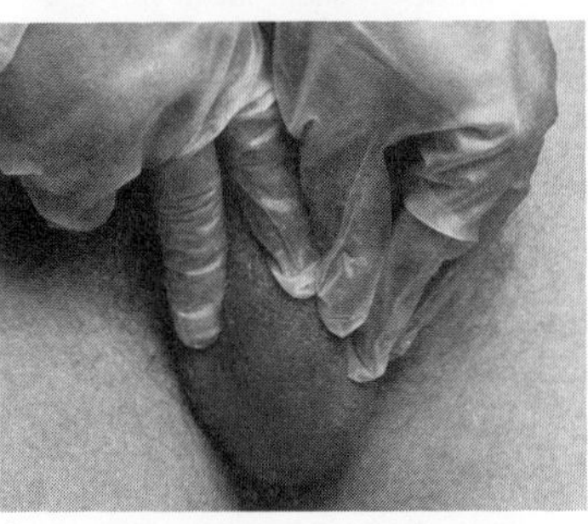

2 Inspect the scrotum's anterior and posterior surfaces. Look for any swelling, nodules, redness, ulceration, or distended veins.

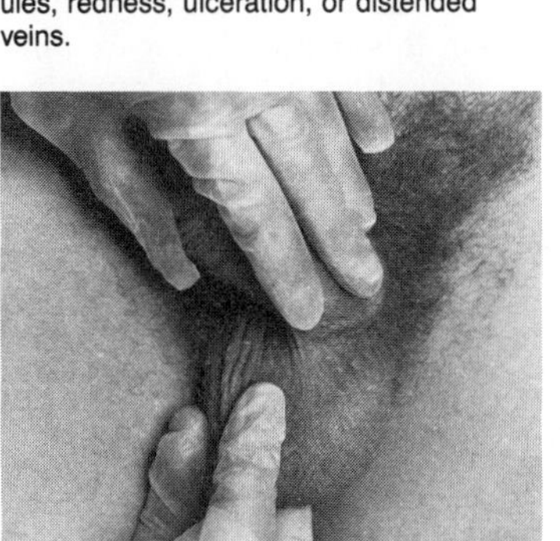

3 Next, gently palpate each testis between your thumb and first two fingers. Note any abnormalities, such as undescended testis, lumps, hardness, atrophy, or softening. Also palpate the epididymis for tenderness, swelling, or induration.

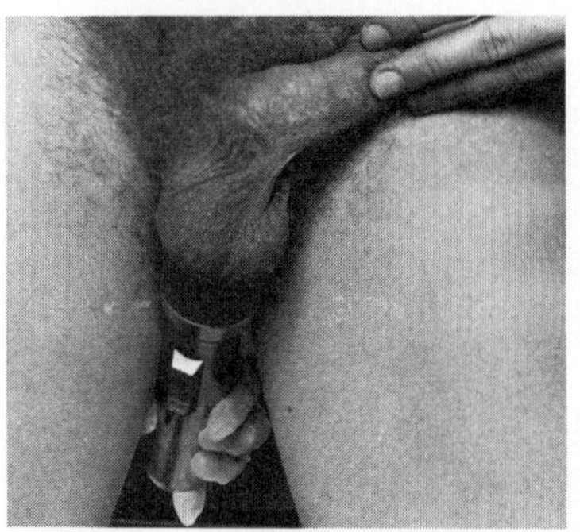

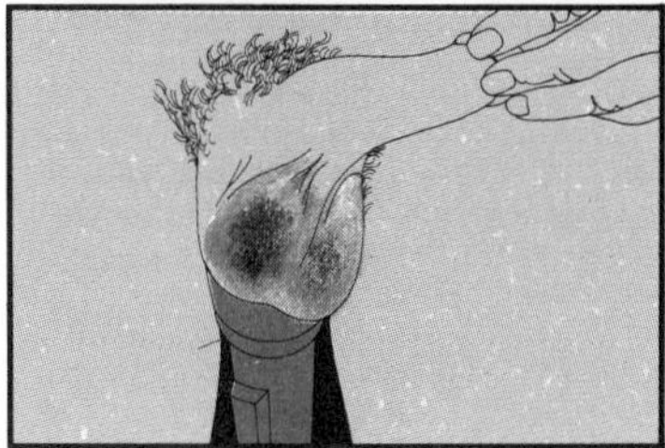

4 If a mass is present, use transillumination to evaluate it. Darken the room, then place a flashlight head flat against the posterior surface of the affected side of the scrotum. Switch on the flashlight, as shown in the inset, and observe the anterior surface. The testis will appear as an opaque shadow, as will any lumps, masses, or blood-filled areas. Transilluminate the opposite side to compare your findings.

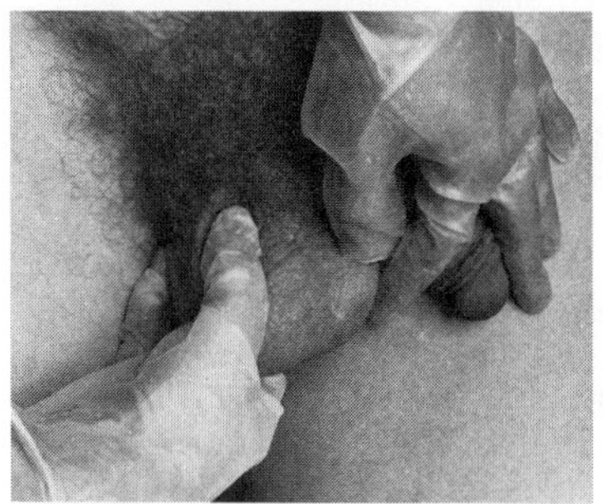

5 Finally, gently grasp each spermatic cord between your thumb and forefinger. Palpate the entire length, from the epididymis to the external inguinal ring, particularly noting any nodules.

PALPATING THE INGUINAL AREA

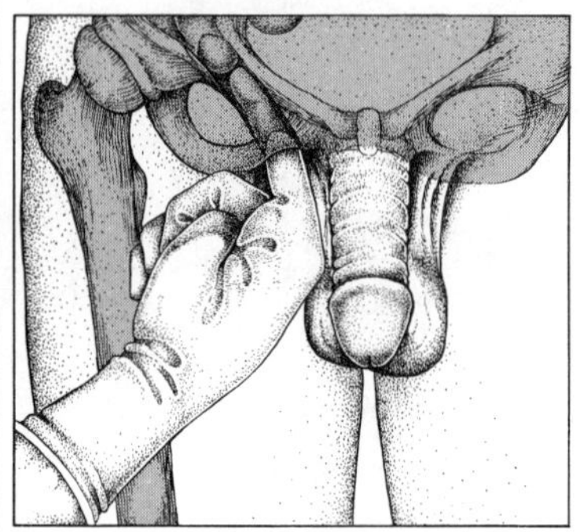

To locate the inguinal area, place your index finger on the distal aspect of the patient's scrotum and push upward. Follow the spermatic cord's course with your index finger until you reach the triangular opening of the external inguinal ring. If possible, gently insert your finger into the inguinal canal and follow its course. While maintaining this finger position, ask your patient to bear down or strain. Note any mass you feel with your finger.

533 Inspecting and palpating the scrotum

To inspect the scrotum, support the patient's penis against his symphysis pubis. The scrotal skin should appear wrinkled. The sac is normally asymmetrical, the left testis hanging about ½″ (about 1 cm) lower in the relaxed scrotum than the right testis. If the patient's right testis hangs lower, make a note of it.

After inspecting the scrotum's anterior surface, be sure to lift it to inspect its posterior surface as well. Note any swelling. Scrotal enlargement may result from a hydrocele, which causes the skin to appear tight and shiny. Also inspect the scrotum for redness, ulcerations, cysts, or distended veins.

Next, gently palpate the scrotum. Begin by palpating each testis between your thumb and first two fingers. Note if the testis isn't present or isn't fully descended into the sac. Normally, testes are the same size. They should feel firm, smooth, and rubbery and move freely in the scrotal sac. Note any atrophy or softening, as well as any hard, irregular areas or lumps. If you find a mass, describe its location, size, consistency, and shape. Also note any tenderness and whether the mass transilluminates (see *Inspecting and Palpating the Scrotum,* page 479).

Now palpate each epididymis, usually located on the posterolateral surface of each testis. Note any tenderness, swelling, or induration. Finally, gently pinch each spermatic cord, which you can feel above the testis. You can readily identify the vas deferens within the cord; it feels noticeably different from the blood vessels and nerves. Using your thumb and forefinger, palpate the entire length of the cord, from the epididymis to the external inguinal ring. Normally, the 3-mm-wide cord feels smooth, round, and resilient. Note any nodular structures that feel like a bag of worms, which may indicate a varicocele—a mass of engorged dilated veins. (A varicocele will collapse slowly when you elevate a supine patient's scrotum.)

534 Examining inguinal and femoral areas

Begin this phase of your examination by inspecting the patient's inguinal and femoral areas, noting any bulges. Ask him to bear down, as though straining at stool. Note any tenderness or masses and whether a mass is reducible. Then, palpate each femoral pulse for possible clues to aortic problems (see Entry 396).

Although you can't palpate the femoral canal, you can estimate its location to help you detect a femoral hernia. Place your right index finger (pointing toward the patient's head) on the patient's right femoral artery, keeping your other fingers close together. Your middle finger will then lie over the femoral vein and your ring finger will lie over the femoral canal. Use your left hand to check the patient's left side.

Next, palpate the lymph nodes in the

inguinal and femoral areas. These freely movable masses usually feel firm. Normally, they're about 0.5 cm in size. Note any tenderness or enlargement. (Be careful not to mistake an enlarged lymph node for a femoral hernia.)

Continue to palpate the patient's entire inguinal area, noting any lumps or bulges. Ask him to bear down as you proceed. Also, as you proceed, ask the patient to cough. Look and palpate for the cough impulse. Then palpate the inguinal ring on each side (see *Palpating the Inguinal Area*). To do this, place your index finger on the neck of the patient's scrotum and gently push upward, unfolding the patient's loose scrotal skin. Use your right index finger for the patient's right side and your left index finger for his left side.

Follow the spermatic cord's course until you reach the triangular opening of the external inguinal ring. (The ring should not be obstructed.) If possible, gently insert your finger into the inguinal canal and follow its course. (If you feel a mass protruding through the external inguinal opening, suspect an inguinal hernia.) With your finger in the inguinal canal, or just at the external ring, ask the patient to bear down and cough. Palpate for any herniating tissue. When assessing your patient for a hernia, remember to examine him in both supine and standing positions.

535 Palpating the prostate gland

Nurses don't routinely perform this assessment technique. If you do perform it, first instruct the patient to urinate. Then, lubricate the index finger of your gloved examining hand. Have

PALPATING THE PROSTATE GLAND

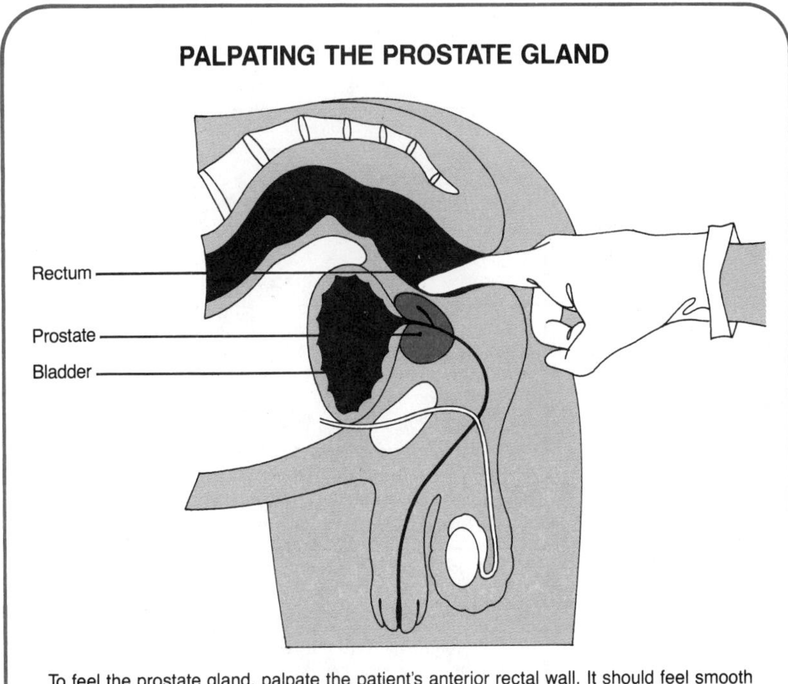

To feel the prostate gland, palpate the patient's anterior rectal wall. It should feel smooth and elastic through the rectal wall mucosa.

The seminal vesicles, which are slightly above the prostate gland on the anterior rectal wall, are not normally palpable unless they're inflamed.

your patient stand at the end of the examining table, with his elbows flexed and his upper body resting on the table. (If he can't stand, position him on the examining table in the left decubitus position, with his knees drawn up to his abdomen, or in the knee-chest position.)

Spread the patient's buttocks apart to expose his anus for examination. Note any lumps, inflammation, or skin tears. Ask him to bear down, to reduce sphincter tension. Gently insert your index finger into his anus. Palpate the anterior rectal wall and then find the prostate gland, located anterior to the wall's mucosa (see *Palpating the Prostate Gland,* page 481). Normally, the prostate doesn't protrude into the rectum; if it does, the gland is inflamed and enlarged.

The prostate should be nontender and feel smooth, firm (but not rocklike), and rubbery through the rectal wall.

Assessment tip: On palpation, the normal prostate gland feels like the mound that forms on the palm at the base of the thumb (thenar eminence) when you clench your fist.

Locate the gland's right and left lateral lobes and the small, shallow groove that divides them. Estimate the prostate's diameter. A hypertrophied prostate gland is usually uniformly enlarged. Note any hard or irregular areas, which

NURSE'S GUIDE TO MALE REPRODUCTIVE SYSTEM DISORDERS

	CHIEF COMPLAINT
INFLAMMATORY OR INFECTIOUS DISEASE	
Orchitis	• *Changes in voiding patterns:* usually none • *Penile discharge:* usually none • *Scrotal or inguinal mass:* unilateral or bilateral scrotal swelling • *Pain or tenderness:* varies from slight discomfort to extreme pain in one or both testes • *Impotence:* precipitated by pain • *Infertility:* possible with severe bilateral infection (mumps)
Prostatitis	• *Changes in voiding patterns:* frequency, urgency; nocturia and hesitancy possible • *Penile discharge:* if condition is acute, thin, watery, blood-streaked semen possible • *Scrotal or inguinal mass:* none • *Pain or tenderness:* dysuria common; possibly low back pain and/or perineal pressure; painful ejaculation possible • *Impotence:* decreased libido and potency possible • *Infertility:* possible
Epididymitis	• *Changes in voiding patterns:* usually none; frequency occurs if urinary tract infection is present • *Penile discharge:* usually none • *Scrotal or inguinal mass:* unilateral or bilateral scrotal swelling • *Pain or tenderness:* intense scrotal pain; may radiate to rectum, lower back, suprapubic region • *Impotence:* precipitated by pain • *Infertility:* possible with severe bilateral infection

may indicate cancer; also note any tenderness or bogginess, which may reflect prostatic inflammation.

The seminal vesicles are slightly above the prostate gland on either side on the anterior rectal wall. Unless they're inflamed, you probably won't be able to palpate them. Finally, perform a complete rectal examination (see Entry 452).

Formulating a diagnostic impression

536 Classifying male reproductive disorders

The most common disorders of the male reproductive system can be classified as *inflammatory* or *infectious diseases, noninflammatory benign processes,* or *malignant diseases.* The first category includes inflammatory or infectious conditions that commonly cause dysuria and pain or tenderness; these symptoms may interfere with sexual function. The second category includes common noninflammatory

HISTORY	PHYSICAL EXAMINATION AND DIAGNOSTIC STUDIES
• Prior infection, especially epididymitis or mumps	• Fever, possibly nausea and vomiting • Inspection reveals reddened scrotal skin, swollen testis. • Palpation reveals warm scrotal skin, tender testis. • Complete blood count reveals elevated WBC count.
• Chronic form commonly occurs in young men. • Prior ascending urinary tract infection common	• Rectal palpation reveals, in acute form, firm, enlarged, tender, boggy prostate gland; in chronic form, enlarged prostate possible, as well as firmness due to prostatic calculi. • Fever and chills possible in acute form. • Third specimen of three- or four-glass urine test contains many WBCs.
• Prior urinary tract infection may be present.	• Fever • Inspection reveals enlarged epididymis, reddened, tender, and swollen scrotal skin. • Palpation reveals warm scrotal skin, painful epididymis. • Complete blood count reveals elevated WBC count; urinalysis may show pyuria.

(continued)

NURSE'S GUIDE TO MALE REPRODUCTIVE SYSTEM DISORDERS *(continued)*

	CHIEF COMPLAINT	
Gonorrhea	• *Changes in voiding patterns:* usually none, but frequency of urination possible • *Penile discharge:* present; thick and yellow-green but may start as milky white • *Scrotal or inguinal mass:* tender; lymphadenopathy possible • *Pain or tenderness:* dysuria • *Impotence:* may be temporary, secondary to dysuria • *Infertility:* present only if untreated (in advanced stage secondary to scar tissue formation in epididymis)	
Syphilitic chancre	• *Changes in voiding patterns:* none in early stage • *Penile discharge:* none • *Scrotal or inguinal mass:* enlarged inguinal lymph nodes possible • *Pain or tenderness:* none • *Impotence:* none • *Infertility:* usually none if detected and treated early	
Genital herpes	• *Changes in voiding patterns:* none • *Penile discharge:* none • *Scrotal or inguinal mass:* tender, enlarged inguinal lymph nodes • *Pain or tenderness:* painful lesions during ulcerative stage; dysuria possible • *Impotence:* none • *Infertility:* usually none	
NONINFLAMMATORY BENIGN PROCESS		
Benign prostatic hypertrophy	• *Changes in voiding patterns:* urinary hesitancy, intermittency with dribbling; reduced urinary stream caliber and force; straining; possibly retention • *Penile discharge:* usually none • *Scrotal or inguinal mass:* none • *Pain or tenderness:* burning on urination with cystitis if accompanied by urinary tract infection • *Impotence:* possible if nerves innervating penis are damaged during open prostatectomy • *Infertility:* common following transurethral prostatectomy due to retrograde ejaculation	
Varicocele	• *Changes in voiding patterns:* none • *Penile discharge:* none • *Scrotal or inguinal mass:* present in scrotum, usually on left side • *Pain or tenderness:* no acute pain or tenderness; some discomfort caused by size of mass • *Impotence:* none • *Infertility:* none	

HISTORY	PHYSICAL EXAMINATION AND DIAGNOSTIC STUDIES
• Sexual exposure within preceding 2 weeks	• Edematous urethral meatus possible • Gram-negative intracellular diplococci on stained smear of urethral exudate • Positive culture on Thayer-Martin medium or equivalent
• Caused by sexual relations with infected partner	• Oval or round indurated ulcer, with raised edge • Dark-field microscopic examination of exudate confirms diagnosis.
• Caused by sexual relations with infected partner	• Fluid-filled lesion usually on the glans penis, penile shaft, or foreskin • Shallow ulcerative lesions, with local redness and swelling when ruptured • Tissue culture may reveal herpes simplex Type 2 in vesical fluid. • Fever common
• Commonly occurs in men over age 50	• Rectal palpation reveals a firm, slightly elastic, enlarged, smooth prostate, with varying degrees of tenderness; rectal mucosa easily glides over hypertrophied gland. • Cystourethroscopy shows prostatic encroachment on the urethra and effects of enlargement on bladder.
• Common in males of high school or college age	• Inspection reveals lower-hanging testis on affected side, pendulous and irregular scrotum. • Palpation reveals soft, irregular mass; enlarged veins make scrotum feel like a bag of worms.

(continued)

NURSE'S GUIDE TO MALE REPRODUCTIVE SYSTEM DISORDERS *(continued)*

	CHIEF COMPLAINT
Hydrocele	• *Changes in voiding patterns:* usually none • *Penile discharge:* none • *Scrotal or inguinal mass:* present in scrotum • *Pain or tenderness:* usually none, except with very large mass • *Impotence:* none • *Infertility:* none
Scrotal hernia	• *Changes in voiding patterns:* none • *Penile discharge:* none • *Scrotal or inguinal mass:* present in scrotum (extension of inguinal hernia) • *Pain or tenderness:* usually none, although mild, aching discomfort possible • *Impotence:* none • *Infertility:* none
MALIGNANT DISEASE	
Cancer of the testis	• *Changes in voiding patterns:* none in early stage • *Penile discharge:* none • *Scrotal or inguinal mass:* testicular mass present • *Pain or tenderness:* usually none until late stages, when accompanied by a feeling of heaviness or an aching or dragging sensation in groin • *Impotence:* psychogenic impotence possible • *Infertility:* none
Cancer of the prostate	• *Changes in voiding patterns:* in later stages, urinary hesitancy, dribbling, and possibly retention • *Penile discharge:* usually none • *Scrotal or inguinal mass:* none • *Pain or tenderness:* low back, hip, and leg pain common in advanced state, caused by metastases to the bones of the pelvis and spine • *Impotence:* follows radical resection of prostate • *Infertility:* follows radical resection of prostate
Cancer of the penis	• *Changes in voiding patterns:* none usually present except in advanced stages • *Penile discharge:* usually not present; bleeding in later stage; purulent drainage with secondary infection possible • *Scrotal or inguinal mass:* enlarged inguinal lymph nodes may be caused by infection or metastasis • *Pain or tenderness:* painful, enlarged regional lymph nodes possible; penile pain in late stage • *Impotence:* usually none • *Infertility:* none

	HISTORY	PHYSICAL EXAMINATION AND DIAGNOSTIC STUDIES
	• Common in infants and adults; prior infection of testis, epididymitis possible	• Inspection reveals smooth, fluctuant mass in scrotum of pyriform or globular shape, with large end above; unable to reduce mass into abdomen; doesn't transmit cough impulse; transilluminates as a translucent mass.
	• Increased intraabdominal pressure may be present on heavy lifting.	• Inspection and palpation reveal inguinoscrotal mass that transmits cough impulse; doesn't transilluminate; possible to reduce mass into abdomen. • Auscultation may detect bowel sounds.
	• Common in men between ages 20 and 40	• Inspection and rectal palpation reveal firm, nontender testicular mass; doesn't transilluminate. • Biopsy confirms diagnosis. • Serum alpha-fetoprotein and beta human chorionic gonadotropin provide important information about tumor type and activity.
	• More common in black men over age 50	• Rectal palpation reveals hard, irregular nodule on posterior prostate; becomes fixed as lesion progresses. • Biopsy confirms diagnosis; serum acid phosphatase level elevated when tumor spreads beyond prostatic capsule.
	• Poor personal hygiene may increase risk; usually occurs in uncircumcised men over age 50	• In early stage, dry, scaly lesion; later, ulceration and necrosis possible. • Biopsy confirms diagnosis. • Inguinal lymph nodes may be enlarged.

(continued)

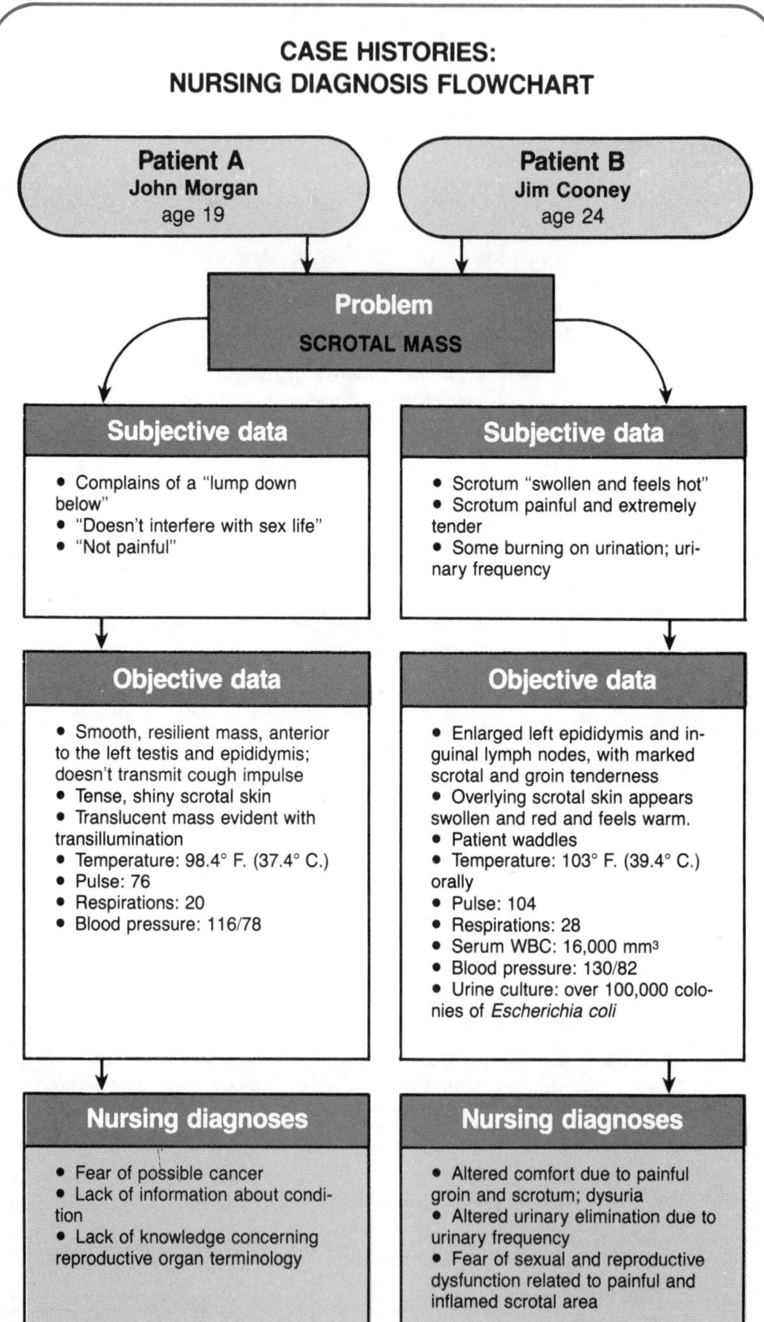
CASE HISTORIES:
NURSING DIAGNOSIS FLOWCHART
Patient A
John Morgan
age 19
Patient B
Jim Cooney
age 24
Problem
SCROTAL MASS
Subjective data
• Complains of a "lump down below"
• "Doesn't interfere with sex life"
• "Not painful"
Subjective data
• Scrotum "swollen and feels hot"
• Scrotum painful and extremely tender
• Some burning on urination; urinary frequency
Objective data
• Smooth, resilient mass, anterior to the left testis and epididymis; doesn't transmit cough impulse
• Tense, shiny scrotal skin
• Translucent mass evident with transillumination
• Temperature: 98.4° F. (37.4° C.)
• Pulse: 76
• Respirations: 20
• Blood pressure: 116/78
Objective data
• Enlarged left epididymis and inguinal lymph nodes, with marked scrotal and groin tenderness
• Overlying scrotal skin appears swollen and red and feels warm.
• Patient waddles
• Temperature: 103° F. (39.4° C.) orally
• Pulse: 104
• Respirations: 28
• Serum WBC: 16,000 mm³
• Blood pressure: 130/82
• Urine culture: over 100,000 colonies of Escherichia coli
Nursing diagnoses
• Fear of possible cancer
• Lack of information about condition
• Lack of knowledge concerning reproductive organ terminology
Nursing diagnoses
• Altered comfort due to painful groin and scrotum; dysuria
• Altered urinary elimination due to urinary frequency
• Fear of sexual and reproductive dysfunction related to painful and inflamed scrotal area

benign processes that cause varying degrees of pain or discomfort, possibly with scrotal masses present. In malignant diseases of the male reproductive system, signs and symptoms vary according to the stage of the disease and the structure involved.

537 Making appropriate nursing diagnoses

Changes in voiding pattern may result from such causes as fluid volume deficit or excess and alterations in bladder capacity. In young men, the most common cause of such changes is urinary tract infection. In older men, the most common cause is benign prostatic hypertrophy, in which the enlarged prostate gland encroaches on the proximal urethra, narrowing its diameter. Signs and symptoms of an enlarged prostate gland include slow onset of urination, a weak and interrupted stream, and increased frequency, leading to nocturia and possibly hematuria. (Late prostatic cancer can produce similar signs and symptoms.) These problems may cause the patient enough anxiety to interfere with his normal sexual performance.

Appropriate nursing diagnoses for a patient who is experiencing changes in voiding pattern include *obstructive urinating pattern, alterations in self-image as a male,* and *sleep disturbance.*

Penile or urethral discharge indicates an inflammation in the terminal male reproductive system and is usually accompanied by dysuria. The causes of such discharges vary, from a sexually transmitted disease to an advanced malignant process. A discharge may affect none or all of the major functions of the male reproductive system (spermatogenesis, regulation of primary and secondary sex characteristics, and sexual performance).

One nursing diagnosis would be *urethral discharge;* other possibilities are *alterations in comfort, anxiety, alterations in cognitive function,* and *alterations in self-image as a male.*

A scrotal or inguinal mass may result from an infectious or malignant process or from a genetic or traumatic event. The origin and size of the mass determine whether it may interfere with any of the major male reproductive functions. Interference with spermatogenesis, and the threat of infertility, would probably produce the greatest anxiety in your patient. (Concerned family members can aggravate the patient's anxiety.) For such a patient, your nursing diagnoses would be *anxiety* and *potential family disruption.* If the process is acute or advanced, your nursing diagnoses would also include *alterations in comfort* and *impaired physical mobility.*

Pain or tenderness may be temporary, localized, and sporadic (as in an acute inflammation) or persistent, widespread, and difficult to relieve (as the result of metastatic disease). If the pain is severe enough, the patient and his family members may not be concerned with other possible problems, such as impaired sexual performance or spermatogenesis, and alterations in hormonal balance. So your nursing diagnoses may vary from mild-to-severe *alterations in comfort* to *hazards of immobility, potential abuse of analgesics,* and *compromised family dynamics.*

Impotence and infertility may occur without associated symptoms or as a result of other disease processes. For instance, patients often dread the end-organ damage of systemic diseases, such as diabetes mellitus and multiple sclerosis, so they may experience psychogenic impotence before physical impairment actually occurs. Some patients display aggressive sexual behavior, looking for reassurance about their sexuality. Such a patient may benefit from your spoken acknowledgment of his frustration. Although impotence is usually temporary, infertility often is not. Your nursing diagnoses may include *alterations in self-image as a male, knowledge deficit, altered family dynamics,* and *anxiety.*

Assessing pediatric patients

538 Growth and sexual development

A boy's penis, scrotum, and testes usually start growing between ages 10 and 13—this is typically the first sign of his sexual maturation. From ages 12 to 15, these structures grow rapidly; by age 17, growth is usually complete. A boy may experience his first ejaculation between ages 11 and 13, but normally, mature sperm aren't produced for another 3 years.

Pubic hair begins to grow, and the boy's voice deepens, between ages 12 and 14. Breast hypertrophy may also occur around this time but usually disappears between ages 14 and 17. Axillary hair may appear between ages 13 and 16; in later adolescence (between ages 15 and 17), chest hair and a beard may develop.

539 Examining a boy's penis and scrotum

If you observe an enlarged scrotum in a boy younger than age 2, suspect a scrotal extension of an inguinal hernia, a hydrocele, or both. (Hydroceles, often associated with inguinal hernias, are common among children in this age-group. To differentiate between the two, remember that hydroceles transilluminate and are neither tender nor reducible.)

When you assess an adolescent boy who is obese, his penis may appear abnormally small. When examining the patient, you may have to retract the fat over the symphysis pubis to properly assess penis size.

Before proceeding to palpate a boy's scrotum, explain what you'll be doing and why. Then make sure he's comfortably warm and as relaxed as possible. (Cold and anxiety may cause his testes to retract so that you can't palpate them.)

Hyperactive cremasteric reflexes commonly cause some patients' testes to retract into the inguinal canal during physical examination (see *The Cremasteric Reflex*). If this happens, locate the testes by milking the inguinal canal with your fingertips. This maneuver should promptly bring normal testes back down into the patient's scrotum. Or, instead of milking the canal, you can have the child squat or sit cross-legged. This position counteracts the cremasteric reflex and increases intraabdominal pressure, which should bring normal testes back down into the scrotum. Examining the child while he is in a warm tub bath also usually brings the testes down (if they're normal). If these techniques are unsuccessful, your patient may have undescended testes.

THE CREMASTERIC REFLEX

The cremaster muscle comprises muscle fiber bands that originate at the lower edge of the abdominal muscles and form muscular loops surrounding the spermatic cord and testis. If you stroke the patient's inner thigh with a sharp object, the corresponding cremaster muscle contracts reflexively, causing elevation of the testis on that side. This is called the *cremasteric reflex*. Presence of the reflex substantiates the integrity of the spinal cord. Because the reflex may be hyperactive in a boy, it should be suppressed before you examine him for undescended testes.

540 Assessing for undescended testes

Undescended testes, or cryptorchidism, occurs when a testis or both testes fail to descend into the scrotum during fetal development. Instead, they remain in the abdomen or inguinal canal or at the external ring. If the testes are bilaterally undescended, the patient will need surgery before puberty, because a testis must be positioned properly in the scrotum for spermatogenesis to occur. Also, the patient runs a greater risk of trauma and testicular cancer if he has an undescended testis.

If you suspect that a boy you're examining has undescended testes, check for an inguinal hernia, which occurs ipsilaterally in many patients. When examining a child for an inguinal hernia, don't rely entirely on his coughing to demonstrate a hernia; it may not increase his intraabdominal pressure sufficiently. Instead, ask him to try to lift a heavy object, such as a footstool, and observe whether this activity demonstrates the hernia. In young children, who can be difficult to examine, you may miss small hernias. A history of intermittent inguinal swelling can be diagnostically important. Remember, too, that many boys with undescended testes were born prematurely; check your patient's history.

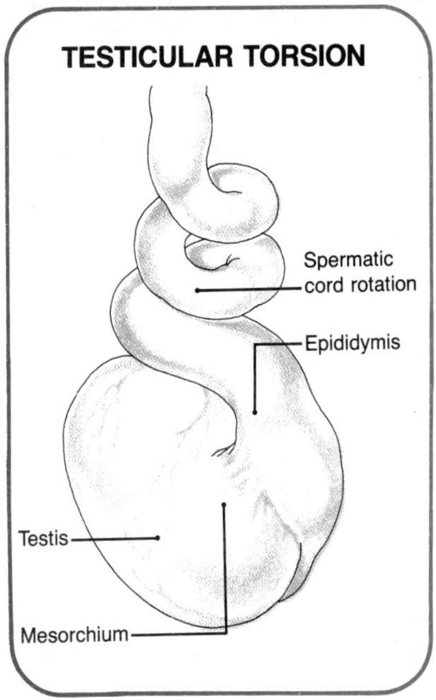

541 How to recognize testicular torsion

This condition, in which the patient's testis rotates spontaneously on its axis, occurs most often during sleep, in boys between ages 12 and 18. The left testis rotates counterclockwise, the right testis, clockwise. Concomitant rotation of the spermatic cord causes testicular strangulation; if untreated, unilateral strangulation leads to testicular infarction, and bilateral strangulation leads to infertility.

If your pediatric patient has testicular torsion, your examination will reveal a twisted or rotated spermatic cord and abnormally elevated testes that are usually warm and swollen (see *Testicular Torsion*). The patient will have severe pain and possibly an elevated temperature. The diagnosis may be confirmed by auscultating the patient's testes for pulses with a Doppler ultrasound stethoscope. In early presentation, if there is no pulsing in the testes because of diminished blood flow, testicular torsion is usually the cause. In later presentation, however, falsely increased pulses may be present because of secondary congestion and inflammation. Accurate assessment of testicular torsion is important, because manual and/or surgical detorsion should be performed as soon as possible.

542 Precocious puberty

A boy with true precocious puberty matures sexually before age 10. This condition may be idiopathic or caused by cerebral lesions. Your examination will reveal secondary sex characteristics and gonadal development.

In pseudoprecocious puberty, secondary sex characteristics become apparent, but gonadal development doesn't occur. Testicular tumor or adrenogenital syndrome can cause this condition. Laboratory tests can help you differentiate true precocious puberty from pseudoprecocious puberty by measuring serum hormone and plasma testosterone levels and by examining ejaculate for spermatozoa. A radiologist can evaluate skull and hand X-rays for bone age.

Assessing geriatric patients

543 Aging and the male reproductive system

The physiologic changes that occur in elderly men include decreased testosterone production that, in turn, may cause a decrease in sexual libido. Among other effects, decreased testosterone production causes the testes to atrophy and soften and decreases sperm production. Normally, the prostate gland enlarges with age and its secretions diminish. Seminal fluid also decreases in volume and becomes less viscous. During intercourse, elderly men experience slower and weaker physiologic reactions. These changes don't necessarily weaken a man's sex drive or lessen his sexual satisfaction.

544 Prostatic hypertrophy

Almost all men over age 50 have some degree of prostatic enlargement. In men with benign prostatic hypertrophy or advanced prostate cancer, however, the gland becomes large enough to compress the urethra and sometimes the bladder, obstructing urinary flow. The cause of benign prostatic hypertrophy is unknown, but evidence points to hormonal changes in elderly men. Possible precipitating factors include neoplastic, inflammatory, metabolic, arteriosclerotic, and nutritional disturbances.

If not treated, benign prostatic hypertrophy can impair renal function, causing such initial signs and symptoms as urinary hesitancy and intermittency, straining, and a reduction in the diameter and force of the urinary stream. As the gland continues to en-

UNDERSTANDING THE EFFECTS OF BENIGN PROSTATIC HYPERTROPHY

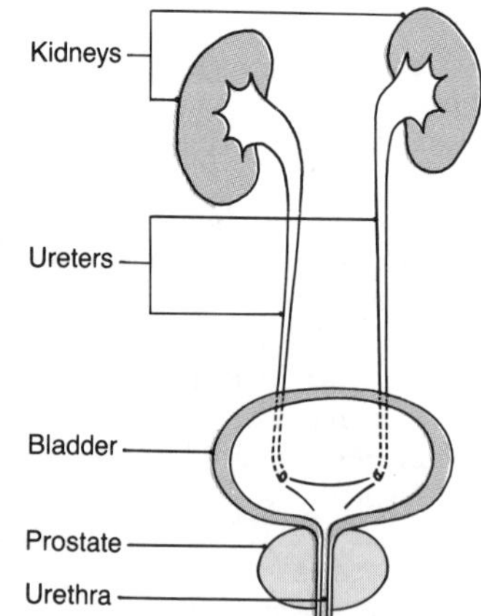

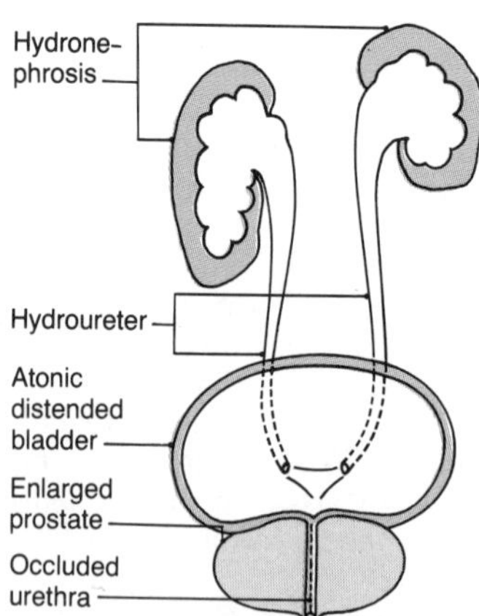

A normal urinary system is shown on the left. The effects of benign prostatic hypertrophy on the urinary system are shown on the right. With this condition, increasing urethral obstruction by the prostate gland results in chronic residual volume after voiding. The accompanying continuous retrograde pressure causes gross enlargement of the urinary system.

large, urinary frequency increases and nocturia occurs, possibly with hematuria. All these signs and symptoms may also be caused by a urinary system disorder (see *Nurse's Guide to Urinary Disorders,* pages 452 to 455).

If your patient does have benign prostatic hypertrophy, you'll probably note nontender and enlarged lateral lobes. These lobes may feel like the thenar eminence of a clenched fist—whereas, in malignant prostatic hypertrophy they feel more like a knuckle. You may not be able to detect an enlarged median lobe, because most of it rests anteriorly. Abdominal palpation and percussion may reveal a midline mass, representing a distended bladder.

UNDERSTANDING THE MALE CLIMACTERIC

Here's a list of the physiologic changes that characterize the male climacteric:

- Erections require more time and stimulation to achieve.
- Erections are not as full or as hard.
- Testosterone production decreases.
- The prostate gland enlarges, and its secretions diminish.
- Seminal fluid decreases.
- Contractions in prostate gland and penile urethra during orgasm vary in length and quality.
- Refractory period following ejaculation may increase from minutes to days.
- Pleasure sensations become less genitally localized and more generalized.

Selected References

Alexander, Mary M., and Brown, Marie Scott. *Pediatric History Taking and Physical Diagnosis for Nurses,* 2nd ed. New York: McGraw-Hill Book Co., 1979.

Barnard, Martha U., et al. *Handbook of Comprehensive Pediatric Nursing.* New York: McGraw-Hill Book Co., 1981.

Bates, Barbara. *A Guide to Physical Examination,* 2nd ed. Philadelphia: J.B. Lippincott Co., 1979.

Beeson, Paul B., et al. *Cecil Textbook of Medicine,* 2 vols, 15th ed. Philadelphia: W.B. Saunders Co., 1979.

DeGowin, Elmer L., and DeGowin, Richard L. *Bedside Diagnostic Examination,* 3rd ed. New York: Macmillan Publishing Co., 1976.

Delp, Mahlon H., and Manning, Robert T., eds. *Major's Physical Diagnosis,* 8th ed. Philadelphia: W.B. Saunders Co., 1975.

Green, J.H., and Silver, P.H.S. *An Introduction to Human Anatomy.* New York: Oxford University Press, 1981.

Guyton, Arthur C. *Textbook of Medical Physiology.* Philadelphia: W.B. Saunders Co., 1981.

Harvey, A. McGehee, et al. *The Principles and Practice of Medicine,* 20th ed. New York: Appleton-Century-Crofts, 1980.

Hudak, Carolyn M., et al. *Clinical Protocols: A Guide for Nurses and Physicians.* Philadelphia: J.B. Lippincott Co., 1976.

Isselbacher, Kurt J., et al., eds. *Harrison's Principles of Internal Medicine,* 9th ed. New York: McGraw-Hill Book Co., 1980.

Malasanos, Lois, et al. *Health Assessment,* 2nd ed. St. Louis: C.V. Mosby Co., 1981.

McClintic, J. Robert. *Physiology of the Human Body,* 2nd ed. New York: John Wiley & Sons, 1978.

Price, Sylvia A., and Wilson, Lorraine M. *Pathophysiology: Clinical Concepts of Disease Processes.* New York: McGraw-Hill Book Co., 1978.

Sana, Josephine, and Judge, Richard D., eds. *Physical Appraisal Methods in Nursing Practice.* Boston: Little, Brown & Co., 1975.

Taylor, Robert B. *A Primer of Clinical Symptoms.* Philadelphia: Harper & Row, 1973.

Thompson, June M., and Bowers, Arden C. *Clinical Manual of Health Assessment.* St. Louis: C.V. Mosby Co., 1980.

Waley, Lucille F., and Wong, Donna L. *Nursing Care of Infants and Children.* St. Louis: C.V. Mosby Co., 1979.

Assessing Your Patients, Nursing Photobook™ Series. Springhouse, Pa.: Intermed Communications, Inc., 1980.

Diseases, Nurse's Reference Library™ Series. Springhouse, Pa.: Intermed Communications, Inc., 1980.

14

KEY POINTS IN THIS CHAPTER

KEY CHARTS IN THIS CHAPTER

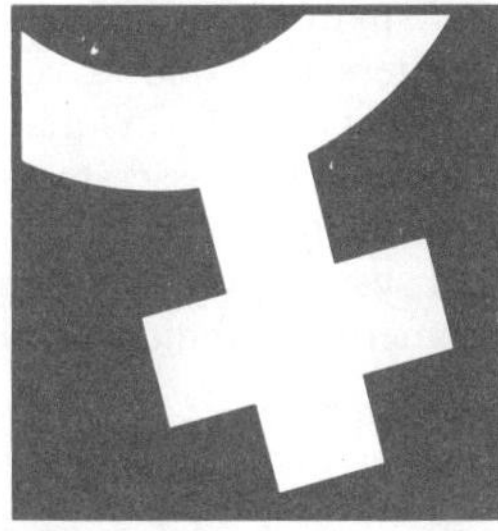

Female Reproductive System

Introduction

545 This system's role and significance

A woman's reproductive system and childbearing capabilities are unique and have physiologic, psychological, and social significance beyond her health concerns. Because of this, probably more women seek health care for matters related to the female reproductive system than for any other category of diseases or disorders. To meet the needs of these patients, you must assess each woman as a total person as well as in relation to the function of her reproductive system.

Physiologically, the female reproductive system is complex and has wide-ranging effects on other body systems. Vaginitis, for example, can lead to a urinary tract infection because of the vagina's proximity to the urethra. During pregnancy, the growing fetus exerts pressure on body organs that can alter GI function. Also, ovarian dysfunction can significantly alter endocrine balance in a woman's body.

Psychosocially, the reproductive function has far-reaching implications beyond its role as the method used to propagate our species. To the individual, it means much more: life passing from parents to offspring so that each generation imparts something of itself to future generations. To a woman, this means that any aberration in normal sexual or reproductive function can affect not only her self-concept but also how society views her.

The social aspects of reproduction can be overwhelming as well. For example, such issues as contraception, artificial insemination, abortion, sexual preference, and unwanted children are constantly before the public. The incidence of sexually transmitted disease and teenage pregnancies continues to rise internationally. To sensitively assess a woman who has concerns about her reproductive system, you need to be aware of these problems and of your patient's attitude, as well as your own, toward them.

546 Special nurse-patient considerations

When you assess a woman's reproductive system, remember that the nurse-patient relationship is delicate. Keep in mind that parental and social attitudes toward sex and the female body as well as your patient's personal experiences influence her ability (and willingness) to discuss her reproductive and sexual problems with you. For example, your caring attitude and assurance of confidentiality will help establish the trust essential to obtaining a complete history. A combination of gentleness and technical skill will enhance your performance of the physical examination. (To assess this system properly, your approach is basically the same as for other body systems: You need a sound knowledge of anatomy and physiology, refined history-taking skills, and the ability to perform sophisticated examination techniques.)

To maintain your patient's confidence, display a mature attitude toward sexual matters that allows you to assess each patient as an individual, without prejudice. Many assessment situations will challenge you, because disorders of this system may occur in unusual, and sometimes tragic, social circumstances.

Reviewing anatomy and physiology

547 Breasts

The prepubescent female's breast tissue is similar to the prepubescent male's, consisting only of branching ducts in fibrous tissue. At puberty, however, the female breasts respond to ovarian production of estrogen and progesterone, causing proliferation of ducts, lobules, and fibrous tissue and accumulations of adipose tissue. Generally, the mature female breast consists of equal parts of glandular tissue, fibrous tissue, and fat. The amount of fat and fibrous tissue, rather than glandular components, determines the size of the mature breast (except during pregnancy and lactation).

The mature breast normally extends from about the second to the sixth rib, overlying the chest muscles. Bands of fibrous tissue (*Cooper's ligaments*) fix the breasts to the chest wall. These ligaments extend from the skin of the breast to the connective tissue covering the muscles of the chest wall.

Glandular breast tissue containing 15 to 20 lobules extends radially from the nipple. The lactiferous ducts from each lobule eventually emerge at the nipple. The nipple's color varies from light pink to dark brown, depending on the complexion; during pregnancy, it's a darker brown. A zone of dark skin (*areola*) encircles the nipple.

Surrounded by fibrous and adipose tissue, the nipple contains many smooth muscle fibers and sensory nerve endings that, when stimulated, cause the nipple to become erect. The breast is extremely responsive to hormonal stimulation. Mild variations in the breast's glandular tissue during the menstrual cycle can cause the breasts to become slightly fuller and more tender during the cycle's middle and later stages.

The breasts have an abundant blood supply and rich lymphatic drainage. Lymphatic channels within the breasts drain into lymph nodes in the axillae and into the mediastinal lymph nodes beneath the sternum.

Breasts are normally similar in size but asymmetrical. However, breasts may not develop uniformly, and one may be somewhat smaller than the other.

548 External female genitalia

The female reproductive system comprises external and internal genitalia. The external genital organs are collectively termed the *vulva,* which includes the mons pubis, the labia majora (outer vulval lips), the labia minora (inner vulval lips), the clitoris, the vaginal vestibule, the hymen, and the greater vestibular (Bartholin's) glands.

549 Vagina and uterus

Internal female genitalia include the vagina, uterus, fallopian tubes, and ovaries. The *vagina* is a distensible fibromuscular channel, about 4″ (10 cm) long, that extends up and back from the vulva to the uterus. The *uterus* is

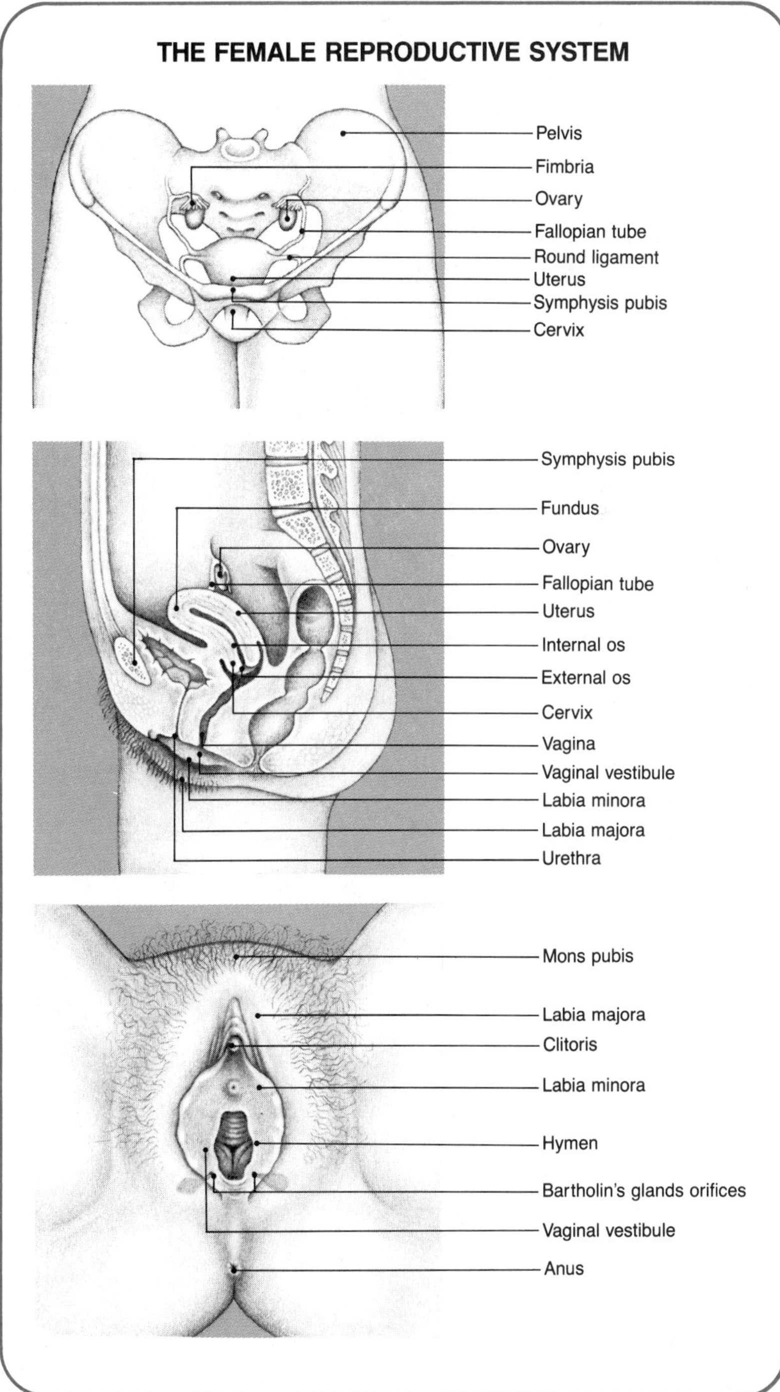
THE FEMALE REPRODUCTIVE SYSTEM
Pelvis
Fimbria
Ovary
Fallopian tube
Round ligament
Uterus
Symphysis pubis
Cervix
Symphysis pubis
Fundus
Ovary
Fallopian tube
Uterus
Internal os
External os
Cervix
Vagina
Vaginal vestibule
Labia minora
Labia majora
Urethra
Mons pubis
Labia majora
Clitoris
Labia minora
Hymen
Bartholin's glands orifices
Vaginal vestibule
Anus

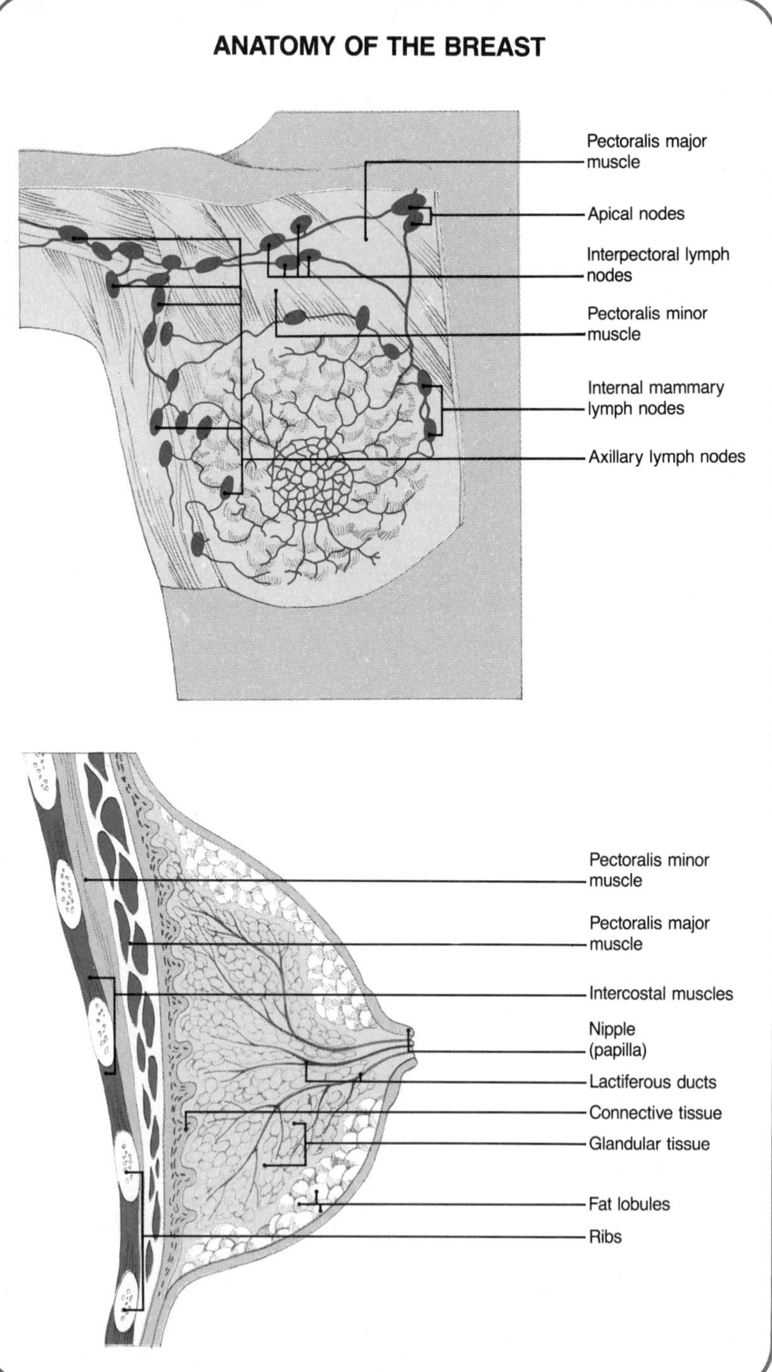
ANATOMY OF THE BREAST
Pectoralis major muscle
Apical nodes
Interpectoral lymph nodes
Pectoralis minor muscle
Internal mammary lymph nodes
Axillary lymph nodes
Pectoralis minor muscle
Pectoralis major muscle
Intercostal muscles
Nipple (papilla)
Lactiferous ducts
Connective tissue
Glandular tissue
Fat lobules
Ribs

a pear-shaped organ, about the size of a fist, suspended in the pelvis. The bulk of the uterus is composed of interlacing bands of smooth muscle (myometrium).

The uterine cavity is roughly triangular and slitlike; it is lined with a glandular mucous membrane called the *endometrium.* This uterine lining undergoes cyclic proliferative and secretory changes and is shed by the uterus with each menstrual period. A layer of *peritoneum,* continuous with the lining of the peritoneal cavity, covers part of the exterior of the uterus.

The *cervix* projects into the vaginal vault. The external opening of the cervical canal, called the *external os,* is normally small and circular. If the cervix has undergone dilatation during childbirth, the external os may appear as a transverse slit.

The point at which the cervical canal becomes continuous with the endometrial cavity is called the *internal os.* The cervical canal is widest at its midportion, narrowing at the external and internal ossa.

Stratified squamous epithelium covers the exterior of the cervix, enabling it to withstand acidic vaginal secretions. A lining of columnar epithelium protects the cervical canal from vaginal acidity.

550 Positions of the uterus

The uterus usually tilts forward, with its anterior wall contacting the dome of the bladder, its posterior surface facing up and slightly back, and its long axis positioned at a right angle to the vagina. This is called the *anterior position.* Normal variations do occur that aren't associated with disease. In *midposition,* for example, the axis of the uterus is in the same plane as the vagina's axis, with the fundus facing directly up. A uterus in the *retroverted position* tilts back, with the fundus projecting posteriorly against the rectum and the cervix located anteriorly to the vagina.

In any position, the uterus normally moves freely on examination. A *fixed* uterus in any position is abnormal and indicates pathology, such as previous infection or endometriosis. These disorders cause adhesions to develop between the uterus and the surrounding tissues, preventing normal mobility.

A normal uterus may exhibit varying degrees of flexion, causing the endometrial cavity to adopt a C-shaped configuration. An anterior bend is called *anteflexion;* a posterior bend, *retroflexion.*

551 Fallopian tubes

Each fallopian tube measures about 4″ (10 cm) in length and extends laterally from the uterine cornu, within the upper free edge of the broad ligament. The distal end of the fallopian tube terminates in delicate fingerlike projections (fimbriae) that aid ovum pickup. Longitudinal folds of ciliated columnar epithelium line each tube. Peristaltic contractions of the tube's musculature, together with currents created by the rhythmic beating of the cilia of the tubal epithelial cells, propel the ovum through the fallopian tube.

552 Ovaries

The ovaries are flattened, ovoid structures suspended from the posterior surface of the broad ligament by a fold of peritoneum. Each ovary measures about 1¼″ to 1½″ (3 to 4 cm) in diameter and contains small follicles and corpora lutea in varying stages of growth and involution.

553 Hormonal function

Ovarian function is mainly regulated by the pituitary gonadotropins follicle-stimulating hormone and luteinizing hormone. In a woman, gonadotropic hormones are secreted cyclically to help regulate the menstrual cycle. (In a man, secretion of gonadotropic hormones occurs continuously.)

UNDERSTANDING THE MENSTRUAL CYCLE

The menstrual cycle works by a series of hormonal peaks and valleys. One cycle usually takes about 28 days and is regulated by negative and positive feedback mechanisms.

- *Menstrual (preovulatory) phase:*

The menstrual cycle starts with menstruation. (The first day of menstruation is considered day 1 of the cycle.) At the beginning of the cycle, low levels of estrogen and progesterone in the bloodstream stimulate the hypothalamus to secrete gonadotropin releasing hormone (GnRH). These releasing factors stimulate the anterior pituitary to secrete follicle-stimulating hormone (FSH) and luteinizing hormone (LH). LH output begins to increase soon after FSH begins to rise.

- *Follicular phase and ovulation:*

LH and FSH act on the ovarian follicle, which secretes estrogen. The rising production of estrogen from the follicle has a negative feedback (decreasing) effect on FSH and a positive feedback (increasing) effect on LH. Estrogen production begins to slack off, the follicle matures, and ovulation occurs.

- *Postovulatory (luteal) phase:*

After ovulation, LH converts the now-ruptured follicle to a corpus luteum. Lutein cells, in the corpus luteum, secrete estrogen and progesterone, which have a negative feedback effect on LH production.

Progesterone secretion prepares the body for pregnancy. If pregnancy does not occur, the negative feedback effect of progesterone on LH production has an adverse effect on the corpus luteum, which becomes less responsive to the effects of LH as it ages. Without continuous LH stimulation, the corpus luteum further ages and regresses, and estrogen and progesterone production decreases until hormone levels are no longer adequate to maintain the endometrium, which is then shed as the menstrual flow.

As estrogen and progesterone levels fall, the hypothalamus is stimulated, causing the cycle to begin again.

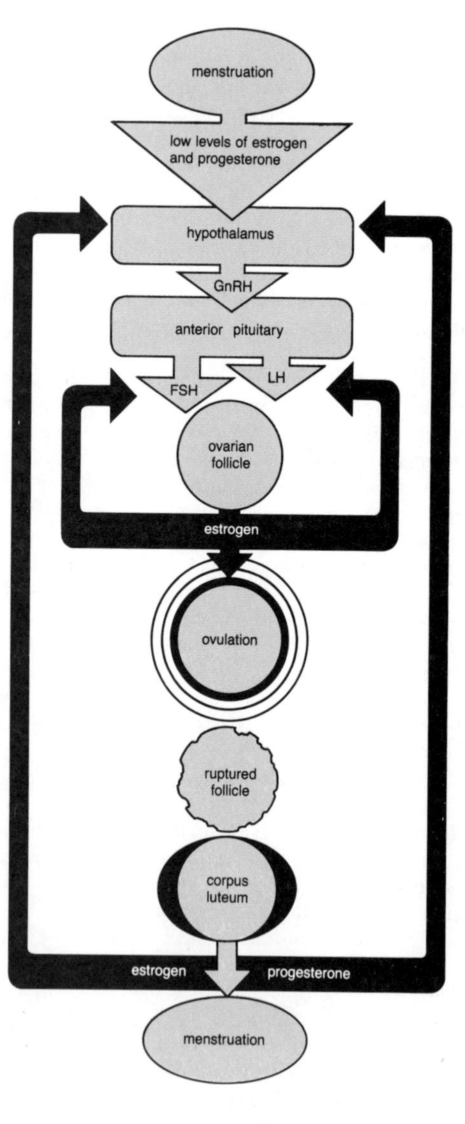

Ovarian hormones include estrogen, produced by the ovarian follicle and the corpus luteum, and progesterone, produced by the corpus luteum. Estrogen is responsible for the development of a woman's secondary sex characteristics, for growth of the endometrium, and for many general metabolic effects not directly related to sexual activity. Progesterone produces secretory changes in the endometrium in preparation for fertilized ovum implantation and helps maintain the implanted ovum.

554 Menstrual cycle

The menstrual cycle can be divided into three phases:
- menstrual (preovulatory) phase
- follicular phase and ovulation
- postovulatory (luteal) phase.

(For more information, see *Understanding the Menstrual Cycle.*)

Collecting appropriate history data

555 Biographical data

When you assess a woman's reproductive system, biographical data are always significant. A woman's race, personal circumstances, and the period of life she's in are related to various normal and abnormal reproductive system developments. Such factors figure significantly in your overall assessment of the patient as well as in your nursing diagnosis. Consider the following points when recording your patient's biographical data:

- ***Age.*** Menarche, the onset of menstruation, usually begins between ages 12 and 13. Girls who begin to menstruate at an earlier-than-normal age are at greater risk of developing breast cancer later in life. Menopause—the period from when the ovaries' ability to produce eggs and estrogen declines until menstruation ultimately ceases—usually begins around age 50. If applicable, record your patient's age

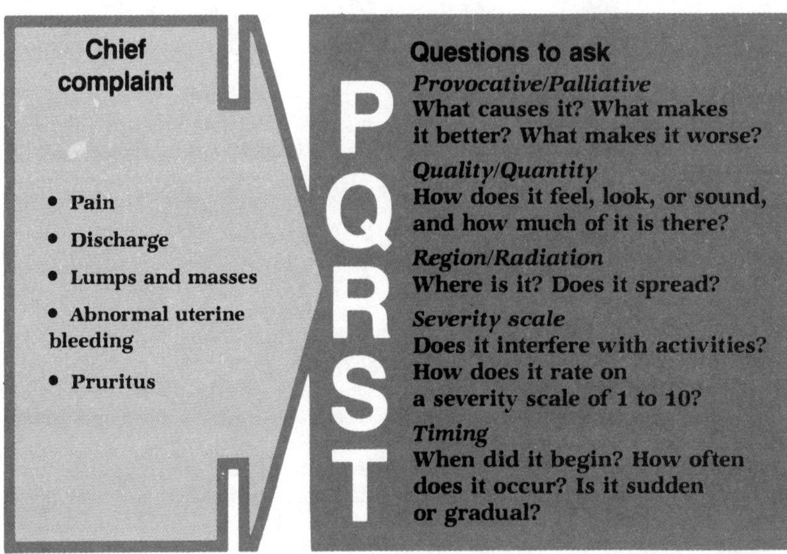

at the end of a 12-month period during which menstruation did not occur.

Women over age 35 are at greater risk of developing breast cancer than younger women. The risk of developing breast cancer (or endometrial cancer) is even greater after menopause. The risk of developing cervical cancer drops markedly after ovulation has stopped.

Sexually transmitted disease is more prevalent in women between ages 12 and 19 than in women who are 20 or older.

• ***Race.*** Whites are more likely to develop breast cancer than blacks. Blacks, however, are about three times more likely to develop benign uterine tumors than whites. Orientals have a low incidence of breast cancer.

556 Chief complaint

The most common chief complaints expressed by women with reproductive system disorders are *pain, discharge, lumps and masses, abnormal uterine bleeding,* and *pruritus.*

Some patients may not have a chief complaint, but they may request a routine Pap smear or breast examination or may ask for information and instruction about contraception.

557 History of present illness

For all chief complaints concerning the female reproductive system or for requests for information or evaluation, be sure to record the following information:

• the date your patient's last menstrual period began
• the date of the menstrual period before her last period
• the duration of her period, or the average number of tampons or sanitary napkins she uses during her period (to determine the amount of her flow)
• the date of her most recent Pap smear and pelvic examination
• the type of contraception she uses, if any
• the date of her most recent douching (because douching can alter Pap smear findings).

This information is vital for evaluating current and future reproductive system problems detected as a result of the history and the physical examination.

Using the PQRST mnemonic device (see page 501), ask the patient to elaborate on her chief complaint. Then, depending on the complaint, explore the history of her present illness by asking the following types of questions:

• ***Pain.*** *Where is the pain located?* Labial or groin pain is often referred from the kidneys; vulvar pain, commonly described as dysuria, usually results from an infectious process. (Because these sites may harbor lesions, consider the possibility of perineal or vulvar lumps.) Lower quadrant pain may be caused by an infectious, malignant, or functional process of supravaginal structures. *Did the pain occur suddenly or gradually?* Sudden pain that quickly reaches maximum intensity suggests a rupture or embolus, or sudden pain may be associated with dyspareunia (painful intercourse). Pain that increases over several days or weeks may be due to ovarian tumor, pelvic congestion, or endometriosis. *How long does the pain last? Is it constant or does it come and go?* Cyclic pain that occurs once a month suggests dysmenorrhea (pain during menstruation) or mittelschmerz (pain during ovulation). *What does the pain feel like?* The words the patient uses to describe the pain can be important in determining its cause. Remember to interpret her description according to her ability to express herself and to her understanding of the pain she's experiencing.

• ***Discharge.*** *When did it start?* Sudden onset may indicate an acute problem or the patient's ignorance of natural discharge, such as postcoital semen. Insidious onset usually indicates chronic inflammation from an infectious or malignant process. *What does it look like? Is there an odor? How much discharge is there?* Vaginal discharge oc-

NURSE'S GUIDE TO SOME DRUGS THAT AFFECT THE FEMALE REPRODUCTIVE SYSTEM

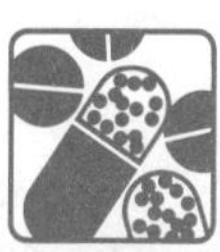

CLASSIFICATION	POSSIBLE SIDE EFFECTS
Antihypertensives	
clonidine hydrochloride (Catapres*) mecamylamine hydrochloride (Inversine)	• Decreased libido
methyldopa (Aldomet*)	• Decreased libido, lactation
Cytotoxics	
busulfan (Myleran*)	• Amenorrhea
calusterone (Methosarb*)	• Clitoral enlargement, virilism, increased libido
cyclophosphamide (Cytoxan*)	• Gonadal suppression (possibly irreversible)
dromostanolone propionate (Drolban)	• Clitoral enlargement, virilism
tamoxifen citrate (Nolvadex*)	• Vaginal discharge and bleeding
thiotepa (Thiotepa*)	• Amenorrhea
Estrogens	
chlorotrianisene (Tace*) conjugated estrogenic substances (Premarin*) esterified estrogens (Estratab) estradiol (Estrace*) estrone (Ogen*) ethinyl estradiol (Estinyl*)	• Breakthrough bleeding, altered menstrual flow, dysmenorrhea, amenorrhea, cervical erosion or abnormal secretions, enlargement of uterine fibromas, vaginal candidiasis, breast changes (tenderness, enlargement, secretions)
dienestrol (Dienestrol cream*)	• Vaginal discharge, uterine bleeding with excessive use, breast tenderness
diethylstilbestrol (DES)	• Breakthrough bleeding, altered menstrual flow, dysmenorrhea, amenorrhea, cervical erosion, altered cervical secretions, enlargement of uterine fibromas, vaginal candidiasis, loss of libido, breast tenderness or enlargement, increased risk of vaginal cancer in female offspring
Oral contraceptives	
estrogen with progestogen (Ortho-Novum*)	• Breakthrough bleeding, dysmenorrhea, amenorrhea, cervical erosion or abnormal secretions, enlargement of uterine fibromas, vaginal candidiasis, breast changes (tenderness, enlargement, secretions)
Progestogens	
dydrogesterone (Gynorest) ethisterone (Progestoral) hydroxyprogesterone caproate (Delalutin*) medroxyprogesterone acetate (Depo-Provera*) norethindrone (Norlutin*) norethindrone acetate (Norlutate*) progesterone (Progestasert*)	• Breakthrough bleeding, dysmenorrhea, amenorrhea, cervical erosion and abnormal secretions, uterine fibromas, vaginal candidiasis, breast changes (tenderness, enlargement, secretion)

(continued)

NURSE'S GUIDE TO SOME DRUGS THAT AFFECT THE FEMALE REPRODUCTIVE SYSTEM (*continued*)

CLASSIFICATION	POSSIBLE SIDE EFFECTS
Psychotherapeutics	
lithium carbonate (Lithane*)	• Decreased libido
Hormones	
dexamethasone (Decadran*) hydrocortisone (Cortef*) thyroid USP (Dathroid) thyrotropin (Thytropar*)	• Menstrual irregularities
Antipsychotics	
chlorpromazine hydrochlorides (Thorazine) perphenazine (Trilafon*) prochlorperazine (Compazine) promazine hydrochloride (Sparine*) thioridazine hydrochloride (Mellaril*) trifluoperazine hydrochloride (Stelazine*)	• Delayed ovulation, menstrual irregularities, changed libido, lactation
haloperidol (Haldol*)	• Menstrual irregularities, increased libido, breast engorgement and lactation
Tranquilizers	
chlordiazepoxide hydrochloride (Librium*)	• Minor menstrual irregularities, decreased libido
diazepam (Valium*)	• Decreased libido
Antidepressants	
amitriptyline hydrochloride (Elavil*) desipramine hydrochloride (Pertofrane*) doxepin hydrochloride (Sinequan*) inipramine hydrochloride (Tofranil*) nortriptyline hydrochloride (Aventyl*) trimipramine maleate (Surmontil)	• Changed libido, breast enlargement and galactorrhea
isocarboxazid (Marplan*)	• Changed libido

*Available in U.S. and Canada. All other products (no symbol) available in U.S. only.

curs in all women with adequate estrogen levels, so some staining is common throughout the menstrual cycle. Excessive staining can be a significant implication of pathology. A marked decrease in the usual amount of discharge may imply a low estrogen level or a vaginal or uterine obstruction. *Does a mucous discharge occur with ovulation?*

Are you using any form of contraception? Evaluate the patient's contraceptive method to distinguish between possible causes of irritation and infection. Oral contraceptives can cause amenorrhea and bleeding. Intrauterine devices can cause heavy menses and cramping and can increase the risk of pelvic inflammatory disease.

Has your sexual partner had an abnormal discharge recently? Both sexual partners usually require treatment for most sexually transmitted infections.

If the patient has a breast discharge, ask whether it's serous or bloody, which may reflect an inflammatory or neoplastic process in the breast. If the discharge is milky, ask the patient about recent pregnancy or abortion and whether she uses oral contraceptives or major tranquilizers. Be sure to question her about headaches or visual problems, because a pituitary neoplasm may be causing the discharge.

• ***Breast lumps and masses.*** *How long has the breast lump been present? Has it changed since you first noticed it? In what way?* Lumps of long duration with little or no recent change are usually benign, whereas new lumps that have undergone obvious changes can indicate cancer. *Is the lump tender?* A tender lump is probably due to an inflammatory or hormonal process. Remember, nipple discharge that concurs with the presence of a mass may indicate cancer (the incidence is at least 50% in women over age 50 when both a discharge and a mass are present). *Have you noticed any other breast lumps?* Women with multiple lumps (fibrocystic disease) are at an increased risk of developing a malignancy in one of the masses.

• ***Perineal or vulvar lump.*** *When did you first notice it?* Some lumps grow slowly and remain asymptomatic until they're quite large. Others are noticed almost immediately because of presenting signs and symptoms, such as pruritus.

Can you feel the lump without touching it? The feeling that a mass is present is often associated with vaginal protuberances secondary to relaxation of pelvic support structures. The patient may liken the sensation of a perineal or vulvar lump to sitting on a ball. *Is it painful?* Discomfort can range from annoying to disabling. *Is it hard?* Hard, nontender lumps suggest malignancy; hard, tender lumps suggest an abscess. Clusters of soft, tender bumps, such as herpes genitalia, may be caused by a sexually transmitted disease.

• ***Missed period.*** *Have you recently had unprotected intercourse? Did you experience an acute illness during the month before the missed period? Have you recently experienced emotional stress, or have you suddenly begun to exercise strenuously?* Most women experience isolated anovulatory cycles during their reproductive years because of functional interference. Acute or chronic disease may also cause a woman to skip a period. Such periodic interruptions in the menstrual cycle are often referred to incorrectly as amenorrhea. Amenorrhea is correctly classified as primary or secondary. *Primary amenorrhea* is the absence of menarche by age 18. *Secondary amenorrhea* is the cessation of established menstruation for at least 3 consecutive months.

• ***Increased menstrual flow.*** *Has the length of your period changed? How many additional tampons or sanitary napkins do you currently use? Has the flow increased gradually or suddenly? Are you passing clots? If so, what size are they?* Determine whether the patient's complaint indicates *metrorrhagia* (sometimes prolonged flow, not occurring at the patient's customary cyclic intervals) or *menorrhagia* (excessive flow of usual duration, occurring at regular cyclic intervals). Remember that reproductive organ lesions cause most episodes of metrorrhagia or menorrhagia.

• ***Spotting.*** *When does spotting usually occur in relation to your period?* Spotting that commonly accompanies ovulation occurs during midcycle. Determine what the patient means by spotting. Does she mean an abnormally small amount of menstrual flow (*hypomenorrhea*)? Or does she mean vaginal bleeding that occurs between normal periods? This condition is correctly termed *metrorrhagia;* it can range from stains to hemorrhages. *Are you using any medications that contain estrogen?* Medications that suppress ovulation can cause spotting and metrorrhagia. *Does the bleeding occur only after intercourse or the use of intravaginal objects?* Trauma or cervical erosion can cause temporary bleeding from the vulva, vagina, or cervical mucosa.

• ***Pruritus.*** Pruritus of the vulval or vaginal mucosa can follow any interruption in the normal production of acidic vaginal secretions. Its effects can range from annoying to debilitating. *Do you use a spray, powder, perfume, antiseptic soap, deodorant, or ointment in the genital area?* The chemicals used in these products can cause vaginal or perineal irritations. *Do you wear tight pants or nylon panties and panty hose?* Tight pants can trap moisture and cause chafing in the perineal area. Nylon panties and panty hose are poor conductors of moisture and air. Perspiration and secretions can accumulate in the perineal area, causing chafing and irritation.

What form of self-treatment have you attempted? Most douching solutions offer only temporary relief and carry the additional hazard of mechanical and chemical interference with vaginal acidity. *Have you used systemic antibiotics recently?* Broad-spectrum antibiotics allow superinfection of the vagina.

558 Past history

Obtain the following information when reviewing your patient's past history:

• ***Pregnancies.*** Note the patient's age at the time of her first pregnancy, the number of pregnancies (gravida #) and deliveries (para #), the weight of each baby, the length of each labor, the type of delivery, and the type of anesthetic used, if any. Describe any miscarriages or abortions, including any complications. Note any health problems that may have occurred during the patient's pregnancies, such as anemia, high blood pressure, mastitis, or toxemia.

Women who are infertile or nulliparous, those who have only one or two children, or those whose first pregnancy occurred after age 35 are at greater risk of developing breast cancer. Women who are nulliparous also have an increased risk of developing endometrial cancer.

• ***Cystic breast disease.*** This disorder increases the chance of developing breast cancer. Note whether the patient had a mammography or biopsy follow-up.

• ***Breast cancer.*** This is the most significant risk factor for future breast malignancies. Record the patient's treatment and follow-up.

• ***Ovarian cysts, uterine tumors, or polyps.*** These are common, usually benign, growths, but they may cause complications. Their presence normally contraindicates use of an intrauterine device.

• ***Other gynecologic, medical, and surgical history.*** Note why the patient sought treatment in the past for any other gynecologic problem. Describe any complications that may have resulted from treatment. If the patient has undergone surgery, note the specific organ or organs operated on or removed. A woman who has had a hysterectomy with a bilateral oophorectomy before age 40 has a reduced risk of developing breast cancer.

• ***Diabetes mellitus.*** This disorder can increase a patient's susceptibility to vaginal fungal infections. Diabetes also requires cautious use of birth control pills and may complicate pregnancy.

• ***Other endocrine diseases.*** Besides diabetes, ask the patient about adrenal, thyroid, and pituitary disorders, which can interfere with the menstrual cycle.

• ***Sexually transmitted diseases.*** Previously adequate treatment of sexually transmitted diseases may no longer be adequate to prevent complications or recurrences. This is because of the development of resistant strains of organisms. Moreover, no known cure exists for herpes genitalis. Remember that the most common complication of sexually transmitted diseases is pelvic inflammatory disease, which can cause sterility secondary to massive scarring or surgery. Also, when you question your patient about these diseases, be prepared to refer to them by their colloquial names (see *Common Names for Some Sexually Transmitted Diseases*), when necessary.

• ***Toxic shock syndrome.*** This disorder, which usually affects women under age 30, tends to recur. It generally occurs in association with continuous use of tampons during the menstrual period. Typical symptoms include sudden onset of high fever, myalgia, vomiting, diarrhea, hypotension (which can lead to shock), and a macular erythematous rash, especially on the palms, fingers, and toes. A change in level of consciousness may also occur.

• ***Trauma.*** Breast or pelvic injuries resulting from rape, assault, or a motor vehicle accident may cause permanent physical and emotional dysfunction.

• ***Musculoskeletal disorders.*** Pelvic deformities from congenital anomalies or arthritis may cause mechanical dysfunction.

• ***Psychiatric disorders.*** Even if the patient has no past history of treatment for a psychiatric disorder, increased stress can cause menstrual irregularities and exacerbate menopausal symptoms.

• ***Radiation exposure.*** Cancer, of course, may develop in any organ exposed to excessive radiation. Ask the patient if she has been X-rayed many times, or if she has undergone any other diagnostic test or received therapy that involved X-rays. Also ask if she works at a job that exposes her to radiation.

559 Family history

Breast cancer on the maternal side of the patient's family doubles her risk of developing it. If the cancer was bilateral, the patient's risk is more than five times the average; if it was bilateral *and* premenopausal, the patient's risk is almost nine times greater than the average.

Diethylstilbestrol is an estrogenic compound used until recently to prevent miscarriages. If your patient's mother used this drug while pregnant with the patient, the risk exists that the patient will develop cervical lesions and vaginal cancer. This may possibly occur even before puberty.

Ask the patient if anyone in her family ever had sickle cell anemia, diabetes mellitus, or thyroid disease. These disorders directly affect the female reproductive system.

COMMON NAMES FOR SOME SEXUALLY TRANSMITTED DISEASES

When you question your patient about these particular diseases, you may have to mention them by their nonmedical as well as their medical names, because she may not know the medical ones.

MEDICAL NAME	COMMONLY USED NAMES
Gonorrhea	GC, clap, gleet, drip, the whites
Syphilis	Lues, siph, bad blood, las bubas, the sore
Herpes genitalis (HSV, HS-2)	Genital herpes, herpes II
Condylomata acuminata	Venereal warts
Trichomoniasis (trichomonal vaginitis)	Tric
Pubic lice	Crabs

560 Psychosocial history

Sexually transmitted diseases occur in women of all socioeconomic levels. Because any woman you assess may have such a disease, inquire tactfully about every female patient's sexual activities. Ask about the gender and number of her partners and about such practices as oral and anal sex. Remember that the incidence of cervical cancer rises with the number of sexual partners a woman has had. Also inquire about stress the woman may encounter at home or at work, which can alter her menstrual cycle.

EMERGENCY

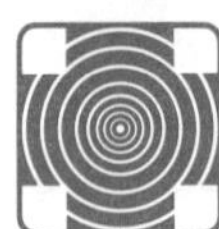

EMERGENCY ASSESSMENT: CARING FOR THE RAPE VICTIM

When dealing with a victim of rape, you can reduce both her trauma and her anxiety by providing effective nursing and psychological care. Follow these guidelines:

- As a first consideration, your hospital should only entrust the rape victim to the care of a nurse and doctor of the same sex as the patient (who's usually female). Place the patient in a treatment area that's quiet, private, and secure. Introduce yourself. Show acceptance for her through eye contact, tone of voice, and (if appropriate) physical contact. Your hospital may have an arrangement with a local rape crisis center. If it does, ask your patient if she'd like to have a rape victim advocate with her during her hospital stay. If your hospital doesn't have such an arrangement, assure the patient that you'll be with her at all times throughout her emergency care.
- Set priorities according to your patient's needs. Physical injuries require immediate attention.
- Do not allow her to drink fluids or to wash her genital area. Explain that such activities would remove any existing semen, which is vital medicolegal evidence.
- After the patient is reasonably calm, explain that the doctor will ask her questions to identify the type of assault made on her. Be open to discussing her feelings and her fears. Demonstrate a nonjudgmental and supportive attitude. You'll find most rape victims have a need to talk.
- Introduce all hospital personnel entering the examination area to the patient.
- Tell the patient what treatment she'll receive: the doctor will perform a head-to-toe physical examination for signs of physical trauma and may order a Pap smear of her vagina, mouth, or rectum; saline suspensions to test for sperm presence; and an acid phosphatase test to determine how recently intercourse took place. The doctor will also order prophylactic antibiotics for sexually transmitted diseases. (When the patient is calm, discuss postcoital contraception, and possible pregnancy, with her.) The police will probably request the patient's articles of clothing as evidence (do not wash or discard them); they may ask you to try to find samples of the assailant's hair and skin tissue by combing the patient's pubic hair and examining her fingernails for deposits. Write down explanations of these procedures and the doctor's orders regarding such things as how often the patient should take antibiotics and when she should be reexamined. She can refer to these later.
- After your patient has been examined and treated, provide her with facilities to wash herself. Also provide mouthwash or a change of clothing, if needed. Before she leaves the hospital, be sure she understands the importance of getting retested for sexually transmitted disease in about 3 weeks, or sooner if symptoms occur. Some patients may require psychiatric referral. Give the rape victim written information about where to go for social, legal, or medical help, if needed.

561 Activities of daily living

As you review your patient's activities of daily living, ask about the following:

- ***Self-assessment techniques.*** *Do you regularly examine your breasts? Have you ever examined your external genitalia for swelling or lumps? Do you watch for vaginal discharge, noting amount, color, odor, and persistence?*
- ***Self-care techniques.*** *Do you wash your hands before inserting a tampon? How long do you wear a tampon? Do you use feminine hygiene products, such as douches? Which products do you use, how frequently do you use them, and why do you use them?* Using these products is often unnecessary and may injure the vaginal mucosa.
- ***Exercise.*** Bicycling, swimming, and other aerobic exercises—although generally healthy practices—are usually contraindicated during treatment of inflammatory disorders and pelvic support problems. If prolonged or strenuous, exercise can cause skipped

periods and secondary amenorrhea.

• ***Tobacco.*** During pregnancy, smoking may increase the risk of fetal abnormalities. When combined with use of birth control pills, smoking increases the risk of myocardial infarction.

• ***Alcohol.*** Drinking during pregnancy may compound the risk of fetal abnormalities. It also reduces the effectiveness of treatment of some sexually transmitted diseases. Excessive alcohol consumption can cause amenorrhea.

• ***Caffeine.*** Coffee, tea, chocolate, and most cola drinks contain moderate to high amounts of caffeine, which may increase the incidence of breast lumps in some women.

562 Review of systems

Ask about the following symptoms as you proceed through a review of your patient's body systems:

• ***General.*** *Have you noticed a recent weight change?* Sudden weight loss or gain can cause menstrual irregularities. *Have you had a fever?* Fever may result from systemic infection secondary to an infection of a reproductive organ. Fever can also induce secondary amenorrhea.

• ***Skin.*** Acute acne, changes in hair texture or distribution, and skin lesions or rashes may result from altered gonadotropin function or systemic infection caused by a sexually transmitted disease or toxic shock syndrome. Hot flashes, sweating, and rapid changes in body temperature can result from withdrawal of estrogen medication or may be associated with menopause.

• ***Nervous.*** Headaches or dizziness may occur with reproductive system infection, estrogen withdrawal or intake, or the use of birth control pills.

• ***Eyes.*** Dry, scratchy eyes and vision changes may result from the use of birth control pills.

• ***Mouth, throat, tongue.*** Rashes, chancres, or sores in the mouth area can be caused by certain sexually transmitted diseases.

• ***Gastrointestinal.*** Anorexia, nausea, vomiting, severe abdominal cramps, and diarrhea or constipation can result from the use of birth control pills, menopause, or systemic infection. Difficulty with bowel movements usually accompanies and aggravates weakening pelvic support structures.

• ***Respiratory.*** Frequent coughing or sneezing can aggravate pelvic support defects.

• ***Cardiovascular.*** Menorrhagia may occur in a patient with congestive heart failure.

• ***Urinary.*** Difficult urination, stress incontinence, or frequent or urgent urination can result from vulvovaginal irritation or inadequate pelvic support.

• ***Musculoskeletal.*** Arthritic pains may accompany toxic shock syndrome and the secondary stages of some sexually transmitted diseases. Estrogen withdrawal decreases bone density, which predisposes women to stress fractures, especially of weight-bearing joints and vertebrae.

• ***Psychological.*** Menstrual and menopausal symptoms can be exacerbated by stress and by functional disorders.

Conducting the physical examination

563 Preliminary considerations

Because of the intimate and invasive nature of breast and pelvic examinations, approach these tasks with the utmost respect for your patient. Protecting her from emotional as well as physical discomfort throughout the examination should be a major concern.

Information you've gathered about your patient during history-taking should help you to understand her self-concept. For example, is she modest about or ashamed of her body? Is she comfortable with the basic language and terminology of the female reproductive system and its functioning? Observe secondary sex characteristics—voice pitch, hair distribution, body odor, musculoskeletal proportions, facial structure, breast development, and skin texture. These observations can provide important physiologic information on the adequacy of the patient's ovarian function.

Begin your preparations for the physical examination by checking state policy, as well as the policy of your facility, concerning chaperone attendance. Female examiners usually work without an attendant, but if the patient requests one—or if she's emotionally disturbed or handicapped in any way—obtain assistance from a staff member. Male examiners should always offer the patient the option of having a female attendant present throughout the examination.

During breast and pelvic examinations, try to keep your patient comfortable and relaxed. Warm hands, for example, increase not only the patient's tolerance of a particular maneuver but also the accuracy of your palpation. Whenever possible, observe your patient's face and hands for signs of discomfort, such as tense facial muscles or clenched fists.

564 Examining your patient's breasts

Use inspection and palpation to examine your patient's breasts. You won't need any special equipment, but you'll need to determine the order in which to palpate the various sections of the breasts. The *spiral, quadrant,* and *spokes/radial* methods are three examples of breast examination patterns (see *Examining Your Patient's Breasts*). Each includes inspection of the nipple, areola, body of the breast, and the tail of the upper outer quadrant of breast tissue, which extends into the axilla. Choose one approach and use it for all breast examinations so that the procedure becomes routine. By doing so, you'll assure a thorough breast inspection for each patient you examine.

Begin the examination with the patient seated so that her breasts are at your eye level. Her arms should be at her sides and her hands should be resting in her lap. Drape only the patient's abdomen, because full anterior and lateral thoracic views are essential. Explain what you'll be doing; then inspect for nipple symmetry, color, contour, venous pattern, and skin integrity. Record all abnormal variations or conditions, such as a scar from a lumpectomy, nipple inversion and dimpling, enlarged pores, and any nipple or areolar discharge. You can distinguish natural asymmetry of the breasts from unilateral edema by inspecting the pores. Edema accentuates or deepens sweat pores, causing the skin of the breast to look like an orange rind. This condition is known as *peau d'orange.*

To detect less obvious abnormalities before you palpate the breasts, have the patient raise her arms over her head and press her palms together. Then, ask her to press her palms into her hips. If the skin of the breasts is attached to the underlying tissues abnormally, you'll note a dimpling or retraction of the skin. For example, a malignant breast tumor can shorten suspensory ligaments, creating traction on the overlying skin. If the patient has unusually full or pendulous breasts, ask her to lean forward while you observe for flattening of the nipple area—another sign of unnatural attachment.

Palpation is usually performed with the patient in the supine position. However, if the patient has a breast mass as a chief complaint or in her past medical history, palpate the breasts when she's seated, as well. Follow this same procedure if the patient is at high risk of developing breast cancer or has pendulous breasts.

Begin breast palpation with the pads of your first and second fingers (some examiners add a third), and move the patient's skin over underlying lymph

EXAMINING YOUR PATIENT'S BREASTS

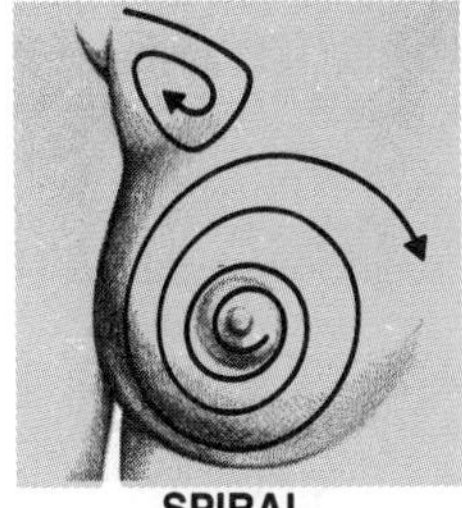
SPIRAL

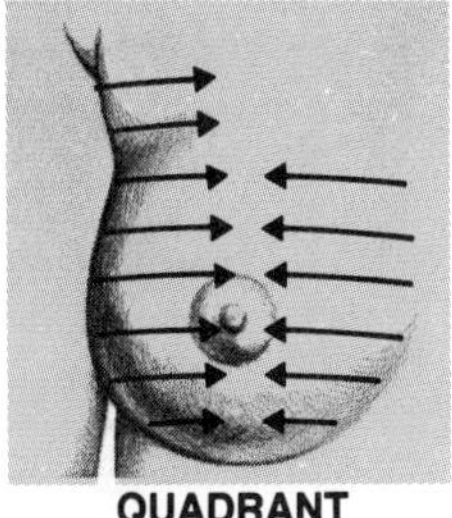
QUADRANT

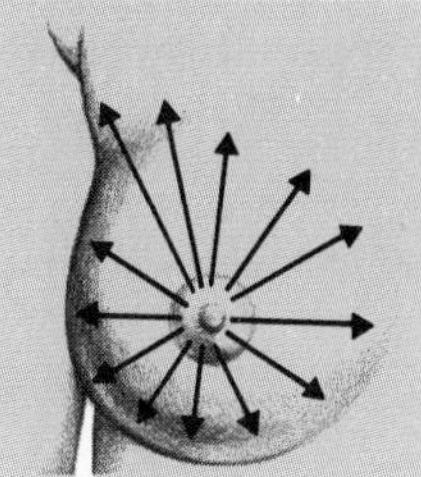
SPOKES/RADIAL

When you examine your patient's breasts, use any of the palpation techniques illustrated here. Also, teach these methods to your patient so she can perform a breast self-examination at home. Encourage her to select one method and to use it routinely.

Obtain printed materials from such organizations as the American Cancer Society. Give them to your patient to reinforce your teaching.

nodes and tissue in a circular motion. Palpate first the axillary, the infraclavicular, and the supraclavicular areas, checking for enlarged or hard lymph nodes, tenderness, and accessory nipples. Because of the breast's abundant lymphatic drainage, a malignant breast tumor spreads first to lymph nodes in the axillae, above the clavicles, and to the mediastinal lymph nodes beneath the sternum. Enlarged axillary and supraclavicular lymph nodes can usually be detected during a physical examination, but enlarged mediastinal lymph nodes are too deeply embedded to be detected this way. You can differentiate an accessory nipple from a nevus by stimulating the accessory nipple's erectile tissue; a nevus will not become erect.

Apply more pressure as you palpate each area. Don't slide or stroke your fingers across the patient's skin—you could miss small nodules.

During palpation, keep normal breast variations in mind. The young breast has a firm elasticity; the middle-aged breast generally feels lobular; the older breast often has a stringy or granular feel. Other normal variations include premenstrual fullness, nodularity, and tenderness.

If the patient has large breasts, place a cushion under one scapula, to shift most of the ipsilateral breast tissue onto the anterior chest wall. This position allows you to feel significant masses more distinctly. You may note a firm transverse ridge of compressed tissue along the breast's lower edge. This is known as the *inframammary ridge*—don't confuse it with a tumor.

Palpate any suspicious areas you found on inspection. Firmly squeeze several inches around an area of altered contour and note the result. Describe any nodule in terms of its location even if you found the nodule in only one patient position: Note its consistency, mobility, size (in metric units), shape, delineation, and tenderness. Gently squeeze each areola and nipple clockwise, noting elasticity, enlarged pores, and discharge. If you detect a discharge, obtain a specimen and send it to the laboratory for cytology examination. Proceed to teach your patient breast self-examination.

565 Preparing for a pelvic examination

A pelvic examination should be conducted in a private area equipped with an examining table with stirrups.

However, situations may arise in which an examining table is unavailable. For example, a visiting nurse may perform this examination in the patient's bedroom. Regardless of the situation, your caring attitude and careful explanation of each technique used during the examination will help the patient relax. Remember, too, that for you to inspect the uterus properly during a pelvic examination, the patient's bladder should be empty.

Assemble the following equipment within your reach:

- tight-fitting disposable gloves
- 1″ (2.5 cm) of water-soluble, sterile lubricating jelly on a paper towel (so you don't have to pick up the tube after the gloves are on)
- opened package of sterile swabs
- cervicovaginal spatula
- glass slides with frosted ends
- culture tubette
- cytologic fixative (hair spray works as well as ethyl-alcohol solutions or commercial sprays)
- several specula (usually medium-sized). If your patient is frightened, very young, or elderly, use a small speculum. If she's obese or multiparous, you may need a large one. Disposable plastic specula provide a more complete view of the vaginal wall coloring than metal specula, but they don't allow complete use of both hands. In addition, plastic specula aren't strong enough to expand the vaginal vault in tense or obese patients and may break; for these patients, the traditional metal speculum—even though follow-up sterilization is necessary—is superior.
- optional equipment, such as a specialized culture medium for gonorrhea (for example, Thayer-Martin medium), laboratory slips, specialized glass slides and coverslips, and a hand mirror for the patient to view her cervix.

Drape the patient's abdomen, pelvis, and breasts with a sheet. You may ask her to wear a hospital gown to cover her breasts. As the woman assumes the lithotomy position, help her by gently flexing her knees and hips and abducting her thighs. When she's properly positioned, place her heels in the stirrups—which should be level with and about 12″ from the front edge of the examining table. Then ask the patient to lift and pull her pelvis, using her arms as leverage, to the front edge of the table. Touch her buttocks with your hand when she reaches the appropriate position.

Place a small pillow under her head. Then instruct her to rest her arms at her sides or on her thorax to give you full access to her relaxed abdomen. To minimize shadows from the patient's legs and your hands during inspection, position a gooseneck lamp nearby.

566 Examination of external genitalia

Put on the disposable gloves and either stand or sit at the foot of the examining table. Some examiners prefer to stand throughout a pelvic examination, but sitting is the most common approach. To help accustom the patient to the inspection, inform her that you will touch her inner thighs as you begin to inspect her vulva and perineum. Note odor, discharge, inflammation, hair type and distribution, any lice or lesions, and the presence of varicosities.

Palpate the labia majora, checking for subcutaneous lesions and tenderness. Then separate the labia majora, checking each specific vulval structure for signs of infection, breaks in tissue integrity, underdeveloped or overdeveloped clitoris, adhesions, neoplasms, and circulatory impairment.

Next, ask the patient to bear down as though she were straining during a bowel movement or during labor. Note any urinary incontinence or bulging of the vaginal vestibule that could indicate an overrelaxed pelvic support system. Note also an unusually tense fourchette, unbroken hymen, urethral abnormalities, or evidence of vaginal irritation or inflammation.

If you notice labial swelling or tenderness, insert your index finger into the posterior introitus and place your thumb along the lateral edge of the swollen or tender labium. Then check the Bartholin's gland by gently squeezing the labium; if discharge from the duct results, culture it.

If the patient's history suggests she may have an inflamed urethra, separate the labia with one hand and insert the water-moistened index finger of your other hand about 2½" (6.4 cm) into the anterior fornix. With the pad of your fingertip, gently press the anterior vaginal wall up into the urethra and pull outward, thus milking the urethra. Use Thayer-Martin medium for any resulting discharge; if Thayer-Martin medium is unavailable, obtain a specimen for Gram's staining.

567 Internal pelvic examination

Some examiners prefer to begin an internal pelvic examination using their fingers instead of a speculum. This allows quick discovery and removal of tampons or other foreign bodies without causing further trauma by an instrument. By using your fingers, you can also detect any deviation from the classic anterior position of the uterus and assess the vagina to determine the

PALPATING YOUR PATIENT'S INTERNAL STRUCTURES

To examine your patient's internal genitalia, follow these instructions:

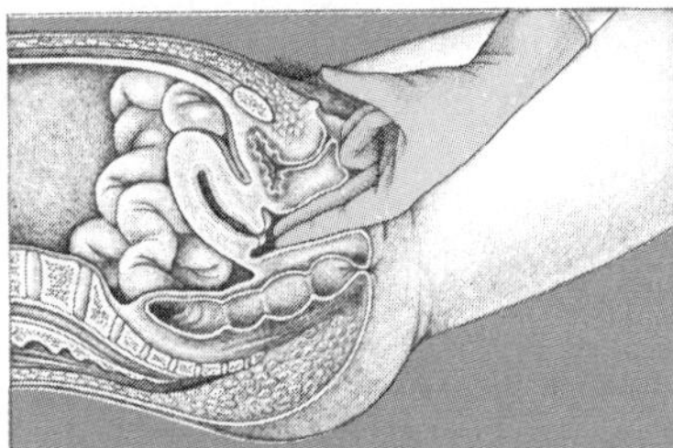

1 To palpate your patient's vagina, insert your fingers using the *palm up* position, as illustrated here. Note any tenderness, nodules, or deviations.

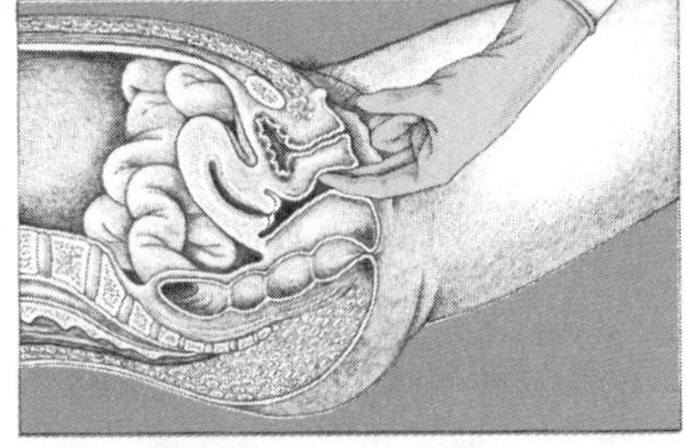

2 To palpate the urethra, sweep your fingers along the anterior vaginal wall, toward the vaginal opening. The urethra should be soft and tubular. Note any discharge or tenderness.

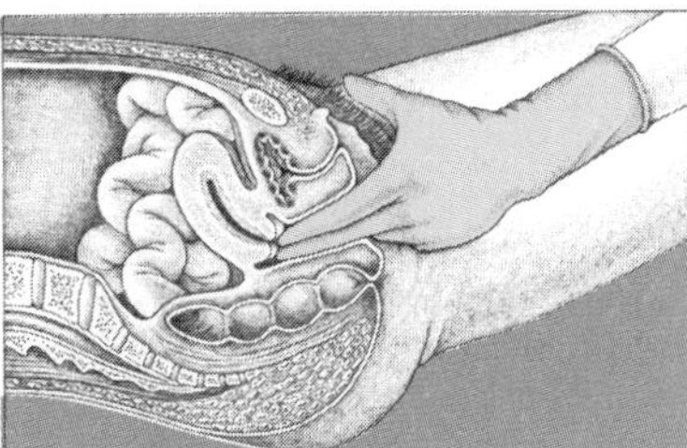

3 To palpate the cervix, sweep your fingers from side to side across the cervix and around the os. The cervix should feel moist, smooth, and firm but resilient and should protrude ½" to 1¼" (1.5 to 3 cm) into the vagina.

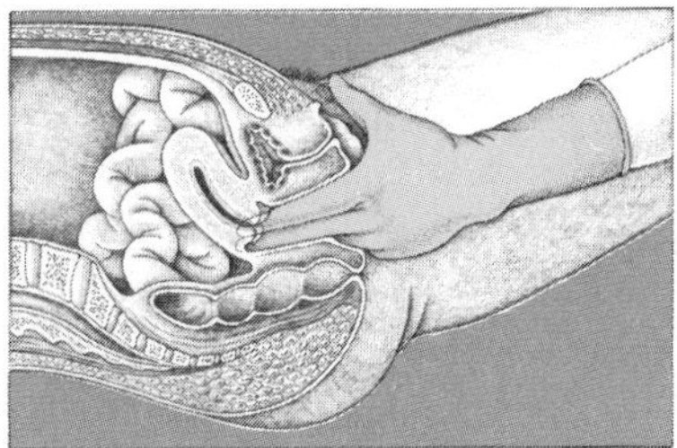

4 To palpate the fornix, place your fingers on the recessed area surrounding the cervix. Gently move the cervix; it should move ½" to ¾" (1.5 to 2 cm) in any direction.

USING A VAGINAL SPECULUM

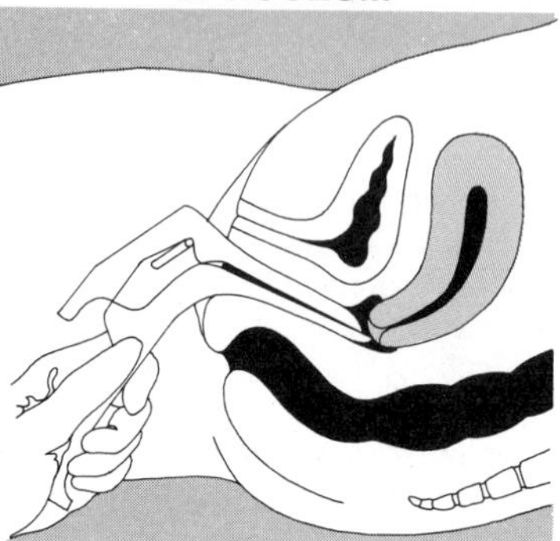

1 To properly insert the speculum into your patient's vagina, begin with the blades pointing down and the speculum handles at a 45° angle to the floor. Gently insert the speculum against the posterior vaginal wall. Move the speculum so the handle is vertical to the floor.

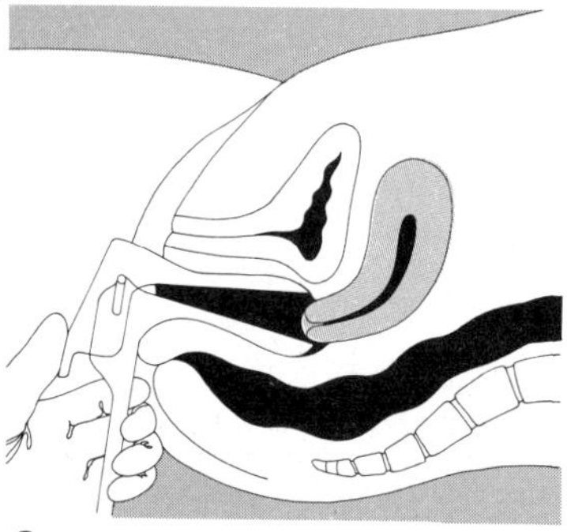

2 When the cervix is in view, open the blades as far as possible and lock them. If the speculum's correctly placed, you should be able to view the cervix.

When you've completed your examination, unlock the speculum blades and close them slowly, as you begin withdrawing the speculum. Before the blades reach the vaginal opening, close them completely. Then, withdraw the speculum from the vagina.

correct speculum size to use—thus preventing unnecessary contamination of equipment. A tense patient may relax more readily if you use your fingers to begin the examination.

For insertion, moisten your index and middle fingers with water rather than a lubricant, which would interfere with cytologic staining. Press your fingers into the posterior wall of the vagina as you insert them. Occasionally, the vagina may accommodate only one finger; in this case, keep your other fingers and thumb enclosed within your palm.

As your fingers enter the vagina, note how the vaginal walls softly engulf them. Record any tenderness or hardness you feel, except for the normally smooth firmness of the cervix on your fingertips when your fingers are almost fully inserted. Normally, the cervix measures about 1¼″ (3 cm) in diameter and should move easily, without causing the patient discomfort. Note any variation in its position. (To continue the examination using palpation only, see *Palpating Your Patient's Internal Structures,* page 513.)

Next, begin withdrawing your fingers, pressing the fingerpads posteriorly against the vagina. With your free hand, obtain the appropriate-sized speculum. Keep your fingers pressed at the posterior edge of the introitus, and ask the patient to bear down again, to relax her perineum. Slowly insert the closed speculum—long blade beneath the shorter one—diagonally into the vagina to avoid direct pressure on the sensitive urethra. (Try to avoid pulling the labial hair into the introitus.) Gently push the blades along the same slant that brought your fingers to the cervix. Then, gradually withdraw your fingers as you increase posterior pressure with the speculum.

When you can no longer advance the speculum, turn the blades horizontally so that the handles are vertical. To open the blades, press the handles together. Then, maneuver the blades until the cervix drops between them. (Locating the cervix is not always easy, but don't become discouraged or impatient.) As you maneuver the blades, note the vaginal rugae and the thick mucosa's multiple transverse ridges exposed between the length of the blades. In an elderly woman, the rugae may be atrophied to a shiny flat surface. Note also the type of discharge on the vaginal walls or on the bottom blade.

When the cervix is in full view, note its shape, color, and mucosal integrity. Examine the os for discharge, lesions, intrauterine device strings, or ectropion; its normal shape depends on whether the woman is nulliparous or multiparous. The cervix should be smooth, round, and rosy-pink, free of ulcerations and nodules. Ovulating discharge should be clear and watery. Slightly bloody discharge is normal just before menstruation. Any other colored discharge is abnormal and needs to be described and cultured.

If the patient's history suggests that she may have a sexually transmitted disease, particularly gonorrhea, first culture any discharge with Thayer-Martin medium. If you are using a metal speculum, lock the thumbscrew to keep the blades in place while you obtain a specimen for culture (see *Using a Vaginal Speculum*).

568 Obtaining a Pap smear

After examining the patient's cervix, obtain a Papanicolaou (Pap) smear, with the speculum still in place. Usually, samples are taken from at least two areas. First, sample the squamous-columnar junction, where abnormalities that may indicate dysplasia or in situ carcinoma first appear. This cel-

OBTAINING A PAP SMEAR

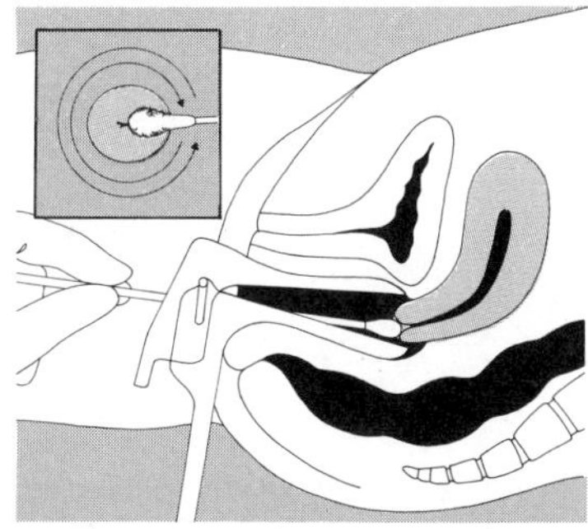

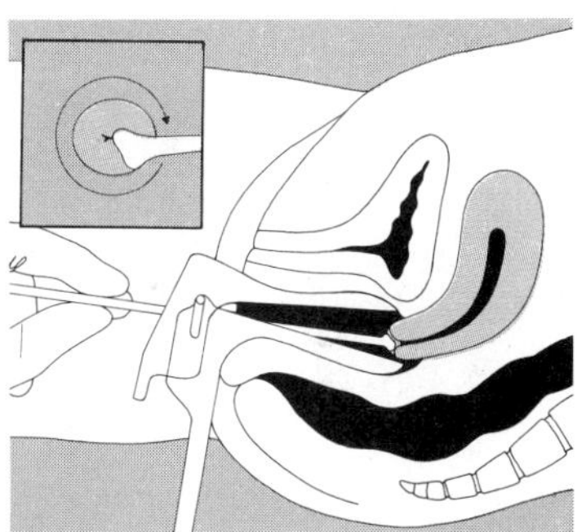

Before you take a Pap smear, review these instructions:

To obtain an endocervical specimen, use a cotton swab, as illustrated on the left. Rotate the swab clockwise and counterclockwise, as shown in the inset. Roll the swab on the properly labeled slide. Then, immediately immerse the slide in fixative.

To take a cervical scrape, use a spatula to obtain the cervical sample, as illustrated on the right. Follow the same guidelines as you would for the endocervical specimen, with these two exceptions: Rotate the spatula only *once* clockwise (as shown in the inset) *and smear* the sample on the properly labeled slide in a single circular motion.

Your institution may categorize laboratory results as follows:

- *Class I:* absence of atypical or abnormal cells
- *Class II:* atypical cytology but no evidence of malignancy (in many cases, the result of a temporary or chronic vaginitis)
- *Class III:* cytology suggestive of but not conclusive for malignancy
- *Class IV:* cytology strongly suggestive of malignancy
- *Class V:* cytology conclusive for malignancy.

If your patient's test result is Class II, Class III, or Class IV, reassure her that this does not necessarily mean she has cancer. Further testing is necessary. But because the Pap test is only an indicator, some doctors prefer to repeat the test. If your patient has vaginitis, defer repeating the test until several days after treatment is completed.

DETERMINING UTERINE POSITIONS

You can accurately determine uterine position while performing a bimanual examination. Use this chart as a guide to evaluate your findings.

	UTERINE POSITION	CERVIX POSITION	PALPABILITY OF BODY AND FUNDUS
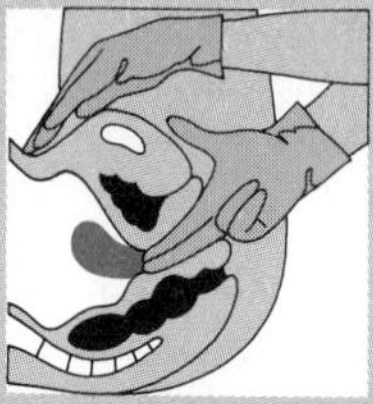	**Anteverted**	Anterior vaginal wall	Palpable with one hand on the patient's abdomen and the fingers of the other hand in her vagina
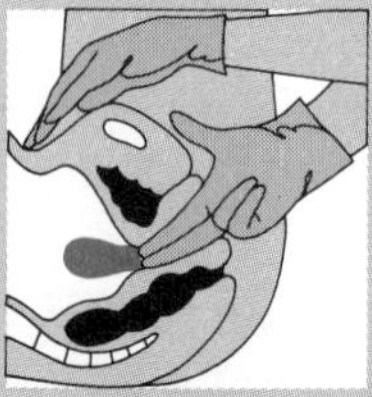	**Midposition**	Vaginal apex	May not be palpable
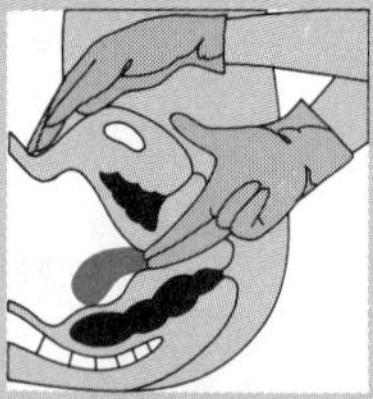	**Retroverted**	Posterior vaginal wall	Not palpable
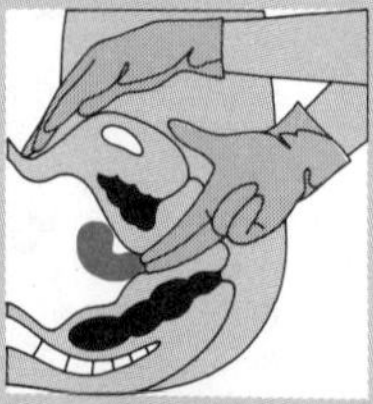	**Anteflexed**	Anterior vaginal wall or apex	Easily palpable (angulation of the isthmus felt in anterior fornix)
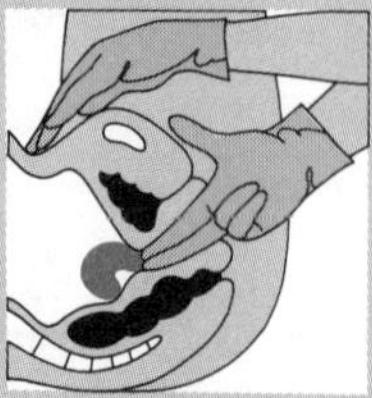	**Retroflexed**	Anterior or posterior vaginal wall or apex	Not palpable

lular sample is called an *endocervical specimen.* You can easily obtain it by inserting a cotton swab, through the speculum, ½" (1 cm) beyond the external os, then rolling it several times between your thumb and index finger. (If you can't insert the swab beyond the external os, adhesions or neoplasms may be obstructing the canal's patency.) Clear cervical mucus should be present on the swab when you remove it. Gently wipe the swab on a glass slide marked *EC* (endocervical). Because cervical cells are fragile, fix the smear immediately with solution or a light, even spray. Then fan the solution dry.

To obtain the second sample, called the *cervical scrape,* press the longer, sculptured tip of the spatula into the external os and turn it clockwise a full revolution. Remove the spatula and gently smear the scraped cellular material on a clean glass slide marked *cerv* (cervical). If a patient has a history of cancer treated by hysterectomy, scrape the surgical stump and note the nature of the scrape on the laboratory slip and on the slide.

With the scrape completed, withdraw the speculum slowly. As the cervix relaxes, release the thumbscrew or allow the blades to close slightly. Again, observe the vaginal walls. Then press the blades posteriorly and diagonally as they close completely. After you've removed the speculum, examine the pool of mucus that will have collected in the bottom blade. If the mucus is colored or odorous, culture it. Inform the patient that she may experience some spotting after the specimens are obtained and that this is normal.

Assessment tip: If your patient is scheduled for a Pap smear but vaginitis is present, defer the Pap smear until a week after treatment is completed. (Acute inflammation from vaginitis can cause a cellular dysplasia that mimics early forms of cancer.)

569 Performing a bimanual examination

You'll usually perform a bimanual (va-

PERFORMING A BIMANUAL VAGINAL EXAMINATION

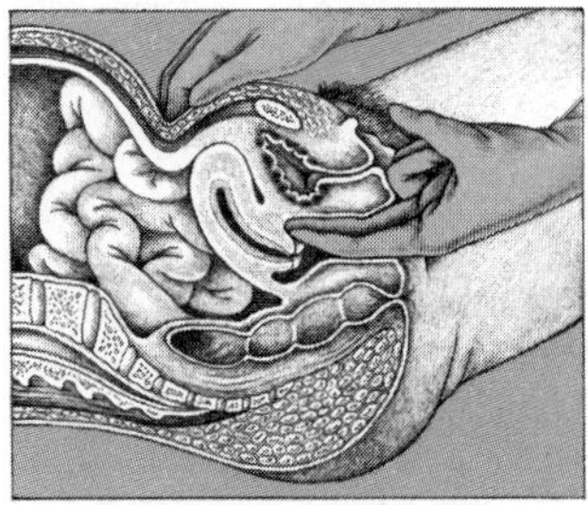

1 To palpate the uterus and anterior fornix, direct your index and middle fingers toward the patient's anterior fornix. In this position you should feel part of the anterior uterine wall. Place your other hand on the abdomen, just above the symphysis pubis, to palpate the posterior uterine wall.

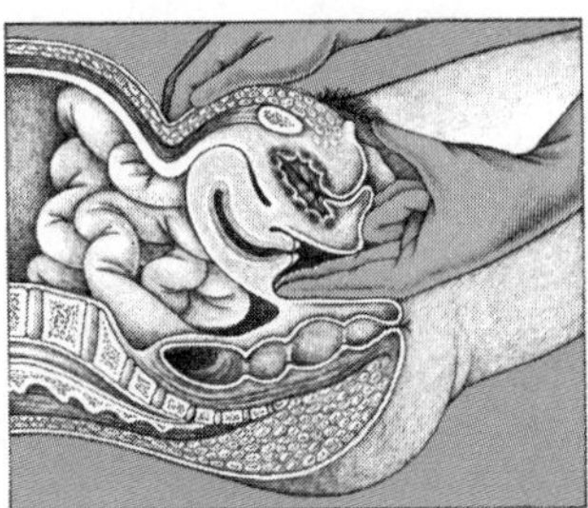

2 To palpate the posterior fornix, direct your index and middle fingers toward the patient's posterior fornix. Press upward and forward so that you can palpate the anterior uterine wall with your abdominally placed hand.

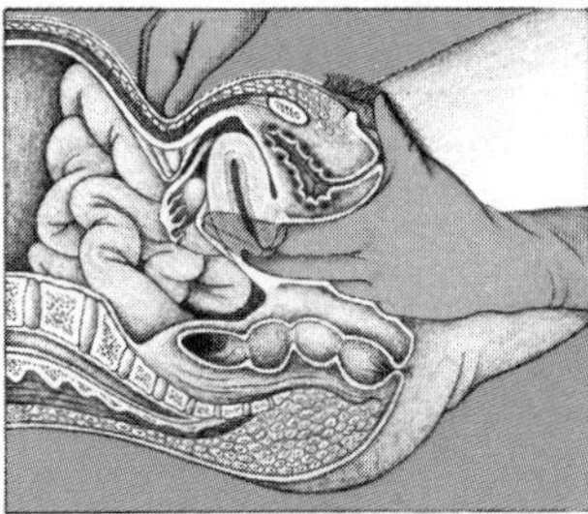

3 To palpate the adnexa, direct your index and middle fingers toward the patient's right lateral fornix and place your other hand on the patient's lower right quadrant. Palpate right and left sides.

ginoabdominal) examination of a patient while standing. To begin, generously lubricate your gloved index and third fingers. (Tell the patient she'll feel an initial cold sensation from the lubricating jelly.) Insert your fingers into the vagina and move them up to the cervix. Explore for tenderness or lesions. First, place your fingers in the anterior fornix (see *Performing a Bimanual Vaginal Examination,* page 517). Then, slip your other hand under the drape, place it on the patient's abdomen, halfway between the umbilicus and the symphysis pubis, and press down toward the cervix. Keep the hand in the patient's vagina aligned with the forearm of your external hand. If your patient is tense, let her press down on her abdomen with her own hand. As she relaxes, place her hand on top of yours as you proceed.

Use your fingers curled on the patient's perineum to press the fingers in the vagina inward and to locate the uterus. The fundus should be smooth, firm, mobile, nontender, and situated midline behind the symphysis pubis. If you can't feel the uterus in this position, direct your fingers into the posterior fornix and again try to palpate the uterus. If the uterus is enlarged, suspect pregnancy or tumors (either necessitates additional laboratory work). If the patient's uterus is retroverted, you may be unable to palpate the fundus through the vagina.

Next, move your external hand to one of the lower abdominal quadrants and the hand in the vagina to the ipsilateral fornix. From this position, check one side of the patient's adnexa (ovaries, fallopian tubes, and supporting tissues). Normally, you can palpate the ovaries if the patient is sufficiently relaxed and not obese. The fallopian tubes and supporting tissue are usually not palpable, and if the woman is 3 to 5 years beyond menopause, her ovaries have probably atrophied and will not be palpable either. If you do feel an ovary in a postmenopausal woman, suspect an ovarian tumor.

Continue your palpation, noting any uterine or adnexal masses and ovarian size, mobility, consistency, and shape. Then, palpate the other side.

Remove your hand from the patient's vagina. (If you suspect gonorrhea, replace your glove with a clean one, to prevent transferring infection from the vagina to the rectum, and lubricate it.) Insert your index finger into the patient's vagina and your third finger into the rectum. (Tell her beforehand that this may stimulate an urge to defecate.) Repeat the bimanual examination, using the rectal finger to palpate the rectovaginal septum, the cul-de-sac, the uterosacral ligaments, and possibly the fundus, if your patient has a retroverted or retroflexed uterus.

Proceed with a rectal examination (see Entries 451 and 452), using your index finger for palpation.

If your patient complains of leg cramps during the examination, slide the table tray forward and place her feet on it. Or, ask her to slide back on the table and rest her feet on its corners.

Formulating a diagnostic impression

570 Classifying gynecologic disorders

The most common disorders of the female reproductive system can be classified into three groups: *inflammatory or infectious diseases, noninflammatory benign lesions,* and *malignant diseases.* Inflammatory or infectious diseases usually produce pain or discomfort, vaginal discharge, and vulvovaginal pruritus. Lumps and varying degrees of pain typically occur with noninflammatory benign lesions. Signs and symptoms of malignant diseases include a lump or mass near the affected organ, abnormal bleeding, and the absence of pain until late in the disease process.

571 Making appropriate nursing diagnoses

Gynecologic disorders produce psychological and physical nursing diagnoses ranging from *fear* and *alterations in coping abilities* to *alterations in comfort* and in *skin integrity*.

Pain is one of the body's responses to tissue damage that can affect the female reproductive system as a result of several processes:

- a mass that exerts pressure on the surrounding tissues (for example, infection, inflammation, or an allergic reaction), which can cause tissue destruction
- overstretching of muscles, ligaments, and skin, as in pelvic support relaxation
- increased vascularization
- excessive sodium and water retention.

The pain and pressure caused by these conditions usually result in *alterations in comfort* for the patient.

Vaginal discharge refers to excessive or abnormal amounts of vulvovaginal secretions. Usually caused by increased or decreased estrogen production, vaginal discharge may also result from a change in the vagina's normal pH, which can lead to an overgrowth of normal bacterial flora. Vaginal discharge can also be caused by such conditions as draining sinuses, weeping lesions, or fistulas, which allow body fluids to enter the vagina.

The character of the vaginal discharge may be pathologically significant. A yellow or green foul-smelling discharge usually implies a sexually transmitted bacterial infection. However, the discharge could be from decomposition of the vaginal mucosa or decreased vaginal mucosal resistance. If frothiness is also apparent, a one-celled organism is probably involved. Gray discharge implies a different bacterial process, and a white discharge—commonly referred to as *leukorrhea*—can reflect either a normal ovulatory effect or abnormal irritation of the cervix. If the discharge is curdlike (resembling cottage cheese) with a sweetish odor, it's usually pathognomonic of a fungus. Red or brown material suggests bleeding.

Breast discharge, which may be endogenous or exogenous, can result from inappropriate lactation, caused by abnormal hormone levels, or from a cyst or malignant tumor.

Both vaginal and breast discharge can cause *alterations in comfort* and in *skin integrity*. If the discharge is copious or malodorous, or stains the patient's clothing, the disorder could cause *alterations in activities of daily living*. In some cases, the patient becomes frustrated by the problem, which may lead to *alterations in coping abilities*.

Lumps and masses may result from a functional process, but this is rare and usually temporary. More common causes include an inflammatory process, blockage of an outflow tract (such as occurs with inflammation of Bartholin's gland), or a tumor. A patient who has difficulty sitting or walking because of a large perineal mass or lump experiences *alterations in comfort* and in *activities of daily living*. In addition, the continued presence and growth of the mass or lump can cause the patient to become anxious and frustrated, resulting in *alterations in coping abilities* and *fear of malignancy*.

Abnormal uterine bleeding can be caused by reproductive disorders (such as the expulsion of the products of conception), changes in hormonal control of the menstrual cycle, tumors, inflammation or trauma, or organic systemic diseases (such as blood dyscrasias). The patient with abnormal uterine bleeding may endure frequent or prolonged menstrual periods, which can cause *alterations in comfort, coping abilities*, and *activities of daily living*

NURSE'S GUIDE TO FEMALE REPRODUCTIVE DISORDERS

	CHIEF COMPLAINT
COMMON INFLAMMATORY AND/OR INFECTIOUS DISORDERS	
***Monilia* (candidiasis)**	• *Discharge:* heavy, with yeasty, sweet odor for preceding 3 to 4 days • *Pain:* dysuria • *Pruritus:* present, with itching
Hemophilus vaginalis	• *Discharge:* fishy odor; gray to yellow-white; soaks through clothing; may last for months • *Pain:* little or none
Trichomoniasis	• *Discharge:* frothy, green-yellow, malodorous, profuse; lasts several days • *Pain:* possible vaginal soreness, burning, dyspareunia • *Pruritus:* vaginal itching
Gonorrhea	• *Discharge:* slight to profuse, purulent • *Pain:* dysuria • *Pruritus:* may be present
Foreign-body vaginitis	• *Discharge:* purulent and fetid, lasting about 1 week • *Pain:* vaginal

	HISTORY	PHYSICAL EXAMINATION AND DIAGNOSTIC STUDIES
	• Predisposing factors include increased emotional stress, birth control pill use, prior pregnancy, diabetes mellitus, antibiotic or steroid therapy, severe illness. • Premenstrual onset • Episodes recur; may lead to chronic cervicitis and erosion. • If untreated, may lead to excoriation and secondary infection.	• White curdlike profuse discharge on vulva, vagina, and cervix; erythema; pruritus; edema of vulvovaginal area • Culture; wet smear with 10% potassium hydroxide to confirm diagnosis
	• Predisposing factors include frequent sexual activity, birth control pill use, frequent douching, sex with partner who doesn't use condom. • Episodes recur, leading to cervical erosion. • If untreated, may lead to contact dermatitis and secondary infection.	• Wet smear (clue cells) identifies organism.
	• Predisposing factors include prior pregnancy, sex with partner who doesn't use condom, close contact with infected person. • Premenstrual onset • Most common in females of childbearing age • Complications may include urinary tract infection, inflammation of Skene's and Bartholin's glands, increased cervical cancer risk.	• Erythema and edema of vulvovagina • Raised petechial lesions (strawberry epithelia) on vagina and cervix • Wet-mount smear of vaginal secretions made with physiologic saline (motile protozoa)
	• Frequent sexual activity is a predisposing factor. • Usually asymptomatic • Most common in females in their teens and 20s • Complications include urethritis, bartholinitis, proctitis, salpingitis, pharyngitis, stomatitis, and conjunctivitis. • If untreated, may lead to systemic infection, including pelvic inflammatory disease, skin eruptions on trunk and legs, arthritis, and tendonitis.	• Urethral meatus may be erythematous and, when milked, may exude pus. • Cervix may be reddened and edematous. • Gram's stain smear for gram-negative diplococci; culture on Thayer-Martin media to confirm diagnosis
	• Predisposing factors include pessary, tampon, or diaphragm use; emotional instability; memory instability; inadequate sex education; use of intravaginal object for sexual pleasure. • Complications include vaginal fistula, cervical erosion, and adhesions.	• Obstructing mass in vagina that causes pain on removal • Possible laceration of cervix or vaginal mucosa • Culture taken

(continued)

NURSE'S GUIDE TO FEMALE REPRODUCTIVE DISORDERS *(continued)*

	CHIEF COMPLAINT	
Atrophic vaginitis	• *Discharge:* follows intercourse or long walks; may go unnoticed by patient • *Pain:* vaginal burning and soreness; postcoital discomfort and dyspareunia possible • *Abnormal uterine bleeding:* spotting possible after douching or after intercourse • *Pruritus:* vaginal itching	
Genital herpes II	• *Discharge:* watery; accompanies appearance of lesions • *Pain:* blisters and/or sores for preceding 1 or 2 days; prodromal symptoms of burning or tingling in genital area possible; *may* be asymptomatic; severe vulval pain following appearance of lesions; severe dysuria or retention possible • *Lumps, masses, ulcerations:* blisters and ulcers covering extensive areas of the vulva and the perianal skin • *Pruritus:* mild itching in genital area preceding eruption of lesions	
Primary syphilis	• *Discharge:* none • *Pain:* none • *Lumps, masses, ulcerations:* solitary, hard, oval ulcer (chancre) on vulva, perineum, labia, cervix, and possibly breasts, fingers, lips, oral mucosa, tongue for several days to weeks • *Pruritus:* none	
Pubic lice	• *Pruritus:* severe itching of genital hair areas for several days	
Bartholinitis (Bartholin adenitis)	• *Pain:* present in Bartholin's gland; reddened, tender overlying skin • *Lumps, masses, ulcerations:* large lump on one side of genitalia for several days	
Chlamydia	• *Discharge:* purulent, rare • *Pain:* dysuria	

	HISTORY	PHYSICAL EXAMINATION AND DIAGNOSTIC STUDIES
	• Predisposing factors include bilateral oophorectomy and cessation of estrogen therapy. • Postmenopausal onset • If untreated, may lead to secondary infection, altered sexual self-esteem, and possibly marital discord and depressive reaction.	• Dry vulva, possibly vulvitis, friable mucosa, few or absent vaginal rugae, pale and shiny vaginal mucosa, and small and tender cervix
	• Most common in women from late teens to early 30s • Predisposing factors include recent gynecologic or lower urinary tract examination, frequent sexual activity, sex with partner who doesn't use condom, recurrent infection. • If untreated, primary lesions persist for 3 to 6 weeks and heal spontaneously. • Symptoms of fever, malaise, or anorexia possible 3 to 7 days after exposure. • Complications include fever; enlarged, tender inguinal lymph nodes; urinary retention, leading to urinary tract infection, cervical cancer; spontaneous abortion or premature delivery; severely infected newborn if delivered vaginally; possibly viremia.	• Cervix may be covered with yellow-gray film; urethra, bladder, and vulva may be exquisitely tender. • Culture of vesicle or ulcer fluid; Tzanck test confirms diagnosis.
	• Frequent sexual activity is a predisposing factor. • May be asymptomatic between stages	• Enlarged inguinal lymph nodes possible • Fluorescent treponemal antibody absorption test and dark-field examination for syphilis
	• Predisposing factors include frequent sexual activity and household history of lice. • Lice transferred primarily by direct contact. • Infection of any hairy part of body possible.	• Oval, light-colored swellings near base of hair shafts; freckled, erythematous, scratched, petechial and/or edematous skin under pubic hair; lice ova (nits) make pubic hair feel bumpy and irregular.
	• Predisposing factors include frequent sexual activity and use of feminine hygiene product. • Abscess or chronic infection possible	• Tender, hot, hard swelling without purulent drainage on posterior labium • Culture taken
	• Predisposing factors include frequent sexual activity and sex with partner who doesn't use condom. • Most common in women in their teens or 20s. • Usually asymptomatic • Complications include trachoma, conjunctivitis, lymphogranuloma venereum, cervical cancer (long-term), salpingitis, newborn conjunctivitis and pneumonia, postpartum endometritis.	• Rough cervical patches; thickened cervix possible but not common • Culture taken; antibody titer urinalysis performed.

(continued)

NURSE'S GUIDE TO FEMALE REPRODUCTIVE DISORDERS *(continued)*

	CHIEF COMPLAINT	
Condylomata acuminata (venereal warts)	• *Pain:* usually painless but pruritic unless warts become infected or irritated by friction; intercourse may be painful if condylomata are large and/or extensive. • *Lumps, masses, ulcerations:* soft warts on perineal and perianal areas	
Acute pelvic inflammatory disease (PID)	• *Discharge:* history of vaginal discharge of variable duration • *Pain:* sharp, bilateral, and cramping, usually in lower quadrants • *Abnormal uterine bleeding:* irregular bleeding and/or longer, heavier menstrual periods	
Toxic shock syndrome (TSS)	• *Pain:* abdominal; myalgia, arthralgia, headache	
Mastitis	• *Pain:* present, accompanied by tenderness in breast • *Lumps, masses, ulcerations:* hard, reddened breast	
COMMON NONINFLAMMATORY BENIGN LESIONS		
Cystocele (several degrees)	• *Pain:* dysuria, with infection, dragging back pain • *Lumps, masses, ulcerations:* fullness at vaginal opening	

HISTORY	PHYSICAL EXAMINATION AND DIAGNOSTIC STUDIES
• May accompany trichomoniasis; resembles vulval cancer • Predisposing factors include frequent sexual activity, birth control pill use, prior pregnancy, massive immunosuppressive therapy, sex with partner who doesn't use condom.	• Inspection reveals soft, wartlike irregularly shaped growths on vulva and perineum and in perianal, vaginal, and/or cervical areas; in advanced stage, cauliflower or deep rose-colored lesions • Dark-field examination of scrapings from wart cells shows marked vascularization of epidermal cells.
• With PID: history of recent abortion, intrauterine device use, sexually transmitted disease, dysuria, severe dysmenorrhea; with acute PID: nausea, vomiting, and elevated temperature, indicating peritoneal involvement or abscess involvement • If untreated and if patient does not succumb to secondary infection, acute PID becomes chronic, with accompanying complications of pelviperitoneal abscess, massive adhesions, and sterility. • PID may be confused with ruptured appendix, degenerating fibroids, ectopic pregnancy, or perforation of gastrointestinal pelvic abscesses caused by uterine perforations.	• Pelvic examination reveals tender cervix; bilateral adnexal enlargement, tenderness, immobility. • Laboratory analysis usually confirms diagnosis; cultured organism is usually *Streptococcus* or *Neisseria gonorrhoeae.*
• History of tampon use during active vaginal bleeding. Early recognition depends on knowledge of patient's history of tampon use and hygiene, last menstrual period, past menstrual history, and previous episodes of TSS • More common in females but can occur in males • May be confused with any viral systemic illness	• Temperature over 102° F. (38.9° C.), nausea, vomiting, hypotension, photophobia, abdominal pain, myalgia, arthralgia, headache • Culture of *Staphylococcus aureus* from vaginal vault
• Usually occurs 3rd or 4th week postpartum; almost always preceded by history of cracked nipples • If untreated, may evolve into breast abscess, with palpable fluctuance and painful axillary lymphadenopathy	• Firm, tender, warm and reddened area apparent in affected breast • Culture usually yields offending organism: *Staphylococcus aureus.*
• Predisposing factors include multiparity, obesity, chronic ascites, prolonged labors, instrument deliveries, chronic cough, heavy-object lifting. • Symptoms may result in social withdrawal, depression • May be asymptomatic	• Inspection reveals soft, reducible, mucosal mass bulging into anterior introitus; with Valsalva's maneuver, the mass increases and urine may squirt or dribble from meatus. • Laboratory tests include urinalysis.

(continued)

NURSE'S GUIDE TO FEMALE REPRODUCTIVE DISORDERS *(continued)*

	CHIEF COMPLAINT
Rectocele (several degrees)	• *Pain:* backaches possible • *Lumps, masses, ulcerations:* fullness at vaginal opening
Prolapsed uterus (several degrees)	• *Pain:* heaviness in pelvis • *Lumps, masses, ulcerations:* feels as if patient's sitting on a ball • *Abnormal uterine bleeding:* menometrorrhagia
Endometriosis	• *Pain:* menstrual; referred to the rectum and lower sacral or coccygeal regions; dyspareunia probable with uterosacral involvement or vaginal extension; pain on defecation with uterosacral involvement or vaginal extension; dysuria possible • *Abnormal uterine bleeding:* excessive, prolonged, or frequent, with no specific pattern
Uterine leiomyomas (fibroids and myomas)	• *Pain:* in pelvic area; accompanied by sensation of weight or dysmenorrhea • *Lumps, masses, ulcerations:* lump in lower abdomen possible; with large tumors, general enlargement of abdomen • *Abnormal uterine bleeding:* excessive menstrual flow and/or irregular bleeding
Functional ovarian cysts (follicle cysts, corpus luteum cysts)	• *Pain:* with large follicle cysts, mild pelvic discomfort, low back pain, or deep dyspareunia possible; with corpus luteum cysts, localized pain and tenderness possible • *Abnormal uterine bleeding:* with follicle cysts, occasional menstrual irregularities; with corpus luteum cysts, delayed menstruation, followed by persistent bleeding
Fibroadenoma of breast	• *Pain:* absent • *Lumps, masses, ulcerations:* well-defined mass or masses found in breast

	HISTORY	PHYSICAL EXAMINATION AND DIAGNOSTIC STUDIES
	• Predisposing factors include multiparity, obesity, chronic ascites, prolonged labors, instrument deliveries, chronic cough, heavy-object lifting. • May be accompanied by chronic constipation, laxative and enema dependency, iatrogenic diarrhea • Most common in postmenopausal women	• Inspection reveals mass bulging into posterior introitus.
	• Predisposing factors include those for cystocele and rectocele, as well as history of sacral nerve disorders, diabetic neuropathy, and pelvic tumors. • Commonly associated with cystocele and rectocele • Commonly accompanied by urinary tract infection, constipation, and painful defecation but may be asymptomatic	• Cervix palpable, closer to introitus, and can be pushed in caudally; in advanced stage, mucosa of exposed mass outside introitus is ulcerated and friable.
	• Most common in women ages 25 to 45 • History of menstrual disturbances • Commonly accompanied by constipation, pain with defecation during menstruation, infertility	• Multiple tender nodules palpable along the uterosacral ligaments or in the rectovaginal septum of the posterior fornix of the vagina. • Diagnosis can be confirmed only by visualization of the lesion; accomplished directly, with external lesions, or by laparotomy or endoscopy with internal lesions. • Uterus may be fixed in retroposition; attempts to move it accompanied by severe pain. • Endometrial cysts present as irregular enlargement of ovary.
	• History of involuntary infertility or repeat spontaneous abortion • Accompanying symptoms include irritability, increased frequency of urination, possibly dysuria, constipation, and occasionally pain on defecation.	• Bimanual examination may reveal one or more nodular outgrowths on the uterine surface or within the uterine wall.
	• Most common in women ages 20 to 40 • May be asymptomatic	• Bimanual palpation may reveal presence of cyst. • Laparoscopy or laporotomy may be performed to confirm diagnosis.
	• Most common in women in their teens or early 20s • Asymptomatic other than mass	• Palpation reveals round, firm, discrete, movable mass, ⅜″ to 2″ (1 to 5 cm) in diameter; usually solitary but may be multiple and bilateral. • Excision necessary for definitive diagnosis.

(continued)

NURSE'S GUIDE TO FEMALE REPRODUCTIVE DISORDERS *(continued)*

	CHIEF COMPLAINT
Fibrocystic disease of the breast (mammary dysplasia, cystic adenosis, chronic cystic disease, cystic mastitis)	• *Discharge:* may be slight • *Pain:* cyst pain and tenderness possible, especially in premenstrual phase of cycle • *Lumps, masses, ulcerations:* thickened, nodular areas in breast (usually bilateral)
Mammary duct ectasia	• *Discharge:* from nipple, accompanied by nipple retraction • *Pain:* in affected areas • *Lumps, masses, ulcerations:* rubbery lesions in breasts; inflammation
COMMON MALIGNANT DISEASES	
Endometrial cancer	• *Pain:* present in later invasive stages of disease • *Abnormal uterine bleeding:* spotting for days to months; may go undetected
Ovarian carcinoma	• *Pain:* abdominal, in later stage of disease • *Lumps, masses, ulcerations:* mass in lower abdomen; may be first indication of disease; ascites possible • *Abnormal uterine bleeding:* irregular or postmenopausal bleeding possible but infrequent
Carcinoma of cervix in situ (preinvasive)	• *Pain:* absent • *Lumps, masses, ulcerations:* absent • *Abnormal uterine bleeding:* absent
Breast cancer	• *Discharge:* from nipple, usually bloody • *Pain:* absent; breast pain possible but infrequent • *Lumps, masses, ulcerations:* lump in breast

as well as *fear.*

Pruritus can be caused by local tissue irritation (from breast or vaginal discharge), an allergic reaction, infectious agents, or systemic diseases, such as diabetes or liver disease, that cause metabolites to accumulate in the skin. Pruritus of the perineum or the breasts

	HISTORY	PHYSICAL EXAMINATION AND DIAGNOSTIC STUDIES
	• Most common in women during productive years • May be exacerbated by caffeine intake	• Palpation of breast reveals single or multiple masses; usually bilateral, mobile, well defined and tender. • Diagnosis established by aspiration of cysts or by biopsy.
	• Most common in early stage menopausal and menopausal women.	• Inspection reveals nipple discharge and, possibly, nipple retraction. • Palpation reveals subareolar ducts as rubbery lesions filled with a pastelike material; enlarged regional lymph nodes possible.
	• History of previous estrogen therapy, nulliparousness, obesity, and possibly diabetes, hypertension, or previous curettage, sterility, or poor fertility • Most common in menopausal or postmenopausal women	• Inspection usually reveals brown stain or red stain on crotch clothing; possibly cervical lesion. • Palpation may reveal uterus or adnexal mass, usually nontender. • Laboratory tests include tissue examination by dilatation and curettage or by section biopsy.
	• History of urinary frequency and constipation possible • Most common in early stage menopausal or postmenopausal, nulliparous women • Usually asymptomatic in early stages • May be secondary site of cancer	• Lower genital tract usually normal, but displaced cervix possible. • Bimanual palpation usually delineates ovarian mass; malignant tumors are partly solid, bilateral.
	• Predisposing factors include sexual activity before age 20, continued exposure to multiple sexual partners, infection, genital herpes. • Usually asymptomatic	• Lesion frequently overlooked; friable cervix and erosions or superficial defect of the ectocervix possible • Laboratory tests include Pap test, colposcopy, microscopic examination of biopsy specimen.
	• Most common in white women of middle or upper socioeconomic class and over age 35, and in those with a family history of breast cancer • History of long menstrual cycles; early menses or late menopause; first pregnancy after age 35; endometrial or ovarian cancer	• Inspection may reveal enlarged, shrunken, or dimpled breast, with nipple erosion, retraction, and/or discharge; abnormality may not be obvious. • Palpation reveals lump, which is usually nontender, firm or hard, irregularly shaped and fixed to skin or fixed to underlying tissues; enlarged surrounding lymph nodes possible. • Laboratory tests include mammography, biopsy, and thermography.

can cause *alterations in comfort.* Constant scratching to relieve the itch can result in *alterations in skin integrity* and *potential for secondary infection.* If the scratching intensifies, particularly in the perineal area, the result could be an *alteration in activities of daily living.*

CASE HISTORIES: NURSING DIAGNOSIS FLOWCHART

Patient A
Martha Sullivan
age 60

Problem
BREAST LUMP

Subjective data

- Discovered a "long lump" in right breast while taking shower last weekend
- Complains of sleeplessness and fatigue since discovery of lump
- No known family history of breast cancer
- Had hysterectomy for fibroids 20 years ago

Objective data

- Anxious
- Elevated systolic blood pressure
- Atrophied, pendulous breasts
- Firm, nontender, thickened ridge within lower quadrants of both breasts
- No dimpling
- No nipple retraction
- No flattening
- No lymphadenopathy
- Pelvic examination within normal limits for age

Nursing diagnoses

- Ineffective coping ability due to stress
- Fear of malignancy
- Lack of knowledge of breast self-examination
- Altered rest-activity pattern due to anxiety

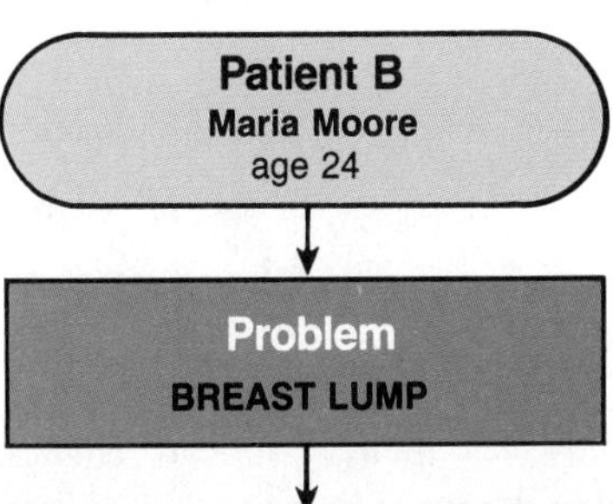

Subjective data

- Boyfriend discovered tender lump in her right breast last month and insisted she have lump checked (patient cannot feel lump)
- Previous menstrual period 3 weeks ago; duration: usual 4 days; tampon use: two or three per day
- Does not know how to perform a breast self-examination
- Maternal aunt had mastectomy at age 40 for cancer
- Used Ortho-Novum 1/50 for 2 years

Objective data

- Slender, relaxed and comfortable with sexuality
- Jokes inappropriately about lump
- Right breast slightly larger than left breast
- Left nipple inverted but easily everted by gentle palpation
- No masses
- No retraction
- No flattening
- No enlarged pores
- No induration
- No discharge
- Multiparous cervix; no sign of yeast infection on pelvic examination

Nursing diagnoses

- Lack of knowledge of normal female physiology
- Anxiety due to family history of breast cancer
- Lack of knowledge of breast self-examination
- Fear of malignancy and deformity
- Ineffective coping: denial
- Disturbance in self-concept due to potential for deformity
- Potential for social isolation if breast is removed

Assessing pediatric patients

572 New assessment approach

In recent years, health-care professionals have come to realize that female infants, children, and adolescents can develop the same gynecologic problems as adult women. Consequently, appropriate assessment of external genitalia during well-baby, well-child, and adolescent examinations is becoming a routine part of pediatric physical examinations. Assessment of your pediatric patient's external genitalia can reveal conditions that necessitate early intervention to prevent serious (and possibly irreversible) damage.

573 The pediatric gynecologic period

The pediatric gynecologic period usually begins during a girl's eighth or ninth year, when signs of sexual maturation become apparent. The mons pubis thickens and begins to grow genital hair, sparsely at first. The clitoris enlarges and the hymen, previously thin and transparent, thickens. The ovaries begin to secrete estrogen, stimulating vulvovaginal tissue. Fat deposits cause the labia majora to enlarge. Sebaceous glands become active. The vagina lengthens—from 1⅘" to 2⅕" (4.5 to 5.5 cm) during early childhood to 3⅕" (8 cm) in the pediatric gynecologic period. By the onset of menarche, the vagina is normally about 4 ⅖" (11 cm) long.

The mucosal lining of the endocervix usually remains unchanged during late childhood. The lining's epithelial growth, which creates the glandular structure of the adult cervix, becomes apparent only after menstruation occurs.

As menarche approaches, the ovaries lengthen and assume an almond shape. Follicular activity occurs during this time, with larger follicles appearing in various stages of development. Although some follicles may become quite large, ovulation doesn't occur. Eventually, the follicles regress.

574 Premenarchal period

During this period, which in most girls spans ages 10 to 12, estrogen secretion by the ovaries creates additional significant changes. The mucosa of the hymen and the vagina become increasingly pink and moist; the vaginal mucosa also thickens. The vaginal lining's rugae begin to develop. Vaginal discharge increases 3 to 12 months before onset of menstruation. The vagina's pH usually ranges from 4.5 to 5.5.

Most girls have significant amounts of a benign discharge during the premenarchal period. However, you may have to perform a microscopic or gynecologic examination, and perhaps obtain cultures, to rule out infection.

Secondary sex characteristics, including breast development, become apparent during the premenarchal period. Changes in fat deposition, especially in the hip area, cause the girl's figure to become rounder. Pubic hair assumes the triangular pattern characteristic of the adult; hair grows in the axillae. And breast development, which can be described in three stages, occurs. In the first stage, the areolae rise and take on their characteristic color, depending on the girl's pigmentation. During the second stage, fat deposition and the growth of glandular structures cause domelike projections. The breasts achieve full development during the third stage, when the nipples project and become erect in response to external stimuli.

575 Early adolescence

Early adolescence begins with onset of menarche (average age 12.9 years) and ends with the first ovulation. This phase usually lasts 3 to 12 months, but it may be as short as 1 month. If a girl ovulates before her first period, technically this phase of adolescence doesn't occur.

As onset of menarche approaches, a girl's vulval skin glands become more active and her vagina lengthens and widens. On pelvic examination, you'll detect anteflexion of the uterus as it widens and grows, developing into an adultlike structure. Some tubal peristalsis may exist, but full progression doesn't occur until ovulation is established.

You can't determine the status of an adolescent girl's fertility unless you use a basal body temperature chart or perform an endometrial biopsy. The unpredictable onset of fertility can create problems for a sexually active adolescent, who may erroneously think she isn't old enough to become pregnant.

576 Educational experience

Your assessment of the adolescent patient should be an educational experience for her. Begin by explaining the examination procedures to the patient and to her parent. (Usually her mother brings her for the examination.) If the patient prefers that her mother not be present during the examination, tactfully ask the mother to leave the room. Use visual aids to supplement your explanations. Most young women are receptive to the idea of viewing their genitalia in a mirror during the examination. You might use one, if appropriate, to teach the patient about female anatomy.

577 Extent of the examination

The extent of a gynecologic examination for a pediatric patient depends on the child's age and her chief complaint. Inspection and palpation of the external genitalia usually suffice for a well-child examination. In some cases, you may also want to include inspection and palpation of her breasts and abdomen. (See Entries 579, 459, and 461.)

Bimanual palpation is never performed on a premenarchal child unless a serious gynecologic problem exists, such as anomalies of the external genitalia, vaginal bleeding (in a girl under age 8), or a possible foreign body in the vagina. It should be done only by a specially prepared nurse or a doctor.

Perform a complete examination on a postmenarchal adolescent if you suspect a gynecologic problem, if the patient is sexually active, if she practices birth control, or if she requests information on contraception.

578 Positioning the pediatric patient

The way you position a child for an assessment of her external genitalia depends mainly on her age. You should also consider other individual factors, such as her size and the extent of her sexual activity. Use the following guidelines:

- *Birth to age 3.* Position the child on the parent's lap, with her back reclining against the parent's chest at a 45° angle. To facilitate your examination, have the parent hold the child's knees against her chest.
- *Ages 3 to 5.* An examining table may be used for a child in this age-group. Position the table with the head at a 30° angle and rest the child against the incline. Have the parent hold the child's knees against her chest.
- *Ages 6 to 15.* The child should lie flat or at a slightly upward angle on an examining table, in a modified lithotomy position—legs flexed at the knees, heels close to the buttocks. Separate the knees so that the genitalia are visible. Have the mother, if present, stand at the head of the table and help the child keep her knees spread.
- *Over age 15.* Use the lithotomy position, as for an adult.

579 How to examine the pediatric patient

When you examine the pediatric patient's breasts, remember that development doesn't actually begin until age 8 or 9. However, you may notice a firm, flat, buttonlike structure beneath the nipples, evidence of initial breast tissue growth.

After warming your hands, palpate the child's abdomen thoroughly. You'll feel the ovaries high in the pelvis. Because of the small pelvic cavity, if an ovarian tumor is present, it will be palpable toward midabdomen.

Before you begin the actual pelvic examination, tell the child to inform you immediately if she experiences any discomfort. First, make a general assessment of the external genitalia, noting any signs of poor perineal hygiene. If a dermatologic condition exists on the external genitalia, consider possible nutritional deficiencies, especially of the B complex vitamins. Begin your examination of the patient's genitalia by inspecting for the presence of pubic hair. Inspect and palpate the labia and clitoris for abnormal size for the child's age and for adhesions and signs of infection. Inspect the urethral meatus for redness, rashes, abnormal positioning (midline is normal), and discharge. Inspect the vaginal introitus for lesions, redness, swelling, rashes, and discharge. For maximum visualization of the introitus, ask the child to cough when you separate her labia. A foul-smelling, blood-streaked purulent discharge may indicate the presence of a foreign body. A domelike, outwardly bulging, purple-red membrane may indicate an imperforate hymen. (The membrane's appearance is caused by the collection of menstrual fluid behind it.) Finally, inspect and, if necessary, palpate the perineum for redness, rashes, and lesions.

If you must inspect the vagina with a speculum, remember that a premenarchal child's vagina is normally short and narrow, and the cervix is flat. Use a pediatric speculum (⅖" to ⅗" or 1 to 1.5 cm wide) for a child or sexually inactive adolescent and a small adult speculum for a sexually active adolescent.

580 Pediatric gynecologic disorders

The following gynecologic disorders occur most commonly among children and adolescents:

• *Nonspecific vulvovaginitis.* This common disorder in premenarchal girls may be caused by a number of conditions, including poor perineal hygiene, respiratory tract infections (a child's hand may carry organisms from the upper respiratory tract to the vaginal area), skin infections and infected wounds, intestinal parasites, and foreign bodies. In most instances, the patient's mother notices the discharge or inflammation and seeks medical attention. The child may also complain of pruritus or dysuria. The vaginal discharge may be scanty or profuse, serous or purulent, but its appearance is not diagnostic.

Vaginitis is also a common complaint in the adolescent. *Candida albicans* is the most common causative organism. Other etiologic factors include birth control pills, deodorants, bactericidal soaps, antibiotics (for acne), and high-carbohydrate diets.

• *Genital injuries.* Most genital injuries are caused by falls, but they may also result from kicking, beating, or sexual assault. When confronted with such an injury in a young girl, inspect for injuries elsewhere on her body. Inspection may reveal vulval contusions and lacerations, vaginal wall lacerations (usually accompanied by vulval injuries), and vaginal hematomas. Depending on the injury, a doctor may order a general anesthetic in order to perform a pelvic examination, urethroscopy, or cystoscopy.

• *Genital tumors.* Although genital tumors in girls under age 14 are uncommon, almost every type of tumor found in women has been reported among girls in this age-group. About 50% of all genital tumors in children are malignant or premalignant. Signs and symptoms of genital tumors include chronic genital ulcer, nontraumatic swelling of the external genitalia, protruding vaginal tissue, bloody discharge, abdominal pain or gross enlargement before age 9, and premature sexual maturation.

• *Precocious puberty.* This condition is characterized by onset of sexual maturation before age 9. Breast development, pubic hair growth, and general acceleration of bodily growth usually precede uterine bleeding by several months. True precocious puberty must be differentiated from *pseudoprecocious puberty.* In true precocious puberty, the ovaries mature and pubertal changes proceed in an orderly manner. In pseudoprecocious puberty, genitalia mature and secondary sex characteristics appear with no corresponding ovarian maturation.

Approximately 85% of all cases of true precocious puberty are caused by early development and activation of the endocrine glands. Other causes include hypothyroidism and central nervous system disorders, such as encephalitis, intracranial neoplasms, McCune-Albright syndrome, and congenital anomalies.

• *Adolescent menstrual problems.* Establishing a regular menstrual cycle often preoccupies teenage girls, who associate it with being normal, feminine, and fertile. An adolescent who hasn't begun to menstruate may feel inadequate and anxious. Careful patient teaching on your part will help dispel her anxiety.

Irregular menstrual function may be accompanied by hemorrhage and resulting anemia. Ask a girl who has this problem how many sanitary napkins or tampons she uses daily and how often she changes them. A complete blood count may be necessary to evaluate blood loss.

An adolescent patient with primary dysmenorrhea usually complains of lower abdominal or back pain during the first 12 to 24 hours of menstruation. Refer such a patient to a doctor for a further evaluation of possible organic problems.

Assessing geriatric patients

581 Physical and emotional changes

Declining estrogen and progesterone levels cause a number of physical changes in an aging woman. Significant emotional changes also take place during the transition from childbearing years to infertility. A postreproductive woman will benefit from counseling and instruction on the changes she'll experience during the latter third of her life. She also needs to know the best way to cope with these changes if she is to continue leading a full and satisfying life.

582 Physical effects of aging

Because a woman's breasts and her internal and external reproductive structures are estrogen-dependent, the aging process takes a more conspicuous toll in the female than in the male. As estrogen levels decrease and menopause approaches, usually at about age 50, the following physiologic changes occur in a woman's reproductive organs:

• *Vulva.* This structure atrophies with age. Changes include pubic hair loss and a flattening of the labia majora. Vulval tissue shrinks, exposing the sensitive area around the urethra and vagina to abrasions and irritation—from undergarments, for example. With age, the introitus also constricts, tissues lose their elasticity, and the epidermis thins from 20 layers to about 5.

• *Vagina.* Atrophy causes the vagina to shorten and the mucous lining to become thin, dry, less elastic, and pale as a result of decreased vascularity. In this state, the vaginal mucosa is highly susceptible to abrasion.

• *Uterus.* After menopause, the uterus atrophies rapidly to half its premenstrual weight. Uterine regression continues until the organ reaches approximately one fourth its premenstrual size. The cervix shrinks and no longer produces mucus for lubrication, and the endometrium and myometrium become thinner.
• *Breasts.* Glandular, supporting, and fatty tissues atrophy. As Cooper's ligaments lose their elasticity, the breasts become pendulous. The nipples decrease in size and become flat and nonerect. Fibrocystic disease that may have been present at menopause usually diminishes and disappears with increasing age. The inframammary ridges become more pronounced.
• *Ovaries.* Ovulation usually stops 1 to 2 years before menopause. As the ovaries reach the end of their productive cycle, they become unresponsive to gonadotropic stimulation.

583 Changes in pelvic support

Relaxation of pelvic support structures is common among postreproductive women. Initial relaxation usually occurs during labor and delivery, but clinical effects often go unnoticed until the process is accelerated by estrogen depletion and loss of connective tissue elasticity and tone, which occurs during menopause. Signs and symptoms include pressure and pulling in the area above the inguinal ligaments, low backache, a feeling of pelvic heaviness, and difficulty in rising from a chair. Urinary stress incontinence may also become a problem if urethrovesical ligaments weaken.

584 History and physical examination

The history questions you'll ask an elderly patient and your physical examination of her reproductive system are basically the same as for a younger woman. However, you'll need to modify your approach to both aspects of the assessment process to deal effectively with the unique problems encountered by elderly women—especially those related to genital atrophy.

A complete gynecologic history of a geriatric patient should include her age at onset of menopause and specific conditions associated with menopause. Did menstrual flow diminish or increase with onset of menopause? Did she experience hot flashes? How long before onset of menopause was her menstrual cycle irregular? Did she notice any psychological changes, such as depression, moodiness, or irritability, as menopause approached?

Also note any bleeding that may have occurred since menopause started. Bleeding that occurs more than 12 months after a woman's last menstrual period must be investigated. If menopause has not yet begun, question your patient about the regularity of her periods. Has the flow recently become lighter or heavier?

Next, tactfully ask the patient about her sexual activity. If she is sexually active, inquire about pain on intercourse and use of lubricant, if any. Also ask if she has symptoms of pelvic relaxation. What are her elimination habits?

When you review an elderly woman's body systems, keep in mind that diminishing estrogen levels can contribute to osteoporosis, a decrease in bone mass that afflicts about 25% of postmenopausal women and results in kyphosis, decreased height, and sometimes fractures.

When you begin the pelvic examination, remember that you may need to use a small speculum because of the decreased vaginal size in older women. To facilitate insertion, dampen the speculum with warm water; don't use a lubricant, because it may alter Pap smear results. Proceed slowly. Abrupt insertion of the speculum can damage sensitive degenerating tissue.

When you perform the bimanual examination, remember that the ovaries normally regress with age, and you may not be able to palpate them.

585 Gynecologic disorders in geriatric patients

The most common gynecologic disorders in postreproductive women are the following:

- *Vulval disorders.* External agents easily damage the vulva's atrophic skin and mucosa, resulting in irritation or abrasions. *Dyspareunia* results or increases when vulval shrinkage reduces the size of the vaginal introitus. Introital distention may cause lacerations (this condition is less common among women who have regular intercourse). Estrogenic cream applied locally may improve the condition. Intense *vulval itching* may result from sensitive vulval mucosa, senile vulvitis, senile vaginitis, urinary incontinence, or poor perineal hygiene. Underlying causes include infection, nutritional deficiency, allergy, trauma, and psychogenic factors.
- *Vaginal disorders.* Estrogen depletion can produce *atrophic* or *senile vaginitis.* Monilial infection may cause superficial vaginal ulcers that will bleed when touched. Monilial infection is often accompanied by diabetes mellitus. As the infection heals, adhesions may develop between the ulcerated areas. *Trichomonas* and *Hemophilus* infections are uncommon in elderly women.
- *Uterine disorders.* Superficial ulceration may develop on an atrophied endometrium, possibly accompanied by spotting or bleeding. (Postmenopausal bleeding may also originate from the cervix, the vagina, or the vulva.) Bleeding that occurs at least 1 year after menopause may indicate a malignant tumor in the uterus.
- *Reproductive cancers.* During the early stages, such cancers are usually asymptomatic. Breast cancer is the most common malignant neoplasm in women. Whereas cervical cancer occurs most often in women between ages 40 and 44, endometrial cancer is most common in women between ages 60 and 64. Ovarian cancer affects more women between ages 65 and 69 than in any other age-group, and the incidence remains high until about age 79.

Selected References

Bates, Barbara. *A Guide to Physical Examination,* 2nd ed. Philadelphia: J.B. Lippincott Co., 1979.

Beeson, Paul B., et al. *Cecil Textbook of Medicine,* 15th ed. Philadelphia: W.B. Saunders, 1979.

Benson, Ralph C., ed. *Current Obstetric and Gynecologic Diagnosis and Treatment,* 2nd ed. Los Altos, Calif.: Lange Medical Publications, 1978.

DeGowin, Elmer L., and DeGowin, Richard L. *Bedside Diagnostic Examination,* 3rd ed. New York: Macmillan Publishing Co., 1976.

Glass, Robert H. *Office Gynecology.* Baltimore: Williams and Wilkins Co., 1976.

Harvey, A.M. *The Principles and Practice of Medicine,* 20th ed. New York: Appleton-Century-Crofts, 1980.

Hogen, Rosemarie. *Human Sexuality: A Nursing Perspective.* New York: Appleton-Century-Crofts, 1980.

Keith, Louis, and Brittain, Jan. *Sexually Transmitted Diseases.* Edited by John P. Wells, translated by A.A. Yuzpe. New York: Irvington Publishing, 1978.

Malasanos, Lois, et al. *Health Assessment,* 2nd ed. St. Louis: C.V. Mosby Co., 1981.

Martin, L. *Health Care of Women.* Philadelphia: J.B. Lippincott Co., 1978.

Novak, Edmund, et al. *Textbook of Gynaecology,* 9th ed. Baltimore: Williams and Wilkins Co., 1975.

Novak, Edmund. *Novak's Gynecologic and Obstetric Pathology: With Clinical and Endocrine Relations.* Philadelphia: W.B. Saunders, 1979.

Pope, Thomas L. "Toxic Shock Syndrome," *The Nurse Practitioner* 6:31, September-October 1981.

Romney, S., et al. *Gynecology and Obstetrics: The Health Care of Women.* New York: McGraw-Hill Book Co., 1975.

Rossman, I., ed. *Clinical Geriatrics,* 2nd ed. New York: J.B. Lippincott, 1979.

Williams, Robert H. *Textbook of Endocrinology,* 6th ed. Philadelphia: W.B. Saunders, 1981.

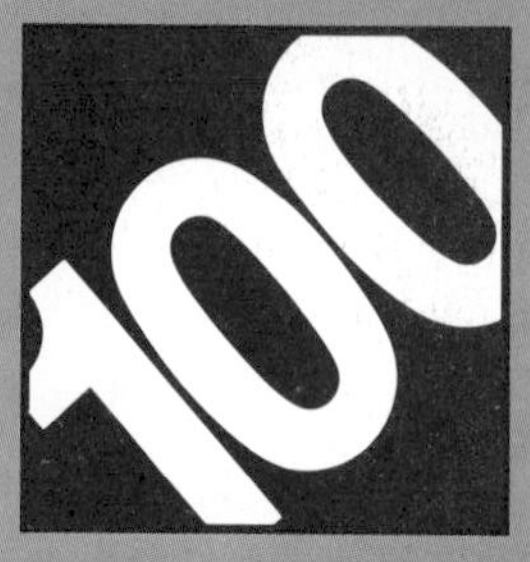

Atlas of One Hundred Common Abnormalities

Introduction

You'll find 100 photographs and illustrations of common abnormalities—most in full color—in the 17 pages that follow. The abnormalities are grouped as follows:

- skin, hair, and nails
- eyes and vision
- ears and hearing
- respiratory system
- cardiovascular system
- gastrointestinal system
- male reproductive system
- female reproductive system
- musculoskeletal system
- endocrine system.

These photographs and illustrations provide a useful guide to recognizing and differentiating some of the disorders you're likely to see in hospitalized patients.

The abnormalities are numbered for identification purposes only; their order has no clinical significance.

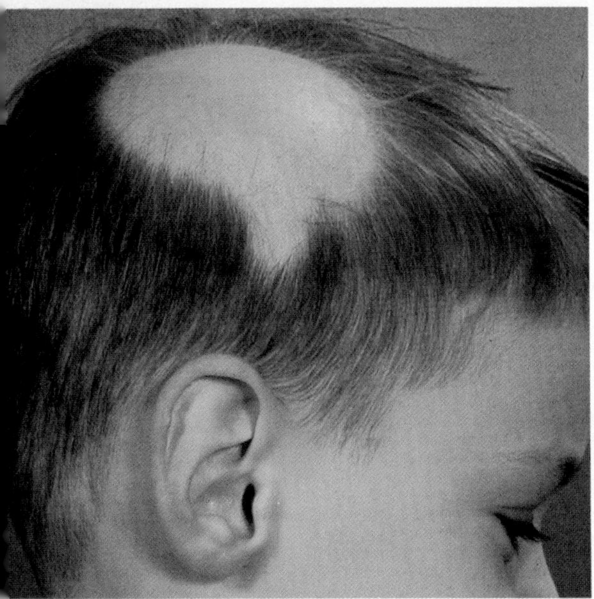

1 Alopecia areata

5 Scabies

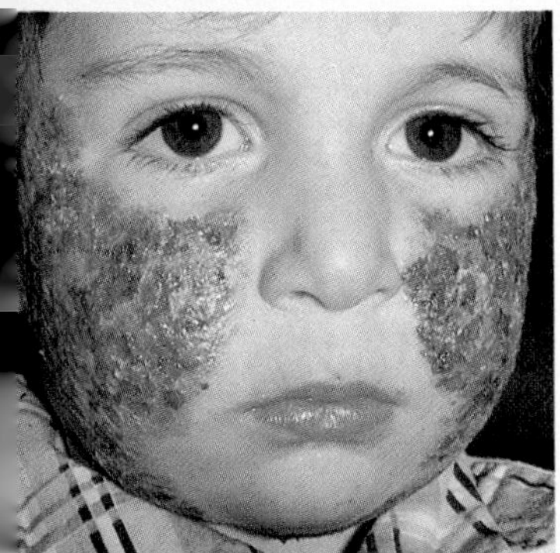

2 Atopic dermatitis

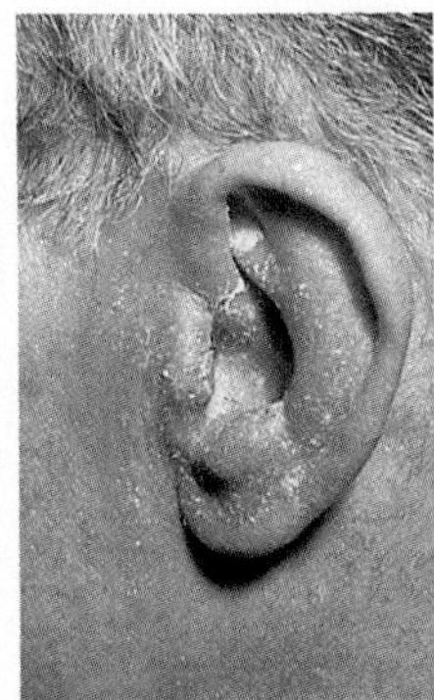

3 Seborrheic dermatitis

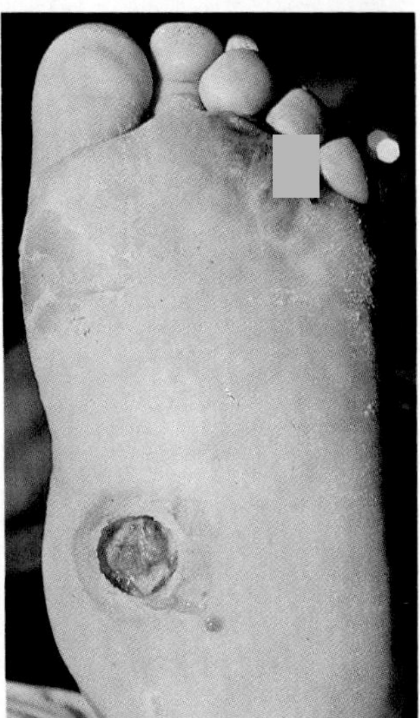

6 Diabetic ulcer

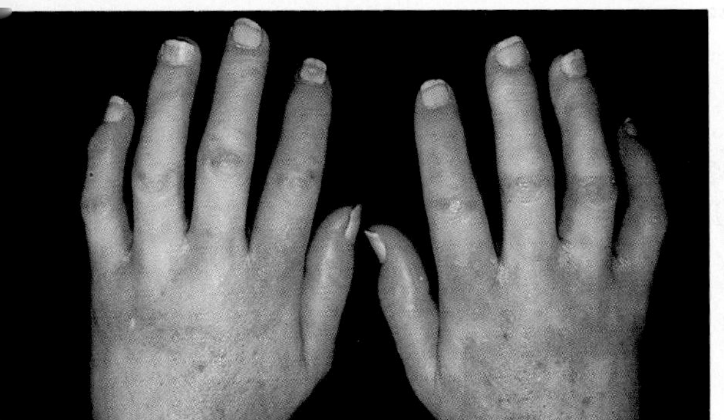

4 Systemic sclerosis

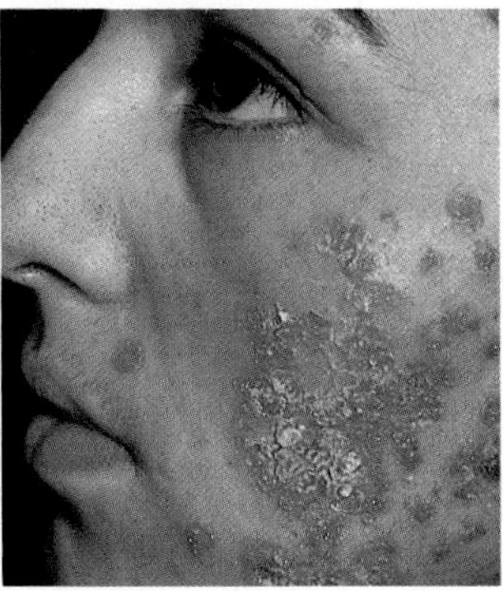

7 Impetigo contagiosa

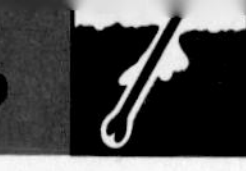

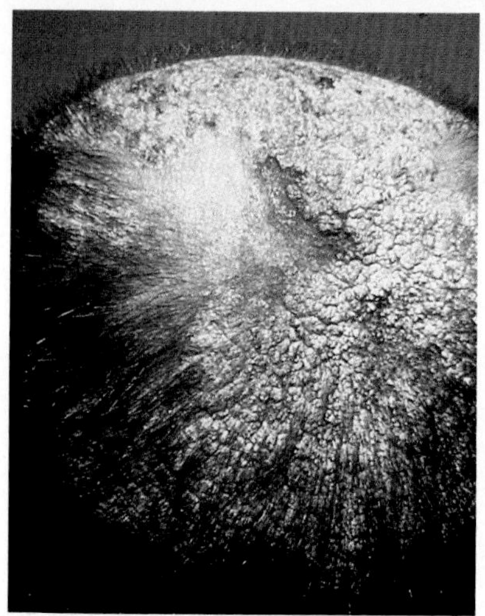

8 Psoriasis

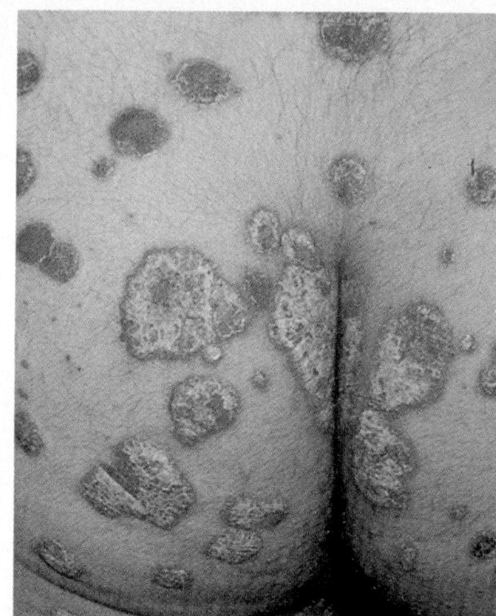

9 Psoriasis

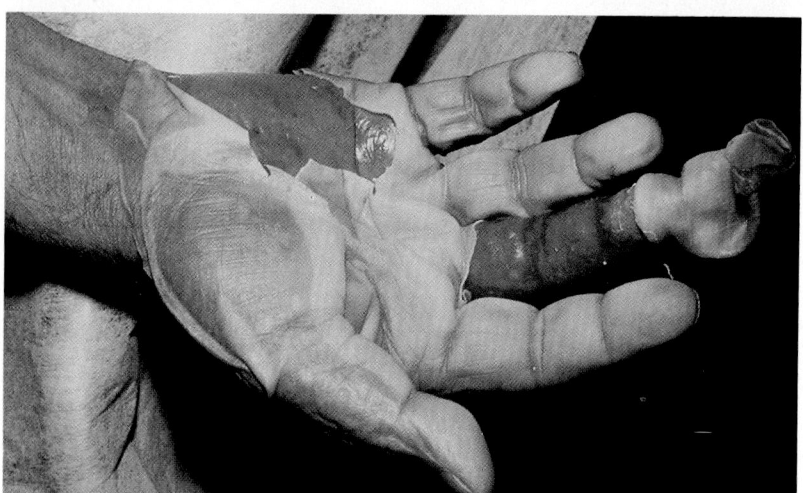

10 Toxic epidermal necrolysis

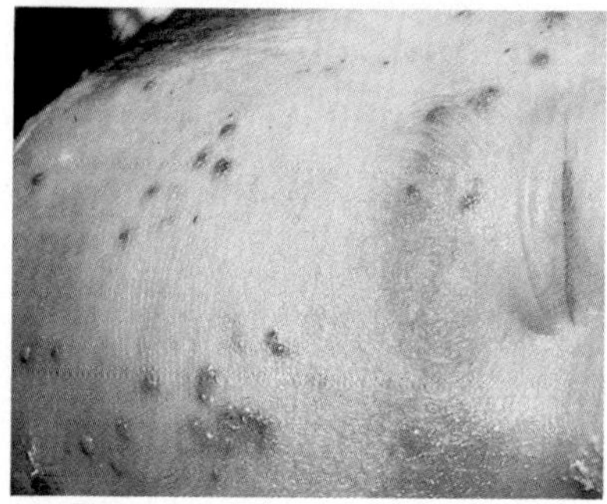

11 Disseminated herpes simplex

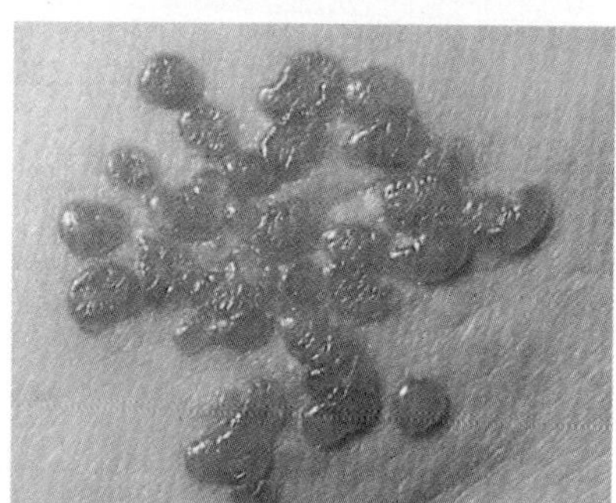

12 Herpes zoster

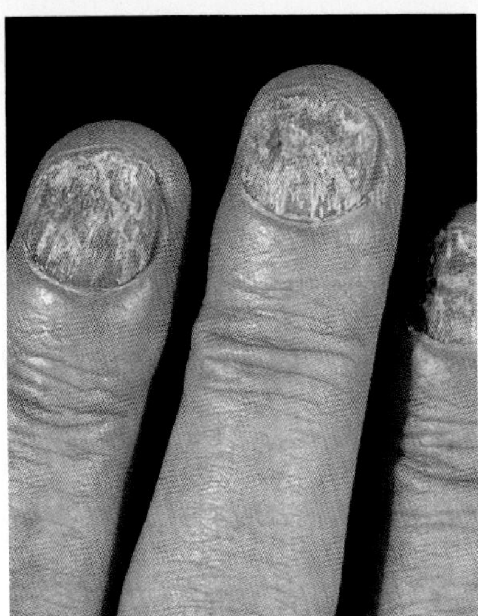
13 Tinea unguium

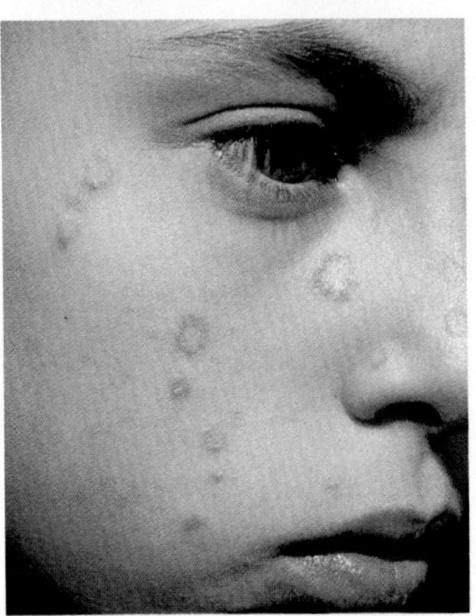
14 Tinea faciale

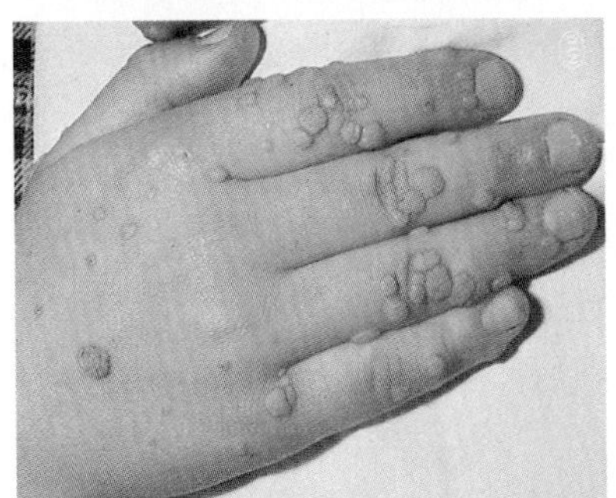
15 Verruca vulgaris

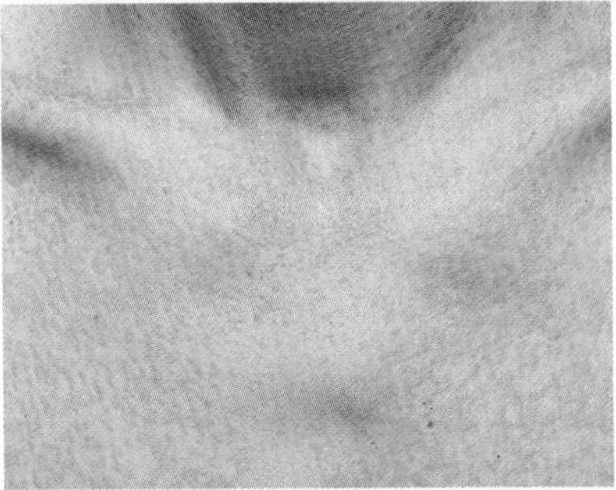
16 Tinea versicolor

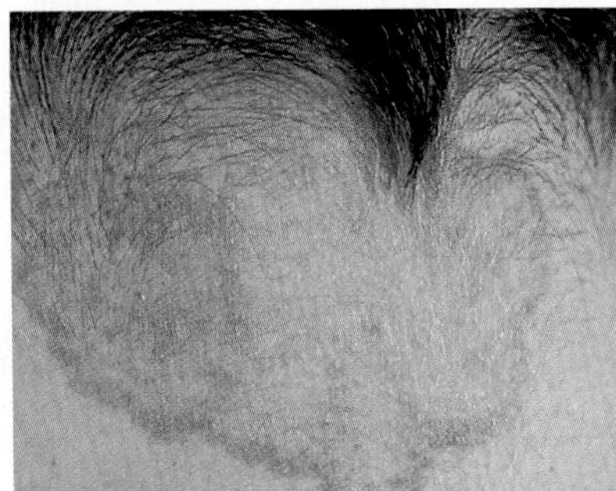
17 Tinea corporis

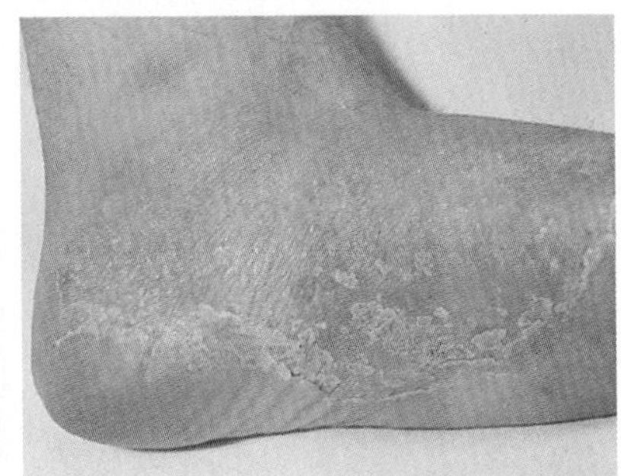
18 Tinea pedis

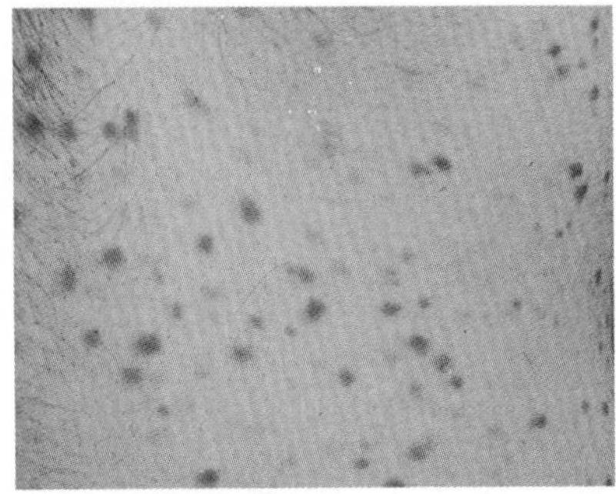
19 Urticaria pigmentosa

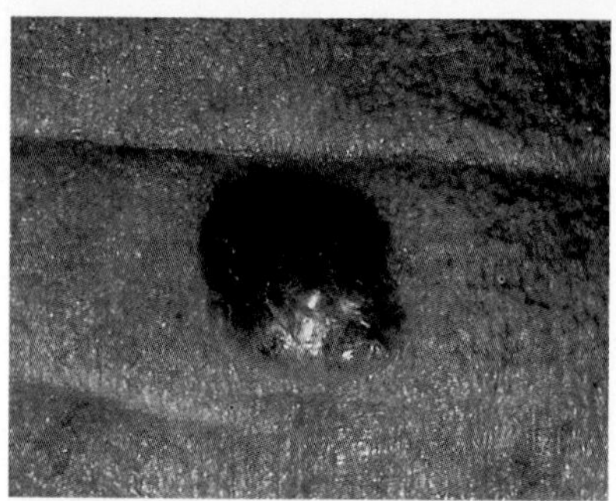

20 Basal cell carcinoma

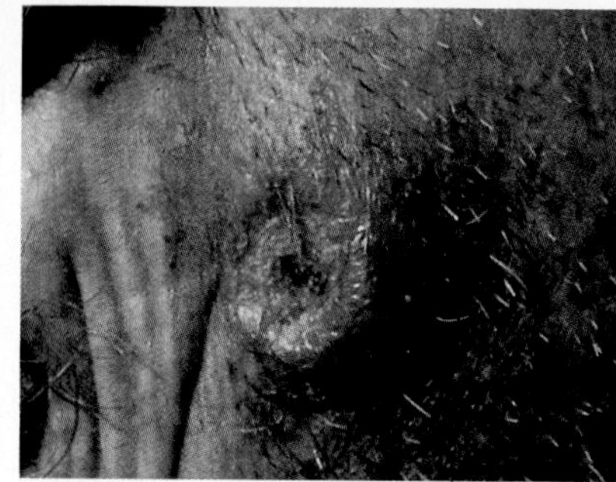

21 Squamous cell carcinoma

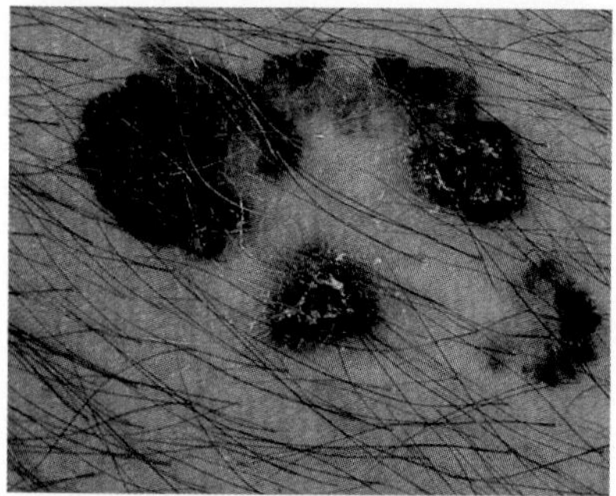

22 Superficial spreading melanoma

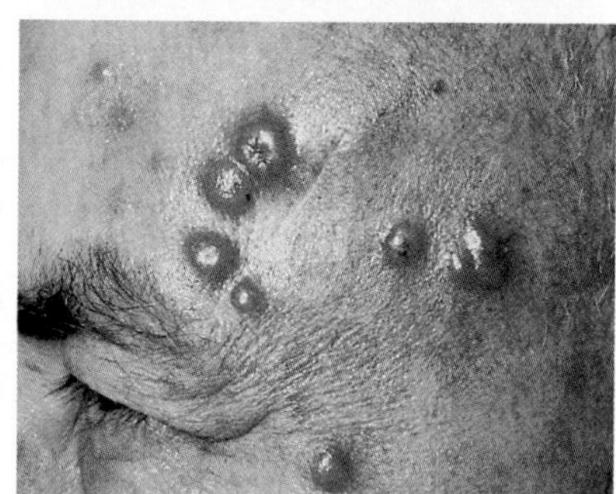

23 Lymphoma

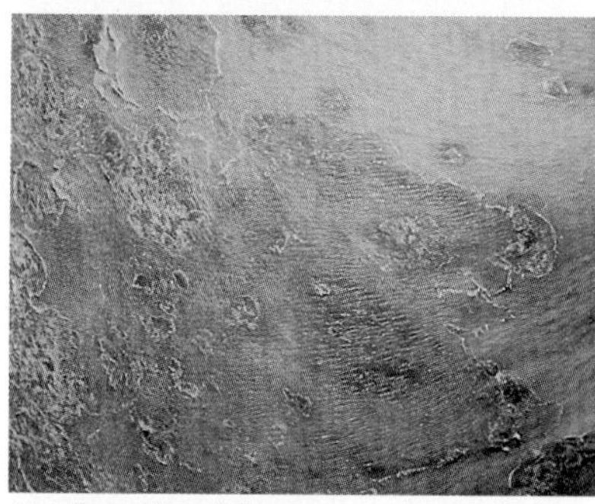

24 Pemphigus foliaceus

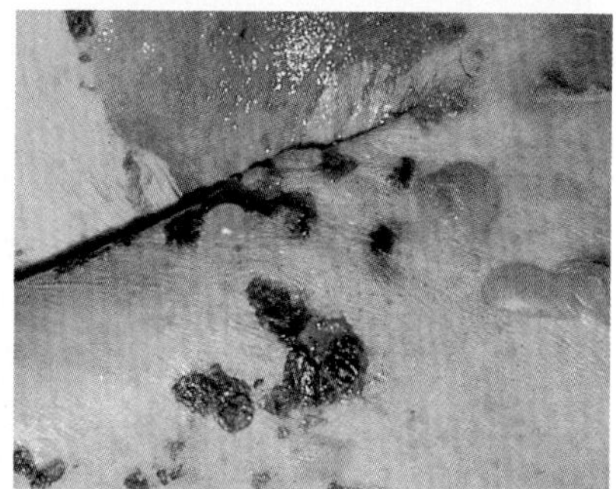

25 Pemphigus vulgaris

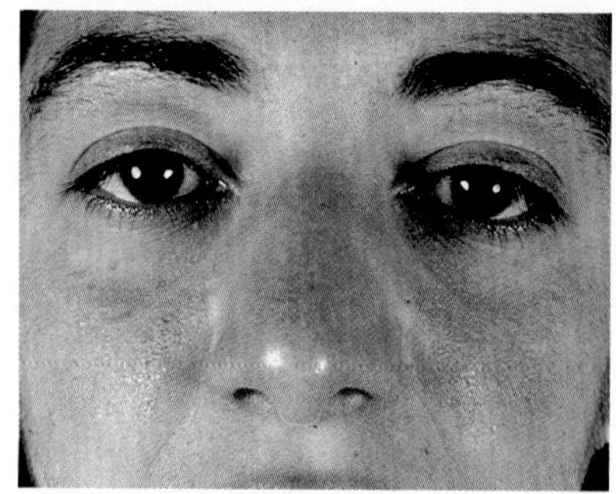

26 Lupus erythematosus

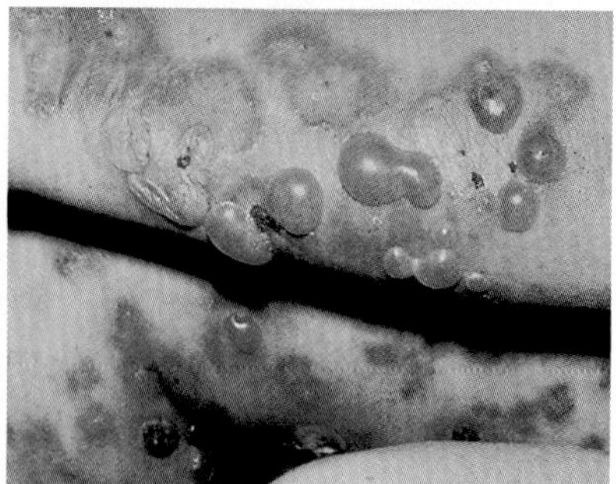

27 Bullous pemphigoid

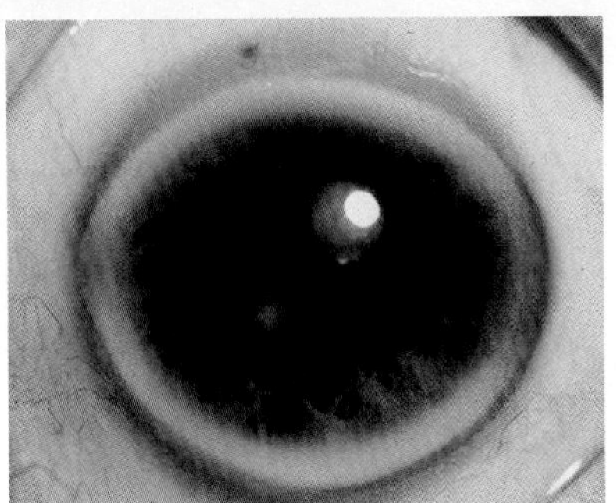

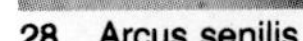

28 Arcus senilis

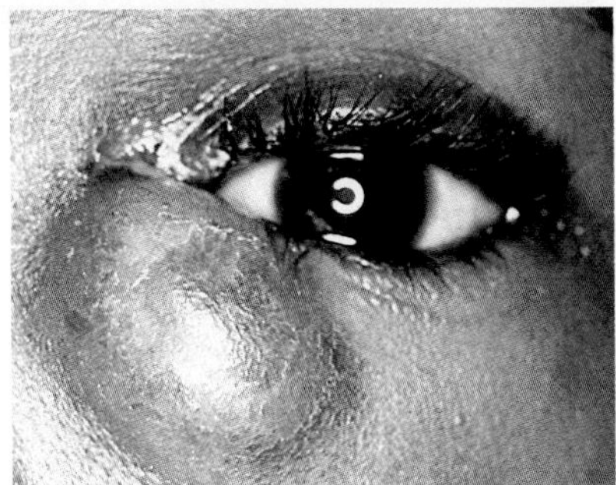

29 Acute dacryocystitis

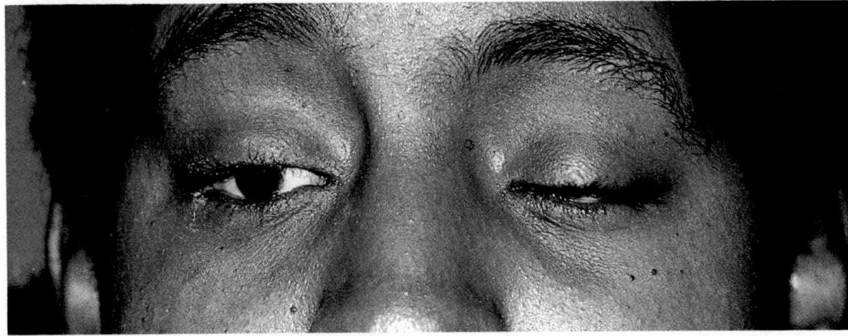

30 Ptosis

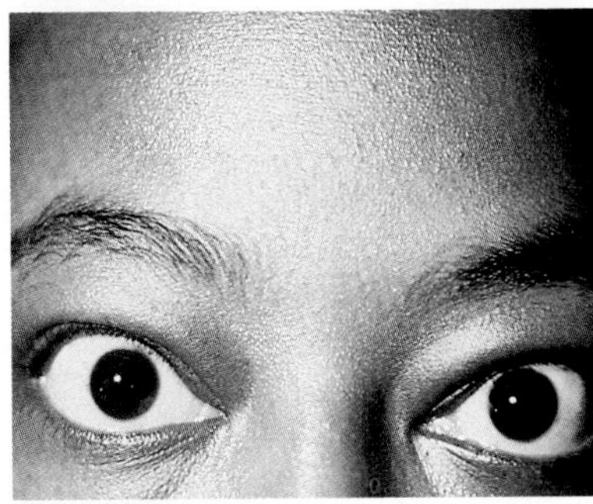

31 Exophthalmos

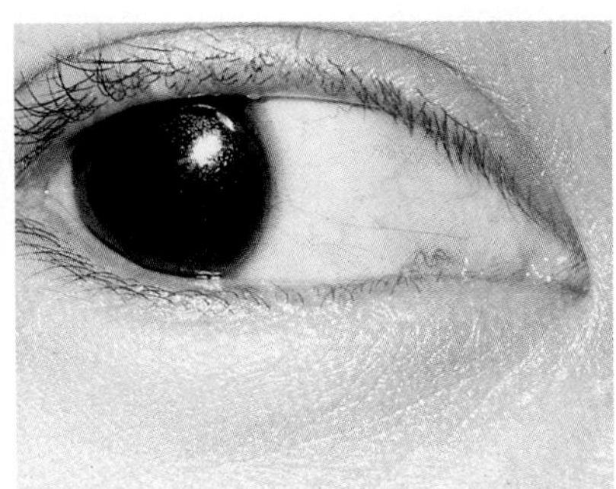

32 Pinguecula

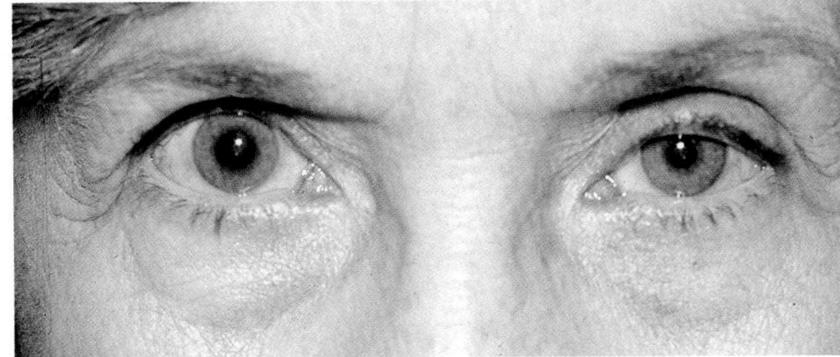

33 Horner's syndrome

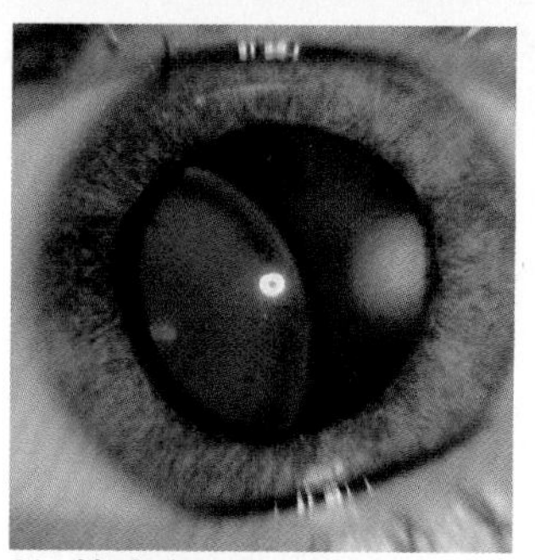
34 Marfan's syndrome

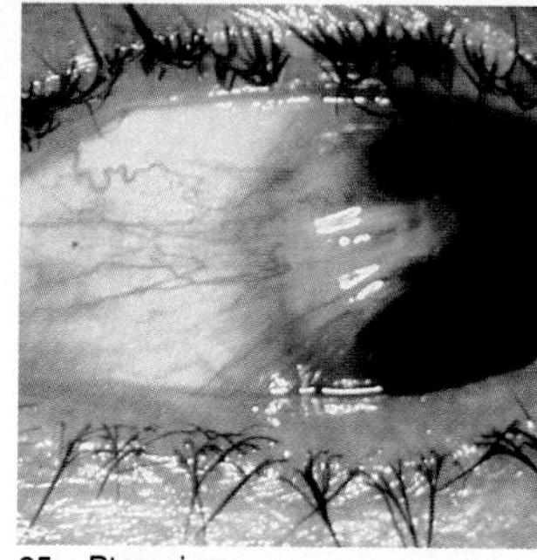
35 Pterygium

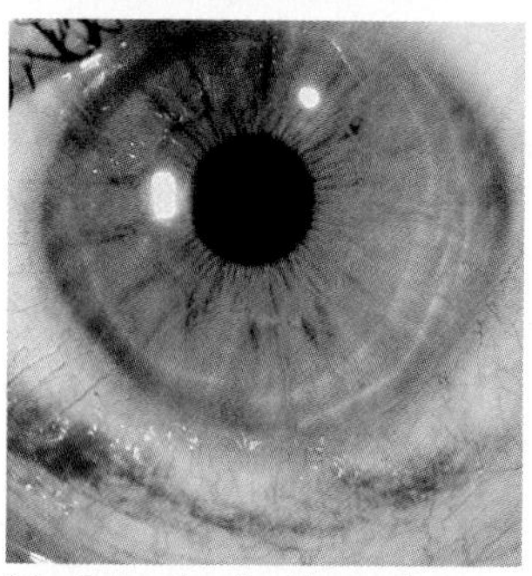
36 Subconjunctival hemorrhage

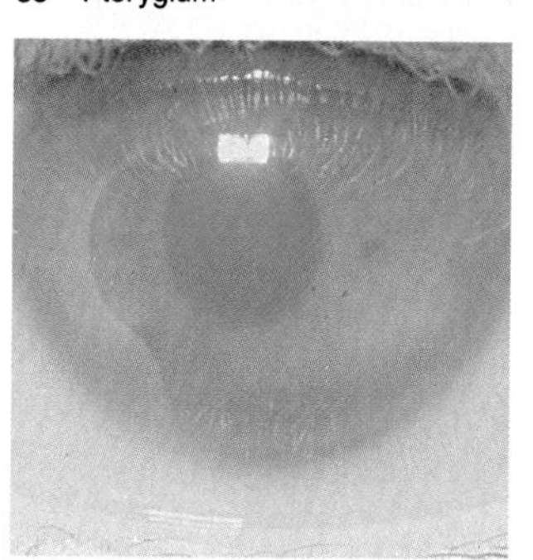
37 Hyphema

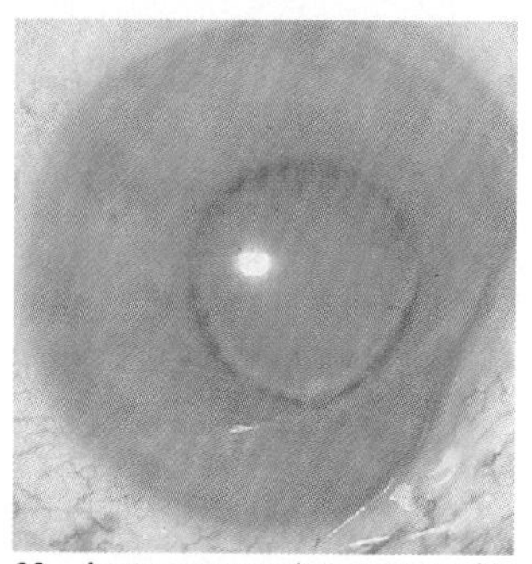
38 Acute nongranulomatous uveitis

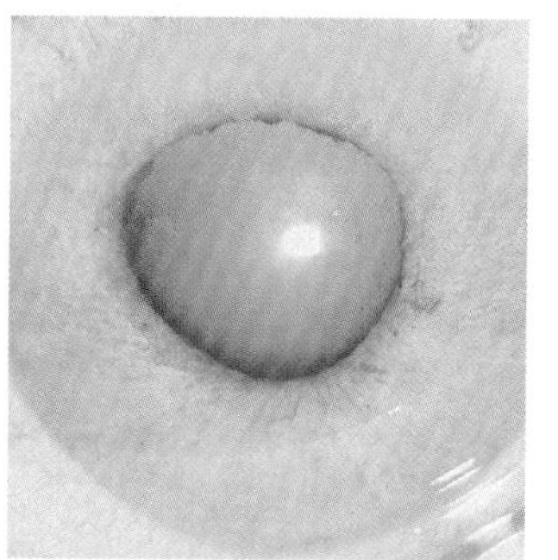
39 Acute glaucoma

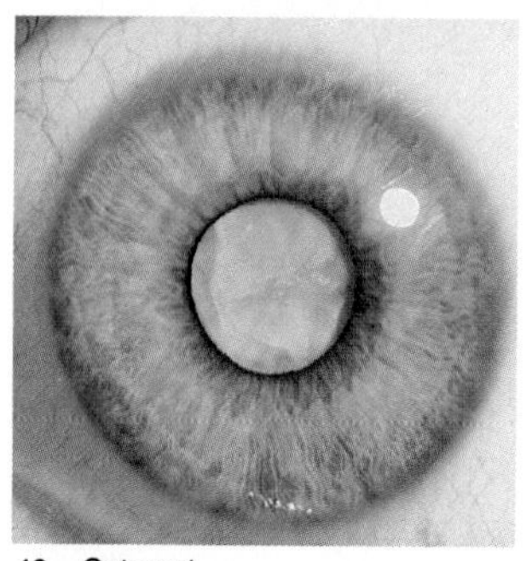
40 Cataract

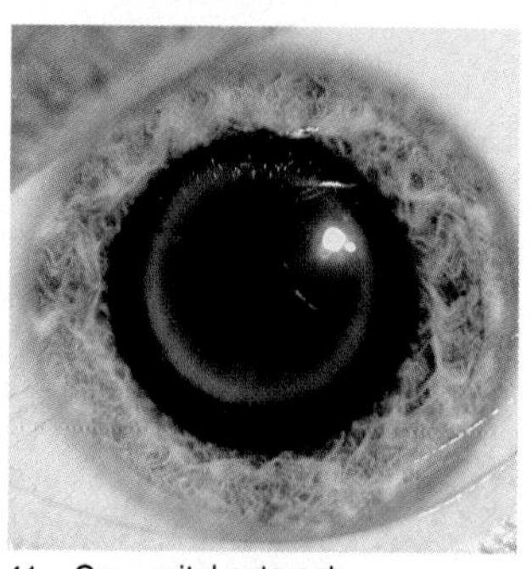
41 Congenital cataract

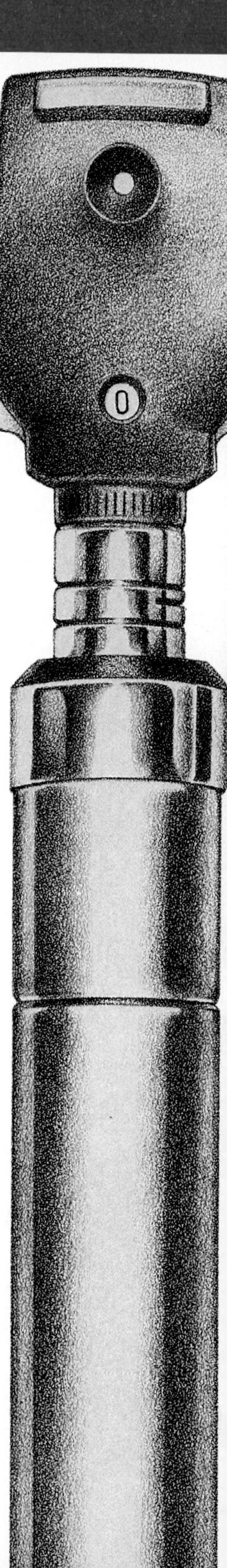

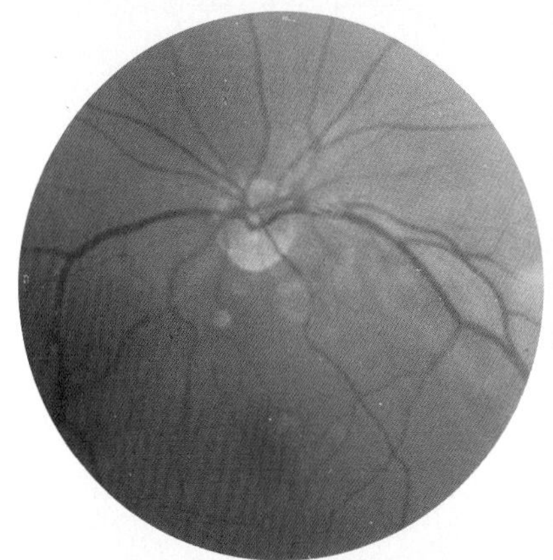

Normal retina

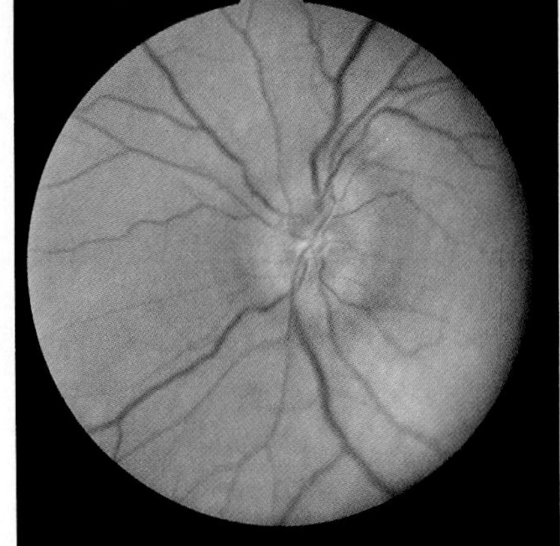

42 Papilledema

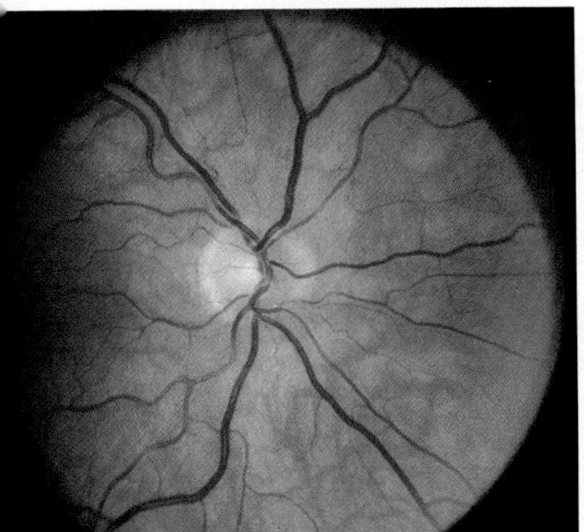

43 Hypertension grade I

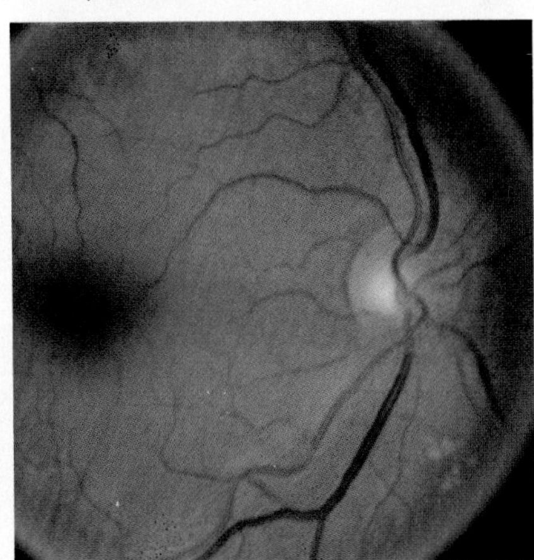

44 Hypertension grade II

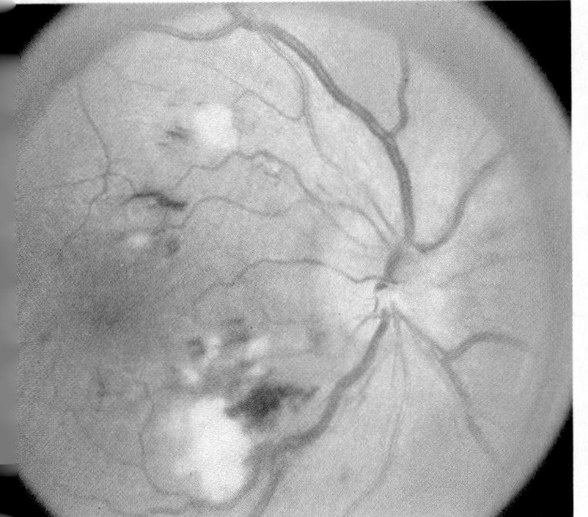

45 Hypertension grade III

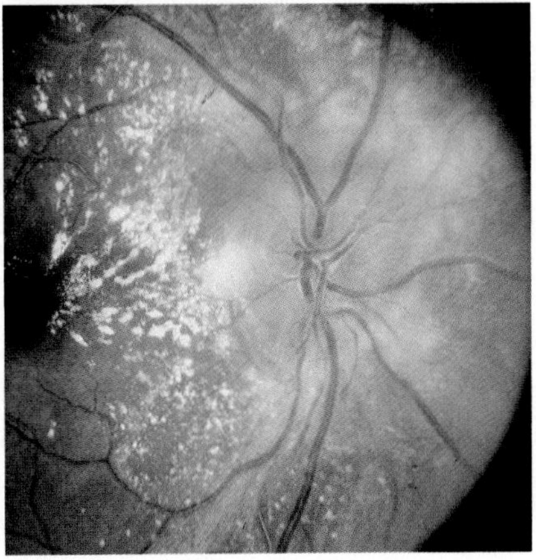

46 Hypertension grade IV

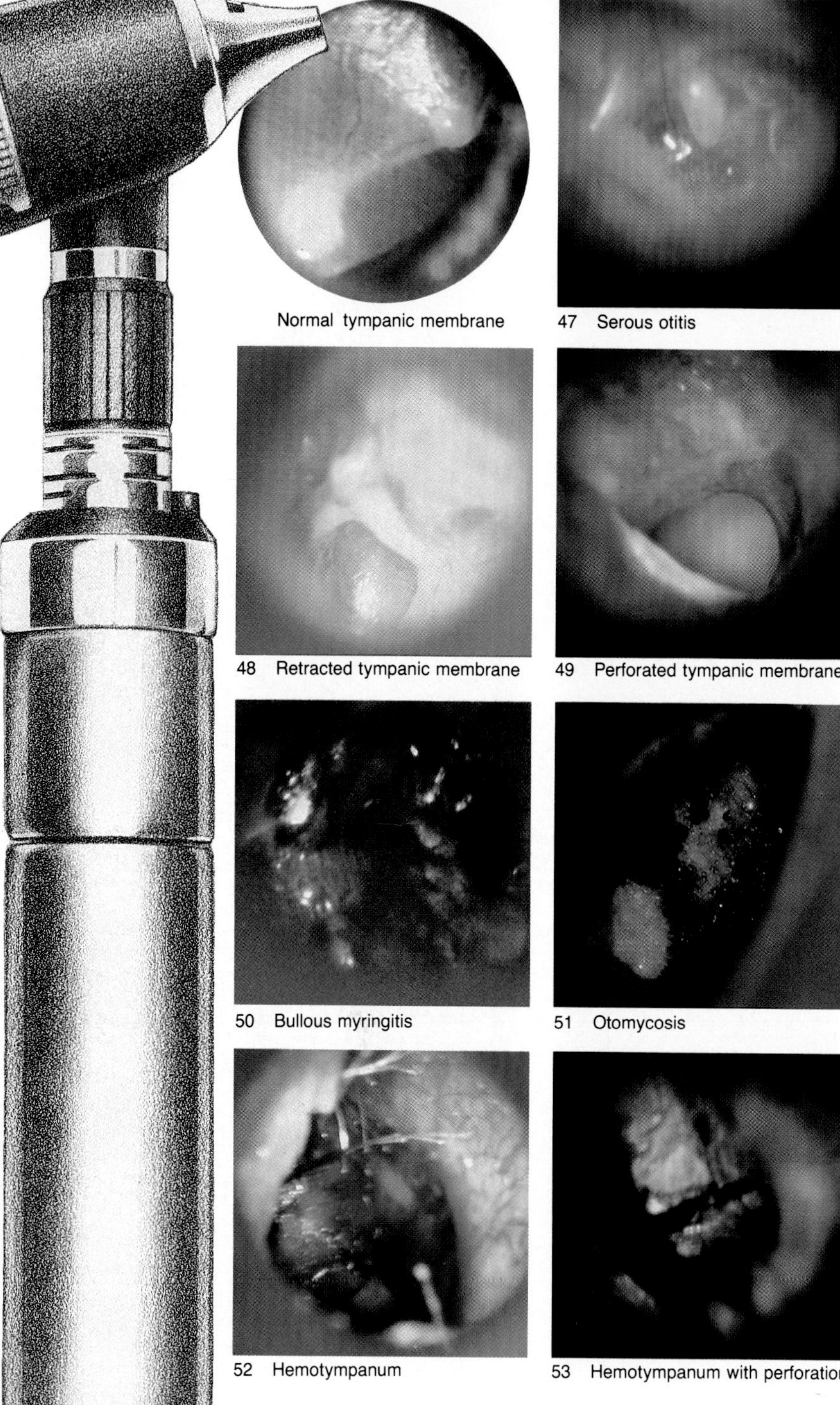

Normal tympanic membrane

47 Serous otitis

48 Retracted tympanic membrane

49 Perforated tympanic membrane

50 Bullous myringitis

51 Otomycosis

52 Hemotympanum

53 Hemotympanum with perforation

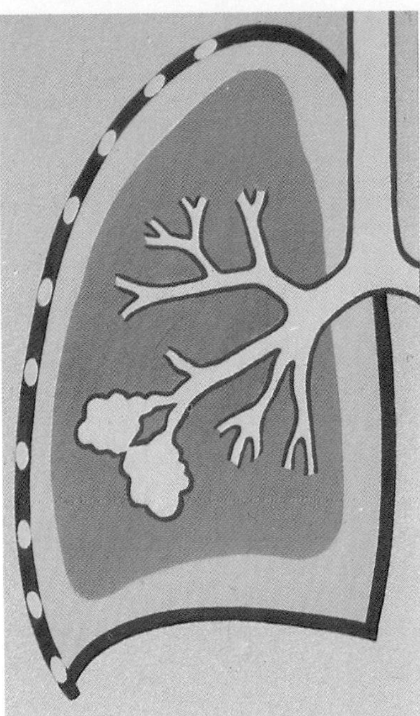

54 Emphysema of the right lung (Hyperinflated alveoli with wall destruction)

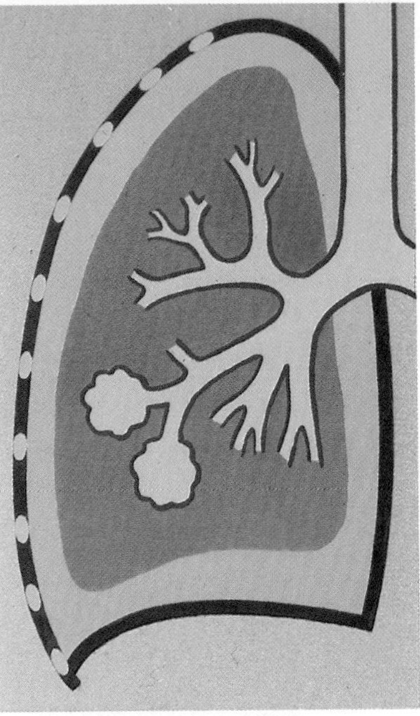

55 Bronchiectasis of the right lung (Hyperinflated bronchial tree and alveoli)

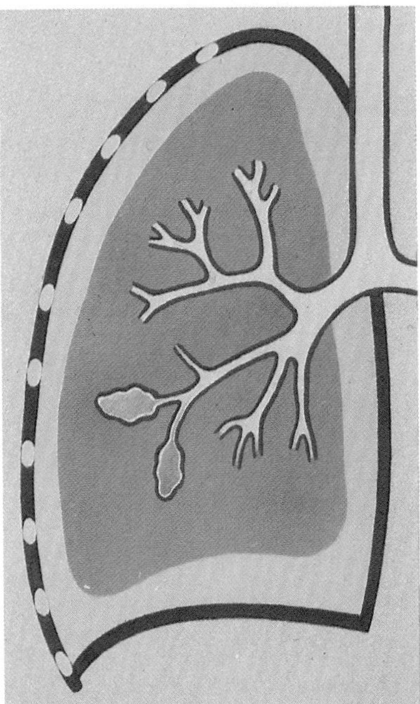

56 Pulmonary consolidation of the right lower lobe (Fluid-filled and deflated alveoli)

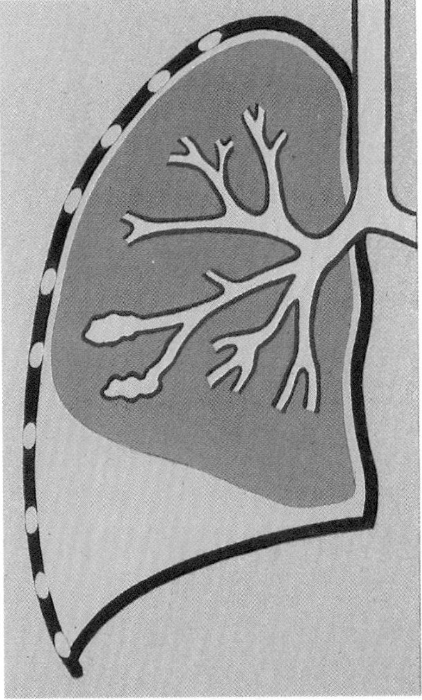

57 Pneumothorax of the right lung (Air-filled pleural space and collapsed alveoli)

58 Laryngeal obstruction: signs and symptoms of asphyxiation (choking, intercostal and supracostal retractions, struggling); commonly caused by edema from severe allergic reaction

59 Tracheal obstruction: signs and symptoms of asphyxiation (choking, intercostal and supracostal retractions, struggling); commonly caused by presence of foreign body

60 Secretion obstruction: signs and symptoms include cough (usually productive), fever; commonly caused by infection

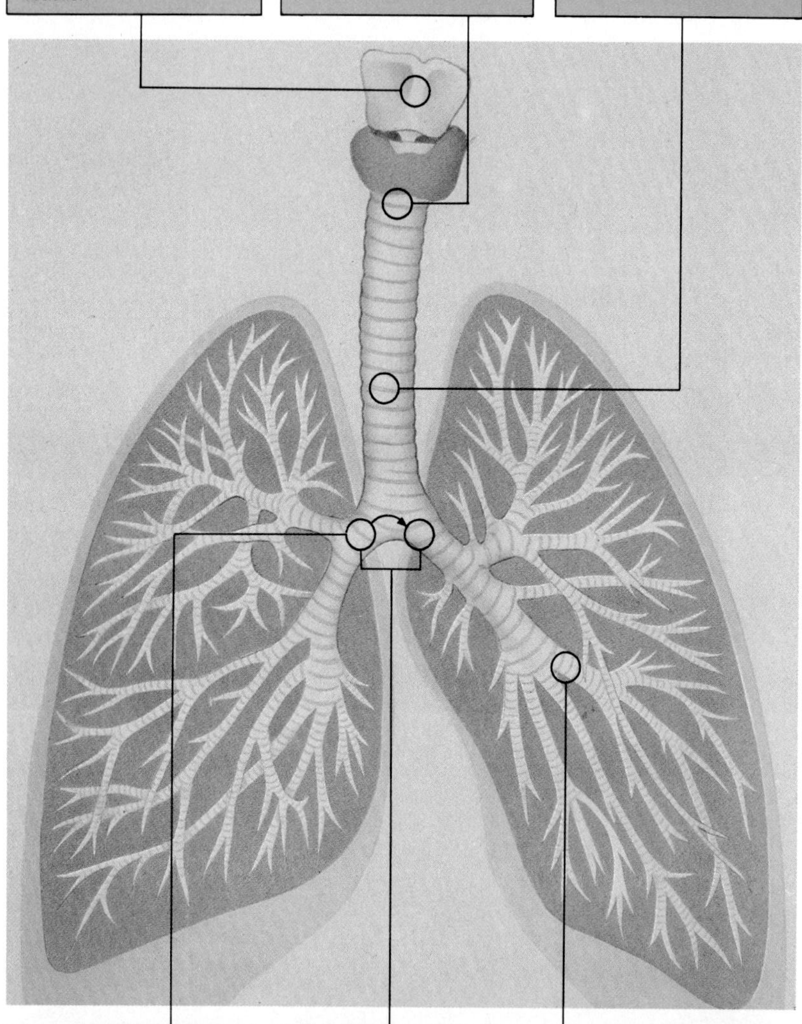

61 Unilateral mainstem bronchial obstruction: signs and symptoms include initial violent cough, followed by asymptomatic period and then chronic cough; commonly caused by presence of foreign body

62 Bilateral mainstem bronchial obstruction: signs and symptoms of asphyxiation if obstruction is total; commonly caused by dislodgement of obstruction from edematous mainstem bronchus to the other

63 Lobar or segmental obstruction: signs and symptoms of unilateral mainstem obstruction occurring over a longer period with less severity; commonly caused by foreign body or secretions

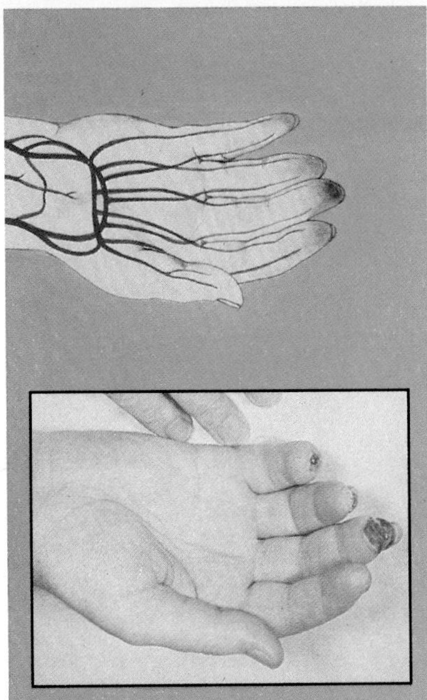

64 Necrosis caused by vasoconstriction of arterial occlusive disease

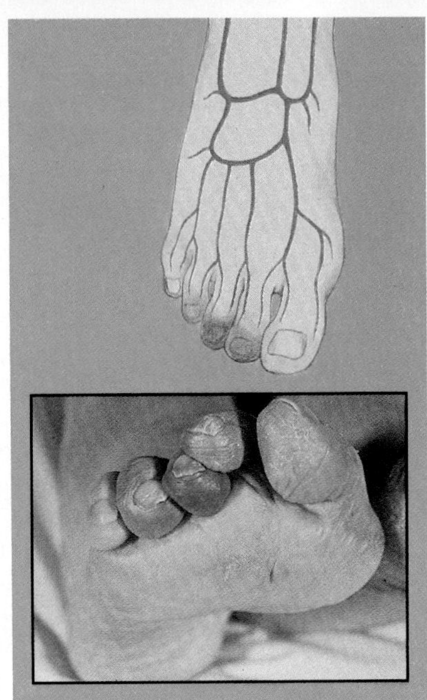

65 Ischemic gangrenous ulcer

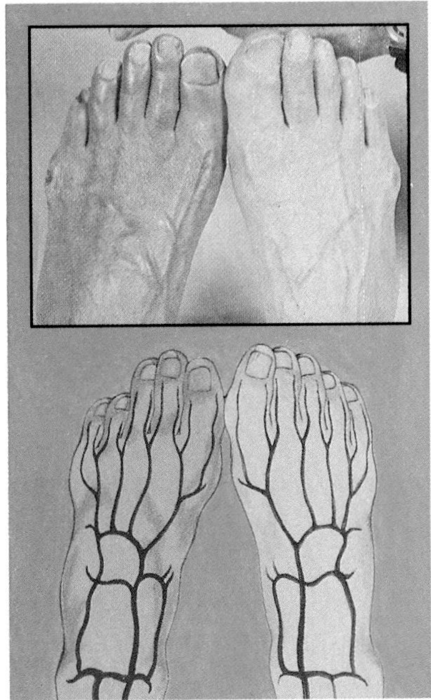

66 Dependent rubor of arterial occlusive disease

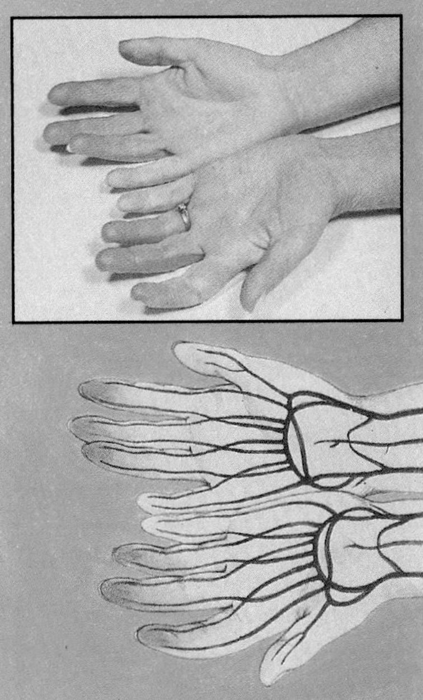

67 Blanching caused by vasospasm of Raynaud's disease

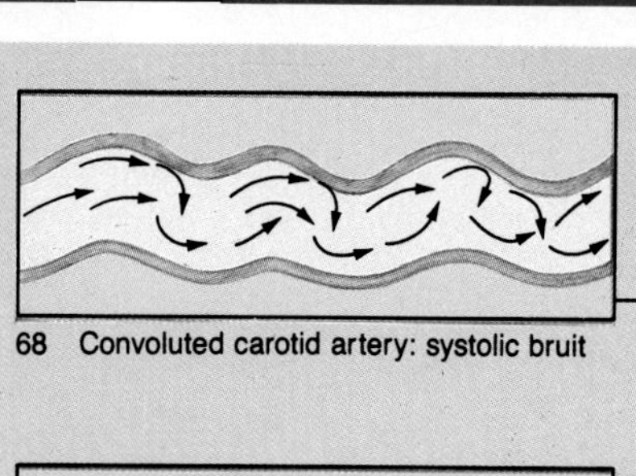
68 Convoluted carotid artery: systolic bruit

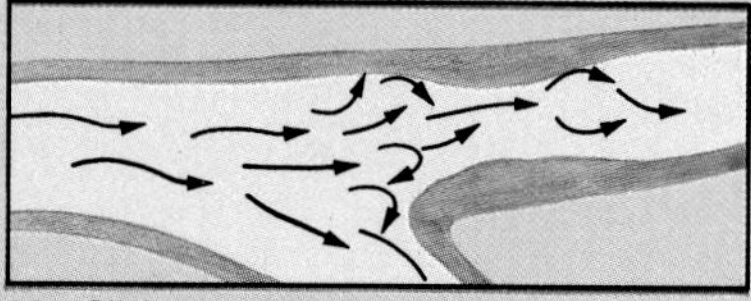
69 Slight arterial stenosis: systolic bruit

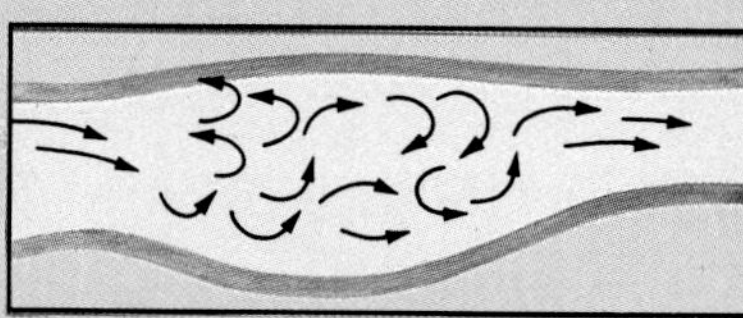
70 Arterial aneurysm: systolic bruit

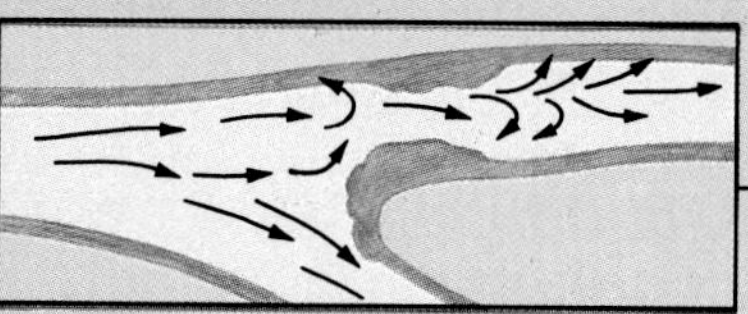
71 Severe arterial stenosis without collateral circulation: diastolic bruit

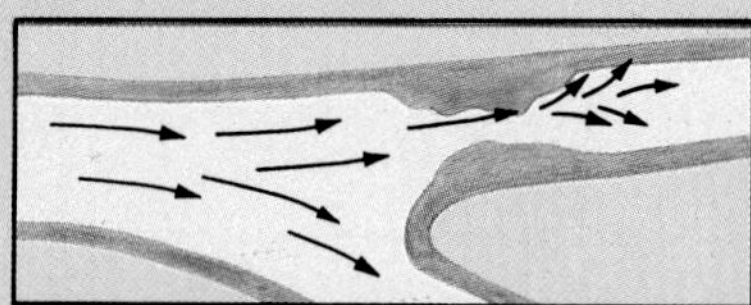
72 Severe arterial stenosis without collateral circulation: systolic bruit

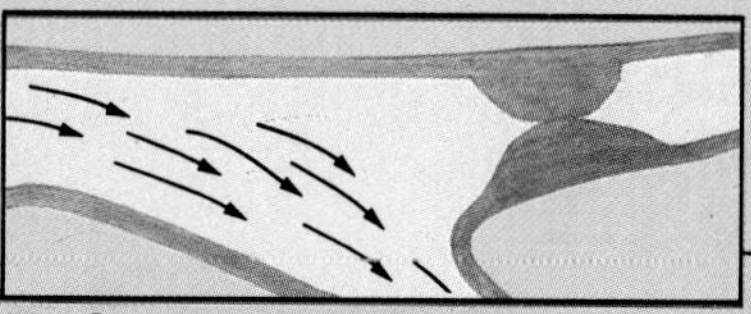
73 Complete arterial obstruction: no bruit

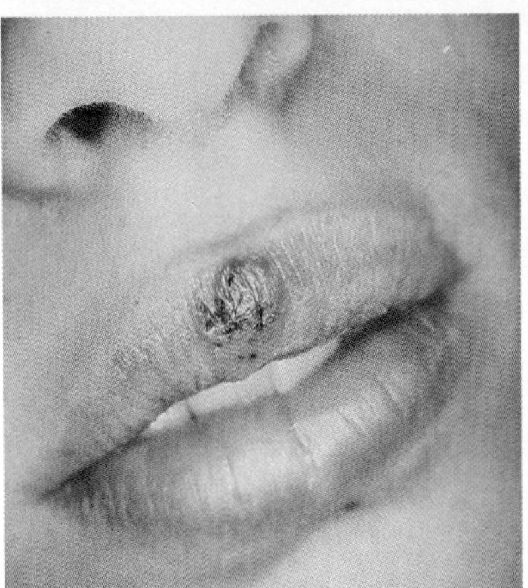
74 Recurrent herpes labialis

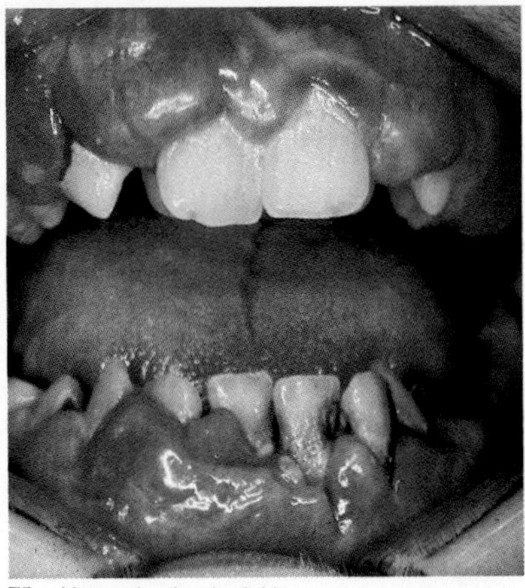
75 Hyperplastic gingivitis

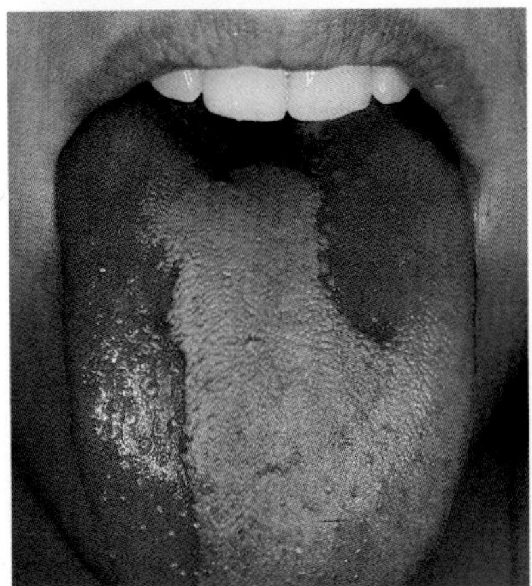
76 Benign migratory glossitis

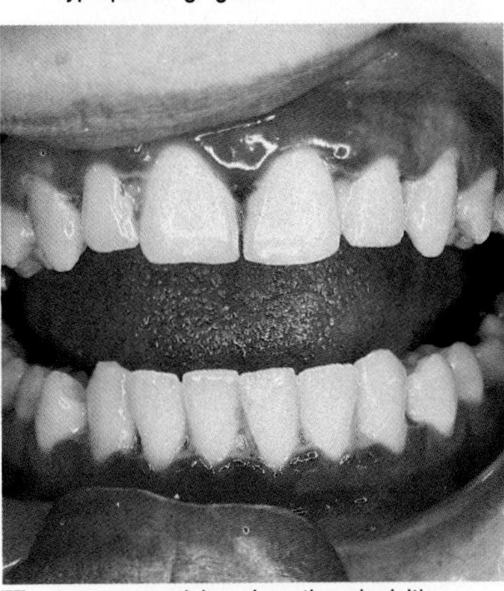
77 Acute necrotizing ulcerative gingivitis

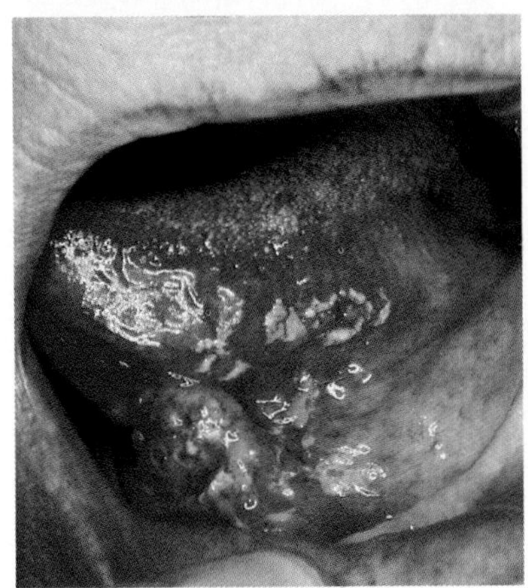
78 Ulcerating carcinoma

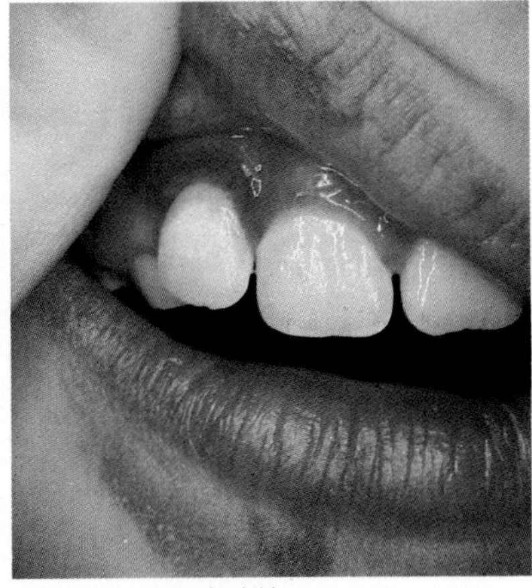
79 Focal acute gingivitis

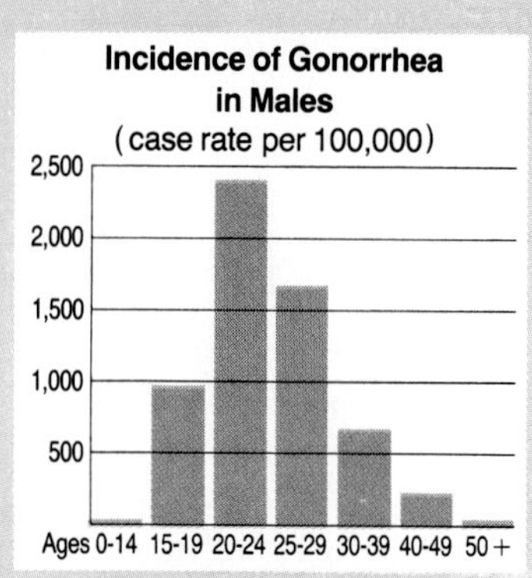

Incidence of Primary and Secondary Syphilis in Males
(case rate per 100,000)

50
40
30
20
10
Ages 0-14 15-19 20-24 25-29 30-39 40-49 50 +

Courtesy: Centers for Disease Control, 1978.

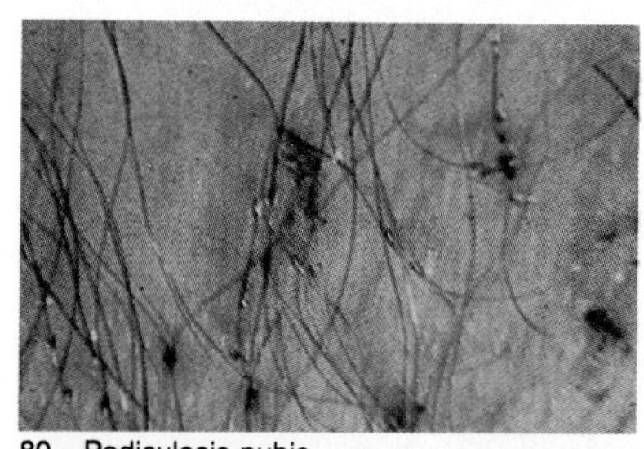
80 Pediculosis pubis

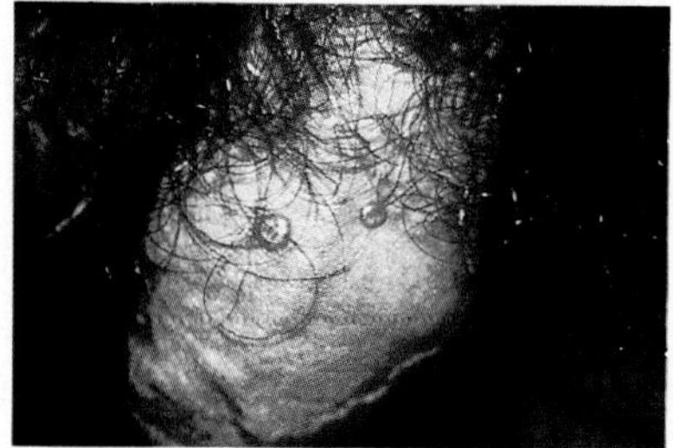
81 Molluscum contagiosum

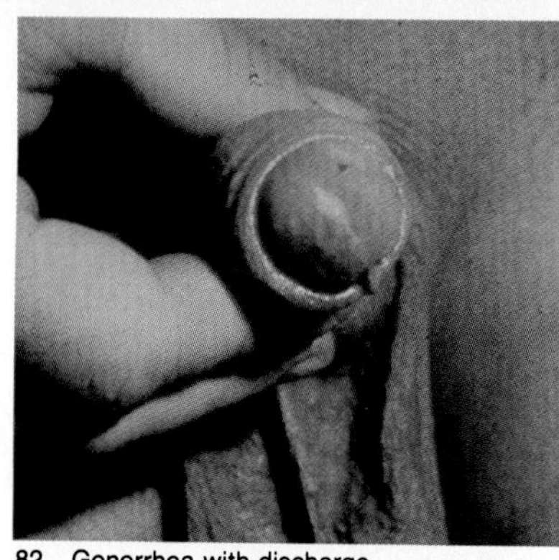
82 Gonorrhea with discharge

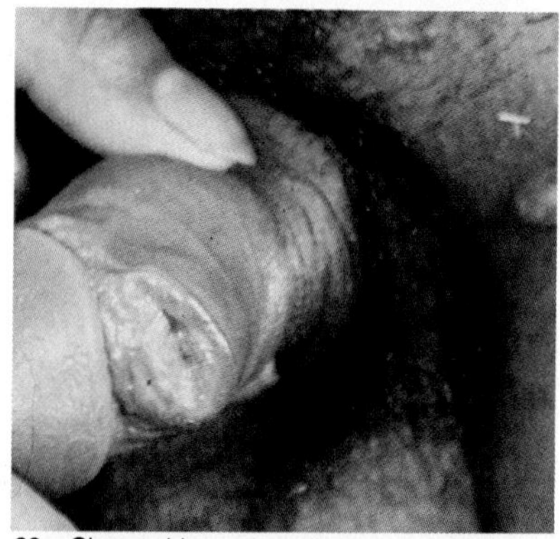
83 Chancroid

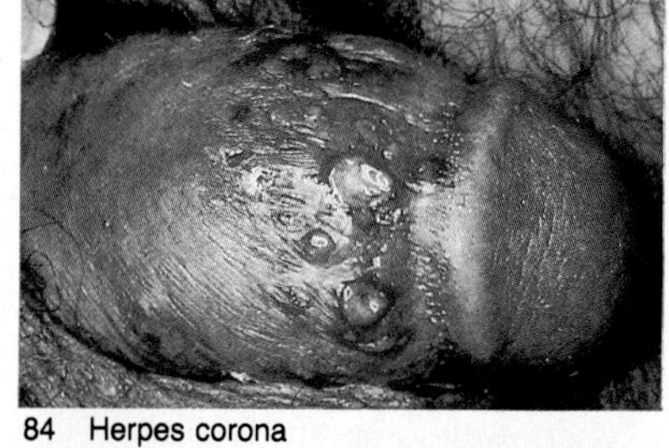
84 Herpes corona

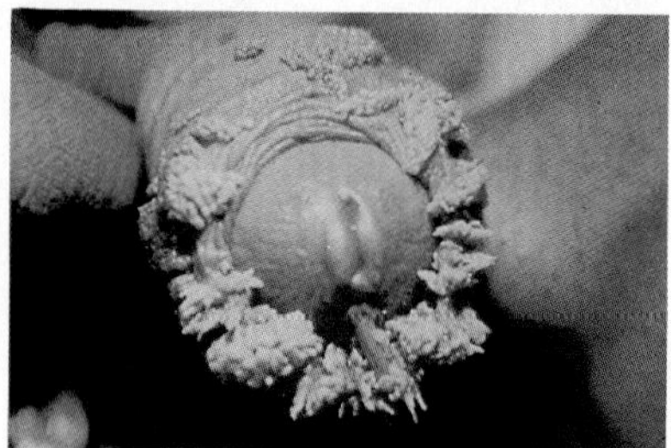
85 Venereal warts

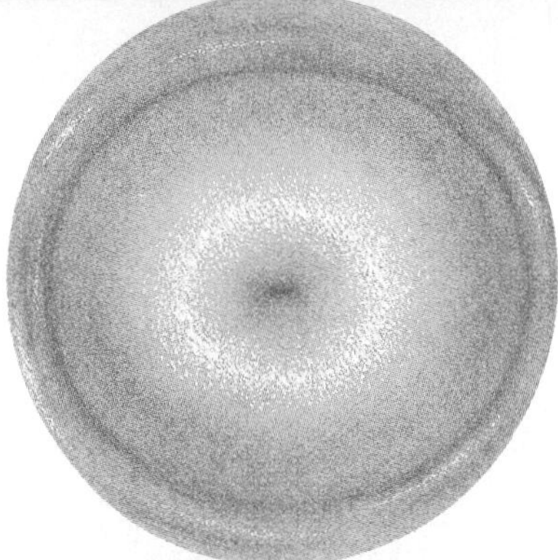
Normal cervical view

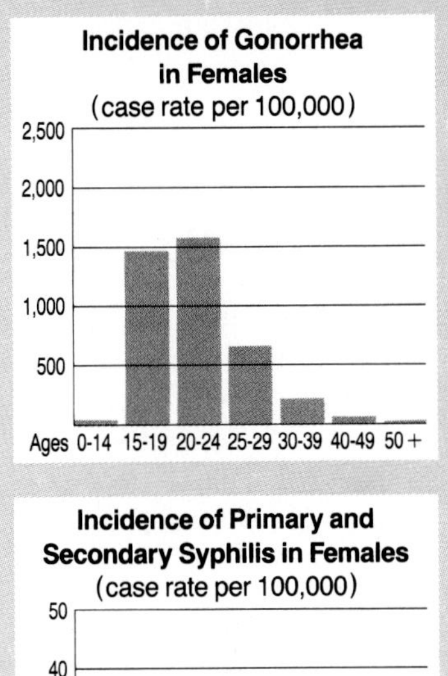

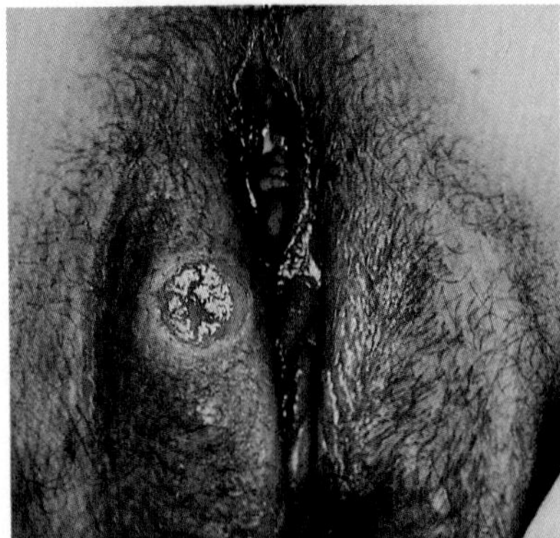
86 Syphilitic chancre of labium majus

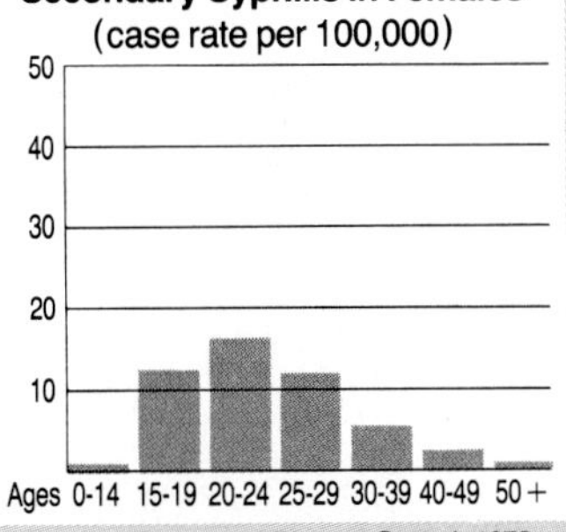

Courtesy: Centers for Disease Control, 1978.

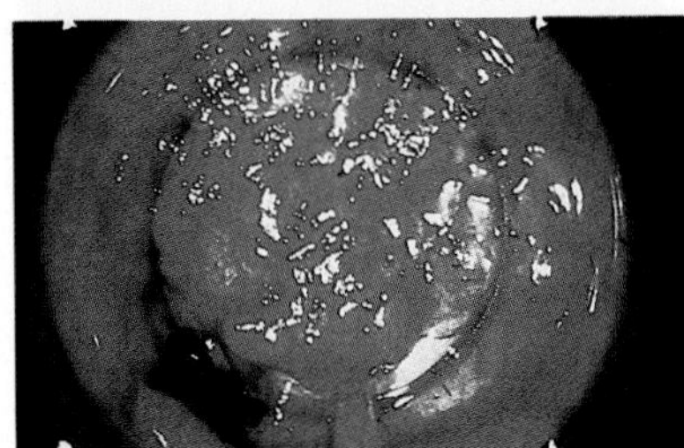
87 Granuloma inguinale

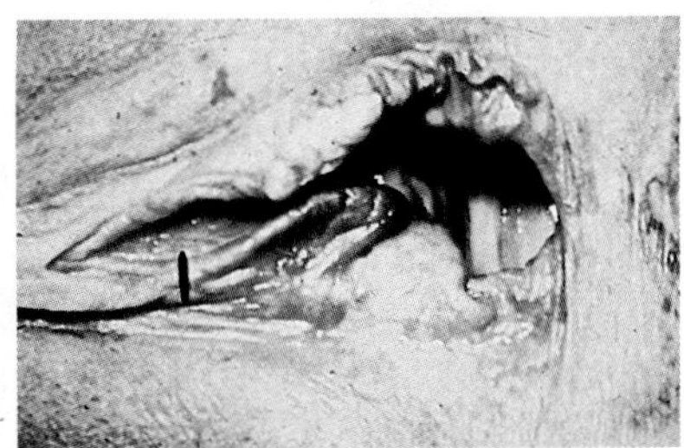
89 Malignant vulvar lesion

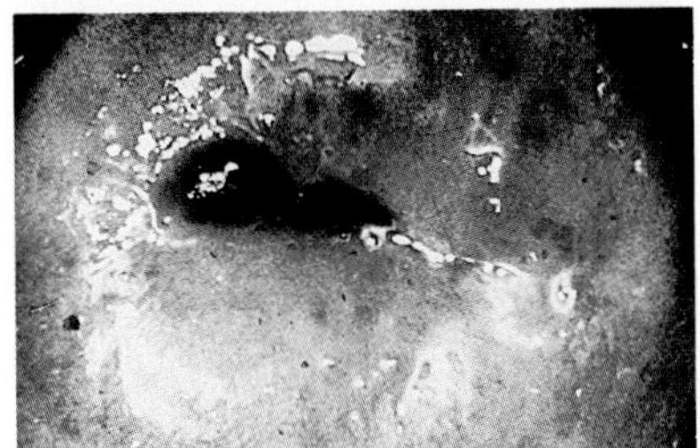
88 Endometriosis

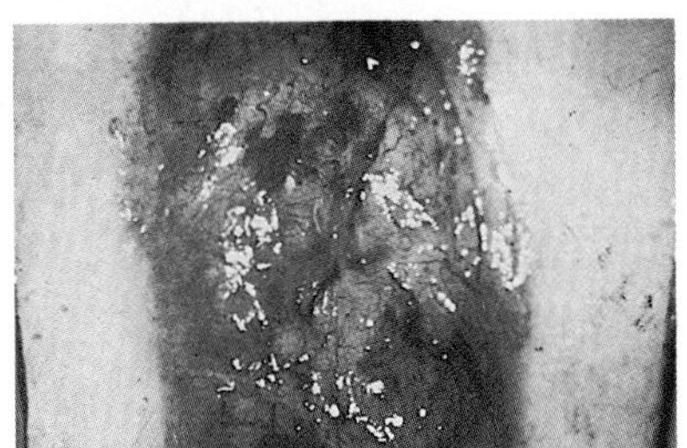
90 Cervical carcinoma

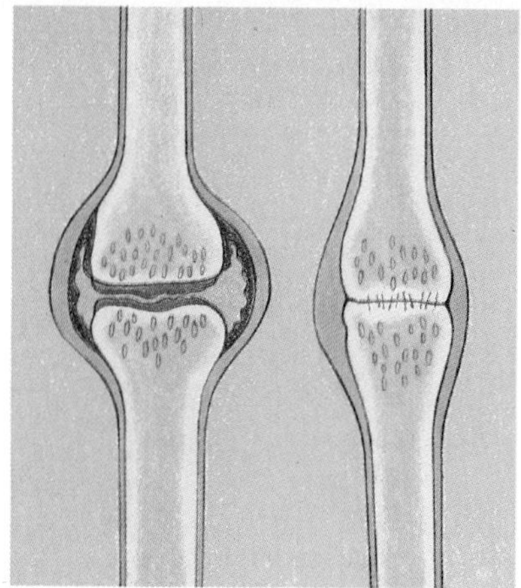

Progressive stages of rheumatoid arthritis

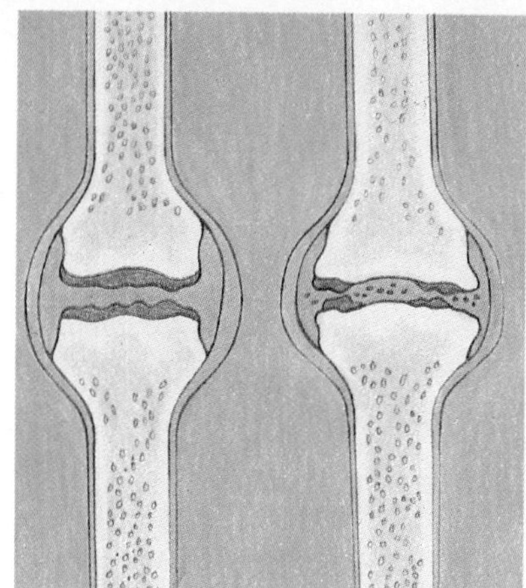

Progressive stages of osteoarthritis

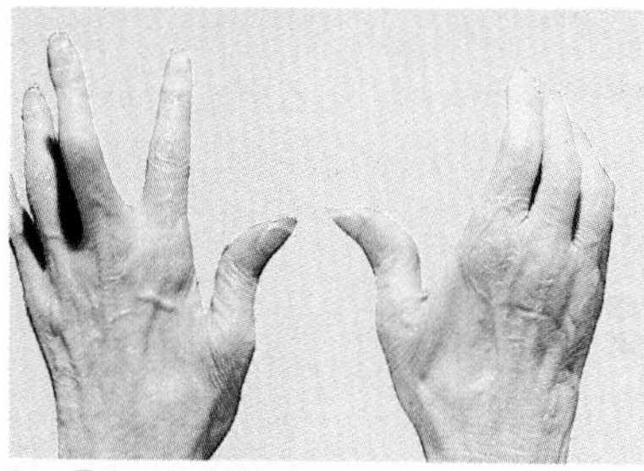

91 Z-thumb deformity

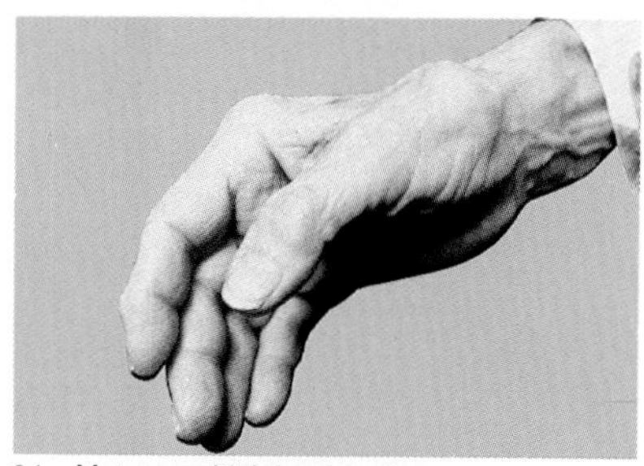

94 Metacarpal joint deformity

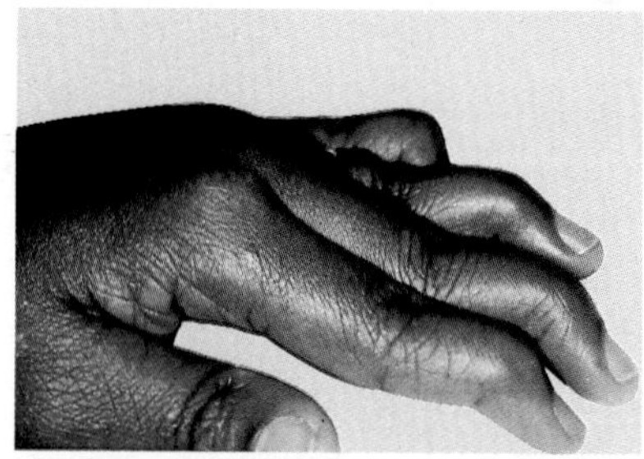

92 Swan neck deformity

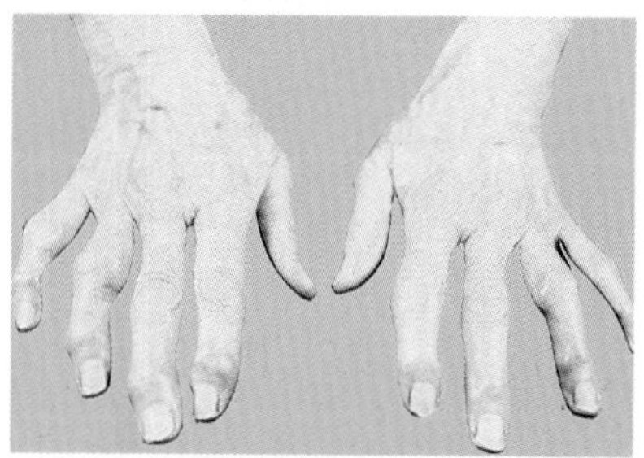

95 Heberden's and Bouchard's nodes

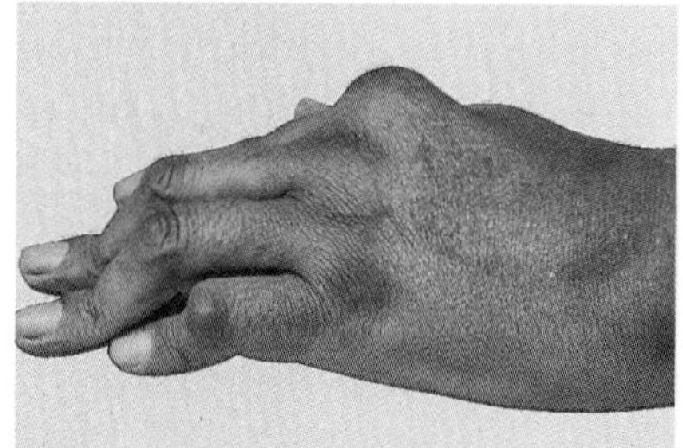

93 Boutonnière deformity

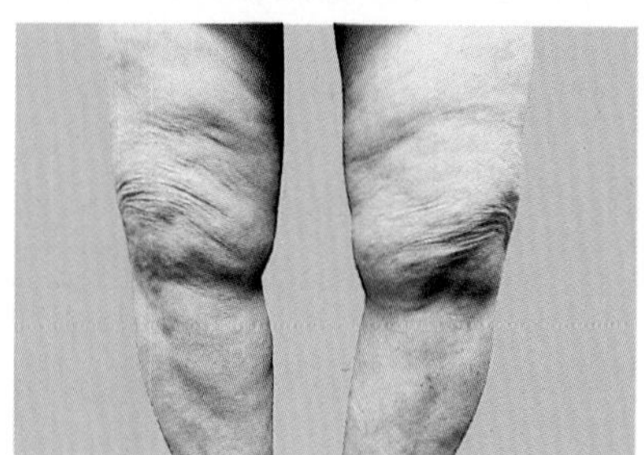

96 Genu varum

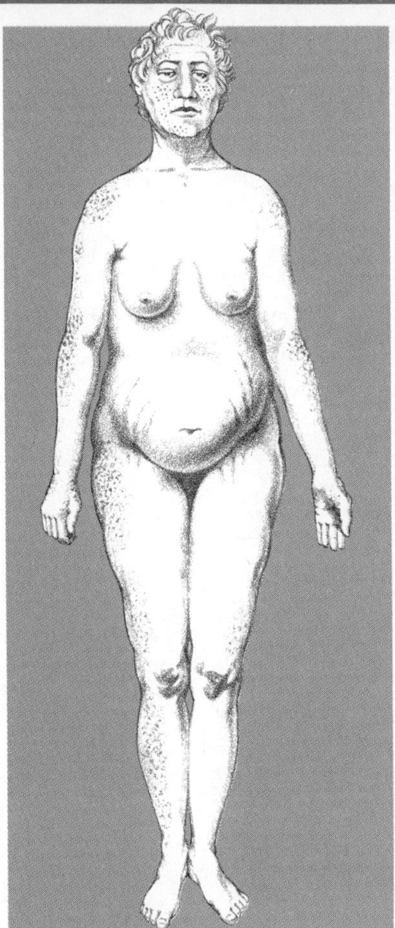

97 Primary myxedema

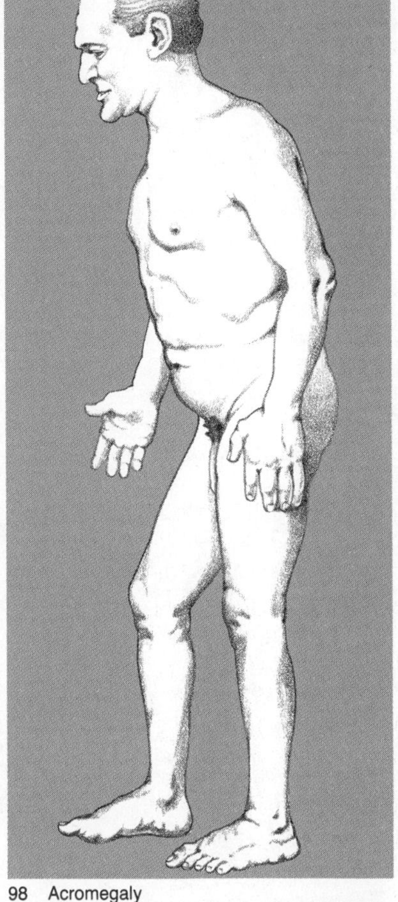

98 Acromegaly

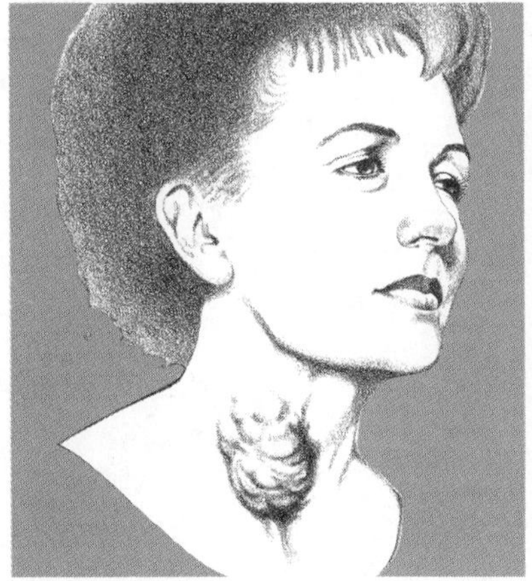

99 Nodular goiter

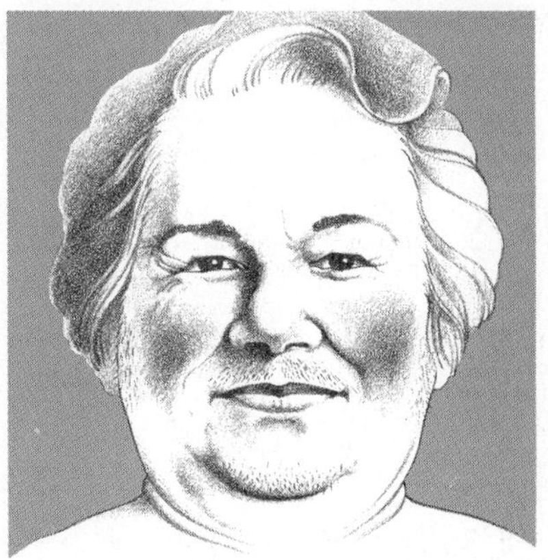

100 Cushing's syndrome

15

KEY POINTS IN THIS CHAPTER

KEY CHARTS IN THIS CHAPTER

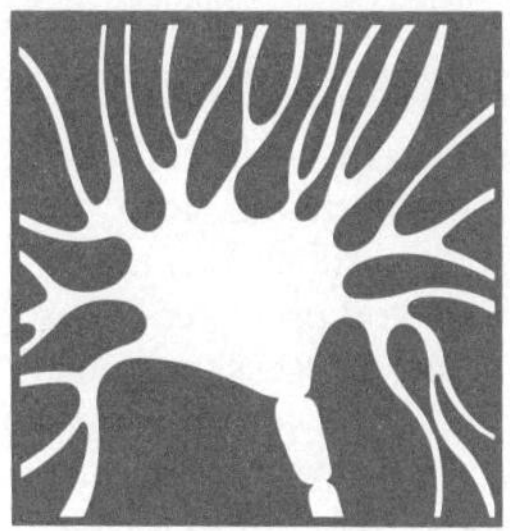

Nervous System

Introduction

586 Approach to neurologic assessment

Advances in neurology and neurosurgery during the 1970s and early 1980s have led to nurses' increased interest and involvement in these fields. Many nurses, however, are still intimidated by assessment of the nervous system. Evaluation of a patient's cerebral function, cranial nerves, sensory and motor functions, and reflexes can seem overwhelming. But the fact is that although tests for neurologic status are extensive, they're also basic and straightforward. They measure a patient's thought processes and coordination, as well as his ability to receive stimuli and respond accordingly. Your daily nursing care may routinely include parts of a neurologic examination. For example, simply conversing with the patient helps you assess his orientation, level of consciousness, and ability to formulate and produce speech. Asking him to describe his pain allows you to test his memory and general knowledge, and having him perform a simple task, such as walking, enables you to evaluate his motor ability.

587 The nervous system's interrelatedness

The implications of neurologic assessment are far-reaching for the patient's nervous system and for his other body systems. The nervous system is related, directly or indirectly, to every other body system. Consequently, patients who suffer from diseases of other body systems can develop related neurologic impairment. Examples of this are the open heart surgery patient who experiences a cerebrovascular accident, the patient whose hip joint infection spreads through his bloodstream and causes a brain abscess, the patient with a cirrhotic liver who develops a metabolic encephalopathy, or the pregnant patient with toxemia. To meet assessment challenges like these, you need to become thoroughly familiar with the nervous system and to master the procedures involved in neurologic assessment. This knowledge and skill will help you identify and assess early signs and symptoms of neurologic dysfunction—which can be life-threatening. You'll also use your knowledge and skill in less critical situations, such as performing neurologic screening during a general physical examination.

Regardless of the clinical circumstances, your findings provide a firm data base for your nursing diagnoses and care plan. Overall, your knowledge of nervous system functioning and appropriate assessment techniques will enhance your patient care and may save some patients from irreversible neurologic damage.

Reviewing anatomy and physiology

588 Nervous system: Structure and function

Structurally, the nervous system is divided into a central nervous system and a peripheral nervous system. The *central nervous system* is composed of the brain and the spinal cord. The major structures of the brain are the cerebrum, the limbic system, and the basal ganglia (telencephalon); the thalamus and hypothalamus (diencephalon); the corpora quadrigemina and the tegmentum and cerebral peduncles (mesencephalon); the pons and cerebellum (metencephalon); the medulla oblongata (myelencephalon); and the reticular activating system.

The spinal cord is divided into five segments: cervical, thoracic, lumbar, sacral, and coccygeal. It contains major ascending and descending nerve tracts, carrying motor and sensory information.

The *peripheral nervous system* consists of the cranial and the spinal nerves. It includes afferent (sensory) and efferent (motor) nerve fibers and *ganglia,* groups of nerve cell bodies located outside the central nervous system.

Functionally, the nervous system is divided into a cerebrospinal (somatic) nervous system and an autonomic (visceral) nervous system. The *somatic nervous system* controls conscious activities, such as perception of the world around us, and voluntary responses to stimuli. The *autonomic nervous system* controls involuntary (smooth) muscles and the functions of glands.

589 Neurons and neuroglia

The functional cell of the nervous system is the *neuron,* a specialized nerve cell that receives and conducts various kinds of stimuli within the body. Neurons have three basic parts: a cell body, an axon, and dendrites. The *cell body,* which contains a nucleus and surrounding cytoplasm, absorbs and metabolizes nutrients and produces energy. The *axon,* a long process extending from the cell body and terminating in branches, conducts nerve impulses *away* from the cell body. *Dendrites* are short, radiating processes extending from the cell body; they carry nerve impulses *toward* the cell body. Most neurons have only one axon but many dendrites.

Most bundles of axons are called *nerve fibers.* (Within the spinal cord or brain, the fibers are called *nerve tracts.*) Axons may be surrounded by a plasma membrane substance—*myelin*—which insulates and protects nerve fibers. The myelin has a series of gaps or constrictions (nodes of Ranvier), which are the noninsulated or conductive areas of the nerve fibers. In myelinated nerves, impulses jump from node to node; they travel continuously along the nerve fiber in unmyelinated nerves. Another layer of sheath cells (Schwann's cells), called the *neurilemma,* covers the myelin. The neurilemma is necessary both for the regeneration of a damaged nerve fiber and for its possible return of function.

The *neuroglia* are the supporting cells of the nervous system. Each type of neuroglia has a specific function. The *ependyma* assists in the production of cerebrospinal fluid. *Astrocytes* form scar tissue (gliosis) to fill cavities following neuron destruction. Astrocytes also play a role in the blood-brain barrier, which consists of capillaries composed of densely packed cells (unlike other capillaries in the body). These glial cells and a continuous membrane surround the capillaries. These structures collectively allow certain substances to pass from the blood into the brain (some rapidly, some slowly); they block passage of other substances. *Oligodendrocytes* form the myelin of the central nervous system, just as Schwann's cells form the neurilemma

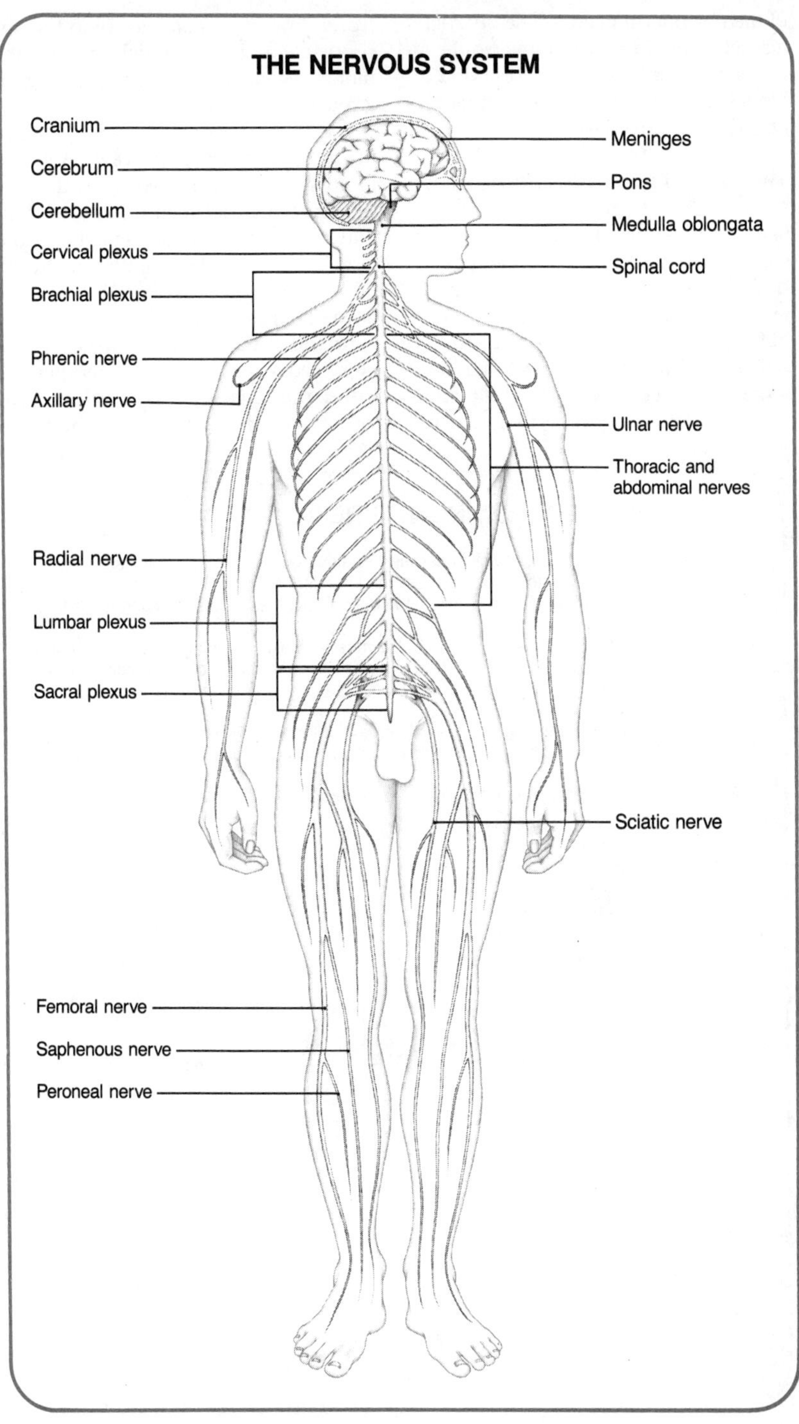
THE NERVOUS SYSTEM
Cranium
Cerebrum
Cerebellum
Cervical plexus
Brachial plexus
Phrenic nerve
Axillary nerve
Radial nerve
Lumbar plexus
Sacral plexus
Femoral nerve
Saphenous nerve
Peroneal nerve
Meninges
Pons
Medulla oblongata
Spinal cord
Ulnar nerve
Thoracic and abdominal nerves
Sciatic nerve

of the peripheral nerves. The *microglia* are relatively inactive in a normal central nervous system. Their function includes phagocytosis in inflammatory and degenerative lesions.

590 Transmission of nerve impulses

Sensory receptors located in the sensory organs and in other tissues of the body supply input into the nervous system. These receptors excite the nerve fibers; the impulse is then transmitted along the sensory pathway to the area where it is integrated. This may stimulate a motor response to form and travel down the motor nerve to the appropriate effector, which causes the motor response to occur in an organ, a muscle, or a gland.

Impulse transmission along nerve fibers is an electrical event. A nerve impulse is carried from a dendrite to the cell body and then on to the axon, which carries it to the dendrite of the next cell. Here the impulse is transmitted chemically across the synapse to the next neuron.

Actual transmission of a nerve impulse from one neuron to another involves the release of a chemical from the end of the axon. This chemical,

FOLLOWING THE REFLEX ARC

To understand the sensory-to-motor transmission path known as the *reflex arc,* study the following sequence of events associated with the knee-jerk reflex:

- The hammer strikes the tendon below the kneecap, which stretches the quadriceps femoris muscle.
- Stretching stimulates peripheral nerves in the muscle, which send impulses through afferent or sensory nerve fibers to the sensory neurons in the dorsal root of the spinal cord.
- The sensory nerve impulse synapses with motor neurons and passes into the ventral root.
- The impulse continues through the spinal nerve and then through the peripheral nerve. It crosses the neuromuscular junction in the quadriceps femoris muscle, where acetylcholine is released.
- Acetylcholine stimulates the muscle to contract, completing the reflex arc.

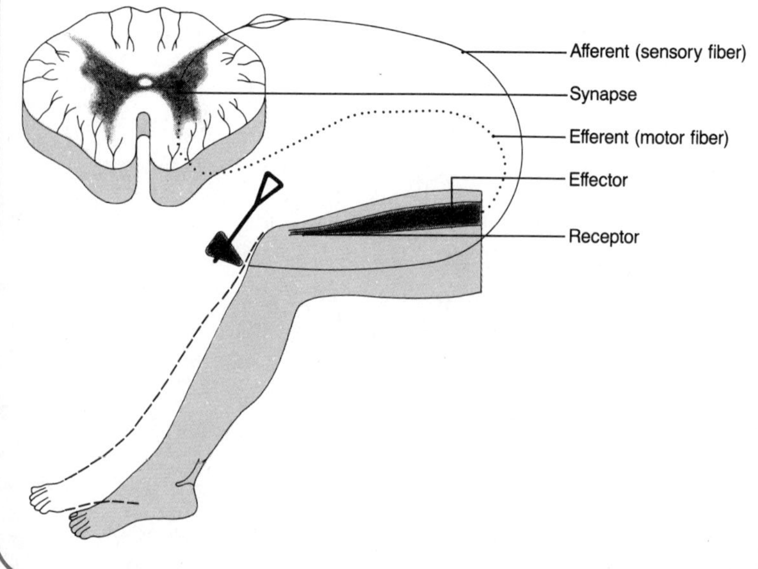

called a *neurotransmitter,* acts as a stimulus to initiate the nerve impulse in the next neuron. Common neurotransmitters are acetylcholine, norepinephrine, dopamine, and serotonin. Cholinesterase is an enzyme released at the neuromuscular junction shortly after acetylcholine is released. It deactivates the remaining acetylcholine, thus preventing reexcitation of the muscle fiber.

591 Spinal cord: Sensory and motor nerves

The spinal cord contains gray matter and white matter. The butterfly-shaped gray matter in the center of the cord contains cell bodies and their processes. The white matter contains myelinated fibers (axons), most of which are ascending or descending.

Impulses enter the spinal cord and are integrated in the gray matter. Then they are either acted on locally, as in a reflex arc, or transmitted to a higher level of the nervous system by way of the ascending tracts in the white matter.

The white matter of the spinal cord contains the motor and the sensory nerve tracts. The major *ascending* sensory tracts are:

- spinothalamic (carries pain and temperature sensation)
- posterior columns (conscious position sense, vibration, and size and shape discrimination)
- spinocerebellar (unconscious position sense).

These tracts terminate mainly in the thalamus; the impulses are then carried to the cerebral cortex.

The major *descending* motor tracts are the *corticospinal* (pyramidal) tract, which carries commands for voluntary movement, and an *extrapyramidal* tract, which combines motor input from higher levels.

All motor activity must be channeled through the *final common pathway,* which consists of cells of gray matter in the spinal cord and axons of the peripheral nervous system. Six levels of information concerning impulse response are channeled through this pathway:

- reflex response, which occurs through the reflex arc at the local spinal cord level
- information from the reticular system in the brain stem, which deals with such visceral activity as breathing, heartbeat, smooth muscle movements, and muscles of balance
- vestibular system, which relates to gravity and acceleration
- extrapyramidal system, which deals with motor integration
- cerebellum, which coordinates all muscle activity
- cerebral cortex, which plans all motor activity.

Most motor fibers of the pyramidal tract cross over (decussate) to the other side at the level of the medulla. This is important in understanding the contralateral and ipsilateral effects produced by lesions of the central nervous system.

592 Cranial nerves

The cranial nerves are so named because they emerge through openings (foramina) in the skull or cranium. They are assigned Roman numerals from I to XII to indicate the sequence in which they emerge from the rostral (head or top) to the caudal (lower or tail) parts of the brain stem. Cranial nerves may have either sensory or motor function, or both. These functions and the muscles or organs innervated by the cranial nerves are shown in *Identifying Cranial Nerves,* page 562.

593 Cerebrum

The cerebrum is divided into two hemispheres, joined by white matter that is composed of bands of nerve fibers, called the *corpus callosum.* In turn, each hemisphere divides into four lobes: *frontal, parietal, temporal,* and *occipital.* Under the frontal and temporal lobes is a fifth lobe, called the *insula.*

IDENTIFYING CRANIAL NERVES

NERVE	ORIGIN	TYPE	FUNCTION(S)
I Olfactory	Olfactory bulb	Sensory	Smell
II Optic	Lateral geniculate body	Sensory	Vision
III Oculomotor	Midbrain	Motor	Eye movement (inward, upward), eyelid elevation, pupil constriction, convergence, consensual reaction
IV Trochlear	Midbrain	Motor	Eye movement (downward, outward)
V Trigeminal	Pons	Motor	Chewing
		Sensory	Sensations of the face, scalp, and teeth
VI Abducens	Pons	Motor	Eye movement (lateral)
VII Facial	Pons	Motor	Facial expressions
		Sensory	Taste (anterior two thirds of tongue), salivation, tearing
VIII Acoustic (cochlear, vestibular)	Pons	Sensory	Hearing, equilibrium
IX Glosso-pharyngeal	Medulla	Motor	Salivation, swallowing
		Sensory	Sensations of the throat and tonsils, taste (posterior one third of tongue)
X Vagus	Medulla	Motor	Swallowing, talking, heart rate, peristalsis
		Sensory	Sensations of the throat, larynx, and viscera
XI Spinal accessory	Medulla	Motor	Shoulder movement, head rotation
XII Hypoglossal	Medulla	Motor	Tongue movement

The surface of the cerebrum—the *cerebral cortex*—consists of gray matter arranged in elevations called *gyri. Sulci* are shallow grooves between gyri. *Fissures* are deep grooves that divide each hemisphere into the various lobes.

The interior of the cerebrum is made up of gray matter and white matter. The white matter is arranged in tracts consisting of nerve fibers, such as the corpus callosum. These tracts provide communication to all parts of the cerebrum, to the rest of the brain, and to the spinal cord.

Each cerebral hemisphere processes information for the opposite side of the body. For example, the left cerebral cortex controls movement of the right hand. Each cerebral lobe also performs specific functions. The posterior part of the *frontal lobe* controls voluntary muscle movement; its anterior part assists in the control of emotions and intellectual activities, such as memory, judgment, ethics, and abstract thinking. Broca's motor speech area is located in the inferior frontal lobe.

The *parietal lobe* receives and interprets sensory impulses—such as pain, heat, cold, pressure, size, shape, texture, and awareness of body parts. The *temporal lobe* receives and interprets auditory and olfactory stimuli. Wernicke's area, which interprets spoken and written words, is located in the posterior part of the superior temporal gyrus. The *occipital lobe* receives and interprets visual stimuli.

The area that initiates all voluntary movement (the precentral gyrus, or motor strip) is located in front of the central sulcus. A general sensory area (postcentral gyrus, or sensory strip) is located behind the central sulcus. The function of the insula is not understood, but it may deal with visceral sensation and motor activity.

594 Basal ganglia and limbic system (lobe)

The basal ganglia and the limbic system are located deep inside each cerebral hemisphere. The basal ganglia play an important role in extrapyramidal function. They integrate voluntary activity, associated movements, and postural adjustments, and they maintain appropriate muscle tone and reflex activity. The limbic system plays a role in sexual behavior, rage, fear reactions, recent memory, alerting processes, feeding behavior, chewing, licking, and swallowing.

595 Diencephalon

The diencephalon, the posterior part of the forebrain, is located between the midbrain and the cerebral hemispheres. The main functional structures in the diencephalon are the thalamus and the hypothalamus.

The *thalamus,* a large oval mass of gray matter at the base of each cerebral hemisphere, acts as a relay and integration center for all types of sensory impulses except olfaction. It plays an important role in transmission of pain impulses, especially burning or aching visceral pain. It also controls some degree of consciousness.

The *hypothalamus* integrates and

CRANIAL NERVE ORIGINS

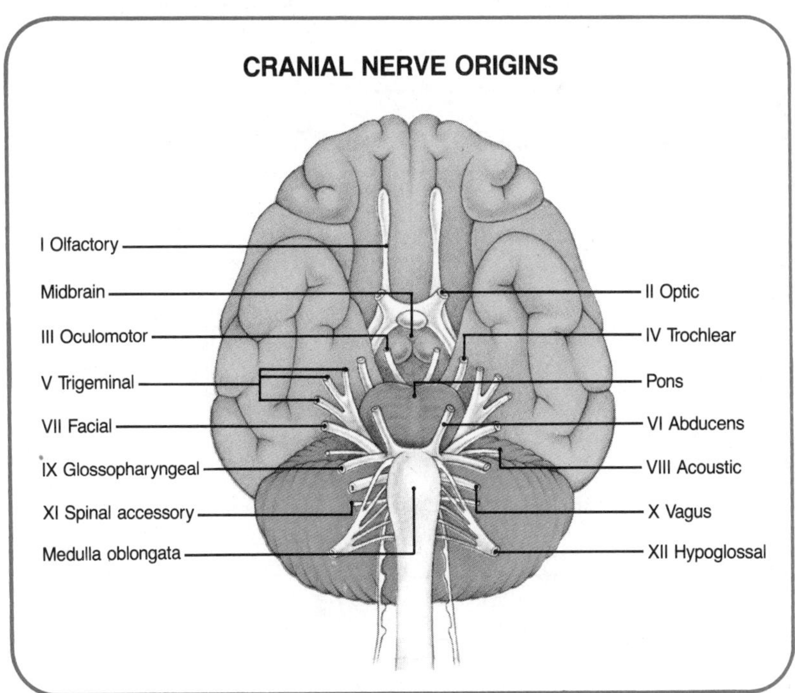

acts on such important information as vital signs, fluid balance, the body's internal temperature, hormonal levels, and other factors that contribute to the body's physical and emotional homeostasis. The epithalamic area contains the *pineal body,* which is usually considered an endocrine gland because it influences the release of gonadotropins through the hypothalamus.

596 Brain stem

The brain stem, the most primitive region of the brain, includes the midbrain, the pons, and the medulla oblongata. Located in the *midbrain* are two massive bundles of nerve tracts (white matter), called *cerebral peduncles;* these peduncles connect the cerebrum with the brain stem and the spinal cord. The corpora quadrigemina, also found in the midbrain, function as a relay station for hearing and play a role in the visual reflex. The *pons,* which lies between the midbrain and the medulla, contains nuclei of certain cranial nerves (see *Identifying Cranial Nerves,* page 562). It also contains the pneumotaxic and apneustic respiratory centers, which control inspiration. The *medulla oblongata,* which lies between the pons and the cervical section of the spinal cord, controls circulation, respiration, and such reflexes as vomiting, sneezing, coughing, swallowing, and hiccuping.

Located on the ventral surface of the medulla oblongata are elevations known as *pyramids.* Motor fibers from the cortex run through these pyramids to the spinal cord, comprising the *pyramidal system,* which controls voluntary action. At the medulla's lower end, about 75% of these fibers cross over to the other side and continue as the lateral corticospinal tract. The fibers that don't cross over continue as the ventral corticospinal tract. This crossover means that most impulses sent to one side of the body originate on the opposite side of the brain.

597 Cerebellum

The cerebellum lies under the posterior parts of the cerebral hemispheres. Its outer surface consists of gray matter;

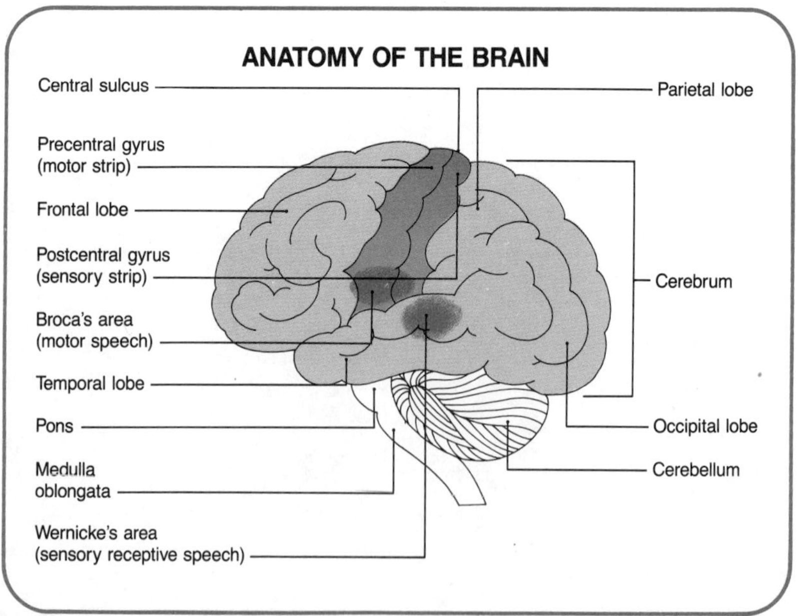

UNDERSTANDING THE BRAIN'S INTERNAL STRUCTURES

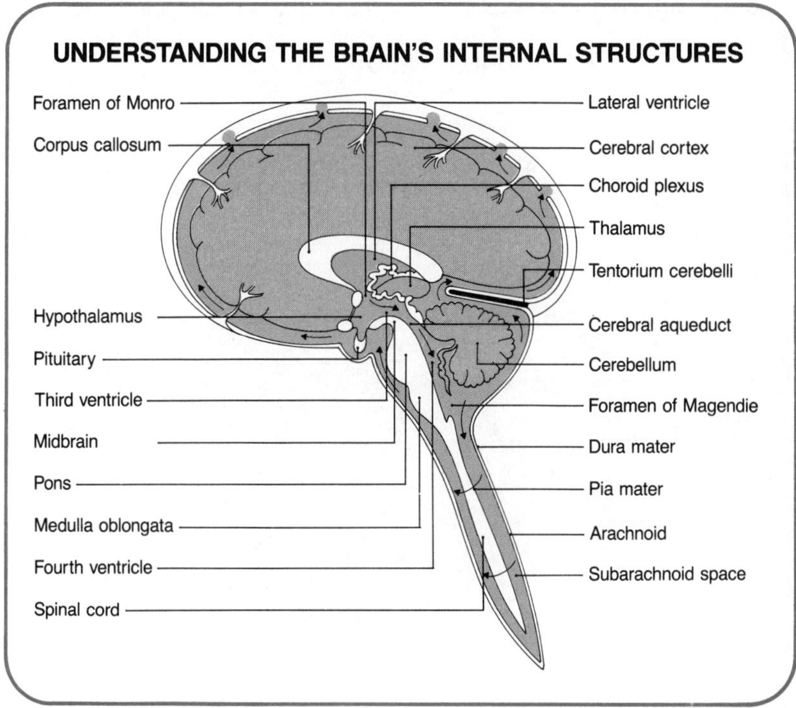

its interior is primarily white matter containing three distinct nuclear masses. The cerebellum is divided into two cerebellar hemispheres, connected by a narrow communicating strip called the *vermis.* It receives proprioceptive impulses from muscles and tendons, information on the body's equilibrium from the vestibular division of the acoustic nerve (CN VIII), and impulses associated with the sensations of touch, vision, and hearing. The cerebellum then correlates all these impulses and directs responses mainly to the cerebral (motor) cortex. The major functions of the cerebellum are coordination of movement, orientation in space, and equilibrium.

598 Protective layers, ventricles, and CSF

Three layers of tissue—collectively called the *meninges*—cover the brain and spinal cord, helping to protect them. The *dura mater,* the thick outer layer, is closest to the skull. It creates two potential spaces: the *epidural* and the *subdural,* which may fill during a pathologic situation, such as arterial bleeding.

The middle layer of the meninges, known as the *arachnoid,* is a thin membrane containing a spidery vascular system. The space under the arachnoid—the *subarachnoid space*—contains cerebrospinal fluid (CSF). The innermost layer, the *pia mater,* is a thin membrane that adheres to the surface of the brain.

The brain contains four cavities, or *ventricles,* where CSF is formed by tiny capillary tufts (choroid plexuses) on the ventricular walls. The CSF fills the ventricles and circulates from them through the subarachnoid space around the brain and the spinal cord. Finally, it returns to the blood from which it was filtered by absorbing through the walls of the arachnoid villi into the venous system. CSF helps support brain

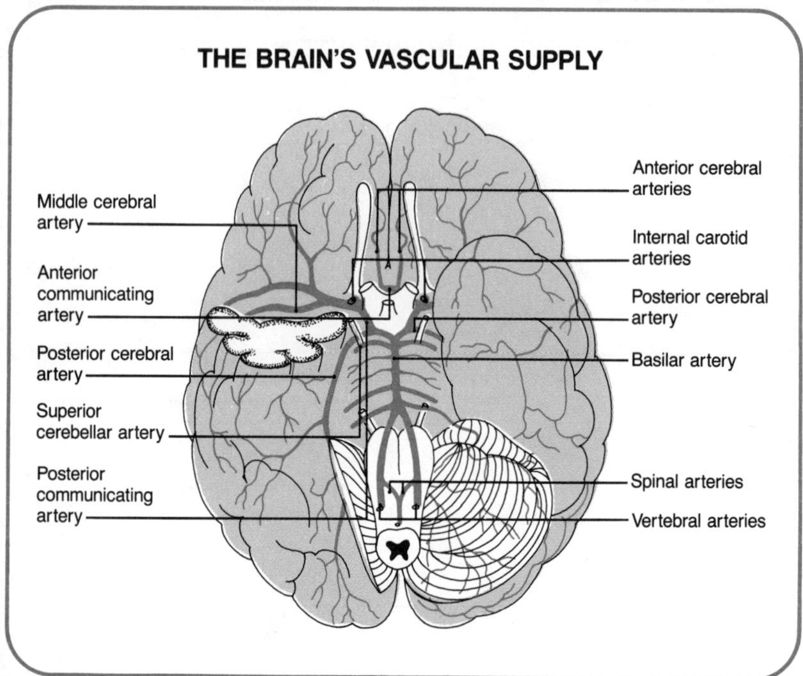

tissues and the spinal cord, cushioning them within their bony cavities.

599 Blood circulation through the CNS

Blood supply to the brain originates from two internal carotid arteries anteriorly and two vertebral arteries posteriorly. The internal carotid arteries branch into cerebral arteries, which supply most of the cerebral hemispheres. The vertebral arteries combine to form the basilar artery, which supplies the brain stem and the cerebellum. This anterior and posterior circulation is joined by communicating arteries to form the *circle of Willis,* which provides an alternate route for blood supply to the brain if obstruction occurs in either the anterior or posterior circulation. Venous drainage of the brain occurs from the top down. Venous blood drains into large sinuses, which eventually empty into the jugular veins. The great cerebral vein that drains the brain's internal portion is a major vein feeding the dural sinuses.

The spinal cord receives blood from the vertebral arteries and the spinal branches of the aorta. Spinal arteries that supply the vertebrae have branches, called *radicular arteries,* that supply the spinal cord. If a radicular artery's blood supply is cut off, damage usually occurs at this level of the spinal cord. One anterior and two posterior longitudinal arteries run along the surface of the spinal cord in the pia mater.

600 Functions of the autonomic nervous system

The autonomic nervous system maintains the body's steady state, without conscious control. This includes regulating such vital functions as temperature, respiration, blood pressure, digestion, and energy metabolism, which are all grouped under the term *homeostasis.* Tissue structures controlled by the autonomic nervous system are smooth muscle and cardiac muscle; organs affected are the heart,

UNDERSTANDING SYMPATHETIC AND PARASYMPATHETIC NERVOUS SYSTEMS

The parasympathetic and sympathetic divisions of the autonomic nervous system play balancing roles in the regulation of the body's cardiac muscles, smooth muscles, and glands. To understand the effects of each division, review the following chart.

You should know that neurotransmitters must be present for any action to take place. The *parasympathetic* division, composed of cholinergic fibers, originates in the cranial area (CN III, VII, IX, and X) and the sacral area (S2 to S4) and uses acetylcholine as its neurotransmitter. The *sympathetic* division, composed of adrenergic fibers, originates in the thoracic area (T1 to T12) and the lumbar area (L1 to L3) and uses epinephrine and norepinephrine as its neurotransmitters.

ORGAN AFFECTED	PARASYMPATHETIC EFFECTS	SYMPATHETIC EFFECTS
Iris	• Contraction of sphincter muscle; pupil constricts	• Contraction of dilator muscle; pupil dilates
Ciliary muscle	• Contraction; accommodation for near vision	• Relaxation; accommodation for distant vision
Lacrimal gland	• Secretion	• Excessive secretion
Salivary glands	• Copious secretion of watery saliva	• Scanty, thick secretion of mucus-rich saliva
Respiratory system		
Trachea/bronchial tree	• Contraction of smooth muscle; decreased diameters and volumes	• Relaxation of smooth muscle; increased diameters and volumes
Blood vessels	• Little effect	• Mildly constricted
Heart		
Rate	• Decreased	• Increased
Stroke volume	• Decreased	• Increased
Cardiac output and blood pressure	• Decreased	• Increased
Coronary vessels	• Constriction	• Dilation
Peripheral blood vessels		
Skeletal muscle	• No innervation	• Dilation
Skin	• No innervation	• Constriction
Visceral organs (except heart and lungs)	• Dilation	• Constriction (may be insignificant)
Stomach		
Wall	• Increased motility	• Decreased motility
Sphincters	• Relaxed	• Contracted
Glands	• Increased secretion	• Decreased secretion
Intestines		
Wall	• Increased motility	• Decreased motility
Sphincters (pyloric, iliocecal, and internal anal)	• Inhibited	• Stimulated
Liver	• Promotes glycogenesis; increases bile secretion	• Promotes glycogenolysis; decreases bile secretion

(continued)

UNDERSTANDING SYMPATHETIC AND PARASYMPATHETIC NERVOUS SYSTEMS *(continued)*

ORGAN AFFECTED	PARASYMPATHETIC EFFECTS	SYMPATHETIC EFFECTS
Pancreas (exocrine and endocrine)	• Increases secretion	• Decreases secretion
Spleen	• Little effect	• Contraction and emptying of stored blood into circulation
Adrenal medulla	• Little effect	• Norepinephrine/ epinephrine secretion
Urinary bladder	• Stimulates wall; relaxes sphincter	• Inhibits wall; contracts sphincter
Uterus	• Little effect	• Inhibits motility of nonpregnant organ; stimulates pregnant organ
Sweat glands	• No innervation	• Increases secretion
Kidneys	• No effect	• Decreased urinary output

Adapted from J. Robert McClintic, *Physiology of the Human Body* (2nd ed.; New York: John Wiley & Sons Publishers, 1978), with permission of the publisher.

blood vessels, irises, hair muscles, thoracic and abdominal organs, and glands.

The autonomic nervous system receives information concerning vital body functions from special chemoreceptors and pressure receptors in blood vessels and internal organs. It's influenced by outside stimuli—such as pain, temperature, and touch—and by special stimuli associated with sight, hearing, smell, and taste. The special receptors transmit messages to the hypothalamus, which in turn stimulates the release of neurohormones or transmitters necessary for a response. The external stimuli indicate danger or pleasure to the body, initiating an autonomic response.

601 Divisions of the autonomic nervous system

The autonomic nervous system is divided into two parts that usually have opposite effects on smooth muscle, cardiac muscle, and glands. One part—the sympathetic division—usually stimulates and the other—the parasympathetic division—usually inhibits. At times, the two parts augment or balance each other. This arrangement provides a fine control of glands and visceral muscle and thus maintains a steady state. The *sympathetic division* of the autonomic nervous system originates in the thoracic (T1 to T12) and upper lumbar (L1 and L2) regions of the spinal cord. When danger threatens, this division controls activities sympathetic, so to speak, to the body's survival. Physical or emotional stress elicits a rapid response from the sympathetic nervous system, producing a combination of responses called the *fight-or-flight reaction.* Sympathetic action takes place through the release of the neurotransmitters epinephrine and norepinephrine, which increase blood and energy supply to vital organs (such as heart, brain, and skeletal muscles) in this emergency response.

UNDERSTANDING CONDUCTION PATHWAYS

Many ascending (sensory) and descending (motor) pathways or tracts run through the central nervous system. Their function is to transmit impulses. Pictured here are a few of the ascending and descending tracts. Look carefully at the location of the tracts. Note the direction in which the impulses travel and where the fibers cross from one side of the spinal cord to the other. The location of these tracts will help you understand how the location of spinal cord disease or injury (lesion) affects different sides of the body.

Sensory pathways

- ***Lateral spinothalamic tract***

  Function: Transmits pain and temperature

  Pathway: Enters the cord and almost immediately crosses to the opposite side, then ascends to the thalamus and to the cerebral cortex (sensory), where the information is interpreted.

  Lesion: Look for loss of pain or temperature sensation below the lesion or on the opposite side of the lesion (contralateral).

- ***Posterior columns***

  Function: Transmit stereognosis (perception of movement, position, form)

  Pathway: Enters the spinal cord and ascends on the same side until it reaches the pyramids in the medulla, where it crosses to the opposite side of the cord and then ascends to the thalamus and cerebral cortex.

  Lesion: Look for ipsilateral loss of muscle and joint sensation of vibration, pressure, and position below the level of the lesion.

Motor pathway

- ***Pyramidal tract*** (also referred to as corticospinal tract or upper motor neuron)

  Function: Transmits motor response to sensory stimuli

  Pathway: Leaves the motor area of the cerebral cortex and extends to the medulla, where it crosses to the opposite side of the cord. It then extends down this side to the ventral (anterior) portion of the spinal cord, where it exits along the motor (afferent) root to the effector muscle for action.

  Lesion: Look for contralateral motor impairment below the level of the lesion.

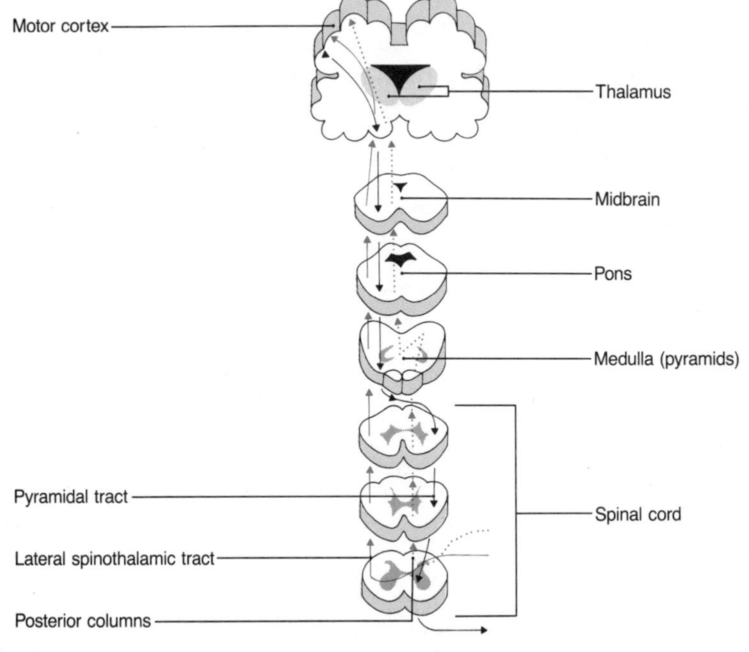

The *parasympathetic division* originates in the cranial region and the sacral portion (S2 to S4) of the spinal cord. For the most part, this division balances the effects of sympathetic stimulation through inhibition of organ function. Parasympathetic action takes place through the release of the neurotransmitter acetylcholine. The parasympathetic response is more localized and slower than the sympathetic responses.

Collecting appropriate history data

602 Biographical data

Although a neurologic disorder can occur at any time in a person's life, some disorders occur most commonly within certain age-groups. For example, the incidence of muscular dystrophies, migraine headaches, and epilepsy is highest among children, adolescents, and young adults. Multiple sclerosis is most prevalent in young adults between ages 20 and 30. Parkinson's disease, Huntington's chorea, amyotrophic lateral sclerosis, and cerebrovascular accident most commonly affect persons over age 40.

603 Chief complaint

The chief complaints most commonly associated with neurologic disorders are *headache/pain, motor disturbances* (including weakness, paresis, and paralysis), *seizures, sensory deviations,* and *altered states of consciousness.*

604 History of present illness

Use the PQRST mnemonic device to help your patient elaborate on his chief complaint. Then, depending on his particular complaint, explore the history of his present illness by asking the following types of questions:

• ***Headache/pain.*** *Is the pain located across your forehead? On one side of your head? At the back of your head and neck?* Pain that emanates from specific areas of the head characterizes certain types of headaches. For example, tension headaches are often located in the occipital area, and migraine pain tends to be unilateral. *Is the pain tight (bandlike), boring, throbbing, steady, or dull?* Headaches can be identified by the quality of pain they produce. A dull, steady pain may indicate a tension (muscle) headache; severe or throbbing pain may indicate a vascular problem, such as a migraine headache. *Is the onset of pain sudden or gradual?* Migraine headaches may develop suddenly, with no warning, but are usually preceded by a prodromal disturbance. Headaches associated with hemorrhage characteristically occur suddenly and with increasing severity. *How long does the pain usually last? Is it continuous or recurrent?* Tension headaches may last from several hours to several days. Migraine headaches may also last this long. Cluster (histamine) headaches last about an hour.

Are the headaches occurring more frequently? A change in headache pattern may signal developing pathology. *Do the headaches occur in the evening? Do you wake up with one during the night? Are the headaches worse when you wake up in the morning?* Although tension headaches usually occur in the evening, a person may awaken in the morning with the headache. Patients who suffer from headaches caused by hypertension, inflammation, or tumors may awaken anytime with the pain. Cluster headaches often awaken the patient a few hours after he has fallen asleep.

Do you see flashing lights or shining

spots or feel tingling, weakness, or numbness immediately before the headache occurs? These are common characteristics of the prodromal (premonitory) neurologic disturbance that frequently precedes a migraine headache.

Does the pain worsen when you cough, sneeze, or bend over? The Valsalva's maneuver may exacerbate a headache caused by an intracranial lesion, such as a subarachnoid hemorrhage.

Do you become nauseated or vomit during the headache? Such gastrointestinal distress may accompany a migraine headache or a brain tumor or hemorrhage. *Have you recently been under a great deal of stress? Are you anxious or depressed?* Headaches that occur daily for a prolonged period may be related to stress or depression.

What medication do you take for the headache? Is it effective? Aspirin is usually ineffective for migraine headaches. *Do other approaches—lying down, applying heat, sleeping—relieve the headache?* Some headaches respond to such techniques.

Would you describe the last headache you experienced as more severe than usual or possibly the worst you've ever had? How a particular headache differs from headaches a patient commonly experiences can give you valuable clues to the cause of his problem.

• ***Motor disturbances.*** *How old were you when you first noticed the problem?* Age is an important factor in identifying motor disturbances, such as epilepsy or parkinsonism. *Did the problem occur suddenly?* Sudden onset may indicate a vascular problem. Gradual onset usually indicates a dystrophy or a tumor. *Is the problem constant or intermittent?* A sign or symptom that is constant may indicate a muscle disorder or dystrophy; one that's intermittent may indicate impaired neuromuscular transmission. *Does the problem occur symmetrically or asymmetrically?* A sign or symptom that presents symmetrically usually indicates a muscle disorder or a peripheral nerve disorder caused by a toxic substance. Asymmetrical presentations usually indicate central nervous system lesions, such as multiple sclerosis, or peripheral nerve disorders from systemic disease.

Do you have difficulty lifting objects, shaving, brushing your hair, walking, or climbing stairs? Such problems may

Chief complaint

- Headache/Pain
- Motor disturbances
- Seizures
- Sensory deviations
- Altered states of consciousness

PQRST

Questions to ask

Provocative/Palliative
What causes it? What makes it better? What makes it worse?

Quality/Quantity
How does it feel, look, or sound, and how much of it is there?

Region/Radiation
Where is it? Does it spread?

Severity scale
Does it interfere with activities? How does it rate on a severity scale of 1 to 10?

Timing
When did it begin? How often does it occur? Is it sudden or gradual?

indicate a myopathy in the proximal muscles of the affected arm or leg. *Do you have difficulty turning doorknobs or picking up pins or similar objects? Do your feet or ankles turn easily, causing you to lose your balance or fall?* Positive responses to these questions may indicate a peripheral nerve disorder (neuropathy). *Does the problem occur after prolonged use of the affected arm or leg? Does it improve after rest?* If so, your patient may have impaired neuromuscular transmission. *Considering the symptoms you've described, would you say you've been more clumsy than weak?* Clumsiness can indicate a problem related to the cerebellum (such as multiple sclerosis) or basal ganglia (such as Parkinson's disease); weakness can indicate a problem in the motor tracts.

Have you experienced tremors? How long? Do the tremors occur only in your hands or throughout your body? Tremors that occur only in the hands may be a sign of thyroid dysfunction, alcoholism, or Parkinson's disease. Tremors of the entire body are typical of anxiety or of delirium tremens, caused by alcoholism. *Do the tremors worsen when you're resting or when you're trying to perform a task?* Tremors that characterize disorders of the cerebellum begin after a voluntary movement and worsen as the movement continues. Tremors of Parkinson's disease characteristically occur when the patient is resting.

• ***Seizures.*** *How old were you when you had your first seizure?* When necessary, obtain information from a family member or friend. In children, seizures are commonly caused by birth injury, infection, epilepsy, or trauma. In adults, seizures can result from tumor, alcoholism, drugs, or trauma. In adults over age 60, vascular disease, tumor, and degenerative disease are possible causes of seizures. *How often do the seizures occur?* Frequency is an important factor in determining treatment.

How would you describe the seizures? Different types of seizures, such as focal motor seizures and petit mal seizures, produce characteristic movements, behavior, and sensory experiences. *Do flashing lights or sounds precipitate seizures?* Some seizures are induced by a certain type of sensory stimulus. *Do your seizures ever occur during times of stress or during alcohol consumption?* These conditions increase the possibility of a seizure. *Can you tell when a seizure is about to occur? Do you see, hear, smell, or feel anything unusual just prior to the seizure?* These characteristic preseizure symptoms or auras can help you identify the location of the disorder. *Do you regain full consciousness slowly or immediately?* Slow recovery can indicate a seizure disorder; immediate recovery, syncope. *What medication do you take for the seizures? Is it effective?* Inadequate therapy could remove the warning aura of seizures or cause undesirable side effects.

• ***Sensory deviations.*** *Do you experience tingling, prickling, or numbness anywhere in your body?* Ask the patient to indicate where on his body he feels the sensations. This will demonstrate the anatomic distribution of the lesion and will help identify the disorder. *Do you have difficulty perceiving pain, temperature changes, or touch?* Certain disorders produce a loss of sensation of any or all of the above.

• ***Altered states of consciousness.*** *How long have you felt confused?* Rapid onset of confusion can indicate metabolic encephalopathy or delirium; gradual onset usually indicates a degenerative disorder. *Does the confusion fluctuate?* This question can help you distinguish between an extracerebral disorder, such as metabolic encephalopathy, and a subdural hematoma caused by intracerebral impairment, such as arteriosclerosis or senile dementia.

If the patient was found unconscious, where was he found? The answer will provide clues to the cause of the unconsciousness—for example, a toxic

NURSE'S GUIDE TO SOME DRUGS THAT AFFECT THE NERVOUS SYSTEM

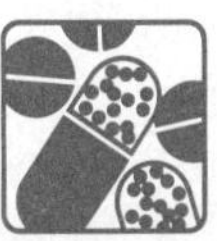

CLASSIFICATION	POSSIBLE SIDE EFFECTS
Adrenergic blockers (sympatholytics) methysergide maleate (Sansert*)	• Vertigo, light-headedness, insomnia, drowsiness, ataxia, hyperesthesia, euphoria, hallucinations
Aminoglycosides All types	• Neuromuscular blockage, headache, lethargy
Anticonvulsants phenytoin sodium (Dilantin Sodium*)	• Headache, ataxia, slurred speech, insomnia, lethargy
Antidepressants amitriptyline hydrochloride (Elavil*) phenelzine sulfate (Nardil*)	• Headache, drowsiness, confusion, tremors
Antihypertensives hydralazine hydrochloride (Apresoline*) methyldopa (Aldomet*)	• Headache, dizziness
Antipsychotics All types	• Extrapyramidal reactions
Antituberculars and antileprotics ethambutol hydrochloride (Myambutol*)	• Headache, dizziness, confusion, peripheral neuritis
streptomycin sulfate	• Transient paresthesias, especially circumoral
Cerebral stimulants All types	• Headache, dizziness, insomnia, tremor, hyperactivity
Cholinergics physostigmine salicylate (Antilirium*)	• Restlessness, twitching, ataxia, sweating
Corticosteroids All types	• Pseudotumor cerebri
Gastrointestinal agents metoclopramide hydrochloride (Reglan**)	• Headache, dizziness, restlessness, drowsiness
Nonnarcotic analgesics and antipyretics indomethacin (Indocin)	• Headache, dizziness, drowsiness, confusion, peripheral neuropathy, convulsions
Psychotherapeutics lithium salts (Lithane*)	• Headache, dizziness, drowsiness, restlessness, tremors, confusion, lethargy, ataxia, epileptiform seizures, blackouts
Spasmolytics theophylline salts (Elixophyllin*)	• Headache, dizziness, restlessness, insomnia, convulsions
Tetracyclines doxycycline hyclate (Vibramycin*) oxytetracycline hydrochloride (Terramycin*)	• Benign intracranial hypertension, dizziness

(*continued*)

NURSE'S GUIDE TO SOME DRUGS THAT AFFECT THE NERVOUS SYSTEM *(continued)*

CLASSIFICATION	POSSIBLE SIDE EFFECTS
Urinary tract germicides	
nitrofurantoin (Furadantin)	• Headache, dizziness, peripheral neuropathy, drowsiness
Vinca alkaloids	
vinblastine sulfate (Velban) vincristine sulfate (Oncovin*)	• Loss of deep tendon reflex, numbness, paresthesias, peripheral neuropathy and neuritis
Miscellaneous	
chloramphenicol (Chloromycetin*)	• Headache, confusion, peripheral neuropathy with prolonged therapy
levodopa (Levopa*)	• Nervousness, fatigue, malaise, choreiform and dystonic movements, psychiatric disturbances, ataxia

* Available in U.S. and Canada. ** Available in Canada only. All other products (no symbol) are available in the U.S. only.

substance, drugs, or alcohol. Did the unconsciousness occur abruptly or gradually? Has the patient's level of consciousness fluctuated? Abrupt loss of consciousness may indicate a vascular accident. Gradual onset could result from metabolic, extracerebral, toxic, or systemic causes. Fluctuating levels of consciousness can signal that systemic hypotension is affecting the brain. Did anything happen to the patient recently that could have exacerbated an existing condition, resulting in unconsciousness? An infection or a break in treatment of an existing condition can result in unconsciousness or coma.

605 Past history

Review the following significant health problems thoroughly when you take your patient's past history:

• ***Head injury.*** Head injury can lead to headache, seizures, or coma from increased pressure, fracture, or intracranial bleeding.

• ***Birth trauma.*** This is a common cause of seizures in children.

• ***Recent infections.*** Ear and sinus infections can cause headaches. Septicemia and pneumonia can cause confusion. Other infections can result in idiopathic polyneuritis.

• ***Cardiovascular disorders.*** In some patients, confusion may be a side effect of treatment with antihypertensives. Systemic hypotension causes reduced cerebral arterial perfusion, resulting in sensory and motor problems.

• ***Respiratory disorders.*** Any severe respiratory disorder can cause hypoxia, leading to confusion and coma.

• ***Thyroid disorders.*** Alterations in thyroid hormone secretions can change a patient's neurologic status. For example, patients suffering from hyperthyroidism commonly experience tremors and extreme overactivity—sometimes to the point of mania. Patients with hypothyroid conditions can experience weakness and coma. Thyroidectomy can result in myxedemic symptoms, including such mental status changes as lethargy and apathy.

• ***Metabolic disorders.*** In a patient with diabetes mellitus, hypoglycemia can result in confusion, seizures, and unconsciousness; hyperglycemia can cause lethargy and coma. Various neuropathies are classic complications of diabetes.

• ***Urinary disorders.*** Chronic renal failure can lead to uremic syndrome, characterized by confusion, convulsions, and coma.
• ***Past neurologic testing.*** The results of a patient's previous brain scan, computerized tomography scan, electroencephalography, skull X-ray, and lumbar puncture can usually provide pertinent information about his present problem.
• ***Psychological disorders.*** Chronic alcoholism and drug abuse can result in convulsions—especially during withdrawal—and produce such changes in a patient's neurologic status as neuropathy, delirium tremens, and confusion. Depression can cause confusion and should be clearly distinguished from organic changes, which sometimes also result in confusion.
• ***Immunizations.*** Inoculations can cause idiopathic polyneuritis.
• ***Drugs.*** Question the patient about his use of over-the-counter drugs for headaches, sleep disorders, and mental disturbances. Improper drug therapy can result in undesirable side effects and may exacerbate symptoms rather than improve them.

606 Family history

Some genetic diseases, such as Huntington's chorea, may be degenerative. Other genetic diseases, such as dystrophies, familial periodic paralysis, and Duchenne's disease, cause muscle weakness. The incidence of seizures is higher among patients whose family history shows idiopathic epilepsy. About 65% of persons suffering from migraine headaches show a family history of the disorder.

607 Psychosocial history

When you assess a patient with a neurologic disorder, consider that his home and work environment may be significant. Recent stress at home or at work and recent emotional disturbances or exposure to toxic substances (such as carbon monoxide, nitrates, or heavy metal fumes) can result in neurologic symptoms or can exacerbate an existing neurologic disorder.

608 Activities of daily living

Your review of the patient's activities of daily living should include questions about drug use. How much does the patient's condition interfere with his daily activities?

609 Review of systems

In your review of systems, ask the patient if he has experienced any of the following signs and symptoms:
• ***Head.*** When associated with fever, a headache and a stiff neck suggest infection or irritation of the meninges. Dizziness may be caused by influenza, high blood pressure, or impaired circulation to the brain.
• ***Eyes.*** Papilledema suggests increased intracranial pressure. Blindness may indicate tumors of the pituitary gland. Glaucoma can produce symptoms—such as headache—similar to those of neurologic disorders.
• ***Respiratory.*** A change in respiratory pattern (rate, depth, regularity) may indicate increasing intracranial pressure.
• ***Musculoskeletal.*** Muscle atrophy occurs in a variety of disorders of the motor cortex. Pain on movement of the spine may be caused by disease of the spinal disks, ligaments, or muscles. Certain signs indicate irritation or infection of the meninges. For example, Brudzinki's sign is positive when the patient's neck is flexed on his chest, causing flexion of both legs and thighs. Kernig's sign occurs when a patient (in the supine position) who has his hip flexed at a right angle cannot extend his leg.
• ***Gastrointestinal.*** Unexpected projectile vomiting may be an indication of increased intracranial pressure.
• ***Reproductive.*** Amenorrhea may be caused by a pituitary tumor.

Conducting the physical examination

610 Preparations

Ask your patient to remove his street clothes or pajamas and put on a hospital gown. (This allows you to inspect the patient's body for symmetry—an essential part of the physical examination—and allows the patient to move freely.) If he appears chilled or tense, drape him with a cloth or blanket, because his discomfort may otherwise interfere with the examination. Make sure you have the necessary examination equipment on hand (see *Preparing for the Neurologic Examination*).

Plan your approach to a neurologic examination, keeping in mind that you can assess several areas at the same time. For example, you can combine assessment of your patient's mental status and speech with history-taking and your general survey, and assessment of several of the cranial nerves with examination of the head and neck. You can also combine inspection of your patient's arms and legs with evaluation of his peripheral vascular and musculoskeletal systems.

611 Preliminary survey

Begin a neurologic examination by performing a general survey of your patient (see Entry 67), which may give you a clue to an underlying disease process. Check the patient's blood pressure and major arterial pulses bilaterally, because increased blood pressure and a decreased pulse rate may be signs of increased intracranial pressure.

Observe the size and shape of the patient's head and jaw. Inspect his nostrils and ear canals for patency (necessary to assess cranial nerves I and VIII, later in the examination). Observe his skin for rash, lesions, discoloration, or scars.

Palpate the patient's cranium for bony abnormalities, lumps, tenderness, and soft areas. Then palpate his carotid and temporal arteries for pulsations. Next, percuss his cranium firmly with your index and middle fingers, and then percuss his sinuses and mastoid processes for tenderness (see Entry 348).

Moving to the patient's neck, auscultate bilaterally for bruits over the carotid artery: The presence of bruits indicates distortion of a blood vessel that could interfere with blood flow to the brain. Assess the patient's neck for suppleness by asking him to place his chin on his chest. He should be able to turn his head easily.

Finally, inspect the patient's spine for deformities, abnormal posture, and unusual hair growth. Palpate the vertebrae for structural abnormalities, pain, and tenderness.

612 Parts of a neurologic examination

Always examine a patient's nervous system in an orderly fashion, beginning with the highest levels of neurologic function and working down to the lowest. For this purpose, the complete examination is usually divided into tests for these five functions: *cerebral, cranial nerve, motor, sensory,* and *reflex*.

613 Testing cerebral function

To assess your patient's cerebral function, briefly evaluate his general appearance and behavior, level of consciousness and orientation, memory, general knowledge, arithmetic skill, and comprehension of abstract relationships and judgment. These tests, collectively known as the *mental status examination* (see Entries 125 to 135), are designed to identify disturbing or abnormal mental processes. Be sure to take into account the patient's age and education. Inappropriate responses to your questions may be caused by these factors rather than by neurologic impairment.

You can perform part of the mental status examination—particularly the tests of orientation to time, person, and place and of memory—as you interview the patient. His subjective responses to your questions will allow you to make objective observations about his mental activity.

614 Level of consciousness and orientation

To determine a person's level of consciousness, note the flow of his speech, the quality of his voice, and the organization and clarity of his thoughts. Ask the patient to respond to such simple commands as "Close your eyes" and "Stick out your tongue." Note how promptly he responds. Also observe for apparent drowsiness or loss of contact.

To determine your patient's orientation to person, place, and time, ask such questions as "What's your name? Where are you? What day is this?" If the patient was transferred several times because of surgery or diagnostic testing, accept a general response—for example, "the hospital"—to your questions about place. Don't expect him to remember his room number.

Assess your patient's ability to remember recent and past (remote) events—a function of the temporal lobe. Ask about past events with which he should be familiar. To test recent memory, show him two or three items and then ask him to recall them a few minutes later.

615 Assessing speech

Speech results from the brain's ability to receive incoming verbal or written information (*receptive process*) and to communicate or send responses (*expressive process*). The brain's interpretation of the message occurs between the receptive and expressive processes.

By assessing the processes involved in speech, you can determine the general areas of dysfunction within the brain. For example, various types of aphasia relate directly to corresponding areas of brain dysfunction. Auditory-receptive aphasia results from temporal lobe dysfunction, whereas the visual-receptive form can be traced to disorders of the parieto-occipital area. Expressive aphasia in the form of an inability to write stems from a dysfunction of the posterior frontal lobe; the oral form of this type of aphasia suggests a problem in the inferoposterior frontal lobes.

To assess the receptive process involved in speech, which includes comprehension of both oral and written symbols, note your patient's response to simple commands when you test his level of consciousness. Then, ask the patient some questions that require an oral response of more than one word. Finally, ask him to read a paragraph from a newspaper and explain it to you in his own words.

PREPARING FOR THE NEUROLOGIC EXAMINATION

Before you begin the neurologic examination, gather this equipment:

- **Transparent millimeter ruler,** to measure pupil size and skin lesions
- **Tuning fork,** to test hearing and vibratory sensation
- **Stethoscope,** to auscultate for bruits
- **Penlight or flashlight,** to test pupillary reflexes
- **Tongue depressors,** to test gag reflex
- **Ophthalmoscope,** to assess eye grounds
- **Otoscope,** to examine ears
- **Toothpaste, tobacco, soap, cloves, or other familiar substances,** to assess sense of smell
- **Sugar, salt, and vinegar or lemon juice,** to assess sense of taste
- **Cotton wisp,** to assess light-touch perception
- **Coins or keys,** to test for tactile agnosia
- **Reflex hammer,** to test deep tendon reflexes
- **Safety pin,** to test pain and pressure perception
- **Test tubes of hot and cold water,** to test temperature perception
- **Snellen chart,** to test visual acuity

EMERGENCY

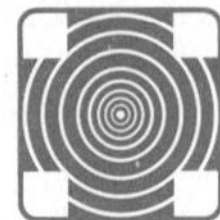

HOW TO PERFORM A NEUROCHECK

Your patient is scheduled for minor surgery. Before surgery, he has a seizure. You need to assess his neurologic status, but you don't have time for a complete neurologic examination. What should you do? Perform a neurocheck. This brief, ongoing evaluation helps you quickly assess a patient's condition and stability and provides information that may indicate neurologic problems. Whenever you note a change in the patient's consciousness level, perform a neurocheck by carefully evaluating the following:

- *Consciousness level:* Does he respond when you talk to him, or do you need to apply light pressure on one of his nail beds to get a response? Use the Glasgow coma scale shown on the opposite page to record your patient's level of consciousness (LOC). With each neurocheck, total the response scores. A total of 7 or less indicates a comatose state. Then, use the terms below to describe his level of consciousness. An altered consciousness level may be the first indication of increased intracranial pressure.

LOC	CHARACTERISTIC RESPONSE
Alert	• Awake • Responds appropriately to auditory, tactile, and visual stimuli; oriented to person, place, and time
Lethargic	• Sleeps often • Arouses easily; responds appropriately
Obtunded	• Aroused by shaking or shouting; responds appropriately • Returns to sleep
Stuporous	• Responds only to painful stimulus • Withdraws finger or pushes your hand away (purposeful movement) • Not completely awake during stimulation
Semicomatose	• Responds only to painful stimulus • Performs reflex movement, such as decerebrate posturing
Comatose	• Shows no response; shows no reflexes • Exhibits flaccid muscle tone in arms and legs

- *Vital signs.* Check your patient's pulse rate, blood pressure, and respirations. Altered vital signs may indicate increased intracranial pressure or neurogenic shock and will help you identify a hemorrhage or tumor.
- *Pupillary reaction.* Evaluate the patient's direct and consensual response to light. Also, measure his pupil size using a pupil gauge like this:

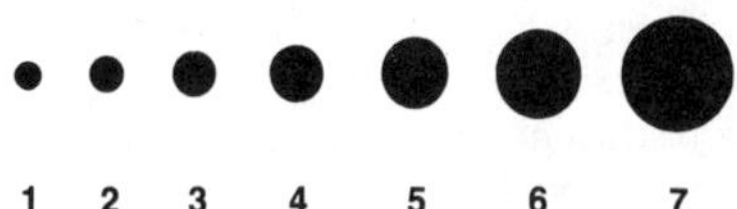

Testing pupillary reaction may help locate a space-occupying brain lesion. Remember, an abnormal pupil reaction occurs on the same side as the lesion (ipsilateral).

- *Motor response.* Test the patient's grip strength, pressure resistance, and ability to move. Evaluating motor response may help locate nerve weakness or damage or a space-occupying lesion. Note, weakness occurs on the side opposite the lesion (contralateral).

Assessing the expressive process in speech also overlaps with testing for level of consciousness. Your patient's speech should be fluent, spontaneous, and clearly enunciated. Remember to judge it according to his native language, education, reading ability, and communication skills. If appropriate, make sure the patient wears his glasses or hearing aid during the examination, so you can record accurate responses.

616 Cranial nerve I: Olfactory

After testing your patient's cerebral function with the mental status examination, begin your assessment of his cranial nerve function. Assess the olfactory nerve first, to determine any loss of smell or differences in the sense of smell between nostrils. Ask the patient to close both eyes and occlude one nostril. Then bring a nonirritating substance with a familiar odor, such as toothpaste or tobacco, near his open nostril and ask him if he smells anything. If he does, ask him to identify it. Then repeat the test on the other nostril. The test should be repeated several times, using a different-smelling substance each time. Because many odors are difficult to identify, consider the patient's olfactory nerve intact if he can perceive at least one odor.

617 Cranial nerve II: Optic

To assess the optic nerve, test your patient's visual acuity and visual fields and examine the fundus of each eye. Your findings should indicate the clarity of each eye's transparent media (cornea, anterior body, lens, and vitreous body), the adequacy of central vision, and the function of nerve fibers from the macula to the occipital cortex.

Before beginning your examination of the optic nerve, inspect the patient's eyes for foreign bodies, cataracts, corneal scarring or inflammation, and conjunctival redness. Then test his visual acuity with a pocket-sized Snellen chart (used for bedside testing) or a newspaper. Because refractive errors aren't particularly significant for neurologic assessment, the patient who wears glasses should be tested both with and without them. Ask the patient to cover one eye and read the smallest line he can on the Snellen chart, or one or two lines of a newspaper story set in small type. Then have the patient cover his other eye and repeat the test.

Normally, a person can read the bedside Snellen chart at 30″ (76 cm). Record the distance at which your patient can read the chart as a fraction of the normal distance. For example, if the patient can only read the chart at 15″ (38 cm), record his visual acuity for that eye as 15/30. To verify your examination, refer to the fractions printed on the eye chart for the smallest line the patient can read.

Visual field testing for a neurologic examination is the same as for an eye examination (see Entry 268). A visual field abnormality may indicate a brain lesion anywhere along the visual pathway, causing damage to all or part of the nerve (see *Identifying Lesions in the Optic Pathway,* page 580). You would

GLASGOW COMA SCALE

TEST	REACTION SCORE
Eyes open	
Spontaneously	4
To speech	3
To pain	2
Not at all	1
Verbal response	
Oriented	5
Confused	4
Inappropriate	3
Incomprehensible	2
None	1
Motor response	
Obeys commands	5
Localizes pain	4
Flexion to pain	3
Extension to pain	2
None	1

also examine the fundus with a direct ophthalmoscope as for an eye examination (see Entry 272).

618 Cranial nerves III, IV, and VI

Cranial nerves III, IV, and VI are usually tested together, because they control the closely coordinated functions of eye movement, pupil constriction, and eyelid elevation. The *oculomotor nerve* (CN III) is responsible for pupillary constriction, elevation of the upper lid, and most eye movements. The *trochlear nerve* (CN IV) makes downward and inward eye movements possible. The *abducens nerve* (CN VI) allows the eyes to move laterally. Your joint assessment of these three nerves should include inspection of the patient's eyes and eyelids and testing for accommodation, direct and consensual pupillary reflexes, and ocular movement.

Begin your assessment of the oculomotor nerve by inspecting the patient's eyes (see Entry 266). Then, with the lights turned down, observe the size, shape, and equality of his pupils (see Entry 271). They should be round and about equal in size. Use a small, bright light source to assess pupillary response by shining the light in one eye and observing for pupil constriction in

IDENTIFYING LESIONS IN THE OPTIC PATHWAY

As you evaluate your patient's vision during the neurologic examination, remember that a lesion anywhere along the optic pathway can cause some degree of blindness. The illustration below shows the specific type of blindness produced by a lesion in the retina, the optic nerve, the optic tract, or the temporal, parietal, or occipital lobe.

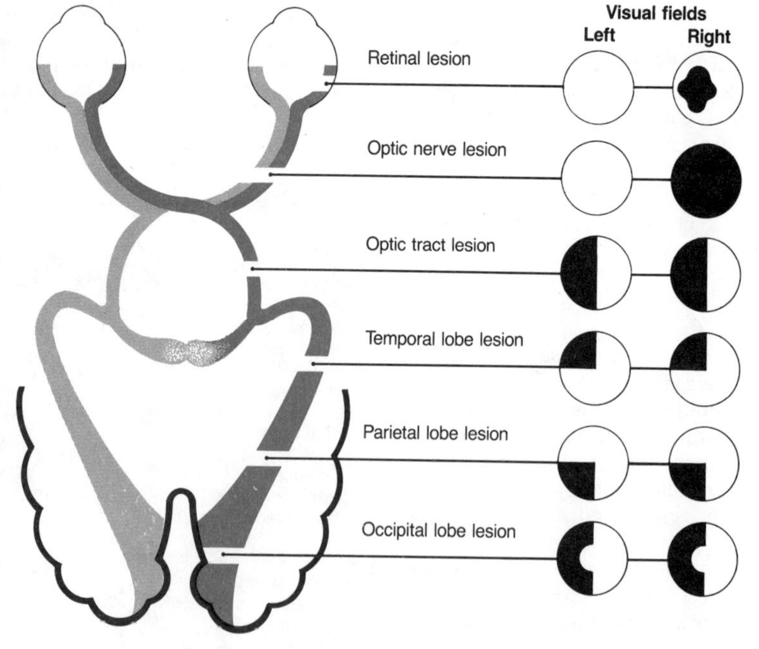

Reprinted with permission from Smith Kline & French Laboratories, *Essentials of the Neurological Examination* (4th ed.; Philadelphia: Smith Kline Corporation, 1962).

this eye (direct response) as well as in the opposite eye (consensual response). Keep in mind that young people normally have larger, more responsive pupils than the elderly.

Assessing the ocular movement function of cranial nerve III allows you to simultaneously evaluate cranial nerves IV and VI. First, observe the patient's eyes at rest, for any obvious deviation. Then ask him to follow an object, such as a pen or pencil, without turning his head. Hold the object about 2′ (60 cm) from the midline of the patient's face and move it to the right. Pause to observe if the patient's eyes are conjugately deviated—positioned in a uniform, parallel fashion—toward the object. Tell your patient to hold his gaze on the object, and ask him if he is experiencing double vision (diplopia). Observe for nystagmus—a rhythmic, bobbing movement of the eyes. Repeat this procedure through the six cardinal fields of gaze (see Entry 267).

619 Cranial nerve V: Trigeminal

The trigeminal nerve is both a sensory and a motor nerve. It supplies sensation to the corneas, nasal and oral mucosa, and facial skin, and also supplies motor function for all muscles of mastication. The sensory division, which predominates, consists of three branches: ophthalmic, maxillary, and mandibular. To test the sensory division, ask the patient to close his eyes; then touch his jaw, cheek, and forehead bilaterally with a cotton wisp (light-touch sensation). Then touch each area with the point of a pin (pain sensation). Ask the patient to compare and describe the sensations on both sides. If you note any abnormality in pain sensation, test for temperature sensation by touching each area first with a test tube containing hot water, then with one containing cold water. Compare sensation on both sides.

Next, test the patient's corneal reflex with a cotton wisp. (If your patient wears contact lenses, ask him to remove them, because they can cause the corneal reflex to appear diminished or absent.) To prevent involuntary blinking, ask the patient to look away. Bring the wisp toward the eye from one side and touch the cornea—not just the sclera—with the point. The normal response is a bilateral blink. Then test the patient's light reflex (see Entry 267).

To test the motor division of the trigeminal nerve, ask the patient to clench his teeth; then palpate the temporal and the masseter muscles bilaterally. Note the strength of the muscles. Next, ask the patient to clench and unclench his jaws several times. Observe for distorted movements or asymmetry. To assess muscle strength, ask the patient to clench his teeth again, while you try to pry his jaws apart against his resistance. Finally, ask the patient to press his jaw laterally against your hand, with his mouth slightly open, as a further test of muscle strength.

620 Cranial nerve VII: Facial

Like the trigeminal nerve, the facial nerve has both sensory and motor functions. Its predominant motor division innervates all facial muscles bilaterally. Some of the expressions controlled by the motor division of the facial nerve include wrinkling the nose, smiling, frowning, closing the eyes, and grimacing. The sensory division is responsible for taste perception on the anterior portion of the tongue.

Begin your assessment of the patient's facial nerve by observing the symmetry of his face. Then ask him to raise and lower his eyebrows. Again observe for symmetry. Next, ask him to close his eyes tightly while you attempt to raise the lids. Finally, ask him to smile, show his teeth, and puff out his cheeks, so you can assess facial muscle strength.

Nurses usually don't perform taste tests on patients. If you do perform these tests, begin by testing the sensory division of the facial nerve. Ask your

EVALUATING ABNORMAL CRANIAL NERVE RESPONSES

NERVE	TEST
I Olfactory	• Have patient identify familiar odors applied to each nostril.
II Optic	• Shine light in affected eye.
	• Shine light in normal eye.
	• Approach patient's eye from side with your hand.
III Oculomotor	• Inspect eye.
	• Shine light in affected eye.
	• Shine light in normal eye.
IV Trochlear	• Have patient follow object without turning his head.
V Trigeminal	*Sensation* • Lightly touch cornea and skin above eye (1-ophthalmic division). • Lightly touch upper lip (2-maxillary division). • Lightly touch lower lip and chin (3-mandibular division).
	Motor • Have patient bite down or chew while you palpate masseter and temporal muscles.
VI Abducens	• Have patient look right and then left.
VII Facial	• Have patient raise and lower eyebrows; close eyes tightly while you attempt to pry eyes open; smile; puff cheeks.
	• Have patient identify tastes.
	• Have patient wrinkle forehead.
VIII Acoustic	• In children and uncooperative patients, clap hands close to patient's ear to elicit a startle reflex.
	• Place tuning fork on middle of patient's forehead (Weber test).
IX Glossopharyngeal	• Have patient identify taste at back of tongue.
	• Apply cotton to soft palate.
X Vagus	• Inspect soft palate and larynx with laryngoscope.

ABNORMAL FINDINGS	POSSIBLE CAUSES
• Anosmia, olfactory hallucinations	• Fracture of cribriform plate or ethmoid area • Olfactory bulb or tract tumor
• Absent direct and consensual pupillary constriction • Present direct and consensual pupillary constriction • Absent blink reflex	• Direct trauma to orbit or globe • Fracture involving optic foramen • Pressure on geniculocalcarine tract • Laceration or intracerebral clot in temporal, parietal, or occipital lobe; rarely from subdural clot
• Dilated pupil, ptosis, eye turns down and out • Absent direct pupil reflex; present consensual reflex • Present direct pupil reflex; absent consensual reflex	• Increased intracranial pressure causing herniating uncus (temporal lobe) on nerve just before it enters cavernous sinus • Fracture involving cavernous sinus
• Eye fails to move down and out	• Pressure on nerve around brain stem from tumor • Fracture of orbit
• Absent sensation of pain and touch; paresthesias • Palpated masseter and temporalis fail to contract	• Tic douloureux caused by sinus or dental problems • Irritation from tumor, aneurysm, meningitis, herpes zoster • Direct injury • Myasthenia gravis
• Affected eye fails to move laterally; diplopia on lateral gaze	• Tumor or trauma at base of brain • Fracture involving cavernous sinus or orbit
• No facial movement, eye remains open, or opens easily, angle of mouth droops, forehead fails to wrinkle • Above responses, loss of taste on anterior two thirds of tongue • No facial movement, forehead fails to wrinkle	• Peripheral laceration or contusion in parotid region; Bell's palsy • Peripheral fracture of temporal bone • Supranuclear, intracerebral clot
• No startle reflex • Sound not heard by involved ear	• Fractures of petrous bone • Ménière's syndrome • Acoustic neuroma
• Loss of taste posterior one third of tongue • Absent sensation on affected side of palate	• Tumor or injury to brain stem • Neck trauma
• Sagging soft palate, deviation of uvula to normal side; gag reflex	• Tumor or injury to brain stem • Neck trauma

(continued)

EVALUATING ABNORMAL CRANIAL NERVE RESPONSES *(continued)*

NERVE	TEST
XI Spinal accessory	• Have patient push chin against your hand.
	• Have patient shrug shoulders.
	• Have patient stretch out hands toward you.
XII Hypoglossal	• Have patient stick out tongue.

patient to stick out his tongue. Then put some sugar on the anterior portion of one side of the tongue. Tell him to keep his tongue out until he's identified the taste. (If he pulls in his tongue prematurely, the test substance will spread to the opposite side, giving inaccurate results.) After he's identified the sugar, have him rinse his mouth. Repeat the procedure on the same side of the tongue, using salt, a sour substance like vinegar or lemon juice, and a bitter substance. Perform the same tests on the other side of the tongue.

For convenience, assess one function of the glossopharyngeal nerve (CN IX) at this time—perception of taste on the posterior third of the tongue. Test this nerve as you did the sensory division of the facial nerve, using a pipette or a swab to apply sweet, salty, sour, and bitter substances. Use a different swab for each substance, and instruct the patient to keep his tongue out during each test. Give the patient a card with the words *sweet, salty, sour,* and *bitter* printed on it, so he can answer your questions without pulling his tongue in to speak. After applying a particular substance, ask him to point to the word that best describes its taste. Instruct the patient to take a sip of water after each test to avoid mixing tastes. Test each substance twice on each side of the patient's tongue.

621 Cranial nerve VIII: Acoustic

The acoustic nerve is a sensory nerve that consists of cochlear and vestibular divisions. The cochlear division is responsible for hearing; the vestibular division governs maintenance of equilibrium, body position, and orientation to space.

To make a gross assessment of the cochlear division, screen for hearing loss by first occluding one of your patient's ears. Then whisper, or rub your fingers together, near his other ear, and ask him if he hears the sound. For a more precise assessment of hearing acuity, use the Weber, Rinne, and Schwabach tests (see Entries 311, 312, and 313).

You wouldn't normally assess the vestibular division of the acoustic nerve as part of a neurologic examination unless your patient's history or physical examination reveals vertigo associated with nausea and vomiting or ataxia. When indicated, a doctor usually assesses this division, using cold water caloric testing.

622 Cranial nerves IX and X

You'll usually test cranial nerves IX and X together, because they're closely associated and similar in function. The motor aspect of the *glossopharyngeal*

ABNORMAL FINDINGS	POSSIBLE CAUSES
• Palpated sternocleidomastoid fails to contract	• Neck trauma • Radical neck surgery • Torticollis
• Palpated upper fibers of trapezius fail to contract	
• Affected arm seems longer; scapula not anchored	
• Tongue protrudes toward affected side; dysarthria	• Neck trauma, usually associated with major vessel damage

Reprinted with permission from *Clinical Symposia* by Cmdr. Frederick E. Jackson (Copyright © 1967, CIA-GEIGY Corporation).

nerve (CN IX) innervates the stylopharyngeus muscle, used in swallowing; it also supplies sensation to the mucous membranes of the pharynx and is responsible for taste perception on the posterior one third of the tongue and for salivation. The *vagus nerve* (CN X) innervates thoracic and abdominal visceral organs; controls swallowing, phonation, and movement of the uvula and soft palate; and supplies sensation to the mucosa of the pharynx, soft palate, and tonsils. The 10th cranial nerve also carries sensory impulses from the gastrointestional tract, the heart, and the lungs. (You'll normally evaluate these functions during the general physical examination.) Begin your assessment of the glossopharyngeal and the vagus nerves by inspecting the patient's soft palate. It should appear symmetrical, with no deviation. When the patient says "Ah," the palate should rise promptly and symmetrically. Note any hoarseness.

To test the palatal reflex, touch the mucous membrane of the soft palate with a swab. The palate should rise promptly on the side touched. Touch the posterior pharyngeal wall with a tongue depressor. The palate will elevate, and the pharyngeal muscles will contract. The patient may feel like he's gagging, a normal reaction known as the *gag reflex*.

623 Cranial nerve XI: Spinal accessory

A motor nerve, the spinal accessory nerve supplies the sternocleidomastoid muscles and the upper portion of the trapezius muscles. To evaluate your patient's spinal accessory nerve, test the strength and bulk of the sternocleidomastoid and the trapezius muscles bilaterally. To assess the sternocleidomastoid muscles, ask your patient to turn his head to the right and hold it in this position while you try to turn it toward the front. You should see the sternocleidomastoid muscles clearly. Inspect and palpate the muscles for fasciculations, weakness, and atrophy. Repeat the procedure with the patient's head turned to the left.

To evaluate the trapezius muscles, ask the patient to shrug his shoulders while you try to hold them down. Then ask him to raise his arms above his head. Inspect and palpate the muscles.

624 Cranial nerve XII: Hypoglossal

This motor nerve is responsible for normal tongue movements involved in swallowing and speech. Assess the hypoglossal nerve by first inspecting the patient's tongue in its normal resting position. Observe for asymmetry, deviation to one side, loss of bulk on one or both sides, and fasciculations. Next, ask the patient to stick out his tongue. It should protrude along the midline. Then, as you hold a tongue depressor against one side of his tongue, ask him to push his tongue against the tongue depressor, to test tongue strength. Repeat with the tongue depressor against the opposite side of the tongue. Finally, ask him to move his tongue rapidly in and out and from side to side.

625 Assessing motor and cerebellar functions

To assess your patient's motor function, observe his gait and posture. Then test the tone and strength of his muscles and his balance and coordination. (For these techniques, see Entries 678, 679, and 687).

To assess your patient's cerebellar functions of balance and coordination,

OBSERVING YOUR PATIENT'S GAIT

During the neurologic examination, observe your patient's gait and note any abnormal characteristics, such as the ones listed below. Your observations may help you pinpoint possible neurologic disorders.

Later, you'll evaluate your patient's gait more extensively, when you assess his musculoskeletal system.

TYPE	CHARACTERISTICS	POSSIBLE DISORDER
Ataxic	Staggering; unsteadiness; inability to remain steady with feet together; tendency to reel to one side	Disease of the cerebellum or posterior columns
Dystonic	Irregular, nondirective movements	Disorder of muscle tone
Dystrophic	Waddling, with legs far apart; weight shifts from side to side; abdomen protrudes; lordosis possible	Weakness or wasting of pelvic girdle (muscular dystrophy); dislocated hip
Hemiplegic	Rigid movements; leg on affected side circles outward, foot drags on floor, arm on same side may be rigidly flexed and does not swing freely; leaning to affected side	Disorder of corticospinal tract
Parkinsonian	Forward-leaning posture, head bent, hips and knees flexed; short, shuffled, rapidly accelerating steps; stiff turns, entire body rotated at once; difficulty starting and stopping	Basal ganglia defects of Parkinson's disease; extrapyramidal tract
Scissors	Short, slow steps, with legs alternately crossing over each other	Spastic paraplegia
Spastic	Short steps, dragging balls of feet	Bilateral lesion of corticospinal tract
Steppage	Exaggerated, high steps, with knees flexed; feet brought down heavily	Footdrop secondary to lower motor neuron lesions

RECOGNIZING ABNORMAL POSTURES

A patient exhibiting any of the three abnormal postures described here may have severe neurologic damage. If your patient assumes any of these postures, alert the doctor immediately.

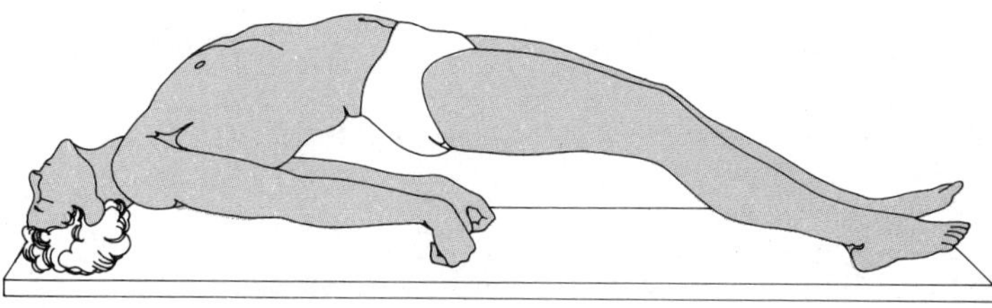

Opisthotonos: characterized by a rigidly arched neck and spine; may indicate meningeal irritation or seizures

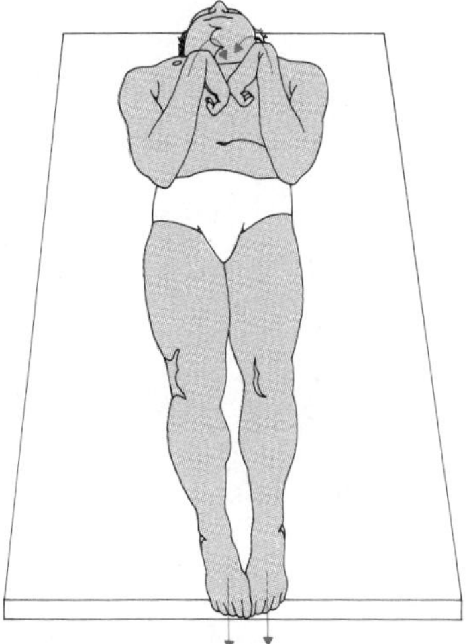

Decorticate posturing: a rigid spine, inwardly flexed arms, extended legs, and plantar flexion; may indicate a lesion at the level of the diencephalon

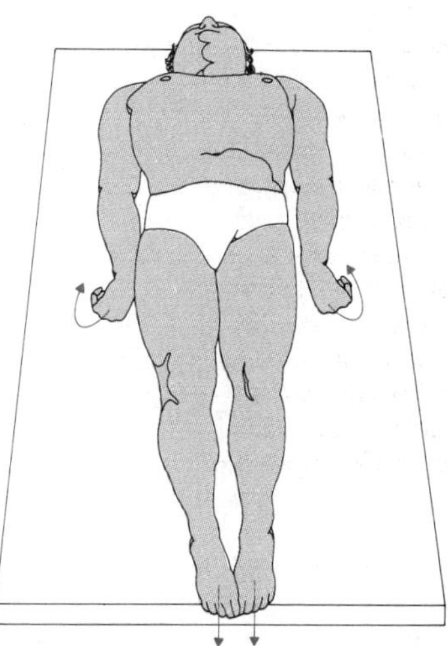

Decerebrate posturing: a rigid and possibly arched spine, rigidly extended arms and legs, and plantar flexion; may indicate a brain stem lesion

test for Romberg's sign (see Entry 314). Then ask the patient to walk heel-to-toe in a straight line with his eyes open (tandem walking). Note any swaying to the right or left. The results of this part of the neurologic examination also reflect the adequacy of the patient's muscle innervation (see *Understanding Muscle Innervation,* page 588).

626 Testing your patient's coordination

These tests evaluate purposeful, fine movements and coordination of the arms and legs. Although the tests themselves aren't complicated, the instructions may be confusing, so show the patient what you expect him to do beforehand. Remember that the patient's

UNDERSTANDING MUSCLE INNERVATION

By testing your patient's motor function, you're also evaluating the adequacy of muscle innervation. Nerve networks supply muscles with the stimuli needed to produce motor functions. This list shows which nerves supply specific muscles and which nerves produce specific reflexes.

MUSCLES OR REFLEXES	INNERVATION
Effector muscles	
Diaphragm, neck	Cervical 1, 2, 3, and 4
Shoulder	Cervical 4, 5, 6, and 7
Arm	Cervical 5, 6, 7, and 8
Finger, hand	Cervical 7 and 8; thoracic 1
Intercostals, abdominal	Thoracic 2 through 12
Hip	Lumbar 4 and 5; sacral 1
Thigh, leg	Lumbar 2, 3, 4, and 5; sacral 1 and 2
Foot	Lumbar 4 and 5; sacral 1
Deep tendon reflexes	
Jaw reflex	Cranial nerve V or nuclei in pons
Biceps reflex	Cervical 5 and 6
Triceps reflex	Cervical 6, 7, and 8
Brachioradialis reflex	Cervical 5 and 6
Patellar reflex (knee reflex)	Lumbar 3 and 4
Achilles reflex (ankle reflex)	Sacral 1 and 2
Superficial reflexes	
Corneal	Cranial nerves V, VII or nuclei in pons
Palate	Cranial nerves IX, X or nuclei in medulla
Pharyngeal (gag)	Cranial nerves IX, X or nuclei in medulla
Upper abdominal	Thoracic 7, 8, 9, and 10
Lower abdominal	Thoracic 11 and 12
Cremasteric	Thoracic 12; lumbar 1
Gluteal	Lumbar 4 through sacral 3
Plantar	Sacral 1 and 2
Babinski	Pyramidal tract

nondominant arm or leg normally won't perform as well as the dominant one. Also, watch for patient fatigue, which may interfere with testing.

With the patient seated facing you, begin assessing his coordination by testing his arms. Ask him to touch each finger rapidly with his thumb, rhythmically pat his leg with his hand, and quickly turn his hand over and back. Have the patient perform each maneuver with each hand for about 30 seconds. Then, ask him to touch your index finger, then his nose, several times. Have him repeat this maneuver with his eyes closed.

To test his leg coordination, ask the patient to tap his foot on the floor or on your palm. Then ask him to place the heel of one foot on his opposite knee and slide the heel down his shin.

As the patient performs all these tests, observe for slowness, tremor, or awkwardness. Does he initiate the movement promptly, or does he hesitate? Does the arm or leg move smoothly and purposefully? Does the arm or leg return to its resting state directly, without extraneous movements?

627 Assessing sensory function

To assess your patient's sensory function, you'll test these five areas of sensation: *pain, touch, vibration, position,* and *discrimination.* Your findings will help you locate the dermatomes where sensations may be absent, decreased, exaggerated, or delayed (see *Identifying Dermatomes,* pages 590 to 591). Make sure your patient is relaxed before beginning the examination. Have him close his eyes during each of the five tests, so he can't see what you're about to do. Because testing every square inch of the patient's body surface is impractical, try to test as many dermatomes as possible by distributing the stimuli over his body. Randomly apply each stimulus, so the patient doesn't anticipate it. Give him time to identify the stimulus and its location.

Note whether the patient perceives the stimulus appropriately and symmetrically. When testing pain and touch, compare distal and proximal parts of the patient's arms and legs. Test vibration and position distally. If you locate a dermatome in which sensation is absent or exaggerated, mark it. Then stimulate a nearby area of greater or lesser sensations, moving away from the suspect dermatome until the patient feels a change.

628 Pain and touch

Use a safety pin to test your patient's pain sensation. Starting at his shoulder, stimulate the skin of the arms, trunk, and legs along dermatomes with the sharp end of the pin. Next, use the blunt end to see if the patient can distinguish between sharp and dull sensations. If he responds normally to the pinpricks, you don't need to test his temperature sensation, because both of these sensations travel along related pathways.

To test the patient's sense of touch, lightly touch his skin along the dermatomes with a piece of cotton. Ask him to tell you where you're touching him each time. Once or twice, pretend you're touching him but don't actually do so—to see whether he can tell the difference. If an area of deficit is present, test from this area upward to a functioning area.

629 Vibration and position

Use a lightly vibrating tuning fork (128 cycles/second) to test your patient's response to vibration. Place it against a bony prominence on each arm and leg, such as the distal joint of a finger or the middle joint of the great toe. Make sure the patient understands he's trying to feel a vibration, not just pressure or touch. To demonstrate the sensation, place the vibrating tuning fork on one of the patient's joints. Then, while the fork is still vibrating on the joint, place your hand on it to stop it and ask the patient if he can feel the difference. If the patient's sense of vibration seems impaired, test more proximal bony prominences, such as the wrists, the elbows, the medial malleoli, the patellas, the anterior superior iliac spine, or the spinous processes.

Next, test the position sense in each arm and leg. Holding one of the patient's fingertips between your thumb and index finger, slowly flex or extend the finger. Ask the patient to tell you when he feels the finger moving and in which direction he thinks it's moving. (Make sure the patient's eyes are closed.) Repeat the maneuver with each great toe. If your patient's position sense seems impaired at the distal joints, test proximal sites until he responds normally.

630 Discrimination

Discrimination testing assesses the ability of the brain's sensory cortex (in the parietal lobe) to interpret and integrate information. You'll perform these tests when the patient's other sensations seem normal, but you'll evaluate the posterior columns more closely. The following tests assess the parietal lobe's ability to interpret these sensations and the posterior column's ability to conduct them.

• *Stereognosis.* Place several small, familiar objects in the patient's hand—keys or coins will do. Ask the patient to identify them, one at a time.

IDENTIFYING DERMATOMES

To document your patient's sensory function, you'll use a body chart, like the one shown here, illustrating cutaneous nerve distribution. The left half of this figure shows the distribution of spinal nerves; the right half shows the distribution of cutaneous fields of peripheral nerves.

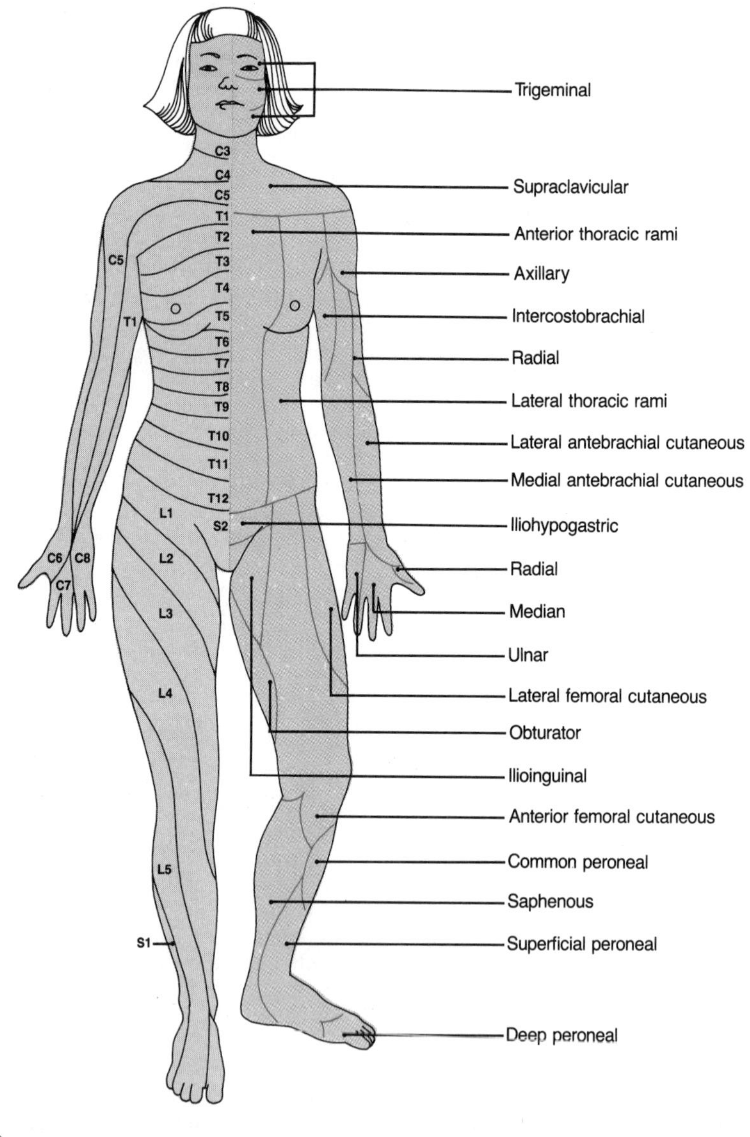

Here's an example of how to document the specific areas tested and the test results: Assume your patient can't feel a pinprick on her right index and middle fingers. Using the chart, you'd document this finding as a loss of pain sensation in the C7 area.

Remember, you may find minor variations in the exact segmental levels, depending on the chart you're using.

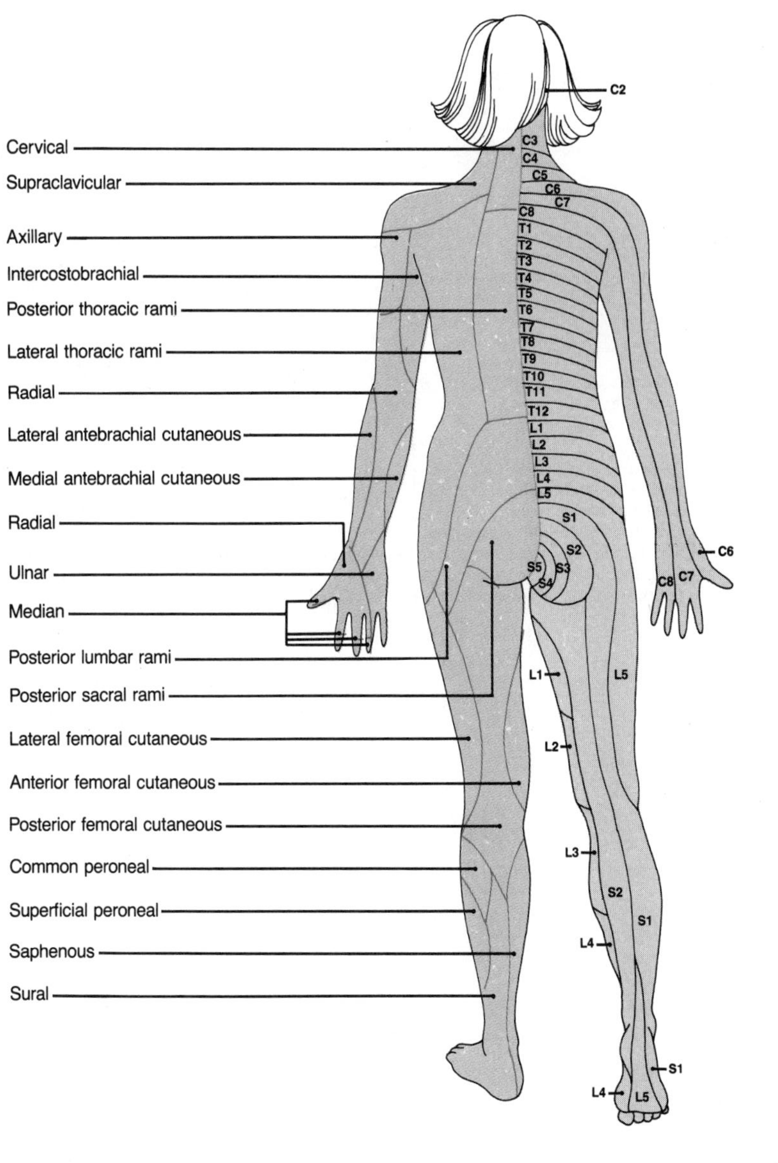

• *Graphesthesia.* With the blunt end of a pen, trace several letters or numbers on each of the patient's palms and ask the patient to identify them.
• *Two-point stimulation.* Prick the patient's fingertip or another body area with two safety pins, held several millimeters apart. Ask the patient if he feels one or two pricks. Repeat the procedure several times, occasionally pricking him with only one pin to test the reliability of his responses. Find the minimal distance at which the patient can discriminate one prick from two, and compare it to normal findings:
—tongue: 1 mm
—fingertips: 2.8 mm
—toes: 3 to 8 mm
—palms: 8 to 12 mm
—chest, forearms: 40 mm
—back: 40 to 70 mm
—upper arms, thighs: 75 mm.
• *Extinction phenomenon.* Prick the patient's skin simultaneously on opposite sides of his body, and ask him if he feels one prick or two. Repeat the procedure several times in different symmetrical areas. Occasionally, apply only one stimulus to test the reliability of the patient's responses.

GRADING REFLEXES

When testing your patient's muscle stretch and superficial reflexes, use the following grading scales:

Muscle stretch reflex grades
0 - absent
1+ - present but diminished
2+ - normal
3+ - increased but not necessarily pathologic
4+ - hyperactive; clonus may also be present

Superficial reflex grades
0 - absent
∓ - equivocal or barely present
+ - normally active

Record the patient's reflex scores by drawing a stick figure and entering the scores at the proper location. The figure shown here indicates normal muscle stretch reflex activity, as well as normal superficial reflex activity over the abdominal area. The *arrows* at the figure's feet indicate normal plantar reflex activity.

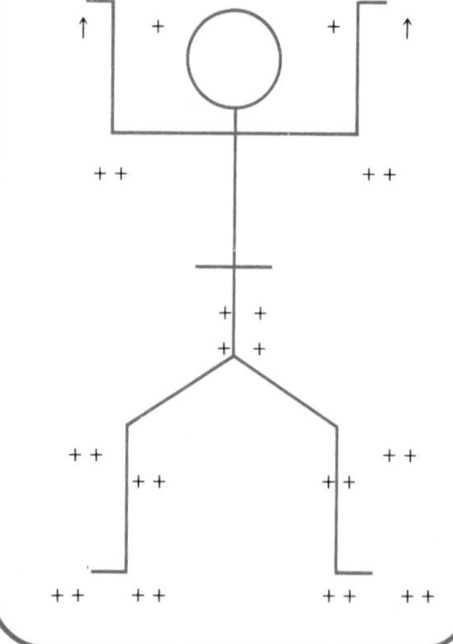

631 Assessing reflexes

Reflexes are divided into two categories: deep tendon and superficial. You elicit deep tendon (or muscle stretch) reflexes when you apply a stimulus to a tendon, a bone, or a joint. You elicit superficial (or cutaneous) reflexes when you apply a stimulus to a skin surface or mucous membrane. Superficial reflexes respond more slowly to stimuli and fatigue more easily than deep tendon reflexes.

Use a percussion hammer—preferably with a soft rubber end—to elicit deep tendon reflexes. To assess superficial reflexes, touch or scratch the patient's skin surface with an object that won't damage the skin, such as a tongue depressor.

For neurologic screening, evaluate only the most significant reflexes. Choose the deep tendon reflexes and the superficial reflexes that you think are most pertinent to your assessment. Test each reflex bilaterally before moving down the patient's body. Compare each reflex response symmetrically as you proceed, using a grading scale. In your notes, indicate the particular scale you used (see *Grading Reflexes*).

632 Common deep tendon reflex tests

The most commonly assessed deep tendon reflexes are as follows:

• *Biceps.* To elicit this reflex, have the patient relax his arm and pronate the forearm slightly, positioned somewhere between flexion and extension. (For best results, ask the patient to rest his elbow in your hand.) Then, percuss the biceps tendon with the reflex hammer. The biceps muscle should contract, followed by flexion of the forearm.

• *Brachioradialis.* Position the patient's forearm in semiflexion and semipronation, resting it either in your hand or on his knee. Tap the styloid process of the radius 1″ to 2″ (2.5 to 5 cm) above the wrist. You should see flexion at the elbow and a simultaneous pronation of the forearm, as well as flexion of the fingers and hand.

• *Triceps.* Position the patient's arm about midway between flexion and extension. If possible, have the patient rest his arm on his thigh or in your hand. Tap the tendon above the insertion on the ulna's olecranon process, 1″ to 2″ above the elbow. The stimulus should elicit muscle contraction of the triceps and elbow extension.

• *Patellar.* Have the patient sit on a table with his legs dangling freely, or have him cross his legs. Place one of your hands over the patient's quadriceps, and use your other hand to tap his tendon just below the patella. A firm tap should draw the patella down and stretch the muscle, causing an extension of the leg at the knee.

• *Achilles.* Have the patient sit on a table with his legs dangling. (If the patient can't sit without support, have him sit or lie in bed.) Flex his leg at the hip and knee, and rotate it externally. If the patient is prone, flex his knee and hip and rotate the leg externally so that it rests on the opposite shin. Then, place your hand under the patient's foot, dorsiflex the ankle, and tap the tendon just above its insertion on the posterior surface of the calcaneus. You should see a plantar flexion of the foot at the ankle.

633 Testing superficial reflexes

The most commonly assessed superficial reflexes are as follows:

• *Upper abdominal.* To test this reflex, have the patient lie down and relax. Move a tongue depressor downward and outward from the tip of his sternum. You can also stroke the area horizontally, moving medially toward the umbilicus. The abdominal muscles should contract, and the umbilicus should deviate toward the stimulus.

• *Lower abdominal.* With the patient lying down, stroke his skin in an upward and outward movement from the symphysis or horizontally in the lower quadrants. The umbilicus should deviate toward the stimulus, along with abdominal contraction.

• *Cremasteric* (males only). Lightly stroke the inner aspect of the upper thigh with a tongue depressor. The testis on the same side as the stimulus should rise.

• *Gluteal.* Stroke the skin over the patient's buttocks, and observe for tense muscles in this area.

• *Plantar.* Firmly stroke the lateral surface of the dorsum of the patient's foot with a test object (the end of a percussion hammer works well). A normal response is plantar flexion of the foot and toes.

• *Pathologic reflex.* Babinski's sign or reflex is the opposite of the normal plantar reflex. When you firmly stroke the lateral aspect of the patient's sole with a blunt object, the great toe extends as the other toes fan out.

634 Tips on reflex testing

Reflexes should be symmetrically equal. If you note a brisk response on one side of the patient's body and an equally brisk response on the other side, the response is probably normal for the patient. Don't be alarmed if you can't elicit a reflex. Approximately 3% to 10% of persons with no central nervous system disease fail to exhibit one or more reflexes.

Remember also that it may be difficult to elicit a particular reflex in an athletic person with firm, well-developed muscles or in a tense, apprehensive person who may be unconsciously bracing his muscles. In these situations, you may need to divert the patient's attention from your test to relax his muscles (*reinforcement*). For example, you might ask the patient to hook his fingers together, then attempt to pull them apart as you test the reflex. Or you could ask the patient to clench his fists, grasp the arm of his chair, look at the ceiling, or take a deep breath. Simply talking to the patient about nonclinical matters as you proceed through the tests can also divert his attention and help him to relax. If you use reinforcement to elicit a reflex response, be sure to document the fact that you have done this. Note it on the patient's grading scale (see *Grading Reflexes*, page 592).

Formulating a diagnostic impression

635 Classifying nervous system disorders

The nervous system controls most body functions—sensory and motor, voluntary and involuntary, conscious and unconscious. Proper functioning of this system depends on sensory, motor, and connector neurons providing pathways for normal transmission of nerve impulses. Also vital are adequate blood and cerebrospinal fluid circulation, integrity of the system's supporting structures, and balanced metabolism.

Disorders of the nervous system are usually classified according to the particular function of the nervous system they affect: disorders in the transmission of nerve impulses, disorders that alter the nervous system's protective structures, disorders affecting arterial or cerebrospinal fluid circulation, and

NURSE'S GUIDE TO NEUROLOGIC DISORDERS

	CHIEF COMPLAINT
DISORDERS IN TRANSMISSION OF NERVE IMPULSES	
Amyotrophic lateral sclerosis (Lou Gehrig's disease)	• *Headache/pain:* pain in arms and legs • *Motor disturbances:* muscle atrophy and weakness, especially in forearms and hands; impaired speech; difficulty chewing, swallowing, and breathing; choking; excessive drooling; urinary frequency, urgency, and difficulty initiating a stream • *Sensory deviations:* paresthesias • *Altered level of consciousness:* depression; crying spells and inappropriate laughter caused by bulbar palsy
Syringomyelia	• *Headache/pain:* painful shoulder • *Motor disturbances:* weakness; hyporeflexia, hyperreflexia, or areflexia; wasting of muscles at level of spinal cord involvement (usually hands and arms); spasticity of lower levels; nystagmus; atrophy and fibrillation of the tongue • *Sensory deviations:* anesthesia in hands or face

disorders of abnormal metabolism (see *Nurse's Guide to Neurologic Disorders*).

636 Making appropriate nursing diagnoses

Headache or pain can signal a number of neurologic disorders. This common symptom occurs when one of the brain's pain-sensitive structures becomes stretched, compressed, dilated, or inflamed. These structures include the meninges; cranial nerves II, III, V, IX, and X; and the large blood vessels in the brain.

Headache or pain can also result from spasm, as in the neck; from unpleasant visual, olfactory, and auditory stimuli; and from psychogenic factors. The symptom is common in patients suffering from disorders that affect arterial or cerebrospinal fluid circulation or from disorders that alter the nervous system's protective structures.

Nursing diagnoses for a patient with headache or pain include *alterations in comfort, sleep pattern disturbances, altered nutrition,* and *fear of the cause of headache or pain.*

Symptoms of motor disturbances—paralysis, paresis, tremors, and abnormal reflexes or movements, for example—can occur in varying degrees in patients with virtually any nervous system disorder. Paralysis may result from an upper or lower motor neuron disorder. Upper motor neuron lesions, in which the reflex arc remains intact, usually cause spastic paralysis. Flaccidity usually occurs in lower motor neuron lesions, which disrupt the reflex arc.

Your nursing diagnoses for the paralyzed patient may include *ineffective coping by patient and family, self-care deficit* (depending on the degree of paralysis), and *alteration in urinary and bowel elimination.* In the case of cervical fractures, *ineffective breathing patterns* may also exist.

Tremors result from lesions in the cerebellar pathways. Involuntary choreiform movements indicate a disease of the basal ganglia, such as Huntington's chorea. Insufficient arterial blood flow to the brain from occlusion or compression results in paresis or paralysis of the body part normally nour-

	HISTORY	PHYSICAL EXAMINATION
	• Onset usually between ages 40 and 70 • Most common in white males • Precipitating factors include nutritional deficiency, vitamin E deficiency (damaging cell membranes), autoimmune disorder, interference with nucleic acid production, acute viral infections, and physical exhaustion.	• Deep tendon reflexes absent; muscle twitches
	• Onset usually between ages 30 and 50 • Symptoms include spontaneous fractures, painless injuries, ulcers from anesthesia; progress irregular (may be in remission for long period)	• Horner's syndrome, nystagmus, knee or shoulder joint deformities, clonus, spasticity, hyperreflexia • Loss of deep tendon reflex, gradual loss of pain and temperature sense

(continued)

NURSE'S GUIDE TO NEUROLOGIC DISORDERS *(continued)*

	CHIEF COMPLAINT
Myasthenia gravis	• *Motor disturbances:* progressive muscle weakness during activity; respiratory muscles affected during crisis; dysarthria; dysphagia • *Sensory deviations:* double vision, weak eye muscles
Polyneuritis	• *Motor disturbances:* leg weakness or paralysis progressing to arms and trunk; weakness most severe in distal extremities and in extensors; footdrop; ataxia; absent leg reflexes; impairment of bowel and bladder function and sphincter control • *Sensory deviations:* paresthesias in hands or feet; anesthesia or hyperesthesia in distal parts of arms and legs; impaired vibratory and kinesthetic sensibilities; nerves sensitive to pressure
Wernicke's encephalopathy	• *Motor disturbances:* ophthalmoplegia, ataxia, nystagmus, tremors • *Seizures:* may occur • *Sensory deviations:* paresthesias of hands and feet • *Altered level of consciousness:* drowsiness; impaired recent memory; unaffected remote, past memory; confabulation; time disorientation; apathy; mild lethargy; occasional frank delirium
Landry's or Guillian-Barré syndrome (acute idiopathic polyneuritis)	• *Motor disturbances:* muscle weakness in legs, extending to arms and face in 24 to 72 hours and progressing to total paralysis and respiratory failure; flaccid quadriplegia possible; cranial nerve paralysis; ocular paralysis in about 25% of cases • *Sensory deviations:* paresthesias vanishing before muscle weakness occurs
Multiple sclerosis (disseminated sclerosis)	• *Motor disturbances:* slurred speech, intention tremor, nystagmus (Charcot's triad), spastic paralysis, poor coordination, loss of proprioception, ataxia, transient muscle weakness, incontinence or retention • *Sensory deviations:* numbness and tingling, vision impairment • *Altered level of consciousness:* euphoria, emotionally unstable
Grand mal seizure (major motor, generalized, tonic clonic)	• *Headache:* present on awakening, possibly accompanied by nausea • *Motor disturbances:* generalized tonic and clonic movements; residual hemiparesis or monoparesis possible • *Seizures:* generalized • *Sensory deviations:* weakness, dizziness, numbness, peculiar sensation • *Altered level of consciousness:* loss of consciousness; mental confusion after awakening, lasting several hours or days

HISTORY	PHYSICAL EXAMINATION
• Onset usually between ages 20 and 40 • Most common in females • Remissions and exacerbations common • Symptoms worsen with emotional stress, prolonged exposure to sunlight or cold	• Deep tendon reflexes present • Double vision, weak eye closure; ptosis; expressionless face; nasal vocal tones; nasal regurgitation of fluids; weak chewing muscles; weak respiratory muscles; weak neck muscles, can't support head; proximal limb weakness (may be asymmetrical)
• Precipitating factors include alcohol abuse, inadequate diet and malnutrition, pregnancy, gastrointestinal disorders, vitamin B deficiency, weight loss. • Common in diabetics over age 50	• Dry, scaly skin on back of wrists and hands, hyperpigmentation of skin, plantar responses absent, abdominal skin reflexes decreased or absent, increased pulse rate possible; reduced or absent patellar and Achilles tendon reflex • Feet tender in diabetics
• Predisposing factors include inadequate diet, low thiamine intake, and alcohol addiction. • Pernicious vomiting possible during pregnancy	• Mental disturbance, retrograde or anterograde amnesia, paralysis of eye movements, ataxia, diplopia, nystagmus, broad-based stance
• Onset at any age • Predisposing factors include recent viral or bacterial infection, surgery, influenza vaccination, Hodgkin's disease, lupus erythematosus, gastroenteritis • Rapid onset of muscular symptoms	• Retinal hemorrhage, sinus tachycardia or bradycardia, choked disk, hypertension, signs of increased intracranial pressure, elevated cerebrospinal fluid pressure, cranial nerve paralysis (VII), symmetrical loss of tendon reflexes, ascending peripheral nerve paralysis or weakness, impaired proprioception, loss of bowel and bladder control, muscle tenderness to pressure
• Most common in young white adults • Higher incidence in northern climate • Genetic tendencies • Initial attack and subsequent relapse may follow acute infections, trauma, vaccination, serum injections, pregnancy, stress.	• Pale optic disk on temporal side, increased deep tendon reflexes, joint contractures and deformities, scanning speech, cranial nerve involvement (vertigo, trigeminal neuralgia), decreased or diminished abdominal reflexes, unsteady gait
• Onset early in life with idiopathic disorder; can occur at any age with secondary disorders, but those associated with fever commonly occur in children. • Predisposing factors include, with idiopathic seizure disorders (epilepsy), familial history of seizures, genetic involvement; with secondary seizure disorders, cerebral palsy, birth injury, infectious diseases, meningitis, encephalitis, cerebral trauma, metabolic disturbances, cerebral edema, carbon monoxide poisoning, insulin shock, anoxia, brain tumor, drug overdose, child abuse, noncompliance with medication regimen	• Shrill cry, pupillary change, loss of consciousness, tonic and clonic movements, tongue-biting, abnormal respiratory pattern (absent during tonic phase), urinary or fecal incontinence, upward deviation of eyes, excessive salivation

(continued)

NURSE'S GUIDE TO NEUROLOGIC DISORDERS *(continued)*

	CHIEF COMPLAINT
Jacksonian seizure (partial motor and partial sensory)	• *Motor disturbances:* focal seizures, lesions of motor cortex or strip (jacksonian motor seizure) • *Seizures:* partial, with no loss of consciousness • *Sensory deviations:* numbness, tingling of one arm or leg or one half of body, auditory alterations (such as ringing noises), lesions of the sensory strip (jacksonian sensory seizure)
Psychomotor seizure (focal)	• *Motor disturbances:* speech disturbance; destructive, aggressive behavior • *Seizures:* temporal lobe dysfunction (behavior disturbance) • *Sensory deviations:* olfactory hallucinations and other sensory manifestations depending on location of focus; feeling of déjà vu and déjà pensé • *Altered level of consciousness:* slower thought processes; altered consciousness; partial amnesia
Extramedullary spinal tumor (neurinomas, meningiomas, sarcomas)	• *Headache/pain:* dull aching and soreness of muscles, mild pain along nerve root • *Motor disturbances:* spastic weakness of muscles below lesion; with severe compression, loss of bladder and bowel control; atrophy of muscles; paraplegia • *Sensory deviations:* paresthesias; impairment of proprioception and cutaneous sensation below lesion; with severe compression, loss of sensation below lesion
Intramedullary spinal tumor (gliomas)	• *Headache/pain:* sharp, tearing, or boring pain, depending on location of tumor; increased by movement and relieved by change of posture • *Motor disturbances:* weakness in one or both legs, clumsiness, shuffling or spastic gait, incontinence • *Sensory deviations:* paresthesias occur after pain diminishes; complete sparing of sensation in legs possible
Intracranial tumors (medulloblastoma, meningioma, astrocytoma, acoustic neuroma, oligodendroma)	• *Headache/pain:* headache; worse in morning; may be accompanied by vomiting • *Motor disturbances:* motor deficits, depending on location of tumor • *Seizures:* generalized or focal, depending on site of tumor • *Sensory deviations:* dependent on pressure on cranial or olfactory nerve • *Altered level of consciousness:* progressive deterioration of intellect; behavior changes possible; decreased level of consciousness with increased intracranial pressure

	HISTORY	PHYSICAL EXAMINATION
	• Predisposing factors include birth injury, trauma, infection, and vascular lesions.	• Clonic twitching begins in one part of body, usually one side of the face or the fingers of one hand, and often progresses from face to hand, to arm, to trunk, to legs on the same side of the body (jacksonian march); if twitching begins in the foot, it may progress reversely through the body; rhythmic clonic movements may affect one area (face, arm, leg) without marching. • Speech loss possible • Sensory deviations may also progress or march through the body. • May progress to a secondary generalized seizure (grand mal)
	• Secondary to birth injury or congenital abnormalities in infants, lesions or trauma in children and adults, arteriosclerosis in adults	• Aura may occur in the form of a hallucination or perceptual illusion • May begin with aura • Characterized by automatisms (patterned behavior): lip-smacking, head-turning, dressing, undressing • Extreme psychotic behavior possible
	• Most common in young and middle-aged adults • Predisposing factors include Hodgkin's disease and metastatic carcinoma. • Symptoms worsened by exertion	• Muscle atrophy and impairment of reflexes, depending on location and extent of injury and amount of time since injury occurred; sensory sparing in some cases; with half the cord compressed, Brown-Séquard syndrome
	• Possible limb heaviness or feeling as though walking on air • Symptoms worsened by exertion	• Overactive leg reflexes, leg weakness, sensory sparing (loss)
	• Medulloblastomas most common in men between ages 50 and 60 • Meningioma most common in women over age 50 • History of present illness includes progressive deterioration of motor function, increasing frequency and duration of headaches, personality changes.	• Signs of increased intracranial pressure: widening pulse pressure and bounding pulse (Cushing's phenomenon), ipsilateral (same side as lesion) pupil dilatation and contralateral (opposite side of lesion) muscle weakness (Weber's syndrome), decreasing level of consciousness, irregular respiratory patterns progressing to respiratory arrest, temperature fluctuation, papilledema, decorticate or decerebrate posturing • Motor and sensory deficits appropriate to affected area

(continued)

NURSE'S GUIDE TO NEUROLOGIC DISORDERS *(continued)*

	CHIEF COMPLAINT	
Spinal cord injury (contusion, compression, complete transection of cord)	• *Motor disturbances:* with contusion and compression, muscle weakness or paralysis; with complete transection, permanent motor paralysis below level of lesion; with upper motor neuron damage, spastic paralysis; with lower motor neuron damage, flaccid paralysis • *Sensory deviations:* related to size of injury and degree of cord shock; absence of perspiration on affected part; with contusion or compression, pain at level of lesion; with complete transection, total sensory loss	
DISORDERS THAT ALTER PROTECTIVE STRUCTURES		
Meningitis	• *Headache:* present, with nausea and vomiting • *Motor disturbances:* exaggerated, symmetrical deep tendon reflexes • *Seizures:* may occur; generalized • *Sensory deviations:* visual disturbances, such as photophobia • *Altered level of consciousness:* irritability, confusion, stupor, or coma	
Brain abscess	• *Headache:* present, with nausea and vomiting • *Motor disturbances:* hemiplegia, speech disturbances, cranial nerve palsies • *Seizures:* focal or generalized • *Sensory deviations:* visual field defect (hemianopia), depending on position of abscess • *Altered level of consciousness:* behavioral changes or loss of consciousness	
Head injury	• *Headache:* varies in intensity and duration; generalized, with nausea and vomiting • *Motor disturbances:* specific to area of injury; dysphagia; dysarthria; paralysis; ataxia • *Sensory deviation:* vertigo, tinnitus worsened by change in posture • *Altered level of consciousness:* unconsciousness varies in depth and duration, depending on severity and area of injury (the more severe the injury, the greater the depth and duration of unconsciousness); confusion after regaining consciousness (the greater the duration of unconsciousness, the greater the incidence of permanent brain damage)	

	HISTORY	PHYSICAL EXAMINATION
	• Auto and motorcycle accidents, athletic injuries (football, diving), falls, gunshot wounds, stab wounds • Cervical injuries most common	• Urinary retention, priapism, perspiration on one side; first 24 to 48 hours, flaccid paralysis, then exaggerated reflexes or spastic paralysis if lower motor neuron remains intact • Specific levels of injury intact and functional loss: with C1 to C2, quadriplegic, no respiratory ability; C3 to C4, quadriplegic, loss of phrenic innervation to diaphragm, absent respirations; C4 to C5, quadriplegic, no arm movements; C5 to C6, quadriplegic, gross arm movements only; C6 to C7, quadriplegic, biceps movement, no triceps movement; C7 to C8, quadriplegic, triceps, no intrinsic muscles of hands; thoracic L1 to L2, arm function intact, loss of some intercostals, and loss of leg, bladder, bowel, sex function; lumbar below L2, motor and sensory loss, impairment of bladder, bowel, sex function according to nerve root damage; sacral, loss of bladder, bowel, sex function
	• Predisposing factors include otitis media, mastoiditis, ruptured brain abscess, sinus infection, hepatitis, tonsillitis, herpes zoster or herpes simplex, bone or skin infection, heart valve or lung infection, skull fracture, recent surgery to head or face, recent viral or bacterial infection, general malaise.	• High- or low-grade fever, rash, sinus arrhythmias, photophobia, nuchal rigidity, opisthotonos, back pain, shock, signs of increased intracranial pressure, positive Brudzinski's and Kernig's signs
	• Predisposing factors include mastoid and nasal sinus disease; bacterial endocarditis; pulmonary, skin, and abdominal infections; head trauma.	• Normal or decreased temperature, papilledema, signs of increased intracranial pressure • Signs similar to those of meningitis, such as nuchal rigidity, positive Brudzinski's and Kernig's signs
	• Some type of fall or accident, such as a vehicular or industrial accident; blow to the head	• Signs of increased intracranial pressure, retrograde and posttraumatic amnesia, hyperthermia, shock, scalp bleeding, evidence of other injuries

(continued)

NURSE'S GUIDE TO NEUROLOGIC DISORDERS *(continued)*

	CHIEF COMPLAINT
Encephalitis	• *Headache:* present • *Motor disturbances:* residual parkinsonian paralysis with acute attack; paralysis; ataxia • *Seizures:* may occur during acute attack; residual seizures in about 60% of cases • *Altered level of consciousness:* lethargy or restlessness progressing to stupor and coma; may remain comatose several days, weeks, or longer after acute phase subsides; personality changes; mental deterioration in about 60% of cases
DISORDERS AFFECTING ARTERIAL OR CEREBROSPINAL FLUID CIRCULATION	
Transient ischemic attack	• *Motor disturbances:* depends on location of ataxia; dizziness; falling; weakness • *Sensory deviations:* numbness, depending on location of affected artery; paresthesias; double vision; fleeting monocular blindness • *Altered level of consciousness:* drowsiness, giddiness, decreased level of consciousness
Cerebrovascular accident	• *Headache/pain:* present, when affecting carotid artery • *Motor disturbances:* when affecting middle cerebral artery, aphasia, dysphasia, contralateral hemiparesis or hemiplegia; when affecting carotid artery, weakness, contralateral paralysis or paresis (especially leg or foot); when affecting vertebral and basilar arteries, contralateral weakness, diplopia, poor coordination, dysphagia, ataxia; when affecting anterior cerebral artery, weakness, loss of coordination, impaired motor function, incontinence; when affecting posterior cerebral artery, contralateral hemiplegia • *Sensory deviations:* when affecting middle cerebral artery, pain and tenderness in affected arm or leg, numbness, tingling; when affecting carotid artery, numbness and sensory changes on opposite side, visual disturbances on same side, transient blindness; when affecting vertebral and basilar arteries, visual field cut, numbness around lips and mouth, dizziness, blindness, deafness; when affecting anterior cerebral artery, numbness of lower leg or foot, impaired vision; when affecting posterior cerebral artery, visual field cut, pain and temperature impairment, cortical blindness • *Altered level of consciousness:* when affecting middle cerebral artery, altered level progressing to coma; when affecting carotid artery, altered level, mental confusion, poor memory; when affecting vertebral and basilar arteries, amnesia, confusion, loss of consciousness; when affecting anterior cerebral artery, confusion, personality changes; when affecting posterior cerebral artery, coma

HISTORY	PHYSICAL EXAMINATION
• Predisposing factors include mosquito bite, measles, chicken pox, mumps, herpesvirus, polio vaccine or virus, syphilis (10 to 25 years after infection).	• Fever, nuchal rigidity, back pain, abnormal EEG, signs of increased intracranial pressure • With history of syphilis, tremors, dysarthria, generalized convulsions, increased deep tendon reflexes, bilateral Babinski's sign; with history of herpes simplex, progressive confusion, recent memory loss, temporal lobe seizures, increased antibody levels to herpes simplex virus; with history of measles virus, memory impairment, seizures, myoclonic jerks, ataxia
• Higher incidence in black men over age 50 • Symptoms include atherosclerosis, transient neurologic deficit lasting seconds to no more than 24 hours; hypertension.	• Normal neurologic examination between episodes
• Precipitating factors include atrial fibrillation, subacute bacterial endocarditis, recent heart valve surgery, lung abscess, tuberculosis, air embolism during abortion, pulmonary trauma, surgery, thrombophlebitis, transient ischemic attack, diabetes mellitus, gout, arteriosclerosis, intracerebral tumors, trauma.	• Labored breathing; rapid pulse rate; fever; nuchal rigidity; evidence of emboli to arms, legs, and intestines and other organs, such as spleen, kidneys, or lungs • When affecting carotid artery, bruits over artery; retinal vessels blanch on pressure

(continued)

NURSE'S GUIDE TO NEUROLOGIC DISORDERS *(continued)*

	CHIEF COMPLAINT	
Arteriovenous malformation	• *Headache:* migraine on side of malformation; accompanied by vomiting • *Motor disturbances:* signs of increased intracranial pressure, depending on area of malformation; paresis and cerebrovascular accident from rupture • *Seizures:* general, focal, or jacksonian; may be first sign of rupture resulting from ischemia • *Sensory deviations:* visual disturbances; sensory loss depending on area involved; symptoms same as hemorrhage from cerebrovascular accident • *Altered level of consciousness:* dementia resulting from brief ischemia	
Cerebral aneurysm and intracerebral or subarachnoid hemorrhage	• *Headache:* sudden, severe headache, with nausea and projectile vomiting • *Motor disturbances:* depends on site of aneurysm and degree of bleeding or ischemia; hemiparesis; aphasia; ataxia; vertigo; syncope; facial weakness • *Seizures:* focal or generalized, depending on area of hemorrhage • *Sensory deviations:* visual impairment with pressure on optic nerve or chiasm; double vision with third, fourth, and fifth cranial nerve compression • *Altered level of consciousness:* stupor to coma, irritability	
Epidural (acute) and subdural (acute and chronic) hematomas	• *Motor disturbances:* hemiplegia or facial weakness on opposite or same side as hematoma; hemiparesis • *Seizures:* generalized • *Altered level of consciousness:* irritability, mental confusion, and progressively decreasing level of consciousness; with chronic form, severe impairment of intellectual faculties	
Migraine (common, hemiplegic, ophthalmoplegic, basilar artery, temporal artery)	• *Headache/pain:* with common migraine, recurrent and severe incapacitating headache (unilateral or bilateral), aura with gastric pain; with hemiplegic or ophthalmoplegic migraine, severe unilateral headache; with basilar artery migraine, severe occipital throbbing headache with vomiting; with temporal artery migraine, throbbing unilateral headache, generalized muscle pain • *Motor disturbances:* with hemiplegic and ophthalmoplegic migraine, extraocular muscle palsy, ptosis, possible permanent third nerve paralysis, hemiplegia; with basilar artery migraine, ataxia, dysarthria • *Sensory deviations:* with common migraine, aura may include visual flashing lights, hemianopsia, visual field defects, numbness, nausea, vomiting, vertigo, sensitivity to light and noise; with hemiplegic and ophthalmoplegic migraine, hemiparesis; with basilar artery migraine, partial vision loss, vertigo, tinnitus, tingling of fingers and toes; with temporal artery migraine, visual loss	

	HISTORY	PHYSICAL EXAMINATION
	• Patient may complain of swishing sensation in head; sudden "stroke" in young patients	• Pulsating exophthalmos from ocular pressure; papilledema; retinal hemorrhage if carotid artery bleeds into cavernous sinus; hydrocephalus if membrane causes pressure on aqueduct of Sylvius; bruits over lesion, which disappear with pressure over ipsilateral carotid artery
	• No symptoms until bleeding or rupture • Precipitating factors include hypertension, oral contraceptives, arteriovenous malformations, family history, recurrent headaches.	• Temperature may reach 102° F. (38.9° C.) or higher; irregular respirations, dilated and fixed pupils, papilledema, retinal hemorrhage, bilateral Babinski's reflex early after rupture, positive Brudzinski's and Kernig's signs, nuchal rigidity, signs of increased intracranial pressure, blood in cerebrospinal fluid
	• Signs occur when hematoma has grown large enough to compromise circulation to the brain (increased intracranial pressure). • With acute form, complaints rapidly develop (within 48 hours). • With chronic form, complaints develop more slowly (within a few days to weeks). • Not all lesions cause signs of increased intracranial pressure (especially chronic).	• Positive Babinski's reflex • Signs of increased intracranial pressure • Epidural hematomas cause a rapid rise in intracranial pressure and should be treated as a surgical emergency.
	• Most common in females • Family history of *sick headache* • Onset usually around age 30 • Predisposing factors include emotional disturbance, fatigue, or anxiety; intense concentration or anxiety; oral contraceptives; menstruation; change in routine; hypothyroidism or hyperthyroidism; food additives; drinking wine or sleeping late. • Temporal artery migraine mostly affects females over age 60.	• With common migraine, tearing, pallor or flushing, perspiration, tachycardia during attack, transitory motor or sensory defects, tenderness and prominent blood vessels on head • With hemiplegic or ophthalmoplegic migraine, ptosis, third cranial nerve dysfunction, hemiplegia • With basilar artery migraine, ataxia • With temporal artery migraine, occasional fever; swollen and tender temporal arteries

(continued)

NURSE'S GUIDE TO NEUROLOGIC DISORDERS *(continued)*

	CHIEF COMPLAINT
Migraine *(continued)*	• *Altered level of consciousness:* with common migraine, aura includes fatigue, depression, anxiety, and euphoria; with temporal artery migraine, confusion, disorientation
Cluster headache	• *Headache/pain:* intense, stabbing eye pain; sudden onset • *Motor disturbances:* drooping eyelids
DISORDERS OF ABNORMAL METABOLISM AND TOXINS	
Tetany (lock jaw)	• *Motor disturbances:* generalized spasms and muscle contractions, stiff neck and back muscles, rigid facial muscles, dysphagia, dysarthria, ptosis, diplopia • *Seizures:* generalized convulsions, paroxysmal tonic syndrome • *Altered level of consciousness:* irritability, restlessness
Lead poisoning	• *Motor disturbances:* paralysis following seizure, cerebellar ataxia, hemiplegia, decerebrate rigidity, facial or oculomotor paralysis • *Seizures:* generalized or focal • *Sensory deviations:* polyneuritis • *Altered level of consciousness:* lethargy, coma, delirium
Botulism	• *Motor disturbances:* ptosis, paralysis of ocular muscles, weakness of trunk and jaw muscles, dysphagia, dysarthria, constipation, urinary retention • *Seizures:* convulsions at terminal stage • *Altered level of consciousness:* mental faculties preserved, but coma terminal
Methyl alcohol ingestion	• *Headache/pain:* headache with nausea and vomiting; abdominal pain • *Motor disturbances:* blurred vision; dizziness • *Sensory deviations:* temporary or permanent blindness • *Altered level of consciousness:* drunkenness, drowsiness, delirium, central nervous system depression leading to coma, respiratory failure, and possible death
Carbon monoxide	• *Headache:* present • *Motor disturbances:* hemiplegia, aphasia, athetoid movements, all transient; may develop parkinsonism in later years • *Sensory deviations:* cortical blindness, multiple neuritis • *Altered level of consciousness:* amnesia after incident, fatigue, mental confusion, seizures, coma, respiratory failure resulting in death

	HISTORY	PHYSICAL EXAMINATION
	• Mostly affects young males • Onset same time each day, usually during evening or one or two hours after falling asleep • Persists nightly from several weeks to several months • Triggered by alcohol • Use of vasodilators, such as nitroglycerin	• Tearing of affected eye; red, runny nose; sweating on affected side of face; Horner's syndrome
	• Predisposing factors include puncture wounds, such as from blank cartridges, fireworks, nails, or splinters; compound fracture; septic abortion; parenteral injections, such as from heroin injections.	• Cyanosis, increased pulse arrhythmias, fluctuating hypotension and hypertension, increased respiratory rates, possible respiratory failure, trismus, rigid facial muscles (sarconic smile), stiff back muscles (opisthotonos); moderate-to-severe spasm, with pain, hyperactive deep tendon reflexes; inability to swallow; aspiration of secretions, fever and excessive perspiration
	• Most common in infants and children • Ingestion of lead paint from crib or wall or from water standing in lead pipe • Exposure to lead (metallic toxins) in the form of fumes from burning batteries, melting lead, or solder	• Symptoms of acute increased intracranial pressure; optic atrophy; anemia; wristdrop, footdrop
	• Symptoms apparent 12 to 48 hours after ingestion of contaminated food (bacterial toxins); may affect several members of same household	• Pupils dilated, no reaction to light; difficulty in convergence of eyes
	• Ingestion of methyl alcohol (wood alcohol) used in solvent, anti-freeze, paint remover, denatured alcohol, such as sterno • Symptoms usually appear 12 to 24 hours after ingestion.	• Visual field defect or loss of vision • Pupils dilated and non-reactive • Arterial blood gases reveal acidosis.
	• Inhalation of automobile exhaust fumes • Defective coal heater in home stove	• Cherry-red skin and mucous membranes • EKG changes • Gradual poisoning may show fever, excessive sweating, decreased exercise tolerance, dyspnea during exertion or rest, signs of increasing intracranial pressure. • Arterial blood gases reveal acidosis.

CASE HISTORIES: NURSING DIAGNOSIS FLOWCHART

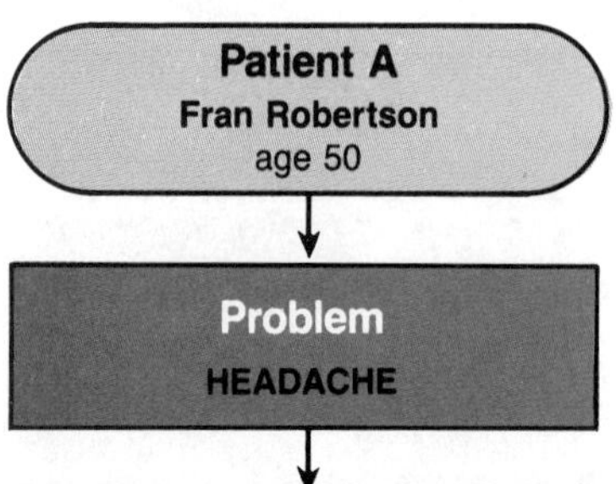

Subjective data

- Sudden onset of severe bilateral, occipital-frontal headache and vomiting
- Headache, lasting 3 days, made worse by coughing
- Headache recurred the afternoon before admission
- Blurred vision in right eye
- No history of hypertension

Objective data

- Alert and oriented
- Temperature: 98.6° F. (37° C.)

III Cranial nerve

- Papilledema, worse in right eye
- Right pupil: 4 mm; no reaction to light or accommodation
- Left pupil: 2 mm; reacts to light
- Ptosis of right eyelid
- Right eye deviates to right

Motor nerves

- Increased deep tendon reflexes
- No sensory deficit
- Nuchal rigidity
- Positive Kernig's and Brudzinski's signs
- Spinal tap shows blood in subarachnoid space
- Arteriography shows aneurysm of right internal carotid artery below junction of posterior communicating artery; narrowing of anterior cerebral artery suggests spasm secondary to blood in subarachnoid space

Nursing diagnoses

- Alterations in comfort due to headache from meningial irritation
- Potential for decreasing level of consciousness, seizures, or death due to continued bleeding of aneurysm and resultant increased intracranial pressure and ischemia
- Stress related to isolation and restricted activity of bed rest and quiet room management
- Fear of dying due to seriousness of problem

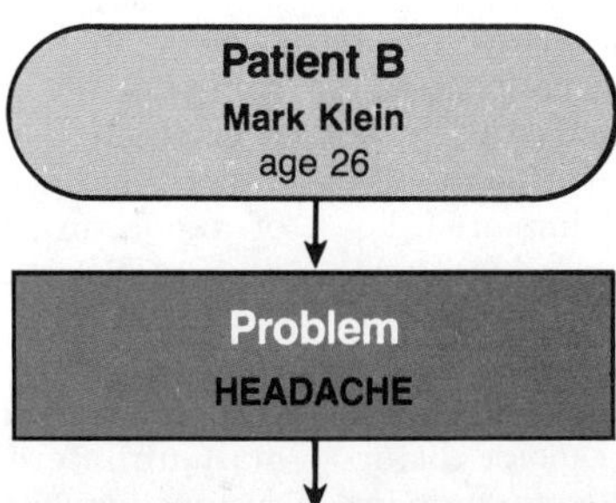

Subjective data

- Severe, constant left frontal headache for 1 week before admission
- Confusion and delirium for 2 days
- Total left-sided facial paralysis for 3 weeks
- Drainage from left ear for 2 days
- Treated for *Staphylococcus aureus* infection of left ear 4 weeks before admission
- Fever

Objective data

- Disoriented; confuses time and sequences of events
- Difficulty with language, calculations, and reading
- Inappropriate emotions
- Temperature: 98.6° F. (37° C.)
- Papilledema and retinal hemorrhage in right eye
- Pupils: equal, round; react to light
- Hearing loss in left ear
- Thick, green, purulent discharge from left ear
- Facial weakness on left side
- Dehydration
- Skull and mastoid X-rays show increased density in left side of mastoid extending to petrous ridge
- Abnormal EEG, slow wave activity in left hemisphere, frontotemporal area

Nursing diagnoses

- Alterations in comfort due to headache caused by intracranial mass
- Potential for transmission of infection from left ear drainage
- Potential for seizure or increasing altered consciousness due to growth of brain abscess
- Alteration in self-image as a result of left-sided facial paralysis

ished by the affected arteries.

Your nursing diagnoses may include *knowledge deficit, fear of body deterioration,* and *progressing self-care deficit.*

Abnormal reflexes usually result from problems involving sensory pathways—from muscles and tendons or from the neuron. When a motor disturbance occurs, gait is impaired, because it's dependent on the normal tone, coordination, and integration of the muscles of his legs and trunk.

If your patient exhibits one or more of these symptoms of a motor disturbance, consider the following nursing diagnoses: *alterations in muscle tone or strength, alterations in effective or purposeful movements,* and *alterations in gait or reflexes.* You might also diagnose *alterations in activities of daily living* (specify activity).

Seizures indicate an underlying disorder that causes the brain to discharge excessive and paroxysmal neural stimuli, which usually originate in the area adjacent to the disease or injury.

The form the seizure takes depends on where the disorder begins and how it spreads. For example, a focal seizure results from focal irritation of part of the motor cortex or strip. It can remain localized, affecting a single muscle or muscle group, or spread to other muscle groups (jacksonian march). Consciousness may be impaired but is usually not lost in a patient having a partial seizure, unless the seizure eventually becomes generalized (secondary generalization). In generalized seizures, the patient loses consciousness because of abnormal electrical activity throughout the brain. Although seizures may occur in all types of nervous system disorders, they're most common in patients with disorders of nerve impulse transmission and in disorders that alter the nervous system's protective structures.

Appropriate nursing diagnoses include *fear and anxiety from anticipation of seizures, fear of bodily harm during the seizure, altered consciousness,* and *ineffective patient or family coping due to public stigma attached to epilepsy.*

Sensory deviations, such as dulling or intensification, are common in patients with peripheral nerve impairment caused by damage to nerve fibers, to cell bodies, or to the myelin sheath. Trauma and ischemia can stop the flow of axoplasm down the nerve fiber, causing distal nerve destruction. Metabolic disorders, such as neuropathies, can change the axoplasm's composition, causing first distal, then proximal, unilateral or bilateral nerve dysfunction.

Lesions of the brain stem's tegmentum may cause loss of pain sensation. Discriminatory sensation loss may indicate a lesion of the posterior column or the sensory cortex. Although present to some degree in each nerve disorder classification, sensory deviations occur primarily in patients with disorders in nerve impulse transmission and in disorders affecting arterial or cerebrospinal fluid circulation.

Nursing diagnoses include *altered sensory perception* (specify sense), *potential for injury,* and *fear of malignancy and death. Sleep pattern disturbances* and *anxiety* may also be appropriate diagnoses if the patient is experiencing intensification.

Altered levels of consciousness result from impaired function in one or more areas of the brain. For a person to maintain consciousness, both neurons and the central reticular activating system must function properly. Metabolic processes must supply the brain with adequate amounts of oxygen and nutrients, such as glucose. Disturbance in any of these functions will alter your patient's level of consciousness.

Altered levels of consciousness occur with disorders that interfere with cerebrospinal fluid circulation, those which cause alterations in the nervous system's protective structures, and those which affect metabolic processes. In such cases, *altered level of consciousness* is the primary nursing diagnosis.

Assessing pediatric patients

637 Special pediatric considerations

When evaluating an infant's or child's nervous system, you'll need to tailor your assessment according to several special considerations. Bear in mind the child's age and behavior, for instance. Is he tired, hungry, irritable, or ill? These factors can affect the child's responses, so be cautious in your overall interpretation of the examination results. With practice, you'll become familiar with the wide range of normal findings in these examinations.

The first step in a successful examination is establishing rapport with the child and his parents. You'll need the parents' help to obtain a patient history. And if you can, discreetly observe the child's interaction with his parents. Allow him to play and climb. Your observations will provide clues about some areas of his development.

Many children are frightened at first, but by turning some of the examination into a game, you can calm a fearful child and establish rapport with him. Remember, you don't need to follow a strict inspection-percussion-palpation-auscultation routine to assess a child's neurologic function. Putting him at ease and observing him in a nonthreatening milieu are more important.

638 The child's neurologic health history

To obtain a thorough health history of a child who may have a neurologic disorder, talk with him (if he's old enough to understand) and his parents. If the child attends a day-care center or has a regular babysitter, talk to the day-care worker or babysitter, too, if possible. Their observations of the child can prove invaluable to your assessment. For an older child, a history of school performance, with reports from the teacher, may be helpful.

Ask questions about the child's health and development from prenatal history to the present. First, inquire about his early development. For instance, did his mother have any diseases or other problems during the pregnancy? Was there any birth trauma or difficulty with the delivery? Did the child have significant jaundice, requiring phototherapy? (See Chapter 20, THE NEONATE.) Did he arrive at developmental milestones, such as sitting up, walking, and talking, at normal ages? (See *Nurse's Guide to Developmental Stages,* pages 98 to 101.)

Ask about childhood diseases and injuries. Has the child experienced any head or nerve injuries? Any headaches, tremors, convulsions, dizziness, fainting spells, or muscle weakness? Is he overly active? Has he ever seen spots before his eyes? At what age did these occur?

Inquire about possible emotional problems. Has the child exhibited any personality change? Has he been lethargic or had hallucinations, delusions, or any unusual cognitive or perceptual experiences? Has he ever experimented with drugs?

Finally, depending on the child's age, ask about school. To determine whether the child is well-adjusted socially, ask if he plays well with other children. Is he aggressive or shy? Does he earn good grades? Does he have any speech or coordination problems?

639 Preparing to examine the child

Although the equipment you'll use for a pediatric neurologic examination is essentially the same as for an adult examination, a few special props might be helpful with young children. For instance, you might use familiar objects—such as blocks, buttons, or bottle caps—to test for tactile agnosia. Try peanut butter or candy to test the child's sense of smell. To assess motor strength and coordination, give the child toys or other objects to play with or give him a pen or pencil and ask him to draw.

640 Assessing the child's head and neck

Because a very young child may be frightened when you try to assess his head and neck, you might want to delay percussion, palpation, and auscultation of his head and neck until later in the examination, when the child feels more comfortable with you. Meanwhile, watch him as he plays or interacts with his parents. Are his head and face symmetrical? Does he appear to have muscle weakness or paralysis? Watch how he cries, laughs, turns his head, and wrinkles his forehead.

To examine a child's cranial bones, gently run your fingers over his head, checking the sutures and fontanelles. Look for fullness, bulging, or swelling, which may indicate an intracranial mass or hydrocephalus. Note the shape and symmetry of his head. Abnormal shape accompanied by prominent bony ridges may indicate craniosynostosis (premature suture closure).

Until a child reaches age 2, measure his head size during every examination. Note any sudden increase in size or failure to grow at a normal rate. Head size changes proportionately throughout maturation (see *How Body Proportions Change*).

If you feel a snapping sensation when you press the child's scalp firmly behind and above the ears (similar to the

HOW BODY PROPORTIONS CHANGE

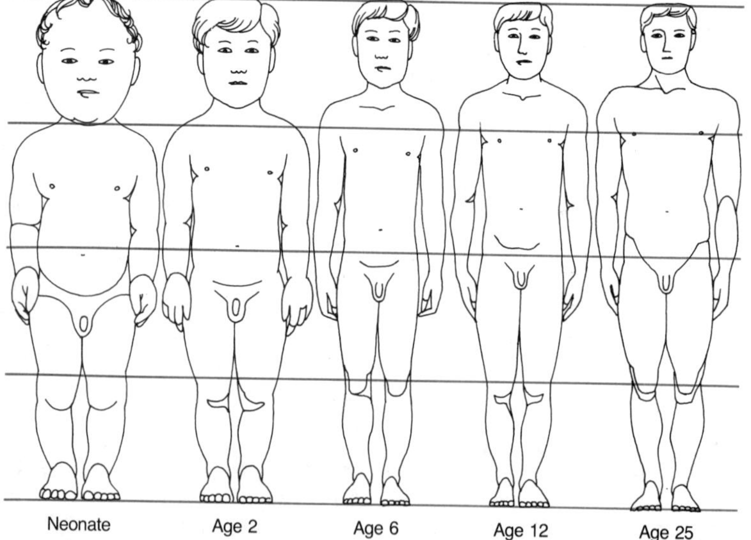

The Stratz chart above shows how the size of a person's head changes in proportion to other areas of the body. During maturation, total head size decreases proportionately and the face elongates. Keep these changes in mind when evaluating the neurologic development of your pediatric patient.

Adapted from William J. Robbins et al., *Growth* (New Haven, Conn.: Yale University Press, 1928), with permission of the publisher.

way a table-tennis ball feels when you press it in), this may indicate craniotabes, a thinning of the outer layer of the skull. Although this thinning is normal at the suture lines, premature infants are susceptible to craniotabes, and such thinning can also be a sign of rickets, syphilis, hypervitaminosis A, or hydrocephalus. A resonant, cracked-pot sound (Macewen's sign), heard when you percuss the parietal bone with your finger, is normal in an infant with open sutures. But if the sutures have closed, this can signal increased intracranial pressure.

If you suspect that a child has an intracranial lesion, hydrocephalus, or decreased brain tissue, transilluminate his skull, using a flashlight fitted with a special rubber ring at the lighted end. Darken the room, and place the light against the child's skull. A small ring of light around the edges of the flashlight is normal, but illumination of the entire cranium is not. If you detect any unusual transparency, refer the child to a doctor.

Next, assess the child's head and neck muscles (see Entry 696). Neck mobility is an important indicator of such neurologic diseases as meningitis. With the child supine, test for nuchal rigidity by cradling his head in your hands. Supporting the weight of his head, move his neck in all directions to assess ease of movement.

641 Assessing a child's cerebral function

A child's cerebral function depends on his age, of course, so you'll need to have an understanding of normal growth and development. A standardized test, such as the Denver Developmental Screening Test, can be helpful for gross screening.

To assess *level of consciousness* in a young child, use motor rather than verbal clues. Is the child lethargic, drowsy, or stuporous? Or, at the opposite extreme, is he hyperactive? When you assess *orientation,* remember that young children are not oriented to time, so only assess their orientation to person or place.

To test a child's *attention span and concentration,* ask him to repeat a series of numbers after you. Generally, a 4-year-old can repeat three numbers; a 5-year-old, four numbers; and a 6-year-old, five numbers. Repeating familiar words, such as *cat* or *dog,* usually holds the interest of a child younger than age 4.

To test a child's *recent memory,* show him a familiar object and tell him that you'll ask him later what it was. Five minutes later, ask him to recall the object.

To test a child's *remote memory,* ask him something like, "What did you have for dinner last night?" Then verify the response with the child's parents.

642 Assessing a child's language development

To assess *receptive speech development,* ask the child to obey simple commands, such as "Sit down" or "Pick up the block." Be careful not to give the child nonverbal clues to your commands. The child's age is important when giving commands. For example, a 3-year-old may fully understand the command but not respond because of shyness or stubbornness.

You can determine a school-age child's ability to comprehend written symbols by asking him to read from a book. Of course, speech can't be tested in infants, but you can evaluate the quality and pitch of an infant's cry. It should be loud and angry-sounding, and it shouldn't be high-pitched.

643 Cranial nerves: Pediatric variations

Assessing the cranial nerves can be difficult in a child under age 2, but you *can* check his symmetry of muscle movement, gaze, sucking strength, and hearing by simple observation. In a child over age 2, assess the cranial nerves as you would an adult's, making the following alterations:

- *CN I* (olfactory). Ask the child to

identify familiar odors, such as peanut butter and chocolate or peppermint candy. For a very young child who may not be able to identify a smell, try a same-different game to determine whether he can distinguish one smell from another.

• *CN II* (optic). You can test a child's

NURSE'S GUIDE TO DEVELOPMENTAL NEUROLOGIC DISORDERS

	CHIEF COMPLAINT
Sydenham's chorea (St. Vitus' dance)	• *Motor disturbances:* sporadic movements of face, trunk, and extremity muscles; incoordination; muscle weakness; facial grimacing; arthritis; arthralgia (growing pains) • *Altered level of consciousness:* restless, emotional instability
Down's syndrome	• *Motor disturbances:* generalized muscular hypotonicity; structural, facial abnormalities • *Altered level of consciousness:* impaired mental capacity
Hydrocephalus	• *Motor disturbances:* spastic movements of arms and legs (more severe in legs), increased tendon reflexes • *Altered level of consciousness:* apathy, lethargy, irritability
Spina bifida	• *Motor disturbances:* weakness, loss of tendon reflexes in legs due to atrophy of leg muscles, gait disturbances, incontinence • *Sensory deviations:* impaired cutaneous and proprioceptive senses in legs
Reye's syndrome	• *Motor disturbances:* In stage I, none; in stage II, hyperactive reflexes; in stage III, decorticate rigidity; in stage IV, decerebrate rigidity, large and fixed pupils; in stage V, loss of deep tendon reflexes, flaccidity • *Seizures:* none, until stage V • *Altered level of consciousness:* in stage I, lethargy; in stage II, coma; in stage III, deepening coma; in stage IV, deep coma
Cerebral palsy (spastic, athetoid, and ataxic forms)	• *Motor disturbances:* In spastic form, hyperactive deep tendon reflexes, rapid alternating muscle contractions and relaxations; in athetoid form, grimacing, dystonia, wormlike movements, sharp and jerky movements before becoming more severe during stress and disappearing during sleep; in ataxic form, muscle weakness, loss of balance and coordination, especially in arms • *Seizures:* in spastic form, seizure disorders possible • *Sensory deviations:* in spastic form, visual and hearing deficits possible • *Altered level of consciousness:* in ataxic form, emotional disorders, mental retardation in about 40% of cases

visual acuity as you would for an adult, but using Allen cards for a very young child or preschooler (see Entry 276). For visual field testing, also follow the procedure for an adult, with one variation: You might want to hold a bright object near the end of your nose to help the young child keep his eyes focused.

	HISTORY	PHYSICAL EXAMINATION AND DIAGNOSTIC STUDIES
	• Onset usually between ages 5 and 15 • Symptoms include rheumatic fever, lack of sleep due to involuntary movements, nightmares; progress over 2 weeks	• Muscle weakness, facial grimacing, no muscle atrophy or contractures
	• Family history of Down's syndrome • Most common in infants born to mothers over age 35 or in firstborn of very young mothers • Growth and development slower than normal	• Gutteral cry; small, round head; flat, occipital, low-set ears; mongoloid slant to eyes; small mouth, with protruding tongue; increased fat pad at nape of neck; short, heavy hands; transverse palmar crease; incomplete Moro's reflex; Brushfield's spots (gray-white specks on iris)
	• Normal head size at birth, increasingly more rapid growth than normal	• Head growth exceeds normal by ½" (1.27 cm) per month; distended scalp veins; full, tense fontanelles; widened cranial sutures; asymmetric appearance of head; setting-sun sign (eyes pushed down in orbit); inability to hold head up; strabismus; cracked-pot sign on skull percussion; high-pitched cry • Skull transilluminates
	• May be asymptomatic • Weakness in legs	• Palpable defect; scoliosis; valgus, varus, or caries deformities of feet, usually unilateral
	• Acute viral infection 1 to 2 days before onset of symptoms • Prodromal symptoms include malaise, cough, earache, rhinorrhea, sore throat	• Vomiting; hyperventilation or respiratory arrest; hyperactive reflexes; absent deep tendon reflexes; decorticate or decerebrate rigidity; large, fixed pupils; rash • Serum ammonia level above 300 mg/100 ml, elevated BUN, elevated liver enzymes (SGOT and SGPT), increased intracranial pressure, prolonged prothrombin time, decreased carbon dioxide pressure (arterial blood gases)
	• Maternal infection, especially rubella • Prenatal radiation, anoxia • Birth difficulties, such as forceps delivery, breech presentation, placenta previa, premature birth • Infection or trauma during infancy, such as brain infection; head trauma; prolonged anoxia	• Underdeveloped affected limbs; hard-to-separate legs; leg crossing, rather than bicycling, when child's lifted from behind; scissors gait; muscle weakness; hyperactive reflexes; contractures; persistent favoring of one hand; nystagmus; dental abnormalities *(continued)*

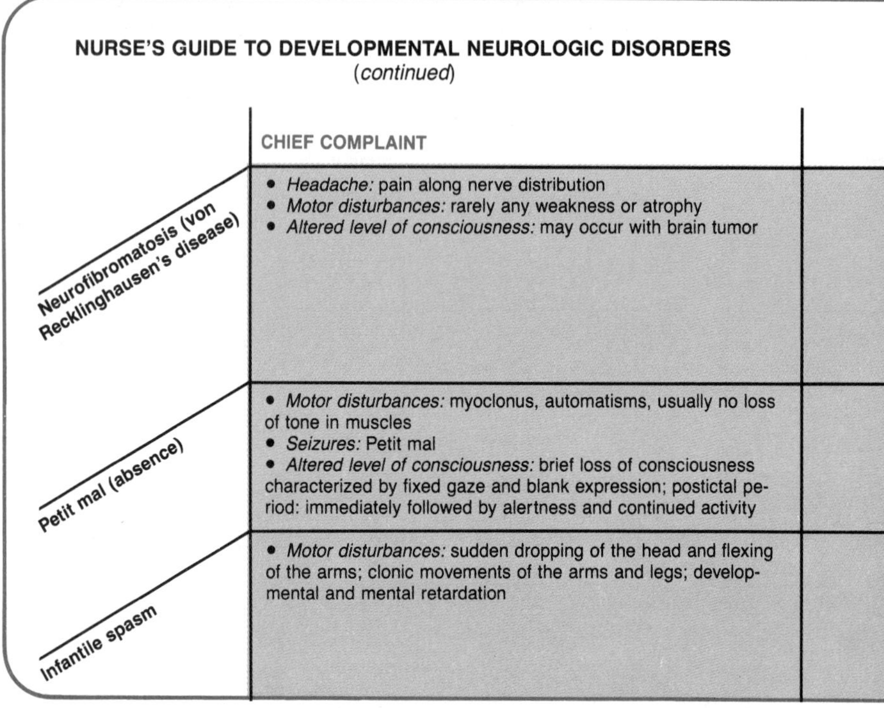

NURSE'S GUIDE TO DEVELOPMENTAL NEUROLOGIC DISORDERS
(continued)

	CHIEF COMPLAINT
Neurofibromatosis (von Recklinghausen's disease)	• *Headache:* pain along nerve distribution • *Motor disturbances:* rarely any weakness or atrophy • *Altered level of consciousness:* may occur with brain tumor
Petit mal (absence)	• *Motor disturbances:* myoclonus, automatisms, usually no loss of tone in muscles • *Seizures:* Petit mal • *Altered level of consciousness:* brief loss of consciousness characterized by fixed gaze and blank expression; postictal period: immediately followed by alertness and continued activity
Infantile spasm	• *Motor disturbances:* sudden dropping of the head and flexing of the arms; clonic movements of the arms and legs; developmental and mental retardation

• *CN V* (trigeminal). Test the sensory division of this nerve as you would for an adult, but make a game out of it by telling the child that a gremlin's going to brush his cheeks, pinch his forehead, and so on. Test the motor division by having the child bite down hard on a tongue depressor as you try to pull it away. At the same time, palpate his jaw muscles for symmetry and contraction strength.
• *CN VII* (facial). Test the muscles controlled by this nerve as you would for an adult, but instead of asking the child to perform certain movements, have him mimic your facial expressions. Test the sensory division of the facial nerve with salt and sugar, as for an adult.
• *CN VIII* (acoustic). Test the cochlear division of the acoustic nerve in a child by checking his hearing acuity and sound conduction (see Entry 322).
• *CN IX, X, XI,* and *XII* (glossopharyngeal, vagus, spinal accessory, hypoglossal). Test these nerves as you would for an adult, using games to facilitate the examination when necessary.

644 Assessing a child's motor function

Assess balance and coordination in a child by watching motor skills, such as dressing and undressing. You can also have him stack blocks, put a bead in a bottle, or draw a cross. Depending on his age, he should be able to draw a cross in two movements, without changing the pencil to his other hand.

A child age 4 should be able to stand on one foot for about 5 seconds, and a child age 6 should be able to do this for 5 seconds with his arms folded across his chest. By age 7, he should be able to do it for 5 seconds with his eyes closed. A child should demonstrate a preference for one-hand dominance before age 12 months.

To evaluate cerebellar function in an infant, observe his coordination during sucking, swallowing, reaching, kick-

HISTORY	PHYSICAL EXAMINATION AND DIAGNOSTIC STUDIES
• Onset may be anytime from childhood to age 50 • Family history of neurofibromatosis—congenital • May be accompanied by meningiomas, gliomas of the central nervous system	• Multiple tumors under the skin of the scalp, arms, legs, trunk, and cranial nerves; pigmentary lesions, café au lait spots; symptoms similar to brain or spinal tumor, depending on tumor's location; overgrowth of skin and of skull and neck tissue; hypertrophy of face, tongue, arms, and legs; skeletal anomalies; bone cysts • Cranial nerve abnormalities if affected
• Idiopathic seizure disorder diagnosed usually between ages 4 and 12; onset rare after age 20 • Predisposing factors include birth injury or developmental defect, acute febrile illness	• Petit mal triad: myoclonic jerks, automatisms, transient absences • May only be characterized by brief staring periods with occasional eye blinks
• Usually lasts until age 4, then possibly changes to generalized seizures	• Brief myoclonic jerks involving entire body • EEG changes

ing, and grasping. (To assess gait and posture in children, as well as muscle strength, see Entries 696 and 697.)

645 Assessing sensory function in a child

Test the sensations of pain, touch, vibration, and temperature in an older child as you would for an adult. (Most of these tests aren't applicable to an infant or very young child. Younger children may respond to pain and touch, but their responses may be unreliable.) Consider the following variations from the adult tests when assessing a child's sense of direction and discrimination:

• *Position.* Children under age 5 usually have no concept of up and down. To test an older child's directional sense, play an up-down game. Ask the child to put out his hand, palm up, close his eyes, and then tell you whether his fingers are up or down as you bend or straighten them. Touch only the sides of the child's fingers, so the weight of your fingers doesn't give him clues.

• *Discrimination.* To test *stereognosis* in a child, ask him to close his eyes, and tell him you'll put one of three objects in his hand (for instance, a bottle cap, a coin, or a button). Then remove the object, and tell the child to open his eyes. Ask him which object it was.

When testing *graphesthesia,* remember that school-age children can usually identify numbers as well as adults. For younger children, use geometric figures or lines (parallel or crossing). Draw the same figure on the child's palms twice, or draw two different figures, and ask the child whether the figures are the same or different. (To make sure the child understands, play the game first with the child watching, then with his eyes closed.) Very young children will probably be difficult to test accurately, because they might not fully understand the concepts of *same* and *different.* Note if an older child consistently fails these tests or seems to do better with one hand.

To test *texture discrimination,* have the child close his eyes and tell you whether a piece of cloth is rough or smooth. Test *two-point discrimination* as you would for an adult, but make a game of it by asking the child to close his eyes and tell you if he feels one or two mosquitoes (pinpricks).

Test the *extinction phenomenon* as you would for an adult. For developmental reasons, this test isn't always accurate in children under age 6. If an older child feels only one sensation when you touch him in two places, he might have a parietal lobe defect.

646 Assessing a child's reflexes

Make a special effort to relax a child when assessing his reflexes. Many children (and some adults) will tighten their muscles, so that testing reflexes is almost impossible. Asking a child to relax usually doesn't work, but having him clench his fingers together and then pull on the count of three (while you tap the tendon) often distracts him, so the appropriate muscles relax. But because this also enhances the reflex, keep in mind that the reflex has been artificially magnified. A positive Babinski's sign may normally be present up to age 2.

647 Hydrocephalus

Children can develop many of the same pathologic conditions of the nervous system as adults: benign and malignant cerebral tumors, cerebral hematomas, spinal cord injuries, seizure disorders, and neurologic infections. With few exceptions, these problems occur in children the same way they do in adults.

Hydrocephalus merits special attention, because it's one of the most easily diagnosed neurologic disorders in both children and adults (although it's less common in adults). This condition results from an imbalance in the production and absorption of cerebrospinal fluid (CSF), which causes excess fluid to accumulate in the brain's ventricular system. CSF pressure is usually elevated, but occasionally it may be almost normal. Hydrocephalus can occur congenitally or result from a birth trauma, an acquired tumor, or a cerebral infection or injury. Acquired hydrocephalus can develop slowly or rapidly, depending on the cause. In severe congenital hydrocephalus, the infant's head may be enlarged at birth, causing a very difficult delivery. The hydrocephalic child may have some neurologic and motor impairment, depending on severity and on treatment. (The child treated with a shunt is prone to bacterial infection.)

648 Down's syndrome

Down's syndrome, a chromosomal disorder also known as trisomy 21, is characterized by specific neurologic deficits. Down's syndrome causes generalized muscular hypotonicity and facial and structural anomalies. (See *Nurse's Guide to Developmental Neurologic Disorders,* pages 614 to 617.) These signs may be apparent in the neonatal phase of development. An infant with Down's syndrome is commonly described as a floppy baby, exhibiting poor muscle tone and posture and an inability to hold his head up. His sucking reflex is usually weak, and his reflexes are generally slow. Brushfield's spots may be found in the iris of the eye. The child develops slowly physically; later testing reveals mild-to-severe mental retardation. Physical examinations throughout childhood and adulthood reveal the same deficits present in the infant: hypotonicity; poor coordination, posture, and balance; and slowed reflexes. He seldom reaches a stature beyond that of a child age 10. Associated cardiac anomalies may be present. The child may have a greater potential to develop infections and acute leukemia. The child with Down's syndrome is usually extremely friendly and restless. He learns activities of daily living slowly.

Assessing geriatric patients

649 Aging's effect on the nervous system

Aging affects the nervous system in many ways. Neurons of the central and peripheral nervous systems undergo degenerative changes. Nerve transmission slows down, causing the elderly person to react sluggishly to external stimuli. After about age 50, a person's brain cells decrease at a rate of about 1% per year. Yet, clinical effects usually aren't noticeable until the aging process is more advanced.

When you test an elderly patient's nervous system, neurologic alterations secondary to changes in other body systems are likely to affect results. Such alterations include sensory receptor changes leading to hearing and vision loss, cerebrovascular dysfunctions, and mental status changes brought on by medications. Other factors that can influence an elderly patient's test responses include fatigue, lack of sleep, depression, hyperactivity, fear, and anxiety. These factors may cause the elderly patient to appear disinterested or preoccupied; he may be slow to respond.

650 Examination findings

When you perform a neurologic examination of an elderly patient, you'll usually detect an alteration in one or more senses (see *Recognizing Neurologic Changes in the Elderly*). The patient may also exhibit akinesia (a slowing of fine finger movements), which makes it difficult for him to perform such maneuvers as the finger-to-nose test. Deep tendon reflexes may be diminished or absent, position sense may be impaired, and vibration detection may be diminished. Gait disturbances are also common (see Entry 700).

651 Neurologic diseases in the elderly

The neurologic disease processes common in elderly persons can result from primary neurologic degenerative changes or can occur secondary to changes in other body systems. *Alzheimer's disease,* which results from progressive brain atrophy, exaggerates the effects of the normal aging process. *Parkinsonism,* which results from degeneration of the basal ganglia, interferes with the extrapyramidal motor system. Decreased production of dopamine, a neurotransmitter, has been associated with this disease process, but the cause is unknown. Physical findings include pill-rolling tremor; slowed, shuffling gait; and posture disturbances (see *Nurse's Guide to Geriatric Neurologic Disorders,* page 620).

Chronic brain syndrome, an organic and irreversible disorder, results in progressive degeneration of memory and intellect. *Acute brain syndrome,* which is usually reversible, may result from dehydration, anemia, or cerebro-

RECOGNIZING NEUROLOGIC CHANGES IN THE ELDERLY

During the neurologic examination of an elderly patient, you may find several sensory alterations. Note the following cranial nerves that may be affected by aging and the alterations produced.

- *Olfactory nerve:* progressive loss of smell
- *Optic nerve:* decreased visual acuity; presbyopia; limited peripheral vision
- *Facial nerve:* decreased perception of all taste, particularly sweet and salty; drooping or relaxation of the mouth, usually unilateral
- *Auditory nerve:* presbycusis or loss of high tones, later generalized to all frequencies
- *Glossopharyngeal nerve:* sluggish or absent gag reflex
- *Hypoglossal nerve:* unilateral tongue weakness (may also be caused by malnutrition or structural [facial] malformation)

NURSE'S GUIDE TO GERIATRIC NEUROLOGIC DISORDERS

	CHIEF COMPLAINT	HISTORY	PHYSICAL EXAMINATION
Parkinson's disease	• *Motor disturbances:* tremor; characteristic rhythmic, unilateral pill-rolling movement involves thumb and forefinger; muscle rigidity; akinesia; inability to initiate and perform volitional motor activities; slow, shuffling Parkinson's gait—may be retropulsive or propulsive; fatigue • *Sensory deviations:* thermal paresthesia, hyperhidrosis, pain in one or both arms • *Altered level of consciousness:* minor intellectual deficit	• Onset usually between ages 50 and 65 • Predisposing factors include family history of parkinsonism; past viral infections, such as influenza • Symptoms include increasing difficulty performing activities of daily living; slow eating and walking; inability to write in script—reversion to printing • Increased tremor during stress or anxiety; tremor decreases with purposeful movement and with sleep	• Resistance to passive movement; postural deformities of arms, legs, and trunk; small, festinating gait; arms fail to swing when walking; cogwheeling; eczema; micrographia; bradykinesia; hand tremor at rest; low, monotone speech pattern
Alzheimer's disease (presenile dementia) and senile dementia	• *Motor disturbances:* expressive and receptive aphasia, echolalia, apraxia, spatial disorientation, repetitive movements, incontinence • *Seizures:* possible • *Altered level of consciousness:* personality changes; progressive dementia; loss of recent memory at first, and then remote memory; decreased attention span; faulty concentration; loss of abstract thinking; restlessness and overactivity	• Most common in women over age 50	• Difficulty comprehending written and verbal speech; slow reflexes; shuffling gait; memory changes; hyperactivity; irritability

vascular accident. Unlike chronic brain syndrome, the patient's history usually shows a relatively recent onset (see Entry 144).

Other disease processes are caused by alterations of other body systems (such as the cardiovascular system) that in turn impair neurologic functioning. *Senile tremor* is a tremor that affects the head and hands but doesn't cause rigidity or bradykinesia. A decreased blood supply to the brain, or cardiac arrhythmia, can lead to *senile epilepsy,* which causes convulsions or loss of consciousness. Interruption in blood supply to the brain stem can cause drop attacks, without loss of consciousness. Gait changes may occur from destruction of the spinal cord's lateral columns.

Selected References

Angevine, Jay B., Jr. *Principles of Neuroanatomy.* New York: Oxford University Press, 1981.

Bakow, Eric D., "Respiratory Care of the Critically Ill Patient with Head Trauma," *Critical Care Quarterly* 2(1):81, 1979.

Barrett-Griesemer, Patricia, et al. "A Guide to Headaches—And How to Relieve Their Pain," *Nursing81* 11:50, April 1981.

Bates, Barbara. *A Guide to Physical Examination,* 2nd ed. Philadelphia: J.B. Lippincott Co., 1979.

Bresnan, Michael, et al. *Pediatric Neurology.* Garden City, NY: Medical Examination Publishing Co., Inc., 1976.

Conway, Barbara L. *Carini and Owens' Neurological and Neurosurgical Nursing,* 7th ed. St. Louis: C.V. Mosby Co., 1978.

Core Curriculum for Neurosurgical Nursing. American Association of Neurosurgical Nurses, 1977.

Davis, Joan, and Mason, Celestine. *Neurologic Critical Care.* New York: Van Nostrand Reinhold Co., 1979.

DeJong, Russell N. *The Neurologic Examination,* 4th ed. Philadelphia: Harper & Row, 1979.

Gady, Debra. "Meningitis in the Pediatric Population," *Nursing Clinics of North America,* vol 15, no 1, March 1980.

Gehrke, Marj. "Identifying Brain Tumors," *Journal of Neurosurgical Nursing* 12:90, June 1980.

Hawken, Margarithe. "Seizures: Etiology, Classification, Intervention," *Journal of Neurosurgical Nursing,* 11:166, September 1979.

Malasanos, Lois, et al. *Health Assessment,* 2nd ed. St. Louis: C.V. Mosby Co., 1980.

Mitchell, P.H., and Irvin, N.J. "Neurological Examination: Nursing Assessment for Nursing Purposes," *Journal of Neurosurgical Nursing* 9:23, March 1977.

Norman, Susan E., and Browne, Thomas R. "Seizure Disorders," *American Journal of Nursing* 81:983, April 1981.

Plum, Fred, and Posner, Jerome, eds. *The Diagnosis of Stupor and Coma,* 3rd ed. Philadelphia: F.A. Davis Co., 1980.

Ramirez, B. "When You're Faced with a Neuro Patient," *RN Magazine* 42:67, January 1979.

Romanes, G.J., ed. *Cunningham's Textbook of Anatomy,* 12th ed. Oxford: Oxford University Press, 1981.

Rusinski, P.S. "Neurological Assessment of the Hemiplegic Patient," *Nurse Practitioner* 4:26, May-June 1979.

Samuels, Martin A. *Manual of Neurologic Therapeutics.* Boston: Little, Brown & Co., 1978.

Simpson, John, and Magee, Kenneth R. *Clinical Evaluation of the Nervous System.* Boston: Little, Brown & Co., 1973.

Snell, Richard. *Clinical Neuroanatomy for Medical Students.* Boston: Little, Brown & Co., 1980.

Swift, Nancy, and Mabel, Robert. *Manual of Neurological Nursing.* Boston: Little, Brown & Co., 1978.

Walleck, C. "Neurological Assessment for Nurses—A Part of the Nursing Process," *Journal of Neurosurgical Nursing* 10:13, March 1978.

Wallhagen, Margaret I., et al. "The Brain Damaged Patient—Approaches to Assessment, Care, and Rehabilitation," *American Journal of Nursing* 79:2117, December 1979.

Wehrmaker, Suzanne, and Wintermute, Joann. *Case Studies in Neurological Nursing.* Boston: Little, Brown & Co., 1978.

Weiner, Howard, L. *Neurology for the House Officer,* 2nd ed., Baltimore: Williams and Wilkins Co., 1978.

Wilson, Susan F. *Neuronursing.* New York: Springer Publishing Co., Inc., 1979.

Young, M. Shelley. "Understanding the Signs of Intracranial Pressure: A Bedside Guide," *Nursing81* 11:59, February 1981.

16

KEY POINTS IN THIS CHAPTER

KEY CHARTS IN THIS CHAPTER

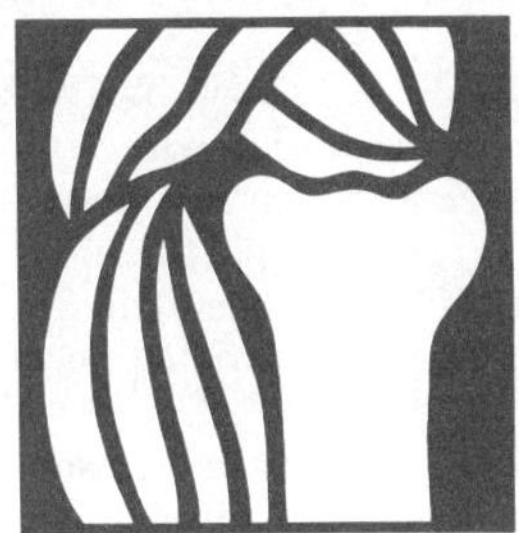

Musculoskeletal System

Introduction

652 Assessing bones, joints, and muscles

To assess a patient's bones, joints, and muscles, you need a thorough understanding of how all the body's systems work together. Why? Because the musculoskeletal system is intricately related to virtually all other body systems and functions. In fact, it's seldom assessed alone; you'll usually evaluate a patient's musculoskeletal system and identify any existing problems in the process of doing a complete physical assessment.

Primary musculoskeletal problems may result from congenital, developmental, neoplastic, infectious, traumatic, or degenerative disorders of the system itself. Disorders of other body systems also can cause musculoskeletal problems for your patient—and assessment problems for you. For example, a cardiovascular disorder or neurologic dysfunction can produce muscle weakness that's difficult to differentiate from a primary musculoskeletal problem, such as differentiating polyneuritis from acute poliomyelitis. Another example: Metabolic and endocrine problems—such as hypervitaminosis D and hypovitaminosis D, juvenile hypothyroidism (cretinism), and hyperparathyroidism or hypoparathyroidism—can affect the growth and nutrition of a patient's bones and muscles.

In nearly all our day-to-day activities, we rely on our ability to move about. When you're examining a patient in whom you've identified a musculoskeletal disorder, try to get a sense of how he perceives his problem and the effect it may have on his life. Remember that the problem may interfere with his social life, his ability to perform his job, or both. If prompt assessment and treatment can't relieve the problem, he faces the possibility of reduced ability to earn a living and to interact with his friends and family—he may even find that his role in the family will change.

Remember, too, that bone structure is an integral part of personal appearance. Bone disease or deformity, or muscle wasting, can change your patient's appearance and negatively affect his self-image. Such a patient needs your support and assurance of continuing care.

One more important consideration to keep in mind is that musculoskeletal assessment is an ongoing process. Once you've identified a patient's musculoskeletal problem, changes that occur after your initial assessment can be as significant as your original findings. So record the initial assessment data completely, clearly, and accurately. Make it a reliable baseline for future evaluation of the patient.

Reviewing anatomy and physiology

653 Musculoskeletal system components

The musculoskeletal system consists of the bones of the human skeleton, the joints, and the muscles. The human skeleton can be divided into two parts: the *axial skeleton,* which includes the bones of the head and trunk, and the *appendicular skeleton,* which includes the bones of the limbs (see *The Musculoskeletal System,* pages 626 to 627).

Bone provides structure, support, and protection for the body. In addition, bones are involved in the production of red blood cells (see Chapter 17, BLOOD-FORMING AND IMMUNE SYSTEMS) and in mineral metabolism, especially of calcium and phosphorus (see Chapter 18, ENDOCRINE SYSTEM). The principal functions of muscles include movement, maintenance of posture, and production of heat.

The functional unit of the musculoskeletal system is the joint, which comprises the capsule (with its synovium, bursae, and synovial fluid) as well as the ligaments, tendons, and skeletal muscles. These structures move and support the bones.

654 Bone composition and classification

All the body's bones are covered by a layer of dense connective tissue called *periosteum,* which contains the bone-producing cells (*osteoblasts*) and the blood vessels, nerves, and lymphatics that supply the bone.

ANATOMY OF BONE

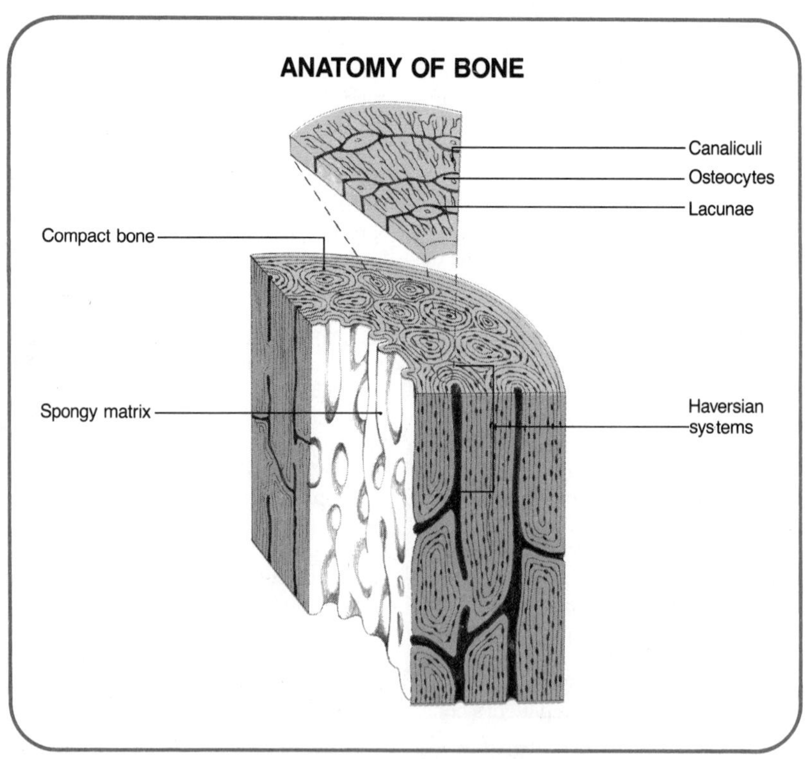

UNDERSTANDING BONE ANATOMY TERMS

TERM	DEFINITION	EXAMPLE
Condyle	A rounded projection at the end of a bone	Condyle of the femur
Crest	A ridge of bone where muscles attach	Iliac crest
Foramen	A hole in a bone through which vessels or nerves pass	Foramen magnum
Fossa	A depression in bone	Olecranon fossa
Head	The rounded end of a bone that fits into a joint	Head of the femur
Meatus	A tube-shaped passageway through a bone	Acoustic meatus
Shaft	The diaphysis, or middle part, of a long bone	Shaft of the femur
Sinus	An air-filled cavity within a bone	Maxillary sinus
Spine (or spinous process)	A sharp prominence where muscles and ligaments attach	Spinous process of a vertebra
Trochanter	Large, blunt processes located below the neck of the femur where muscles attach	Greater trochanter
Tubercle	A small, rounded projection where muscles and ligaments attach	Zygomatic tubercle
Tuberosity	A large, broad, rough process where muscles and ligaments attach	Ischial tuberosity

Bone is composed of very hard, dense tissue that basically is made up of an outer compact layer and an inner spongy matrix (see *Anatomy of Bone*). The functional unit of the outer bone layer is the *haversian system*. Each distinct unit contains a tiny central canal that carries blood vessels and nourishes the living bone cells (called *osteocytes*). The osteocytes are contained within lacunae. Canaliculi extend from each of the lacunae, connect the lacunae with the central haversian canal, and provide nourishment to the osteocytes.

The function of the osteocytes is to maintain the inner bone matrix. The inner matrix consists of collagen fibers with deposits of calcium salts, magnesium, and sodium—minerals that are constantly being stored or mobilized to meet the body's needs.

Bones are classified according to their shape. *Long bones,* such as the femur and humerus, consist of a hollow shaft and expanded ends. *Flat bones,* such as the cranium and sternum, are thin and may be slightly curved. A third classification, *short bones,* includes bones that are more cubical in shape, such as the wrist and ankle. Other types of bones, such as the spinal column and the jaw, are called *irregular bones* because of their varied shapes. In addition to shape, bones are usually identified according to a variety of other characteristics and some special terms (see *Understanding Bone Anatomy Terms*).

655 Bone formation and growth

Bone is formed by ossification of cartilage. Two types of ossification—in-

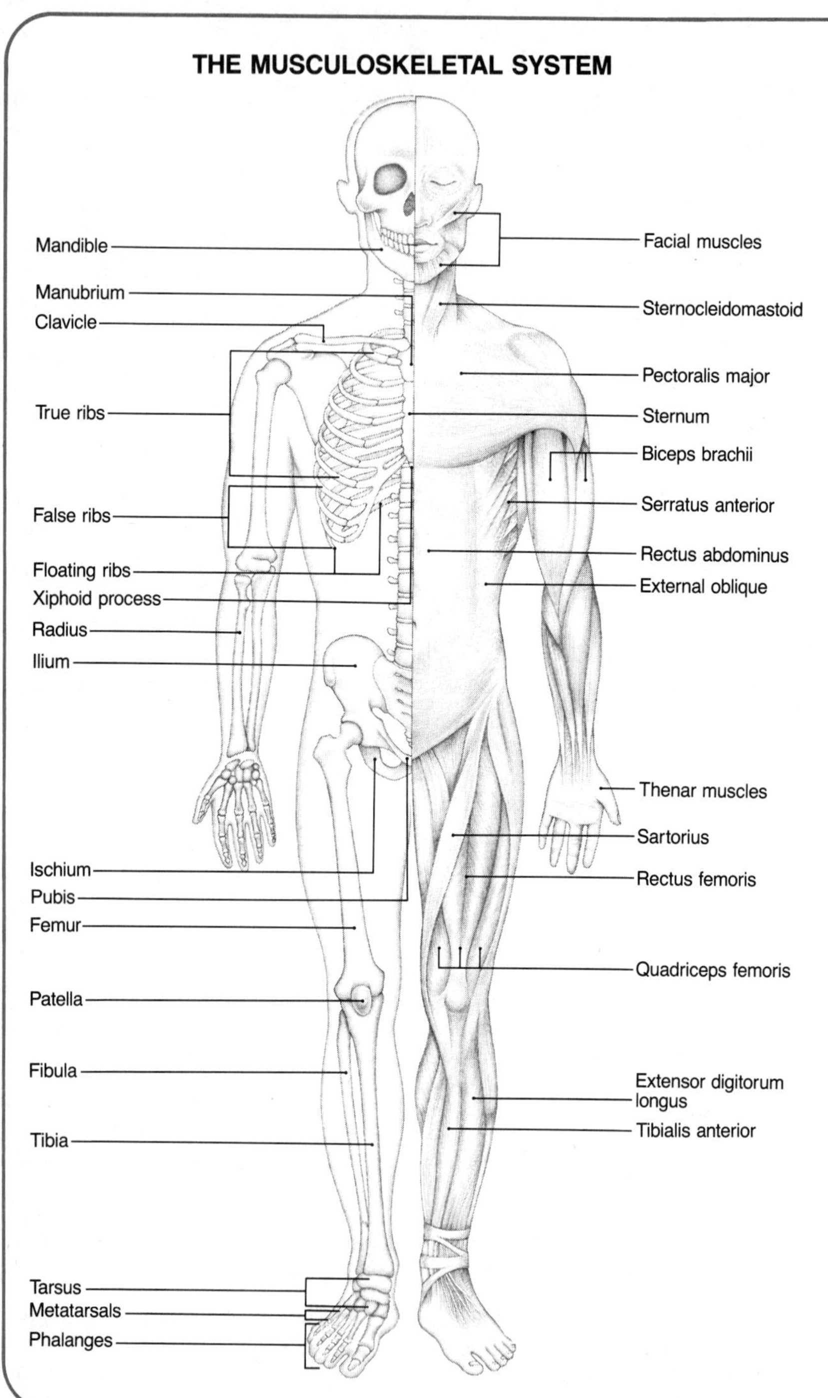
THE MUSCULOSKELETAL SYSTEM
Mandible
Manubrium
Clavicle
True ribs
False ribs
Floating ribs
Xiphoid process
Radius
Ilium
Ischium
Pubis
Femur
Patella
Fibula
Tibia
Tarsus
Metatarsals
Phalanges
Facial muscles
Sternocleidomastoid
Pectoralis major
Sternum
Biceps brachii
Serratus anterior
Rectus abdominus
External oblique
Thenar muscles
Sartorius
Rectus femoris
Quadriceps femoris
Extensor digitorum longus
Tibialis anterior

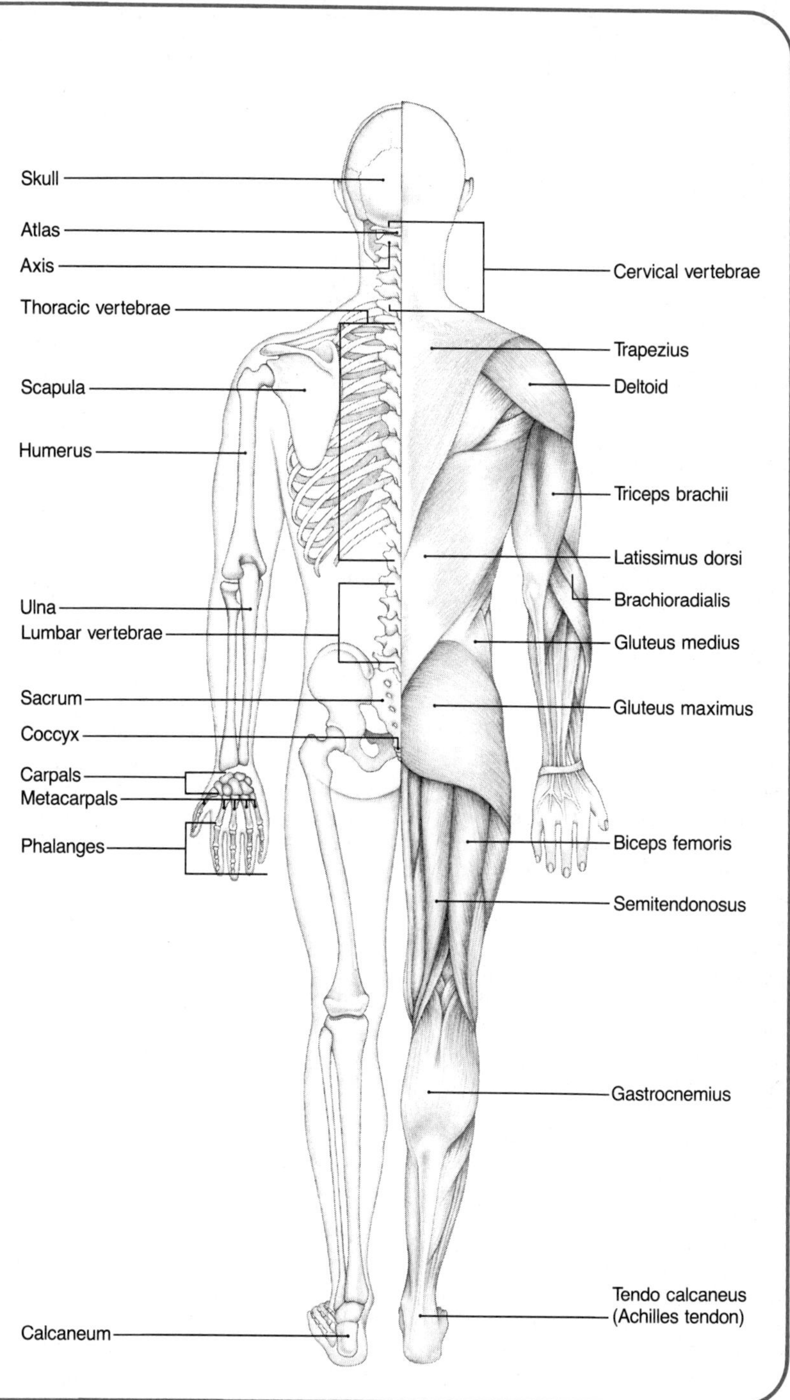
Skull
Atlas
Axis
Thoracic vertebrae
Scapula
Humerus
Ulna
Lumbar vertebrae
Sacrum
Coccyx
Carpals
Metacarpals
Phalanges
Calcaneum
Cervical vertebrae
Trapezius
Deltoid
Triceps brachii
Latissimus dorsi
Brachioradialis
Gluteus medius
Gluteus maximus
Biceps femoris
Semitendonosus
Gastrocnemius
Tendo calcaneus
(Achilles tendon)

UNDERSTANDING OSSIFICATION STAGES

Ossification, or bone formation, can be classified as intramembranous or endochondral. *Intramembranous ossification* is the process that forms the flat, irregular, and short bones as well as the epiphyses of long bones. *Endochondral ossification* is the process that forms the diaphyses of long bones.

Intramembranous ossification occurs in these stages:

- Mesenchymal cells cluster in a fibrous membrane. Cells become osteoblasts.
- Osteoblasts secrete a collagenous fiber matrix in which calcium salt deposits form, resulting in calcification. Osteoblasts surrounded by the collagenous fiber matrix are called *trabeculae*.
- Trabeculae fuse and become trapped in lacunae. Trapped cells are called *osteocytes*.
- Osteocytes do not fuse into solid sheets. Instead, the spaces between them become filled with bone marrow.
- Osteocytes and bone marrow are surrounded by periosteum, forming true spongy bone.
- Maturation continues until the surface becomes solid, dense, and compact.

Endochondral ossification occurs in these stages:

- A cartilage model is present.
- A change in pH activates the chondrocytes and lacunae to hypertrophy and cause calcium salt deposit formation, resulting in cartilage calcification.
- Mesenchymal cells in the perichondrium become osteoblasts.
- Osteoblasts produce osteocytes, which form a shell of bone, the periosteum, on the outer layer of the spicules of calcified cartilage.
- The calcified cartilage is excavated and removed. Blood vessels grow into these excavated spaces. If the bone is long enough, the excavated spaces run together, forming bone marrow cavities.
- The cartilage model grows in length at the epiphyses. Secondary ossification sites grow at proximal epiphyses, where spongy bone develops.
- The distal epiphyses ossify after birth.
- A layer of hyaline cartilage remains on the outside of the epiphyses as articular cartilage. A plate of cartilage also remains between the epiphyses and diaphysis, allowing bone to grow until early adulthood.

tramembranous and endochondral—take place. *Intramembranous ossification* forms the spongy bone found in flat, short, and irregular bones and in the epiphyses of long bones. With maturation, the surface of these bones is restructured into dense compact bone. *Endochondral ossification* forms the compact bone found in the diaphysis of long bones (see *Understanding Ossification Stages*).

Bone is constantly being eroded by osteoclasts and built up by osteoblasts, a process that strengthens the bone and allows growth in bone diameter. This process is influenced by vitamin D, parathyroid hormone, and thyrocalcitonin. Production of new bone also increases and decreases, depending on the amount of stress on the bone. Growth in bone length occurs at the line of cartilage between the epiphysis and diaphysis of long bones (the epiphyseal plate); this process continues until early adulthood.

656 Bones of the head and neck

Bones of the head and neck include the skull, the mandible, and the cervical vertebrae (see *Anatomy of the Vertebral Column*, pages 630 to 631). The skull bones, which fuse after birth, form the cranial cavity containing the brain and the pituitary gland. They also form the bony orbits, which house the eyes, and several special structures, such as the nasal cavities, the temporal and infratemporal fossae, and the hard palate. The mandible contains the lower teeth and articulates with the skull at the temporomandibular joint.

The neck contains seven cervical vertebrae. The top vertebra, called the *atlas*, articulates with the occipital condyles of the skull. Unlike most of the cervical vertebrae, it doesn't have a body or spinous process. The second cervical vertebra, the *axis*, is characterized by its odontoid process, which articulates with the atlas. The remaining cervical vertebrae have holes in their transverse processes (foramina transversarii), for the transmission of vertebral arteries, and short bifid spinous processes. The seventh cervical vertebra has a longer, prominent spinous process (vertebra prominens) that can be palpated at the neck's posterior base when the head is bent forward.

657 Bones of the upper limb

The bones of the upper limb include those of the shoulder girdle (scapula and clavicle), the arm (humerus), the forearm (radius and ulna), the wrist (carpus), and the hand (metacarpals and phalanges).

The scapula, or shoulder-blade, is a thin, triangular bone supported by muscles against the second and seventh ribs. The clavicle, or collarbone, extends laterally between the manubrium of the sternum and the acromial process of the scapula, forming the acromioclavicular joint. The clavicle serves as a strut between the axial skeleton and the upper limb and is held firmly in place by ligaments.

The humerus is the single long bone of the upper arm. Its proximal end, or head, articulates with the glenoid cavity of the scapula to form the glenohumeral (shoulder) joint. The distal end articulates with the ulna and radius of the forearm. The radius rotates around a vertical axis to carry the hand over and back—actions called pronation and supination, respectively. The ulna, unlike the radius, is largest proximally and narrows dramatically at its distal end. Its proximal end forms the tip of the elbow.

Eight carpal bones, roughly ar-

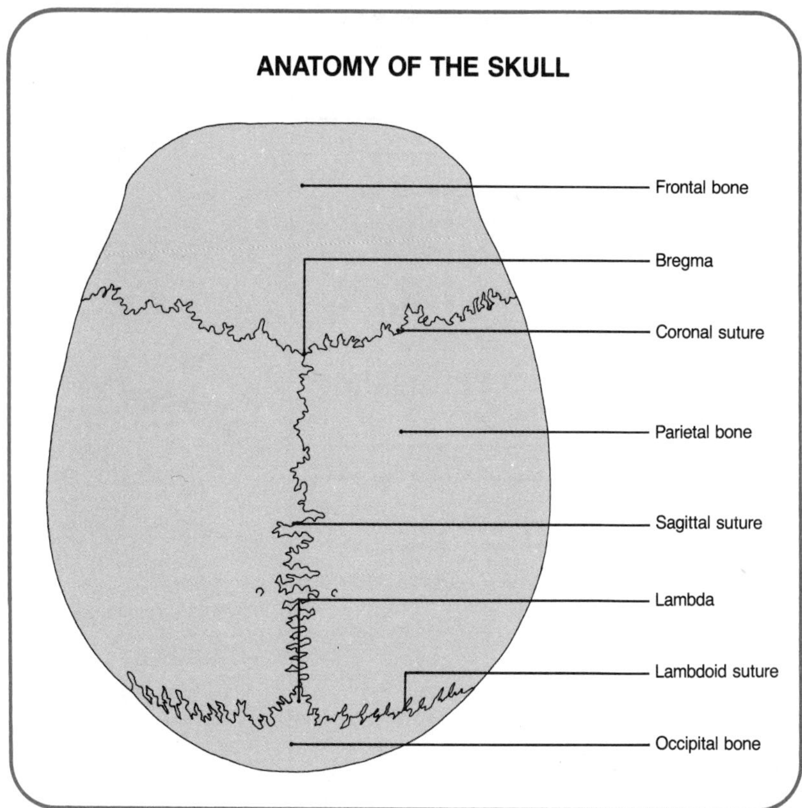

ANATOMY OF THE VERTEBRAL COLUMN

1. Atlas

Anterior tubercle
Superior articular surface
Foramen transversarium
Facet for dens
Posterior tubercle

2. Axis

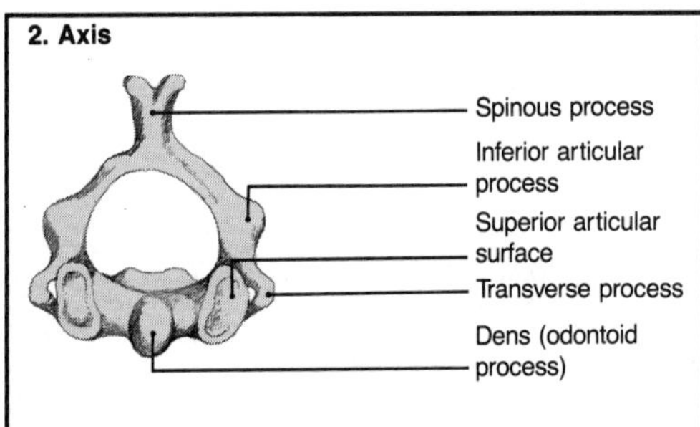

3. Cervical vertebrae

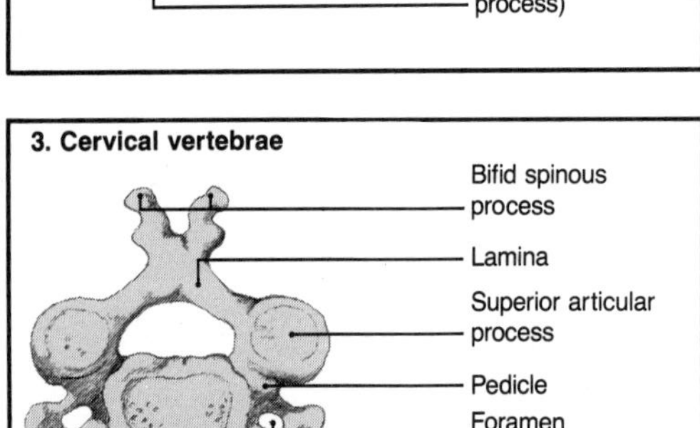

4. Thoracic vertebrae

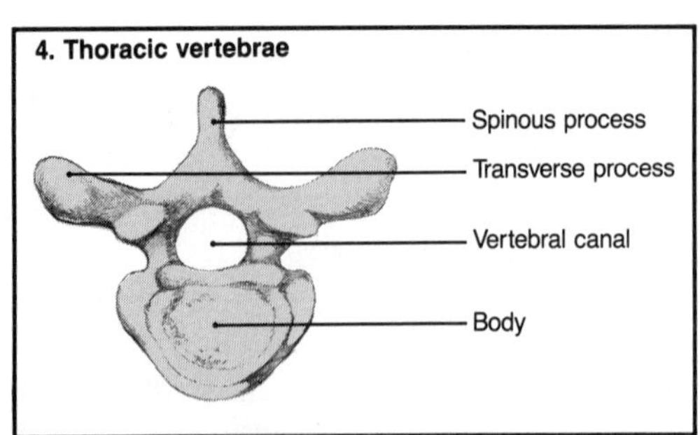

Vertebral column from behind

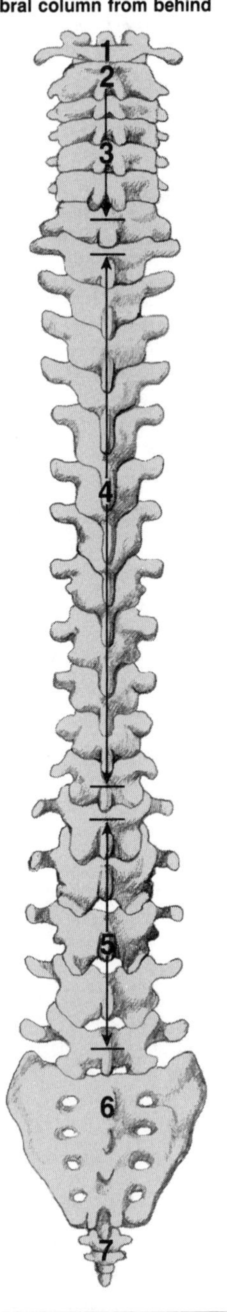

Vertebral column, left lateral view

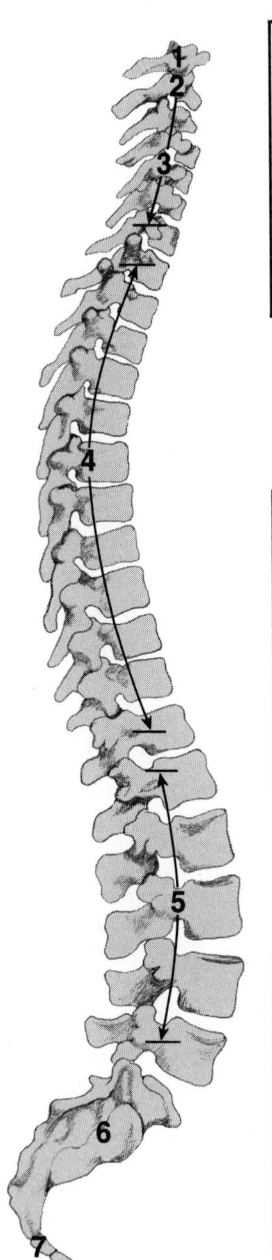

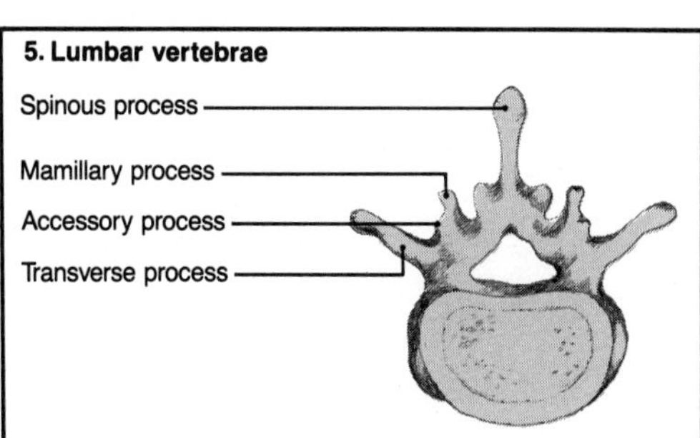

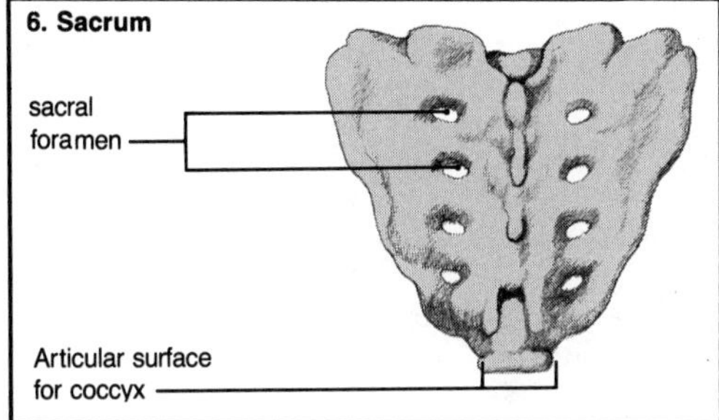

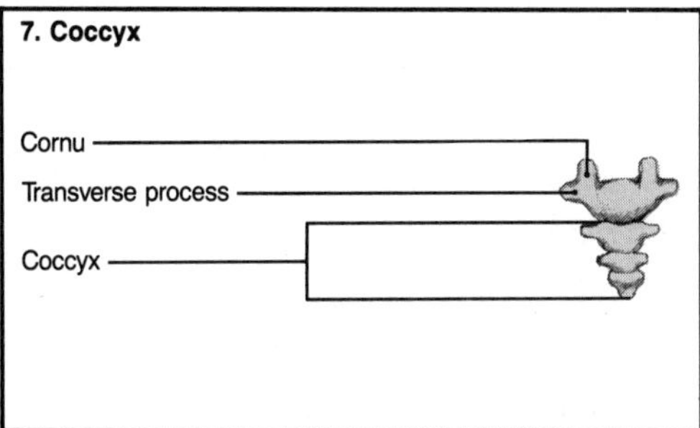

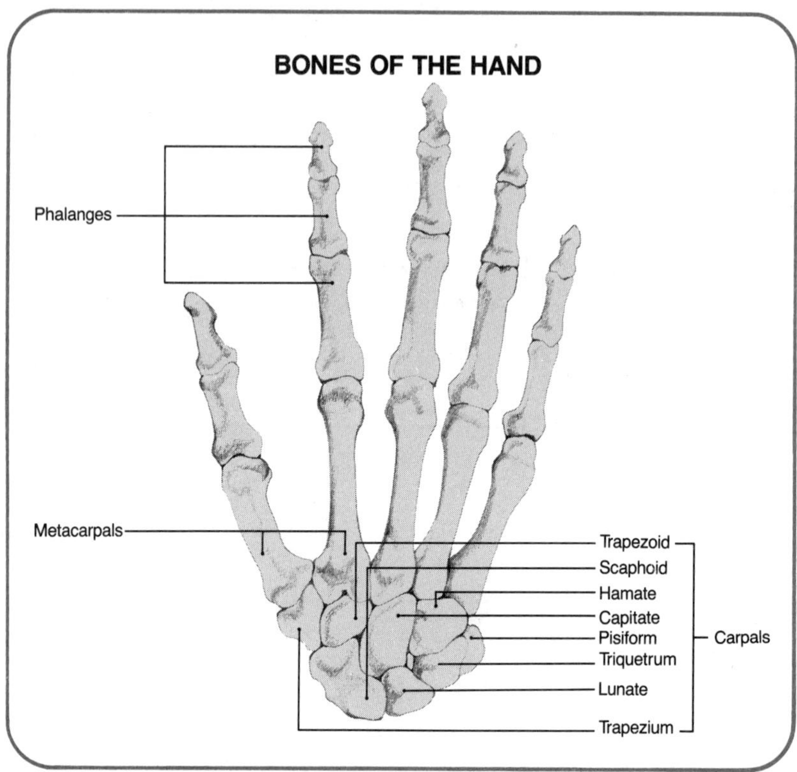

ranged in two rows of four bones each, make up the wrist, or carpus. Five metacarpal bones connect the carpus to the phalanges. The thumb has two phalanges (a proximal and a distal), whereas each of the other fingers has three (a proximal, a middle, and a distal).

658 Bones of the trunk

The bones of the trunk include the thoracic vertebrae, the ribs, the sternum, and the lumbar vertebrae. The 12 thoracic vertebrae have long, slanted, tapering spinous processes, which overlap the adjacent vertebrae, and facets that articulate with the ribs. Each side of the body contains 12 ribs. A typical rib has a head that articulates with the thoracic vertebrae, a neck, and a curving shaft that bends around the thoracic wall.

The first seven pairs of ribs (1 to 7 on each side) are called *true ribs* because they articulate directly with the sternum through individual costal cartilages. The remaining five pairs (ribs 8 to 12) are *false ribs:* the costal cartilages of ribs 8, 9, and 10 join to form the costal arch, which attaches to the seventh costal cartilage. The two lowest ribs, called *floating ribs,* end freely (they're not attached to the sternum).

The sternum consists of the manubrium, the body, and the xiphoid process. The manubrium, the uppermost portion of the sternum, articulates with the medial ends of the clavicles and with the first costal cartilage and the upper half of the second. Its upper border, called the jugular notch, is concave; you can palpate it between the two sternoclavicular joints. The body of the sternum is a thin, flat, elongated plate of bone below the manubrium.

It receives the second through the sixth costal cartilages. The sternal angle, a palpable transverse ridge, lies between the manubrium and body of the sternum. It marks the level of the second rib and costal cartilage; the second intercostal space is directly under it. The xiphoid process, the lowest and smallest part of the sternum, varies in shape and is commonly bifid. It has no direct rib attachment, but on its superior angle a notch—corresponding to the notch on the inferior angle of the body of the sternum—receives the seventh costal cartilage.

The five lumbar vertebrae, designed for weight bearing, are the largest vertebrae in the body. Unlike the cervical and thoracic vertebrae, their articular processes are placed for limited movement.

659 Pelvic bones

The pelvic bones include the ilium, the ischium, the pubis, the sacrum, and the coccyx. The two iliac bones have large winglike *crests* that extend superiorly. The ischium is L-shaped and extends to the pubis (see Entry 781).

The point where the ilium, ischium, and pubis join laterally is the *acetabulum,* the socket that holds the head of the femur. The sacrum consists of five fused vertebrae that narrow progressively and form a wedge. The coccyx, or tailbone, is formed by the fusion of vertebrae, usually four.

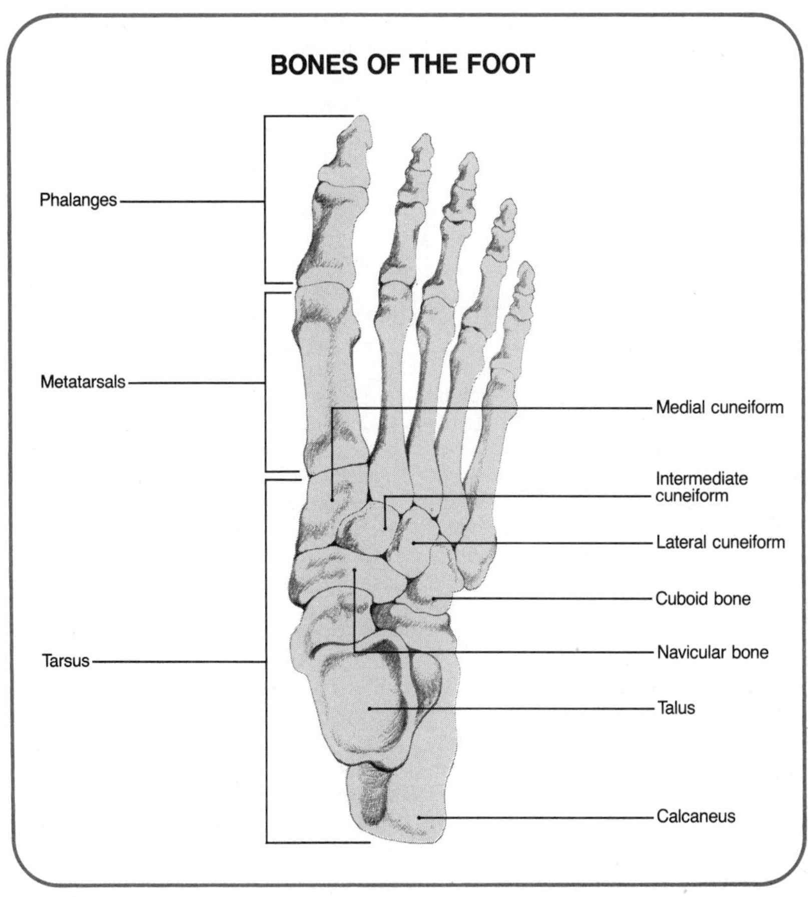

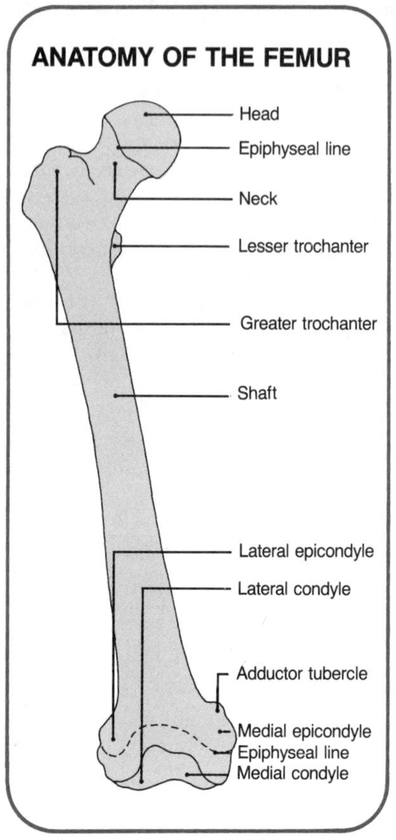

660 Bones of the lower limb

The bones of the lower limb include those of the thigh (femur), leg (tibia and fibula), and foot (tarsus, metatarsals, and phalanges). Also, a large sesamoid bone, the *patella,* is associated with the knee. The femur articulates proximally with the acetabulum of the pelvis. Between the femoral head and shaft is the narrow neck, which allows free movement of the femur. The tibia, or shin bone, is a strong, weight-bearing bone that articulates with the femur proximally and with the talus, or ankle bone, distally. The fibula, which lies lateral to the tibia, bears no direct weight because it doesn't articulate with the femur. Like the tibia, it also articulates distally with the talus.

The tarsus consists of seven bones that, along with ligaments, maintain the foot arches. Each foot contains five metatarsal bones, larger versions of the hand's metacarpal bones. Like the thumb, the great toe has two phalanges; the other toes, like the fingers, have three each.

661 Joints: Structure and function

Joints are the areas where rigid body components connect, thus holding the skeleton together. They may be movable or immovable. Joints are classified as fibrous, cartilaginous, or synovial. *Fibrous joints* (synarthroses) permanently unite structures; the sutures between the skull bones, for example, are fibrous joints. *Cartilaginous joints* (amphiarthroses), such as the pubic symphysis, are united by cartilage and are therefore slightly movable. The third classification, *synovial joints* (diarthroses), is the most common type of joint, a freely movable articulation. A synovial joint can take one of several forms: ball-and-socket, hinge, pivot, condyloid, gliding, or saddle (see *Identifying the Types of Joints*). For the types of joint motion produced by muscle contraction, see *Types of Joint Movement,* page 636.

662 Skeletal muscles

Unlike cardiac and smooth muscles, skeletal muscles are voluntarily controlled, with various modes of action. Each muscle fiber consists of a plasma membrane (sarcolemma) that encloses a fluid (sarcoplasm) containing many striated myofibrils. Muscle contraction begins when a nerve impulse from the central nervous system spreads along the sarcolemma and enters the muscle fiber. This impulse increases the fiber's permeability to calcium. As calcium enters the motor end plate, acetylcholine is released. This causes the muscle membrane to become permeable to sodium. As sodium moves into the muscle fiber, the change in electric potential causes the muscle to contract.

IDENTIFYING THE TYPES OF JOINTS

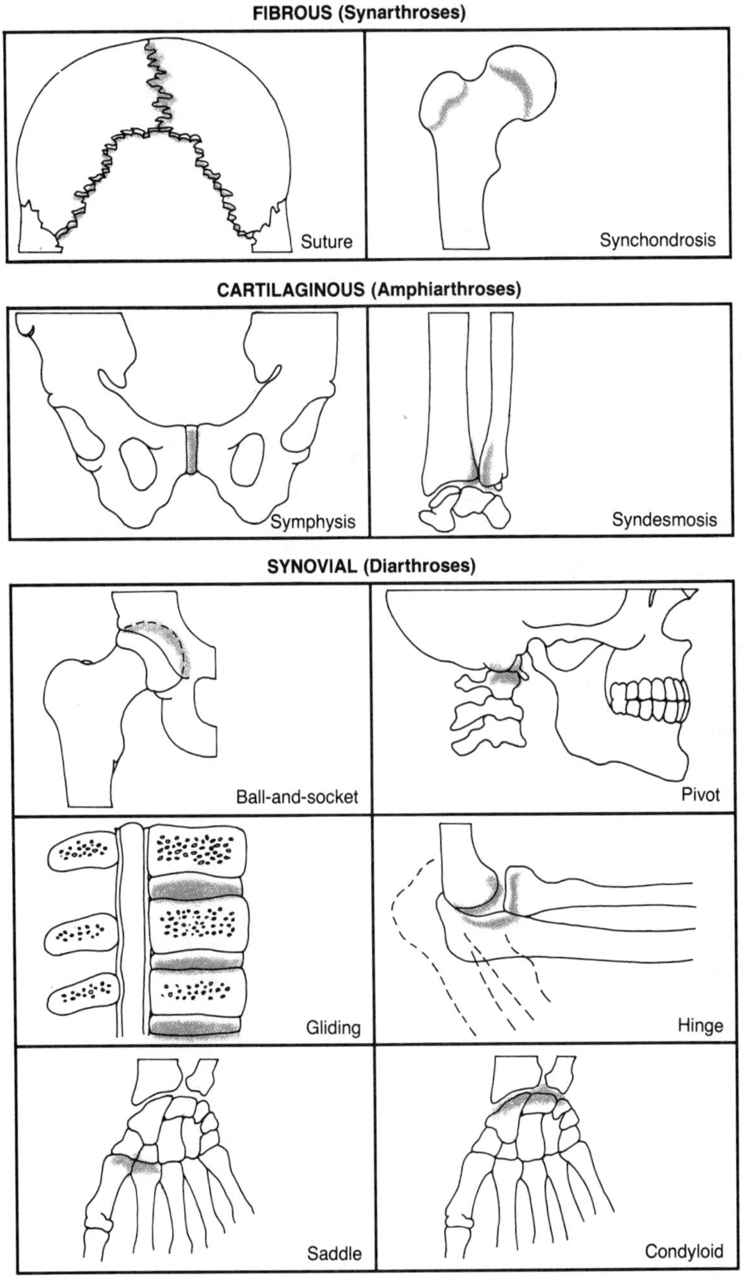

FIBROUS (Synarthroses)

Suture

Synchondrosis

CARTILAGINOUS (Amphiarthroses)

Symphysis

Syndesmosis

SYNOVIAL (Diarthroses)

Ball-and-socket

Pivot

Gliding

Hinge

Saddle

Condyloid

TYPES OF JOINT MOVEMENT

Abduction: drawing away from the median plane or axial line of a limb

Adduction: drawing toward the median plane or axial line of a limb

Inversion: turning inward

Eversion: turning outward

Pronation: facing downward or, with the hand, turning the palm backward or downward

Supination: facing upward or, with the hand, turning the palm forward or upward

Internal rotation: turning on an axis medially

External rotation: turning on an axis laterally

Extension: straightening

Flexion: bending

Circumduction: moving in a circle

Contraction takes place when filaments of actin slide between myosin filaments. Bands of these filaments, located in the sarcomere, give skeletal muscle its striated appearance. As the filaments slide over one another, they cause the sarcomere to shorten; it lengthens as they relax.

663 Head and neck muscles

The facial muscles are those of the scalp, anterior neck, and face. Innervated by the seventh cranial (or facial) nerve (CN VII), these muscles help express a person's emotions, such as when he frowns, opens his eyes wide in surprise, or smiles. Unlike most muscles, facial muscles don't originate from or insert on bone; rather, they lie in subcutaneous tissue and insert on the skin.

Various groups of neck muscles work constantly during a person's waking hours to support and move the head. The long, bilateral *sternocleidomastoids* flex and turn the head. The *strap muscles* are associated with the hyoid bone and the thyroid cartilage, which they depress and stabilize. The *laryngeal muscles* move the vocal cords; the *prevertebral muscles* control the cervical spine. Other neck muscles are the *scalenes,* which insert on the upper ribs and act as accessory muscles of respiration; the *temporal* and *infratemporal fossae muscles;* the *muscles of the tongue* and *floor of the mouth;* and the *muscles of the middle ear, palate,* and *pharynx.*

The muscles involved in visceral functions—such as swallowing, chewing, and talking—and in some cardiac, gastric, and respiratory functions are largely supplied by cranial nerves (primarily V, VII, X, and XI). Cervical spinal nerves mainly innervate the muscles that act on the spinal column to move the head, neck, and chest.

664 Back muscles

The back contains two kinds of muscles—*superficial* and *deep.* The primary superficial muscles are the *trapezius,* used in shrugging the shoulders, and the *latissimus dorsi,* which permits extension of the arm. The eleventh cranial nerve (CN XI) innervates the trapezius; a branch of the brachial plexus (spinal nerves) supplies the latissimus dorsi. Deep muscles, more numerous and more complicated than superficial muscles, act on the spine, primarily during extension of the trunk. Usually segmental, deep muscles extend posteriorly from the sacrum and ilium to the vertebrae; they also work between different vertebrae or between vertebrae and ribs. They are the only muscles of the body innervated by dorsal primary rami of the spinal nerves. (All other muscles are supplied by ventral primary rami or cranial nerves.)

665 Muscles of the upper limb

The muscles of the upper limb are those of the scapula, arm, forearm, and hand. All scapular muscles originate from the scapula, insert on the humerus, and receive nerve impulses from ventral primary rami of the fifth and sixth cervical vertebrae (C5 and C6), through branches of the brachial plexus.

The six *scapular muscles* abduct the upper limb, or rotate the humerus medially or laterally around a vertical axis. Four of these muscles and tendons form the rotator cuff, which strengthens the shoulder joint. The upper arm between the shoulder and elbow contains three muscles anteriorly and one posteriorly. The anterior muscles primarily flex the forearm, although they can flex and adduct the entire arm. The long posterior muscle, the *triceps brachii,* is a powerful extensor of the forearm. It originates from the scapula and humerus and inserts on the olecranon process of the ulna.

The forearm, that portion of the upper limb between the elbow and wrist, contains 8 muscles anteriorly and 12 posteriorly. The anterior muscles primarily flex the wrist and fingers and pronate the hand. Most of these muscles are supplied by the median nerve. The posterior muscles extend the wrist and fingers and supinate the hand. One of these muscles aids in extending the forearm; another helps flex the elbow. They are innervated by the radial and posterior interosseous nerves.

The hand contains many small muscles between the metacarpals or anterior to them. The *thenar muscles* (innervated by the median and ulnar nerves) flex, abduct, and adduct the thumb and oppose the palmar surface of the thumb to the palmar surfaces of the fingers. The *hypothenar muscles* (innervated by the ulnar nerve) flex, abduct, and oppose the little finger. The *palmar* and *dorsal interossei,* located between the metacarpals, respectively adduct and abduct the fingers. The four small *lumbrical muscles* run from the long flexor tendons to the extensor expansion on the dorsum of the fingers. Innervated by the ulnar and median nerves, they control fine finger movements. When they contract, the lumbricals flex the metacarpophalangeal joints and straighten the interphalangeal joints, resulting in the *z* position in which the fingers are straight but flexed at the metacarpophalangeal joints—the position required for writing or painting.

666 Thoracic and abdominal muscles

The primary thoracic muscles are the pectoralis major and minor and the intercostals. The large *pectoralis major* covers the chest anteriorly and inserts on the humerus. It serves as a powerful adductor and flexor of the arm. The *pectoralis minor* lies beneath the pectoralis major and inserts on the scapula's coracoid process. Branches of the brachial plexus innervate both.

Three layers of *intercostal muscles* extend between the ribs, acting as muscles of respiration and protecting underlying organs. Intercostal nerves, the ventral rami of the thoracic spinal nerves, supply these muscles.

The major abdominal muscles are the *external* and *internal obliques, transversus,* and *rectus abdominis.* These muscles compress the abdominal contents and flex the spinal column. The *psoas major* and the *iliacus,* muscles of the pelvic girdle, act as flexors of the hip joint (see Entry 423).

667 Muscles of the lower limb

The muscles of the lower limb are those of the buttock, thigh, leg, and foot. Larger than the muscles of the upper limb, they are nevertheless similar in structure and function, with two notable exceptions—the elbow flexes anteriorly whereas the knee flexes posteriorly, and the great toe is positioned medially whereas the thumb is positioned laterally.

The buttock's muscles consist primarily of the gluteus maximus, the gluteus medius, and the gluteus minimus, plus several smaller muscles that rotate the femur. The *gluteus maximus,* a powerful climbing muscle, makes up most of the buttock's muscle mass. The *gluteus medius* and *gluteus minimus* abduct and rotate the thigh. When one leg is raised off the ground, as in normal walking, the opposite gluteus medius and gluteus minimus contract to stabilize the pelvis so that it doesn't sag on the side that is not bearing any weight.

The thigh muscles are divided into three groups. The *anterior thigh muscles,* primarily the *quadriceps femoris,* flex the thigh and extend the knee, as in kicking. They are innervated by the femoral nerve. The second group comprises the *medial thigh muscles,* which are adductors. These muscles are innervated primarily by the obturator nerve. The *posterior muscles* (hamstrings)—the third group, innervated by the sciatic nerve—extend the thigh and flex the knee.

The lower leg, that portion of the limb between the knee and the ankle, is controlled by anterior, posterior, and lateral muscles. The *anterior muscles* primarily dorsiflex the foot (raise its angle closer to the leg) and invert it (turn the sole inward). The *posterior muscles* plantar flex the foot (depress the sole). The *gastrocnemius* also flexes the knee, providing the propelling force in walking or running. The *lateral muscles* evert the foot (turn the sole outward). The muscles are innervated by the tibial and peroneal nerves (branches of the sciatic nerve).

The muscles of the foot are similar to those of the hand, except that the feet don't have *opponens muscles,* which explains why we can't touch the plantar surfaces of our toes together. However, the foot does have two muscles not found in the hand: the *flexor accessorius,* which straightens the pull of the long flexors, and the *extensor digitorum brevis* on the dorsum of the foot, which helps with the extension of the phalanges of the middle three toes. The foot muscles are innervated by the medial and lateral plantar branches of the tibial nerve.

668 Musculoskeletal system blood supply

Generally, the artery closest to a muscle supplies it with blood. Arteries enter bone through small *nutrient foramina* to nourish its interior. Deep veins drain these structures.

Many joints of the body have *collateral circulation,* which allows blood to bypass primary arterial channels when they become occluded. This is particularly true of movable joints, such as the elbow, wrist, knee, and foot. If the elbow, for example, is tightly flexed for a long time (as might occur during sleep or unconsciousness), blood can bypass the impeded main channel through one or more collateral channels. Otherwise, the forearm and hand might become ischemic.

Collecting appropriate history data

669 Biographical data

Your patient's age and sex may prove significant in assessment of a suspected musculoskeletal disorder. For example, osteoarthritis occurs in approximately 85% of people over age 70. Reiter's syndrome most commonly afflicts men between ages 20 and 40, whereas carpal tunnel syndrome and osteoporosis occur most often in postmenopausal women. Osteogenic sarcoma rarely occurs after age 40. Approximately 90% of patients with ankylosing spondylitis are men.

670 Chief complaint

The most common chief complaints associated with the musculoskeletal system are *pain, joint stiffness, redness and swelling, deformity and immobility,* and *sensory changes.*

671 History of present illness

Using the PQRST mnemonic device (see page 640), ask the patient to elaborate on his chief complaint. Then, depending on the complaint, explore the history of the present illness by asking the following types of questions:

• ***Pain.*** *Can you point to its exact location?* Deep, poorly localized pain usually indicates damage to blood vessels, fascia, joints, or periosteum. *Would you describe the pain as an ache? A constant throbbing?* Pain arising in bones is often described as throbbing. A patient will usually characterize muscle and joint pain as an ache.

Does the pain worsen with movement? With temperature changes? When you're carrying something heavy? Pain that increases with motion indicates a joint disorder. The pain of degenerative joint disease of the hip occurs with weight-bearing. Leg pain that worsens with standing, walking, or exercise and that persists for longer than 10 minutes after the patient stops the activity is probably caused by a degenerative hip or knee joint problem. Bending or lifting can elicit leg or back pain in a patient with a herniated lumbar disk. Pain associated with carpal tunnel syndrome worsens after extensive use of the hands. Cold and damp weather increases osteoarthritis pain.

Is the pain worse at any particular time of day? The pain caused by inflammation of the tendons and bursae may become intolerable at night. Joint discomfort from degenerative disease is often most intense at the end of the day. *Is the pain relieved by rest?* Pain from most forms of degenerative joint disease is relieved by rest. *Does aspirin relieve the pain?* Aspirin relieves joint pain caused by inflammation. *Have you recently fallen or been injured?* Trauma causes such injuries as fractures, torn ligaments, and back problems.

• ***Joint stiffness.*** *Which of your joints feel stiff? How many joints would you say are involved?* The patient's answers will help you identify the cause of his problem. *Does stiffness and pain in your joints stop for extended periods, maybe several weeks, and then recur?* Certain joint diseases, such as ankylosing spondylitis, are characterized by patterns of exacerbation and remission.

Is the stiffness severe when you wake up in the morning? How long after that does it last? In a patient with degenerative joint disease, inactivity during sleep causes stiffness that diminishes with joint use during the day. *Is the stiffness relieved or aggravated by temperature changes?* Heat relieves joint stiffness by alleviating muscle spasms. In a traumatic joint injury, however, heat applied immediately after the injury may aggravate stiffness by increasing bleeding into the joint. Generally, failure to use the joint and exposure to cold and dampness exacerbate joint stiffness.

Is the stiffness accompanied by locking of the joint? Can you feel or hear the bones rubbing together? Locking indicates poor bone alignment within the joint. Crepitus can occur in a fracture or from destruction of the joint's cushioning structures.

• ***Redness and swelling.*** *How long have you had the swelling? Did pain occur at the same time?* Edema and pain often occur simultaneously in traumatic injuries to muscles and bones. They are also present simultaneously in certain forms of bursitis, such as housemaid's knee. Swelling associated with degenerative joint disease can occur weeks or months after the pain, because of proliferative changes in cartilage and bone. *Does the swelling limit motion?* Swelling of soft tissue over a joint may act as a splint and immobilize it. Swelling within a joint also inhibits motion.

Does rest or elevation relieve the swelling? Elevation relieves swelling from a fresh injury because it facilitates blood return and prevents fluid from pooling in the extremity. *Has a cast or splint been removed from the affected part recently?* This may have

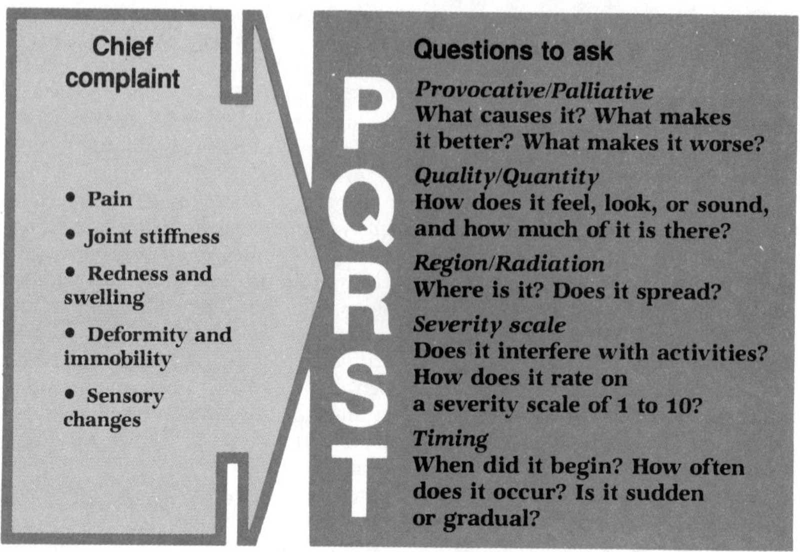

caused the swelling, because the loss of muscle tone that normally occurs in a casted extremity impairs venous blood return. *Did the affected area ever appear red or feel warm?* Redness and warmth are signs of acute inflammation, infection, or recent trauma. These signs don't usually occur in degenerative joint disease.

• ***Deformity and immobility.*** *Did you notice the deformity recently, or has it been gradually increasing in size?* A slow-growing mass may be a tumor. Gradual bony enlargement of a joint causes deformity.

Does the deformity limit your movement? Is it always present, or is it more evident at certain times, such as after you've been active or when your body's in a particular position? In a patient with degenerative joint disease, movement limitation depends on the joints involved and the progression of the disease. A patient with contracture of the hand, for example, can't extend his fingers. *Does the deformity or limitations of movement interfere with your daily activities? In what specific ways have you had to alter your routine because of these restrictions?* Knowledge of how the patient carries out his daily activities helps you determine how the deformity affects his ability to function.

Do you need, or prefer to use, any support equipment, such as crutches or elastic bandages? This information will give you a general idea of the severity of the patient's limitation of movement.

• ***Sensory changes.*** *Have you noticed any loss of feeling? Is it associated with pain?* Swelling can put pressure on a nerve, causing a loss of sensation in the area distal to the affected site. Compression of nerves or of blood vessels by a tumor or fracture also can cause a loss of feeling. Sensory changes sometimes accompany arm or hand pain.

672 Past history

Focus on the following relevant health problems when reviewing your patient's past history:

• ***Endocrine disorders.*** *Diabetes mellitus* can predispose the patient to development of degenerative joint disease.

• ***Blood dyscrasias.*** *Hemophilia* and *sickle cell anemia* can cause bleeding into a patient's joints and muscles, leading to pain, swelling, tenderness,

DRUGS

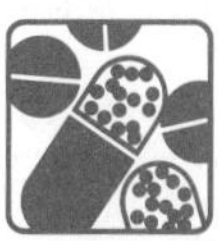

NURSE'S GUIDE TO SOME DRUGS THAT AFFECT THE MUSCULOSKELETAL SYSTEM

CLASSIFICATION	POSSIBLE SIDE EFFECTS
Anticoagulants	
heparin sodium (Hepalean**, Lipo-Hepin)	• Arthralgia
Anticonvulsants	
mephenytoin (Mesantoin*)	• Choreiform movements, ataxia, dysarthria, polyarthropathy
paraldehyde (Paral)	• Muscle irritation
phensuximide (Milontin*)	• Muscle weakness, ataxia
phenytoin sodium [extended] (Dilantin*)	• Osteomalacia, ataxia, twitching
Antifungals	
amphotericin B (Fungizone*)	• Arthralgia, myalgia, muscle weakness secondary to hypokalemia
Antilipemics	
clofibrate (Atromid-S*)	• Myalgia, arthralgia, polyphagia
Antimalarials	
chloroquine hydrochloride (Aralen HCl)	• Neuromyopathy
Corticosteroids	
betamethasone (Celestone*) prednisone (Colisone**)	• Muscle weakness, myopathy, osteoporosis, pathologic fractures, aseptic necrosis of femoral and humeral heads
cortisone acetate (Cortone Acetate*) hydrocortisone (Cortef*)	• Myopathy, muscle weakness, osteoporosis, compression, and pathologic fractures
Diuretics	
chlorothiazide (Diuril*)	• Gout, muscle spasm
Oral contraceptives	
estrogen with progestogen (Demulen*)	• Myopathy, myalgia, leg cramp
Penicillins	
carbenicillin disodium (Geopen)	• Neuromuscular irritability
penicillin G procaine (Wycillin*)	• Arthralgia

*Available in U.S. and Canada. **Available in Canada only. All other products (no symbol) available in U.S. only.

and possibly permanent deformity.

• ***Skin or autoimmune disease.*** *Psoriasis* may precede the onset of psoriatic arthritis. *Systemic lupus erythematosus* may cause joint deformities.

• ***Previous injuries.*** Repeated trauma resulting in damage to cartilage can cause degenerative changes in a young person identical to those caused by degenerative joint disease in an older person.

• ***Drugs.*** Many drugs can affect the musculoskeletal system (see *Nurse's Guide to Some Drugs That Affect the Musculoskeletal System*). For example, an anticoagulant overdose can cause hemarthrosis, and the use of corticosteroids can precipitate avascular necrosis of the head of the femur, predisposing the patient to septic arthritis. And discontinuing corticosteroid therapy too rapidly can cause arthralgia.

673 Family history

A number of musculoskeletal disorders, including ankylosing spondylitis, gout, and the development of Heberden's nodes in distal interphalangeal osteoarthritis, may be inherited. All forms of muscular dystrophy are inherited. Of patients with psoriatic arthritis, about 30% have a family history of psoriasis.

674 Psychosocial history

Find out if your patient's *occupation* requires any heavy lifting or strenuous activity, because this can lead to muscle strain, rotator cuff tears, and degenerative vertebral disk disorders. Occupations that involve long-distance driving or long hours of standing may also cause lower back pain.

675 Activities of daily living

Without realizing it, your patient may be damaging parts of his musculoskeletal system. For instance, poor alignment of the vertebrae caused by *poor posture* strains the spinal column. And *walking* in high-heeled shoes can cause contracture of the Achilles tendon. *Habitually carrying heavy objects,* such as a well-filled shoulder bag or attaché case, or photographic gear, can place uneven pressure on a person's spinal column.

Other important considerations to keep in mind when reviewing your patient's activities of daily living are *diet* and *exercise.* Poor calcium intake can lead to bone decalcification, and subsequent fractures and lack of exercise can cause both bone decalcification and muscle atrophy. Certainly a sedentary life-style results in poor muscle tone and an increased susceptibility to muscle strain. But sporadic exercise can be harmful, too, overworking poorly toned muscles and causing sustained muscle contraction or spasm.

Contact sports, such as football and hockey, can lead to skeletal, joint, or soft tissue trauma; improper landing on the heels while jogging can damage the Achilles tendon. *Racquet sports,* such as tennis (or any other activity that requires a forceful grasp, wrist extension against resistance, or frequent rotation of the forearm), can cause joint pain.

676 Review of systems

Focus on the following signs and symptoms when reviewing your patient's body systems:

• ***Skin.*** Skin changes can be significant in helping identify musculoskeletal disease. For example, dry skin often occurs over the thumb and first two fingers of a patient with carpal tunnel syndrome. Skin lesions occur with Reiter's syndrome.

• ***Eyes.*** Conjunctivitis can be a symptom of Reiter's syndrome. Nongranulomatous uveitus may accompany ankylosing spondylitis.

• ***Gastrointestinal.*** Weight loss may occur in association with a neoplasm, and weight gain can aggravate degenerative joint disease. Chronic diarrhea may accompany arthritis associated with colitis and other gastrointestinal disorders.

• ***Genitourinary.*** Pain or burning with urination and urethral discharge are symptoms of Reiter's syndrome and gonococcal arthritis. A patient with a herniated lumbar disk sometimes has difficulty urinating.

• ***Cardiovascular.*** Tachycardia and hypertension may accompany gout. Carditis and aortic regurgitation may accompany Reiter's syndrome.

Conducting the physical examination

677 Preparations

During a musculoskeletal examination, at various times the patient will sit, stand, lie down, walk, and bend over. So the examination room should be large enough for him to move around. If possible, examine the patient under natural light (or lighting that simulates natural light). This lets you observe skin color changes and swelling without the distortion that artificial light causes.

Make sure the room temperature and the examination table are comfortably warm, because temperature extremes can change the patient's skin color (and make him uncomfortable). Air-conditioning and tobacco smoke also can affect skin color. Finally, help your patient to relax for the examination.

The equipment you'll need for examining the patient's musculoskeletal system includes a metal or cloth tape measure, for measuring limb circumference and chest expansion, and a goniometer—a flexible protractor—for measuring range of motion in degrees (see *Using a Goniometer*). The patient should remove all clothing except underpants and wear a hospital gown.

678 Examination sequence and techniques

Begin your examination with general observation of the patient. Then proceed with a head-to-toe musculoskeletal assessment, systematically examining specific body parts. Check for gross abnormalities during the early stages of your assessment. For example, observe your patient's posture, build, and muscular development and bulk as he walks into the room. During the examination, observe the position of the different parts of his body at rest and when he moves.

Organize the examination so that it progresses smoothly, with minimal position changes for the patient. A good way to do this is to begin with the patient sitting on the edge of the examination table, so you can examine his head, neck, shoulders, and upper extremities. Then examine his chest, back, ilium, and gait with him standing and, later, walking. Finally, have the patient lie supine on the table while you examine his hips, knees, ankles, and feet.

Inspection and palpation are the principal techniques you'll use to examine a patient's musculoskeletal system. Inspect and palpate each body part; then test its range of motion and muscle strength. Examine each muscle and joint bilaterally, comparing both sides of the patient's body for equality of size, shape, color, and strength. (Remember that both sides of his body must be in the same position—for example, both arms extended—for you to compare them.)

You may auscultate to assess a vascular abnormality or bone crepitation; percussion may help you to assess fluid in a joint or to elicit tenderness.

USING A GONIOMETER

To measure your patient's range of motion, use a goniometer, or flexible protractor, such as the one shown here. Place the center, or zero point, on the joint to be measured, in this case, the lateral epicondyle of the humerus. Place the axis (the immovable part of the goniometer) perpendicular to the plane of motion. Use the movable arm to mark the degrees.

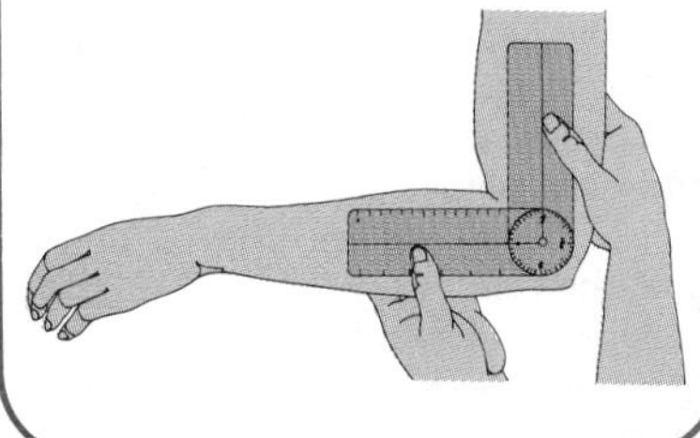

RECORDING MUSCLE STRENGTH

To record your patient's muscle strength, use this rating scale:

5/5: Patient moves joint through full range of motion (ROM) against normal resistance and gravity

4/5: Patient completes full ROM against moderate resistance and gravity

3/5: Patient completes full ROM against gravity only

2/5: Patient completes full ROM with gravity eliminated

1/5: Patient's attempt at muscle contraction is palpable, but limb doesn't move

0/5: Patient makes no visible or palpable muscle contraction; muscle is paralyzed

679 Range of motion and muscle strength

After you've inspected and palpated each body part with the patient at rest, test its active and passive range of motion. During passive range-of-motion testing, assess the patient's muscle tone by feeling the muscles' movements under your hand. This adds to the information you obtained during your earlier palpation, when you felt the muscles at rest.

Next, test the strength of various muscle group functions, such as shoulder elevation and elbow flexion and extension. (Before you begin muscle strength tests, find out whether the patient is right- or left-handed, because the dominant arm is usually stronger.) To test the strength of each muscle group, ask the patient to perform active range of motion again as you apply resistance to his movements. Note the strength that the patient exerts against your resistance. If the muscle group is weak, you should lessen your resistance or provide no resistance to permit more accurate assessment. If necessary, position the patient's extremity so that he doesn't have to resist gravity, and repeat the test.

Record your findings according to a five-point scale—developed to minimize subjective interpretations of test findings (see *Recording Muscle Strength*). Remember to test your patient's symmetrical muscles consecutively so that you can compare their strength.

680 Examining the head and neck

First, inspect the patient's face for evidence of trauma and swelling and for symmetry. The mandible should be in the midline, not shifted to the right or left. Next, palpate the temporomandibular joint. Tenderness may indicate poor occlusion or trauma. If you note any tenderness over the temporomandibular joint, palpate the maxillary buccal mucosa posterior to the molars. This will cause pain if there is spasm of the pterygoid muscles caused by improper temporomandibular joint alignment.

To test range of motion, ask the patient to open his mouth so you can insert three fingers sideways. This distance should be 1″ to 2″ (2.5 to 5 cm). Observe this movement for smoothness, and check that the mandible maintains its midline position when it's opened. To test mandible muscle strength, place your hand under the patient's chin and ask him to open his mouth while you apply resistance.

Inspect the front, back, and sides of his neck, noting any abnormalities. Also look for symmetry of the neck muscles, and note any masses. Palpate the spinous processes of the cervical vertebrae and the supraclavicular fossae for any tenderness, swelling, or nodules.

Test the neck's range of motion by asking the patient to place his chin on his chest. Then hold the chin in the midline and raise the patient's head so that he's looking at the ceiling. Also ask the patient to touch his chin to each shoulder. Finally, ask him to try touching each ear to the ipsilateral shoulder. Test the patient's neck muscle strength by applying resistance with your hand as he tries to perform each motion a second time.

RANGE OF MOTION OF THE NECK AND SHOULDER

This chart features some of the most common range-of-motion tests you'll perform passively and actively with your patient. Note that the ranges indicated are normals.

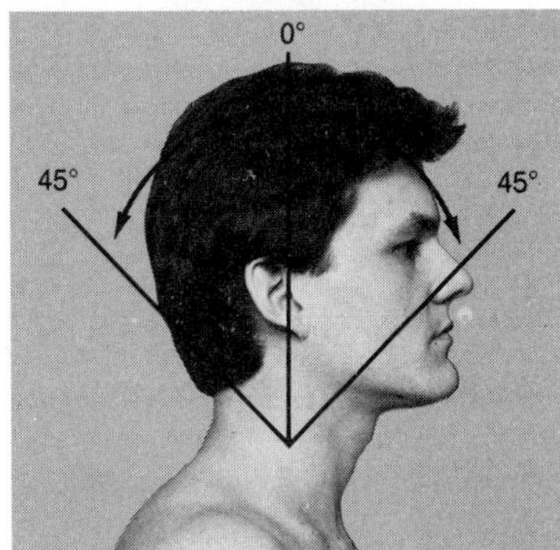

Neck: Flexion and extension

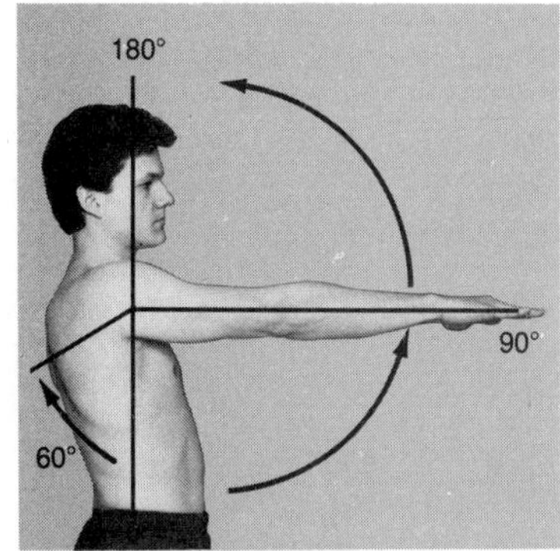

Shoulder: Forward flexion and backward extension

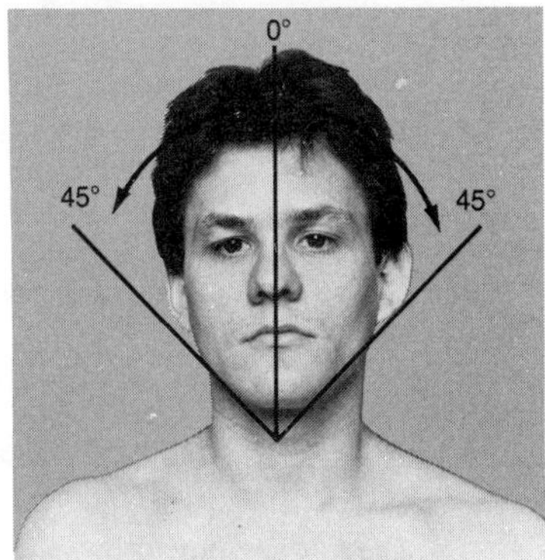

Lateral bending

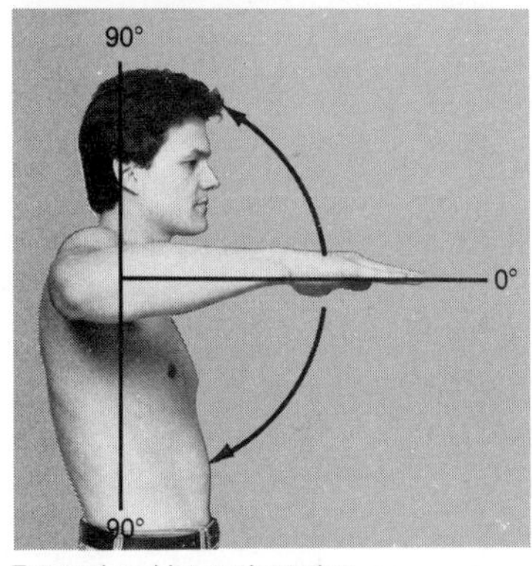

External and internal rotation

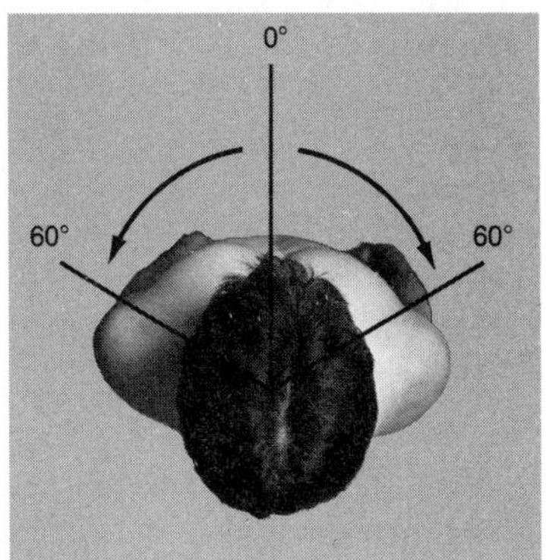

Rotation

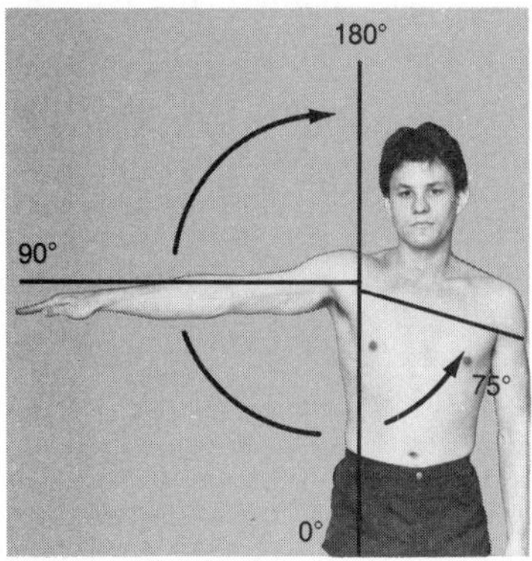

Abduction and adduction

RANGE OF MOTION OF THE ELBOW AND WRIST

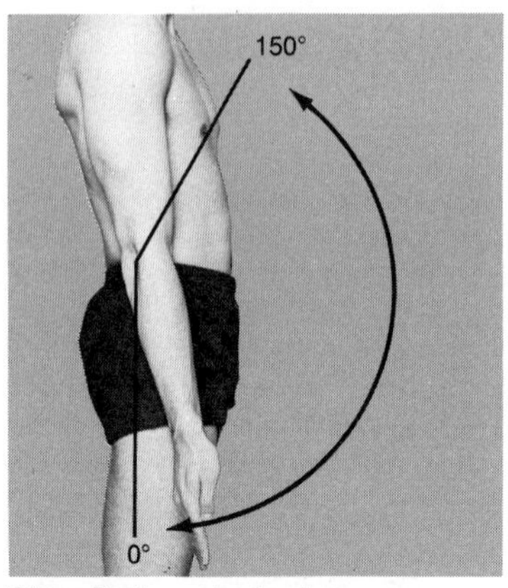

Elbow: Flexion and extension

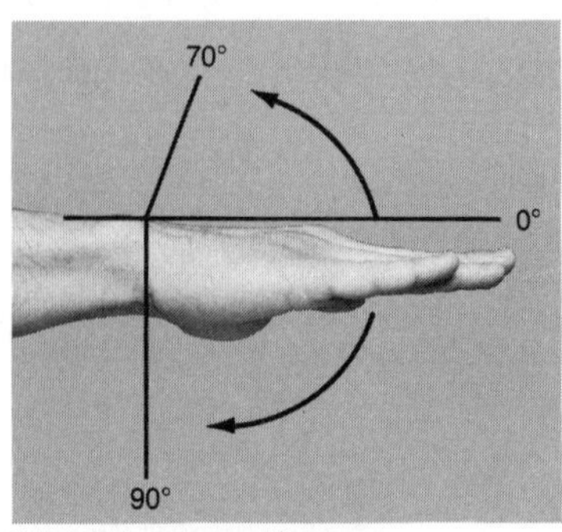

Wrist: Extension and flexion

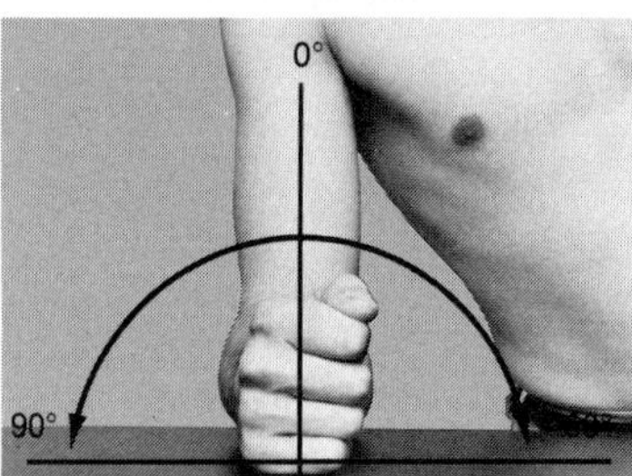

Supination and pronation

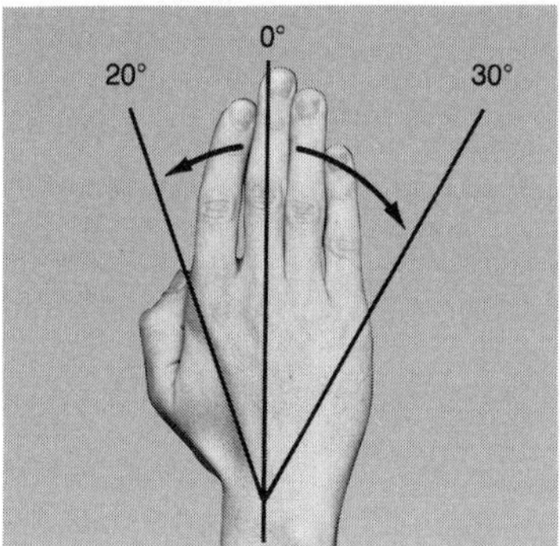

Radial and ulnar deviation

681 Assessing the shoulders

Inspect and compare the patient's shoulders, noting bony or muscular asymmetry, muscle atrophy, and any deformities. Compare his clavicles for symmetrical alignment. Inspect the deltoid muscle for atrophy, for prominence of the greater tuberosity of the humerus, and for the presence of hollows in the muscle (indicating displacement of the humerus).

Have the patient extend his arms and throw his shoulders back. Inspect the scapulae, checking for equal height and distance from the spinal column. Palpate the shoulders with the palmar surfaces of your fingers to locate bony landmarks; note any crepitus or tenderness. Using your entire hand, palpate the shoulder muscles for firmness and symmetry of size.

Range-of-motion testing of the patient's shoulders should include active and passive movement through forward flexion, backward extension, horizontal flexion and extension, abduction, and adduction. Test the rotator cuff muscles by passively abducting the extended arm to 90° and having the patient lower his arm slowly. If the patient has a rotator cuff tear, the arm will fall abruptly. A subluxated acromioclavicular joint may result from a sports injury, or it may occur in a patient with a paralyzed arm and shoulder that are poorly supported. If you note any tenderness during range-of-motion testing of this joint, test it by having the patient place his right hand on his left shoulder and lean forward. Then apply pressure to the distal end of the right clavicle. If the joint is subluxated, this maneuver will cause pain and abnormal movement of the clavicle. Repeat the procedure with the patient's other shoulder.

Test the trapezius muscle for strength by asking the patient to shrug his shoulders while you try to hold them down.

682 How to examine the elbows

For inspection, flex each of the patient's elbows to 90°. Compare the two elbows, noting any difference between the elbow joint angles when the patient holds his arms in passive extension. Check for redness, swelling, or a change in the contour of the joint or muscles.

RANGE OF MOTION OF THE THUMB

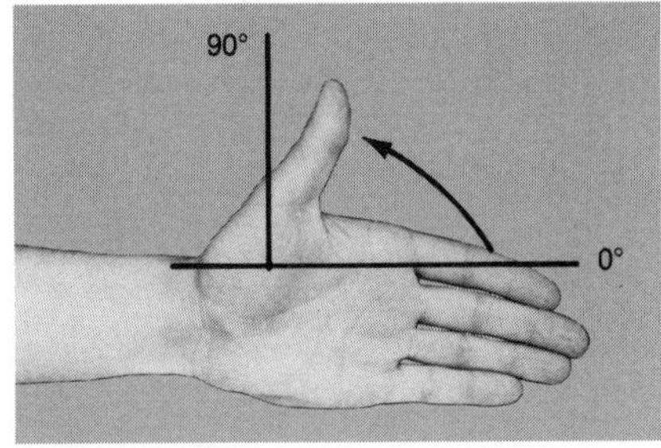

Thumb: Extension

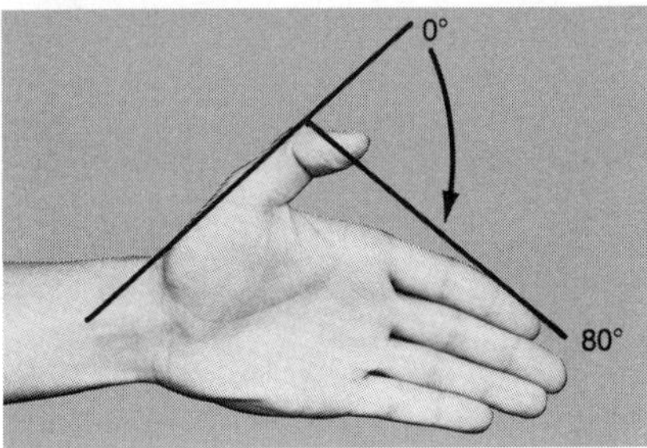

Interphalangeal thumb joint: Flexion

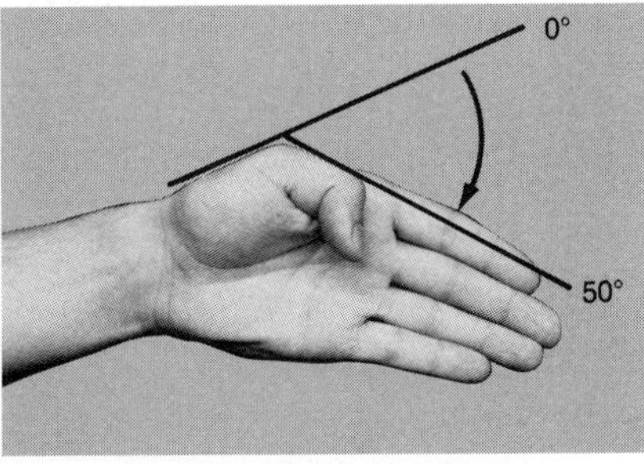

Metacarpophalangeal thumb joint: Flexion

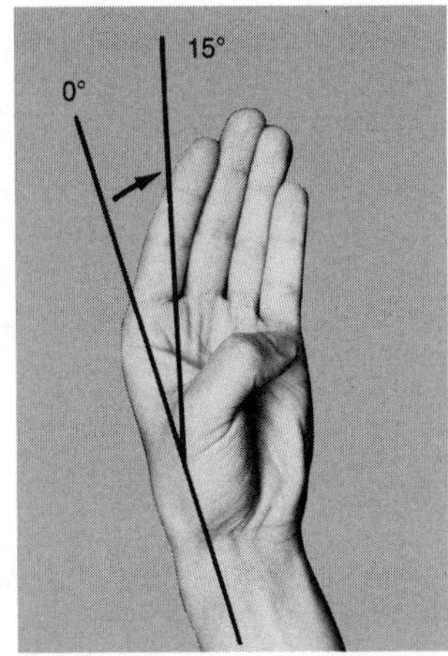

Carpometacarpal thumb joint: Flexion

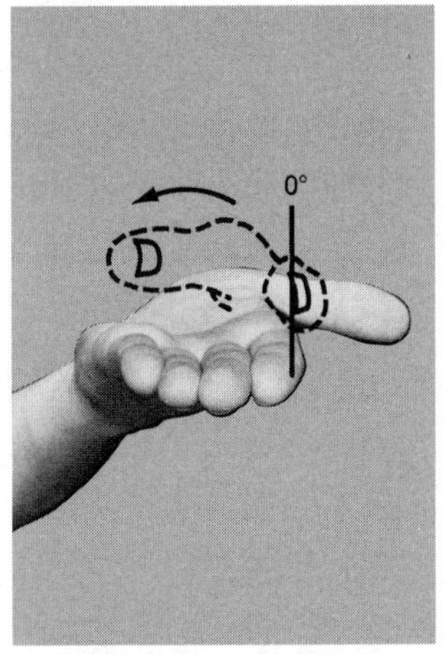

Thumb: Abduction and rotation

RANGE OF MOTION OF THE FINGERS

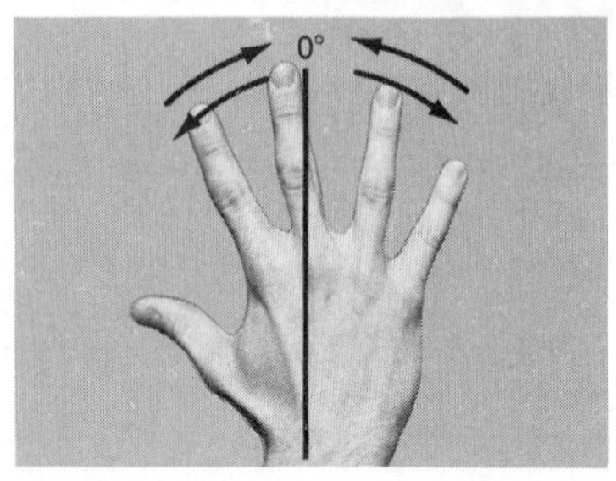

Fingers: Abduction and adduction

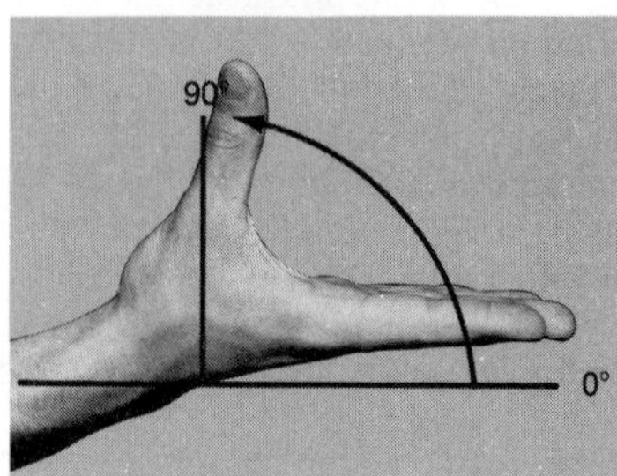

Fingers: Circumduction

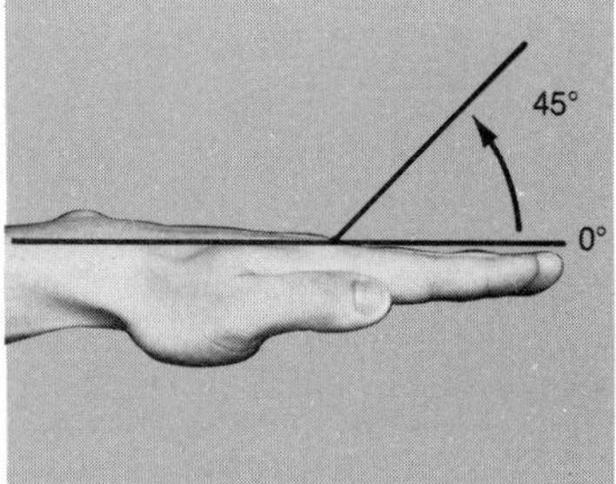

Metacarpophalangeal joint: Extension

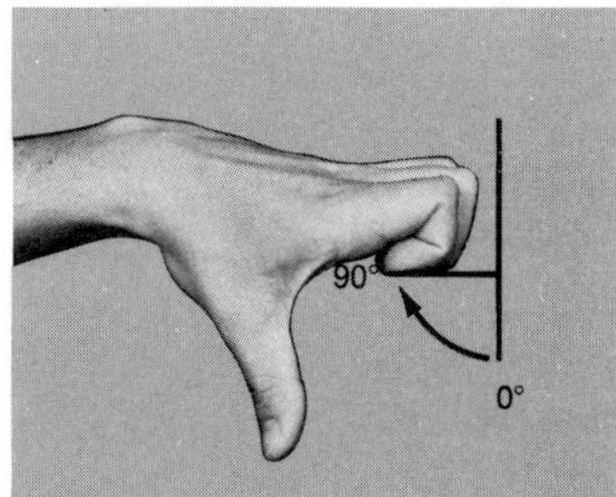

Distal interphalangeal joint: Flexion

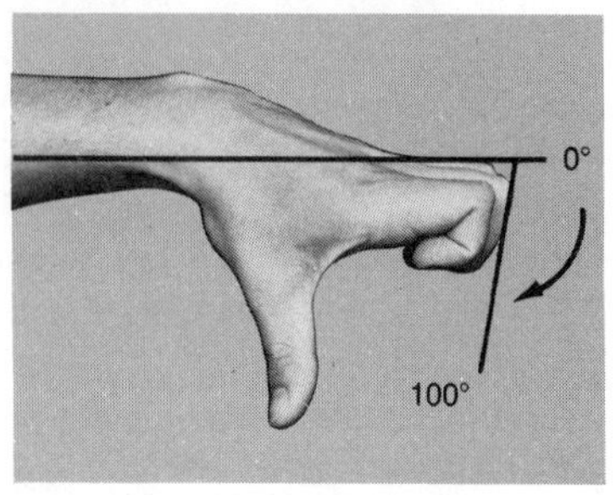

Proximal interphalangeal joint: Flexion

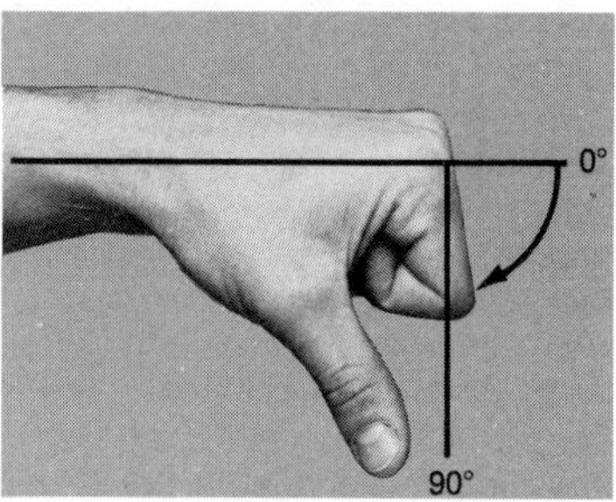

Metacarpophalangeal joint: Flexion

Palpate each elbow with the tips of your fingers, checking for subcutaneous nodules, bogginess, and enlargement of the supracondylar lymph nodes, which normally aren't palpable (see Entry 725). (They are located just above the epicondyles; if you can palpate them, the patient may have an infection below the elbow.)

For range-of-motion testing, the patient should be able to demonstrate flexion, extension, supination, and pronation. Some people can hyperextend their elbows from 5° to 15°; this is usually a normal finding.

683 Evaluating the wrists

Inspect each of the patient's wrists for contour, and compare the two for symmetry. Also observe for thickening of the flexor tendon sheath of the median nerve, a sign of carpal tunnel syndrome. This may be seen on inspection of the palmar surface of the wrist. Then, using a circular motion, palpate the radial and ulnar styloid processes with the palmar surfaces of your fingers. Use two hands, with your thumbs on one side of the wrist and your fingers on the other. The styloid processes should be firm and nontender. Palpate the hollow on the radial side of each wrist, between the patient's thumb and index finger, by asking him to extend his thumb away from the fingers. He shouldn't feel any discomfort. For range-of-motion testing, remember that ulnar deviation is greatest with the wrist in supination.

Further testing for carpal tunnel syndrome is accomplished by holding the patient's wrist in flexion for 60 seconds. If he experiences Phalen's sign (numbness and paresthesia over the palmar surface of the hand, the first three fingers, and half of the fourth), the test is positive for carpal tunnel syndrome. A second test for carpal tunnel syndrome is positive if you can elicit Tinel's sign (a tingling sensation on the palmar aspect of the wrist). This may be done by tapping over the median nerve on the palmar surface of the patient's wrist.

684 How to assess the hands and fingers

Inspect your patient's hands, checking that they're about the same size. Inspect the thenar and hypothenar eminences for atrophy, which decreases the palmar depression. Thenar atrophy results from compression of the median nerve, as in a patient with carpal tunnel syndrome. Ulnar nerve disorders cause hypothenar atrophy.

Next, observe the contour of the metacarpophalangeal joints, and check the patient's hands and fingers for nodules, redness, swelling, deformities, and webbing between the fingers. Palpate the bony landmarks and the joints for tenderness, nodules, or bogginess. Soft hollows between the tendons indicate muscular atrophy. Now palpate the metacarpophalangeal joints. Normally, you'll feel depressions between them, but in some disorders (such as inflammatory or degenerative joint diseases) these depressions may disappear.

In range-of-motion testing, note any difficulty the patient has in flexing his thumb; de Quervain's disease can cause this finding. Perform Finkelstein's test by asking the patient to clench his fingers over his thumb. Then forcefully push the base of his thumb toward the ulna. If this maneuver causes pain on the radial side of his thumb, or toward the elbow on the radial side, the test is positive for chronic stenosing tenosynovitis. To assess muscle strength, apply resistance to the fingers as the patient tries to flex them, extend them, spread them, and bring them together. You can also assess general muscle strength by shaking hands with the patient.

685 Examining the back and chest

Ask the patient to stand with his back and buttocks exposed. Inspect the spinal column's curvature from both posterior and lateral views. In severe scoliosis, the chest becomes flattened on the side of the lateral deviation, and the opposite side, viewed posteriorly, becomes pronounced. Also, the scapulae become prominent, and the shoulders may not be level. Lordosis, an exaggerated lumbar curvature, occurs when the patient's abdomen protrudes or when the stomach muscles are weak, as in obesity or advanced pregnancy. Arthritis or muscle spasm may cause a loss of normal spinal curvature.

Ask the patient to bend over as far as he can. Muscular structures on both sides of the spine should be symmetrical in size, contour, and position. Postural kyphosis (accentuation of the convex thoracic curve) disappears when the patient bends over to touch his toes. The hump (razor back) deformity of scoliosis, caused by posterior protrusion of the ribs on the convex side of the spine, is also more apparent when the patient bends over.

Palpate the spinous processes and paravertebral muscles, noting any tenderness or swelling. Also palpate the paravertebral muscles, with the flat of your hand, to detect muscle hardening from spasm. To assess muscle strength, note any difficulty the patient has in performing range of motion for normal movements of the spinal column—including flexion, extension, hyperextension, lateral bending, and rotation. Measure his chest expansion using the technique described in Entry 351.

RANGE OF MOTION OF THE BACK

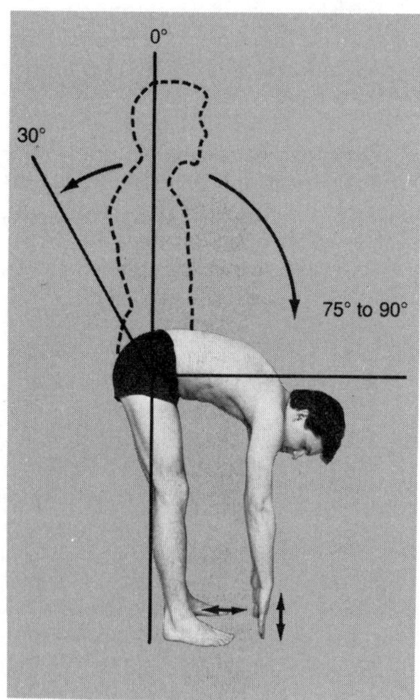

Extension and flexion

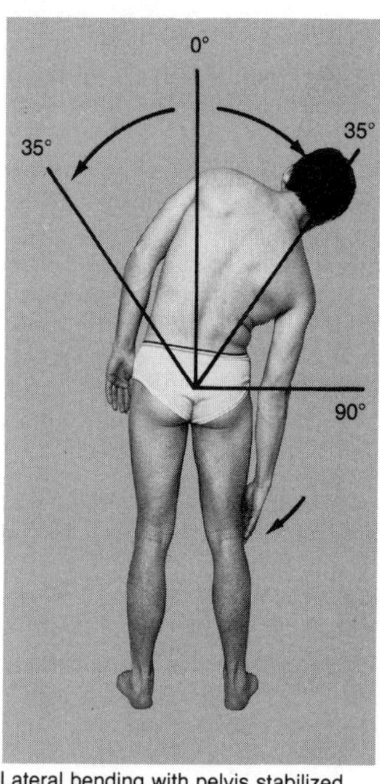

Lateral bending with pelvis stabilized

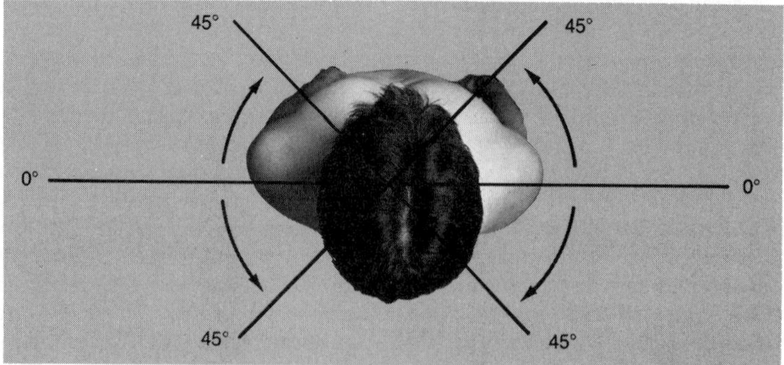

Rotation with pelvis stabilized

ASSESSING THE ILIAC CRESTS

Place your fingers on the iliac crests and extend your thumbs, as shown. You should be able to draw an imaginary straight line from crest to crest. Consider a tilting line abnormal. It may indicate spinal curvature, unequal leg length, or muscle weakness.

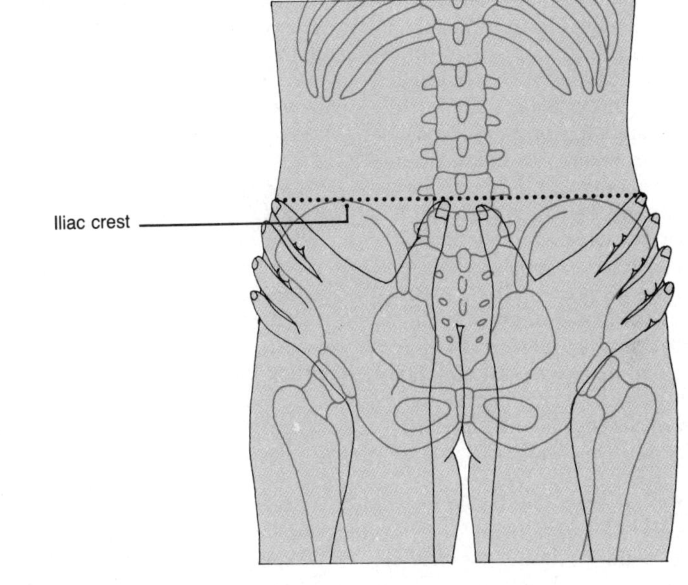

686 Assessing the iliac crests

With the patient positioned so that your eyes are level with his pelvis, inspect the contour of his legs. Then observe his pelvis from the back. Place your fingers on the iliac crests and extend your thumbs in a straight line across the patient's back. Then draw an imaginary line from crest to crest. (The line should be straight.) Tilting may be from abnormal curvature of the spine, a muscle disorder, or unequal leg length. Observe the buttocks' muscles for symmetry. Asymmetry may be caused by congenital hip dislocation, scoliosis, muscle atrophy, or unequal leg length.

687 Assessing gait and posture

Observe the patient as he sits, stands, and walks naturally. Gait varies from person to person, but normally you'll notice a certain rhythm to a person's walk. Ask the patient to walk about 20 steps and turn around. As he walks, observe his posture, his footing, his balance, the swing of his arms, his stride length, the rhythm to his walk, and any associated movements. A distance of 2″ to 4″ (5 to 10 cm) should separate his heels when he walks, and his stride length should be about 15″, depending on his height. His arms should swing freely at his sides, he should be well balanced, and his posture should be erect. When he turns, his face and head should turn before the rest of his body.

Gait abnormalities suggest such problems as hip dislocation or ankylosis. The Trendelenburg gait—in which the patient's trunk lists to one side, producing a distinctive waddle with each step—is a sign of unilateral hip dislocation.

After observing his gait, ask the patient to walk in a straight line, heel to toe. If the patient can't do this, perform the Romberg test. (Stand close to him to protect him if he loses his balance.) Have the patient stand unsupported with his arms at his sides, his feet together, and his eyes open. If he can do this, have him maintain this position but close his eyes. Normally, he should sway only slightly. If he's ataxic as a result of a cerebellar problem, he won't be able to maintain his balance with his eyes open or closed. If he maintains his balance with his eyes open but not when they're closed, he may have difficulty with his position sense—a positive Romberg's sign. If the patient is able to walk in a straight line and is reasonably healthy, ask him to hop in place on each foot. Successful completion of this task indicates normal motor function of the legs as well as normal cerebellar function and position sense.

688 Testing the hips

Have the patient climb onto the examination table and lie supine. Note any trouble he has in doing this. Then, with his legs aligned symmetrically, measure the length of each from the anterior superior iliac spine to the medial malleolus. The legs should be equal in length.

To check for a flexion deformity of the hips, perform the *Thomas test.* Flex one of the patient's hips by bending his knee toward his chest. Any hip flexion on the opposite side indicates a flexion deformity of that hip. If the patient experiences any pain, he may have a pelvic fracture (see *Range of Motion of the Hip and Knee*).

With the patient still on his back, perform the *straight-leg–raising test* to check for a herniated disk. Raise one leg from behind the heel until the patient complains of pain. Then dorsiflex the foot. Repeat the procedure with the other leg and compare the results. You should be able to raise both legs to 90° of hip flexion without causing pain (see *Range of Motion of the Hip and Knee*).

Pain behind the knees can indicate tight hamstrings; back pain can indicate pressure on the lumbosacral nerve roots from a herniated disk. Also while the patient is supine, test hip rotation by rocking each of his legs from side to side. Watch the patella and foot each time, to estimate range of motion. If this maneuver causes pain, carefully and gently carry out other range-of-motion and muscle-strength tests.

689 Inspecting and palpating the thighs

With the patient supine on the examination table, inspect his thighs for contour and symmetry. Measure their circumferences with a tape measure at the same level on each leg. The dominant leg may normally measure up to ⅜″ (1 cm) larger. Palpate the thigh muscles with the palmar surfaces of your fingers, starting at the uppermost aspect of each thigh and moving lengthwise in a circular motion to cover the anterior, posterior, medial, and lateral aspects. The thigh muscles should be firm and continuous from the point of origin to insertion.

690 Knee assessment

With the patient supine on the examination table, inspect his knee alignment and contour. Note any deformities, such as knock-knees (genu valgum) or bowlegs (genu varum)—both most apparent with the patient standing. Observe the quadriceps muscle for atrophy, and look for absence of the normal hollows around the patella. Then palpate each knee by placing your thumb and forefinger over the suprapatellar pouch on both sides of the quadriceps. Note any thickening, bogginess, or tenderness of the synovial membrane. Also note any bony enlargement around the knee joint. With the other hand, palpate each side of the patella and the area over the tibiofemoral joint space, again noting any thickening, tenderness, fluid, or bogginess. Then palpate

RANGE OF MOTION OF THE HIP AND KNEE

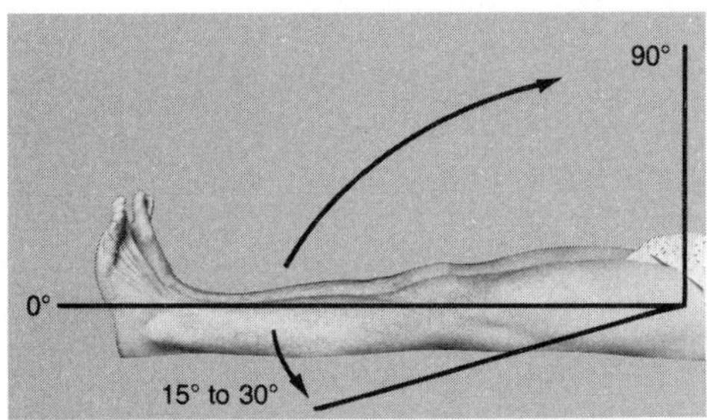

Hip: Flexion and extension with knee straight

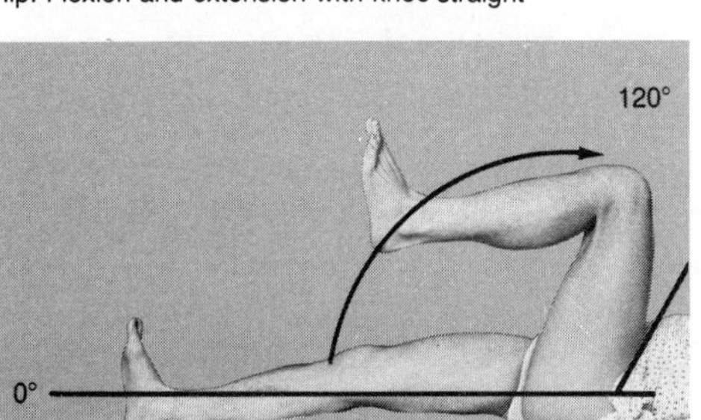

Hip: Flexion with knee flexed

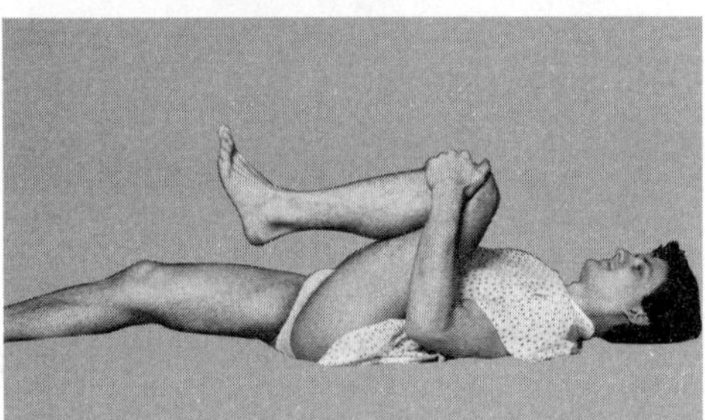
Thomas test for flexion contractures (Bend patient's knee toward chest to flex one hip.)

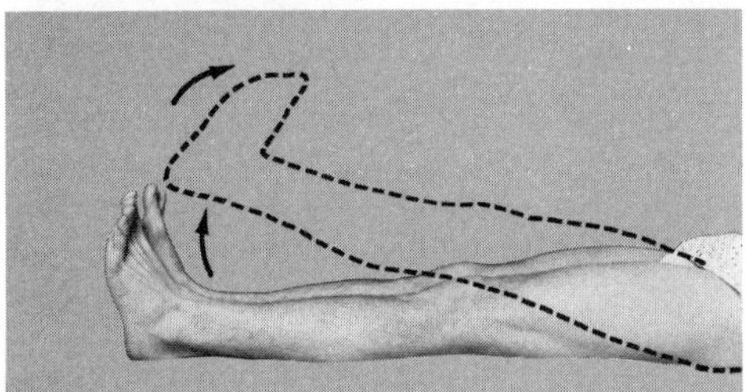
Straight-leg–raising test for herniated disk (Raise leg from behind the heel until he complains of pain, then dorsiflex the foot.)

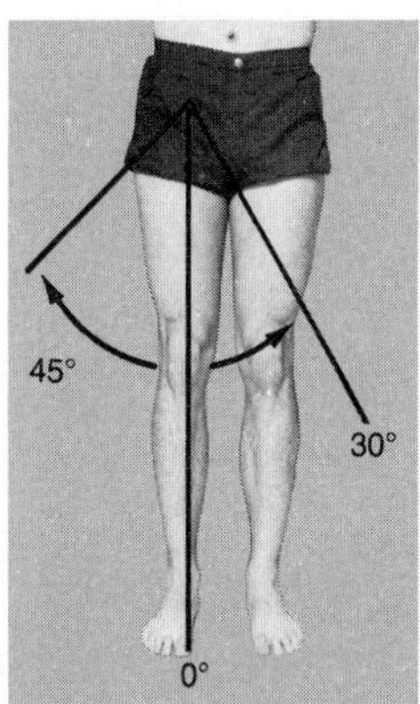

Hip: Abduction and adduction

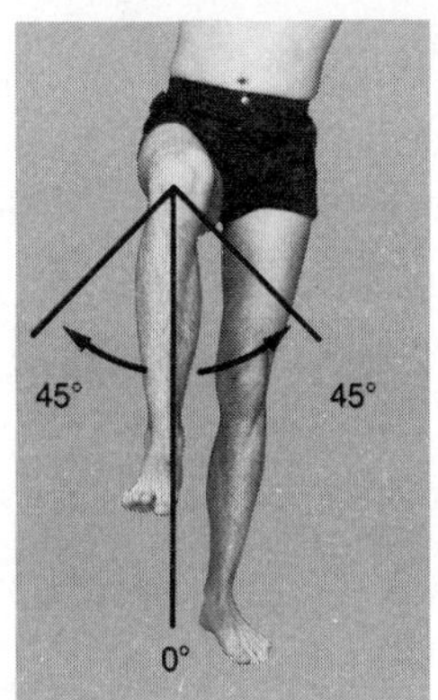

Hip: Internal and external rotation

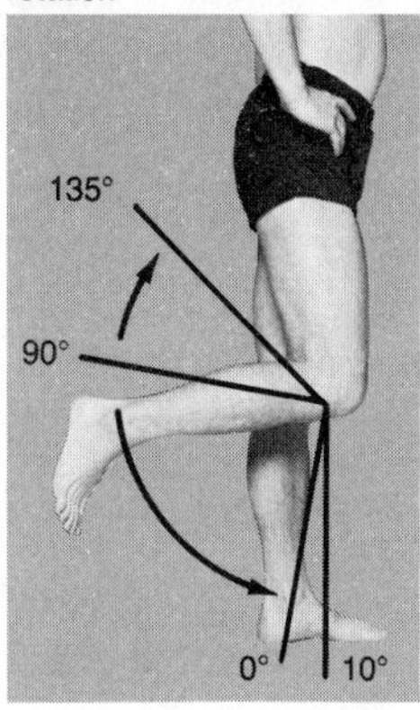

Knee: Flexion and extension

the popliteal space to check for swelling or cysts. Test each knee for full range of motion.

To test the muscle strength of the patient's hamstrings, have the patient alternately cross and uncross his legs. Then, you can test the quadriceps by trying to bend the patient's leg at the knee while he tries to hold it stiff. If you suspect any abnormality, assess the knee further (for more information, see *Testing Stability and Obstruction in the Knee*).

691 Examining the ankles and feet

Inspect the patient's ankles and feet for swelling, redness, nodules, and other deformities. Check the arch of each foot, and look for any toe deformities. Note any skin changes. Check the position of the ankles, noting whether the medial malleolus angles in or out abnormally. Also note any edema, calluses, bunions, corns, ingrown toenails, plantar warts, trophic ulcers, hair loss, or unusual pigmentation.

RANGE OF MOTION OF THE ANKLES, FEET, AND TOES

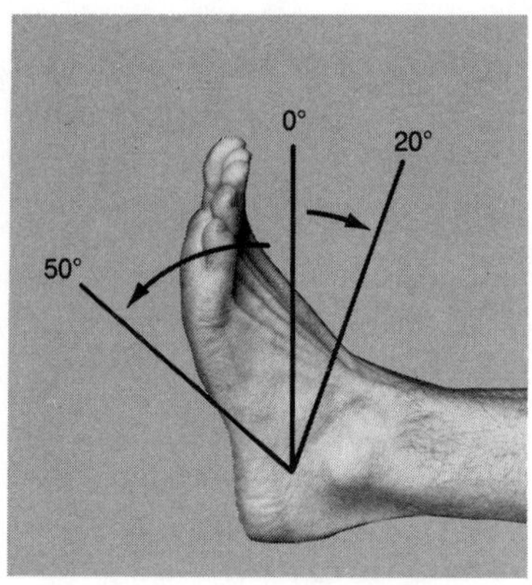

Ankle: Dorsiflexion and plantar flexion

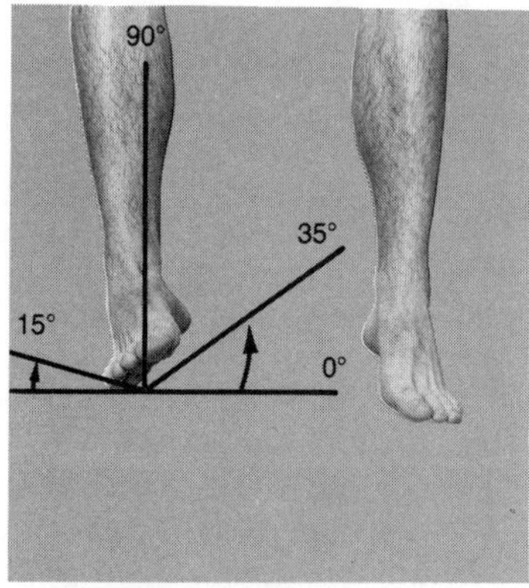

Foot: Inversion and eversion

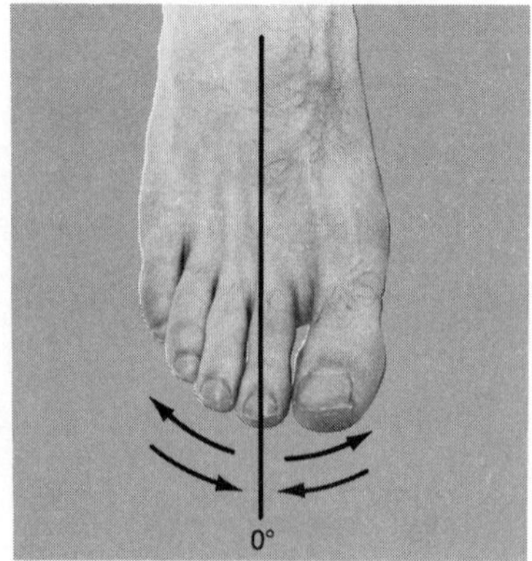

Toes: Abduction and adduction

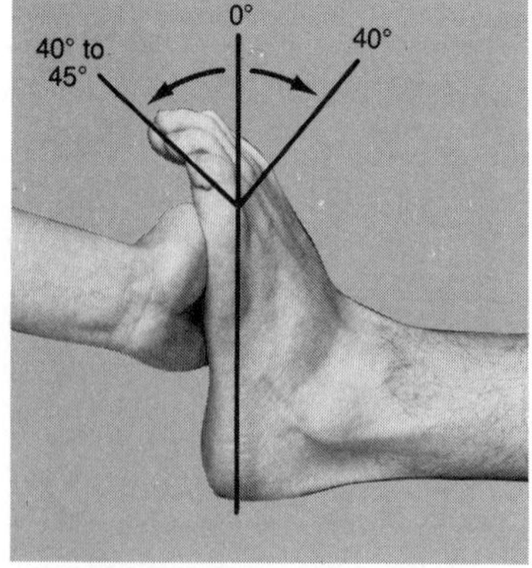

First metatarsophalangeal joint: Flexion and extension

TESTING STABILITY AND OBSTRUCTION IN THE KNEE

TEST	TECHNIQUE	RESULTS
Ballottement	Grasp thigh just above knee to force fluid into space between patella and femur. Push patella sharply against femur.	If patella bounces back quickly, this indicates fluid presence.
Bulge sign	With palm of hand, milk knee upward two to three times to displace fluid. Then, tap knee just behind lateral margin. Watch for bulge of returning fluid to form.	If bulge appears on side opposite to pressure, this indicates fluid presence.
Collateral ligament integrity	Stabilize knee with one hand on medial side of femur. Push laterally and then medially on tibia.	If tibia slides medially, this indicates a tear or weakness in medial collateral ligament. If tibia slides laterally, this indicates a tear or weakness in lateral collateral ligament.
Cruciate ligament integrity	Flex knee to 90°. Stabilize foot. Grasp lower leg and try pushing backward and then pulling forward.	If tibia slides backward, this indicates a tear or weakness in posterior cruciate ligament. If tibia slides forward, this indicates a tear or weakness in anterior cruciate ligament.
McMurray sign	Flex knee completely, moving foot close to buttock. Put one hand on knee, placing thumb and index fingers on either side of joint space. With other hand, hold heel and rotate foot and lower leg laterally. Keeping leg rotated, extend the knee to a 90° angle. Repeat the procedure, rotating the foot and lower leg medially.	If click is heard and felt, this indicates meniscal tears.

Palpate the bony and muscular structures of the patient's ankles and feet as follows: Hold each foot behind the ankle with one hand and palpate with the fingertips of your other hand. Palpate the metatarsophalangeal joints and the metatarsal heads on the sole of each foot by compressing each joint. Test his ankles and toes for full range of motion.

Formulating a diagnostic impression

692 Classifying musculoskeletal disorders

Compromise of bone integrity by disease or trauma may interrupt the *skeletal system's* vital functions of body support, protection, and movement, reducing the patient's ability to take an active part in his daily activities. Blood cell production and mineral metabolism may also be affected.

The *muscular system*, besides its role in heat production, supports the skeletal system, facilitating body move-

NURSE'S GUIDE TO MUSCULOSKELETAL DISORDERS

BONE INTEGRITY DISRUPTIONS	CHIEF COMPLAINT
Osteoarthritis	• *Pain:* during inclement weather; worse after exposure to cold, exercise, or weight-bearing; relieved by rest • *Joint stiffness:* transient stiffness worse in morning or after inactivity; affects weight-bearing joints • *Swelling and redness:* joints swollen and tender but not red or hot • *Deformity and immobility:* Heberden's nodes in distal joints; Bouchard's nodes in proximal joints; flexion contracture possible
Gout	• *Pain:* present, severe; worse after high purine food ingestion; frequently nocturnal; onset usually sudden • *Joint stiffness:* joint immobility caused by pain and swelling • *Swelling and redness:* red, or cyanotic tense, hot skin over affected swollen joint; in acute form, usually monoarticular • *Deformity and immobility:* painless tophi (urate deposits) in external ears, hands, elbows, and knees; can't bear weight on affected limb
Reiter's syndrome	• *Pain:* present • *Joint stiffness:* present, usually in sacroiliac joint and sometimes in foot, knee, or ankle joints; weight-bearing joint involvement usually asymmetrical • *Swelling and redness:* signs of acute inflammation • *Deformity and immobility:* presence depends on extent of arthritis that is part of Reiter's syndrome
Ankylosing spondylitis (Marie-Strümpell disease)	• *Pain:* begins as lower back ache that radiates down thighs • *Joint stiffness:* decreased joint mobility and muscle stiffness • *Swelling and redness:* present, resembling rheumatoid arthritis, synovitis • *Deformity and immobility:* progressively limited back movement and chest expansion; in severe cases, fusion of entire spine
Osteomyelitis	• *Pain:* present in affected joint with movement • *Joint stiffness:* restricted movement caused by pain • *Swelling and redness:* onset of swelling in 1 to 2 days; inflammation; increased fluid in joint • *Deformity and immobility:* joint may be immobilized by pain
Osteoporosis	• *Pain:* possible; symptom of fracture or vertebral collapse; aggravated by movement • *Deformity and immobility:* fractures of involved bones; collapse of vertebrae; increasing kyphosis or dowager's hump possible

	HISTORY	PHYSICAL EXAMINATION AND DIAGNOSTIC STUDIES
	• Onset usually after age 55 • Moderate to severe disease more common in postmenopausal women • Predisposing factors include joint damage from trauma, infection, or stress; dietary calcium deficiency; history of arthritis in one or both parents; occupation.	• Decreased range of motion; altered bone contour; bony enlargement; malaligned joints; no systemic manifestations; crepitation on motion • Diagnostic studies include X-rays of affected joints.
	• Predisposing factors include renal disease, family history of gout, disorders that cause alterations in purine metabolism or decreased renal clearance of uric acid.	• Altered bone contour; elevated blood pressure; tachycardia; fever; nephrolithiasis; renal failure; thickened, wrinkled, desquamated skin • Diagnostic studies include uric acid levels; complete blood count; synovial fluid analysis; arthroscopy.
	• More common in young men • Recent sexual activity • Cause unknown	• Limited range of motion • Lesions of mucous membranes, oral and genital skin, and nails; resembles psoriasis; lesions with yellow vesicles on soles and palms; low-grade fever; conjunctivitis; urethritis • Diagnostic studies include synovial fluid analysis.
	• Most common in male children and young male adults ages 10 to 30 • Familial disorder; genetic predisposition	• Decreased spinal range of motion; abnormal vertebrae alignment; flattened lumbar curve; exaggerated thoracic curvature; decreased chest expansion; cardiac complication with long-standing disease; atrophy of trunk muscles; fever; fatigue; weight loss • Diagnostic studies include X-rays and HLA antigen studies.
	• Predisposing factors include recent infection, surgery, fracture, puncture wound, bites, prolonged drug addiction. • Sudden onset	• Limited range of motion; unequal limb circumferences; local necrosis or lesion on skin surface; fever; chills; malaise • Diagnostic studies include blood cultures and X-rays.
	• Predisposing factors include endocrine disorders, excessive cigarette smoking, chronic low dietary calcium intake, malabsorption, prolonged immobility. • Most common in postmenopausal women	• Evidence of healed fracture; loss of height; wedging of dorsal vertebrae or anterior vertebrae • Diagnostic studies include X-rays and bone densitometry measurements.

(continued)

NURSE'S GUIDE TO MUSCULOSKELETAL DISORDERS *(continued)*

	CHIEF COMPLAINT	
Paget's disease	• *Pain:* present in deep bone • *Joint stiffness:* present, as in rheumatoid arthritis • *Swelling and redness:* increased heat in affected area from increased vascularity • *Deformity and immobility:* bowing of long bones; kyphosis; frequent fractures with slight trauma • *Sensory changes:* headaches, deafness, vertigo, tinnitus, or other sensory changes possible; caused by bony growth that compresses nerves	
Osteogenic sarcoma	• *Pain:* persistent and progressive; local at first, then diffuse; bone tenderness • *Joint stiffness:* if tumor is located in joint • *Swelling and redness:* present in area of tumor; appears gradually as tumor grows; variable swelling; local heat • *Deformity and immobility:* pathological fractures; limited movement of affected part	
Cervical disk herniation	• *Pain:* present in neck, shoulder, or arm; exact distribution depends on which nerve route is compressed; increases with neck flexion and rotation; paroxysmal • *Deformity and immobility:* limited neck range of motion; muscle (biceps) weakness • *Sensory changes:* paresthesia and sensory loss over neck, shoulder, arm, and/or hand, depending on specific nerve root involvement	
Herniated lumbosacral disk (lower back pain)	• *Pain:* present with coughing, sneezing, straining, bending, or lifting; increases with sitting; occurs over dermatome for that specific disk; accompanied by mild or severe low back, buttock, or leg pain; may be associated with spasms • *Joint stiffness:* inflexible spine • *Deformity and immobility:* muscle atrophy of affected extremities • *Sensory changes:* decreased sensation, paresthesias; absent reflexes over dermatomes; voiding or defecating difficulties, particularly urinary retention	
Scoliosis	• *Pain:* present; radiates from back to extremities • *Joint stiffness:* hip or knee flexion contractures • *Deformity and immobility:* rib cage deformity; hamstring tightness; the higher the location of the scoliosis, the more severe the deformity • *Sensory changes:* decreased sensation to lower extremities	
Kyphosis	• *Pain:* present in back; radiates to legs • *Joint stiffness:* stiff back • *Deformity and immobility:* round back in thoracic region; lordotic curve; hamstring tightness • *Sensory changes:* decreased sensation in lower legs	

	HISTORY	PHYSICAL EXAMINATION AND DIAGNOSTIC STUDIES
	• Predisposing factors include recent deafness, family history of Paget's disease, cardiovascular and pulmonary disease. • Most common in men	• Altered bone contour; waddling gait; increased head size • Diagnostic studies include blood tests for increased calcium and alkaline phosphatase; bone scan; X-rays.
	• Peak incidence at age 20 • More common in males • Accompanying factors include weight loss. • Predisposing factors include history of Paget's disease, exposure to radiation, trauma.	• Decreased range of motion; unequal limb circumferences; venous engorgement; anemia • Diagnostic studies include biopsy and X-rays.
	• Recent neck trauma or forceful hyperextension	• Cough, sneeze, or strain (downward pressure on head) in hyperextended position causes pain; diminished biceps or triceps jerk • Diagnostic studies include X-rays, myelography, computerized tomography scan.
	• Predisposing factors include recent spinal trauma, heavy lifting, or occupational stress on back; lack of exercise; weight gain; degenerative changes.	• Decreased spinal range of motion; unequal limb circumferences; abnormal posture; scoliosis; abnormal leg reflexes; diminished ankle or knee jerk; positive straight-leg–raising test (limited ability to straight-raise leg) • Diagnostic studies include X-rays and myelography.
	• Predisposing factors include genetic history of scoliosis, poliomyelitis, congenital abnormalities.	• Limited spinal range of motion; fatigued or tired back; hair patches, dimples, and pigmentation on back; decreased chest expansion; impaired pulmonary or cardiac function (hypoxia, cyanosis, chronic obstructive pulmonary disease); one scapula, breast, or flank more prominent than other; shoulders and hips not level • Diagnostic studies include X-rays.
	• Compression fracture of thoracic vertebrae is a predisposing factor. • Recent spinal trauma, osteoporosis, chronic arthritis, tuberculosis	• Limited spinal range of motion; decreased pulmonary function • Diagnostic studies include X-rays.

(continued)

NURSE'S GUIDE TO MUSCULOSKELETAL DISORDERS *(continued)*

	CHIEF COMPLAINT
Fracture	• *Pain:* intensity increases until fragments are set • *Joint stiffness:* may be present with fracture near joint; crepitation • *Swelling and redness:* varying degrees of swelling and bleeding into tissues • *Deformity and immobility:* bone deformity; bone may project through skin; lost function of fractured part • *Sensory changes:* if nerves severed, bleeding and swelling cause pressure on nerves; if large vessel severed, blood loss to fractured part
SUPPORTIVE-STRUCTURES DISORDERS	
Temporomandibular joint syndrome	• *Pain:* facial, localized in ear or jaw; may extend to neck and shoulders; present on yawning or chewing, or with headache • *Joint stiffness:* limited jaw movement, especially in morning • *Swelling and redness:* swelling over joint • *Deformity and immobility:* can lead to malocclusion
Spasmodic torticollis	• *Pain:* present with neck movement in trapezius, sternocleidomastoid, and other neck muscles; sudden or gradual onset; worsens under stress • *Joint stiffness:* stiff neck caused by muscle spasm • *Deformity and immobility:* muscle spasms cause head rotation to opposite side and flexion to same side
Adhesive capsulitis (frozen shoulder)	• *Pain:* localized tenderness over biceps; worsens at night because of pressure while sleeping; aggravated by extremes in shoulder movement • *Joint stiffness:* shoulder stiffness • *Swelling and redness:* inflammation of capsule of scapulohumeral joint • *Deformity and immobility:* limited mobility
Bursitis	• *Pain:* severe on movement; in chronic form, nagging, intermittent pain possible • *Joint stiffness:* inflammation of bursae and calcific deposits in subdeltoid, olecranon (miners' elbow), trochanteric, or prepatellar (housemaid's knee) bursae • *Swelling and redness:* over affected joint
Carpal tunnel syndrome	• *Pain:* worsens after manual activity or at night; radiates up arm; may be intermittent or constant • *Swelling and redness:* soft tissue swelling possible • *Deformity and immobility:* inability to oppose thumb and little finger • *Sensory changes:* numbness, burning, or tingling on palmar surface (may be initial symptom)

HISTORY	PHYSICAL EXAMINATION AND DIAGNOSTIC STUDIES
• Direct trauma • Indirect trauma above or below fracture • Predisposing factors include repeated stress, osteogenic sarcoma, osteoporosis, Paget's disease, hematopoietic diseases, nutritional deficiencies.	• Bone contour defect, abnormal bone motion, possibly shock • Diagnostic studies include X-rays.
• Trauma, causing dislocation of joint • Osteoarthritis	• Joint clicks when mouth opens; limited range of motion
• Difficult birth is a predisposing factor. • Accompanying disorders include eye imbalance or defects, psychogenic problems, spinal or muscular defects. • Most common in adults ages 30 to 60	• Possible neck muscle spasms, which pull head forcibly to one side • Asymmetry of head and neck
• Predisposing factors include recent trauma to distal part of arm requiring shoulder immobilization; hemiplegia; cardiac disease; mastectomy.	• Decreased shoulder range of motion; shoulder tenderness on palpation • Diagnostic studies include X-rays.
• Predisposing factors include recent trauma to joint, occupational stress to joint, rheumatoid arthritis, gout, infection.	• Decreased range of motion in affected joint
• Predisposing factors include trauma or injury to wrist, rheumatoid arthritis, gout, myxedema, diabetes mellitus, leukemia, acromegaly, edema associated with pregnancy. • Most common in postmenopausal women and in women in advanced pregnancy	• Atrophy of thenar eminences; positive Tinel's sign (tingling present with wrist percussion); positive Phalen's sign (tingling with sustained wrist flexion); muscle weakness; dryness of skin over thumb and first two fingers • Diagnostic studies may include electromyography.

(continued)

NURSE'S GUIDE TO MUSCULOSKELETAL DISORDERS *(continued)*

	CHIEF COMPLAINT	
Tenosynovitis	• *Pain:* insidious or precipitated by strenuous activity; may radiate • *Joint stiffness:* joint locking possible; inflammation common • *Swelling and redness:* local swelling	
Ganglion	• *Pain:* continuous aching aggravated by joint motion • *Joint stiffness:* present • *Swelling and redness:* gradual swelling over joint increased with extensive use of affected extremity; tense or fluctuant, rounded, nontender • *Deformity and immobility:* nodule over joint; weak fingers and joints next to ganglion, if connected to tendon sheath	
Slipped femoral epiphysis (epiphyseal coxa vara)	• *Pain:* groin discomfort; subsides with rest; hip or knee aches; becomes intense in chronic phase • *Joint stiffness:* stiff hip joint • *Deformity and immobility:* limp; increases with fatigue; affected limb eventually becomes shorter	
Meniscal tear	• *Pain:* acute pain or localized tenderness • *Swelling and redness:* local swelling • *Deformity and immobility:* muscle atrophy of quadriceps muscle above knee; inability to straighten knee	
Ligamental tear	• *Pain:* tenderness on palpation • *Joint stiffness:* sensation of slight catching • *Swelling and redness:* fluid around knee, swelling, ecchymosis • *Deformity and immobility:* excessive tibia motion at anterior and posterior femur • *Sensory changes:* weakness, instability	
Morton's neuroma	• *Pain:* severe, between third and fourth toes • *Swelling and redness:* swelling between third and fourth toes • *Sensory changes:* burning, numbness, and paresthesias between toes	
Lower back strain	• *Pain:* acute and severe, or chronic, less severe, and aching; localized pain; may radiate • *Joint stiffness:* may be present • *Swelling and redness:* swelling caused by hemorrhage into tissues	
Sprain	• *Pain:* varying degrees over involved joint • *Joint stiffness:* present • *Swelling and redness:* soft tissue swelling; superficial bruise • *Deformity and immobility:* limited range of motion • *Sensory changes:* can be seen in cervical sprain	

	HISTORY	PHYSICAL EXAMINATION AND DIAGNOSTIC STUDIES
	• Predisposing factors include injury or surgery of involved joint. • Most common in women in early 40s	• Decreased range of motion; pain on palpation
	• May occur after trauma, weight gain, compression • Disappears and recurs • Onset between adolescence and age 50 • Most common in women	• Limited range of motion of affected joint; palpable nodule more prominent on flexion, less prominent on extension
	• Predisposing factors include hip trauma, obesity. • Most common in boys ages 10 to 17 • Insidious onset • Occurs during rapid skeletal growth	• Muscle spasms; limited hip abduction, with internal rotation and flexion; abnormal waddling gait • Diagnostic studies include X-rays.
	• Predisposing factors include twisting injury or direct blow to knee, repeated squatting or kneeling. • Most common in athletes	• Unequal knee contour; positive McMurray sign; blood in joint space
	• Popping sound heard when injury occurred; trauma to knee • Most common in athletes	• Unstable knee joint; abnormal knee range of motion; point tenderness; changed knee joint contour
	• Difficulty walking long distances; foot requires frequent massage • Use of high-heeled shoes • Most common in women	• None
	• Muscle suddenly forced beyond capacity; trauma; degenerative disk disease; continued mechanical strain; pregnancy	• Tenderness with firm pressure; bruise; muscle spasm; inflammation; decreased range of motion
	• Sudden twisting injury	• Edema and discoloration around joint; no X-ray changes except soft tissue swelling; tenderness over joint

(continued)

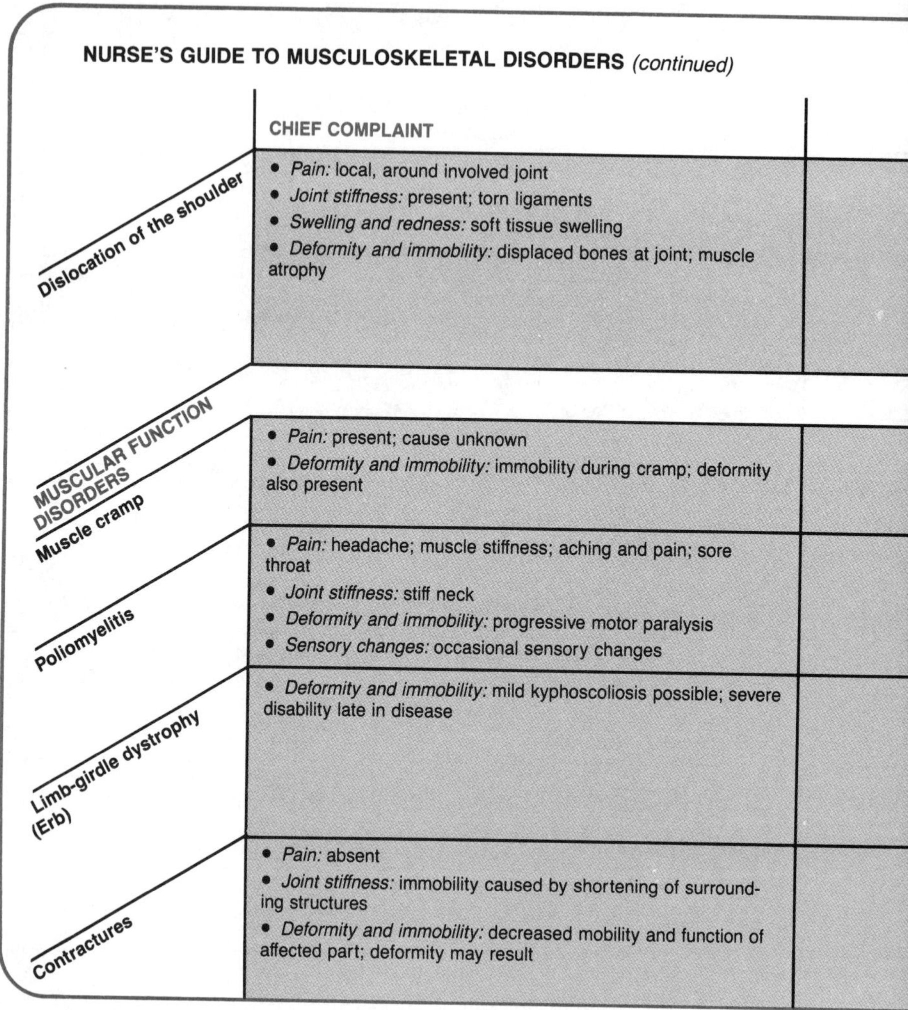

NURSE'S GUIDE TO MUSCULOSKELETAL DISORDERS *(continued)*

	CHIEF COMPLAINT
Dislocation of the shoulder	• *Pain:* local, around involved joint • *Joint stiffness:* present; torn ligaments • *Swelling and redness:* soft tissue swelling • *Deformity and immobility:* displaced bones at joint; muscle atrophy
MUSCULAR FUNCTION DISORDERS	
Muscle cramp	• *Pain:* present; cause unknown • *Deformity and immobility:* immobility during cramp; deformity also present
Poliomyelitis	• *Pain:* headache; muscle stiffness; aching and pain; sore throat • *Joint stiffness:* stiff neck • *Deformity and immobility:* progressive motor paralysis • *Sensory changes:* occasional sensory changes
Limb-girdle dystrophy (Erb)	• *Deformity and immobility:* mild kyphoscoliosis possible; severe disability late in disease
Contractures	• *Pain:* absent • *Joint stiffness:* immobility caused by shortening of surrounding structures • *Deformity and immobility:* decreased mobility and function of affected part; deformity may result

ment and maintaining posture. It is composed of skeletal muscles (muscles attached to bones).

Musculoskeletal disorders may be classified in three categories: disorders that disrupt bone integrity, disorders of the supportive structures of bone, and disorders of muscle function (see *Nurse's Guide to Musculoskeletal Disorders*).

693 Making appropriate nursing diagnoses

Pain is present sometime in most musculoskeletal problems. Musculoskeletal pain commonly results from chemical, thermal, or mechanical processes that stimulate nerve endings in pain-sensitive tissues. Inflammatory pain-producing processes may be triggered by trauma, infection, or irritation. Swelling produces increased local pressure, which causes pain. Pain also results from alterations in musculoskeletal structures (for example, cysts and tumors) that cause pressure on nerves.

A nursing diagnosis for a patient

HISTORY	PHYSICAL EXAMINATION AND DIAGNOSTIC STUDIES
• Traumatic injury • Predisposing factors include congenital changes in skeletal contour, weakness of musculature, past history of dislocation. • May reduce itself, or recur • Most common in young adults, athletes	• Decreased range of motion; altered joint configuration; changed extremity length
• Common during pregnancy and in athletes • Usually occurs at night after strenuous activity	• Muscle is visibly and palpably tight; fasciculations; excessive sweating • Diagnostic studies include electromyography.
• Most common in infants, children, and young adults • Usually occurs in midsummer or fall	• Low-grade fever; nausea, vomiting, diarrhea, constipation; muscles tender on palpation; diminished or absent deep tendon reflexes • Diagnostic studies include examination of spinal fluid.
• Most common in adults ages 20 to 30 • Inherited • Rate of progression and severity are variable	• Primarily involves shoulder and pelvic girdle muscles; peculiar gait; muscle weakness; muscle contractions; muscle fasciculations; occasionally pseudohypertrophy of other muscles; may lead to respiratory and cardiac muscle involvement • Diagnostic studies include muscle biopsy, serum enzymes, electromyography.
• Trauma, infection, nerve lesions, result of immobilization	• Shortening of skin, muscle, or ligaments; flexion of joint

with musculoskeletal pain is *alterations in comfort. Fear of debilitation* from the cause of the pain may also be an appropriate nursing diagnosis.

Joint stiffness can be caused by inflammation, soft tissue swelling, muscle spasm, misalignment, or bony deformity. Inflammatory conditions, such as bursitis, cause soft tissues to swell and act as a splint, obstructing joint flexion. Vertebral column stiffness may be caused by synovitis of the involved spinal joints. Disruptions in joint structure can also cause stiffness. Joint stiffness primarily occurs in disorders of the supportive structures of bones and disorders of bone integrity.

Possible nursing diagnoses for joint stiffness include *impaired mobility, self-care deficit,* and *alterations in comfort.*

Swelling and erythema that occur over a bone may be caused by inflammation from trauma, degenerative disease, or infection. Joint swelling may result from inflammation of the synovium or hemorrhage into the joint.

Transfer of fluid and cells from the bloodstream to the interstitial tissues

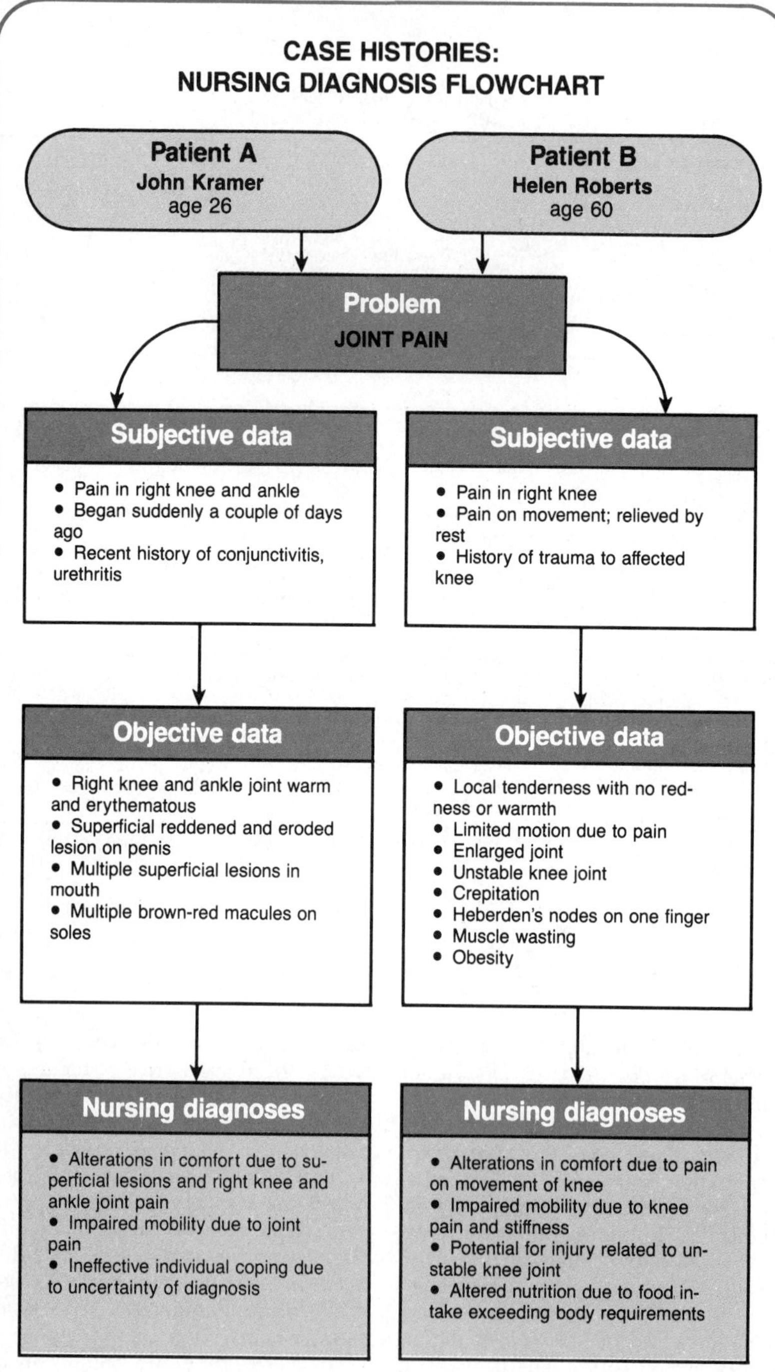
CASE HISTORIES:
NURSING DIAGNOSIS FLOWCHART
Patient A
John Kramer
age 26
Patient B
Helen Roberts
age 60
Problem
JOINT PAIN
Subjective data
• Pain in right knee and ankle
• Began suddenly a couple of days ago
• Recent history of conjunctivitis, urethritis
Subjective data
• Pain in right knee
• Pain on movement; relieved by rest
• History of trauma to affected knee
Objective data
• Right knee and ankle joint warm and erythematous
• Superficial reddened and eroded lesion on penis
• Multiple superficial lesions in mouth
• Multiple brown-red macules on soles
Objective data
• Local tenderness with no redness or warmth
• Limited motion due to pain
• Enlarged joint
• Unstable knee joint
• Crepitation
• Heberden's nodes on one finger
• Muscle wasting
• Obesity
Nursing diagnoses
• Alterations in comfort due to superficial lesions and right knee and ankle joint pain
• Impaired mobility due to joint pain
• Ineffective individual coping due to uncertainty of diagnosis
Nursing diagnoses
• Alterations in comfort due to pain on movement of knee
• Impaired mobility due to knee pain and stiffness
• Potential for injury related to unstable knee joint
• Altered nutrition due to food intake exceeding body requirements

causes soft tissue swelling. This may be caused by trauma-induced inflammation or abscess formation. Swelling accompanied by erythema and heat is usually caused by an acute inflammatory process. The erythema is caused by dilatation of the arterioles in the area. This dilatation releases more blood into the microcirculation, causing capillaries to become congested and producing an erythematous area on the skin. Swelling and erythema occur principally in disorders of the supporting structures of bone.

Nursing diagnoses for these patients include *alterations in comfort, potential for injury,* and possibly *disturbance in self-concept.*

Trauma, such as a fracture, can cause misalignment of a bone or joint, resulting in a musculoskeletal deformity. Congenital diseases, such as scoliosis, that result in abnormal bone curvatures, and bone tumors that create a mass or deterioration of bone, can also cause deformity. Degenerative disease deformities are caused largely by bony overgrowth and loss of articular cartilage. Motion limitations may be intentional, because of pain, or may be due to joint-space narrowing. They may also result from disuse of the joint. Misalignment of bones (fractures) and disruption of articulating surfaces (for example, by trauma, bony overgrowth, or inflammation) result in varying degrees of immobility. Deformity and immobility may be present in disorders of supportive structures of bone, disorders of bone integrity, and disorders of muscle function.

Nursing diagnoses include *disturbance in self-concept, impaired mobility,* and possibly a *knowledge deficit of correct posture and/or body mechanics.*

Sensory changes, such as paresthesias, numbness, tingling, and decreased sensation, can occur in a body part when sufficient pressure is placed on a nerve (or nerve root) to interfere with the conduction of nerve impulses. Some causes of this include swelling, inflammation, overgrowth of bone, tumors, or cysts. Tingling and prickling paresthesias also result from excitation of sensory nerve fibers, as in severe muscle cramps. Numbness and tingling also result from a decrease in blood circulating to an area distal to an obstruction.

Appropriate nursing diagnoses for these patients are *potential for injury* and *sensory perceptual alterations.*

UNDERSTANDING CAST SYNDROME

If your patient's had spinal surgery and is now in a body cast or jacket, be alert for the signs and symptoms of cast syndrome. These include nausea, vomiting, abdominal pressure and pain, dehydration, and alkalosis. Cast syndrome probably results from this series of events: hyperextension of the spine accentuates lumbar lordosis, which compresses the third portion of the duodenum between the superior mesenteric artery anteriorly, and the aorta and vertebral column posteriorly. Untreated cast syndrome may be fatal. Remember, cast syndrome may develop several weeks or months after cast application.

UNDERSTANDING FAT EMBOLISM

If you're caring for a patient who's fractured an arm or a leg, be alert to the possibility of fat embolism formation. This potentially fatal complication often follows trauma, because a traumatic event causes the release of catecholamines, which mobilize fatty acids. These fatty acids can develop into fat emboli and lodge in the lungs or even the brain. This condition usually occurs within 24 hours after the fracture, but may occur up to 3 days after.

Suspect fat embolism if your patient shows any of these signs and symptoms: a chest and shoulder petechial rash, apprehension, sweating, fever, tachycardia, pallor, dyspnea, pulmonary effusion, cyanosis, convulsions, or coma.

Arterial blood gas studies will show low Po_2, and a chest X-ray may exhibit a typical snowstorm pattern of infiltrates, scattered over the lungs.

Assessing pediatric patients

694 A child's musculoskeletal development

Physical growth and maturation are important indicators of the musculoskeletal system's competence. Growth data reveal age uniformities that are quantifiable, predictable, and useful in evaluating a child's relative health status. For example, children normally learn to walk between ages 9 and 15 months. By age 4, most children can hop on one foot.

Various tools for measuring normal development are available. For example, growth charts for height help you determine if a child's skeletal growth is normal (see Chapter 5, ASSESSING NUTRITIONAL STATUS). The Denver Developmental Screening Test measures a child's motor skills. Between birth and adulthood the skeleton triples in size, with normal growth spurts during infancy and adolescence.

Because a child's bones are growing, osteogenic activity is greater than in an adult. A child's bones are also more porous and flexible than an adult's. This is why greenstick fractures occur most commonly in children, and why a child's bones heal more rapidly than an adult's.

Only one concave (C-shaped) spinal curve, the *primary* curve, is present at birth; the *secondary*, or compensatory, curves, which give the spine its characteristic S shape, develop later. The cervical curve appears at about age 3 to 4 months, when the infant begins to hold up his head. The lumbar curve appears when the child is walking, at around age 12 to 18 months. (See *Comparing Adult and Child Lumbar Curvature.*)

A child's muscular development, closely related to his nervous system development, proceeds from the simple to the complex. For example, a child will be able to hit an object with his hand before he is able to pick it up with his fingers.

695 History-taking considerations

When you're taking the past history of a child with a suspected musculoskeletal disorder, obtain information on his *immunizations* and on *past problems* he's experienced. A history of repeated fractures, muscle strains or sprains, painful joints, clumsiness, lack of coordination, abnormal gait, or restricted movements may indicate a musculoskeletal problem. A developmental history includes the ages when the child reached *major motor-development milestones;* this information will also help you determine if he has a musculoskeletal disorder. For an infant, some of these milestones include his age when he held up his head, rolled over, sat unassisted, and walked alone. Motor milestones for an older child include his age when he first ran, jumped, walked up stairs, and pedaled a tricycle.

During the family history, ask if any family member has experienced a musculoskeletal disease, such as arthritis or muscular dystrophy. Find out if the child's mother took any *medications* during the pregnancy. Certain drugs—such as streptomycin, tetracycline, meprobamate, and androgens and estrogens—can cause defects in fetal bone formation. Also ask if the mother has diabetes mellitus, which can predispose her child to hypoplasia of the femur.

When reviewing activities of daily living, ask the parent about the child's usual daily *diet* and *recreational activities.* Calcium deficiencies can cause osteoporosis in children. Sports that involve throwing, such as baseball, may cause epiphyseal separation of the shoulder or wrist, especially at puberty.

COMPARING ADULT AND CHILD LUMBAR CURVATURE

Whereas accentuated lumbar curvature in the adult (as shown on the left) is abnormal, the same condition is normal in the child up to age 4 (as shown on the right).

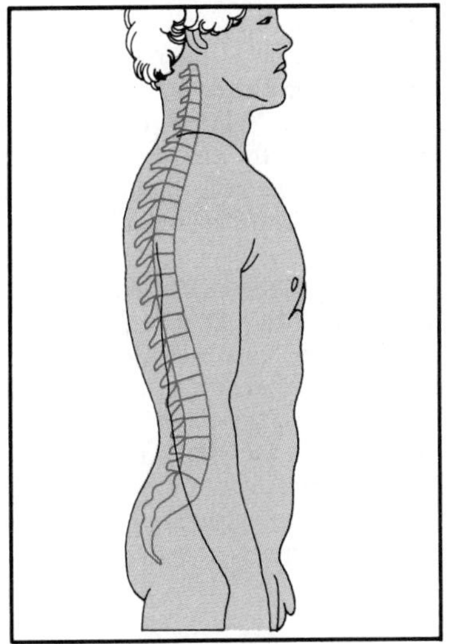

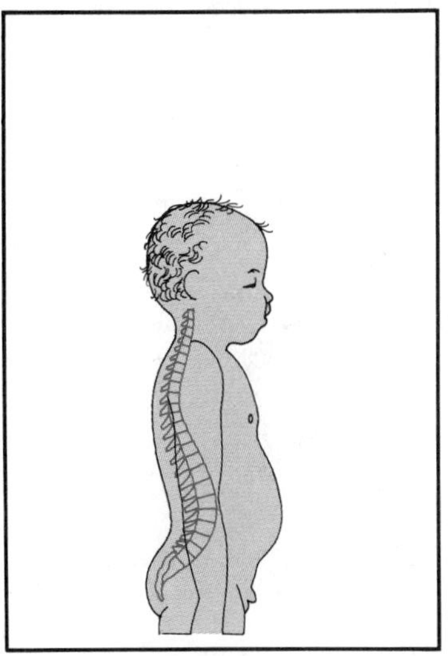

696 Musculoskeletal assessment

You can perform much of the testing of a child's range of motion, muscle strength, and gait while playing with him or watching him run, jump, sit, and climb. In infants and toddlers, you'll obviously assess only passive movements for range-of-motion testing. For children who are able to follow instructions and can do active range-of-motion movements, demonstrate what you want the child to do and ask him to mimic you. Observe the child's muscles for size, symmetry, strength, tone, and abnormal movements.

Test muscle strength in a preschool or school-age child as you would test it in an adult, by having the child push against your hands or your arms. To check muscle strength in a toddler or in an infant who is not yet able to understand directions, observe his sucking as well as his general motor activity.

697 Evaluating a child's spine and gait

Check your patient's spine for scoliosis, kyphosis, and lordosis. If the child has scoliosis (most commonly seen in girls), differentiate between the functional and the structural type. Ask the child to bend over and touch her toes without bending her knees. (You'll get a better view of her spine if you squat to inspect it.) Functional scoliosis (also known as *postural scoliosis*) disappears with this maneuver, whereas structural scoliosis remains—and often becomes accentuated. Also, in structural scoliosis, one shoulder may appear higher than the other when the child bends over. Kyphosis and lordosis (which follows as a compensatory mechanism) most often result from poor posture.

To check a child's gait, balance, and stance, ask him to walk, run, and skip away from you and then return.

Assessment tip: If your patient's a toddler, remember that he won't want

IDENTIFYING COMMON SPINE ABNORMALITIES

When examining the spine of the pediatric or adolescent patient, look for these common abnormalities:

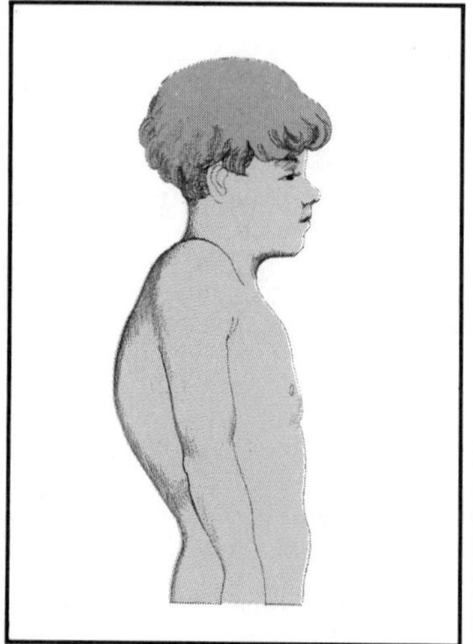

Kyphosis (rounded shoulders and exaggerated posterior chest convexity)

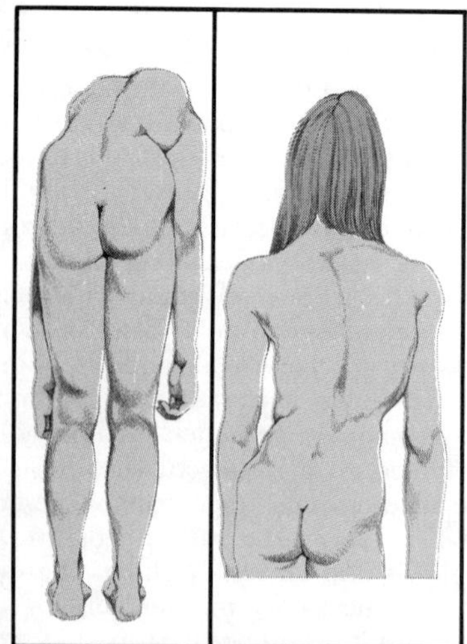

Scoliosis (thoracic or lumbar spine curving laterally to left or right in an S shape, particularly evident when the patient bends over)

to walk *away* from his parents, but he will walk *toward* them. So to assess his gait, put the child down several yards away from his parents.

Keep developmental changes in a child's gait in mind, so you don't mistake them for abnormal conditions. For instance, a new walker (ages 12 to 18 months) normally has a wide-based gait with poor balance, whereas a preschooler usually has a narrow-based stance with enough balance to stand on one leg for a few seconds.

698 Examining a child's hips and legs

Inspect the child's gluteal folds for asymmetry, which may indicate a dislocated hip. If hip dislocation is a possibility, test for Ortolani's sign (see *Assessing Hip Dislocation,* page 793).

Observe the child's legs for shape, length, symmetry, and alignment. *Genu varum* (bowlegs) is common in children between ages 1½ and 2½; *genu valgum* (knock-knees) is common in preschoolers. If these conditions do not improve over time or are excessive, evaluate the child for a tibial torsion (an internal or external rotation of the tibia). To test for bowlegs, have the child stand straight with his ankles touching. In this position, the knees shouldn't be more than 1" (2.5 cm) apart. To test a child for knock-knees, have him stand straight with his knees touching. The ankles shouldn't be more than 1" (2.5 cm) apart in this position. Also, look at the pattern of wear on the child's shoes: wear on the outside of the heel suggests bowlegs; on the inside, knock-knees.

Next, observe the child's feet for *clubfoot* (talipes equinovarus); *outward-turned toes* (toeing out, or pes valgus), and *pigeon toes* (toeing in, or pes varus).

Finally, test the child for tibial torsion. One way to do this is to have him lie on his back with his knees flexed so that the feet are flat on the table, in a vertical line with his knees. Place your thumb and index fingers on the

UNDERSTANDING TIBIAL TORSION

Tibial torsion, or twisting of the tibia, is the most common orthopedic disorder in toddlers. Here are two common causes:

- *External tibial torsion* can be seen in *toeing-out*—when the foot points out while the knee remains straight. This condition may be a normal finding, correcting itself by the time the child is age 1 to 1½. If it persists, the child may be sitting for prolonged periods with his buttocks flat on the floor and his knees and ankles flexed, also flat on the floor.
- *Internal tibial torsion* can be seen in *toeing-in* (or pigeon-toeing)—when the foot points in while the knee remains straight. Internal tibial torsion may be a normal finding, correcting itself when the child is age 2 to 4. If it persists, the child may be sitting on his feet.

To test for tibial torsion, draw a line from the patient's anterior superior iliac crest through the patella to the floor. Normally, the line will intersect the second toe; intersecting the fourth or fifth toe indicates internal tibial torsion. If it intersects the arch of the foot instead of the toes, external tibial torsion is present. Record tibial torsion by measuring the degree of deviation from the norm. External tibial torsion deviation may range from +10° (mild) to +30° (severe). Internal tibial torsion deviation may range from −10° (mild) to −30° (severe).

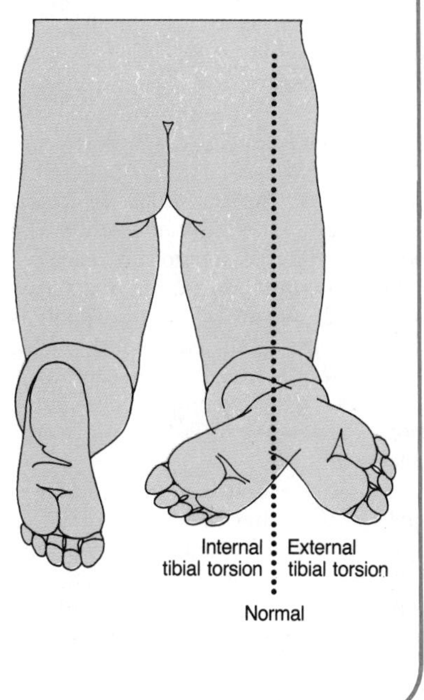

lateral and medial malleoli of both feet. In an infant, the four malleoli should be parallel to the table. In an older child, the external malleoli may normally rotate up to 20°.

699 Common childhood disorders

Because children's growing bones are somewhat flexible, *greenstick fractures* (incomplete fractures with angulation caused by disruption of the periosteum on one side of a bone) are common. Also known as an *infraperiosteal fracture,* this type of injury may be present whenever a child has bone pain accompanied by swelling and deformity.

Subluxation of the radius or shoulder sometimes results when an adult picks up or swings a child by the hands. In *subluxation of the radius,* the patient has elbow or wrist pain worsened by passive range of motion in all positions except supination. Shoulder pain accompanied by swelling and refusal to move the arm suggests *shoulder subluxation.*

Always be alert to the possibility that a child has been physically abused. Such a child usually will have multiple bone injuries, in different stages of repair, and may have other serious injuries, such as a subdural hematoma.

Necrosis of the head of the femur, known as *Perthes disease,* occurs in children (usually boys) between ages 5 and 10. Clinically, the patient presents with a limp and with hip pain (often referred to the knee). Motion is restricted only on abduction and rotation.

Muscular dystrophy is an inherited disease characterized by progressive weakness from muscle atrophy. Skeletal muscle is primarily involved, but cardiac involvement can also occur. One of the first symptoms of Duchenne's form of muscular dystrophy, which occurs only in boys, is pelvic girdle weakness that causes toe-walking, falling, and waddling that begin as soon as the child starts to walk. The disease progresses throughout childhood. By adolescence, the child is usually confined to a wheelchair. The Landouzy-Déjerine form of muscular dystrophy affects boys and girls, and usually first becomes apparent in adolescence. Most commonly, the first symptom is shoulder girdle weakness. Progression is slower than in Duchenne's form of the disease, with some children ultimately becoming disabled and others being scarcely aware of any symptoms throughout life.

Scoliosis, which is most common in girls, is an S-shaped lateral curvature of the spine that becomes apparent during periods of spinal growth, such as pubescence. In a child with scoliosis, one shoulder is elevated, one hip may be prominent, or the spinal curve itself may be noticeable. Of the two types of scoliosis, the most serious is *structural scoliosis,* caused by changes in the shape of the vertebrae or thorax. *Postural* or *functional* scoliosis is caused by poor posture.

Slipped femoral epiphysis is a disorder that occurs during epiphyseal closure, which marks the completion of skeletal growth. In this disorder, the femoral epiphysis gradually slips upward, often causing a slight limp on the affected side. Pain in the hip, sometimes referred to the knee, occurs as the disorder worsens, along with abduction and internal rotation of the affected limb.

Osteosarcoma (osteogenic sarcoma) is the most common primary malignant bone tumor of childhood. Although it may occur in other locations, osteosarcoma usually involves the end of a long bone—commonly the lower end of the femur or upper end of the tibia or humerus. Pain and swelling are the principal symptoms of this life-threatening disorder.

Assessing geriatric patients

700 Musculoskeletal changes in the elderly

The most apparent musculoskeletal change in elderly persons is decreasing height. This results from exaggerated spinal curvatures and narrowing intervertebral spaces, which shorten the person's trunk and make his arms appear relatively long. Other changes include decreased muscle mass (which may result in muscle weakness), and a decrease in collagen formation that causes loss of resilience and elasticity in joints and supporting structures. Aging's effect on the geriatric patient's nervous system may cause difficulty in tandem walking. Usually the person walks with shorter steps and a wider leg stance to achieve better balance and stable weight distribution.

701 Special history questions

Biographical data are significant for the elderly, because osteoporosis most commonly occurs after age 50.

If your patient's *chief complaint* is pain associated with a fall, determine if the pain preceded the fall. Pain present before a fall may indicate a pathologic fracture. Also, ask if your patient has noticed any vision or coordination changes that may make him more susceptible to falling.

When recording the patient's *past history,* determine if he's had asthma (treatment with steroids can lead to osteoporosis), arthritis (which produces joint instability), or pernicious anemia (inadequate absorption of vitamin B_{12} in pernicious anemia leads to loss of vibratory sensation and proprioception, resulting in falls). Cancer of the breast, prostate, thyroid, kidney, or bladder may metastasize to bone. Hyperparathyroidism leads to bone decalcification and osteoporosis. Hormone imbalance can result in postmenopausal osteoporosis.

During the *activities of daily living* portion of the history, ask your patient if he's decreased his activities recently. *Inactivity* increases the risk of osteoporosis. Also ask your patient to describe his usual *diet.* Elderly persons often have an inadequate calcium intake, which can cause osteoporosis and muscle weakness.

702 Physical examination findings

Your examination of an elderly patient with a suspected musculoskeletal disorder is the same as for a younger adult. But older patients may need more time or assistance with such tests as range of motion or gait assessment, because of muscle weakness and decreased coordination. Disorders of motor and sensory function—manifested by muscle weakness, spasticity, tremors, rigidity, and various types of sensory disturbances—are common in the elderly. Damaging falls may result from difficulty in maintaining equilibrium and from uncertain gait. Be sure to differentiate gait changes caused by joint disability, pain, or stiffness from those caused by neurologic impairment or another disorder. Bone softening from demineralization (senile osteoporosis) causes abnormal susceptibility to major fractures. Most patients over age 60 have some degree of degenerative joint disease, which causes joint pain and limits spinal motion.

Selected References

Alexander, Mary M., and Brown, Marie Scott. *Pediatric History Taking and Physical Diagnosis for Nurses,* 2nd ed. New York: McGraw-Hill Book Co., 1979.

Bates, Barbara. *A Guide to Physical Examination,* 2nd ed. Philadelphia: J.B. Lippincott Co., 1979.

Brashear, H. Robert, and Raney, R. Beverly. *Shand's Handbook of Orthopaedic Surgery,* 9th ed. St. Louis: C.V. Mosby Co., 1978.

Burns, Kenneth R., and Johnson, Patricia J. *Health Assessment in Clinical Practice.* Englewood Cliffs, N.J.: Prentice-Hall, Inc., 1980.

Cohen, Stephen, and Viellion, Gigi. "Patient Assessment: Examining Joints of the Upper and Lower Extremities," *American Journal of Nursing* 81:763, April 1981.

DeGowin, Elmer L., and DeGowin, Richard L. *Bedside Diagnostic Examination,* 3rd ed. New York: Macmillan Publishing Co., 1976.

Feldman, Frieda. *Radiology, Pathology, and Immunology of Bones and Joints.* New York: Appleton-Century-Crofts, 1978.

Harrison's Principles of Internal Medicine. New York: McGraw-Hill Book Co., 1980.

Hilt, Nancy E., and Cogburn, Shirley B. *Manual of Orthopedics.* St. Louis: C.V. Mosby Co., 1980.

Hilt, Nancy E., and Schmitt, E. William, Jr. *Pediatric Orthopedic Nursing.* St. Louis: C.V. Mosby Co., 1975.

Iversen, Larry D., and Clawson, D. Kay. *Manual of Acute Orthopaedic Therapeutics.* Boston: Little, Brown & Co., 1977.

Judge, Richard D., and Zuidema, George D., eds. *Methods of Clinical Examination: A Physiologic Approach.* Boston: Little, Brown & Co., 1974.

Krupp, Marcus A., and Chatton, Milton J., eds. *Current Medical Diagnosis and Treatment,* rev. ed. Los Altos, Calif.: Lange Medical Publications, 1980.

Malasanos, Lois, et al. *Health Assessment,* 2nd ed. St. Louis: C.V. Mosby Co., 1981.

O'Connor, Richard L. *Arthroscopy.* Philadelphia: J.B. Lippincott Co., 1977.

Watanabe, M., et al. *Atlas of Arthroscopy,* 3rd ed. New York: Springer-Verlag, 1979.

17

KEY POINTS IN THIS CHAPTER

KEY CHARTS IN THIS CHAPTER

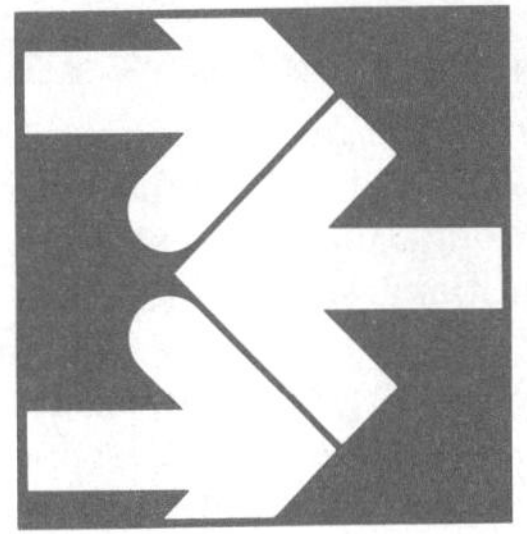

Blood-forming and Immune Systems

Introduction

703 These systems' challenges

Most systems of the body are composed of groups of organs. In contrast, the blood-forming system is made up of bone marrow and blood cells. The immune system is made up primarily of billions of cells that circulate throughout the cardiovascular system, as well as other structures—such as lymph nodes—distributed throughout the body. This means that the blood-forming and immune systems can directly affect—and are affected by—every organ system. Although some blood-forming and immune disorders cause hallmark signs and symptoms (such as the butterfly rash of systemic lupus erythematosus or the plethora of polycythemia), detecting other problems in these systems can provide you with a real challenge.

You'll want to be especially careful and thorough when taking your patient's history, because nonspecific symptoms from blood-forming and immune disorders can appear in any body system. A complete patient history may suggest a pattern that will lead you to suspect a blood-forming or immune disorder. An example might be a patient's chief complaint of shortness of breath. Without the complete history, you might simply examine the patient's respiratory or cardiovascular system and overlook the possibility that anemia is his primary problem.

Study of the immune system—the body's defense mechanism against disease processes and traumatic events—is one of the most rapidly growing areas in medicine. The past 20 years have produced significant advances in our understanding of this complex mechanism, but much remains unclear. We know, for example, that alterations in immunity occur in such disorders as allergies and primary immunodeficiencies. But in such disorders as rheumatoid arthritis, scleroderma, and systemic lupus erythematosus, the origins and significance of the alterations in immunity are unknown, although theories abound.

Here's a question that continues to intrigue researchers: Why, in certain disorders, does the body produce antibodies against its own tissue proteins? Study of these autoantibodies' development has become one of the last frontiers in our knowledge of the human body. The answers to this question will give us information about recognized autoimmune disorders, such as rheumatoid arthritis and systemic lupus erythematosus, and may also reveal the origins of such disorders as myasthenia gravis, diabetes mellitus, and cancer. The answers may even reveal the origins of the aging process.

Reviewing anatomy and physiology

704 Blood: Functions and components

Blood continuously circulates through the cardiovascular system, performing many essential functions. It transports oxygen, carbon dioxide, hormones, and enzymes to and from body cells. Blood also maintains homeostasis (by regulating fluid volume, pH, and body temperature) and provides protection against injurious agents by transporting important factors to the injury site and initiating vascular changes to concentrate and release them.

Circulating components of the blood-clotting mechanism prevent blood loss. Without these components, the slightest injury could result in fatal hemorrhage.

The major components of blood are *plasma* and the *formed elements.* Plasma is the liquid intercellular component that constitutes a little more than half of total blood volume. It carries formed elements—erythrocytes (red blood cells), leukocytes (white blood cells), and platelets (thrombocytes)—through the cardiovascular system. Of the three, erythrocytes far outnumber the other two. The ratio of erythrocytes to leukocytes, for example, is about 1,000:1.

705 Erythrocytes

Erythrocytes (red blood cells, or RBCs) are part of the blood-forming system. They are formed through a process called *erythropoiesis.* In the fetus, erythropoiesis starts in the yolk sac at about the third week. This process is gradually taken over by the liver and spleen and—after the 20th week of gestation—the red bone marrow. In an adult, erythrocyte production takes place only in the marrow of the ribs, sternum, iliac crest, cranium, and (to a lesser extent) vertebral bodies. However, the rest of the bone marrow retains its ability to form erythrocytes and will produce them in extremely stressful conditions, such as blood dyscrasias.

The genesis of an erythrocyte occurs when the stem cell or hemocytoblast produces a daughter cell that differentiates into an erythroblast, which eventually synthesizes hemoglobin. As the hemoglobin concentration increases, the immature RBC nucleus grows smaller and is eventually pushed out of the cell. The cell continues to develop into an erythrocyte, which enters the capillaries from the bone marrow.

The mature erythrocyte is a biconcave disk about 7.7 microns in diameter, with a life span of about 120 days. Erythropoiesis keeps the erythrocyte count high enough for adequate oxygen supply and low enough for unimpaired blood flow. This steady production of mature erythrocytes requires various nutritional substances, such as iron, vitamin B_{12}, folic acid, and amino acids.

The primary function of erythrocytes is to carry hemoglobin, which transports oxygen from the lungs to body tissues. Hemoglobin also transports carbon dioxide and water from the cells to the lungs. The erythrocytes act as an acid-base buffer. (Hemoglobin and the erythrocytes are buffering compounds that help keep the pH of the blood within the appropriate range, 7.35 to 7.45.) When an erythrocyte reaches the end of its life span, reticuloendothelial cells break down its hemoglobin into iron, globin, and the bile pigment bilirubin. Most of the iron is returned to the bone marrow for new hemoglobin formation. Iron in excess of the need for new red blood cells is stored as either hemoglobin or hemosiderin in the cells of the reticuloendothelial system. The globin's amino acids are used in protein synthesis, and the bilirubin is excreted, primarily in bile.

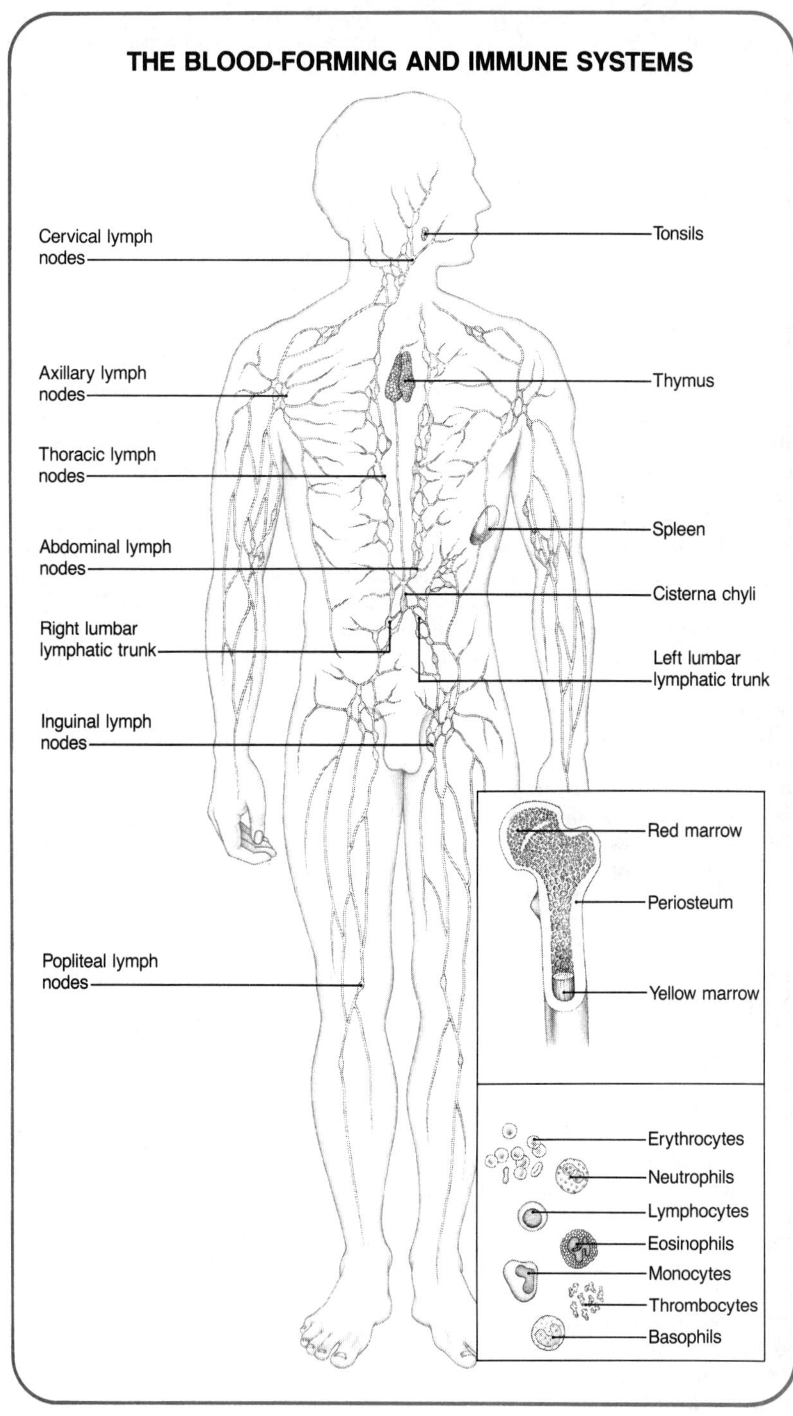
THE BLOOD-FORMING AND IMMUNE SYSTEMS
Cervical lymph nodes
Tonsils
Axillary lymph nodes
Thymus
Thoracic lymph nodes
Spleen
Abdominal lymph nodes
Cisterna chyli
Right lumbar lymphatic trunk
Left lumbar lymphatic trunk
Inguinal lymph nodes
Popliteal lymph nodes
Red marrow
Periosteum
Yellow marrow
Erythrocytes
Neutrophils
Lymphocytes
Eosinophils
Monocytes
Thrombocytes
Basophils

706 Leukocytes

Leukocytes (white blood cells, or WBCs) are nucleated cells derived from stem cells. Unlike erythrocytes, leukocytes contain no hemoglobin. Leukocytes are a functional part of the immune system and fall into two categories: *granulocytes* (also called *polymorphonuclear leukocytes* or *PMNs*) and *nongranulocytes.* Granulocytes in turn are divided into neutrophils, eosinophils, and basophils. Nongranulocytes are divided into lymphocytes and monocytes.

The primary function of PMNs is to protect the body from invading agents. In the inflammatory process, an injury causing inflammation first triggers the release of histamine into the surrounding fluid. This causes both increased blood flow to the injury site and greater capillary permeability, which allows large amounts of fluid and protein to leak into the tissues. The extracellular area then becomes edematous. Neutrophils and, later, monocytes migrate through the capillary walls into the affected tissue. Then the neutrophils and large monocytes begin engulfing bacteria and necrotic tissue (phagocytosis). After this role is completed, the involved leukocytes die.

After several days of this process, a cavity forms in the inflamed area, and necrotic tissue, dead neutrophils, and macrophages form pus.

707 Platelets

Platelets (thrombocytes), anuclear circulating fragments of the megakaryocyte (a very large cell derived from the undifferentiated stem cell) with a life span of only about 10 days, release clotting factors to induce coagulation (see *Understanding Blood Clot Formation*). Blood vessel injury triggers the release of *serotonin,* a vasoconstrictor that reduces blood flow and facilitates hemostasis. Platelets then begin adhering to the wound site and releasing their clotting factors, leading to the formation of fibrin strands. These strands trap erythrocytes, forming a clot. Platelets also aid in clot retraction and induce vascular contraction.

708 Lymphatic system

The lymphatic system consists of capillaries, vessels, ducts, and nodes. Its primary functions are to drain tissue fluid and to carry proteins and large particulate matter from the tissue spaces into the circulatory system.

The lymphatic capillaries carry *lymph*—a fluid containing proteins, leukocytes, and a few platelets and erythrocytes—from tissue spaces to the lymphatic vessels. The three major lymphatic vessels are the *left lumbar, right lumbar,* and *intestinal* trunks. The left and right lumbar trunks carry lymph from the legs, pelvis, kidneys, adrenals, and deep abdomen. The intestinal trunk carries lymph from the stomach, spleen, liver, and small intestine. These vessels, which are similar to the veins, contain valves that permit lymph flow in one direction only—toward the thoracic cavity, where the two lymphatic ducts (the right lymphatic and the thoracic) are located.

The *right lymphatic* duct joins the venous system at the junction of the right internal jugular and subclavian veins. This duct drains lymph from the right side of the liver's upper lobe; the right lung and pleura; the right side of the heart, head, and neck; and the right arm. The *thoracic* duct originates in the abdomen at the cisterna chyli, a sac beneath the diaphragm that receives lymph from the major lymphatic vessels. This duct enters the circulatory system where the left internal jugular joins the subclavian vein. It drains lymph from the legs; the abdomen; the left side of the thorax, head, and neck; and the left arm.

Lymph nodes are small oval bodies located along the course of the lymphatic vessels. Consisting of lymphatic tissue enclosed by connective tissue, these nodes—both deep and superficial—appear in clusters. They produce

UNDERSTANDING BLOOD CLOT FORMATION

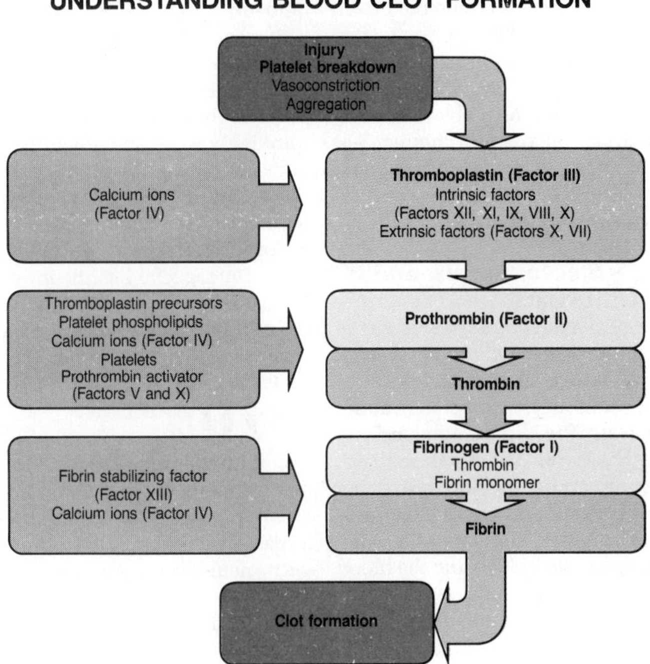

Basically, blood clot formation occurs in three steps:

1 A vascular injury triggers smooth muscle spasm; serotonin, epinephrine, and lipoprotein are released, and blood vessels contract. Together, these events constitute vasoconstriction.

Next, platelets come into contact with the ruptured vessel wall or traumatized blood. They secrete adenosine diphosphate, which causes the platelets to break down, become sticky, and form what's called a platelet plug. This plug prevents further blood loss from the wound.

Then, the platelets and the injured tissue, in the presence of calcium ions (Factor IV), activate the thromboplastin. Thromboplastin precursors, platelet phospholipids, calcium ions, and prothrombin activators (Factors V and X) all must be present for thromboplastin to initiate the next step—the conversion of prothrombin.

2 For blood to coagulate, either an *extrinsic* mechanism (an injury to a blood vessel or outside tissue) or an *intrinsic* mechanism (trauma within the blood itself) must be activated. As you can see from the above flowchart, each mechanism's action involves specific factors in clot formation.

Plasma coagulation factors (by way of either intrinsic or extrinsic pathways) activate prothrombin activator to convert prothrombin to thrombin. If an extrinsic mechanism's activated, Factors X, VII, and V are released. If an intrinsic mechanism's activated, Factors XII, XI, IX, VIII, X, and V are released.

3 Thrombin acts progressively on fibrinogen, forming a fibrin monomer. This monomer forms into long fibrin threads, too weak by themselves to hold the clot. Thrombin then acts on a substance, fibrin stabilizing factor (Factor XIII), which in the presence of calcium ions forms strong fibrin threads that cross-link. In this fibrin mesh, erythrocytes, platelets, and plasma attach—and a stable clot is formed.

lymphocytes (which help produce immunity to diseases and transplanted tissue) and release them into the blood; lymph nodes also filter products from inflammatory and malignant lesions.

Because the lymphatic system lacks a contractile apparatus, lymph movement depends on such mechanisms as massage from arteries and skeletal muscles; intestinal peristalsis; and respiratory pressure changes.

709 Spleen, tonsils, and thymus

The spleen, tonsils, and thymus aid in the function of the lymphatic system. The *spleen* is an oval, soft, and vascular organ, located in the upper left abdomen beneath the diaphragm and behind the lower ribs and costal cartilage. Its many functions include destroying old erythrocytes and producing antibodies. The spleen also acts as a blood reservoir and filter, cleansing the blood of microorganisms.

The *tonsils*—palatine, adenoid, and lingual—provide a protective barrier for the mouth, throat, larynx, trachea, and lungs (see *Anatomy of the Tonsils*). Composed of lymphoid tissue, the tonsils also aid in the development of immune bodies.

The two-lobed *thymus*—a flat, pinkish-gray gland—lies in the chest anterior to the aorta and posterior to the sternum. It is where *T lymphocytes,* which are primarily important in the delayed hypersensitivity reaction, mature. During fetal life, the thymus serves as the primary source of lymphocytes. After birth, its growth slows, and atrophy occurs by adulthood.

710 Immunity

Immunity, innate or acquired, is the body's capacity to prevent tissue and organ damage by resisting invading organisms and toxins. *Innate immunity* includes phagocytosis of bacteria by leukocytes and reticuloendothelial cells, skin resistance to invading or-

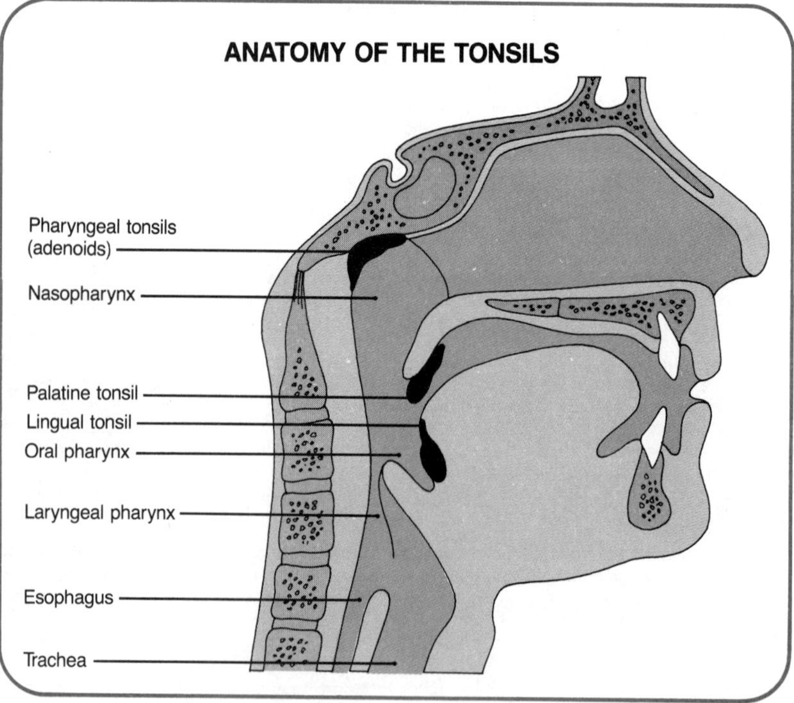

ganisms, and the destruction of organisms by acids secreted in the stomach and by chemicals in the blood.

Antibodies with the ability to bind antigens are known as *immunoglobulins*. These are divided into five classes, based on their individual structures and functions. The symbol for immunoglobulins is *Ig*, and each class is designated by a letter—IgA, IgD, IgE, IgG, and IgM.

Acquired immunity can be humoral or cellular. In *humoral immunity*, the antibodies are specific to an antigen. The stem cells develop into the lymphocytes (immature B cells). These migrate to the lymph nodes, liver, and spleen. They bind with an antigen, and their antibodies become specific for that antigen. Activated B cells form clones with two cell lines. Some become plasma cells and are secreted into the blood to fight the antigen through the release of their surface antibodies. Some (memory cells) are stored in the lymph nodes for future use. When the same antigen is again encountered, the memory cells activate.

Cellular immunity refers to the production and release of T lymphocytes sensitized to a specific foreign substance or antigen. In cellular immunity, stem cells from the embryonic yolk sac seed the thymus and develop into T cells. T cells migrate to the lymph nodes, where they may come in contact with an antigen that they can bind with, thus becoming sensitized T cells. Some T cells kill the invading cell directly by releasing a lymphotoxin (a poison) against the cell. Other T cells attract macrophages into the area and promote the phagocytosis of the invading cell.

When antibodies bind with a specific antigen, they form the *antigen-antibody complex*. This complex renders the antigen harmless. This may occur in any of several different ways:

- If the antigen is a toxin, the antigen-antibody complex neutralizes it.
- The antigen-antibody complex can cause agglutination of invader cells.

UNDERSTANDING BLOOD GROUP COMPATIBILITIES

In blood transfusions, the donor's blood must be compatible with the recipient's blood. If it isn't, the results can be fatal. That's why precise blood typing and cross-matching are essential. Use this chart as a guide when determining blood group compatibility.

RECIPIENT	COMPATIBLE BLOOD GROUP
A	A, O
B	B, O
AB	A, B, AB, O
O	O

- The antigen-antibody complex can change the shape of the antibody slightly to expose complement-binding sites. These initiate activity that releases enzymes, which destroy the invading cells.

Acquired immunity can be broken down into types that include:

- *active immunity*—antibody production by the body in response to vaccination or the contraction of a disease
- *passive immunity*—injection of an antibody into the body from another person or animal, for example, a tetanus toxoid
- *passive-active immunity*—antibody and antigen injection that triggers antibody production
- *active-passive immunity*—antibody injection during antigen exposure to reduce severity (for instance, a gamma globulin injection).

711 Blood groups

Erythrocytes contain genetically determined antigens (*agglutinogens*) on their surface. The presence or absence of the agglutinogens determines the classification of the A-B-O blood groups. Each person has one of four possible blood groups: A only, B only, A and B, or neither A nor B. Between ages 2 and 8 months, a person develops antibodies in his plasma (called *agglutinins*), which correspond to the agglutinogen not present in his blood (see *Understanding Blood Group Compatibilities,* page 681).

Before a transfusion, donor and recipient blood must be typed and crossmatched. If the two types of blood aren't compatible, the red blood cells agglutinate and the procedure can be fatal to the recipient. For instance, a person with type A blood can't receive type B, because type A contains the agglutinin anti-B. Type O blood is called the *universal donor* because it contains no agglutinogens; type AB is the *universal recipient* because it has no antibodies.

The Rh system consists of eight genotypes of Rh antigens, called *Rh factor,* which are divided into two blood groups: Rh positive and Rh negative. *Rh positive* indicates blood with the Rh antigen on the erythrocytes; *Rh negative* blood has no antigen. When Rh positive blood is transfused into an Rh negative person, anti-Rh antibodies will develop (the recipient becomes immunized). Subsequent transfusions with Rh positive blood will lead to a transfusion reaction (agglutination of the donor blood by the recipient's blood).

Additional genetic variations exist that produce antigens—examples are M, N, Lewis, and Hr. Transfusion reactions from these antigens rarely occur, except in individuals who receive transfusions frequently.

Collecting appropriate history data

712 Biographical data

Biographical information—particularly *age, sex, race,* and *ethnic background*—will assist you in your assessment, because some blood-forming and immune conditions occur more frequently in certain groups of people than in others. For instance, certain autoimmune diseases appear more often in women—especially young women—than in men. Sickle cell anemia occurs primarily in blacks and less frequently in Mediterranean, Middle Eastern, and Asian peoples. Pernicious anemia occurs most frequently in Northern Europeans.

713 Chief complaint

The most common chief complaints regarding blood-forming and immune disorders are *abnormal bleeding, lymphadenopathy, fatigue and weakness, fever,* and *joint pain.*

714 History of present illness

Using the PQRST mnemonic device, ask your patient to elaborate on his chief complaint. Then, depending on the chief complaint, explore the history of the patient's present illness by asking him the following types of questions:

• ***Abnormal bleeding.*** *Have you experienced any unusual blood loss? For instance, have you passed black stool, bloody urine, or unusually heavy menses?* Excessive blood loss may result in anemia. *Do you have frequent nosebleeds? Do you frequently notice bruises on your skin but can't recall their cause?* A platelet or clotting mechanism deficiency can result in bruises from minimal pressure or slight bumps. *Do you bleed for a long time when you cut your finger or have your teeth cleaned?* Such excessive bleeding suggests a defective clotting mechanism. *Do you start bleeding for no apparent reason? Does bleeding after injury start slowly and last a long time?* All these

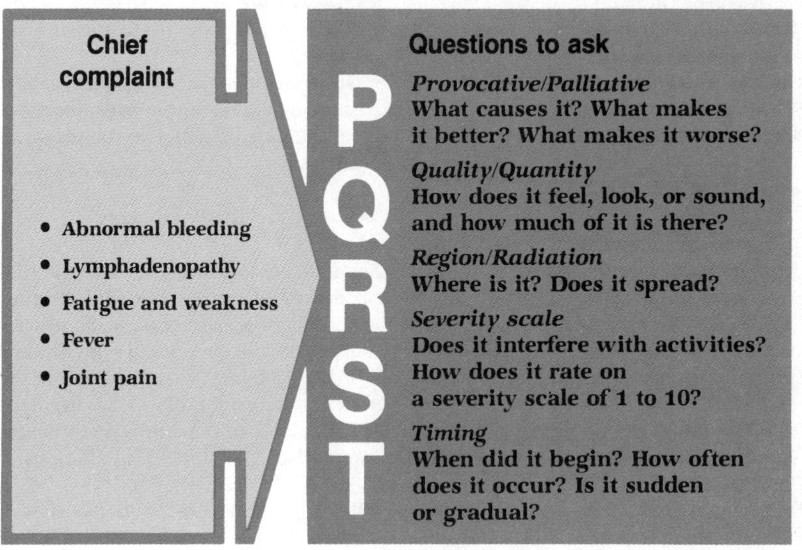

signs and symptoms are indicative of vascular, platelet, or coagulation disorders.

• ***Lymphadenopathy.*** *Do you have swelling in your neck, armpit, or groin? Are the swollen areas sore, hard, or red? When did you first notice the swelling? Is it on one side, or both?* Enlarged lymph nodes may indicate an inflammatory process, an infection, or the elevated lymphocyte production characteristic of certain leukemias. Enlargement from a primary lymphatic tumor usually isn't painful. Hodgkin's disease, however, may be accompanied by red, tender, enlarged lymph nodes. A large mass may indicate a lymphoma. Ask if a biopsy has ever been done on one of these lymph nodes. This may indicate a previously diagnosed malignancy.

• ***Fatigue and weakness.*** *Do you feel tired all the time, or only during exertion? Do you nap during the day? How many hours do you sleep at night? Are you experiencing weakness? Is the weakness more noticeable on one side? Is it adjacent to joints? Did it develop gradually? Is the weakness persistent? Were you ever told you were anemic?* Fatigue and weakness on exertion can suggest moderate anemia; extreme or constant fatigue and weakness can occur in a patient with severe anemia (or with neuropathy from an autoimmune disease).

• ***Fever.*** *How long have you had a fever? Does your temperature drop to normal at all during the day?* Intermittent fevers occur with lymphomas. *Do you have periods of fever alternating with periods of normal temperature?* (Recurrent fever occurs in Hodgkin's disease.) *Do you have frequent fevers?* Fever from frequent infections may suggest a poorly functioning immune system. It may also suggest rapid cell proliferation. *Do you perspire excessively with the fever? When you look in the mirror, does your face appear flushed?* These symptoms usually accompany an infection.

• ***Joint pain.*** *Do you have joint pain? Which joints are affected? Did the joint pain occur in several joints at the same time? Did it affect additional joints? Did swelling, redness, or warmth appear with the pain? Are the joints painful when you're resting? Do you have early-morning stiffness?* Pain in the knees, wrists, or hands may indicate an autoimmune process or hemarthrosis from a blood disorder. *Do your bones ache?* Aching bones may result from the pressure of expanding bone marrow. *How do you relieve the pain?* Heat application or salicylates relieve pain from an inflammatory process.

715 Past history

Focus on the following relevant medical conditions when reviewing your patient's past history:

- ***Surgery.*** *Gastric surgery* decreases the level of instrinsic factor needed for vitamin B_{12} absorption. *Bilateral nephrectomy* may produce a diminished erythropoietin level. *Hepatic surgery* may reduce the formation of coagulation factors.
- ***Sore throats.*** Frequent sore throats may indicate poor resistance to infection.
- ***Blood donation refusals.*** A patient rejected as a blood donor may have long-standing anemia or a history of hepatitis or of jaundice with an undetermined cause.
- ***Blood transfusions.*** A history of blood transfusions may give you a clue to anemia. Try to determine the reason for the transfusions, how many units were given, and the patient's reaction, if any.
- ***Autoimmune diseases.*** The presence of one autoimmune disease can predispose a person to others.
- ***Immunizations.*** A history of the patient's immunizations is essential.
- ***Allergies.*** Ask the patient about known allergies to such substances as foods, drugs, insects, or environmental pollutants. Multiple allergies are common.
- ***Asthma.*** A history of asthma may indicate immunopathology.
- ***Radiation therapy.*** Radiation therapy can cause decreased blood cell production.
- ***Medications.*** A history of taking prescribed medications may indicate previous immune and blood-forming disorders. Also, note that certain drugs can produce side effects in the blood-forming and immune systems (see *Nurse's Guide to Some Drugs That Affect the Blood-forming and Immune Systems*).
- ***Gastrointestinal.*** A patient's past history of peptic ulcer with excessive bleeding may be a clue to the presence of anemia.

716 Family history

Some blood-forming and immune disorders demonstrate familial tendencies. Others are hereditary. So always determine if your patient's family has a history of anemias, cancers in the system, abnormal bleeding problems (particularly in male relatives), or immune disorders, including allergies.

717 Psychosocial history

Increased *stress* may reduce a patient's resistance to infection and can trigger an autoimmune disease. *Exposure to chemicals*—such as industrial cleaning fluids, glues used in some hobbies, or insecticides used in gardening or farming—may cause blood dyscrasias.

718 Activities of daily living

When recording your patient's activities of daily living, focus on his *diet* (see Entry 173). Specifically, determine his typical daily diet and inquire about idiosyncratic, religious, or cultural dietary restrictions. Also, ask about recent significant dietary changes and weight loss.

Poor nutrition can greatly affect a person's immune system. For example, a severely protein-deficient diet can result in lymphoid tissue atrophy, diminished antibody response, fewer circulating T cells, and impaired cellular immunity. Although infection increases the need for nutrients and caloric intake, it may paradoxically cause anorexia. Also ask about the patient's alcohol consumption. If it's excessive, he may have nutritional deficits. Ask, too, about exercise and rest patterns. Problems associated with these daily

NURSE'S GUIDE TO SOME DRUGS THAT AFFECT THE BLOOD-FORMING AND IMMUNE SYSTEMS

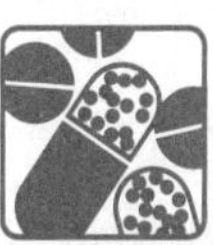

CLASSIFICATION	POSSIBLE SIDE EFFECTS
Antiarrhythmics	
procainamide hydrochloride (Pronestyl*)	• Thrombocytopenia, agranulocytosis, hemolytic anemia, increased ANA titer
propranolol hydrochloride (Inderal*)	• Eosinophilia, thrombocytopenia, agranulocytosis
Anticonvulsants	
carbamazepine (Tegretol)	• Aplastic anemia, agranulocytosis, eosinophilia, leukocytosis, thrombocytopenia
mephenytoin (Mesantoin*)	• Leukopenia, neutropenia, agranulocytosis, thrombocytopenia, pancytopenia, eosinophilia
phenytoin (Dilantin*)	• Thrombocytopenia, leukopenia, agranulocytosis, pancytopenia, lymphadenopathy, megaloblastic anemia
Antidepressants	
imipramine hydrochloride (Tofranil*)	• Agranulocytosis, thrombocytopenia, eosinophilia
Antidiabetic agents	
chlorpropamide (Diabinese*)	• Bone marrow aplasia
Antihypertensives	
methyldopa (Aldomet*)	• Hemolytic anemia, reversible granulocytopenia, thrombocytopenia
Alkylating agents	
chlorambucil (Leukeran)	• Leukopenia, thrombocytopenia, anemia, myelosuppression
cyclophosphamide (Cytoxan*)	• Leukopenia, thrombocytopenia, anemia
Vinca alkaloids	
vincristine sulfate (Oncovin*)	• Mild anemia, leukopenia, thrombocytopenia
Antipsychotics	
chlorpromazine hydrochloride (Chlorprom**, Thorazine)	• Transient leukopenia, agranulocytosis
Diuretics	
furosemide (Lasix*) hydrochlorothiazide (Hydro-diuril*)	• Leukopenia, aplastic anemia, thrombocytopenia, agranulocytosis
Nonsteroidal anti-inflammatory agents	
indomethacin (Indocid**, Indocin)	• Hemolytic anemia, aplastic anemia, agranulocytosis, leukopenia, thrombocytopenic purpura, iron deficiency anemia
oxyphenbutazone (Oxalid, Tandearil) phenylbutazone (Butazolidin*)	• Fatal aplastic anemia, agranulocytosis, leukopenia, thrombocytopenia, hemolytic anemia
Uncategorized drugs	
levodopa (Levopa*)	• Hemolytic anemia

*Available in U.S. and Canada. **Available in Canada only. All other products (no symbol) available in U.S. only.

activities may give you a clue to a blood-forming or immune disorder.

719 Review of systems

• ***General.*** *Frequent illness* suggests immunologic problems.

• ***Skin.*** An anemic patient may have pale, sallow, or clammy skin. Anemia can also cause nail changes (brittleness, ridges, flattening). Subcutaneous nodules may indicate an autoimmune disorder. Characteristic skin rashes, such as the butterfly rash of systemic lupus erythematosus, accompany some autoimmune disorders.

• ***Eyes.*** *Keratitis* and *retinal hemorrhages* may be present in patients with clotting and autoimmune disorders.

• ***Mouth.*** A *sore throat, a sore and burning tongue, dysarthria,* or *dysphagia* suggests (among other things) infection or inflammation. Mouth ulcers may indicate anemia or an immune disorder.

• ***Cardiovascular.*** *Tachycardia* may result from the blood's reduced ability to carry oxygen.

• ***Respiratory.*** *Wheezing* or *rhinitis* can indicate an allergic response. *Dyspnea* or *orthopnea* may suggest anemia or connective tissue disease.

• ***Genitourinary.*** Hematuria can occur in some anemias and in advanced autoimmune disease. Pernicious anemia can cause *incontinence* and *impotence.*

• ***Gastrointestinal.*** *Nausea* or *appetite loss* may result from infection, an inflammatory process, or advanced autoimmune disease.

• ***Neurologic.*** If the patient has difficulty walking or experiences a *pins-and-needles* sensation, he may have a vitamin B_{12} deficiency, resulting in pernicious anemia. Central nervous system complications of systemic lupus erythematosus may cause emotional instability, headaches, irritability, and depression.

Conducting the physical examination

720 Preparations

During the physical examination, your patient will alternate between sitting and lying down, so adjust the examining table to an appropriate height for both positions. Ensure proper lighting for skin inspection—a key part of blood-forming and immune assessment (see Entry 223). Remember, if lighting produces a glare, you may not be able to detect subtle color changes. Before starting the examination, give your patient the opportunity to urinate, because you'll be doing deep abdominal palpation.

Be sure to explain the purpose of the examination to the patient, and tell him what you'll be doing before starting each procedure. Have the necessary equipment ready—stethoscope, sphygmomanometer, ophthalmoscope, scale, and measuring tape.

721 General physical status

Because signs and symptoms of blood-forming and immune disorders are often nonspecific, a thorough observation of your patient's general physical status is essential (see Entry 67). Inspect his general appearance and note if he looks acutely ill. Observe his face for flushing, profuse perspiration, or grimacing (as if he's in pain). Then observe for indications of chronic illness, including dehydration, pallor, emaciation, and listlessness.

Does your patient look his stated age? Chronic disease and nutritional deficiencies associated with blood-forming and immune problems may make a patient look older than he is.

Next, weigh the patient and measure his height. Compare his weight to the

TESTS FOR BLOOD COMPOSITION, PRODUCTION, AND FUNCTION

Overall composition

- *Peripheral blood smear* shows maturity and morphologic characteristics of blood elements and determines qualitative abnormalities.
- *Complete blood count (CBC)* determines the actual number of blood elements in relation to volume and quantifies abnormalities.
- *Bone marrow aspiration* or *biopsy* allows evaluation of hematopoiesis by showing blood elements and precursors, and abnormal or malignant cells.

RBC function

- *Hematocrit (HCT)* (packed cell volume) measures the percentage of RBCs per fluid volume of whole blood.
- *Hemoglobin (Hgb)* measures the amount (grams) of hemoglobin per 100 ml of blood, to determine oxygen-carrying capacity.
- *Reticulocyte count* allows assessment of RBC production by determining concentration of this early erythrocyte precursor.
- *Schilling test* determines absorption of vitamin B_{12} (necessary for erythropoiesis) by measuring excretion of radioactive B_{12} in the urine.
- *Mean corpuscular volume (MCV)* describes the red cell in terms of size.
- *Mean corpuscular hemoglobin (MCH)* determines average amount of hemoglobin per RBC.
- *Mean corpuscular hemoglobin concentration (MCHC)* establishes average hemoglobin concentration in 100 ml of packed RBCs.
- *Serum bilirubin* measures liver function and extravascular RBC hemolysis.
- *Sugar-water test* assesses the susceptibility of RBCs to hemolyze with complement.
- *Direct Coombs' test* demonstrates the presence of IgG antibodies (such as antibodies to Rh factor) and/or complement on circulating RBCs.
- *Indirect Coombs' test*, a two-step test, detects the presence of IgG antibodies on RBCs in the serum.
- *Sideroblast test* detects stainable iron (available for hemoglobin synthesis) in normoblastic RBCs.

Hemostasis

- *Platelet count* determines number of platelets.
- *Prothrombin time (Quick's test, pro time, PT)* aids evaluation of thrombin generation (extrinsic clotting mechanism).
- *Partial thromboplastin time (PTT)* aids evaluation of the adequacy of plasma-clotting factors (intrinsic clotting mechanism).
- *Thrombin time* detects abnormalities in thrombin fibrinogen reaction.
- *Activated partial thromboplastin time (APTT)* aids assessment of plasma-clotting factors (except factors VII and XIII) in the intrinsic clotting mechanism.

WBC function

- *WBC count, differential* establishes quantity and maturity of WBC elements (neutrophils [called polymorphonuclear granulocytes or bands], basophils, eosinophils, lymphocytes, monocytes).

Plasma

- *Erythrocyte sedimentation rate (ESR)* measures rate of RBCs settling from plasma and may reflect infection.
- *Electrophoresis of serum proteins* determines amount of various serum proteins (classified by mobility in response to an electrical field).
- *Immunoelectrophoresis of serum proteins* separates and classifies serum antibodies (immunoglobins) through specific antisera.
- *Fibrinogen (Factor I)* measures this coagulation factor in plasma.

ideal for his height, bone structure, and build (see Entries 177, 179, 180, 182). Weight loss may result from anorexia and gastrointestinal problems associated with blood-forming or immune conditions. If your patient appears undernourished or cachectic (see Entry 184), assess him for chronic disease.

Next, inspect your patient for abnormal body posture, movements, or gait; these can indicate joint, spinal, or neurologic changes.

Finally, record your patient's vital signs (see Entry 68). Changes in blood pressure, pulse, and temperature may indicate infection, inflammation, elevated metabolic rate, or fluid and electrolyte disturbances—all possibly indicative of blood-forming or immune disorders.

722 General mental status

Observe your patient's behavior to assess his mood (see Entry 128). Of course, a chronically ill patient, regardless of the nature of his disorder, may be depressed or angry. But irritability, confusion, hallucinations, or other symptoms of psychosis (such as paranoid thinking) may occur with immune disorders, particularly systemic lupus erythematosus. Forgetfulness and sleeplessness may occur with anemia. Slowed responses or a poor attention span can result from either blood-forming or immune disorders.

723 Assessing skin color and integrity

Inspect your patient's skin color, noting any pallor, cyanosis, or jaundice (see Entry 224). Pallor can result from decreased hemoglobin content. Cyanosis suggests excessive deoxygenated hemoglobin in cutaneous blood vessels caused by hypoxia, which appears in some anemias. Cyanosis or pallor in a patient's fingers or toes may result from Raynaud's phenomenon, seen in some autoimmune diseases.

Examine the patient's face, conjunctivae, hands, and feet for ruddy cyanosis or plethora (red, florid complexion), which appear in polycythemia. Then, inspect for erythema, a possible sign of local inflammation or fever (see Entry 228).

Look for jaundice in the patient's sclerae, mucous membranes, and skin. For dark-skinned patients, also inspect the buccal mucosa, palms of the hands, and soles of the feet. For an edematous patient, examine the inner forearm for jaundice. An elevated bilirubin level may be secondary to increased erythrocyte hemolysis—a problem that may be hereditary or acquired. (Remember, excessive intake of carrots or yellow vegetables may cause yellow skin but will not cause color change in the sclerae or mucous membranes.)

If you suspect a clotting abnormality, inspect the patient's skin for purpuric lesions, which result most commonly from thrombocytopenia. These lesions can vary in size (see Entry 228). For dark-skinned patients, assess the oral mucosa or conjunctivae for petechiae or ecchymoses. As blood is reabsorbed, skin color changes from yellow to yellow green. (These two skin changes are difficult to detect in dark-skinned patients.) Also, inspect for such abnormalities as telangiectasias, and note their location.

Assess skin integrity, noting if the patient has any signs of infection, such as abnormal temperature, wound drainage, poor wound healing, or ulceration (see Entry 233). Check for rashes; among many possible causes, a rash can indicate autoimmune disease. Certain autoimmune diseases have uniquely characteristic rashes—the butterfly rash of systemic lupus erythematosus, the heliotrope rash of dermatomyositis. So be sure to note the rash's distribution.

724 Examining hair and nails

Inspect your patient's hair growth patterns, noting any alopecia on the arms, legs, or head (see Entry 229). Remember, alopecia patches may occur in systemic lupus erythematosus.

Inspect the patient's nails and note any abnormalities (see Entry 231). Specifically, note any longitudinal striation, which is associated with anemia, or koilonychia (also called *spoon nail*), which is characteristic of iron deficiency anemia. Look for platyonychia (abnormally broad or flat nails), which may precede development of koilonychia, and for onycholysis or loosening of the nails. Then, inspect for nail clubbing, indicative of chronic hypoxia—which can result from a blood-forming or immune disorder. (See *Understanding Nail Abnormalities,* pages 188 to 189.)

725 Assessing lymph nodes

Normally, you'll inspect and palpate

PALPATING NECK NODES

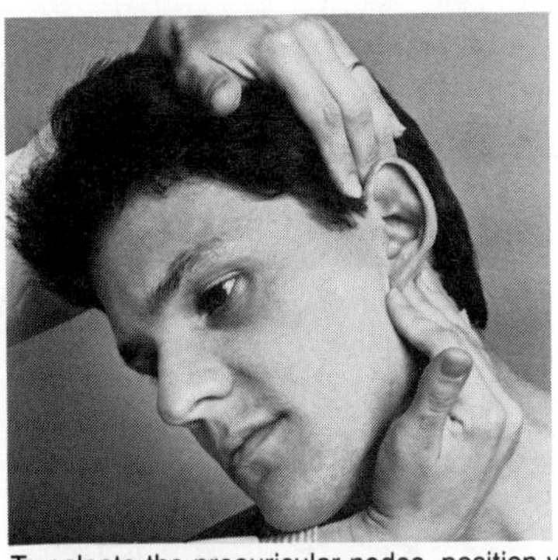

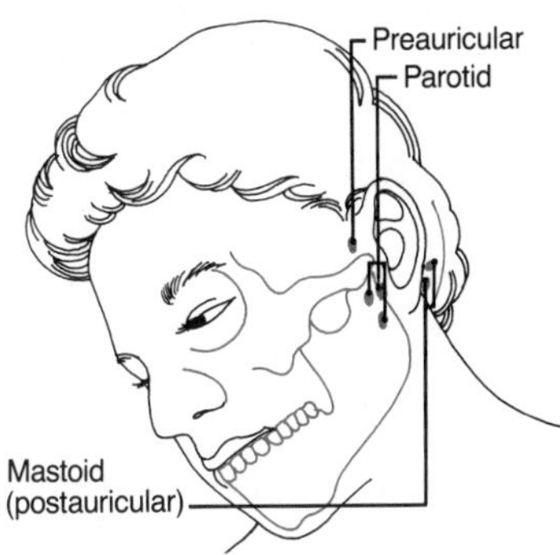

To palpate the preauricular nodes, position your fingers as shown here.

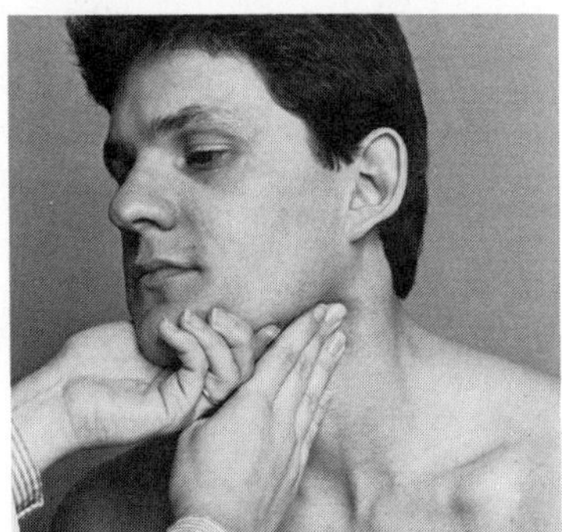

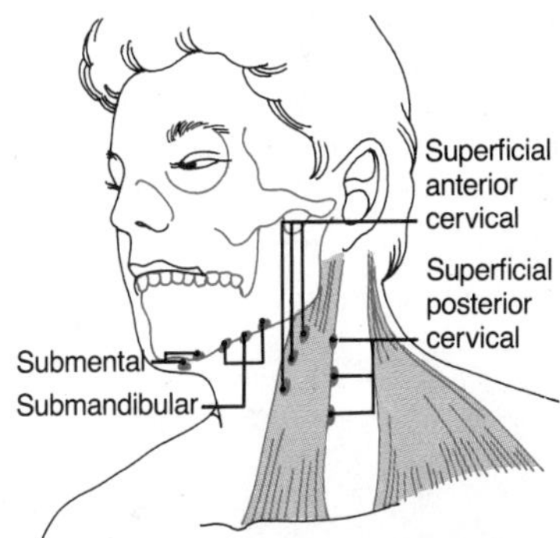

To palpate the submandibular, submental, and cervical nodes, position your fingers as shown here. Palpate over the mandibular surface and continue moving up and down the entire neck. You can flex the head forward or to the side being examined to relax the tissues and make enlarged nodes more palpable.

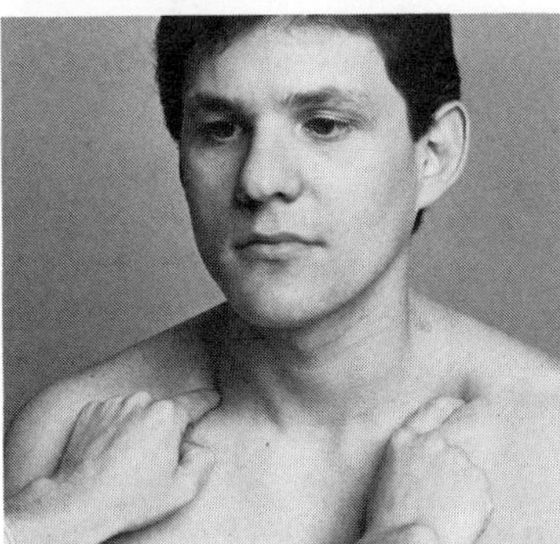

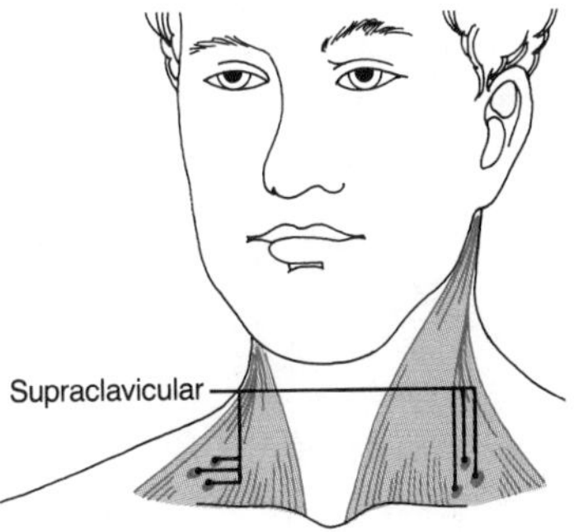

To palpate the supraclavicular nodes, first encourage your patient to relax, so his clavicles drop. Flex his head slightly forward with your free hand, to relax the soft tissues of his anterior neck. Then, hook your left index finger over the clavicle lateral to the sternocleidomastoid muscle. Rotate your finger deeply into this area to feel these nodes.

the patient's neck, axillary, epitrochlear, and inguinal lymph nodes as you examine the areas of the body. First inspect the skin over the nodes, noting any color abnormalities or obvious enlargements. Then palpate the nodes, using your finger pads to move skin over the area. (When you're palpating the nodes in the patient's neck, he should be sitting.) To palpate axillary nodes, the patient should remain sitting or be supine, with his right arm relaxed. Use your nondominant hand to support his right arm and put your other hand as high in his right axilla as possible. Palpate against the chest wall for the lateral, anterior, posterior, central, and subclavian nodes. Use the same procedure for the patient's left axilla. For the epitrochlear nodes, palpate the medial area of his elbow. For the inguinal nodes, palpate below the inguinal ligament and along the upper saphenous vein. As you palpate all nodes, note their size, consistency (hard or soft), and whether they're fixed or movable, tender or painless.

Red streaks in the skin, palpable nodes, and lymphedema may indicate a lymphatic disorder. Enlarged (palpable) nodes suggest current or previous inflammation. Nodes covered by red-streaked skin suggest acute lymphadenitis (you'll usually see an obvious infection site). Hard nodes may suggest a tumor. General lymphadenopathy can indicate an inflammatory or neoplastic process.

726 Examining your patient's eyes

Inspect your patient's eyelids for signs of infection or inflammation—such as edema, redness, or lesions (see Entry 266). Note the eyes' position and alignment, and check the conjunctivae for

PALPATING AXILLARY NODES

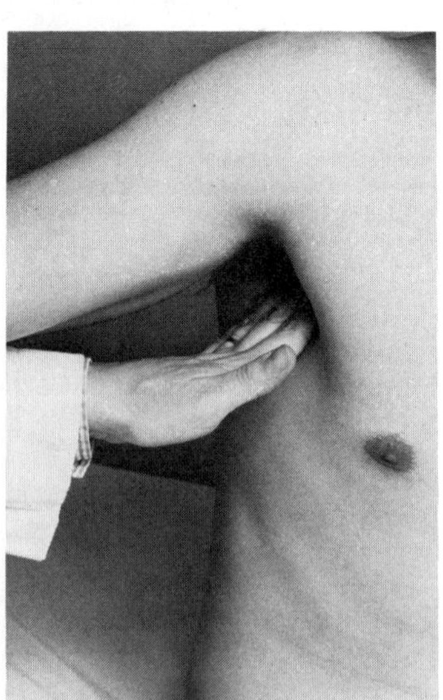

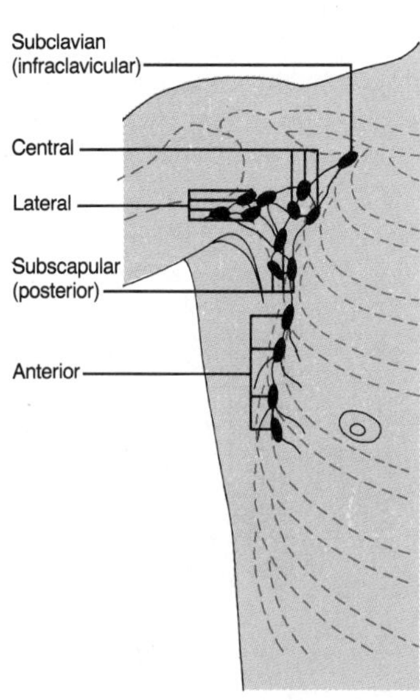

To palpate the axillary nodes, gently press the soft tissues against the chest wall and the muscles surrounding the axilla (the pectoral muscles, latissimus dorsi, subscapularis, and serratus anterior muscles).

engorged or enlarged vessels. (Keratoconjunctivitis, as well as iritis and scleritis, may accompany rheumatoid arthritis.) Then use the ophthalmoscope to examine the patient's retinas (see Entry 272). Vessel tortuosity may result from sickle cell anemia; hemorrhage or infiltration can suggest, among other possibilities, hemorrhagic leukemia, vasculitis, or thrombocytopenia.

727 Inspecting the mouth

Inspect your patient's buccal mucosa, lips, gums, teeth, tongue, and palate (see Entries 434 to 438). Red mucous membranes may result from polycythemia; an enlarged tongue from multiple myeloma (among other possible disorders); absence of papillae from pernicious anemia; and purpuras and telangiectasias from bleeding disorders. Tonsillar hypertrophy appears in lymphomas; gingival hypertrophy that makes teeth look sunken may result from myelogenous leukemia. (*Note:* These changes occur in chronic, not acute, neoplastic diseases.) Oral nasopharyngeal ulcers may accompany systemic lupus erythematosus.

728 Cardiovascular/respiratory assessment

Auscultate the patient's precordium for heart murmurs (see Entry 392). Ventricular enlargement and apical systolic murmurs may result from severe anemia. Mitral, aortic, and pulmonic murmurs can occur in sickle cell anemia. Tachycardia may also occur in some anemias. Congestive heart failure or pericardial effusions may develop in a patient with systemic lupus erythematosus or rheumatoid arthritis.

Next, inspect your patient's peripheral circulation. Raynaud's phenomenon may occur in some patients with autoimmune diseases.

Assess the patient's chest carefully (see Chapter 9, RESPIRATORY SYSTEM). First, note any signs of respiratory distress, particularly dyspnea, coughing, or cyanosis. These can be associated with a blood-forming or immune disorder. Auscultation may detect wheezing—a possible sign of allergy or asthma. Percussion and auscultation may reveal a pleural effusion; a patient with rheumatoid arthritis or systemic lupus erythematosus may develop this condition.

729 Abdominal examination

Place your patient in the supine position, with a pillow under his head. Then percuss and palpate his liver (see Entry 448). Next, percuss the left upper quadrant to examine his spleen. Normally, percussion in this area will produce a dull note between the sixth and tenth ribs just posterior to the midaxillary line. (Always place your percussion finger—pleximeter—between the ribs to avoid eliciting a dull note from the bone.) The gastric bubble, which creates a tympanic note, is near the spleen, so isolating the dull splenic note requires careful comparison (see Entry 94).

Normally, a patient's spleen cannot be palpated unless it's enlarged. An enlarged spleen is usually tender (this finding is most common in acute disorders), so when percussion is difficult, use light palpation to detect tenderness. Hepatomegaly and splenomegaly may result from congestion caused by cell overproduction (as in polycythemia or leukemia) or from excessive demand for defective cell destruction (as in hemolytic anemias).

730 Neuromuscular assessment

Test your patient's range of motion, particularly the joints of his hands, wrists, and knees (see Entries 683, 684, and 690). Systemic lupus erythematosus, rheumatoid arthritis, or hemarthrosis can limit a patient's range of motion and cause joint enlargement. Note any joints that are inflamed, erythematous, swollen, or asymmetrical.

Also test your patient's equilibrium

PALPATING AND PERCUSSING THE SPLEEN

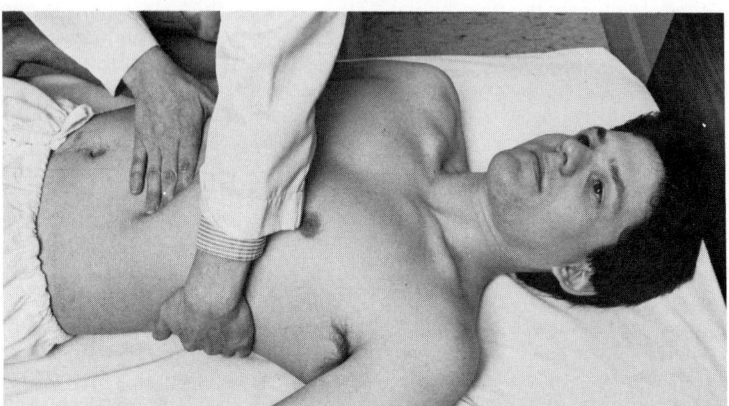

To palpate your patient's spleen properly, place him in the supine position. Approach him from his right side and reach over him, as shown here. With your left hand, support his lower left rib cage and move it forward. Place your right hand below the left costal margin and press inward.

Tell your patient to take a deep breath. You may be able to feel the edge of the spleen as the patient slowly exhales. Note: Usually you cannot palpate the spleen unless the person is very thin. If you can feel your patient's spleen on inspiration and expiration, it's probably enlarged. In such a patient, the spleen may extend into the left lower quadrant and even across the midline.

When you percuss your patient's spleen, you should hear normal dullness between the 6th and 10th ribs, posterior to the midaxillary line. If splenic dullness can be heard over a larger area than normal, suspect splenic enlargement. In such a patient, you should percuss the spleen in the lowest interspace in the anterior axillary line.

and observe for Romberg's sign (see Entry 314). Hemorrhage, cellular infiltration, or metabolic abnormalities from blood-forming disorders can affect the central and peripheral nervous systems.

Be sure to assess the patient for neuropathies, which may occur with systemic lupus erythematosus and rheumatoid arthritis. If the patient's history or your other assessment findings indicate the need for a more extensive neurologic examination, see Entries 611 to 634.

Formulating a diagnostic impression

731 Classifying these disorders

The primary functions of the blood-forming and immune systems are to transport oxygen and regulate homeostasis. Oxygen transportation depends on normal levels of circulating erythrocytes and proper synthesis of hemoglobin. Homeostasis regulation also relies on normal production and retention of other blood components—such as leukocytes, platelets, and lymphocytes—and their protection against invading substances and blood loss.

Disorders affecting the blood-

forming and immune systems can be classified as follows (see *Nurse's Guide to Blood-forming and Immune Disorders,* pages 694 to 699):
- *disorders altering oxygen transportation* by impaired production of erythrocytes, increased destruction of erythrocytes, or altered hemoglobin synthesis and structure
- *disorders increasing cell proliferation,* which causes bone marrow or lymphoid tissue hyperplasia
- *disorders causing immune complex accumulation* in vascular or basement membranes, resulting in localized tissue inflammation.

732 Making appropriate nursing diagnoses

Abnormal bleeding can result from vascular defects, platelet disorders (alterations in function or number), or coagulation factor abnormalities (these can be hereditary or due to some other disease process). This symptom predisposes your patient to *potential for injury (hemorrhage)* and *fear of potentially fatal bleeding.*

Lymphadenopathy may result from increased production of lymphocytes or reticuloendothelial cells or from the infiltration of cells not normally present. This symptom may be generalized (involving three or more node groups) or localized. Generalized lymphadenopathy may be caused by an inflammatory process, such as a bacterial or viral infection, a connective tissue disease, an endocrine disorder, or a neoplasm (including lymphomas and

TYPES OF IMMUNE DISORDERS

TYPE	DESCRIPTION	EXAMPLE
Immunodeficiency	Deficiency in phagocytosis, immunoglobulin production, cellular functioning, or a combination of these	• *Primary:* DiGeorge's syndrome • *Secondary:* Immunosuppression caused by radiation or chemotherapy
Gammopathy	Abnormal production of high levels of dysfunctional gamma globulins	• Multiple myeloma, macroglobulinemia
Hypersensitivity (allergy)	Exaggerated or inappropriate response to sensitizing antigens, classified as follows:	
	Type I (anaphylactic): Humoral mediation (IgE binds to mast cells); immediate onset	• Hay fever, allergic asthma, anaphylactic shock caused by allergies to, for example, penicillin or contrast medium
	Type II (cytotoxic): Humoral mediation (IgG or IgM binds to cell surface antigen); immediate onset	• Transfusion reactions
	Type III (immune complex): Humoral mediation (IgG or IgM forms complex with soluble antigen); immediate onset	• Serum sickness, acute glomerulonephritis
	Type IV (cell-mediated): Cellular mediation (T cells and macrophages cause tissue destruction); delayed onset	• Graft rejection, reaction to tubercle bacillus
Autoimmunity	Altered discrimination between self and nonself, causing immunologic attack on self antigens	• Pernicious anemia, systemic lupus erythematosus, rheumatoid arthritis, myasthenia gravis

NURSE'S GUIDE TO BLOOD-FORMING AND IMMUNE DISORDERS

	CHIEF COMPLAINT
OXYGEN TRANSPORTATION DISORDERS	
Iron deficiency anemia	• *Fatigue and weakness:* present; increases with anemia's severity
Pernicious anemia	• *Fatigue and weakness:* present, accompanied by lightheadedness
Aplastic anemia	• *Abnormal bleeding:* mild bleeding from nose, gums, vagina, or gastrointestinal tract • *Fatigue and weakness:* mild and progressive • *Fever:* may be present
Hemolytic anemias	• *Fatigue and weakness:* present, variable

HISTORY	PHYSICAL EXAMINATION AND DIAGNOSTIC STUDIES
• Predisposing factors include poor nutrition; chronic blood loss from ulcers, gastritis, or excessive menstruation. • Signs and symptoms include headache, shortness of breath, pica (craving odd things to eat, such as starch or clay). • Most common in children, female adolescents, and women in their reproductive years	• Tachycardia, functional systolic murmur, slight cardiac and liver enlargement, spoon-shaped nails, poor skin turgor, stomatitis, pallor, ankle edema, menstrual disturbances • Diagnostic studies include complete blood count, measurement of serum iron level, possibly bone marrow biopsy; guaiac test performed to detect presence of occult blood in stool.
• Predisposing factors include immune disorders, positive family history. • Signs and symptoms: gastrointestinal system—digestion disturbances, nausea, vomiting, diarrhea, constipation, anorexia; central nervous system—neuritis, peripheral numbness and paresthesias, impaired coordination and movement, light-headedness, altered vision; cardiovascular system—palpitations, dyspnea, orthopnea • Insidious onset; progresses slowly	• Pallor, slightly icteric skin and eyes, rapid pulse rate, cardiomegaly and possibly systolic murmur, slight hepatosplenomegaly, positive Romberg and Babinski reflexes, altered mental status • Diagnostic studies include gastric analysis for decreased acid and pepsin secretion, bone marrow aspiration, complete blood count, assay for serum vitamin B_{12}, Schilling test.
• Predisposing factors include use of medication, such as chloramphenicol or benzene derivatives, that suppresses bone marrow; therapeutic X-rays; infectious hepatitis. • Insidious onset	• Pallor, ecchymoses, petechiae • Diagnostic studies include complete blood count, measurement of serum iron level, total iron-binding capacity, bone marrow biopsy.
• Predisposing factors include chronic immune-related illness, such as systemic lupus erythematosus; neoplastic disease; recent cardiac trauma; use of such drugs as amphotericin; toxin or poison ingestion; blood transfusion incompatibility; positive family history.	• Mild jaundice, pallor • Orthostatic hypotension, tachycardia, some cardiac murmurs • Splenomegaly possible • Diagnostic studies include complete blood count, bone marrow biopsy, Coombs' test, urine test for urobilinogen. *(continued)*

NURSE'S GUIDE TO BLOOD-FORMING AND IMMUNE DISORDERS *(continued)*

	CHIEF COMPLAINT
Sickle cell anemia	• *Fatigue and weakness:* may be present • *Fever:* present • *Joint pain:* may be severe and involve multiple joints
CELL PROLIFERATION DISORDERS	
Primary polycythemia (polycythemia vera)	• *Abnormal bleeding:* nosebleeds, spontaneous bruising, bleeding ulcers • *Fatigue and weakness:* present • *Joint pain:* may be present
Acute leukemia	• *Abnormal bleeding:* nose and gum bleeding, easy bruising, prolonged menses • *Lymphadenopathy:* present; may be generalized or primarily involve cervical nodes • *Fatigue and weakness:* present; severity depends on extent of illness • *Fever:* may be high or low grade
Chronic leukemia	• *Abnormal bleeding:* rare • *Lymphadenopathy:* may be present • *Fatigue and weakness:* may be present; characterized by vague feeling of malaise and fatigue • *Fever:* low grade and unexplained in lymphocytic leukemia
Hodgkin's disease	• *Lymphadenopathy:* asymmetrical enlargement usually involves cervical nodes, but occasionally involves axillary or inguinal or femoral nodes • *Fever:* may be present

	HISTORY	PHYSICAL EXAMINATION AND DIAGNOSTIC STUDIES
	• Recurrent infections caused by increased susceptibility • Inherited genes from both parents • Signs and symptoms include dyspnea, aching bones, chest pain. • Infection, stress, dehydration, and conditions that provoke hypoxia may provoke periodic crisis. • Most common in blacks of African descent	• Asthenic habitus with disproportionately long arms and legs in adulthood; retarded growth; delayed sexual maturity; tachycardia, cardiomegaly, and systolic murmurs; pulmonary infarctions; hepatomegaly leading to cirrhosis; jaundice, pallor; joint swelling; ischemic leg ulcers • Diagnostic studies include hemoglobin electrophoresis, liver biopsy, stained blood smear showing sickle cells, complete blood count.
	• Signs and symptoms include headaches; dizziness, tinnitus, and vertigo; blurred vision; pruritus; chest pain; dyspnea; gastrointestinal distress; intermittent claudication. • May be asymptomatic in early stages • Most common in Jewish males from middle to old age	• Plethora or ruddy cyanosis of face, hands, and mucous membranes; ecchymoses; engorged conjunctival and retinal veins on ophthalmoscopic examination; enlarged, firm, and nontender spleen; hypertension, thrombosis, or emboli • Diagnostic studies include complete blood count, bone marrow biopsy, and analysis of arterial blood gases.
	• Exposure to radiation or benzene derivatives is a predisposing factor. • Signs and symptoms include headache, tinnitus, shortness of breath, chills, recurrent infections, abdominal or bone pain.	• Petechiae, ecchymoses, purpura, pallor, edema, splenomegaly, retinal hemorrhages on ophthalmoscopic examination • Diagnostic studies include complete blood count with differential and bone marrow aspiration and biopsy.
	• Predisposing factors include exposure to therapeutic or accidental radiation or to such chemicals as benzene or alkalyzing agents. • Signs and symptoms include anorexia, weight loss, bone tenderness.	• Splenomegaly, hepatomegaly, edema, anemia; in lymphocytic leukemia, papular or vesicular skin lesions, herpes zoster, collapsed vertebrae • Increased white blood cell count with proliferation of one type of white cell (depends on type of leukemia) • Further diagnostic studies include complete blood count with differential count and bone marrow aspiration or biopsy.
	• Signs and symptoms include generalized and severe pruritus; anorexia and weight loss in advanced stage. • 50% of cases occur in persons aged 20 to 40.	• Enlarged, rubbery, painless nodes; splenomegaly; anemia • Symptoms depend on nodes affected and disease stage. • Diagnostic studies include lymphangiography; lymph node, bone marrow, liver, and spleen biopsies; blood tests (Coombs', complete blood count, erythrocyte sedimentation rate, alkaline phosphatase); chest X-ray; staging laparotomy, gallium scan, ultrasound of abdomen. *(continued)*

NURSE'S GUIDE TO BLOOD-FORMING AND IMMUNE DISORDERS *(continued)*

	CHIEF COMPLAINT
Multiple myeloma	• *Abnormal bleeding:* may be present • *Fatigue and weakness:* present; possibly severe • *Fever:* present
IMMUNE COMPLEX DISORDERS	
Systemic lupus erythematosus	• *Abnormal bleeding:* heavy menses possible • *Lymphadenopathy:* enlargement without tenderness • *Fatigue and weakness:* present • *Fever:* present • *Joint pain:* arthralgia common in fingers, hands, wrists, ankles, and knees; deformities possible
Rheumatoid arthritis	• *Abnormal bleeding:* easy bruising in long-standing disease • *Lymphadenopathy:* generalized, or present only in the nodes proximal to the involved peripheral joints • *Fatigue and weakness:* generalized • *Fever:* may rise to 100.4° F. (38° C.) • *Joint pain:* joint stiffness and swelling; in advanced stages, deformities; vague arthralgias and myalgias; limited ROM
Systemic sclerosis (scleroderma)	• *Abnormal bleeding:* present, in gastrointestinal tract • *Fatigue and weakness:* vague fatigue and weakness • *Fever:* rare, may reflect concurrent problem • *Joint pain:* diffuse aching and stiffness, polyarticular arthritis; deformities and immobility caused by skin encasement
Polymyositis/dermatomyositis	• *Fatigue and weakness:* insidious onset in proximal muscles of hips and neck • *Fever:* possibly low grade, intermittent, appearing after development of muscle weakness • *Joint pain:* arthralgia

HISTORY	PHYSICAL EXAMINATION AND DIAGNOSTIC STUDIES
• Signs and symptoms: mild, transient skeletal pain progressing to severe back, rib, or extremity pain; decreased urinary output; anorexia and weight loss; repeated bacterial infections • Most common in middle-aged and elderly men	• Bone deformities from demineralization and pathologic fractures may occur as disease progresses. • Anemia, possible hepatosplenomegaly, renal insufficiency, peripheral neuropathy • Diagnostic studies include complete blood count, bone marrow aspiration, urine tests for protein and calcium, serum electrophoresis for protein, skeletal survey, intravenous pyelography.
• Predisposing factors include genetic disorder, viral infections. • Signs and symptoms include weight loss, anorexia, malaise, muscle pain, cough. • Most common in females aged 10 to 35	• Butterfly rash with blush and swelling or scaly maculopapular rash on cheeks and bridge of nose; pigmentation changes; patchy alopecia; pleural effusion; pericarditis; myocarditis; nephritis; Raynaud's phenomenon; hepatomegaly; convulsive disorders; mental status changes • Diagnostic studies include antinuclear antibody test, Coombs' test, rheumatoid factor LE-cell test, skin and renal biopsy.
• Insidious or acute onset • Most common in women aged 40 to 50	• Keratoconjunctivitis sicca; increased warmth, tenderness and swelling of involved joints; rheumatoid nodules possible; skin ulcers; muscle atrophy; pleural effusion possible • Diagnostic studies include erythrocyte sedimentation rate, latex agglutination test for rheumatoid factor, antinuclear antibody test, synovial fluid analysis, joint X-rays.
• History of Raynaud's phenomenon may occur shortly before skin changes or may precede them by many years. • Signs and symptoms include weight loss (may be profound) and exertional dyspnea, dysphagia, heartburn. • Most common in women aged 20 to 50 • Family history rare	• Raynaud's phenomenon; thickened edematous skin that becomes waxy, taut, and atrophic; pigmentation changes; telangiectasias; pulmonary interstitial fibrosis; progressive cardiac involvement; progressive renal failure • Diagnostic studies include erythrocyte sedimentation rate, rheumatoid factor, antinuclear antibody test, skin biopsy, gastrointestinal X-rays, hand X-rays.
• Predisposing factors include respiratory or obscure systemic illnesses, neoplastic lesions, other connective tissue diseases. However, first symptoms may develop during excellent health. • Signs and symptoms include myalgias, dysphagia, anorexia, weight loss, dyspnea, photosensitivity. • Most common in females aged 5 to 15 and 45 to 60	• Raynaud's phenomenon: dusky erythema over face, shoulders, and arms; heliotrope rash over eyelids; scaling maculopapular lesions over bony prominences; contractures • Diagnostic studies include erythrocyte sedimentation rate, complete blood count, serum enzymes, rheumatoid factor, electromyography, muscle biopsy.

CASE HISTORIES: NURSING DIAGNOSIS FLOWCHART

Patient A
Sharon Hall
age 30

Patient B
John Kratz
age 7

Problem
JOINT PAIN

Patient A

Subjective data

- "My ankles are so stiff and sore, especially in the morning."
- Constant fatigue; can't complete normal tasks
- Poor appetite; lost 6 lb (2.7 kg) in past 3 weeks

Objective data

- Height: 67″ (170 cm); weight: 109 lb (49 kg)
- Hyperextended distal phalanges; flexed proximal phalanges
- Several subcutaneous nodules on joints
- Thin, shiny skin over slightly edematous knees
- Red blood count decreased; white blood count 13,000 μl

Nursing diagnoses

- Alterations in comfort due to painful and swollen joints
- Impaired mobility due to discomfort and limited range of motion in legs and feet
- Disturbance in self-concept due to inability to perform activities of daily living
- Altered nutrition due to anorexia, causing weight loss

Patient B

Subjective data

- On admission, patient said he fell from bicycle that afternoon
- Pain in right knee
- Some soreness in right wrist
- Mother reports John has frequent nosebleeds and a cousin has a bleeding disorder

Objective data

- Height 50″ (127 cm), weight: 55 lb (24.7 kg).
- Edematous, warm right knee; limited movement
- Blood oozing from abrasions on ulnar border of right hand
- Ecchymotic areas around right knee, outer ankle, and hand
- Prolonged partial thromboplastin time

Nursing diagnoses

- Alterations in comfort due to knee pain possibly caused by hemarthrosis
- Impaired mobility due to right knee discomfort
- Potential for injury due to bleeding tendencies

leukemias). Localized lymphadenopathy most commonly results from infection or trauma affecting the drained area. Possible nursing diagnoses include *alterations in comfort, impairment of skin integrity (potential or actual) from an inflammatory process,* and *fear of an unknown disease or the possibility of cancer.* Depending on the size and location of the enlarged nodes, you may also diagnose *disturbance in self-concept* and *impaired mobility.*

Fatigue and weakness commonly result from anemia or an autoimmune disease. Fatigue can be caused by the extra energy a person's body expends to fight an infectious process. In a patient with anemia, fatigue on exertion can result from decreased oxygen transport to the muscles. Peripheral neuropathy can cause weakness. These symptoms may result in *potential for injury from falling, self-care deficit,* and *disturbance in self-concept.* Anorexia, which often accompanies fatigue and weakness, may produce *alterations in nutrition.*

Fever, which may result from infection or dehydration, is caused by neutrophils and macrophages, which synthesize and release endogenous pyrogens. These act on the thermoregulatory centers of the central nervous system to produce the fever. Fever can cause a *fluid volume deficit* and *alterations in comfort.* High fever may cause *alterations in thought processes.* Physical limitations from fever can produce *ineffective coping mechanisms* and *self-care deficit.*

Joint pain from an autoimmune disorder may result from an accumulation of inflammatory cells in the synovial tissue and fluid. Hemarthrosis, which may be caused by bleeding disorders, produces pressure, pain, and decreased mobility as the joint increases in size and the skin becomes taut. Pain from a blood-forming or immune disorder requires a nursing diagnosis of *alterations in comfort.* Additional diagnoses are *impaired physical mobility, impaired home maintenance management,* and *self-care deficit.*

Assessing pediatric patients

733 Developing immunity and blood production

The neonate's immune system depends on passive immunity acquired from the mother transplacentally. This means that the infant is susceptible to infectious diseases the mother hasn't had. And as his passive immunity diminishes, the infant may experience repeated infections until his own immune system matures. Development of his own immunity begins during the first few months after birth, when bone marrow and the reticuloendothelial system mature.

Immunity may also be acquired in other ways. Breast-feeding, for instance, introduces special immunoglobulins into the gastrointestinal tract. And immunizations also fortify the body's immune system.

Because an infant can't conjugate bilirubin and excrete it into bile as rapidly as occurs in an older child, his elevated bilirubin level may produce physiologic jaundice.

734 The child's health history

When recording the health history of a child with a suspected blood-forming disorder, check for anemia by asking the parents if the child has had the common signs and symptoms—pallor, fatigue, failure to gain weight, malaise, and lethargy. If you suspect a clotting disorder, determine if the family has a history of abnormal bleeding tendencies. Make sure you ask the patient's mother about obstetric bleeding complications, and note any history

IDENTIFYING BLOOD-FORMING AND IMMUNE DISORDERS IN CHILDREN

DISORDER	SIGNS AND SYMPTOMS
Hemophilia	• Abnormal bleeding that may be mild, moderate, or severe and can include hemarthrosis, leading to ankylosis of involved joints • Hemorrhage into soft tissue or viscera • Muscle atrophy
Thalassemia (Cooley's anemia)	• Severe anemia, pallor • Jaundice • Hepatosplenomegaly • Mongoloid facies, prominent upper teeth • Retarded growth and sexual maturity • Irritability
Schönlein-Henoch purpura	• Erythematous maculopapular lesions on face, arms, trunk, and legs that become petechial and purpuric; may be accompanied by pruritus and paresthesia • Arthralgia with mild arthritis • Abdominal pain, constipation, vomiting, and gastrointestinal bleeding • Hematuria, azotemia • Headache • Hypertension • Fever, malaise
Juvenile rheumatoid arthritis	• Fever, occasional chills, malaise • Red macular rash on face, trunk, extremities • Arthralgia, joint stiffness, swelling and mild warmth with some limitation of movement of involved joints • Hepatosplenomegaly, abdominal pain • Lymphadenopathy • Pleurisy, dyspnea • Pericarditis, tachycardia • Growth disturbances possible
Allergic rhinitis (hay fever)	• Sneezing, coughing, wheezing, dyspnea • Edema of mucous membranes • Red, weepy conjunctiva • Itchy eyes, nose, ears, and palate; rhinorrhea
Asthma	• Tight, nonproductive coughing and wheezing • Tachypnea and dyspnea (with accessory muscle use), barrel chest possible • Abdominal pain • Profuse perspiration

of Rh incompatibility.

When recording past history, determine if the child has any known congenital abnormalities. Ask about a history of past infections. Continual severe infections may suggest thymic deficiency or bone marrow dysfunction. Thoroughly document any history of allergic conditions. Remember, a child is more susceptible to allergies than an adult. Also, record a complete immunization history.

Ask about a family history of infections and allergic or autoimmune disorders, because these may suggest a pattern of immune deficiencies. If you're

HISTORY	DIAGNOSTIC STUDIES
• Cyclic disorder; symptom-free periods alternate with repeated hemorrhages; noticeable during infancy • Family history of disorder in maternal male relatives • Occurs almost exclusively in males.	• Partial thromboplastin time • Factor assay
• Poor eating habits noticeable at ages 6 to 12 months • Most common in persons of Mediterranean ancestry. • Family history of disorder	• X-rays • Hemoglobin electrophoresis • Hematocrit
• Predisposing factors include respiratory tract infections and food and drug allergies. • Most common in children aged 2 to 8 and in males.	• Bleeding time, tourniquet test • Erythrocyte sedimentation rate • Complete blood count
• Most common in children aged 2 to 5 and 9 to 12.	• Antinuclear antibody test • Erythrocyte sedimentation rate
• Strong family history • Seasonal • Usually not seen before age 4.	• Skin tests for allergies
• Family history of allergies or asthma • Noticeable before age 5.	• Complete blood count • Chest X-ray • Pulmonary function tests

assessing a bottle-fed baby, ask the mother if she uses an iron-fortified formula.

735 Pediatric examination considerations

The physical examination for a child with a suspected blood-forming or immune disorder is the same as for an adult, but normal findings are different. In a child under age 12, normal lymph nodes are often palpable. You may feel normal cervical and inguinal nodes ranging in size from about 3 mm across to as much as 1 cm across. Moderate numbers of nodes that are cool, firm, movable, and painless indicate past infection. Palpable cervical nodes of this description, for example, can suggest a past respiratory infection.

You may be able to palpate a normal liver and spleen in a child. Usually you'll feel the liver edge 1 to 2 cm below the right costal margin. (If it extends further than 3 cm, the liver may be enlarged; this finding calls for further investigation.) In some normal children, the liver doesn't extend below the costal margin and so won't be palpable. If you are able to palpate a child's spleen, normally you should just feel the tip—anything more than that is abnormal. Use percussion to determine liver size. The child's liver and spleen should not be tender.

The normal range for laboratory values is wider in children than in adults (see APPENDIX).

736 Common disorders in children

Immune problems affecting children fall into three categories: immune deficiencies, autoimmune diseases, and allergies (see *Identifying Blood-forming and Immune Disorders in Children,* pages 702 to 703). A child's—and his family's—history of infections may indicate a pattern suggesting an immunodeficiency. About 5 to 6 viral infections a year is normal for an infant; about 8 to 12 is average for school-age children. However, two serious bacterial infections in a 2-year period, especially beginning in infancy, can indicate an immune dysfunction.

Certain autoimmune disorders that affect both adults and children have signs and symptoms, severity, and incidence that differ for the two age-groups. For instance, childhood systemic lupus erythematosus is usually more acute and severe than the form that occurs in adults. Schönlein-Henoch purpura is the most prevalent type of vasculitis in children. Juvenile rheumatoid arthritis—unlike adult rheumatoid arthritis—doesn't usually cause permanent joint damage. When it does cause permanent joint damage, the damage occurs much later in the disease process.

The most common problems in children are allergies, especially such respiratory allergies as rhinitis and asthma. In fact, asthma remains the leading cause of chronic illness in children, particularly of school age.

Many hematologic problems—including the anemias, leukemias, and clotting disorders—begin during childhood (see *Identifying Blood-forming and Immune Disorders in Children,* pages 702 to 703). Hereditary anemias usually diagnosed during childhood include sickle cell anemia and thalassemia. The most common hematologic problem in children, as well as the most common form of anemia, is iron deficiency anemia.

Acute leukemias are the most common types of cancer in children. Clotting disorders, including hemophilia and von Willebrand's disease, affect both children and adults but are usually detected early in life.

Assessing geriatric patients

737 Effects of physiologic changes

Immune system function starts declining at sexual maturity and continues to decline with age. As an elderly person's immune system begins losing its ability to differentiate between self and non-self, the incidence of autoimmune disease increases. The immune system also begins losing its ability to recognize and destroy mutant cells; this inability presumably accounts for the increased incidence of cancer among older persons. Decreased antibody response in the elderly makes them more susceptible to infection. Tonsillar atrophy and lymphadenopathy commonly occur in older persons.

Total and differential leukocyte counts don't change significantly with age. However, some persons over age 65 may exhibit a slight decrease in the range of a normal leukocyte count. When this happens, the number of B cells and total lymphocytes decreases, and T cells decrease in number and become less effective.

As a person ages, fatty bone marrow replaces some active blood-forming marrow—first in the long bones and later in the flat bones. The altered bone marrow can't increase erythrocyte production as readily as before in response to such stimuli as hormones, anoxia, hemorrhage, and hemolysis. With age, vitamin B_{12} absorption may also diminish, resulting in reduced erythrocyte mass and decreased hemoglobin and hematocrit.

738 History and examination

Older patients have virtually the same signs and symptoms of blood-forming and immune disorders as younger adults, although cerebral and cardiac effects may be more pronounced. Ask if your elderly patient experiences joint pain, weakness, or fatigue. Does he take walks? If so, for how long? Does he have any difficulty using his hands? Ask about current medications, and note which ones produce side effects similar to signs and symptoms of blood-forming and immune disorders. For instance, digitalis may cause anorexia, nausea, and vomiting, and aspirin can produce mucosal irritation and gastrointestinal bleeding.

Determine your patient's typical daily diet (see Entry 173). Also ask if he lives alone and cooks for himself. Because of limited income, limited resources, and decreased mobility, older patients may have diets deficient in protein, calcium, and iron—nutrients essential to the blood-forming process. Even with an adequate diet, nutrients may not be absorbed because of excessive laxative use or may not be metabolized because of fewer enzymes. (About 40% of people over age 60 have iron deficiency anemia.)

Physical assessment of the geriatric patient is the same as for the younger adult. However, when evaluating vital signs, remember that the elderly patient has a reduced febrile response to infection.

Selected References

Birney, Margaret H. "Pernicious Anemia" and "Iron Deficiency Anemia," in *Diseases*, Nurse's Reference Library™ Series. Springhouse, Pa.: Intermed Communications, Inc., 1981.

Guyton, Arthur C. *Textbook of Medical Physiology*, 5th ed. Philadelphia: W.B. Saunders Co., 1981.

Harrison's Principles of Internal Medicine. New York: McGraw-Hill Book Co., 1980.

Levitt, D.Z. "Multiple Myeloma," *American Journal of Nursing* 81:1345, July 1981.

Lind, Mary. "The Immunologic Assessment: A Nursing Focus," *Heart & Lung: The Journal of Critical Care* 9:658, July-August 1980.

Maslow, William C., et al. *Practical Diagnosis: Hematologic Disease.* Boston: Houghton Mifflin Professional Publishing, 1980.

Stiehm, E. Richard, and Fulginiti, Vincent A. *Immunologic Disorders in Infants and Children*, 2nd ed. Philadelphia: W.B. Saunders Co., 1980.

Vaughan, Victor C., III, et al. *Nelson Textbook of Pediatrics*, 11th ed. Philadelphia: W.B. Saunders Co., 1979.

Williams, William J., et al. *Hematology*, 2nd ed. New York: McGraw-Hill Book Co., 1977.

Zurier, R.B. "Systemic Lupus Erythematosus," *Hospital Practice* 14:45, August 1979.

18

KEY POINTS IN THIS CHAPTER

KEY CHARTS IN THIS CHAPTER

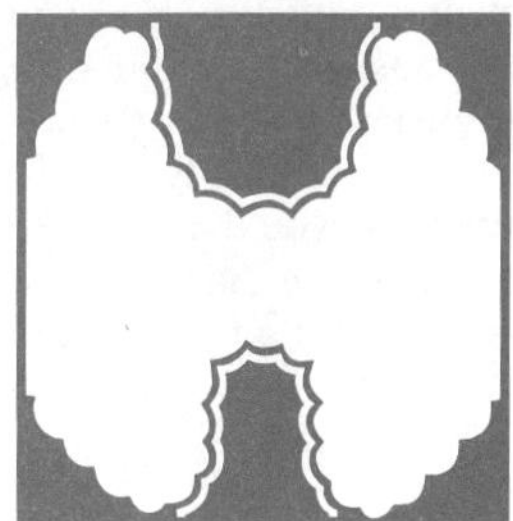

Endocrine System

Introduction

739 Why assess the endocrine system?

In contrast to the current view of endocrinology as a fascinating and highly respected area of study, only 50 to 60 years ago little was known about hormones and their actions. As a result, persons with hormonal abnormalities received little or no medical treatment. As our knowledge of endocrinology has expanded, so has the opportunity for effective patient care—and for the nurse to play an important role in assessing this system.

The endocrine system functions primarily as the regulatory system for the entire body. It consists of eight glands that produce hormones—powerful chemicals that profoundly affect our lives. Hormones influence a person's growth and development, physical appearance, body functions, and emotional status. A disorder or imbalance of the endocrine system, therefore, affects not only a person's body functions but also his physical and emotional well-being.

Some endocrine disorders, such as pituitary dwarfism, can severely limit the affected person's ability to live a normal life. Although such a patient's mental maturity may be unaffected by his condition, his abnormally short stature sets him apart from the rest of society.

Other endocrine disorders are less physically obvious but have serious health implications. A patient with diabetes mellitus may have hypertension, severe renal problems, and eye problems that can lead to blindness. The sooner a patient's endocrine disorder is detected and treated, the better chance he will have to live a normal life. You may play a vital part in this aspect of patient care. As a nurse, you commonly spend more time with patients than doctors do. If you know how to assess the endocrine system properly, you may be able to identify subtle abnormalities that signal a patient's problems with this system.

740 Recognizing endocrine problems

When assessing a patient's endocrine system, remember that it affects many, if not all, of the other body systems. In fact, you should evaluate the endocrine system when you assess any of a patient's body systems. Why? Because, for instance, an endocrine disorder may cause cardiovascular, reproductive, or nervous system signs and symptoms. Be aware of the obvious signs and symptoms that characterize endocrine disorders. Here are two examples: A patient with symptoms of nervousness, apprehension, and emotional instability may be having an anxiety attack—

or he may be suffering from hyperthyroidism. If you're knowledgeable about endocrine disorders, you'll consider the possibility that this patient has one if you find that his hands are warm and moist. (This contrasts with the cold, moist extremities of a patient who's anxious.) Or, if you're performing a physical assessment and you find many ecchymoses on the patient's skin, you might routinely suspect an injury or some vascular disorder. But again, if you have a working knowledge of endocrine dysfunction, you'll also note whether or not the patient has a round, bloated (moon) face and a heavy trunk with thin arms and legs—characteristic signs of an endocrine disorder.

Reviewing anatomy and physiology

741 Endocrine system

The endocrine glands are one of two major groups of glands in the body. The digestive and salivary glands compose the larger group, called *exocrine* glands because they discharge their secretions directly onto an epithelial surface through an excretory duct (*exo* means outward). Conversely, the *endocrine* glands (*endo* means within) discharge their secretions—six hormones—directly into the bloodstream to regulate body functions.

Negative feedback controls hormonal secretion: Once a hormone achieves its physiologic effect on the target organ, information travels back to the producing gland to inhibit further secretion. When an inadequate amount of hormone is secreted, negative feedback causes the producing gland to release more.

The endocrine system includes the pituitary, thyroid, parathyroid, adrenal, thymus, and pineal glands, the islet cells of the pancreas, and the gonads (ovaries or testes). Remember that endocrine glands aren't the only sites of hormone production; specialized cells in other organs also secrete hormones. The kidneys, for example, produce erythropoietin, and the cells of the gastric and duodenal mucosa produce gastrin. But these hormone-producing cells aren't part of the endocrine system.

742 Pituitary gland

The pituitary—a small, pea-shaped gland located at the base of the brain—hangs at the end of a narrow stalk that connects it to the hypothalamus directly above. The gland sits in a small depression within the sphenoid bone, called the *sella turcica,* or *pituitary fossa.* Located near the pituitary is the optic chiasm, where nerve fibers from both eyes cross as they convey impulses to the brain.

The pituitary consists of an anterior lobe, a posterior lobe, and a small, rudimentary intermediate lobe that's actually part of the anterior lobe. The anterior and the posterior lobes differ not only in their embryologic origin but also in their structure and the way they interact with the hypothalamus.

The *anterior pituitary* consists of cords of epithelial cells, including eosinophils, basophils, and chromophobes. Many of these cells contain granules of stored hormone. The hypothalamus communicates with the anterior lobe through a specialized network of blood vessels called the *portal system.* Capillaries around the hypothalamus merge into larger vessels that travel down the pituitary stalk and eventually become capillaries again around the cells of the anterior lobe. Through this vascular pathway, *releasing hormones* from the hypothalamus reach the anterior pituitary cells, stimulating them to secrete hormones. Each anterior pituitary hormone has a releasing hormone in the hypothalamus. Only some of these hormones

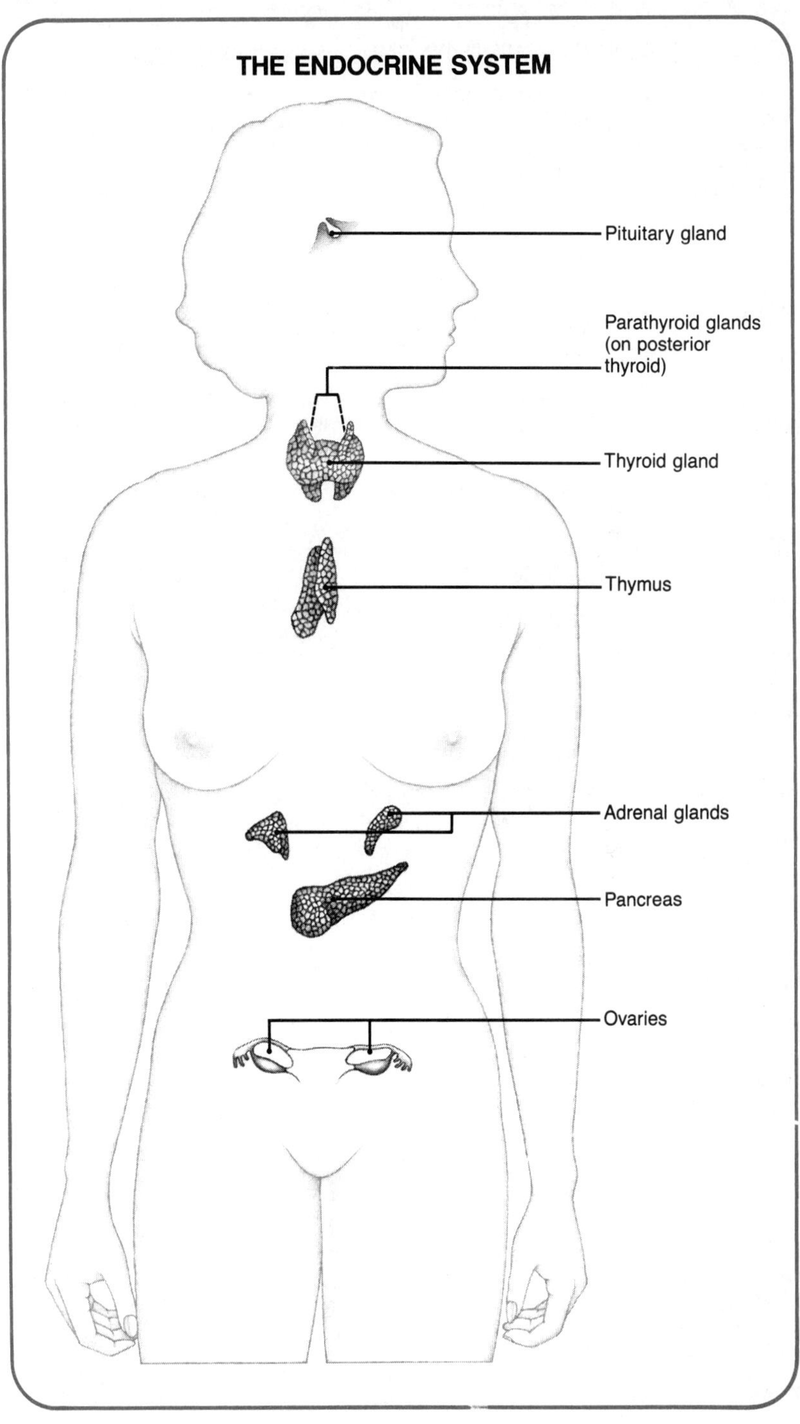
THE ENDOCRINE SYSTEM
Pituitary gland
Parathyroid glands (on posterior thyroid)
Thyroid gland
Thymus
Adrenal glands
Pancreas
Ovaries

NURSE'S GUIDE TO ENDOCRINE FUNCTION

GLAND	HORMONE SECRETED	TARGET STRUCTURE	PRIMARY FUNCTION
Anterior pituitary	Growth hormone	Bones, muscles, organs	Promotes growth and retention of nitrogen for protein metabolism
	Thyroid-stimulating hormone	Thyroid	Promotes growth and function of thyroid; controls release of thyroxine
	Adrenocorticotropic hormone	Adrenal cortex	Promotes growth and function of adrenal cortex
	Follicle-stimulating hormone	Ovaries and seminiferous tubules	Promotes development of ovaries, secretion of estrogen, and sperm maturation
	Luteinizing hormone	Ovaries	Promotes maturation of ovaries, ovulation, and secretion of progesterone
	Interstitial cell–stimulating hormone	Testes	Promotes secretion of testosterone
	Prolactin	Breasts and corpus luteum	Maintains corpus luteum; promotes secretion of progesterone and milk
Posterior pituitary	Antidiuretic hormone	Renal tubules	Promotes reabsorption of water
	Oxytocin	Uterus	Contracts pregnant uterus
Thyroid	Thyroxine	All tissues	Regulates metabolic rate
	Calcitonin	Bone, renal tubules	Maintains serum calcium levels, bone remodeling
Parathyroids	Parathyroid hormone	Gastrointestinal tract, bone, renal proximal tubules	Activates bone calcification; maintains serum calcium levels
Adrenal cortex	Glucocorticoids (cortisol)	All tissues	Metabolizes carbohydrates, fats, and proteins; acts as an anti-inflammatory
	Mineralocorticoids (aldosterone)	Primarily renal distal tubules	Balances sodium, potassium, and water concentrations
Adrenal medulla	Epinephrine, norepinephrine	Adrenergic receptors	Controls vasoconstriction
Pancreas	Insulin	Throughout body	Increases anabolism of carbohydrates; lowers blood glucose
	Glucagon	Throughout body	Elevates blood glucose

have corresponding hypothalamic inhibitory hormones.

The *posterior pituitary,* made up of nerve fibers and specialized cells that resemble nerve cells, connects more directly to the hypothalamus than does the anterior lobe. Nerve cell bodies in the hypothalamus send their axons down the pituitary stalk to establish direct contact with the cells in the posterior lobe. Hormones produced by the hypothalamus travel down the nerve axons to the posterior lobe; here they're stored and released, as needed, in response to nerve impulses from the hypothalamus. Thus, the posterior pituitary, unlike the anterior lobe, stores—but doesn't actually produce—the hormones it releases.

743 Pituitary hormones

The pituitary gland secretes nine principal hormones. Its anterior lobe secretes six: growth hormone (GH), prolactin, thyroid-stimulating hormone (TSH), adrenocorticotropic hormone (ACTH), follicle-stimulating hormone (FSH), and luteinizing hormone (LH). *GH* has many functions, all related to general tissue growth. *Prolactin* maintains the corpus luteum and secretion of progesterone. It also promotes breast milk secretion, provided the breast has been stimulated previously by estrogen and progesterone. *TSH* triggers the secretion of thyroid hormone. *ACTH* stimulates the adrenal glands to produce and secrete adrenocortical hormones; it mainly affects the glucocorticoids that control carbohydrate, fat, and protein metabolism. *FSH* and *LH,* known as the *gonadotropic hormones,* regulate the growth and maturation of germ cells and control sex hormone production by the gonads.

The pituitary's posterior lobe secretes antidiuretic hormone (ADH) and oxytocin—two hormones produced in the hypothalamus but stored in the posterior pituitary. *ADH* affects the permeability of the renal collecting tubules, causing them to absorb more water so that a more concentrated urine is excreted. *Oxytocin* stimulates uterine contractions and contributes to milk release from lactating breasts. The intermediate lobe secretes *melanocyte-stimulating hormone* (MSH), which darkens the skin but has no critical function.

744 Thyroid gland

The thyroid gland consists of two lateral lobes, each measuring about 1½" (4 cm) from top to bottom and ¾" (2 cm) in width. An isthmus connects the two lobes in the middle. The thyroid is located in the lower part of the neck and overlies the trachea with the isthmus below the cricoid cartilage and the lateral lobes along the lower margins of the thyroid cartilage. A fibrous capsule surrounds the gland, and loose connective tissue fixes it to the trachea. Consequently, the thyroid moves with the larynx and the trachea during swallowing. The lower portions of the sternocleidomastoid muscles partially cover the lateral lobes.

Histologically, the thyroid gland consists of minute, spherical vesicles

LOCATING PARATHYROID GLANDS

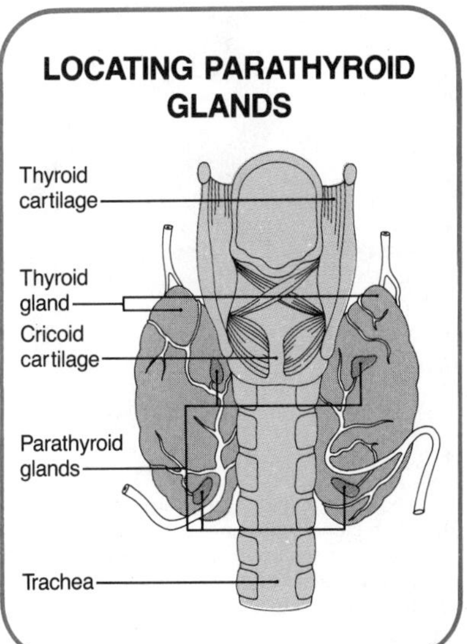

called *thyroid follicles*. These follicles synthesize the two thyroid hormones—triiodothyronine (T_3) and thyroxine (T_4)—under the influence of thyroid-stimulating hormone. T_3 and T_4 control the rate of the body's metabolic processes and influence growth and development. The thyroid also contains small groups of slightly larger cells, located adjacent to the follicles. These *parafollicular cells* secrete a hormone called *calcitonin,* which lowers ionized calcium levels in the blood.

745 Parathyroid glands

The parathyroids are four small glands, only a few millimeters in diameter, located on the posterior surface of the thyroid gland's lateral lobes. Their location varies from person to person because of migration during embryonic development.

The parathyroid glands secrete *parathyroid hormone* (PTH). This hormone regulates the ionized calcium and phosphate levels in the blood by controlling calcium and phosphate release from bone, calcium and phosphate absorption from the intestine, and the rate of calcium and phosphate excretion from the kidneys. PTH causes loss of phosphate in the urine at the same time as it causes increased renal tubular reabsorption of calcium. Control of PTH secretion is by a feedback mechanism involving the extracellular fluid concentration of calcium ions. If calcium levels fall, the parathyroids secrete more PTH than usual; if calcium levels rise, PTH secretion decreases. (Calcitonin, which has the opposite effect of PTH on calcium metabolism, plays only a minor role in the regulation of blood calcium levels.)

746 Adrenal glands

The adrenals are paired, triangular glands that sit atop the kidneys. Each gland weighs only a few grams, measures about 1¼" (3 cm) in diameter,

ANATOMY OF THE ADRENAL GLANDS

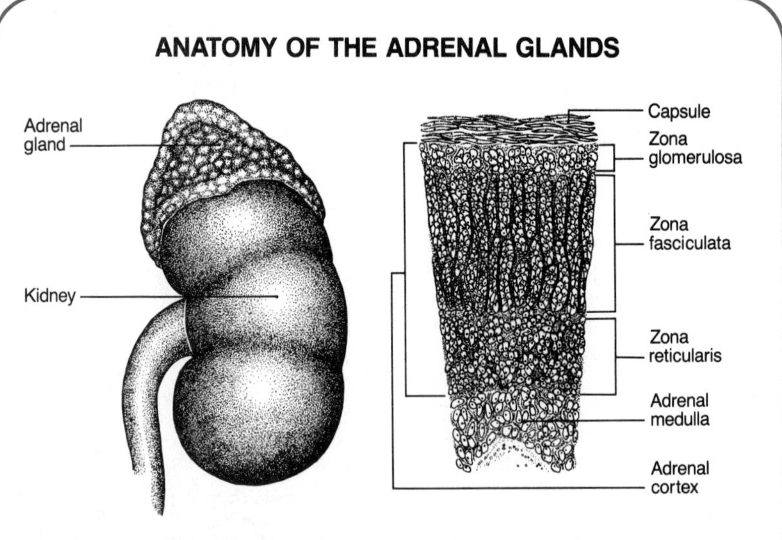

The adrenal glands are paired structures located retroperitoneally, one atop each kidney. Each gland consists of the cortex, composed of three layers, and the medulla, as shown in the cross section on the right. The outer layer of the cortex, the zona glomerulosa, produces aldosterone; the first inner layer, the zona fasciculata, produces cortisol; and the medulla stores catecholamines (epinephrine and norepinephrine).

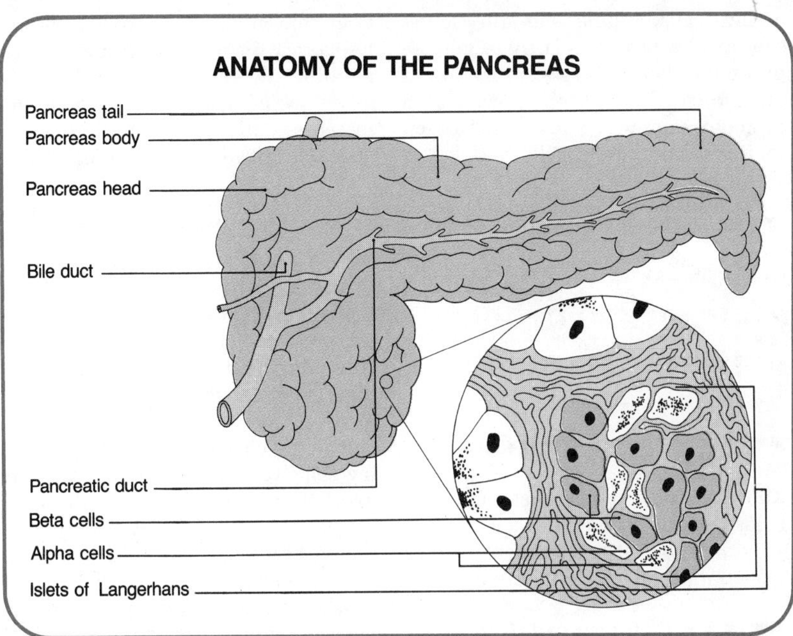

and consists of two separate structures—the adrenal cortex and the adrenal medulla.

The *adrenal cortex,* the major part of the gland, produces three kinds of steroid hormones: glucocorticoids, mineralocorticoids, and small amounts of both male and female sex hormones. *Glucocorticoids* control carbohydrate metabolism, promote gluconeogenesis, deplete tissue protein, raise blood glucose levels, and suppress inflammatory processes. Cortisol is the principal glucocorticoid. *Mineralocorticoids* regulate electrolyte and water balance by promoting sodium and water absorption and potassium excretion by the renal tubules. Aldosterone is the principal mineralocorticoid. The small amounts of *sex hormones* produced by the adrenals are normally insignificant compared to those produced by the gonads (see Entries 522 and 553).

The *adrenal medulla* secretes epinephrine and norepinephrine, known as *catecholamines.* Released on stimulation by the sympathetic nervous system, catecholamines prepare the body to respond to stress—primarily by accelerating the heart rate, increasing blood pressure, and mobilizing glucose and fatty acids to provide energy (see *How the Body Reacts to Stress,* page 108).

747 Pancreas

The pancreas functions primarily as an exocrine gland. As an exocrine gland, it's involved in food digestion; as an endocrine gland, it's involved in secretion of vital hormones. The endocrine part of the pancreas consists of more than a million tiny clusters of alpha, beta, and delta cells, known collectively as the *islets of Langerhans. Alpha cells,* which make up about 20% of the total, secrete glucagon, a hormone that raises blood glucose levels. *Beta cells,* the most numerous type (about 75% of the total), secrete insulin, which lowers blood glucose levels. As the chief hormone secreted by the islets, insulin regulates carbohydrate metabolism and influences protein and fat metabolism. It acts mainly on liver cells, muscle, and adipose tissue. Insulin promotes entry of glucose into the cells and favors utilization of glucose as a source of energy. It also promotes storage of glucose as glycogen in liver and muscle cells and favors both conversion of glucose to fat and fat storage in adipose tissue. The remaining 5% of the islet cells—*delta cells*—secrete gastrin, a hormone that increases gastric secretion but doesn't affect carbohydrate metabolism.

Collecting appropriate history data

748 Biographical data

Knowing your patient's *age* and *race* helps you determine if variations in growth, pubertal development, or hair distribution are within normal limits.

749 Chief complaint

The most common chief complaints regarding endocrine disorders are *fatigue and weakness, weight changes, abnormalities of sexual maturity or function, mental status changes,* and *polyuria and polydipsia.*

750 History of present illness

Using the PQRST mnemonic device, ask your patient to elaborate on his chief complaint. (*Note:* Remember that these chief complaints may be related to an endocrine disturbance or they may be psychogenic. Careful questioning helps you differentiate between the two.) Then, depending on the complaint, explore the history of his present illness by asking the following types of questions:

• ***Fatigue and weakness.*** *Is your fatigue constant or intermittent? If it's intermittent, when does it occur—when you wake up in the morning or at the end of the day? Do you feel more tired after strenuous exercise? What makes you feel better—rest?* Fatigue is a nonspecific complaint that occurs in both organic and psychological illnesses.

Chief complaint

- **Fatigue/weakness**
- **Weight changes**
- **Abnormalities of sexual maturity or function**
- **Mental status changes**
- **Polyuria/polydipsia**

P Q R S T

Questions to ask

Provocative/Palliative
What causes it? What makes it better? What makes it worse?

Quality/Quantity
How does it feel, look, or sound, and how much of it is there?

Region/Radiation
Where is it? Does it spread?

Severity scale
Does it interfere with activities? How does it rate on a severity scale of 1 to 10?

Timing
When did it begin? How often does it occur? Is it sudden or gradual?

Fatigue from organic causes is intermittent—worse at the end of the day and after exercise, better in the morning and after rest. *Is your feeling of weakness generalized or localized?* In many cases, generalized weakness indicates systemic illness, such as an endocrine disorder; localized weakness may suggest a neurologic disorder. *Do you feel numbness or tingling in your arms or legs?* These sensations may indicate peripheral neuropathy, which occurs in some endocrine disorders.

• ***Weight changes.*** *How much do you usually weigh? What's the most you've ever weighed? The least?* Use these figures as baselines. *How long were you gaining (or losing) weight? Are you still gaining (or losing) weight? Has your weight gain (or loss) been intentional?* Answers to these questions should help you determine if the patient's weight changes are from an organic disorder or from overeating (or strict dieting). *What is your daily food intake, including alcoholic beverages?* (See Entry 173.) *Has your appetite increased or decreased? If it has decreased, is the decrease constant or are you intermittently hungry?* Persistent loss of appetite suggests an organic cause; intermittent loss of appetite may indicate a psychogenic problem, such as depression. *Are you eating more but losing weight?* This condition may result from an endocrine disorder.

• ***Abnormalities of sexual maturity or function.*** If your patient is a woman, ask the following types of questions: *At what age did you begin to menstruate? Describe the volume of your normal flow; for instance, is it heavy? How many days does your period usually last? When did you have your last normal period? How many periods have you missed? Could you be pregnant? Are you under a great deal of stress?* Severe stress can cause amenorrhea. *Did your periods resume normally after childbirth?* Unless the patient is breast-feeding her child, nonresumption of menstruation may indicate an endocrine disorder.

Ask both male and female patients: *Has your sexual desire increased or decreased? When did this change occur? How often do you normally experience sexual desire? Has your breast size changed?* Endocrine disorders can cause breast enlargement, especially in men. Make sure such enlargement isn't from weight gain. *Have your breasts been secreting milk?* Lactation from an endocrine disorder can occur in both men and women.

• ***Mental status changes.*** *Do you have difficulty coping with your problems? Are you nervous? All the time? Do you have difficulty sitting still? Are these feelings triggered by specific events?* Endocrine disorders can cause nervous behavior or emotional lability. *Have you been feeling confused recently? How long have you felt this way? Was the onset quick or gradual? Is the feeling constant or intermittent? Have you had similar episodes before?* Confusion caused by endocrine disorders has a quick onset and is usually intermittent. *Do you have difficulty sleeping? For instance, do you have trouble falling asleep or staying asleep? How long have you been having difficulty sleeping? How many hours do you sleep? How is this different from your usual pattern? Do you feel you have to sleep during the day? Are you sleepy all day? How long have you felt this way? Do you wake up refreshed?* Changes in sleep patterns may result from endocrine disorders. Certain endocrine disorders may produce hallucinations and delusions, so note any reference to thought disorders during your conversation with the patient.

• ***Polyuria and polydipsia.*** *How long have you been passing large quantities of urine? Was the onset sudden or gradual? How many times a day do you urinate? Do you pass large quantities of urine every time you urinate or only sometimes?* Varying amounts suggest dysuria, not polyuria. *Do you wake up at night to urinate?* This may suggest a urinary tract disorder instead of an endocrine disorder.

Is your thirst insatiable? Is it constant or variable? Do you prefer ice-cold fluids? A preference for ice-cold fluids may suggest an endocrine disorder; no preference may indicate psychogenic polydipsia. *How much fluid do you now drink? How much did you formerly drink? If you're deprived of fluid, do you urinate less frequently?* Answers to these questions help you distinguish the compulsive drinker from a patient with polydipsia caused by an endocrine condition.

751 Past history

When recording your patient's past history for assessment of a suspected endocrine condition, focus on these key areas:

• ***Trauma.*** Repeated fractures may indicate adrenal or parathyroid problems; fracture at the base of the skull may cause midbrain injury, resulting in pituitary and hypothalamus dysfunction. *Fright, stress,* or *trauma* may precipitate diabetes insipidus.

• ***Surgical procedures.*** *Bilateral oophorectomy* results in decreased estrogen and progesterone production, leading to signs and symptoms of the climacteric, such as amenorrhea. *Neck surgery* may cause thyroid function abnormalities. *Partial or total adrenalectomy* may result in adrenal crisis. *Hypophysectomy* impairs regulation of fluid volume by antidiuretic hormone. Also, the stress from any surgery can precipitate endocrine disorders, such as pheochromocytoma.

• ***Obstetric history.*** *Gestational diabetes mellitus* may indicate impending diabetes mellitus, as may giving birth to an infant weighing more than 10 lb (4.5 kg).

• ***Drugs.*** *Prescribed and over-the-counter medications for sleep problems, diet, or anxiety* may mask or simulate symptoms of endocrine disorders (see *Nurse's Guide to Some Drugs That May Affect the Endocrine System*).

• ***General.*** *Unexplained neuromuscular disorders* and such nonspecific symptoms as nervousness, fatigue, and weakness may indicate underlying hyperthyroidism. Thyroid test results may reveal previous thyroid problems. *Long-standing obesity* contributes to the development of diabetes mellitus. *Irradiation* can cause glandular atrophy. *Meningitis* or *encephalitis* can cause hypothalamic disturbances.

752 Family history

Because certain endocrine disorders are inherited and others have strong familial tendencies, a thorough *family history* is essential. Ask your patient if anyone in his family is (or was) obese, or has had *diabetes mellitus, thyroid disease,* or *hypertension.* Diabetes mellitus (particularly Type II, or the non–insulin-dependent form) has an especially strong familial tendency. Thyroid conditions, such as goiter, also show familial tendencies. *Pheochromocytoma* may result from an autosomal dominant trait. *Delayed puberty* recurs in certain families; in women, this condition causes primary amenorrhea.

753 Psychosocial history

The most important aspect of your patient's psychosocial history is *environment,* because iodine deficiency in local water and food may cause thyroid enlargement.

754 Activities of daily living

When recording your patient's activities of daily living for endocrine assessment, be sure to ask about his *diet.* Specifically, determine whether he has any unusual eating habits. For instance, does your patient routinely follow a strict, limited, or fad-food diet? Adolescent girls often diet unnecessarily and may develop severe nutritional deficiencies and extreme weight loss, which can cause amenorrhea.

Also, determine whether your patient takes *drugs* or drinks *alcohol* reg-

NURSE'S GUIDE TO SOME DRUGS THAT MAY AFFECT THE ENDOCRINE SYSTEM

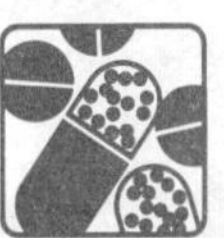

CLASSIFICATION	POSSIBLE SIDE EFFECTS
Antipsychotics	
chlorpromazine hydrochloride (Thorazine) haloperidol (Haldol*)	• In males, gynecomastia; in females, menstrual irregularities, hyperprolactinemia, weight gain
Miscellaneous psychotherapeutics	
lithium carbonate (Lithane*)	• Transient hyperglycemia, goiter, hypothyroidism, hyponatremia, drying and thinning of hair
Antidepressants	
desipramine hydrochloride (Norpramin*)	• Sweating, weight gain
tranylcypromine sulfate (Parnate*)	• Changed libido, impotence, peripheral edema, sweating, weight changes
Nonsteroidal anti-inflammatory agents	
phenylbutazone (Butazolidin*)	• Hyperglycemia, toxic and nontoxic goiter
tolmetin sodium (Tolectin*)	• Sodium retention, edema
Antidiabetics	
chlorpropamide (Diabinese*)	• Prolonged hypoglycemia, dilutional hyponatremia
tolbutamide (Orinase*)	• Hypoglycemia
Estrogens	
diethylstilbestrol (DES)	• Hyperglycemia, hypercalcemia, hirsutism or hair loss; in males, gynecomastia, testicular atrophy; in females, dysmenorrhea, amenorrhea
esterified estrogen (Estabs)	• Hyperglycemia, hypercalcemia, hirsutism or hair loss, oily skin; in males, testicular atrophy, gynecomastia; in females, breakthrough bleeding, breast changes (tenderness, enlargement, secretion), altered menstrual flow, dysmenorrhea, amenorrhea
Oral contraceptives	
estrogen with progestogen (Enovid)	• Changes in appetite, weight gain, breakthrough bleeding, amenorrhea, hyperglycemia, hypercalcemia, oily skin, breast changes (tenderness, enlargement, secretion)
Heavy metal antagonists	
dimercaprol (BAL in Oil*)	• Decreased iodine uptake, sweating
Alkylating agents	
busulfan (Myleran*)	• Amenorrhea, gynecomastia, testicular atrophy, addisonian-like wasting syndrome, alopecia
cyclophosphamide (Cytoxan*)	• Gonadal suppression, sterility, syndrome of inappropriate antidiuretic hormone secretion, alopecia

(continued)

NURSE'S GUIDE TO SOME DRUGS THAT MAY AFFECT THE ENDOCRINE SYSTEM (*continued*)

CLASSIFICATION	POSSIBLE SIDE EFFECTS
Diuretics	
chlorothiazide (Diuril*)	• Hypokalemia, hyperglycemia, and impairment of glucose tolerance; fluid and electrolyte imbalances, including dilutional hyponatremia, hyperchloremia
mannitol (Osmitrol*)	• Fluid and electrolyte imbalances, water intoxication, cellular dehydration
spironolactone (Aldactone*)	• Anorexia, hyperkalemia, dehydration, hyponatremia; in males, gynecomastia; in females, breast soreness, menstrual disturbances

*Available in U.S. and Canada. All other products (no symbol) available in U.S. only.

ularly. If he does, ask how much and how often. Intoxication or withdrawal from drugs or alcohol can produce signs and symptoms that mimic endocrine disorders.

755 Review of systems

When recording the review of systems, ask your patient about the following symptoms:

• ***General.*** *Frequent infections* can occur in a patient with diabetes mellitus, because sugar-rich body fluids make infection control difficult. Also, protein depletion decreases resistance.

• ***Skin.*** *Hirsutism* occurs with ovarian and adrenocortical disorders that result in increased androgen production. *Excessive hair loss* may be an autoimmune response. *Loss of axillary and pubic hair* may result from a pituitary disorder. Episodes of *flushing* and *diaphoresis* may occur in association with *abnormal heat intolerance,* a classic complaint of patients with hyperthyroidism. *Abnormal cold intolerance* may indicate hypothyroidism.

• ***Eyes.*** *Exophthalmos* is present in endocrine disorders involving the thyroid. *Partial loss of vision* may indicate a pituitary tumor.

• ***Mouth and throat.*** *Hoarseness* can indicate laryngeal nerve compression from a tumor or, in women, excessive androgen production. *Difficulty swallowing* may be the result of compression or displacement of the esophagus by an enlarged thyroid gland.

• ***Cardiovascular.*** *Orthostatic hypotension* occurs in adrenal disorders. *Palpitations* with sweating and flushing may result from the hormonal imbalances of an endocrine disorder, such as hyperthyroidism, or possibly from an adrenal tumor that increases epinephrine production. *Leg swelling* from congestive heart failure or myxedema occurs in patients with thyroid disorders.

• ***Nervous.*** *Tremors* during periods of sustained posture (for instance, when a patient holds his arm out in front of his body for a period of time) may occur in patients with thyroid disorders. *Paresthesia* may result from peripheral neuropathies associated with certain endocrine disorders.

• ***Musculoskeletal.*** *Arthralgia, bone pain,* and *extremity enlargement* may result from disorders of the growth process.

• ***Respiratory.*** *Stridor* or *dyspnea* may occur in the patient with an enlarged thyroid gland that compresses his trachea.

• ***Gastrointestinal.*** *Frequent loose bowel movements* may accompany hyperthyroidism; *constipation* may accompany hypothyroidism.

Conducting the physical examination

756 Considerations and techniques

Remember that because of the endocrine system's interrelationship with all other body systems, physical assessment of a patient's endocrine function consists of a complete evaluation of his body. Make sure the lighting in the examining room is adequate, because your assessment depends primarily on inspection. (To examine the patient's thyroid gland, you'll also use palpation and auscultation.)

757 General health status

Begin your assessment of the endocrine system by focusing on the patient's general physical appearance and emotional status. Often, during the initial moments of patient contact, an astute nurse can recognize the effects of major endocrine disorders, such as hyperthyroidism, hypothyroidism, myxedema, dwarfism, and acromegaly.

Observe the patient's apparent state of health, and note any signs of distress. Assess general body development—height and weight, body build and posture, and proportion of body parts. Note the distribution of body fat, too. In men, fat tissue should be distributed evenly over the entire body. In women, fat tissue normally concentrates in the shoulders, breasts, buttocks, inner thighs, and pubic symphysis. (In men and women who are obese, excessive fat accumulates in these same areas.) In endocrine assessment, you must distinguish between the fat distribution of obesity and that of Cushing's syndrome: In a patient with Cushing's syndrome, fat is concentrated on the face, neck, interscapular area, trunk, and pelvic girdle.

While you talk with your patient, assess his activity level. Does he move briskly or are his movements extremely slow? The former may indicate hyperthyroidism; the latter, hypothyroidism. Note his speech—its coherence, quality, and speed. The patient with hyperthyroidism can't get his words out fast enough; the patient with myxedema sounds hoarse and slurs his words.

Next, assess your patient's *vital signs* (see Entry 68). Take his blood pressure in both arms. Hypertension occurs in many endocrine disorders, particularly pheochromocytoma and Cushing's syndrome. Hyperthyroidism causes systolic blood pressure elevations. Arrhythmias may accompany metabolic disturbances. When taking a patient's apical pulse, note its quality and character. In an adult, a heart rate below 60 or above 100 beats/minute may suggest thyroid disease. Deep, rapid respirations (Kussmaul's respirations) may indicate diabetic ketoacidosis.

758 Assessing your patient's skin

Focus first on skin color (see Entry 224). Observe for hyperpigmentation, both generalized and localized, on the patient's exposed areas and at pressure points. Remember, hyperpigmentation can range from tan to brown. When assessing pigmentation, consider racial and ethnic variations. For example, hyperpigmented gums are normal in blacks but may indicate Addison's disease in whites. Also, observe the patient for areas of hypopigmentation (vitiligo), which may be associated with Addison's disease, thyroid disorders, or diabetes mellitus. You can distinguish yellow pigmentation caused by myxedema from jaundice by inspecting the patient's sclerae. Jaundice causes yellowing of the sclerae; myxedema doesn't.

Next, examine the patient's skin for hydration and texture (see Entries 225 and 226). Dry, rough skin may be a sign of hypothyroidism or dehydration;

smooth, flushed skin can accompany hyperthyroidism. Observe for areas of lipoatrophy and wasting, which may appear at injection sites in patients with diabetes mellitus. Easy bruising may be associated with the tissue breakdown of Cushing's syndrome. Skin lesions and ulcerations commonly appear in patients with diabetes mellitus. Also look for poor wound healing, which is associated with the peripheral circulation problems characteristic of some endocrine disorders, such as diabetes mellitus.

759 Examining nails and hair

Observe your patient's nails, noting color, shape, and quality (see Entry 231). Thick, brittle nails may suggest hypothyroidism; thin, brittle nails may result from hyperthyroidism. Separation of the nail from the bed, beginning at the nail edge, may suggest a thyroid disorder. Increased nail pigmentation occurs in Addison's disease.

Inspect the patient's hair for abnormalities (see Entry 229). Note the amount of scalp and body hair. Check for abnormal patterns of hair loss or hair growth; if your patient is a woman, note any excessive facial, chest, or abdominal hair (hirsutism). Remember to consider racial and ethnic variations in texture and distribution of hair.

Note the texture of the patient's hair by inspecting and touching it. Fine, soft, silky hair is characteristic of hyperthyroidism, in contrast to the coarse, dry, brittle hair you'll find in patients with hypothyroidism.

Observe for hair thinning or loss on the outer eyebrows, axillae, and genitalia in both men and women.

760 How to examine the face and neck

Carefully inspect your patient's face. First, study his expression. Does he stare and look alarmed? Or, is his expression dull and apathetic? Note any coarsening of facial features, such as his nose, lips, and ears, and check for a prominent forehead and protruding lower jaw. These are possible signs of a growth abnormality. *Moon face* is a sign of Cushing's syndrome. Also observe for facial edema, especially around the patient's eyes. With your index finger, apply firm pressure to this area and watch for pitting. Nonpitting facial edema, especially if accompanied by periorbital edema, may indicate hypothyroidism.

After observing your patient's entire face, carefully inspect his eyes. Observe their position and alignment. Be especially alert for abnormal protrusion of the eyeball with obvious lid retraction (exophthalmos), which may indicate increased thyroid function.

Test extraocular movements through the six cardinal fields of gaze (see Entry 267). Note any evidence of extraocular muscle paralysis or reduced function, which can develop secondary to diabetic neuropathy or thyroid dysfunction. Test for eye convergence, which is usually poor in a patient with hypothyroidism. Inspect the relation of the upper eyelids to the eyeballs as the patient moves his eyes to gaze upward and then down. Lid lag—a margin of white sclera between the upper lid and the iris as the patient's gaze moves down—may indicate hyperthyroidism.

Use the Snellen chart to test your patient's visual acuity (see Entry 263). Then test his visual fields (see Entry 268). Some endocrine disorders, such as pituitary tumors, may cause visual field defects and reduced visual acuity.

Using an oblique light source, inspect for opacities in the cornea and the lens of your patient's eye. Premature cataracts may appear in a patient with diabetes or hypoparathyroidism. When performing a funduscopic examination, be alert for microaneurysms (tiny red spots), hemorrhages (large, slightly irregular red spots), and exudates (yellow spots), which are characteristic of diabetic retinopathy. Watch for arteriolar narrowing, which may be present in a patient with long-term hyperten-

PALPATING THE THYROID GLAND: TWO APPROACHES

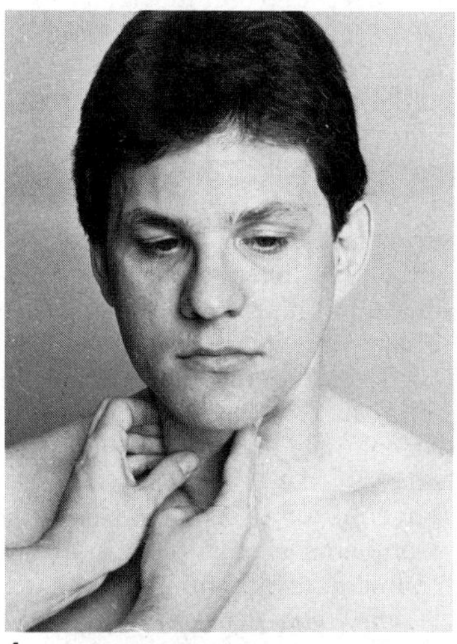
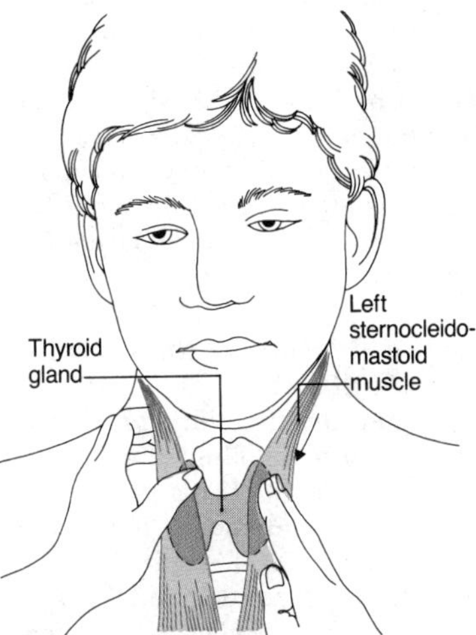

1 When palpating from the front, here's how to position your hands. The nurse in this photograph is palpating the right thyroid lobe.

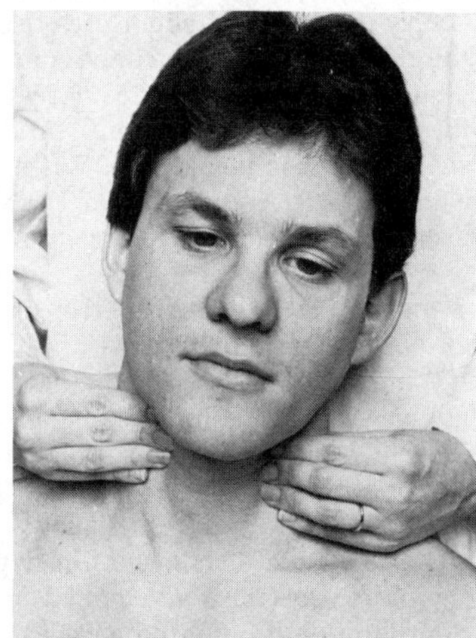
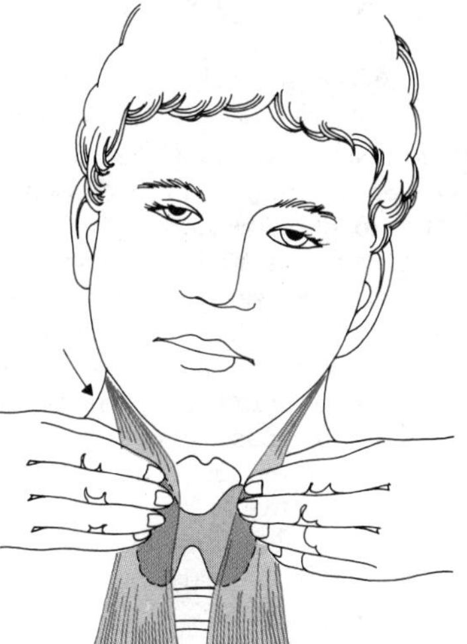

2 When palpating from the rear, position your hands this way. The nurse shown here is palpating the left thyroid lobe.

sion associated with pheochromocytoma and Cushing's syndrome.

Next, examine the patient's mouth. Inspect the buccal mucosa for color and condition. Look for patchy, brown pigmentation of the gums, a possible sign of Addison's disease. Inspect the tongue for color, size, and tremors. (An enlarged tongue is associated with myxedema.) Note the patient's breath odor;

if it smells fruity, like acetone, he may be in diabetic ketoacidosis.

Carefully inspect the patient's neck. First, move any hair and clothing away from his neck to check contour and symmetry. Then, observe his slightly extended neck for visible signs of thyroid enlargement or asymmetry. Note how the thyroid gland moves when the patient swallows. Ask him if he has difficulty swallowing, and if he has any hoarseness or neck pain.

761 Palpating the thyroid gland

To examine the thyroid, stand facing the patient or behind him, and ask him to lower his chin. (This relaxes the neck muscles and makes the examination easier.)

Palpate the thyroid gland for size, shape, symmetry, tenderness, and nodules. When palpating from the front, use your index and middle fingers to feel for the thyroid isthmus, below the cricoid cartilage, as the patient swallows. (Swallowing raises the larynx, the trachea, and the thyroid gland—but not the lymph nodes and other structures.) To palpate one lobe at a time, ask the patient to flex his neck slightly to the side you're examining. To palpate the right lobe, use your right hand to move the thyroid cartilage slightly to the right. Then, grasp the sternocleidomastoid muscle with your left hand (tips of index and middle fingers behind the muscle, thumb in front), and try to palpate for the right lobe of the thyroid between your fingers. To palpate the left lobe, use your left hand to move the thyroid cartilage and your right hand to palpate.

To palpate the thyroid from behind the patient, gently place the fingers of both hands on either side of the trachea, just below the thyroid cartilage. Try to feel the thyroid isthmus as your patient swallows. While you're palpating one lobe at a time, ask the patient to flex his neck to the side being examined. To feel for the right lobe, use your left hand to move the thyroid cartilage to the right. Grasp the sternocleidomastoid muscle with your right hand, while placing your middle fingers deep into and in front of the muscle. For the left lobe, use your right hand to move the cartilage to the left and your left hand to palpate. (See *Palpating the Thyroid Gland: Two Approaches,* page 721.)

In most patients, you won't feel the thyroid gland, but you may feel the isthmus. (You may see or feel a normal thyroid in a patient with a thin neck.) When you do palpate a large mass, don't confuse thick neck musculature with an enlarged thyroid or goiter. An enlarged thyroid may feel finely lobulated, like a well-defined organ. Thyroid nodules feel like a knot, protuberance, or swelling. A firm, fixed nodule may be a tumor.

When you detect an enlarged thyroid, perform Kocher's test to determine if it's compressing the patient's trachea. Ask your patient to inspire deeply as you apply slight pressure on the gland's lateral lobes. If the enlarged gland is causing tracheal compression, the pressure you apply will produce stridor on deep inspiration. When you elicit a positive response to Kocher's test, observe your patient for dyspnea.

762 Auscultating the thyroid gland

If you palpate an enlarged thyroid, auscultate the gland for systolic bruits. Place the stethoscope's diaphragm over one of the thyroid's lateral lobes. Then listen carefully for a bruit—a low, soft, rushing sound. This occurs in hyperthyroidism because accelerated blood flow through the thyroid arteries produces vibrations. (You may have to ask the patient to hold his breath and not swallow, so tracheal sounds don't interfere with your auscultation.) To distinguish a bruit from a venous hum, listen for the rushing sound, then gently occlude the jugular vein with your fingers on the side you're auscultating and listen again. A venous hum disappears during venous compression.

USING LABORATORY TESTS TO ASSESS ENDOCRINE FUNCTION

Familiarize yourself with the following tests; they're used to determine your patient's hormone or gland function.

ORGAN	LABORATORY TEST	PURPOSE
Thyroid	Serum triiodothyronine (T_3)	• Measures T_3 levels in the blood • Detects hyperthyroidism
	Serum thyroxine (T_4)	• Measures T_4 levels in the blood • Detects hyperthyroidism
	Serum thyroid-stimulating hormone (TSH)	• Measures TSH levels in the blood • Detects hypothyroidism
	Antithyroglobulin antibodies and antithyroid microsomal antibodies	• Detects antibody titers indicative of thyroid inflammation (Hashimoto's disease)
	Radioactive iodine (^{123}I) uptake	• Detects thyroid hypofunction and hyperfunction
	T_3 resin uptake	• Evaluates thyroxine binding to plasma proteins
	Thyroid scan	• Evaluates functional capacity of thyroid nodules • Detects thyroid nodules or tumors
	Thyroid ultrasonography	• Evaluates anatomic characteristics of thyroid nodules • Detects solid or cystic masses in the thyroid
Parathyroid glands	Parathyroid function tests: parathyroid hormone and calcium levels	• Measures parathyroid hormone and calcium levels in the blood • Detects hyperparathyroidism
Adrenal glands	Plasma cortisol	• Determines the release of cortisol from the adrenals • Detects abnormalities in cortisol secretion—hyperfunction (Cushing's syndrome) or hypofunction (Addison's disease)
	17-hydroxycorticosteroids	• Measures steroid levels in urine • Detects hyperadrenocorticism
	17-ketosteroids	• Measures steroid levels in urine • Detects hyperadrenocorticism
	Dexamethasone suppression test	• Measures suppression of adrenocorticotropic hormone production in conjunction with serum cortisone levels or 17-hydroxycorticosteroids • Detects Cushing's syndrome
	Urine metanephrine	• Detects pheochromocytoma

(continued)

USING LABORATORY TESTS TO ASSESS ENDOCRINE FUNCTION *(continued)*

ORGAN	LABORATORY TEST	PURPOSE
Adrenal glands *(continued)*	Plasma catecholamines (epinephrine and norepinephrine)	• Evaluates adrenal medullary function • Detects pheochromocytoma
	Urine vanillylmandelic acid	• Detects pheochromocytoma • Measures catecholamines
Pituitary	Serum growth hormone	• Detects hyperpituitarism (gigantism and acromegaly)
	Prolactin levels	• Measures prolactin secretion • Detects pituitary tumors causing galactorrhea
	Insulin tolerance test or insulin stress test	• Measures growth hormone, which should increase as blood glucose decreases • Detects hypopituitarism
	Metyrapone test	• Measures adrenocorticotropic hormone production
Pancreas	Fasting blood sugar	• Measures blood glucose levels
	Glucose tolerance test	• Measures blood glucose levels • Detects decreased tolerance to glucose, as seen in diabetes mellitus and Cushing's syndrome • Detects increased tolerance to glucose, as seen in hypothyroidism, Addison's disease, and hypopituitarism

763 Breast, abdomen, and genitalia examination

Inspect your patient's breasts for areas of hyperpigmentation, especially the nipples and skin creases. Note the presence of purple-red striae, which may occur in a patient with Cushing's syndrome. If you suspect an endocrine disorder characterized by galactorrhea (such as a pituitary dysfunction), milk the breasts and note the character of the drainage. (You may ask your patient to do this, for the sake of comfort.)

Inspect the patient's abdomen for abnormalities associated with endocrine disorders. Observe the abdominal contour and the distribution of fat, and look carefully at the skin, noting any purple-red striae. If your patient is a woman, observe for abdominal hair distribution.

Next, inspect the patient's external genitalia for sexual maturation, particularly the size of the testes or clitoris. Small testes may indicate hypogonadism; an enlarged clitoris suggests virilization. Also note the amount and distribution of pubic hair (see Entries 532 and 566).

764 Musculoskeletal assessment

Inspect the size and proportions of your patient's body. Extremely short stature suggests dwarfism; disproportionate body parts, such as enlarged hands or feet, may be caused by excessive amounts of growth hormone, as in acromegaly.

Next, inspect the patient's vertebral column for such deformities as an enlarged disk or kyphosis, which may appear in acromegaly and hyperparathyroidism (see Entry 685). Observe the joints for enlargement and deformity, and use range-of-motion tests to check for stiffness and pain (see Entries 679 to 691). All these signs and symptoms can result from hypothyroidism. Inspect the patient's muscles for atrophy and tremors. Atrophy occurs in Cushing's syndrome and hyperthyroidism, and tremors may also indicate hyperthyroidism.

765 Neurologic examination

Assess your patient's sensitivity to pain, touch, and vibration, and his position sense (see Entries 628 and 629). Sensory loss may occur in diabetic neuropathy; paresthesias can result from hypothyroidism, diabetes, and acromegaly. Note any loss of motor function. Wristdrop or ankledrop may signal extreme diabetic neuropathy.

Assess deep tendon reflexes (see Entry 632) in your patient, noting any evidence of hyperreflexia with delayed relaxation—associated with hyperthyroidism and hypoparathyroidism. Hyporeflexia, especially with ankle jerk, may occur in a patient with hypothyroidism or diabetic neuropathy.

Keep in mind that alterations in consciousness, including coma, may result from uncontrolled diabetes or myxedema.

766 Testing for hypocalcemic tetany

You can determine if your patient has hypocalcemic tetany (a rapid drop in serum calcium levels from hypoparathyroidism or parathyroid gland removal) by testing for Trousseau's sign and Chvostek's sign. To check for Trousseau's sign, apply a blood pressure cuff to the patient's arm just above the antecubital area. Inflate the cuff until you've occluded the blood supply to his arm. If this procedure precipitates carpal spasm (finger contractions and inability to open the hand), Trousseau's sign is positive. Test for Chvostek's sign by tapping one finger in front of the patient's ear at the angle of the jaw, over the facial nerve. If contracture of the lateral facial muscles results, Chvostek's sign is positive.

767 Further diagnostic tests

Your initial impressions should serve primarily as indications for further investigation. Diagnostic tests provide you with important additional information. They're especially significant in differentiating endocrine disorders from disorders affecting other body systems—which may cause many of the same signs and symptoms. These tests include blood and urine analyses, scanning, and tissue biopsy. Laboratory tests that measure blood and urine levels of various hormones can determine if a gland or a feedback mechanism is functioning properly in your patient (see *Using Laboratory Tests to Assess Endocrine Function*). Tests can be performed for each endocrine gland and hormone.

Formulating a diagnostic impression

768 Classifying endocrine disorders

The functions of the endocrine system include regulating growth and development, responding to stress and injury, regulating reproduction, and maintaining ionic homeostasis and energy metabolism. Hormones, synthesized and secreted by endocrine glands and transported to target tissues, control these essential functions. All endocrine disorders alter hormonal synthesis or secretion and result in a

NURSE'S GUIDE TO ENDOCRINE DISORDERS

	CHIEF COMPLAINT	
DEFICIENT HORMONE SECRETION		
Pituitary tumor	• *Abnormalities of sexual maturity or function:* decreased libido; amenorrhea; impotence; changes in amount of sexual hair (such as beard and pubic) • *Mental status changes:* in advanced stages, drowsiness, stupor, convulsions, mental aberrations	
Hypopituitarism	• *Fatigue/weakness:* lethargy; easy fatigability • *Weight changes:* may occur (usually loss) • *Abnormalities of sexual maturity or function:* general loss of secondary sex characteristics; amenorrhea • *Mental status changes:* somnolence, coma	
Diabetes insipidus	• *Fatigue/weakness:* may be present • *Weight changes:* weight loss may be profound because of water loss; anorexia • *Mental status changes:* irritability; apathy • *Polyuria/polydipsia:* present, may be severe; nocturia; preference for cold drinks	
Hypothyroidism	• *Fatigue/weakness:* present, accompanied by lethargy; need for increased amount of sleep • *Weight changes:* weight gain • *Abnormalities of sexual maturity or function:* diminished sexual functioning; menorrhagia; impotence • *Mental status changes:* abnormal tranquillity possible; answers to questions may be inappropriate; slowing of cognitive ability; depression	
Myxedema (severe)	• *Fatigue/weakness:* present, accompanied by lethargy; need for increased amount of sleep • *Weight changes:* weight gain, decreased appetite • *Abnormalities of sexual maturity or function:* diminished sexual functioning; menorrhagia; impotence • *Mental status changes:* in extreme cases, coma, overt psychosis possible	
Multinodal goiter	• Usual chief complaints of endocrine disorders not present	
Thyroiditis (chronic form: Hashimoto's thyroiditis)	• *Fatigue/weakness:* fatigue possible; malaise	

HISTORY	PHYSICAL EXAMINATION AND DIAGNOSTIC STUDIES
• Neurologic symptoms	• Visual field and visual acuity defects, skin changes, headache, intolerance to cold, increased intracranial pressure • Diagnostic studies include skull X-rays, computerized tomography, and carotid angiography.
• Predisposing factors include congenital abnormalities, acute infections, vascular problems, and pituitary tumor.	• Skin changes, such as discoloration (yellow), wrinkling, thinning, drying; slow pulse rate; hypotension; decreased growth; genital atrophy; loss of teeth; brittle nails; anorexia; constipation • Diagnostic studies include complete blood count, serum thyroxine, serum triiodothyronine, and urine 17-ketogenic steroids. Test results show decrease in one of pituitary hormones (rarely more than one).
• Onset may be insidious or sudden. • Predisposing factors include fright and head injury or tumors.	• Dry skin, poor turgor, headache • Diagnostic studies include plasma osmolality and dehydration tests.
• Predisposing factors include surgery or use of radioiodine to treat hyperthyroidism. • Onset usually insidious.	• Sparse (especially at eyebrows), brittle, coarse hair; muscle stiffness; diminished hearing; sensitivity to cold; constipation; hoarseness • Diagnostic studies include serum thyroxine, serum triiodothyronine, and basal metabolic rates.
• Predisposing factors include long-standing hypothyroidism, exposure to cold, use of respiratory depressants, such as anesthetics.	• Hypothyroidism symptoms continue. • Dry, scaling, cool, yellow-orange, thickened skin; dull, expressionless face; hypothermia; heart enlarged; rate lowered; edema, especially periorbital; thickened tongue; decreased deep tendon reflexes • Diagnostic studies include serum thyroxine, serum triiodothyronine, and basal metabolic rates.
• Most common in women • Patient may be asymptomatic for years. • Predisposing factors include iodine deficiency, familial history of disorder.	• Tenderness and visible enlargement of neck; respiratory difficulty, stridor, sensation of choking, hoarseness • Diagnostic studies include serum thyroxine and ^{123}I.
• Predisposing factors include family history of thyroiditis, Graves' disease, myxedema. • Onset is insidious. • Patient may be asymptomatic except for palpable gland and high titer; believed to be autoimmune disorder.	• Symptoms of hypothyroidism possible • Enlarged thyroid (two to five times normal size; typically feels rubbery; lobular pyramidal lobe usually prominent); may experience choking feeling, swallowing difficulty, and sensation of local pressure. • Diagnostic studies include antithyroglobulin antibody test and/or microsomal antigens. *(continued)*

NURSE'S GUIDE TO ENDOCRINE DISORDERS *(continued)*

	CHIEF COMPLAINT	
Addison's disease (primary adrenal insufficiency)	• *Fatigue/weakness:* slow, progressing fatigue and weakness • *Weight changes:* weight loss caused by poor appetite, food idiosyncrasies, nausea, vomiting, diarrhea • *Abnormalities of sexual maturity or function:* loss of secondary sex characteristics and libido in females • *Mental status changes:* depression, irritability, restlessness	
Diabetes mellitus	• *Fatigue/weakness:* fatigue possible; loss of strength • *Weight changes:* weight loss; in chronic illness, bloating, fullness • *Abnormalities of sexual maturity or function:* impotency in males • *Polyuria/polydipsia:* present; classic symptoms of diabetes mellitus	
Hypoparathyroidism	• *Fatigue/weakness:* lethargy • *Mental status changes:* irritability, emotional lability, impaired memory, confusion, depression, changes in level of consciousness	
EXCESSIVE HORMONE SECRETION		
Syndrome of inappropriate hypersecretion of antidiuretic hormone	• *Fatigue/weakness:* weakness, lethargy • *Weight changes:* weight gain • *Mental status changes:* confusion, possibly progressing to convulsions and coma	
Acromegaly	• *Fatigue/weakness:* progressive weakness • *Abnormalities of sexual maturity or function:* in early stages, increased libido, hypertrophy of genitalia; in later stages, decreased libido, galactorrhea, amenorrhea, impotence, deepening voice • *Mental status changes:* emotional instability • *Polyuria/polydipsia:* polydipsia present	
Thyroid tumors	• May present with none of the usual chief complaints of thyrotoxicosis or of endocrine disorders	

HISTORY	PHYSICAL EXAMINATION AND DIAGNOSTIC STUDIES
• Onset is insidious. • Predisposing factors include history of tuberculosis, treatment with exogenous steroids, and family history of adrenal insufficiency.	• Fasting hypoglycemia; hypotension and syncope; poor coordination; blue-gray hyperpigmentation on exposed areas of body and mucous membranes, occasionally with vitiligo; abdominal pain; salt craving from hyponatremia • Diagnostic studies include plasma cortisol and urine 17-ketogenic steroids.
• Predisposing factors include long-standing obesity, pancreatic disease, history in females of delivering large infants, and family history of diabetes. • In Type II, mild symptoms may be long-standing.	• Dry skin and mucous membranes, polyphagia, blurred vision, light-headedness, pruritus • In chronic illness, intermittent claudication, especially of feet; pain; paresthesia; hyperpigmentation; xanthomas; poor healing; microaneurysms and exudates in eyes; decreased sensation to pain and temperature; lipodystrophy (from repeated insulin injections); gastrointestinal hyperactivity; decreased perspiration; decreased reflexes • Diagnostic studies include fasting blood sugar and glucose tolerance tests.
• Predisposing factors include injury to or removal of thyroid (parathyroids taken with thyroid).	• Tetany (numbness; tingling in fingers, toes, and around lips), cyanosis; Chvostek's sign, laryngeal stridor, dyspnea; papilledema (sometimes associated with increased intracranial pressure); malformed, pitted nails; thinning hair, alopecia; coarse, dry skin; dysplasia of tooth enamel; diplopia, cataracts, eyes sensitive to light; convulsions, abdominal pain, nausea, vomiting; EKG changes • Diagnostic studies include serum electrolytes, primarily calcium.
• Predisposing factors include cancer (most commonly bronchogenic), head injury, meningitis, encephalitis, brain abscess, cerebrovascular accident, neurosurgery to midbrain, tuberculosis.	• Retention of fluids • Diagnostic studies include BUN, serum creatinine, urine sodium, serum osmolality, serum antidiuretic hormone.
• Insidious onset in third decade of life • Continued increase in hat, glove, shoe size after puberty • Rapid growth spurt or growth in adult life	• Face broadened; overgrowth of lips, nose, tongue, jaw, forehead; pain and stiffness in fingers and toes; increased pigmentation of skin; deep, thick skin creases; excessive sweating; increased facial hair; edema; hypertension; enlarged internal organs: heart, liver, spleen, glands (especially pancreas); polyphagia; headache, visual disturbances, paresthesia • Diagnostic studies include X-rays and glucose tolerance test for growth hormone.
• Predisposing factors include radiation for thymic enlargement and congenital metabolic defects.	• Hoarseness; pain in neck area, difficulty swallowing; enlarged cervical lymph nodes • In thyrotoxicosis, tachycardia, heart failure, vascular collapse, hyperthermia • Diagnostic studies include ^{123}I scan, biopsy, serum thyroxine, and serum triiodothyronine.

(continued)

NURSE'S GUIDE TO ENDOCRINE DISORDERS *(continued)*

	CHIEF COMPLAINT
Hyperthyroidism (thyrotoxicosis)	• *Fatigue/weakness:* weakness present and prominent, increased fatigue; muscle atrophy • *Weight changes:* decreased subcutaneous fat; weight loss despite increase in appetite • *Abnormalities of sexual maturity or function:* short and scanty menstrual periods; decreased fertility; possibly temporal recession of hairline in females • *Mental status changes:* anxiety; nervousness; difficulty concentrating; agitation; paranoid tendencies • *Polyuria/polydipsia:* polyuria possible, with increased thirst
Cushing's syndrome	• *Fatigue/weakness:* present, loss of muscle mass • *Weight changes:* weight gain; distribution of fat increases on neck, face, abdomen, girdle • *Abnormalities of sexual maturity or function:* hirsutism; clitoral hypertrophy; amenorrhea; gynecomastia in males • *Mental status changes:* irritability, emotional lability, depression, psychosis • *Polyuria/polydipsia:* may be present with other symptoms of diabetes mellitus
Adrenal virilizing syndromes	• *Abnormalities of sexual maturity or function:* reversal of primary and secondary sex characteristics, scanty menstrual periods, amenorrhea, increased sexual drive
Pheochromocytomas (tumors of adrenal medulla)	• *Fatigue/weakness:* malaise • *Weight changes:* weight loss • *Mental status changes:* nervousness; apprehension; feelings of impending doom (prodrome of attack)
Primary aldosteronism	• *Fatigue/weakness:* muscle weakness; fatigue • *Polyuria/polydipsia:* polyuria present; polydipsia possible
Fasting hypoglycemia	• *Fatigue/weakness:* lethargy, weakness, paralysis • *Weight changes:* weight gain • *Mental status changes:* inability to concentrate; changes in sensorium; irritability; inappropriate affect
Hyperparathyroidism	• *Fatigue/weakness:* weakness, fatigability • *Weight changes:* weight loss, anorexia • *Mental status changes:* difficulty concentrating; disorientation; delirium; psychosis; confusion; stupor; coma • *Polyuria/polydipsia:* polyuria may cause polydipsia

	HISTORY	PHYSICAL EXAMINATION AND DIAGNOSTIC STUDIES
	• Predisposing factors include recent emotional crisis, infection, physical stress, family history of Graves' disease. • Relatively common disorder; symptoms depend on severity of disorder.	• Fine, moist palmar erythema; thin and brittle hair and nails; palpable thyroid; systolic bruit over thyroid; possibly tender supraclavicular lymph nodes; palpitations, tachycardia, paroxysmal atrial tachycardia; increased heat production, with excessive perspiration and decreased tolerance to heat; exophthalmos and lid lag characteristic of Graves' disease; pretibial edema; insomnia; fine tremors, exaggerated reflexes • Diagnostic studies include serum thyroxine and serum triiodothyronine.
	• Predisposing factors include steroid treatment and adrenal tumors. • Most common in women	• Hypertension; osteoporosis, spontaneous fractures, height reduction, backache; purple striae on arms, breasts, abdomen, and thighs; petechial hemorrhage, excessive bruising; decreased healing ability • Diagnostic studies include serum electrolytes, plasma cortisol, and urine 17-hydroxycorticosteroids.
	• May be congenital or acquired • Most common in women • Difficult to detect in postpubertal males • Congenital syndromes are believed to be caused by mutant autosomal recessive genes.	• Hirsutism of face, body, and extremities; thinning of hair, temporal baldness; deepening of voice, Adam's apple enlargement; acne, increased sebum production; development of male habitus, increased muscle mass, and increased strength; breast and uterus atrophy, enlargement of clitoris • Diagnostic studies include 17-ketosteroids and 17-hydroxycorticosteroids in urine; dexamethasone suppression test; testosterone levels; adrenal tomography and adrenal angiography.
	• Familial incidence most common between ages 40 and 60 • Sudden emotion or physical changes may precipitate attack.	• Hypertension, dyspnea, paresthesias, tetany, blurred vision, severe and throbbing headache, palpitations (possibly intense), profuse sweating, nausea, vomiting, anorexia, abdominal pain, pallor
	• Most common in women between ages 30 and 50 • Predisposing factors include use of oral contraceptives.	• Hypertension, headache, ventricular enlargement, cardiac arrhythmias, hypokalemia • Diagnostic studies include serum electrolytes and urine 17-hydroxycorticosteroids.
	• Predisposing factors include liver disease, family history of diabetes mellitus, and use of alcohol, propranolol, and salicylate. • Most common between ages 40 and 60	• Tachycardia, trembling, blurred vision, pallor, paresthesias, palpitations, diaphoresis, decreased coordination, nausea, vomiting, headache • May lead to convulsions • Diagnostic studies include glucose tolerance and fasting blood sugar tests.
	• May vary in degree from asymptomatic, insidious onset to rapid onset with severe symptoms • Chronic renal disease • Rickets • Osteomalacia may lead to compensatory hyperparathyroidism.	• Cardiac irregularities; anemia; enlarged head; pathologic fractures; hypotonia of muscles; altered reflexes; decreased hearing; ataxic gait; renal symptoms, such as urinary tract infections, pyelonephritis, renal colic; severe headache; bone pain; epigastric pain; nausea; vomiting; pancreatitis; hoarseness; paresthesias for vibration • Diagnostic studies include serum electrolytes and radioimmunoassay for parathyroid hormone.

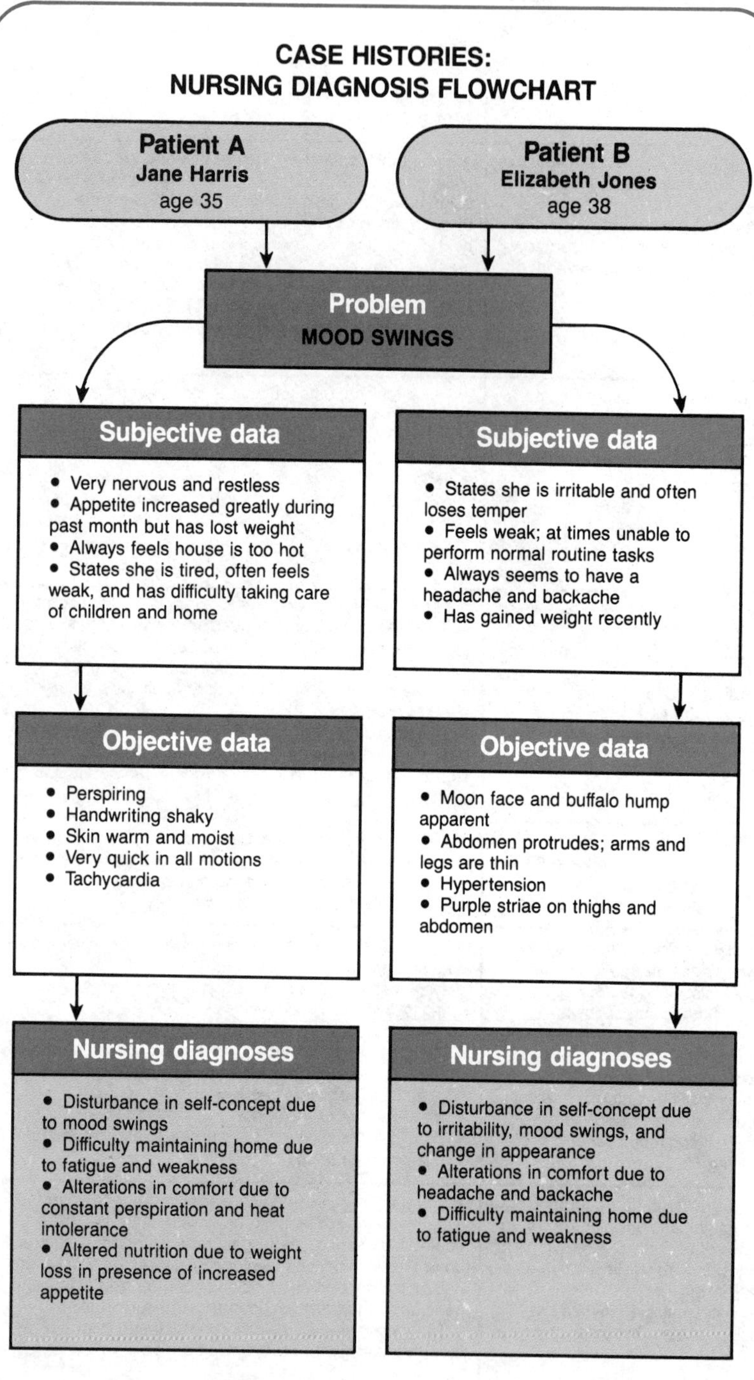
CASE HISTORIES:
NURSING DIAGNOSIS FLOWCHART
Patient A
Jane Harris
age 35
Patient B
Elizabeth Jones
age 38
Problem
MOOD SWINGS
Subjective data
• Very nervous and restless
• Appetite increased greatly during past month but has lost weight
• Always feels house is too hot
• States she is tired, often feels weak, and has difficulty taking care of children and home
Subjective data
• States she is irritable and often loses temper
• Feels weak; at times unable to perform normal routine tasks
• Always seems to have a headache and backache
• Has gained weight recently
Objective data
• Perspiring
• Handwriting shaky
• Skin warm and moist
• Very quick in all motions
• Tachycardia
Objective data
• Moon face and buffalo hump apparent
• Abdomen protrudes; arms and legs are thin
• Hypertension
• Purple striae on thighs and abdomen
Nursing diagnoses
• Disturbance in self-concept due to mood swings
• Difficulty maintaining home due to fatigue and weakness
• Alterations in comfort due to constant perspiration and heat intolerance
• Altered nutrition due to weight loss in presence of increased appetite
Nursing diagnoses
• Disturbance in self-concept due to irritability, mood swings, and change in appearance
• Alterations in comfort due to headache and backache
• Difficulty maintaining home due to fatigue and weakness

hyperfunctioning or hypofunctioning gland. Thus, endocrine disorders can be functionally divided into two categories: those causing excessive hormonal secretion and those causing deficient hormonal secretion.

769 Making appropriate nursing diagnoses

Fatigue and weakness are nonspecific symptoms, occurring in disorders of many body systems. In endocrine disorders, they may result from excessive or deficient hormonal secretion by any of several glands. For instance, diminished thyroxine secretion (in hypothyroidism) alters protein, fat, and carbohydrate metabolism, causing fatigue, and also decreases muscle tone, causing weakness. In contrast, hypersecretion of growth hormone (in acromegaly) causes rapid muscle development and increased metabolism, which eventually deplete energy stores and cause fatigue and weakness. Appropriate nursing diagnoses for a patient with these symptoms may include *impaired physical mobility, impaired home maintenance management,* and *ineffective rest-activity pattern.*

Weight changes can result from alterations in fat or fluid balance, depending on the gland and hormone affected. The pituitary, thyroid, adrenal, and sex hormones influence fat distribution and deposition. In a patient with Cushing's syndrome (adrenal hyperfunction), excessive cortisol secretion stimulates appetite and frees glucose for fat synthesis. This causes excessive fat deposition in the patient's face, neck, trunk, and abdomen. In a patient with hypothyroidism, decreased thyroxine leads to a diminished metabolic rate and reduced nutrient use, and the patient gains weight. Reduced cortisol levels in adrenal insufficiency (Addison's disease) result in appetite loss, impaired gluconeogenesis, and fat mobilization: All cause weight loss. The increased metabolic rate in hyperthyroidism causes accelerated use of nutrients, decreased fat, and weight loss—even though the patient's appetite increases.

Fluid balance alterations may also result in weight changes. Hormonal secretion that produces water and sodium retention causes weight gain; hormonal secretion resulting in water and sodium depletion produces weight loss.

Nursing diagnoses for weight changes may include *fluid volume deficits* or *potential for fluid volume excess, alterations in nutrition,* and *disturbance in self-concept from change in body weight.*

Abnormalities of sexual maturity or function result from disturbances in hormonal secretion from the pituitary, the adrenals, and the gonads. Deficient gonadotropin secretion by the pituitary results in delayed or arrested sexual development. Postpubertal gonadotropin deficiency—especially when accompanied by reduced thyroid and adrenal secretion—results in gradual recession of secondary sex characteristics, decreased libido, and infertility. Excessive gonadotropin secretion causes precocious puberty and exaggeration of secondary sex characteristics. Possible nursing diagnoses for abnormalities of sexual maturity or function include *sexual dysfunction, disturbance in self-concept, ineffective individual coping, role disturbance,* and *alterations in family dynamics.*

Mental status changes range from confusion, disorientation, and stupor to impaired concentration, nervousness, and psychosis. Any of these changes may result directly or indirectly from altered hormonal secretion. Excessive secretion of thyroid hormone causes cellular hypermetabolism, leading to impaired concentration, increased cerebration, and nervousness. Deficient cortisol secretion from the adrenals produces reduced cerebration and a diminished ability to respond to stress. Mental status changes may also result from the fluid and electrolyte imbalances, acidosis, and blood sugar level elevations or reductions that occur

EMERGENCY

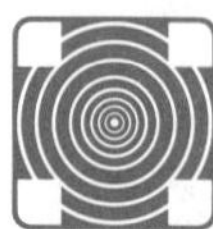

NURSE'S GUIDE TO LIFE-THREATENING DIABETIC COMPLICATIONS

COMPLICATIONS	SYMPTOMS
Diabetic ketoacidosis (DKA)	• Anorexia, nausea, vomiting, polyuria, weakness, malaise, Kussmaul's respirations, abdominal pain, hyperglycemia (blood sugar from 400 to 800 mg/100 ml); if untreated, may lead to drowsiness, stupor, coma
Hyperglycemic hyperosmolar nonketotic coma (HHNK)	• Vomiting, diarrhea, tachycardia, rapid breathing, volume depletion, focal motor seizures, transient hemiplegia, severe hyperglycemia (blood sugar about 1,000 mg/100 ml), possibly leading to stupor and coma
Insulin shock (hypoglycemia)	• Sweating; tremors; increased blood pressure, pulse rate, respirations; headache; confusion; incoordination; blood sugar 50 mg/100 ml or less; can lead to convulsions, coma

in endocrine disorders.

Depending on your patient's specific problem, nursing diagnoses for mental status changes may include: *alterations in thought processes sensory perceptual alterations, ineffective individual coping, alterations in family dynamics, impaired home maintenance management, sleep pattern disturbances, memory deficits, role disturbance,* and *social isolation.*

Polyuria and polydipsia may result from diabetes insipidus or diabetes mellitus. In diabetes insipidus, diuresis is precipitated by insufficient antidiuretic hormone secretion, which reduces the ability of the distal renal tubules to reabsorb water. The resulting dehydration causes polydipsia. In diabetes mellitus, the elevated blood sugar level causes polyuria. When the blood sugar level exceeds the renal threshold for reabsorption, glycosuria results. Hyperglycemia osmotically pulls water from the cells, causing diuresis; polydipsia results from the dehydration. Your nursing diagnoses for polyuria and polydipsia may include *potential or actual fluid volume deficits, knowledge deficit concerning hyperglycemia,* and *alterations in patterns of urinary elimination.*

Assessing pediatric patients

770 Special history-taking considerations

When you assess a child's endocrine function, your findings may be critical in the early detection of abnormalities or disorders. (Remember, endocrine dysfunction can occur even at birth and cause permanent physical and mental damage.) Although many endocrine disorders present the same signs and symptoms in children as in adults, some have manifestations unique to children. Perhaps the most common

CAUSE	INSULIN LEVELS	MORTALITY
• Cessation of insulin, or physical or emotional stress • Occurs predominantly in Type I diabetes (insulin-dependent)	• Zero	• In known diabetics, approximately 5% (most commonly due to late treatment)
• Stress, burns, steroids, diuretics • Severe dehydration from sustained hyperglycemic diuresis in which patient cannot sustain adequate fluid levels • Occurs predominantly in Type II diabetes (non–insulin-dependent)	• Low (some residual ability to secrete insulin)	• About 50%; treatment may be complicated by patient's age and debilitated state
• Too much insulin, too little food, excessive physical activity	• High	• Prognosis satisfactory when treated immediately; prolonged hypoglycemia can lead to permanent central nervous system damage

signs and symptoms of endocrine abnormalities in children are growth and developmental disturbances. However, these disturbances are often so subtle that only a thorough physical examination will reveal them. Parents may want their child examined because he's restless or doing poorly in school.

Common signs and symptoms for a neonate or infant include feeding problems, constipation, jaundice, hypothermia, or somnolence. With an older child, ask the parent or child to describe the child's activities on a typical day; this will help you distinguish a so-called quiet child from a child who's always tired and inactive and who may have decreased endocrine function. A quiet child will sit quietly and read; in the same circumstances, a child with endocrine problems will usually lie down and sleep. Review of daily activities can also help distinguish active children from hyperactive children: An active child can sit quietly to play or watch television, whereas a hyperactive child cannot do this.

When you evaluate a child, obtain a thorough family history from one or both parents, because many endocrine disorders are hereditary—such as diabetes mellitus and thyroid problems—or show a familial tendency—such as delayed or precocious puberty. Remember that an older child or adolescent can probably give you a more accurate history of his physical growth and sexual development than his parents can, so interview the child, too, when this is possible.

771 Evaluating growth and development

Childhood endocrine problems usually cause growth and developmental abnormalities that may acutely embarrass an older child or adolescent. For this reason, try to examine a child who's in this age range without his parents present.

Measure the child's height and weight. Height (in relation to age) and weight (in relation to stature and age) provide important indices of growth (see *Using Pediatric Growth Grids,* pages 164 and 165). Poor weight gain with little or

DISTINGUISHING BETWEEN TYPE I AND TYPE II DIABETES

TYPE I (INSULIN-DEPENDENT)	TYPE II (NON–INSULIN-DEPENDENT)
Age at onset: usually before age 20	*Age at onset:* usually after age 30
Type of onset: abrupt	*Type of onset:* gradual
Symptoms: polydipsia, polyuria, appetite increase, weight loss, endogenous insulin absent, lethargy	*Symptoms:* sometimes none; endogenous insulin present
Stability: wide fluctuations of blood glucose, with marked sensitivity to diet, exercise, and insulin	*Stability:* usually easily controlled if patient adheres to a proper diet
Disease control: difficult	*Disease control:* less difficult
Need for insulin: needed by all	*Need for insulin:* needed by only 20% to 30%; usually diet-controlled
Need for oral hypoglycemic: not indicated	*Need for oral hypoglycemic:* useful for about 40% of patients

no increase in height may indicate a lack of growth hormone. Hyperthyroidism can cause weight loss.

Some endocrine disorders selectively affect trunk or extremity growth. Check segmental measurements against those considered normal for the child's age and sex.

Also, test the child for age-related skills. If he's very young, for example, observe for such behavior as holding his head up, sitting, or walking. If your patient hasn't reached developmental milestones for his age, suspect physical or mental retardation, possibly of endocrine origin.

In your physical examination, always inspect the child's face to determine if his facial appearance correlates with his age. In cretinism, for example, a child retains his infantile facial appearance. When inspecting his mouth, check if the number of teeth corresponds with normal expectations for the child's age. Delayed eruption of teeth occurs in hypothyroidism and hypopituitarism. Normally, you'll examine a young child's thyroid gland by placing him in the supine position.

Throughout the physical examination—and especially when you're examining the child's breasts, abdomen, and genitalia—inspect for the developmental signs of precocious puberty. Suspect delayed puberty if a child who's reached mid-adolescence has none of the physical changes associated with puberty. As described in Entry 776, endocrine dysfunction can cause both precocious and delayed puberty. Further diagnostic tests to confirm endocrine dysfunction are just as essential in a child as in an adult.

772 Growth hormone abnormalities

Growth hormone secretion fluctuates from day to day (it increases during exercise, for example) and over long periods. Accelerations of growth hormone production seem to result in the growth spurts noted on standard growth charts for children. Growth hormone deficiency can lead to dwarfism; excessive growth hormone production can result in gigantism in a prepubescent child or acromegaly in one who is older.

773 Signs and symptoms of thyroid dysfunction

In newborns, hypothermia, persistent neonatal jaundice, high birth weight from postmaturity, or posterior fontanelle enlargement suggest congenital hypothyroidism or cretinism. If the diagnosis of cretinism is not made at birth, the infant will gradually develop other signs and symptoms. These include failure to thrive, feeding problems, constipation, hoarse cry, somnolence, dry skin, poor abdominal tone, umbilical hernia, a puffy face, and an enlarged tongue. Hypothyroidism that begins in childhood can delay growth as well as mental and sexual development. Consider that an older child may have juvenile hypothyroidism if he's slightly overweight (but not obese), has retained the naso-orbital configuration of a young child, has experienced delayed eruption of permanent teeth, or performs intellectual tasks poorly.

Childhood hyperthyroidism (most commonly occurring in school-age girls) can cause serious and even fatal acceleration in body metabolism. Signs and symptoms of this disorder during childhood include restlessness, hyperactivity, and a short attention span, as well as the classic adult symptoms. Children with this condition often fall into the upper percentile for height and the lower percentile for weight in comparison with standard growth charts.

774 Insulin disorders in children

Insulin is essential to a child's growth and development because it regulates blood glucose levels and plays a vital role in carbohydrate, fat, and protein metabolism, thus promoting the effects of other hormones that stimulate growth. *Type I diabetes mellitus* (caused by lack of insulin secretion from the islets of Langerhans in the pancreas) usually occurs in older children and adolescents. Children commonly experience an abrupt onset precipitated by some form of stress, such as infection or emotional upset. The earliest sign of this disease in children may be weight loss or growth retardation. Other signs and symptoms are similar to those of Type II diabetes mellitus. (See *Distinguishing Between Type I and Type II Diabetes.*)

775 Cushing's syndrome

Suspect Cushing's syndrome in children with exogenous obesity, especially if they show glucose intolerance and striae. Certain types of drug therapy (for example, synthetic corticosteroids, such as prednisone) may also result in high cortisol levels and produce the same signs and symptoms as those of Cushing's syndrome if the drug is used for a long time.

Typical assessment findings in a child with Cushing's syndrome (usually caused by a malignant tumor of the adrenal cortex) include an increased cortisol level, which causes obesity and hypertension; obesity, with accumulations of fat on the cheeks and chin and little fat on the extremities; red face, especially cheeks; signs of abnormal masculinization or feminization, from overproduction of androgen or estrogen; and purple striae appearing on hips, abdomen, and thighs.

776 Disturbances of sexual maturation

A child's precocious sexual maturation or delayed sexual maturation can indicate abnormal function of his hypothalamus, pituitary, adrenals, or gonads. Hypopituitarism, pituitary tumors, and adrenal and gonadal tumors can affect the onset of puberty. In addition, such endocrine problems as hypothyroidism can prevent sexual maturation by slowing the entire growth process.

Precocious puberty is usually defined as the appearance of secondary sex characteristics in a girl before age 8 and in a boy before age 9.

Puberty is considered to be delayed if secondary sex characteristics are not apparent before age 13 in girls and age 14 in boys, or if more than 5 years have elapsed between the first physical signs of puberty and onset of menarche in girls or completion of genital growth in boys.

Assessing geriatric patients

777 Endocrine signs and symptoms

Many endocrine disorders cause signs and symptoms in the elderly that are similar to changes that normally occur with aging. For this reason, these disorders are easily overlooked during assessment. In an adult patient with hypothyroidism, for example, mental status changes and physical deterioration—including weight loss, dry skin, and hair loss—occur. Yet these same signs and symptoms characterize the normal aging process.

Other endocrine abnormalities may complicate your assessment because their signs and symptoms are different in the elderly than in other age-groups. Hyperthyroidism, for example, usually causes nervousness and anxiety, but a few geriatric patients may instead experience depression or apathy (a condition known as *apathetic hyperthyroidism of the elderly*). And an elderly patient with Graves' disease may initially have signs and symptoms of congestive heart failure or atrial fibrillation rather than the classic manifestations associated with this disorder.

RECOGNIZING HORMONAL CHANGES DUE TO AGING

Use this chart as a guide to hormonal changes in the elderly.

HORMONE	SERUM CONCENTRATION
Growth hormone*	No change
Thyroid-stimulating hormone*	No change
Thyroxine	No change
Triiodothyronine	Decreases
Parathyroid hormone	Decreases
Cortisol	No change
Adrenal androgens*	Decreases
Aldosterone	Decreases
Insulin*	No change
Glucagon	No change

*Decreasing response to stimulation

778 Normal variations in endocrine function

A very common and important endocrine change in the elderly is a decreased ability to tolerate stress. The most obvious and serious indication of this diminished stress response occurs in glucose metabolism. Normally, fasting blood sugar levels aren't significantly different in young and old adults. But when stress stimulates an older person's pancreas, the blood sugar concentration increase is greater and lasts longer than in a younger adult. This decreased glucose tolerance occurs as a normal part of aging, so keep it in mind when you're evaluating an elderly patient for possible diabetes.

During menopause, a normal part of the aging process in women (see Entries 581 and 582), ovarian senescence causes permanent cessation of menstrual activity. Changes in endocrine function during menopause vary from woman to woman, but normally estrogen levels diminish and follicle-stimulating hormone production increases. This estrogen deficiency may result in either or both of two key metabolic effects: coronary thrombosis and osteoporosis. Remember, too, that some symptoms characteristic of menopause (such as depression, insomnia, headaches, fatigue, palpitations, and irritability) may also be associated with endocrine disorders. In men, the climacteric stage causes a decrease in testosterone levels and in seminal fluid production (see Entry 544).

Selected References

Alexander, M., and Brown, M.S. *Pediatric History Taking and Physical Diagnosis for Nurses,* 2nd ed. New York: McGraw-Hill Book Co., 1979.

Bates, Barbara. *A Guide to Physical Examination,* 2nd ed. Philadelphia: J.B. Lippincott Co., 1979.

Beeson, Paul B., et al. *Cecil Textbook of Medicine,* 15th ed. Philadelphia: W.B. Saunders Co., 1979.

Carnevali, Doris L., ed. *Nursing Management for the Elderly.* Philadelphia: J.B. Lippincott Co., 1979.

Carotenuto, R., and Bullock, J. *Physical Assessment of the Gerontologic Client.* Philadelphia: F.A. Davis Co., 1981.

Conn, Howard F., and Conn, Rex B., Jr. *Current Diagnosis,* 6th ed. Philadelphia: W.B. Saunders Co., 1980.

DeGroot,Leslie J., ed. *Endocrinology,* 3 vols. New York: Grune and Stratton, Inc., 1979.

Garofano, Catherine D., et al. "Helping Diabetics Live With Their Neuropathies," *Nursing80* 10:42, June 1980.

Guyton, Arthur C., *Textbook of Medical Physiology,* 6th ed. Philadelphia: W.B. Saunders Co., 1981.

Harvey, A. McGehee, et al. *The Principles and Practice of Medicine,* 20th ed. New York: Appleton-Century-Crofts, 1980.

Hillman, Robert. *Clinical Skills: Interviewing, History Taking, and Physical Diagnosis.* New York: McGraw-Hill Book Co., 1981.

Isselbacher, Kurt J., et al., ed. *Harrison's Principles of Internal Medicine.* 9th ed. New York: McGraw-Hill Book Co., 1980.

Krueger, J., and Ray, J. *Endocrine Problems in Nursing.* St. Louis: C.V. Mosby Co., 1976.

Krupp, Marcus A., and Chatton, Milton J., eds. *Current Medical Diagnosis and Treatment,* rev. ed. Los Altos, Calif.: Lange Medical Publications, 1980.

Malasanos, Lois, et al. *Health Assessment,* 2nd ed. St. Louis: C.V. Mosby Co., 1981.

Netter, Frank H. *Endocrine System and Selected Metabolic Diseases,* vol. 4 in *The CIBA Collection of Medical Illustrations.* Summit, N.J.: CIBA Pharmaceutical Co., 1974.

Price, S., and Wilson, L. *Pathophysiology: Clinical Concepts of Disease Processes.* New York: McGraw-Hill Book Co., 1978.

Sana, J., and Judge, R., eds. *Physical Appraisal Methods in Nursing Practice.* Boston: Little, Brown & Co., 1975.

Sanford, S.F. "Dysfunction of the Adrenal Gland: Physiologic Considerations and Nursing Problems," *Nursing Clinics of North America* 15:481, September 1980.

Sciarra, John J., ed. *Gynecology and Obstetrics,* vol. 1. Philadelphia: Harper & Row, annual revision.

Seedor, Marie M. *The Physical Assessment: A Programmed Unit in the Fundamentals of Nursing,* New York: Teachers College Press, 1980.

Solomon, B.L. "The Hypothalamus and the Pituitary Gland: An Overview," *Nursing Clinics of North America* 15:435, September 1980.

Taylor, Robert B. *A Primer of Clinical Symptoms.* New York: Harper & Row, 1973.

Vaughan, Victor C., III, et al., eds. *Nelson Textbook of Pediatrics,* 11th ed. Philadelphia: W.B. Saunders Co., 1979.

Vinicor, F., and Cooper, J. "Early Recognition of Endocrine Disorders," *Hospital Medicine* 15:38, December 1979.

Wake, M., and Brensinger, J.F. "The Nurse's Role in Hypothyroidism," *Nursing Clinics of North America* 15:453, September 1980.

Watts, N., and Keffer, J. *Practical Endocrine Diagnosis,* 2nd ed. Philadelphia: Lea and Febiger, 1978.

Williams, Robert H., ed. *Textbook of Endocrinology,* 5th ed. Philadelphia: W.B. Saunders Co., 1974.

19

KEY POINTS IN THIS CHAPTER

KEY CHARTS IN THIS CHAPTER

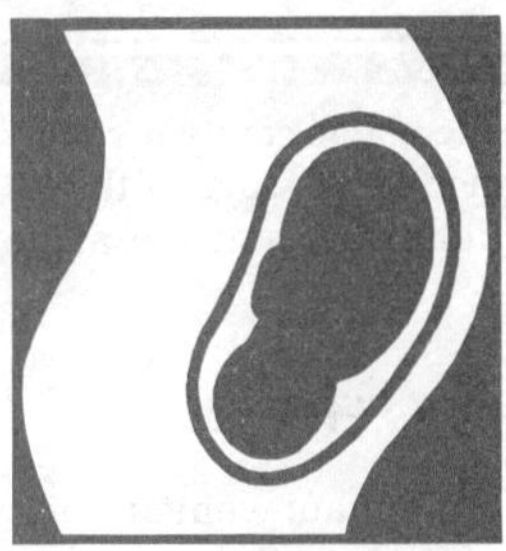

The Pregnant Patient

Introduction

779 Challenges of patient care in pregnancy

Your assessment of a pregnant patient can be challenging and exciting. If you know how to thoroughly evaluate a woman's health during pregnancy, you can implement an individualized plan of prenatal care that will help secure a positive outcome for both mother and child.

Pregnancy affects a woman's entire body, so make your assessment comprehensive. Begin with the common complaints of pregnancy and a complete assessment of each body system. Evaluate the patient's emotional stability, including her acceptance of the pregnancy, her preparation for parenthood, and the pregnancy's impact on the family.

Always assess a pregnant patient within the context of the *maternal-fetal unit.* Although mother and child have separate and distinct needs, their interdependent relationship means that factors influencing the mother's health may affect the health of the fetus, and alterations in fetal well-being may influence the mother's physical and emotional health.

Educating your patient about her pregnancy is as fundamental to the relationship the two of you share as the ongoing assessment you perform at each prenatal visit. Your initial assessment may indicate that the woman should modify some of her health practices in such areas as diet, rest, exercise, alcohol intake, and smoking. Help her to evaluate her health habits and to change any that may be harmful to her or her baby. You may also want to recommend support services that will enhance her well-being and the family's during the pregnancy and after the birth of the baby.

780 Providing emotional support

The support you provide as your patient adjusts to the physical and emotional changes of pregnancy is extremely important. For example, the pregnant woman's increasing weight and altered body image, as well as changes in her body functions, can make her very anxious. Or, the woman accustomed to being in control of her feelings may be frustrated and even frightened by the mood swings that commonly accompany pregnancy. Pregnancy should be a time of happy anticipation for a woman. But financial, medical, or family problems can make her pregnancy seem burdensome. Your encouragement and guidance, as well as appropriate referral to other members of the health-care team, will play a significant role in helping your patient cope with her concerns.

Reviewing anatomy and physiology

781 Female pelvis

The female pelvis is a bony, basin-shaped structure that encloses the pelvic organs and provides a supportive arch for distribution of weight to the legs. It consists of the sacrum, the coccyx, and two innominate, or hip, bones (see *Anatomy of the Pelvis*, page 744).

The *sacrum* is a large triangular bone with a concave ventral surface, formed by the fusion of the five sacral vertebrae. Its lower surface connects to the *coccyx;* several small coccygeal vertebrae, fused together, create this rudimentary structure. The *hip bones* form the side and anterior walls of the pelvis. They join anteriorly at the symphysis pubis. The sacroiliac joints link them with the sacrum posteriorly.

Each hip bone is actually composed of three separate bones: the ilium, the ischium, and the pubis. In the adult, these bones fuse at the acetabulum, the cup-shaped socket of the hip joint that receives the head of the femur.

The *ilium,* the largest of the bones, forms the upper part of the hip bone. Its expanded, fanlike upper end forms the *iliac crest,* which you can easily feel by placing your hand on your patient's hip. The *ischium* lies below and behind the acetabulum. You can palpate its most prominent feature, the large broad ischial tuberosity, deep in the buttock. The ischial spine, a sharp triangular process, projects posteriorly and medially from the ischium.

The C-shaped *pubis* forms the front wall of the pelvis. Its upper extension joins with the acetabulum; its lower extension fuses with the ischium, forming the *subpubic arch.*

A woman's pelvic bones are thinner and lighter than a man's. The opening of her pelvis—the *pelvic inlet*—is larger than a man's, the pelvic cavity is roomier (to accommodate passage of the fetus during childbirth), and the angle is wider.

782 Pelvic capacity

Estimation of a pregnant woman's pelvic capacity depends on several measurements (see *Pelvic Measurements,* page 746). The measurements associated with the pelvic inlet are the anteroposterior diameters and the transverse diameter. The *anteroposterior diameters of the pelvic inlet* are:

- the *true conjugate*—the distance from the sacral promontory to the top of the symphysis pubis
- the *obstetric conjugate*—the distance from the middle of the sacral promontory to approximately ½″ (1 cm) below the pubic crest (the middle of the symphysis pubis). It is through this diameter that the fetus must descend.
- the *diagonal conjugate*—the distance from the sacral promontory to the inferior margin of the symphysis pubis.

The *transverse diameter of the pelvic inlet* is the widest side-to-side area located off the exact center of the pelvic inlet, nearer to the sacral promontory than to the symphysis pubis.

In the midpelvis, the *interspinous diameter* is important. It's the distance between the two ischial spines (the narrowest part of the midpelvis).

The diameters of the pelvic outlet are:

- the *anteroposterior diameter of the pelvic outlet*—the distance from the lower border of the symphysis pubis to the tip of the sacrum
- the *transverse diameter of the pelvic outlet* (the intertuberous diameter)—the distance between the inner surfaces of the ischial tuberosities (see *Comparing Pelvic Types,* page 745).

783 Pelvic muscles

Pelvic muscles are grouped as follows:

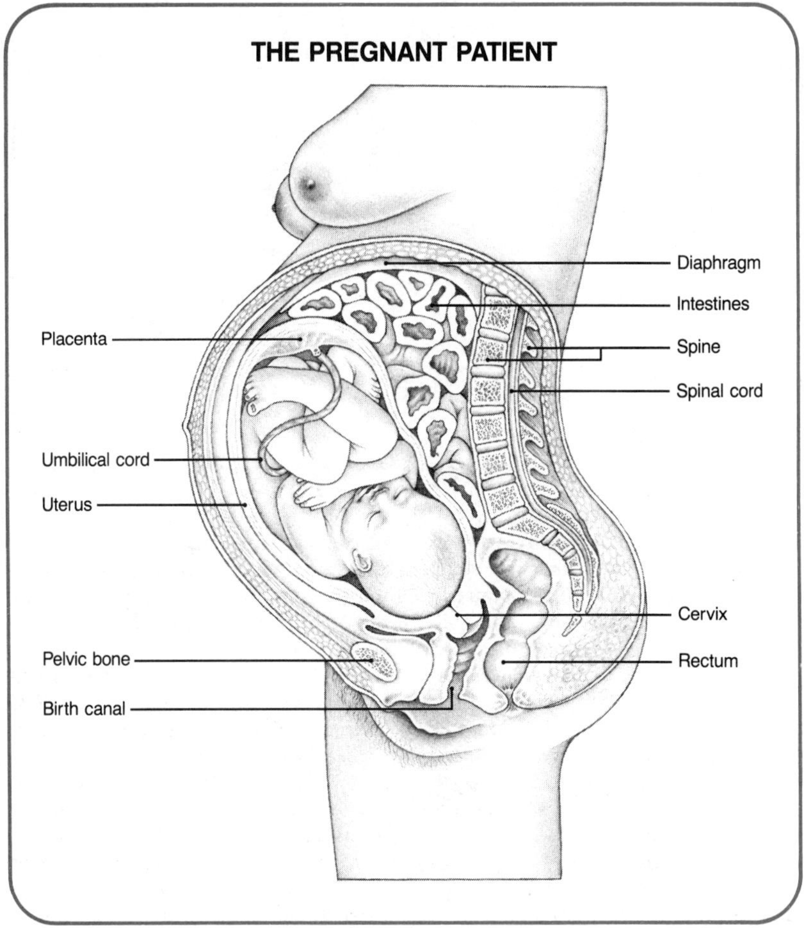

• *Group I:* These are the muscles that line the lateral pelvic walls. They include the piriformis and obturator internus muscles.
• *Group II:* This is the muscle group that forms the muscular sling that supports the pelvic organs. The levator ani and coccygeus muscles belong to this category.
• *Group III:* Lying between the lower extension of the pubis and associated with the external genitalia, these muscles are represented by the bulbospongiosus, the ischiocavernosus, and the superficial transverse perineal. (For more information, see *Muscles of the Pelvic Floor,* page 747.)

784 Fertilization

At ovulation, the mature ovarian follicle discharges its ovum, which promptly moves into the fallopian tube. Cilia propel the ovum down the tube, aided by rhythmic contractions of smooth muscle in the tubal wall. For fertilization to occur, the sperm must penetrate the *zona pellucida,* a homogeneous membrane surrounding the ovum. The *head cap* (acrosome), a thin membrane covering the sperm head, contains the enzymes necessary to do this. The sperm and egg nuclei then fuse, restoring the full complement of 46 chromosomes, to become a *zygote.*

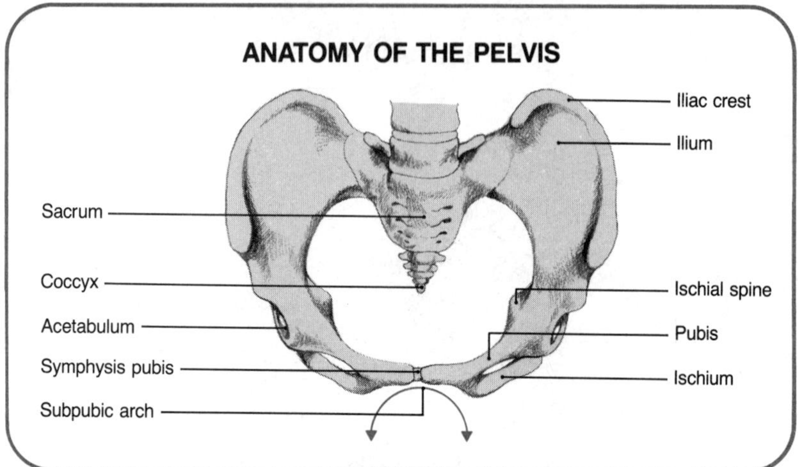

785 Early development and implantation

Shortly after fertilization, the zygote begins moving down the fallopian tube toward the endometrium. Along the way, it undergoes a series of mitotic divisions (known as *cleavage*); the first division is completed about 30 hours after fertilization. These divisions convert the zygote into a little ball of cells called a *morula,* which reaches the endometrial cavity about 3 days after fertilization.

Inside the endometrial cavity, the morula's core begins to fill with fluid and becomes a *blastocyst.* This structure has two parts: the *trophoblast,* a rim of cells that form the fetal membranes and help create the placenta, and the *inner cell mass,* a cluster of cells within the trophoblast that form the embryo.

For several days, the blastocyst lies freely in the endometrial cavity. Then the zona pellucida degenerates, exposing the underlying trophoblast, which responds by proliferating and invading the endometrium. Gradually the blastocyst burrows into the endometrium until it lies completely beneath its surface. The site of penetration then seals over. This process, known as *implantation,* is complete about 1 week after fertilization.

786 Embryonic development

Soon after implantation, the embryo—which contains the beginnings of all major body structures—begins to develop from the blastocyst's inner cell mass. First the inner cell mass turns into a three-layered *embryonic disk.* Then an *amniotic sac* forms on one side of the disk, and a *yolk sac* forms on the other side. The blastocyst cavity enclosing the disk and sacs acquires a lining of connective tissue. The entire structure is called a *chorionic vesicle.* It has a wall, the *chorion,* and fingerlike projections of trophoblast called *chorionic villi.*

As the vesicle develops, it flexes and becomes cylindrical. During the flexion process, the amniotic sac surrounds the embryo and grows with it. Eventually, the sac completely fills the chorionic cavity and fuses with the chorion.

Formative blood vessels within the growing villi attach to other rudimentary vessels in the chorion's connective tissue lining and in the *body stalk*—the band of tissue that connects the embryo to the chorion. (The body stalk later becomes the umbilical cord.) When the embryo's heart starts to beat, blood begins to flow through this network of vessels—from the embryo through the body stalk, to the chorion, into the villi, and back to the embryo. This marks the beginning of *fetoplacental circulation* and occurs about 22 days after fertilization.

787 Placenta formation and structure

Placenta formation begins during the third week of embryonic development, at the site of implantation. At term, the disk-shaped placenta measures about 6″ to 8″ (15 to 20 cm) in diameter and weighs 14 to 21 oz (400 to 600 g), or about one sixth the normal weight of the newborn.

During pregnancy, the endometrium of the pregnant uterus, called the *decidua,* thickens to about ⅜″ (1 cm). This is the maternal portion of the placenta. The chorionic villi form spaces in the base of the decidua. These spaces fill with maternal blood, and the villi proliferate and form the *chorion frondosum,* the placenta's fetal component. The placental layer closest to the fetus is called the *amnion.* The developing placenta is divided into compartments, called *cotyledons,* in which the vascular systems formed by the villi become the junction of the maternal and fetal layers. This junction becomes the site of maternal-fetal transfer of gases and nutrients.

The umbilical cord develops from the body stalk. It extends from the fetal umbilicus to the placenta's fetal surface. White, moist, and amnion-covered, the cord is ⅜″ to 1″ (1 to 2.5 cm) in diameter, with an average length of 22″ (55 cm) at term.

COMPARING PELVIC TYPES

Illustrated here are the four basic pelvic types—gynecoid, anthropoid, android, and platypelloid.

You'll find that most women's pelves are combinations of two types, although characteristics of one type—such as the gynecoid, the most common in women—usually predominate. The woman with a gynecoid or anthropoid pelvis is likely to have an uncomplicated labor and delivery. The woman with a predominantly android or platypelloid pelvis may require delivery by cesarean section.

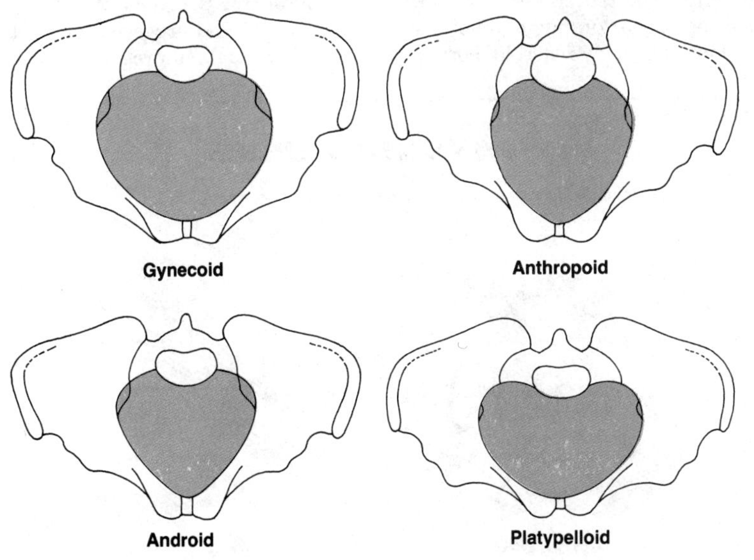

788 Blood circulation in the placenta

The placenta has two kinds of blood circulation. *Fetoplacental circulation* delivers deoxygenated blood from the fetus through the umbilical arteries into the chorionic villi. It also carries oxygenated blood rich in nutrients to the fetus through the umbilical vein. *Uteroplacental circulation* delivers oxygenated maternal blood into the large vascular network called the *intervillous spaces*. After circulating around the villi through the intervillous spaces, the blood flows back into veins that enter the basal part of the placenta adjacent to the uterine arteries.

The maternal and fetal circulations don't normally mix within the placenta, but they do remain in close contact. This allows the transfer of oxygen and nutrients from maternal blood in the intervillous spaces to fetal blood in the villi, and it permits transport of fetal waste products to the maternal blood for elimination.

789 Placenta's endocrine function

Along with nourishing and sustaining the fetus, the placenta acts as an endocrine organ, producing two protein hormones and two steroid hormones. The protein hormones are *human chorionic gonadotropin* (HCG) and *human placental lactogen* (HPL), also called *human chorionic somatomammotropin* (HCS). The steroid hormones are *estrogen* and *progesterone*. The placenta also produces a thyroid-stimulating hormone called *human chorionic thyrotropin* (HCT), but its significance in pregnancy is not yet clear.

The function of HCG is to stimulate the corpus luteum to increase secretion of estrogen and progesterone. HCG levels begin to rise soon after conception. Levels rise rapidly and peak about the time of the second missed period. After the first trimester, HCG production declines.

HPL, which is similar to pituitary growth hormone, stimulates maternal metabolism of proteins and fats. This ensures adequate amino acid and fatty acid production to supply the growing fetus. HPL also stimulates maternal breast growth. Levels of this hormone rise progressively throughout pregnancy.

HCT stimulates the thyroid, accounting in part for the hyperplasia of that gland during pregnancy.

Estrogen and progesterone levels increase throughout pregnancy. The pla-

PELVIC MEASUREMENTS

The measurements indicated here are used to estimate pelvic capacity.

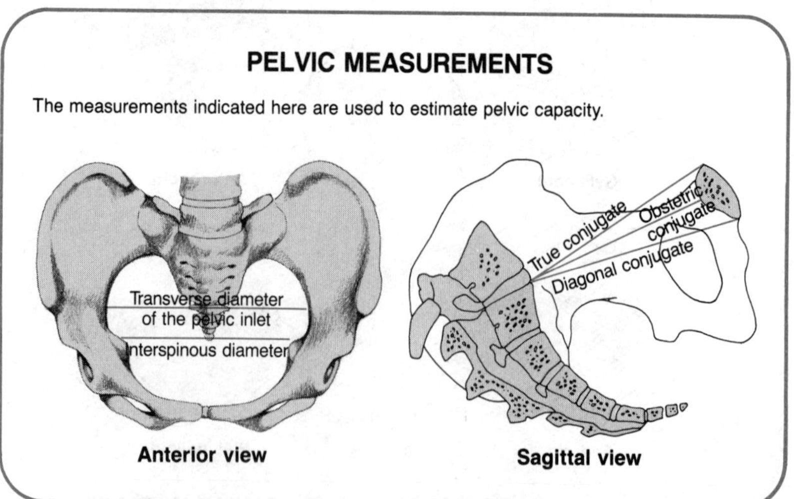

MUSCLES OF THE PELVIC FLOOR

The illustration on the top shows the pelvic floor muscles that line the lateral pelvic walls and support the pelvic organs, as viewed from above. The illustration on the bottom shows the pelvic floor muscles associated with external genitalia, as viewed from below.

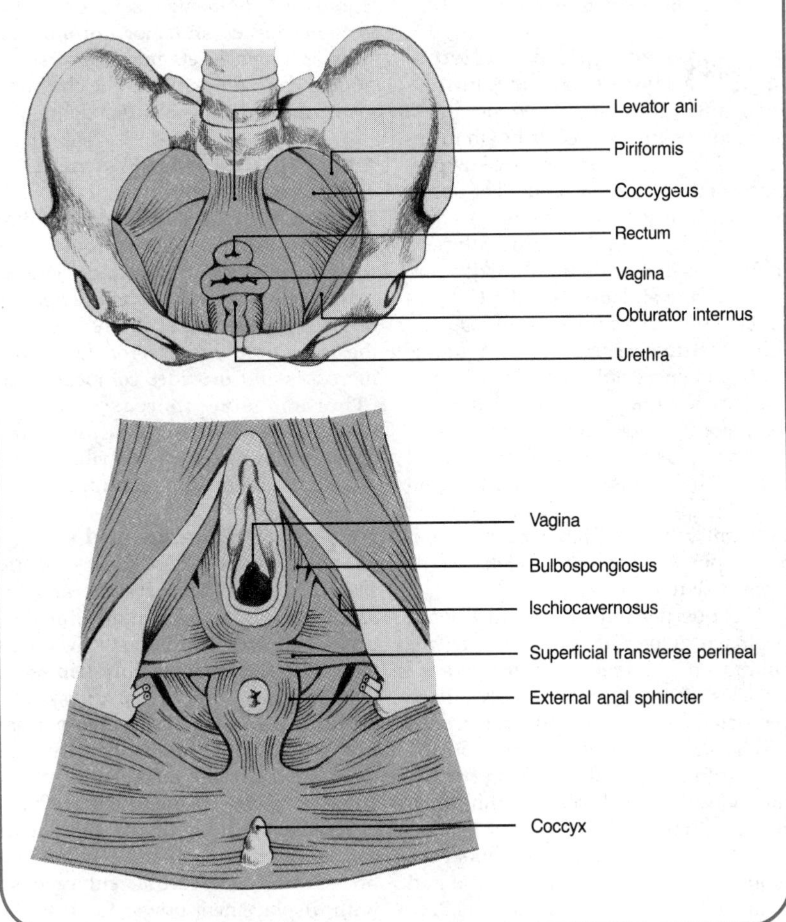

centa synthesizes estrogen and progesterone. The fetal adrenal glands and the uteroplacental circulation supply the many precursor steroid compounds required to produce them. Estrogen produces enlargement of the pregnant woman's uterus, breasts, and breast glandular tissue. It also plays a significant part in increasing vascularity and vasodilation at the end of pregnancy.

Because the fetal adrenal glands supply most of the estrogen precursors, a progressively rising output throughout pregnancy reflects fetal well-being; declining estrogen production may indicate fetal distress or failing placental function.

Progesterone must be present for implantation to occur, and it maintains pregnancy by inhibiting myometrial contractility. It also increases secretions in the fallopian tubes and uterus to provide nutrients to the developing embryo. The condition of the fetus doesn't affect progesterone levels. Normally, the placenta produces large amounts of progesterone, which reach 250 mg a day near term.

790 Reproductive system changes in pregnancy

Soon after the first missed period, a pregnant woman's breasts begin to enlarge due to hormone-induced hyperplasia of the glandular tissue. The uterus progressively softens and enlarges during pregnancy. As the uterus enlarges, it distends the abdominal cavity and stretches the abdominal wall. The umbilicus may become everted. During this time, the cervical mucous glands undergo hypertrophy, and the mucosal folds become thick and prominent. Large amounts of thick mucus, secreted by the hyperplastic glands, fill the cervical canal. The uterus, cervix, and vagina also become more vascular during pregnancy. The vagina, normally pink, turns purple-blue (Chadwick's sign) from vascular engorgement.

The puerperium is a 6- to 8-week postpartum period during which involution of the uterus occurs and the muscles of the vagina and pelvic floor recover their tone. A moderate vaginal discharge, called *lochia*, occurs during this period. Red at first (lochia rubra), on about the fourth postpartum day it becomes pale pink and watery (lochia serosa) and remains so until about the tenth day, when it becomes white and creamy (lochia alba). This discharge gradually subsides, disappearing within a few weeks. Lactation also occurs during the puerperium. For 2 to 3 days after delivery the mother's breasts secrete colostrum; then, true milk production begins.

791 Skin changes during pregnancy

Increased secretion of melanocyte-stimulating hormone from the pituitary gland causes a generalized increase in skin pigment during pregnancy. The most conspicuous early manifestation of this change is darkening of the areolae. Sometimes the woman's facial skin develops irregular areas of dark pigmentation, called *chloasma*. Pigmented skin nevi also become darker and more prominent. High estrogen levels may cause small angiomas on the skin over the chest and arms; these disappear after delivery.

792 Respiratory system changes

The growing uterus displaces the diaphragm upward, which tends to hinder the mother's respiration and increase her respiratory rate. But vital capacity doesn't change significantly, because the transverse diameter of the thorax increases and provides compensation. (Thoracic size increases due to hormone-mediated relaxation of the ligaments connecting the ribs to the vertebral column and sternum.)

793 Pregnancy and the cardiovascular system

Blood pressure, both systolic and diastolic, tends to fall slightly in midpregnancy and then rise to the woman's normal level during the third trimester. Consider any rise above 30 mm systolic or 15 mm diastolic from her normal pressure abnormal. Normally, the woman's heart rate increases by about 10 beats/minute during pregnancy; exaggerated splitting of the first heart sounds, murmurs in the jugular and breast areas, and cardiac enlargement with displacement upward and to the left are also normal findings. White blood cell count, which varies during pregnancy, is usually within a range of 5,000 to 12,000/ml.

Blood volume—both red cell and plasma—increases during pregnancy by as much as 1,500 ml. As plasma volume expands, the concentration of red cells falls, stimulating the bone marrow to increase red cell production—and also causing a hemodilution effect, because the rise in plasma volume exceeds the compensatory increase in red cells.

Venous pressure in legs and feet increases during pregnancy, because the enlarging uterus compresses the pelvic veins and impedes venous return. This venous compression also contributes to dependent edema and to varicose veins in the legs and vulva.

794 Gastrointestinal changes in pregnancy

The exact cause of nausea and vomiting (morning sickness) during pregnancy is unknown. This may be among the first signs and symptoms the pregnant patient experiences. Increased progesterone levels during pregnancy cause relaxation of the smooth muscles of the gastrointestinal (GI) and biliary tracts. Among other effects, this results in decreased colon motility that predisposes the woman to constipation and hemorrhoids. Hemorrhoids are caused by constipation that leads to increased pressure in veins below the enlarged uterus. Decreased stomach emptying time and reflux of stomach contents, resulting in heartburn (pyrosis), may be additional results of GI tract smooth-muscle relaxation.

The high estrogen level characteristic of pregnancy promotes increased excretion of cholesterol in the bile. The resulting cholesterol-supersaturated bile, coupled with stasis of bile in the gallbladder (caused by relaxation of the smooth muscle of the gallbladder), leads to the precipitation of cholesterol crystals from the bile and may predispose the patient to gallstones.

795 Effects on the urinary system

During the first trimester the enlarging uterus puts pressure on the bladder, resulting in urinary frequency. Pressure is relieved in the second trimester, when the uterus becomes an abdominal organ. Late in pregnancy, engagement of the presenting part exerts pressure on the bladder. The bladder becomes concave, and its capacity is greatly reduced.

Some dilatation of the ureters and the renal calices and pelves is common in pregnancy. It probably occurs because the enlarged uterus compresses the ureter against the pelvic brim. Urine drainage is commonly impeded; this can lead to urinary stasis and predispose the woman to urinary tract infection.

796 Musculoskeletal system changes

A pregnant woman's enlarging uterus displaces her center of gravity forward, causing an increased lumbar lordosis (necessary to maintain balance). Enlarging breasts may cause kyphosis. Increased elasticity of connective and collagen tissue—caused by the increase in circulating steroid sex hormones during pregnancy—results in slight relaxation of the pelvic joints.

Collecting appropriate history data

797 Biographical data

Biographical data are especially pertinent to your assessment of a pregnant patient. Before recording this information, assure your patient that it will be kept confidential. Here are some guidelines and points to follow in this part of your patient's health history:

- *Name.* During the initial interview, address the patient as *Ms.* ______. Never assume—even if the patient has given pregnancy as the reason for her visit—that she is married.
- *Age.* Your patient's exact age is important in determining the possibility of a high-risk pregnancy. Reproductive

risks are greater among adolescents under age 15 and women over age 35. The adolescent patient runs a whole gamut of serious risks: increased incidence of low–birth-weight and premature infants, preeclampsia, anemia, prolonged labor, and cephalopelvic disproportion. Expectant mothers over age 35 are at risk for placenta previa, abruptio placentae, hydatidiform mole, and vascular, neoplastic, and degenerative diseases, as well as for having fraternal twins or infants with genetic abnormalities, especially Down's syndrome (trisomy 21).

• *Race.* Black pregnant women should be screened for sickle cell trait; Jewish women of Eastern European ancestry, for Tay-Sachs disease.

• *Religion.* A woman's religious affiliation may affect her health practices during pregnancy and could predispose her to complications. For example, an Amish woman may not be immunized against rubella. Seventh-Day Adventists traditionally exclude dairy products from their diets.

• *Marital status.* Your patient's marital status may help you identify her family support systems, sexual practices, and possible stress factors.

• *Occupation.* If your patient is working in a high-risk environment (one that exposes her to such hazards as chemicals, inhalants, or radiation), inform her of the risks and consequences for her pregnancy and discuss the possibility of a transfer.

• *Education.* Your patient's educational experiences—both formal and informal—may influence her attitude toward pregnancy, the adequacy of her prenatal care and nutritional status, her knowledge of infant care, and the psychosocial changes that accompany childbirth and the parenting years.

798 Chief complaint

If the patient hasn't specified pregnancy as the reason for her visit, you may want to be cautious about suggesting pregnancy as the reason—unless you've obtained a positive pregnancy test or other supportive data. To obtain the most helpful information, allow the patient to explain the reason for her visit in her own words. (Her explanation for seeking obstetric evaluation may also suggest her degree of acceptance of a possible pregnancy.) She may have specific complaints, such as *bleed-*

Chief complaint

• **Bleeding changes**

• **Nausea, with or without vomiting**

• **Urinary disturbances**

• **Fluid retention**

P Q R S T

Questions to ask

Provocative/Palliative
What causes it? What makes it better? What makes it worse?

Quality/Quantity
How does it feel, look, or sound, and how much of it is there?

Region/Radiation
Where is it? Does it spread?

Severity scale
Does it interfere with activities? How does it rate on a severity scale of 1 to 10?

Timing
When did it begin? How often does it occur? Is it sudden or gradual?

ing changes (including amenorrhea and vaginal bleeding disorders), *nausea* (with or without vomiting), *urinary disturbances,* or *fluid retention.* You'll investigate these complaints to determine if she's pregnant and to identify pregnancy-related disorders.

799 History of presenting symptoms

Using the PQRST mnemonic device, ask the patient to elaborate on her complaint. Then, depending on the complaint, explore the history of the presenting symptoms with the following types of questions:

• ***Bleeding changes (amenorrhea).*** *When was your last menstrual period?* If the patient has difficulty recalling, refer to a calendar and try to prompt her memory with landmark dates, such as holidays. Consider the possibility of pregnancy when a woman who has regular menses abruptly misses a period. Consider it likely if the woman has missed two consecutive periods. *Was your last period "normal"? How long did the period last? Was the flow lighter than usual?* Although amenorrhea is the usual condition in a well-established pregnancy, a few women may report periodic bleeding for several months. Usually this bleeding is lighter and lasts for a shorter time than a normal menstrual flow. *Have you recently experienced an illness or unusual stress?* Recent illness, rapid or excessive weight loss, or change in daily routine may contribute to amenorrhea.

• ***Bleeding changes (vaginal bleeding disorders).*** *What specific events preceded the bleeding?* Sexual intercourse or a vaginal examination may traumatize the cervix. Exposure to infection or disease may precipitate a spontaneous abortion. Trauma can cause abruptio placentae. *When in your pregnancy did the bleeding begin?* Spontaneous abortion is a major cause of bleeding during the first 20 weeks of pregnancy. Bleeding that occurs later in the pregnancy can indicate such disorders as placenta previa or abruptio placentae. The bleeding may also be the *bloody show* that signifies the onset of labor. *Is the bleeding accompanied by pain and/or cramping?* Pain usually accompanies ectopic pregnancy, abruptio placentae, and spontaneous abortion. Hydatidiform mole, placenta previa, and spontaneous abortion caused by cervical incompetence are usually painless.

• ***Nausea (with or without vomiting).*** *When did the nausea begin?* Nausea and/or vomiting associated with pregnancy usually begins about 6 weeks after the woman's last menstrual period, when hormone levels are high. *When does the nausea and/or vomiting occur?* Nausea associated with pregnancy often occurs in the morning hours when the stomach is empty. However, it may persist throughout the day or evening. *What relieves the nausea?* Women generally report that nausea is relieved by eating dry crackers or toast in the morning and frequent small meals throughout the day (for example, six small meals instead of three large ones). However, the symptoms usually disappear through the normal course of pregnancy after 12 to 16 weeks. *Are you able to tolerate any food at all?* Severe nausea and vomiting, with little or no tolerance of food, may indicate hyperemesis gravidarum. *Have medical problems or stressful situations preceded the nausea?* You know that nausea is a universal symptom that can indicate many underlying problems, such as stress or physiologic disorders.

• ***Urinary disturbances.*** *Have your bladder habits changed recently? When did the urinary disturbances begin?* Pregnant women commonly experience urinary frequency with urgency, particularly during the first and third trimesters of pregnancy.

Have you noticed other urinary changes? Painful urination, foul-smelling or cloudy urine, color changes, and bladder tenderness may indicate a urinary tract infection.

• ***Fluid retention.*** *Have you noticed any swelling? Do your rings fit more tightly? Are your eyelids puffy?* Edema of the hands and face may indicate preeclampsia. Dependent edema of the feet and ankles, especially in late pregnancy, is common. *Is this your first pregnancy?* Preeclampsia occurs most often with first pregnancies, but its symptoms may occur in later pregnancies if predisposing factors exist, such as diabetes mellitus, multiple gestation, fetal hydrops, hydatidiform mole, or underlying chronic vascular disease. *What decreases the swelling?* A woman may get relief by lying on her side, commonly the left. Decreasing or eliminating intake of salty foods may also help physiologic edema. *What other changes have you noticed?* Visual disturbances, headache, and epigastric and right upper quadrant pain may indicate progressive preeclampsia; refer the patient promptly.

800 Past gynecologic history

Explore your patient's gynecologic history with the following types of questions:

• ***Menstrual history.*** *When did your last menstrual period begin? How many days passed between your last two periods? What is the usual amount and duration of menstrual flow?* Based on this information, you can calculate your patient's estimated date of confinement, using Nägele's rule: *first day of last normal menstrual period, minus three months, plus seven days.* Because Nägele's rule is based on a 28-day cycle, you may need to vary the calculation for a woman whose menstrual cycle is irregular, prolonged, or shortened.

Age of menarche is important when determining pregnancy risks in adolescents. Pregnancy that occurs within 3 years of menarche indicates an increased risk of mortality, morbidity, and a newborn who's small for his gestational age. Keep in mind that pregnancy can also occur before regular menses are established. (For information on how to take a complete menstrual history, see Entries 555 to 562.)

• ***Contraceptive history.*** *What form of contraception do you use? How long have you used it? Are you satisfied with the method?* Pregnancy that results from contraceptive failure needs special consideration to ensure the patient's medical and emotional well-being. For example, birth control pills taken in the first trimester can be teratogenic. If your patient has used an intrauterine device, refer her to her obstetrician to have it removed promptly upon verification of pregnancy. This will avoid the risk of spontaneous abortion in the second trimester.

• ***Sexual history.*** *When did you begin your sexual activity? How frequently do you engage in sexual activity? Are you experiencing any difficulties?* Knowledge of the patient's sexual activity will inform you about her sexual knowledge and guide your patient teaching during her pregnancy. Don't assume that every pregnant woman is well-informed about sex.

Your patient's sexual desire may decrease during the first trimester, a common occurrence that may be attributed to the increased fatigue, nausea, and vomiting that most women experience then. During the second trimester, however, sexual desire often returns because of feelings of well-being and resolution of the first trimester's signs and symptoms. Alterations in comfort and additional psychophysiologic changes may decrease sexual desire again during the third trimester.

801 Past obstetric history

If your patient is a multigravida, you'll want to know about any complications that affected her previous pregnancies. A woman who has delivered one or more very large infants (more than 9 lb, or 4 kg), or who has a history of recurrent *Monilia* infections or unexplained unsuccessful pregnancies, should be screened for diabetes. A history of recurrent second-trimester abortions may indicate an incompetent cervix. A woman with a history of urinary tract infections in previous pregnancies will usually have this problem with every pregnancy. Be especially careful when you evaluate a woman whose pregnancies have been complicated by hypertension.

Always record your patient's obstetric history chronologically. Use a single-digit gravida number (G) to reflect the number of times the woman's been pregnant, followed by a four-digit para number (P), which tells you about the outcomes of the pregnancies. The para digits represent the number of full-term births (greater than 37 weeks' gestation), premature births (less than 37 weeks' gestation), abortions before 20 weeks, and living children. (The first letter of each word in *Florida Power And Light* may help you remember the order of the para digits.) For example, "G-2/P-1-0-1-1" represents a patient who's been pregnant twice, has had one full-term birth, no premature births, one abortion (before 20 weeks), and one living child.

An abbreviated but less informative version reflects only the gravida and para numbers and the number of abortions. For example, "G-3, P-2, Ab-1" represents a patient who's been pregnant three times, has had two deliveries after 20 weeks' gestation, and one abortion. (For other types of information that you should include in a complete obstetric history, see *Taking the Obstetric History*.)

802 Past medical and family history

In this part of the history, ask the patient about previous medical problems that may be exacerbated by her pregnancy. For example, displacement of the stomach by the gravid uterus, along with relaxation of the cardiac sphincter and decreased gastric motility caused by increased progesterone, may augment symptoms of peptic ulcer disease, such as gastric reflux.

Find out whether the woman is taking any medications, including over-the-counter drugs. Most drugs cross the placenta and reach the fetus. The patient's doctor must carefully evaluate her medications, weighing the benefits of each drug against its risk to the fetus.

Also inquire about medical problems that may jeopardize the pregnancy. Maternal hypertension increases the risk of abruptio placentae. Preeclampsia occurs more often in women with essential hypertension, renal disease, or diabetes. In addition, diabetes can worsen during pregnancy and harm both mother and fetus.

Rubella infection during the first trimester may have teratogenic effects on the developing fetus. A pregnant woman with a history of genital herpes should be watched closely for any signs of active disease, because she may transmit the disease to her infant if she doesn't deliver by cesarean section.

Other problems that you should ask your pregnant patient about are: cardiac disorders, chronic obstructive pulmonary disease, tuberculosis, sexually transmitted disease, phlebitis, epilepsy, urinary tract infections, gall-

TAKING THE OBSTETRIC HISTORY

When taking your pregnant patient's obstetric history, ask her about the following:

- History of infertility
- Genital tract anomalies
- Full-term pregnancies
- Preterm pregnancies
- Abortions
- Birthplace, weight, and condition of infants
- Type of delivery
- Medications used during pregnancy
- Complications during previous pregnancies and labors
- Duration of labor
- Rh of previous babies
- Postpartum problems the mother experienced after previous pregnancies
- Problems with previous infants during first several days after birth.

bladder disease, malignancies, alcoholism, smoking, drug addiction, and psychiatric problems.

A family history of varicose veins is important; some people have an inherited weakness in blood vessel walls that may become evident during pregnancy. Preeclampsia and eclampsia also have familial tendencies. Also ask about a family history of multiple births and congenital diseases or deformities. Sex-linked disorders may be attributed to the father. Some fetal congenital anomalies have been traced to paternal exposure to environmental hazards.

803 Activities of daily living

Talk with your patient about the following aspects of her daily life, which may affect the course of her pregnancy:

• *Nutrition.* Pregnancy places additional nutritional demands on a woman's body. Remember, a woman's health during pregnancy is influenced by her nutritional status prior to pregnancy as well as her nutrition during pregnancy. Carefully assess your patient's food preferences, any ethnic dietary practices, allergies, food intolerances, and present diet. (See Chapter 5, ASSESSING NUTRITIONAL STATUS.)

• *Exercise.* Exercise does not need to be limited in an uncomplicated pregnancy. If your patient exercised regularly before she became pregnant, she probably can continue. Don't advise a pregnant patient to start a new exercise program, such as jogging, however. Make sure the patient understands that she must get adequate rest whether she exercises or not.

• *Travel.* Travel during an uncomplicated pregnancy isn't harmful. If the patient must take lengthy trips, instruct her to exercise intermittently while traveling—for example, by walking every two hours. Advise her not to travel extensively during the final weeks of her pregnancy; she should stay close to her doctor and a hospital in case complications develop.

• *Personal hygiene.* Good personal hygiene habits can help prevent complications, such as infections, and help the woman feel more comfortable during her pregnancy. She should be careful, during bathing, to avoid falling. This is a greater hazard than usual in the final weeks of pregnancy, when the woman's enlarged uterus shifts her body's center of gravity. Douching, especially with a hand-held syringe, is contraindicated. Increased pressure from the syringe may dislodge her mucous plug.

• *Sexual activity.* Usually, a pregnant woman may have sexual intercourse without harming the fetus if she has no vaginal bleeding or pain and shows no signs of a ruptured membrane.

• *Smoking.* Small infants are more frequently born to mothers who smoke, and strong evidence exists that a mother who smokes is more likely to have an unsuccessful pregnancy.

• *Alcohol.* Excessive intake of alcoholic beverages during pregnancy may produce fetal alcohol syndrome in the newborn. Children of alcoholic mothers may also experience growth retardation and other related problems. No safe level of alcohol intake during pregnancy has been identified, so avoiding alcoholic beverages during pregnancy is the best precaution.

• *Drugs.* Chronic use of such drugs as amphetamines, barbiturates, and opium derivatives is harmful to the fetus. Low birth weight, intrauterine fetal distress, and withdrawal symptoms after birth are some of the common problems seen in infants of mothers who use these drugs.

• *Pets.* A pregnant woman shouldn't empty a cat's litter box, because the litter can harbor toxoplasmosis.

804 Review of systems

Conduct a complete review of systems to determine if your patient has any health disorders coexisting with her pregnancy. Also, ask her if she has any of the following signs and symptoms

EMERGENCY

IDENTIFYING DANGER SIGNS

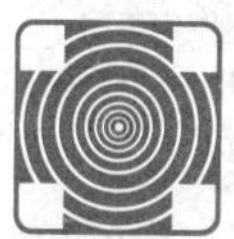

If your patient reports any of the following, notify the doctor immediately. These signs and symptoms *may* pose a threat to the course of the pregnancy and to the mother's health.

SIGN OR SYMPTOM	POSSIBLE INDICATION
Dyspnea	• Impending cardiac decompensation, premature separation of the placenta, excessive amniotic fluid accumulation, or pulmonary embolus
Persistent or recurring headache	• Pregnancy-induced hypertension
Persistent nausea and vomiting	• Hyperemesis gravidarum or systemic infection
Vision changes (flashing lights, dots before eyes, dimming or blurring of vision)	• Pregnancy-induced hypertension
Dizziness when not supine	• Hypoglycemia, anemia, or cardiac arrhythmias
Abdominal pain	• Ectopic pregnancy, abruptio placentae, or uterine rupture
Edema of the face and hands	• Pregnancy-induced hypertension
Cessation of fetal movement	• Fetal death
Vaginal bleeding	• Placenta previa, abruptio placentae, or spontaneous abortion
Sudden escape of fluid from the vagina	• Premature ruptured membranes

that may result from the physiologic changes of pregnancy (see *Identifying Danger Signs*):

• *Metabolic. Weight changes* and *easy fatigability* are common during the early stages of pregnancy, possibly because of a fall in metabolic rate.

• *Skin. Pruritus* is the most common skin complaint during pregnancy. It may be localized to the abdomen or vulva or may spread over the body. The cause is unknown.

• *Ears.* Pregnancy may cause *impaired hearing.* The patient may complain that her ears feel as if they're stuffed with cotton. Occasionally, a pregnant woman's impaired hearing is caused by blocked eustachian tubes.

• *Nose. Altered sense of smell* and *nasal stuffiness* may occur. These signs and symptoms may be vasomotor in origin or may be associated with the mucosal hyperemia that occurs during pregnancy.

• *Mouth.* A pregnant woman may experience *increased gingival bleeding* when she brushes her teeth, secondary to increased estrogen levels.

• *Cardiovascular.* Uterine pressure during pregnancy may inhibit venous return and reduce cardiac output, causing *faintness* and *dizziness* when the woman's in the supine position. Pregnant women often complain of *headaches* in early pregnancy. Severe headache, especially after the 20th week of gestation, may be a sign of preeclampsia.

• *Respiratory.* Hyperventilation may result from increased progesterone levels.

• *Gastrointestinal.* During early pregnancy, increased progesterone levels relax smooth muscles throughout the gastrointestinal system, often causing *nausea* and *vomiting.* Heartburn may result from abnormal gastroesophageal sphincter activity, which permits reflux of gastric fluids. Flatulence, constipation, and hemorrhoids are also common complaints.

• *Reproductive.* Hormonal stimulation during pregnancy typically causes *breast tenderness, sensitivity, tingling,* and *engorgement. Vaginal discharge (leukorrhea)* and *itching* may occur during pregnancy. This often begins during the first trimester, when hormonal influences cause hyperplasia of the vaginal mucosa and increased secretion of mucus by the endocervical glands. These symptoms may also signal vaginitis, especially from *Monilia;* this type occurs more commonly in pregnancy. *Dyspareunia* may result from pelvic congestion, uterine pressure, vulval varicosities, or psychogenic causes, such as fear of hurting the baby.

• *Musculoskeletal. Backache* is a common complaint of pregnancy. It may be due to kyphosis and slouching caused by enlarging breasts and/or lumbar lordosis, which occurs as the uterus enlarges.

• *Psychological. Mood changes, sleeplessness,* and *irritability* may result from the physical signs and symptoms of the first trimester—such as fatigue, nausea, and vomiting. Emotional stress associated with pregnancy may also cause these signs and symptoms.

Conducting the physical examination

805 Scheduling antepartal care

The antepartal period in pregnancy ranges from the first day of the woman's last menstrual period to the start of true labor. The period of time is usually divided into trimesters: weeks 1 to 12 constituting the first trimester; weeks 13 to 27, the second trimester; and weeks 28 to 40, the third trimester. Antepartal-care visits are usually scheduled every 4 weeks for the first 32 weeks of pregnancy; every 2 weeks until week 36 of pregnancy; then weekly until delivery, which usually occurs between weeks 38 and 42.

An early first visit followed by regular visits will help assure a successful pregnancy. Women with known risk factors or who develop complications during the course of pregnancy require more frequent visits.

806 First visit: General survey

On the patient's first visit, perform a complete physical examination, noting any of the normal changes of pregnancy as described in Entries 790 through 796. Then continue with the first visit examination, described in Entries 807 through 810.

807 Examining the breasts

As you inspect and palpate the woman's breasts (see Entry 564), you'll note some normal variations, including increased size and nodularity during the first 20 weeks. This marked and rapid breast hypertrophy may cause *striae* (stretch marks) to appear. The woman may complain of a tingling sensation or breast heaviness during the first and third trimesters. Nipples and areolae usually darken, and superficial veins may dilate. The tubercles of Montgomery usually enlarge; colostrum may appear after the 12th week. Around the 20th week of pregnancy, you'll note the secondary areola—a series of pale spots that surround the primary areola. In multiparas, the breasts are usually less firm.

808 Examining the abdomen

Other than routine examination of the abdomen (see Entry 443), initial abdominal examination of the pregnant woman includes inspection for such normal changes of pregnancy as linea nigra—darkened skin in the abdominal midline. If the pregnancy is sufficiently advanced (usually by the 12th week), palpate for fetal height and position, and auscultate for fetal heart tones (see *Measuring Fundal Height,* page 758).

In early pregnancy, the umbilicus is usually deeply indented, but it becomes more shallow as the pregnancy progresses. At term, the umbilicus is usually level with or protruding from the surface of the abdomen. You may also hear uterine souffle—a soft, blowing sound caused by blood pulsating through the placenta. It occurs at the same rate as the maternal pulse. If the woman's pregnancy is sufficiently advanced, check fetal heartbeats with an ultrasonic stethoscope (at 10 to 12 weeks' gestation) or fetoscope (at 16 weeks' gestation). Fetal heartbeats should range between 120 and 160 beats/minute.

809 Examining the pelvis

Begin pelvic examination of the pregnant patient by inspecting her external and internal genitalia (see Entries 566 and 567). Keep in mind several normal deviations that occur during pregnancy. The labia majora are usually loose and pigmented; the vagina, which appears pink or dark pink at the start of pregnancy, turns purple-blue by the 8th to 12th week.

During the first 4 weeks of gestation, the cervix becomes enlarged in the anteroposterior diameter. At 4 to 6 weeks' gestation, softening of the uterine isthmus occurs (Hegar's sign). By the 8th week, the cervix is uniformly softened (Goodell's sign), and Ladin's sign, a soft area of the uterus near the junction

PRESUMPTIVE, PROBABLE, AND POSITIVE SIGNS OF PREGNANCY

Your pregnancy diagnosis depends on *presumptive* signs and symptoms (those which you or your patient recognize), *probable* signs and symptoms (evidence of pregnancy that you find during the physical examination), and *positive* signs (confirming diagnostic indications usually not apparent until the 4th month of pregnancy).

PRESUMPTIVE SIGNS	PROBABLE SIGNS	POSITIVE SIGNS
• Amenorrhea • Nausea, with or without vomiting • Frequent urination • Breast changes • Discoloration of vaginal mucosa • Increased skin pigmentation and abdominal striae • Fatigue • Quickening	• Uterine enlargement • Softening of the uterine isthmus (Hegar's sign) • Changes in the shape of the uterus • Softening of the cervix (Goodell's sign) • Purplish or bluish color of upper vagina and cervix (Chadwick's sign) • Braxton Hicks contractions • Palpation of fetal parts • Positive pregnancy test results for human chorionic gonadotropin in urine or serum	• Identification of fetal heart sounds • Palpation of active fetal movements • Identification of the fetal skeleton by radiology or sonography

of the uterine body and the cervix, occurs as well. The cervix appears blue. (See *Nurse's Guide to Pregnancy Assessment,* page 761.)

The pear-shaped uterus, which normally is mobile within the pelvis and has a smooth surface, is located at the upper end of the vagina during early pregnancy. By the 8th week of pregnancy, it becomes globular and is often anteflexed against the bladder.

After completing your examination of the patient's pelvic organs, estimate the capacity of her pelvis by taking several pelvic measurements, both internal and external, as discussed in Entry 782 and in *Taking Pelvimetry Measurements.* You can take these measurements when you first examine the pregnant woman's pelvis. Remember, however, that the pelvic ligaments are more relaxed in the late stages of pregnancy. If you wait until then to take your patient's pelvic measurements,

MEASURING FUNDAL HEIGHT

By estimating your patient's uterine size, you can evaluate the fetus' gestational age. How? By measuring fundal height. Between the 18th and 32nd weeks of pregnancy, the fundal height in centimeters equals the fetus' gestational age in weeks. Say your patient's at 24 weeks' gestation; her fundal height should be about 24 cm. Remember, though, that fundal height measurements taken late in pregnancy may not be accurate, because fetal weight variations can distort your reading.

To measure fundal height, follow these steps. With your patient lying flat, place the end of a tape measure at the level of her symphysis pubis. Stretch the tape to the top of the uterine fundus. Record this measurement. Another method of determining fundal height involves using three landmarks: the symphysis pubis, the umbilicus, and the xiphoid process. At 16 weeks, the fundus can be found halfway between the symphysis pubis and the umbilicus. At 20 to 22 weeks, the fundus is at the umbilicus. At 36 weeks, the fundus is at the xiphoid process.

Choose one method of determining fundal height, and use it consistently throughout the patient's pregnancy. Depending on your clinical setting, you may measure with calipers. Remember: Such factors in your patient as a full bladder, amniotic fluid volume, obesity, or tension may affect fundal height measurement.

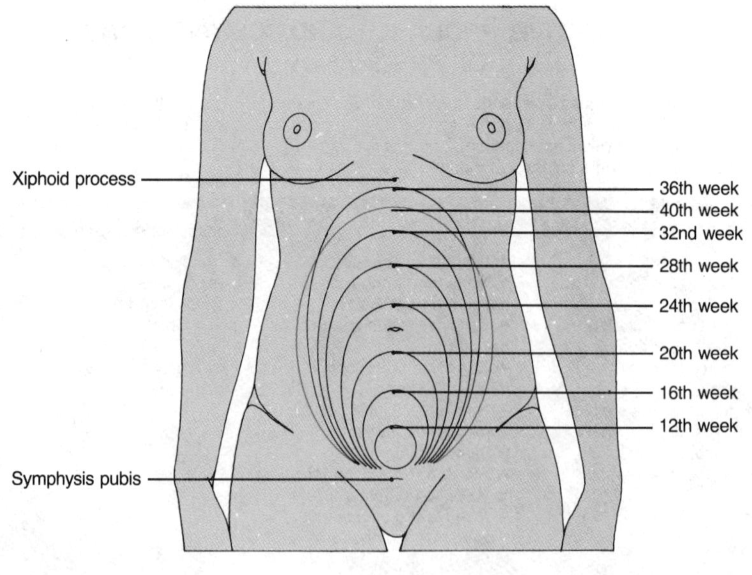

TAKING PELVIMETRY MEASUREMENTS

To estimate pelvic capacity, measure the subpubic arch, intertuberous diameter, interspinous diameter, and diagonal conjugate. Ask the patient to void first. Explain that she may feel discomfort during the procedure but that you'll be very careful.

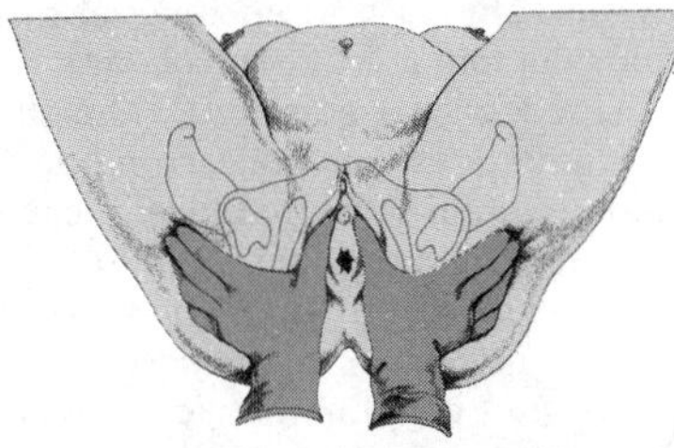

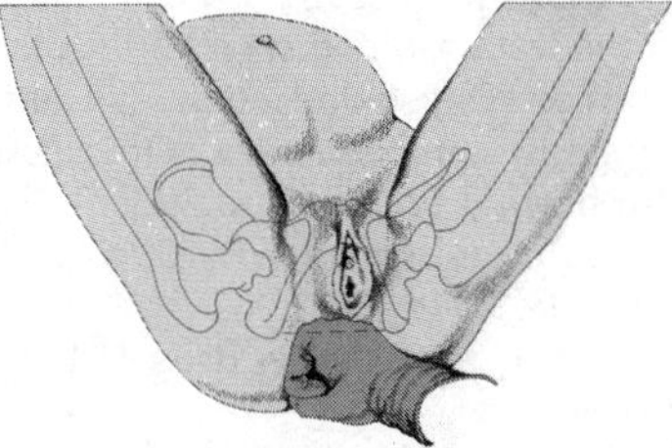

Pelvic outlet measurements: To palpate the subpubic arch—the inferior margin of the symphysis pubis—and to estimate its angle, turn your hands horizontally and place the thumbs in the arch, as shown on the left. Both thumbs should fit comfortably, forming an angle slightly more than 90°. A narrower subpubic angle may cause dystocia.

To estimate the intertuberous, or transverse, diameter, first clench your fist and measure the width of your knuckles. Then, insert the fist between the ischial tuberosities, as shown on the right. If the knuckles are a width of 8 cm or more and fit comfortably, the diameter is adequate. You may use a Thom's pelvimeter to take this measurement.

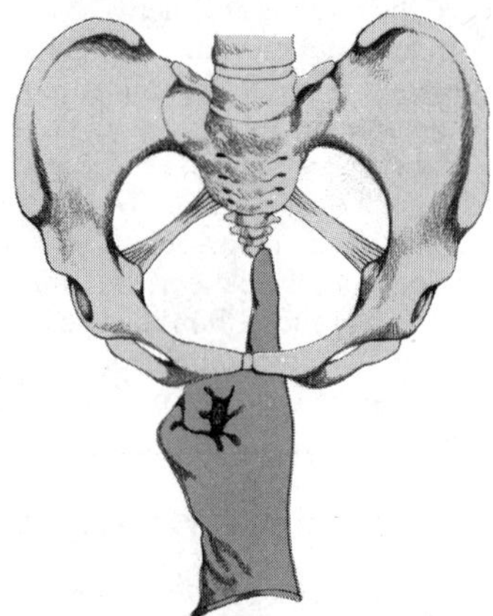

Midpelvis measurement: The interspinous diameter cannot actually be measured. But an estimate of midpelvic capacity can be made by inserting the examining finger or fingers into the vagina and palpating the ischial spines (they should be blunt), the side walls of the pelvis above and below the ischial spines (they should be straight and parallel), the sacrospinous ligament (it should be 2.5 to 3 fingerbreadths long), and the sacrum from below upward (it should be concave and hollow; you should be able to feel only the last three sacral vertebrae without indenting the perineum). Finally, gently palpate the coccyx. It should move easily.

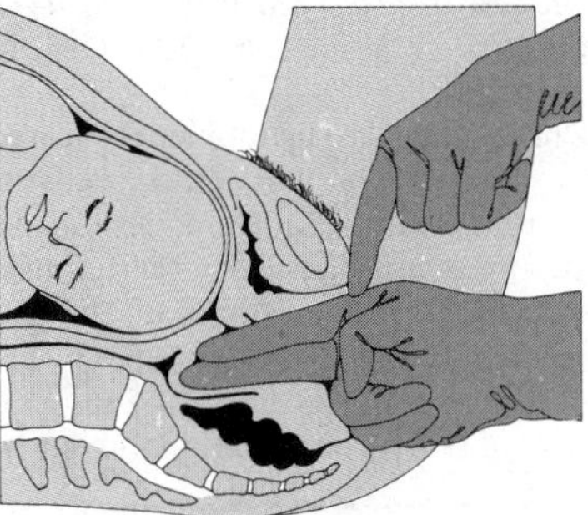

Pelvic inlet measurement: Measurement of the diagonal conjugate may cause your patient the most discomfort. Insert two fingers into the vagina. Attempt to reach the sacral promontory by indenting the perineum with the knuckles of your third and fourth fingers and then walking your fingers up the sacrum to the promontory. If you feel the promontory, maintain contact with it while raising your hand until it touches the lower margin of the symphysis pubis. With the other hand, mark this point as shown in the illustration. Withdraw the hand from the vagina and measure the distance from the tip of your finger to the point you marked. The measurement should be 11.5 cm or more. If you cannot reach the promontory, assume that the diameter is adequate.

To obtain the obstetric conjugate, usually 10 cm, subtract 1.5 cm from the measurement of the diagonal conjugate.

she'll be more comfortable during the procedure, and she'll tolerate it better.

810 Laboratory tests for pregnancy

The first laboratory tests performed for a pregnant patient are the pregnancy test, the test for blood type and Rh factor, a complete blood count, an antibody screen, and a Pap test. Other tests (with normal findings) include:

- hemoglobin/hematocrit—12 to 16 g/dl blood/42% ± 5
- serologic test for syphilis (STS)—nonreactive
- gonorrhea culture (GC)—negative
- urinalysis—negative protein; small amount of glucose; pale yellow in color; negative RBC, WBC, casts; specific gravity of 1.015 to 1.025; and pH of 4.6 to 8.0
- rubella titer, most commonly the hemagglutination-inhibition test—a ratio greater than 1:6 indicates immunity.

Chest X-rays are usually not required for a pregnant patient. But if you suspect tuberculosis, administer the tuberculin skin test. Other tests that may be necessary, depending on the patient's race and symptomatology, are sickle cell trait testing, vaginal cultures, and postprandial blood sugar testing (see *Understanding Immunologic Pregnancy Testing*).

811 Return visits

During each of your patient's return visits, always take an interval history of symptomatology (see *Nurse's Guide to Pregnancy Assessment*). This should include questions concerning any abdominal pain, vaginal bleeding, headache, or urinary tract pain. Record the patient's weight and blood pressure; check her urine for glucose and protein; and examine her for edema, especially of the face and hands, which may indicate preeclampsia. Also be sure to document the first occurrence of quickening (fetal movement) as indicated by the patient, usually around the 16th to 20th weeks. At each visit thereafter, check with the patient to be sure the fetus is still active.

If your patient fails to gain weight, this may result in an unfavorable outcome for the pregnancy. Excessive weight gain (more than 2 lb or 0.9 kg per week) may result from excessive caloric intake or preeclampsia. An elevation from the patient's baseline blood pressure of more than 30 mm systolic/15 mm diastolic is abnormal. The presence of protein in the urine is also ab-

UNDERSTANDING IMMUNOLOGIC PREGNANCY TESTING

Immunologic pregnancy testing is based on the detection of human chorionic gonadotropin (hCG) in urine, using the result of an antibody-antigen reaction. The routine immunologic tests currently in use are the 2-hour test-tube test and the 2-minute slide test. A more sensitive method, known as radioimmunoassay, specifically tests for the beta subunit of hCG in blood samples. The beta-subunit assay has the advantage of being able to detect a pregnancy soon after conception, even before the first period is missed, but it is more expensive than routine immunologic tests and takes 24 hours to complete.

Remember, a positive pregnancy test is only a probable indication of pregnancy. The test results should always be verified by a follow-up physical examination. A woman whose pregnancy test is negative but who continues to experience signs and symptoms of pregnancy should have the test repeated within 10 days.

Other factors that contribute to a false negative reading are the use of dilute or old urine and conditions in pregnancy accompanied by low levels of hCG, for example, ectopic pregnancy or spontaneous abortion. A false positive reading may occur with hematuria, proteinuria, malignancies, menopause, cysts of the corpus luteum, a pelvic abscess, or the ingestion of methyldopa, large doses of aspirin, methadone, promethazine, and psychotropic drugs.

NURSE'S GUIDE TO PREGNANCY ASSESSMENT

GESTATIONAL AGE	NORMAL CHANGES OF PREGNANCY
First trimester	
Weeks 1 to 4	• Amenorrhea occurs • Breast changes begin • Immunologic pregnancy tests become positive: radioimmunoassay test is positive a few days after implantation; urine hCG test is positive 10 to 14 days after occurrence of amenorrhea • Nausea and vomiting begin, between the 4th and 6th week
Weeks 5 to 8	• Goodell's sign occurs (softening of cervix) • Ladin's sign occurs (softening of uterine isthmus) • Hegar's sign occurs (softening of lower uterine segment) • Chadwick's sign appears (purple-blue vagina and cervix) • McDonald's sign appears (easy flexion of the fundus over the cervix) • Braun von Fernwald's sign occurs (irregular softening and enlargement of the uterine fundus at the site of implantation) • Piskacek's sign may occur (asymmetrical softening and enlargement of the uterus) • Cervical mucous plug forms • Uterine shape changes from pear to globular • Urinary frequency and urgency occurs
Weeks 9 to 12	• Fetal heartbeat detected using ultrasonic stethoscope • Nausea, vomiting, and urinary frequency and urgency lessen • By 12 weeks, uterus palpable just above symphysis pubis
Second trimester	
Weeks 13 to 17	• Mother gains approximately 10 to 12 lb (4.5 to 5.4 kg) during second trimester • Uterine souffle heard on auscultation • Mother's heartbeat increases approximately 10 beats between 14 and 30 weeks' gestation. Rate is maintained until 40 weeks' gestation. • By the 16th week, mother's thyroid gland enlarges by approximately 25%, and the uterine fundus is palpable halfway between the symphysis and umbilicus • Maternal recognition of fetal movements, or quickening, occurs between 16 and 20 weeks' gestation
Weeks 18 to 22	• Uterine fundus palpable just below umbilicus • Fetal heartbeats heard with fetoscope at 20 weeks' gestation • Fetal rebound or ballottement possible
Weeks 23 to 27	• Umbilicus appears level with abdominal skin • Striae gravidarum usually apparent • Uterine fundus palpable at umbilicus • Shape of uterus changes from globular to ovoid • Braxton Hicks contractions start
Third trimester	
Weeks 28 to 31	• Mother gains approximately 8 to 10 lb (3.6 to 4.5 kg) in third trimester • Uterine wall feels soft and yielding • Uterine fundus is halfway between umbilicus and xiphoid process • Fetal outline palpable • Fetus very mobile and may be found in any position

(continued)

NURSE'S GUIDE TO PREGNANCY ASSESSMENT *(continued)*

GESTATIONAL AGE	NORMAL CHANGES OF PREGNANCY
Weeks 32 to 35	• Mother may experience heartburn • Striae gravidarum becomes more evident • Fundal height measurement no longer accurate indication of gestational age • Uterine fundus palpable just below the xiphoid process • Braxton Hicks contractions increase in frequency and intensity • Mother may experience shortness of breath
Weeks 36 to 40	• Umbilicus protrudes • Varicosities, if present, become very pronounced • Ankle edema evident • Urinary frequency recurs • Engagement, or lightening, occurs • Mucous plug expelled • Cervix effacement and dilatation begin

normal and may indicate preeclampsia.

Perform abdominal palpation on your patient to determine fundal height and fetal position and presentation (see *Measuring Fundal Height,* page 758, and *Performing Leopold's Maneuvers*). Also check the correlation between fetal growth and estimated gestational age. Fetal position may vary during the pregnancy, but the position of the fetus for labor is usually apparent by week 36.

Auscultate the fetal heart for rate and location. For best results, auscultate through the fetus' back.

Perform the bimanual palpation and a vaginal examination only if indicated. Repeat the hemoglobin/hematocrit test at 28 to 32 weeks' gestation and, if appropriate, the STS and GC tests at 36 weeks. If your patient is Rh negative, repeat the antibody screen test at about 28, 32, and 36 weeks' gestation.

812 Examining your patient near term

Generally, the patient will return for an examination every week during the last four weeks of pregnancy. She'll probably be especially anxious to know when she'll have her baby. Let her know that you can determine whether preparatory events are occurring, but that you can't predict when labor will begin.

During this stage of the pregnancy, continue to monitor fetal heart tones and movement. The fetus should continue to move during the last few weeks: If the fetus is unusually quiet, notify the doctor immediately (see *Assessing Fetal Well-being,* page 764).

During each visit, palpate the patient's uterus for Braxton Hicks contractions, which should now occur more frequently; they also should be more intense and last longer. For each contraction, you'll feel a tightening of the fundal region that moves downward in a wavelike motion and ends with a pulling or tugging near the cervix. The patient usually has at least one internal vaginal examination during the last four weeks of pregnancy.

813 The final internal examination

To perform the internal examination at this stage of pregnancy, you needn't place the patient in stirrups or use a speculum. Instead, using a sterile glove and lubricant, insert two fingers into her vagina and locate the cervix. Note

PERFORMING LEOPOLD'S MANEUVERS

Before auscultating the fetal heart rate, you'll need to determine fetal position. This is important because you will be able to hear fetal heartbeats most clearly through the fetal back. To determine fetal position, perform Leopold's maneuvers, described here. Begin by having the patient empty her bladder. Position her supine, with her abdomen exposed. To perform the first three maneuvers, stand to either side of the patient and face her. For the fourth maneuver, reverse your position and face the patient's feet.

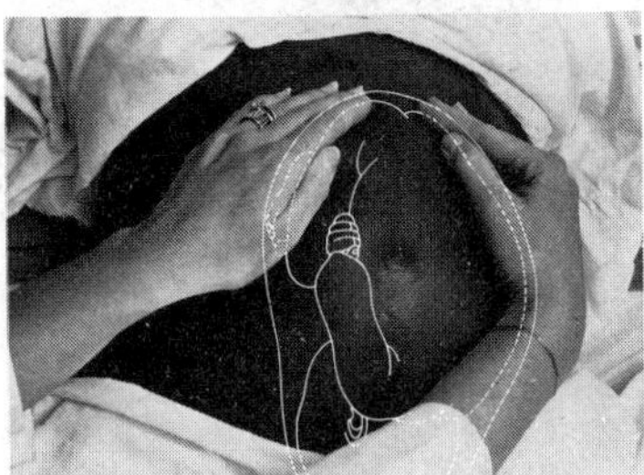

First maneuver: Place your hands on the patient's abdomen, curling your fingers around her uterine fundus. If the fetus is in a vertex position, you'll feel an irregularly shaped, soft object—the buttocks. If the fetus is in a breech position, you'll feel a hard, round, movable object—the head.

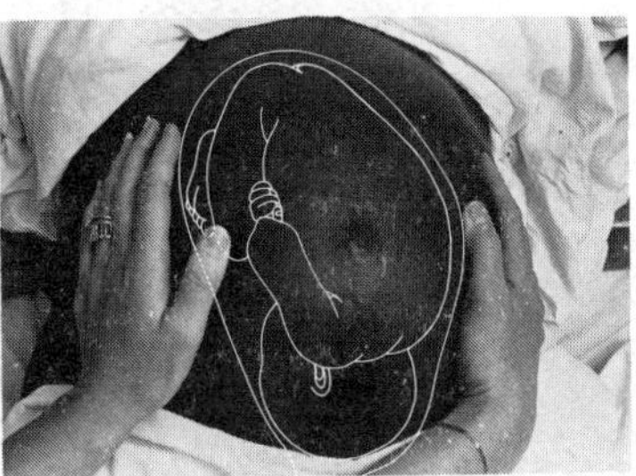

Second maneuver: Next, move your hands down the sides of the patient's abdomen, and apply firm, even inward pressure with the palms. Note whether you feel the fetal back on the patient's left side or right side and whether it's directed anteriorly, transversely, or posteriorly. If the fetus is vertex, you'll feel a smooth, hard surface on one side—the back. On the other side, you'll feel lumps and knobs—the knees, hands, feet, and elbows. If the fetus is breech, you may not be able to feel the back.

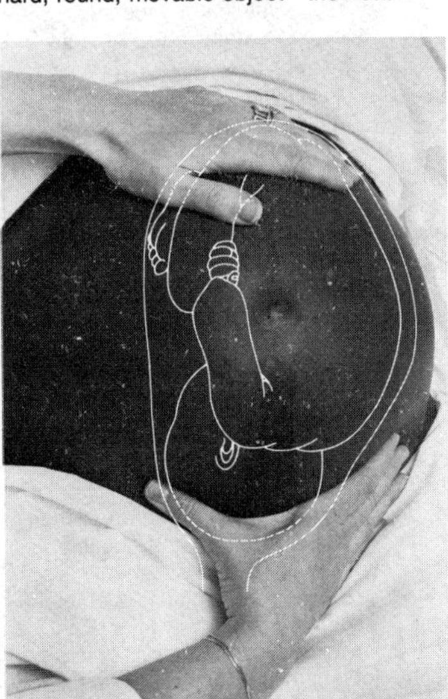

Third maneuver: Now spread apart your thumb and fingers of one hand and place them just above the patient's symphysis pubis. Bring your fingers together. If the fetus is vertex and hasn't descended, you'll feel the head; if the fetus has descended, you'll feel a less distinct mass.

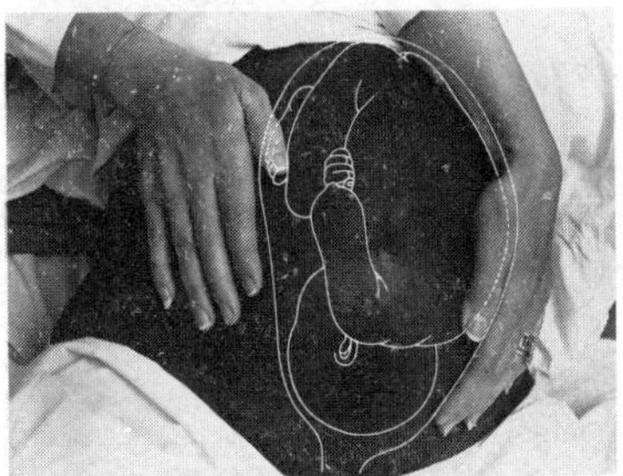

Fourth maneuver: Place your hands on both sides of her lower abdomen. Apply gentle pressure with the fingers of each hand, sliding your hands down toward the symphysis pubis. If the head presents, one hand's descent will be stopped by the cephalic prominence. The other hand will descend unobstructed more deeply. If the fetus is in the vertex position, you'll feel the cephalic prominence on the same side as the small parts. In face presentation, you'll feel the cephalic prominence on the same side as the back. If the fetus is engaged, you can't feel the cephalic prominence.

its softness, the percentage of effacement, and the degree of cervical dilatation.

Assessment Tip: Note that some cervical effacement and dilatation may precede labor, but often these changes do not occur until active uterine contractions have begun.

Effacement, evaluated in percentages, is the obliteration or shortening of the cervical canal from an approximate length of 4⁄5″ (2 cm) to a structure

ASSESSING FETAL WELL-BEING

TEST	DESCRIPTION	USES AND INDICATIONS
Ultrasound	An ultrasonic transducer, placed on the mother's abdomen, transmits high-frequency sound waves. These pass through the abdominal wall, deflect off the fetus, and bounce back to the transducer, where they're translated into a visual image on a monitoring screen.	• Early identification of pregnancy • Biparietal diameter measurement • Placental localization • Placental anomalies • Intrauterine device detection • Identification of multiple gestation • Fetal position and presentation • Fetal anomalies • Demonstration of hydramnios and oligohydramnios • Fetal death • Detection of incomplete or missed abortion • Observation of fetal cardiac activity and breathing movements
Estriol measurement	The placenta converts fetal adrenal precursors to estriol, which enters the mother's blood and urine in measurable amounts. For correct interpretation of estriol values, serial measurements should be performed. In general, rising estriol levels are a positive indicator of fetal well-being; falling levels are a negative indicator. Chronically low estriol levels may indicate intrauterine growth retardation.	• Evaluation of placental function and fetal well-being. • Taken especially in situations involving high-risk conditions, such as maternal diabetes or hypertensive diseases, postmature pregnancy, intrauterine growth retardation syndrome, poor obstetric history, or late antepartal care
Amniocentesis	A sample of amniotic fluid is aspirated for diagnostic tests, which are indicative of fetal well-being. After an adequate pocket of amniotic fluid is localized with sonography, a needle is inserted into the patient's abdomen, through the uterus, and into the amniotic sac to aspirate a sample of the amniotic fluid.	• Assessment of fetal maturity, especially with premature labor or when planning a cesarean section of a patient with a questionable estimated date of confinement • Biochemical monitoring of fetal well-being, especially in an Rh-isoimmunized pregnancy or if other fetal hemolytic disease is suspected • Prenatal diagnosis of genetic disorders, especially if maternal age is advanced (over 35) or a history of chromosomal abnormalities in previous pregnancies, in parents, or in close family members exists

MEASURING FETAL STATION

To identify the level of the presenting fetal part in the birth canal during the vaginal examination, use the scale shown here. First, locate the ischial spines, zero station. Then locate the presenting fetal part, usually the head. Compare this level with the level of the ischial spine. Zero station indicates engagement. At −5 and −4 the fetus is floating; at −1 the fetus is fixed but still not engaged. Positive station measurements mean that the presenting part is low and delivery is imminent.

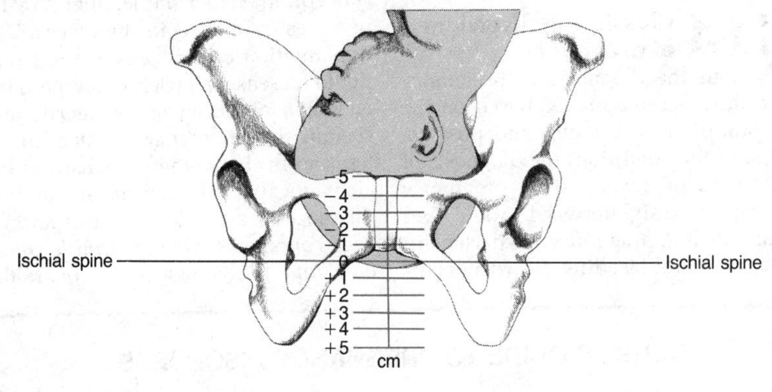

in which the canal is replaced by a circular opening with paper-thin edges. *Dilatation* is the progressive enlargement of the external os to 10 cm. You can judge dilatation by the number of fingertips you can rest comfortably in the external os. Record this in centimeters, not the number of fingertips.

Also determine whether the presenting part of the fetus is properly positioned, or engaged. Approximately two weeks before delivery, primigravidas generally experience *lightening*, the descent of the fetus' presenting part through the inlet of the pelvic canal. Multigravidas usually experience this during labor. You determine this engagement in relation to the level of the ischial spines—the *zero* station. Locate the ischial spines and estimate the descent of the fetus' presenting part. If the presenting part is above the ischial spines, it is not engaged (this is called *floating* and is assigned a negative station number that reflects the number of centimeters the presenting part is above the ischial spines, which are considered station zero). If the presenting part is below the ischial spines, it is engaged and a positive number is assigned to indicate how far, in centimeters, the presenting part lies below station zero. Station measurements are especially important for evaluating the progress of the patient's labor.

Finally, locate the membranes, which feel like tough, rubbery balloons. Sometimes, you can feel them bulging through the cervical os. Determine whether they've ruptured. Also find out if the pink-tinged mucous plug that has protected the developing fetus has been expelled (*bloody show*)—a reliable sign that labor is imminent.

IMPENDING-LABOR SIGNS

Signs of impending labor that every pregnant woman should know are:

- Uterine contractions increasing in frequency, duration, and intensity
- Bloody show
- Mucous plug expulsion
- Membrane rupture

Formulating a diagnostic impression

814 Classifying disorders of pregnancy

Although the diagnosis of pregnancy is a fairly simple matter based on the presumptive, probable, and positive signs of the condition, the diagnosis of disorders associated with pregnancy is not as straightforward. You'll find that, during pregnancy, hypertensive disorders and bleeding disorders commonly occur (see *Nurse's Guide to Pregnancy Disorders*).

815 Making appropriate nursing diagnoses

Amenorrhea normally occurs after conception, when the fertilized ovum becomes implanted in the uterus. The implantation causes progesterone output to increase in order to maintain the endometrial lining of the uterus and sustain the pregnancy. If such an alteration in the woman's menstrual cycle is unexpected, appropriate nursing diagnoses may include *lack of knowledge concerning normal female anatomy and physiology* and *fear.* If the

NURSE'S GUIDE TO PREGNANCY DISORDERS

HYPERTENSIVE DISORDERS	HISTORY AND CHIEF COMPLAINTS
Gestational edema	• Signs and symptoms include generalized fluid accumulation after 12 hours of bed rest.
Chronic hypertensive disease	• History of hypertension before pregnancy, and/or hypertension apparent before 20th week of gestation • No history of neoplastic trophoblastic disease or persistent hypertension after 6 weeks postpartum in previous pregnancies
Gestational hypertension	• No past history of hypertension
Gestational proteinuria	• No history of hypertension, edema, renal infection, or known renovascular disease
Preeclampsia	• Occurs after 20th week of gestation. May appear earlier with an advanced hydatidiform mole or with extensive molar change; most common in primigravidas, especially older women and pregnant adolescents • Family history of preeclampsia or eclampsia • Signs and symptoms include visual disturbances, ranging from blurred vision to blindness in extreme cases, and headache (usually mild; uncommon). • May be asymptomatic except for elevated blood pressure • With severe preeclampsia, signs and symptoms include nausea, vomiting, irritability, severe frontal headache, epigastric or right upper quadrant pain (usually a sign of impending convulsion), and respiratory distress suggesting pulmonary edema.

pregnancy is unwanted, the woman may resent the pregnancy or try to deny it, conditions that may ultimately affect the parent-child relationship. For these patients, appropriate nursing diagnoses might include *disturbance in self-concept* and *noncompliant attitude that delays diagnosis and care.*

A number of conditions may cause periodic vaginal bleeding during the first several months of pregnancy, including friability of the cervix, implantation bleeding, or discontinuation of oral contraceptives. Reproductive tract trauma or separation of the placenta from the site of implantation can cause bleeding. Vaginal bleeding during pregnancy can also be caused by lesions of the cervix, cervicitis, cervical polyps, a spontaneous abortion, an ectopic pregnancy, or a hydatidiform mole. A woman's apprehension over such bleeding may be appropriately diagnosed as *fear of possible loss of the fetus.* If the bleeding is severe, it may adversely affect uteroplacental perfusion and cause the fetus to abort. In this situation an appropriate nursing diagnosis might be *anticipatory grief.*

The nausea and vomiting that often occur during pregnancy are associated with hormonal changes, but the exact cause of these symptoms is unknown. Emotional stress can exacerbate these problems. Excessive vomiting can deplete a woman's essential minerals, nutrients, and fluids and interfere with adequate fetal nourishment. Appropri-

	PHYSICAL EXAMINATION AND DIAGNOSTIC STUDIES
	• Edema (+1 pitting) • Weight gain of 5 lb (2.25 kg) or more in 1 week with or without edema after bed rest
	• Systolic blood pressure: 100 mmHg or greater, or rise of 30 mmHg or greater from baseline pressure • Diastolic blood pressure: 90 mmHg or greater, or rise of 15 mmHg or greater from baseline pressure
	• May not occur until the first 24 hours postpartum and disappears within 10 days postpartum • Blood pressure as described in chronic hypertensive disease; usually discovered on physical examination during latter half of pregnancy • No other signs of preeclampsia or hypertensive vascular disease
	• Urine protein level increased by 0.3 g/liter in 24-hour period, or 1 g/liter in two different specimens collected at least 6 hours apart
	• Edema evidenced by puffiness of fingers and swollen eyelids; becomes generalized and is also apparent in sacral area and abdominal wall; sudden excessive weight gain; hypertension; proteinuria • With severe preeclampsia, increased blood pressure (160/100 mmHg) that does not decrease with bed rest; proteinuria (urine protein increased 5 g in 24 hours, +3 or +4), oliguria (urinary output reduced by 500 ml or more in 24 hours); increased serum creatine, cerebral disturbances, hyperaflexia (3 to 4+/4+, clonus), cyanosis, severe thrombocytopenia, hepatocellular damage

(continued)

NURSE'S GUIDE TO PREGNANCY DISORDERS (*continued*)

	HISTORY AND CHIEF COMPLAINTS
Eclampsia	• Most common in last trimester • Family history of preeclampsia or eclampsia • Signs and symptoms usually preceded by preeclampsia; in the absence of neurologic diseases, convulsions at onset • Respiratory distress
Superimposed preeclampsia or eclampsia	• Predisposing factors include chronic hypertensive vascular disease or renal disease. • May occur early in pregnancy and progress to eclampsia
BLEEDING DISORDERS	
Placenta previa (total, partial, marginal, or low-lying)	• Higher incidence in women over age 35 and in multiparas; tendency for recurrence • Bleeding may begin at any time during pregnancy, with no warning, but usually occurs after 24 weeks. • Signs and symptoms include painless, bright red vaginal bleeding; intermittent, slight, or in gushes.
Abruptio placentae (mild, moderate, or severe)	• Most commonly occurs after 20 weeks • Higher incidence in women over age 35 • Predisposing factors include high parity, previous abruptio placentae, hypertension, inferior vena cava compression, folic acid deficiency, abdominal trauma, sudden uterine compression, short umbilical cord. • Signs and symptoms include mild to moderate abdominal pain and vaginal bleeding.
Hydatidiform mole	• Highest incidence in women over age 45 • Predisposing factors include previous mole (found in only 2% of the population) and low-protein diet. • Signs and symptoms include excessive nausea and vomiting and uterine bleeding (from spotting to profuse hemorrhage).
Spontaneous abortion (threatened, inevitable, complete, incomplete, missed, habitual)	• Usually occurs around 12th week or not later than 20th week • Signs and symptoms include cramps, backache, vaginal bleeding; patient may complain of "not feeling pregnant anymore"; sudden gush of fluid from vagina occurs in inevitable abortion.
Ectopic pregnancy	• History of endosalpingitis, adhesions in the fallopian tubes, or uterine or adnexal mass • Signs and symptoms include lower abdominal pain (may be stabbing, sharp, or dull; unilateral or bilateral, constant or intermittent), nausea, vomiting, amenorrhea in about 75% of patients; vaginal spotting or bleeding possible in tubal pregnancy

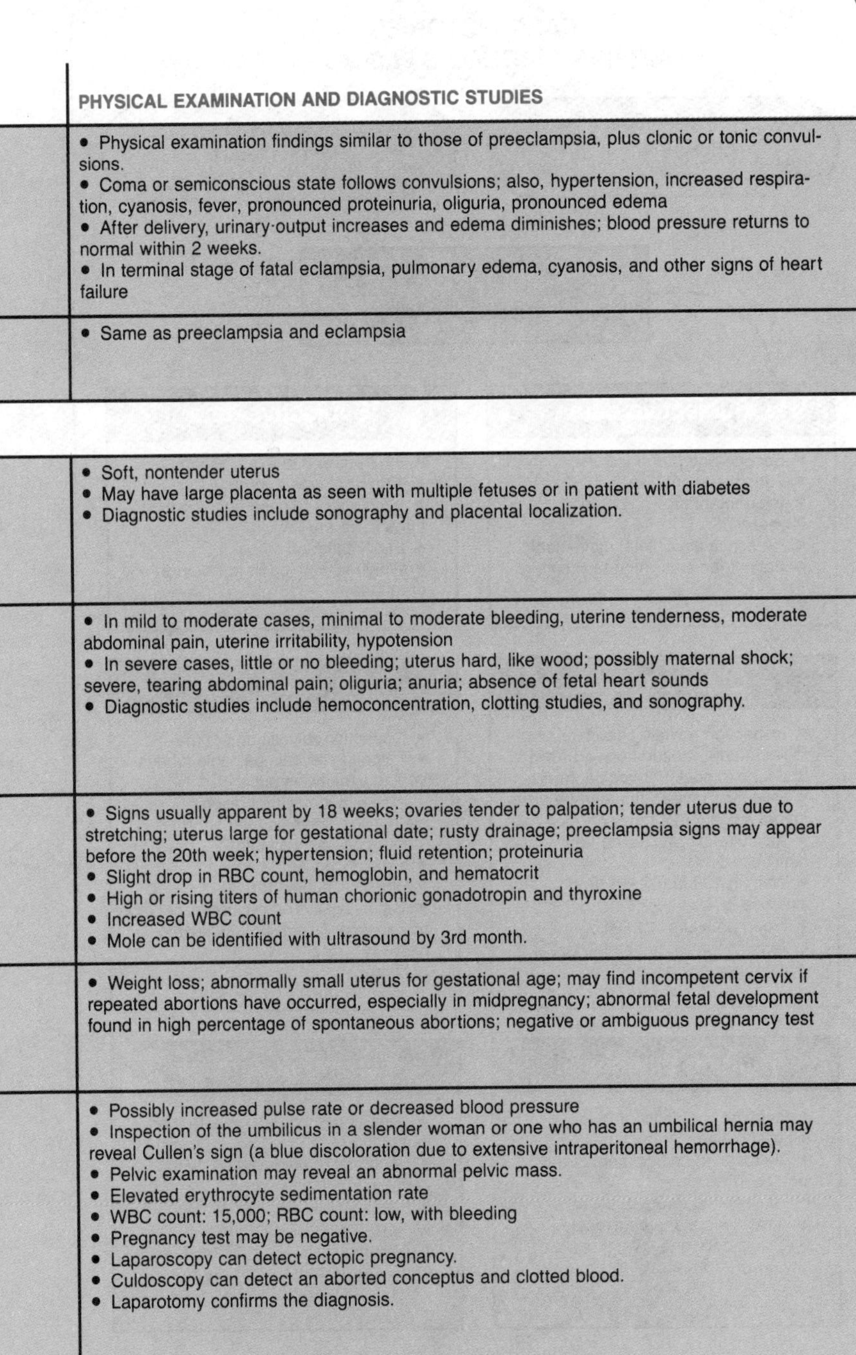

	PHYSICAL EXAMINATION AND DIAGNOSTIC STUDIES
	• Physical examination findings similar to those of preeclampsia, plus clonic or tonic convulsions. • Coma or semiconscious state follows convulsions; also, hypertension, increased respiration, cyanosis, fever, pronounced proteinuria, oliguria, pronounced edema • After delivery, urinary-output increases and edema diminishes; blood pressure returns to normal within 2 weeks. • In terminal stage of fatal eclampsia, pulmonary edema, cyanosis, and other signs of heart failure
	• Same as preeclampsia and eclampsia
	• Soft, nontender uterus • May have large placenta as seen with multiple fetuses or in patient with diabetes • Diagnostic studies include sonography and placental localization.
	• In mild to moderate cases, minimal to moderate bleeding, uterine tenderness, moderate abdominal pain, uterine irritability, hypotension • In severe cases, little or no bleeding; uterus hard, like wood; possibly maternal shock; severe, tearing abdominal pain; oliguria; anuria; absence of fetal heart sounds • Diagnostic studies include hemoconcentration, clotting studies, and sonography.
	• Signs usually apparent by 18 weeks; ovaries tender to palpation; tender uterus due to stretching; uterus large for gestational date; rusty drainage; preeclampsia signs may appear before the 20th week; hypertension; fluid retention; proteinuria • Slight drop in RBC count, hemoglobin, and hematocrit • High or rising titers of human chorionic gonadotropin and thyroxine • Increased WBC count • Mole can be identified with ultrasound by 3rd month.
	• Weight loss; abnormally small uterus for gestational age; may find incompetent cervix if repeated abortions have occurred, especially in midpregnancy; abnormal fetal development found in high percentage of spontaneous abortions; negative or ambiguous pregnancy test
	• Possibly increased pulse rate or decreased blood pressure • Inspection of the umbilicus in a slender woman or one who has an umbilical hernia may reveal Cullen's sign (a blue discoloration due to extensive intraperitoneal hemorrhage). • Pelvic examination may reveal an abnormal pelvic mass. • Elevated erythrocyte sedimentation rate • WBC count: 15,000; RBC count: low, with bleeding • Pregnancy test may be negative. • Laparoscopy can detect ectopic pregnancy. • Culdoscopy can detect an aborted conceptus and clotted blood. • Laparotomy confirms the diagnosis.

CASE HISTORIES: NURSING DIAGNOSIS FLOWCHART

Patient A
Mary Snyder
age 36

Patient B
Pam Reinhart
age 24

Problem
NAUSEA AND VOMITING

Patient A

Subjective data

- Second antepartal visit
- 20th gestational week
- Intermittent brown spotting for 2 weeks
- No sensation of fetal movement
- Patient feels she's gotten "so big"

Objective data

- Inspection reveals periorbital and facial edema, closed cervix, brown drainage in posterior vaginal fornix.
- Palpation reveals nontender uterus, fundal height of 24 cm (6 cm increase).
- Auscultation reveals no fetal heart tones.
- Weight: 138 lb (62 kg) (8 lb increase in 4 weeks)
- Blood pressure: 138/94
- Tests: negative urine glucose, +2 protein, hemoglobin 9.5

Nursing diagnoses

- Fluid volume deficit due to excessive nausea and vomiting
- Alteration in self-concept due to increased weight
- Fear related to the absence of fetal movement and heartbeat
- Anticipatory grief over possible fetal loss

Patient B

Subjective data

- First antepartal examination
- 11th gestational week
- Intermittent nausea and vomiting throughout the day
- Easily fatigued
- Weighed 120 lb (54 kg) before pregnancy

Objective data

- Inspection reveals no edema.
- Palpation reveals palpable fundus behind symphysis pubis.
- Auscultation with ultrasonic stethoscope reveals fetal heart tones: 140 beats/minute
- Weight: 117 lb (53 kg)
- Blood pressure: 120/80
- Tests: negative urine glucose, negative protein, specific gravity 1.030, hemoglobin 10

Nursing diagnoses

- Alteration in nutrition due to food intolerance
- Decrease in fluid volume due to nausea and vomiting
- Fear that she's unable to supply fetus with adequate nutrition
- Alteration in self-concept related to feeling of losing bodily control

ate nursing diagnoses for these conditions include *alteration in nutritional requirements, decrease in fluid volume due to vomiting,* and *fear that she is unable to provide necessary nourishment for optimal fetal development.* If the woman is accustomed to maintaining firm control over her body and its functions, she may experience an *alteration in self-concept.*

Urinary frequency during the first trimester is the result of hyperemia, which affects all pelvic organs, and uterine enlargement, which exerts pressure on the bladder. In midpregnancy the problem diminishes because the uterus becomes an abdominal organ. During the last trimester, urinary frequency occurs as the presenting part of the fetus descends into the pelvis and compresses the bladder. Because nocturia is usually an outcome of this, *sleep disturbances* may be an appropriate diagnosis. *Alteration in patterns of urinary elimination* is another appropriate nursing diagnosis.

Urinary tract infections can result from a number of causes, including decreased bladder tone; decreased urine flow time; decreased peristalsis of ureters; dilatation of the ureters and renal pelves; bladder catheterizations; and glycosuria, which provides a favorable medium for bacteria growth. Undetected urinary tract infections may develop into pyelonephritis. In addition to the nursing diagnoses cited above, *alterations in comfort* occur with urinary tract infections.

Dependent edema of the feet and ankles is usually caused by uterine compression of the pelvic veins and inferior vena cava. This retards blood flow and increases venous pressure in the legs, forcing fluid into the interstitial tissues. An appropriate nursing diagnosis might be *alteration in fluid volume.* If preeclampsia develops, your nursing diagnosis should indicate an *alteration in uteroplacental perfusion* (see *Case Histories: Nursing Diagnosis Flowchart*).

Selected References

Bash, Deborah M., and Gold, Winifred A. *The Nurse and the Childbearing Family.* New York: John Wiley & Sons, 1981.

Blair, Carole L., and Salerno, Elizabeth M. *The Expanding Family: Childbearing.* Boston: Little, Brown & Co., 1976.

Butnaurescu, G. F. *Perinatal Nursing,* 2 vols. New York: John Wiley & Sons, 1978.

Clark, Ann L., et al. *Childbearing: A Nursing Perspective,* 2nd ed. Philadelphia: F.A. Davis Co., 1979.

Gibbs, R.S., and Gibbs, C.E. *Ambulatory Obstetrics: A Clinical Guide.* New York: John Wiley & Sons, 1979.

Ingalls, A. Joy, and Salerno, M. Constance. *Maternal and Child Health Nursing,* 4th ed. St. Louis: C.V. Mosby Co., 1979.

Jensen, Margaret, and Bobak, Irene. *Handbook of Maternity Care: A Guide for Nursing Practice.* St. Louis: C.V. Mosby Co., 1980.

Malasanos, Lois, et al. *Health Assessment,* 2nd ed. St. Louis: C.V. Mosby Co., 1981.

Martin, Leonide L. *Health Care of Women.* Philadelphia: J.B. Lippincott Co., 1978.

Neeson, Jean D., and Stockdale, Connie R. *The Practitioner's Handbook of Ambulatory OB-GYN.* New York: John Wiley & Sons, 1981.

Olds, Sally. *Obstetric Nursing.* Reading, Mass.: Addison-Wesley Publishing Co., Inc., 1980.

Pritchard, Jack A., and MacDonald, Paul C. *Williams Obstetrics,* 16th ed. New York: Appleton-Century-Crofts, 1980.

Romney, Seymour, et al., eds. *Gynecology and Obstetrics: The Health Care of Women,* 2nd ed. New York: McGraw-Hill Book Co., 1980.

Tucker, Susan M., and Bryant, Sandra. *Fetal Monitoring and Fetal Assessment in High Risk Pregnancy.* St. Louis: C.V. Mosby Co., 1978.

Varney, Helen. *Nurse-Midwifery.* Boston: Blackwell Scientific Publications Inc., 1980.

20

KEY POINTS IN THIS CHAPTER

KEY CHARTS IN THIS CHAPTER

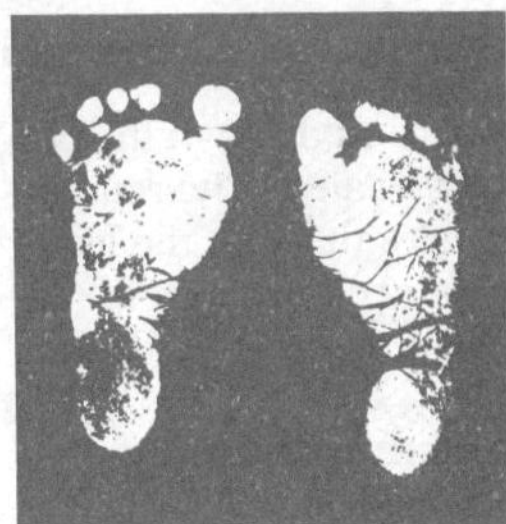

The Neonate

Introduction

816 Your role in neonatal assessment

Assessing the neonate in the delivery room involves swift and critical appraisal of his transition to extrauterine life—a transition accompanied by rapid physiologic changes and numerous adaptations, all necessary for survival. In a very short period (usually seconds), the neonate's external surroundings change from warm, dark, relatively quiet, and fluid-enveloped to cold, dry, noisy, and bright. Internally, he switches to totally different respiratory and circulatory systems. Hepatic and renal functions, blood oxygen saturation, and numerous metabolic processes are altered.

Probably no other 24-hour period in an individual's life is so important as the neonate's first day of adjustment to extrauterine existence. One half of all neonatal deaths (those occurring within the first 28 days of life) take place within these first 24 hours. Because this transition is so critical, it calls for the earliest possible detection of any problems that could threaten the neonate's survival and well-being.

Neonatal assessment is an ongoing process that begins in the delivery room and continues for the duration of the neonate's nursery stay. The nurse is usually the first health-care professional to examine the neonate in the delivery room. To conduct such an examination, you need to know how to calculate an Apgar score and how to make general—but crucial—observations about the neonate's appearance and behavior. This information, coupled with pertinent maternal and fetal history data, provides an initial data base for nursery personnel and pediatricians to use during subsequent examinations.

The first *thorough* examination of the neonate takes place in the nursery, usually within 24 hours of his birth. This examination must be comprehensive, covering all body systems. You must know how to determine his gestational age and status, which are extremely important in evaluating his condition. Until recently, newborn infants below a certain weight were classified as premature and treated similarly. Health-care professionals now realize that some low–birth-weight infants are actually full-term infants who, for various reasons, didn't grow as much as expected in utero. This distinction is vital, because the kind of care—including diet—a premature infant should get may be inappropriate for a full-term but low-weight infant.

By providing the neonate with the best care possible you can make an important contribution to his start on a healthy life.

Reviewing anatomy and physiology

817 Fetal circulation

To understand the anatomy and physiology of the neonate, you must first review the phenomenon of fetal circulation. During pregnancy, the fetus receives oxygenated blood from the placenta through the umbilical vein. The umbilical vein continues into the *ductus venosus,* which lies on the inferior surface of the liver. The ductus venosus shunts this oxygenated blood to the inferior vena cava (see *Understanding Fetal Circulation*). The blood then travels into the right atrium of the fetal heart. A rudimentary valve, or flap, directs most of the blood through the opening between the atria (*foramen ovale*) into the left atrium, bypassing the right ventricle and the airless lungs. From the left atrium the blood flows down into the left ventricle, up into the aorta, and on to the carotid and subclavian arteries to nourish the upper body.

Venous blood from the head returns to the superior vena cava through the brachiocephalic veins and passes into the right atrium, where it mixes with the oxygenated blood coming from the inferior vena cava. The inferior vena cava also returns some unoxygenated blood from the lower body. The two streams of blood (oxygenated and unoxygenated) don't mix significantly, and the oxygen content remains adequate. Some of the blood in the right atrium flows into the right ventricle and on into the pulmonary trunk. It bypasses the airless lungs and enters the aorta through the *ductus arteriosus,* a thick artery that joins the left branch of the pulmonary trunk to the aorta, distal to the origin of the aortic arch's three branches. The aorta carries the majority of the blood to the two umbilical arteries and through the placenta to be reoxygenated. The remaining blood circulates through the lower body and then returns through the inferior vena cava.

818 Cardiopulmonary conversion

When the neonate takes his first breath, air rushes into his lungs. The remaining fetal pulmonary fluid is swallowed, or absorbed by the lymphatic system. As the infant's lungs expand and air reaches terminal lung spaces, pulmonary vascular resistance falls and pulmonary circulation begins. The shunts that bypassed the lungs now close, so blood can flow through the heart and lungs. After birth, the heart functions as a dual pump. The right heart receives venous blood and pumps it to the lungs. The left heart receives oxygenated blood from the lungs and pumps it throughout the body. At about age 2 months, the intraabdominal part of the umbilical vein and the ductus venosus become continuous fibrous cords—the *ligamentum teres hepates* and the *ligamentum venosum.*

When the infant's lungs expand, pulmonary vascular resistance decreases and pulmonary blood flow increases. This causes an increase in blood return to the left atrium, making left atrial pressure greater than right atrial pressure. This pressure change prevents the flow of blood from the right atrium to the left atrium (low pressure to high pressure). In response, the two shutterlike flanges between the atria overlap and eventually adhere, closing the foramen ovale and leaving a shallow depression called the *fossa ovalis* in the interatrial septum. (Anatomic closure should occur by age 1.) After the foramen ovale closes, blood from the right atrium must flow into the right ventricle and then into the pulmonary artery, because of decreased peripheral vascular resistance. The large volume of blood held in the placenta during fetal life increases the infant's circulating volume and systemic pressure after birth. Aortic pressure rises and prevents blood flow from the pulmonary artery through the ductus arteriosus into the aorta, as in fetal circulation. Within a few hours, the lack of blood flow through the ductus arteriosus causes its muscular walls to contract and close off this shunt, permitting blood pumped by the right ventricle to circulate through the lungs. The ductus arteriosus becomes a fibrous band, the *ligamentum arteriosum,* which connects the first part of the left pulmonary artery to the aortic arch. (Anatomic closure should occur between ages 1 and 4 months.)

819 Musculoskeletal and nervous systems

Compared to an adult, the full-term neonate is top-heavy: His large head contrasts markedly with his trunk. In fact, head circumference is larger than chest circumference. His arms are well

UNDERSTANDING FETAL CIRCULATION

Note the structures involved in fetal circulation, especially the umbilical vein, ductus venosus, foramen ovale, ductus arteriosus, and umbilical arteries. Shortly after birth, the umbilical vein, ductus venosus, ductus arteriosus, and umbilical arteries functionally close to adjust pulmonary blood circulation. Within 3 months, the foramen ovale also functionally closes, adjusting to the changing blood pressure between the right and left atria.

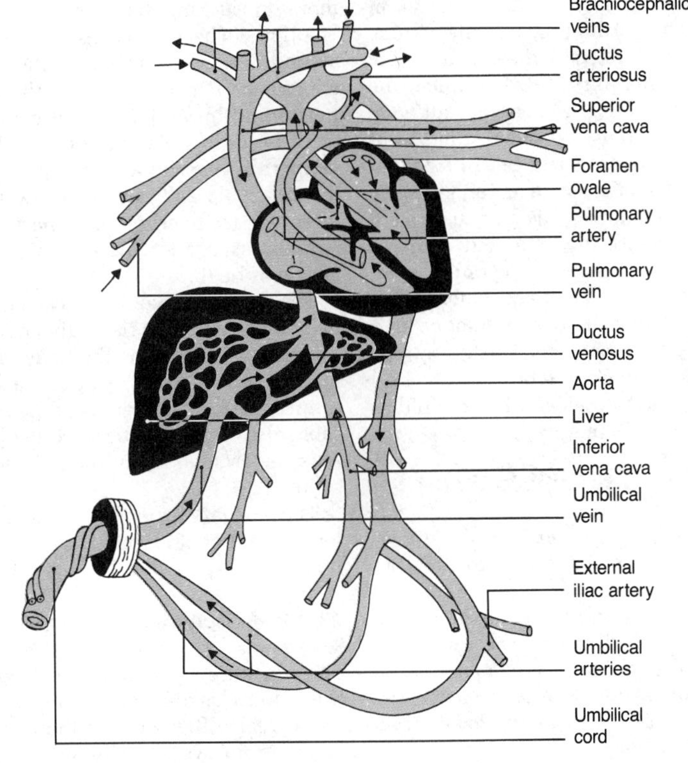

developed, but they move atactically because of his nervous system's immaturity. He can flex and hyperextend his fingers. The grasping reflex is remarkably strong, but many months must pass before his hands become the infant's chief tactile organs. Until then, the neonate uses his lips to feel and his hands to bring objects to his mouth for close examination.

The neonate's leg musculature is poorly developed. At birth the legs remain in the fetal position of flexion. The legs may assume this position while at rest up to age 6 months. Not until the child begins to walk and run will his legs become firm and muscular.

The neonate's vertebral column is C-shaped. Secondary curvature won't develop until the infant is able to raise his head and, later, to crawl and walk.

The neonate's whole body seems to respond to nervous stimulation, as in the Moro (startle) reflex. Many of these generalized reflexes disappear a few months after birth. For instance, the startle reflex begins as an overall body reaction to noise or other stimuli but gradually becomes less generalized and should disappear by age 4 months. As the infant matures, his nervous system becomes more differentiated, and his neurologic behavior becomes more predictable. By about age 3 months, he has more muscle tone. Mentation and motor system behavior (including gait coordination and sensory function) continue to develop until the child is neurologically mature.

820 Neonatal skull and face

The most striking feature of the neonatal skull is the disproportion between the cranium and the facial skeleton. The cranium appears large compared to the face. The roundness of the neonatal skull, as compared with the adult skull, occurs primarily because facial bones grow slower than cranial bones.

The bones that make up the skull, or cranial vault, are ossified at birth but are still mobile. This permits the cranial molding that usually occurs during delivery. The sutures connecting the cranial bones are not closed as in the adult skull, leaving areas called fontanelles. The coronal suture separates the frontal bone from the parietal bones, and the sagittal suture separates the right and left parietal bones. The diamond-shaped area where these sutures will eventually meet is the anterior fontanelle. This fontanelle usually closes when the neonate is about age 18 months. The lamboid suture separates the parietal and temporal bones from the occipital bone. The triangular area where the sagittal and lamboid sutures will eventually meet is the posterior fontanelle. It closes by age 2 months.

The muscles of facial expression are well developed at birth but are oriented more to sucking than to expressing emotion. (The first is instinctive; the second develops with stimulation and experience.) In the neonate, the temporomandibular joint's main movement is sliding. The masseter and the temporalis muscles are small, because the infant doesn't need to chew until after his teeth erupt. The paranasal sinuses, except for the ethmoids, are absent at birth.

The neonate's mandible is separated by a midline fibrous tissue that ossifies by about age 1. Later, the body of the mandible lengthens to accommodate erupting teeth. The ramus of the mandible also lengthens, because the jaws must separate to allow room for tooth eruption.

The neonate's mouth is small. His tongue is flat and relatively large at birth.

821 Sensory organs

The neonate's eyeballs and their associated muscles are well developed and are scarcely different from those of the adult. Eyebrows are absent or scant, but lashes are present on upper and

IDENTIFYING FONTANELLES AND SUTURES

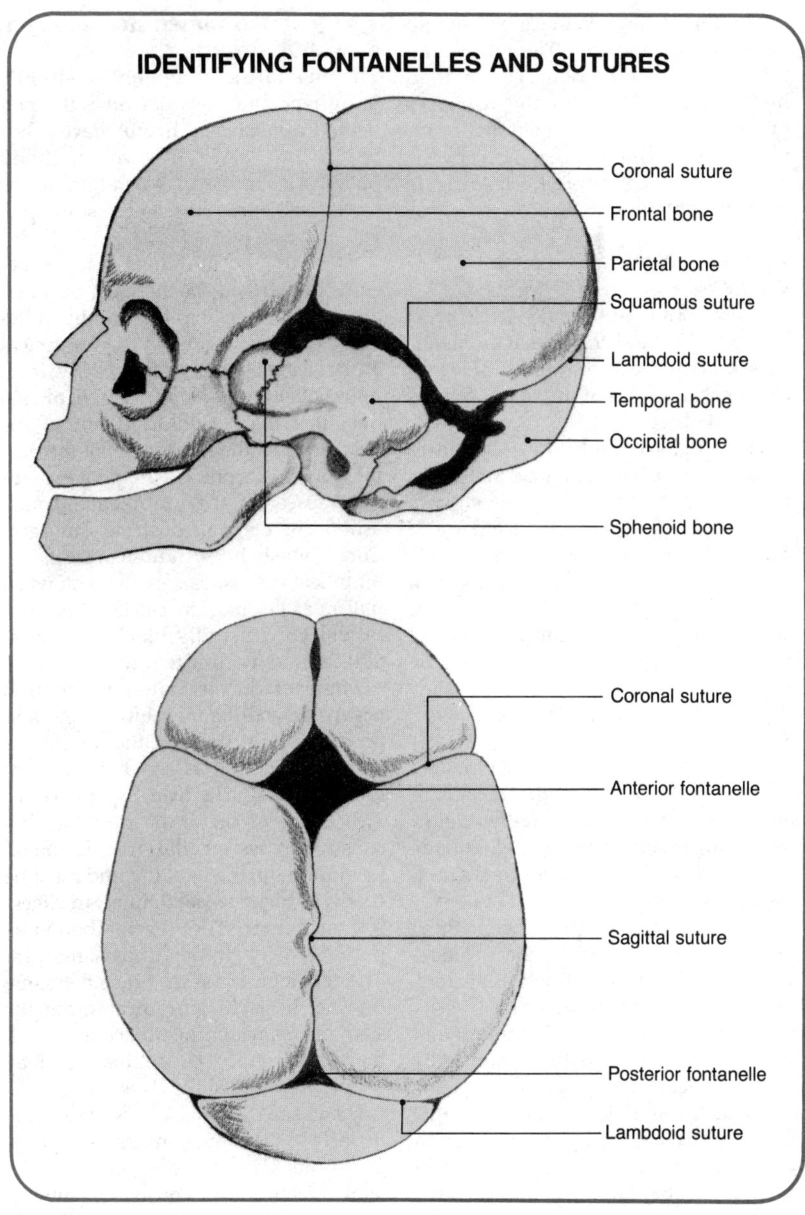

lower lids. Because the lower face is so small, the eyes appear large.

The nasal septum is largely cartilage, because little ossification has occurred. The external nasal cartilage is poorly developed and the nose appears broad and flat, with widely spaced nostrils. Cilia are not visible. The neonate is an obligate nose breather. Kiesselbach's area, the network of small blood vessels located at the anterior part of the nasal septum, is well supplied with blood. Later, it becomes the potential site of epistaxis.

The top of the neonate's ear should be level with the eye. The eustachian tube is short and more horizontal than in the adult. At birth, the neonate's middle ear is usually filled with amniotic fluid, which is displaced by air after breathing begins. Hearing is present at birth.

822 Neck and throat

The newborn infant has no visible neck; his lower jaw and chin touch his shoulders and thorax. Gradually, his neck elongates and his chin loses contact with his chest.

The epiglottis and larynx lie closer to the tongue's base in the neonate than in the adult. They descend slowly, reaching adult levels only after age 7. The larynx is about two or three vertebrae higher in the neonate than in the adult. By age 1, the vocal cords are only 5 mm long. The laryngeal tonsil is present at birth.

823 Thoracic cavity

The neonate's chest is nearly circular, whereas an adult's is oval. The ribs in an infant lie more horizontally than in the adult, causing the rib cage to ride higher, which makes the neonate's neck appear shorter.

The mediastinum occupies one third of the thoracic cavity in the neonate. The large thymus, destined to atrophy at puberty, extends from the lower neck through the superior mediastinum and into the anterior mediastinum. The neonate's heart has essentially the same shape as the adult's. A major anatomic difference is that the right and left myocardia of the neonate's heart are approximately the same thickness. (In the adult heart, the left ventricle has a thicker muscular wall than the right ventricle.) The shape and lobe division of the neonate's lungs are similar to those of the adult. After birth, the neonate's bronchioles and alveolar ducts develop further and the alveoli increase rapidly in size and number.

824 Abdomen and internal organs

The neonate's abdomen is slightly prominent but does not have the potbellied appearance it will have when he's a little older. The young child's potbelly is caused by a combination of a relatively large liver and a small pelvis.

At birth, the umbilical arteries become obliterated for the most part and are transformed into the umbilical ligaments (urachus). The superior vesical and internal iliac arteries arise from their remnants. The left umbilical vein becomes the round ligament of the liver, joining the left branch of the portal vein. A fibrous elastic ring eventually closes off the umbilical opening around its deep, or posterior, margin. The ring shrinks tightly around the umbilical vessels, closing them off when placental circulation ceases. The umbilical cord usually blackens, dries, and falls off within two weeks.

Many of the neonate's abdominal organs have different relative sizes and positions than those of the adult. The liver, colon, and adrenal glands are large. At birth, the liver is proportionately twice as big as in the adult, because it plays a vital role in blood formation during fetal life and must be ready at birth to participate in digestive processes. The inferior border is palpable below the right costal margin. The left lobe is large, often the same size as the right lobe, preventing the stomach from coming into contact with the diaphragm. The gallbladder may be situated under the liver.

During his first 24 hours, a neonate usually passes meconium—a pasty, green-black stool that collects in the fetal intestine and consists of mucus, desquamated epithelial cells, lanugo hair, and vernix caseosa. The green color is the result of bile secreted by the liver during the fourth month of gestation.

The adrenal glands have a thick cortex containing a fetal or transitional zone, which begins to disappear a few weeks after birth. They are relatively large at birth, each weighing about ¼ oz (7 g). They're this large because they need to produce important corticosteroid hormones needed for development during early life.

The neonate's stomach lies to the left of the midline. Its cardiac portion lies at the level of the tenth thoracic vertebra, and its pyloric portion is located at the level of the first lumbar vertebra. The neonate's spleen is small; accessory spleens sometimes develop.

The neonate's kidneys have little perirenal fat and therefore lie close to the peritoneum, where they are more susceptible to injury than in the adult. The bladder is capable of holding 100 ml of urine but averages about 50 ml.

825 Genitalia

The male neonate usually has a large scrotum and a small penis. The penis consists of three cylindrical bodies enclosed in several layers of fascia and covered with skin. One body (the corpus spongiosum) contains the urethra, which passes through the prostate gland and the urogenital diaphragm before entering the penis. The other two bodies (the corpora cavernosa) are composed of erectile tissue. The testes usually descend into the scrotum by the time of birth.

The female neonate's uterus is cylindrical and usually lies vertically in the pelvis. A crescentric fold of vascularized tissue—the hymen—may partially or completely cover the vaginal orifice. The labia majora and labia minora may be large or swollen as a result of maternal hormones. Smegma (a cheesy secretion from sebaceous glands) may be found in both the male and the female neonate.

Collecting appropriate history data

826 Biographical data

Record the neonate's approximate gestational age based on obstetric tests (see Entry 810). Then determine gestational age based on your findings during the physical examination (see *How to Estimate Gestational Age,* page 789). Compare these estimates, bearing in mind that examination techniques for establishing gestational age are more reliable than obstetric tests.

827 Chief signs and symptoms

The most common chief signs and symptoms in neonates are *skin color changes, neurologic changes, respiratory distress, altered heart rate,* and *gastrointestinal abnormalities.*

828 History of present illness

If the neonate shows any of the chief signs and symptoms while he's in the nursery, use the PQRST mnemonic device (see page 780) as a guideline to record complete information. If signs and symptoms develop after the neonate's discharged from the nursery, use PQRST when asking the neonate's parents to elaborate on the problem.

• ***Skin color changes.*** *Cyanosis* or *pallor* may indicate an alteration in cardiovascular or respiratory function. Central cyanosis necessitates immediate attention. Because neonates have a high percentage of fetal hemoglobin, which is capable of carrying about 25% more oxygen than adult hemoglobin, central cyanosis doesn't develop until PO_2 is very low, between 30 and 44 mmHg. Pallor may occur with a decreased hemoglobin level, as in anemia. Jaundice occurring in the first 24 hours of life can indicate true hemolytic disease, such as Rh incompatibility from erythroblastosis fetalis.

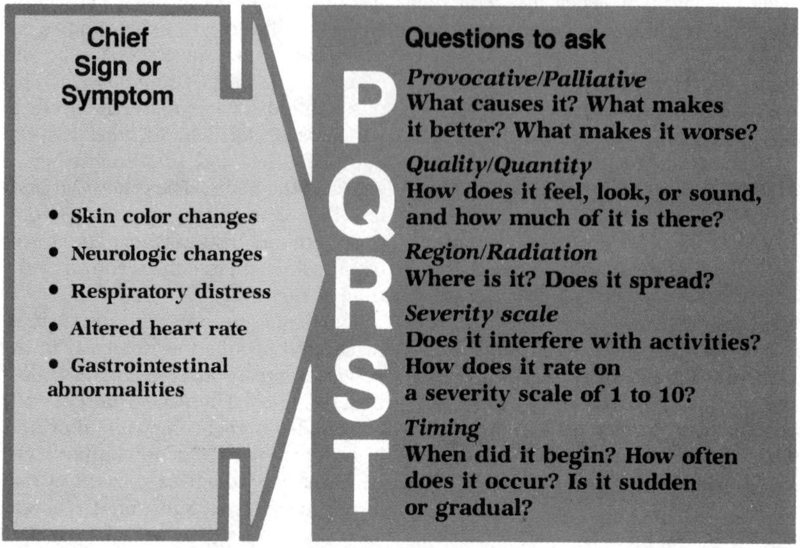

Chief Sign or Symptom		Questions to ask
• Skin color changes • Neurologic changes • Respiratory distress • Altered heart rate • Gastrointestinal abnormalities	P	*Provocative/Palliative* **What causes it? What makes it better? What makes it worse?**
	Q	*Quality/Quantity* **How does it feel, look, or sound, and how much of it is there?**
	R	*Region/Radiation* **Where is it? Does it spread?**
	S	*Severity scale* **Does it interfere with activities? How does it rate on a severity scale of 1 to 10?**
	T	*Timing* **When did it begin? How often does it occur? Is it sudden or gradual?**

Jaundice occurring on the second or third day may be considered physiologic jaundice (*icterus neonatorum*), which isn't uncommon but may require further evaluation. The neonate's body may exhibit a complete division of color into a pale side and a red side (harlequin color change). This is usually temporary and of little significance to neonatal well-being.

• ***Neurologic changes.*** *Lethargy, irritability, hypertonia* or *hypotonia, tremors,* or *seizures* may indicate an alteration in neurologic function. Maternal drug addiction may lead to these signs and symptoms as the neonate experiences withdrawal. Hypoglycemia can also cause these signs and symptoms.

• ***Respiratory distress.*** *Apnea* for more than 10 seconds, as well as *dyspnea, tachypnea, grunting, nasal flaring, sternal retractions,* and *wheezing,* can indicate a life-threatening problem. Examples of possible underlying conditions are infant respiratory distress syndrome and pneumonia. These conditions require immediate intervention.

• ***Altered heart rate.*** *Bradycardia* or *tachycardia* can indicate severe oxygenation problems from cardiac, respiratory, or neurologic disorders.

• ***Gastrointestinal abnormalities.*** *Abdominal distention* and *vomiting* (especially of bile-stained substances) may reflect intestinal obstruction. *Failure to pass meconium* could indicate that the enervation of the distal colon is absent (Hirschsprung's disease); another possible cause is imperforate anus. *Feeding problems* accompanied by *dyspnea* may indicate obstruction of the posterior nares (choanal atresia), tracheoesophageal fistula, or such cardiovascular disorders as congestive heart failure or atrial or ventricular septal defects.

829 Past history

A neonate's past history includes information about his health status before the examination. This could take only a matter of minutes, for an evaluation performed in the nursery, or may cover up to 27 days if the neonate is seen after discharge. Obtain information from family members about any known *congenital anomalies* and other problems.

The neonate's past history, especially

during the first few critical days of life, also includes the following maternal history aspects:

- ***Maternal age.*** The mother's age, the outcome of the pregnancy, and the neonate's health can be directly related. Mothers younger than age 20 experience more difficulties than older mothers. Some common maternal problems that affect the fetus directly are excessive weight gain, preeclampsia, and prolonged labor. Neonates born to mothers in this age-group are more likely to have a low birth weight, especially if the mother's nutritional status is poor.

  The incidence of trisomy 21 (Down's syndrome) rises if the mother is over age 35. Other fetal malformations (musculoskeletal disorders, cardiovascular defects, gastrointestinal abnormalities, and central nervous system anomalies) are also more common in neonates born to mothers over age 35.
- ***Drugs.*** Both over-the-counter and prescription drugs taken by a woman during pregnancy may be passed to the fetus transplacentally (see *Nurse's Guide to Some Drugs with Possible Teratogenic Effects,* pages 783 to 784). Neonates of drug-addicted mothers are at greater risk of being born with congenital anomalies, particularly extremity malformations. These neonates are usually premature and exhibit signs and symptoms of withdrawal, such as tremors, agitation, and seizures, shortly after delivery.
- ***Alcohol.*** Excessive consumption of alcohol in early pregnancy can produce congenital anomalies involving the heart, face, and extremities, and can retard fetal growth. Alcohol consumption before delivery can cause toxic symptoms in the neonate. Because alcohol is a central nervous system depressant, it can interfere with the neonate's cardiopulmonary adaptation.
- ***Smoking.*** Neonates born to women who smoked cigarettes during pregnancy are more likely to be underweight.
- ***Infections.*** Because of its inadequate immunologic system, the fetus is susceptible to many organisms. For example, rubella contracted by the mother during the first trimester can cause retarded intrauterine growth and congenital malformations in the neonate, including cardiac defects. Among infections transmitted during delivery, maternal gonorrhea can cause *ophthalmia neonatorum* and a monilial infection can cause *thrush.* Such infections usually have less severe consequences—although more serious infections, such as herpes simplex virus, can be fatal to the neonate.
- ***Diseases and disorders.*** Many pathologic maternal conditions, such as diabetes mellitus, chronic hypertension, cardiac disease, thyroid imbalance, preeclampsia, or eclampsia, can cause problems for the neonate. Observe the neonate of a diabetic mother for neonatal hypoglycemia, hyperbilirubinemia, hypocalcemia, and idiopathic respiratory distress syndrome. Congenital malformations, including skeletal and ventricular septal defects, are three times more likely to occur if the mother is diabetic. For neonates born to mothers with hyperthyroidism, a serum thyroxine measurement should be performed at birth, and the neonate should be observed closely during the first 2 weeks of life for signs and symptoms of hyperthyroidism. The neonate whose mother has hypothyroidism can have a congenital goiter or cretinism. These neonates also have a high incidence of congenital abnormalities. The manifestations of preeclampsia or eclampsia are mainly maternal; however, the fetus in such cases is also at risk. If maternal hypertension accompanies either of these disorders, fetal growth may be retarded. The neonate may develop hypermagnesemia if the mother is treated with magnesium sulfate.
- ***Prenatal care.*** Neonates born to mothers who didn't have adequate prenatal care are more likely to have complications.

830 Labor and delivery history

Labor and delivery cause great stress to every neonate. Uterine contractions exert extreme pressure on the fetus at the same time that the fetus meets resistance from pelvic structures. It must also withstand brief periods of hypoxia, caused by decreased circulation during uterine contractions. This traumatic process occurs in all vaginal deliveries. For some neonates, vaginal birth may be even more dangerous, and cesarean delivery may be employed to reduce the risk.

When recording a neonate's prenatal history, consider the following complications and their effects:

• ***Premature labor.*** Labor that occurs before the 37th week of gestation endangers the neonate, because his major body systems, notably the respiratory system, are immature compared with the functional requirements for extrauterine survival. His ability to store and regulate body heat is also impaired.

• ***Premature membrane rupture.*** This can cause an infection in the neonate from amniotic fluid reaching the tracheobronchial tree. Infection transmitted through the cord vessels can also produce fetal sepsis.

• ***Dysfunctional labor pattern.*** In hyperactive labor, the unusually strong contractions and rapid progression can cause cerebral trauma. In hypoactive labor, the long birth process and prolonged pressure on the fetal head can result in a cephalhematoma, caput succedaneum (fetal scalp edema), or excessive molding of cranial bones.

• ***Abnormal fetal presentation.*** Malpresentation can injure the neonate. Brow presentation can tear the tentorium, compress the head and neck, and damage the trachea and larynx. Face presentation can cause caput succedaneum, neck swelling, and petechiae and ecchymoses of the facial skin's superficial layers. Breech presentation can result in cervical cord injury, intracranial hemorrhage, brachial plexus palsy, arm fracture, ecchymosis and edema of the presenting part, and kidney, liver, and spleen hemorrhage. Also, the neonate may remain in the breech posture for some time after delivery. A frank breech presentation, for example, results in extended legs and abducted, fully rotated thighs.

• ***Analgesics and anesthetics.*** If administered to the mother during labor and delivery, a large amount of anesthetic or such drugs as meperidine, morphine sulfate, and secobarbital cross the placental barrier and may cause respiratory depression in the neonate and decrease his responsiveness and feeding ability.

831 Family history

When recording a neonate's family history, ask the parents about congenital defects or genetically transmitted diseases, previous multiple births, infant deaths (including stillbirths and abortions), and family members' general health (ask about such diseases as diabetes or epilepsy).

832 Psychosocial history

Record pertinent information about the neonate's family. For example, determine what arrangements have been made at home for the neonate's care. Ask the mother if she anticipates any financial or family problems. Encourage her to discuss any emotional concerns or life-style conflicts she may have relating to the care and health of the neonate. When appropriate, determine what effects, if any, the family's religious practices may have on the care the neonate will receive at home.

833 Activities of daily living

If the neonate has been brought back for care after being discharged from the nursery, ask the mother about *feeding patterns* as well as the color and consistency of his feces.

DRUGS

NURSE'S GUIDE TO SOME DRUGS WITH POSSIBLE TERATOGENIC EFFECTS

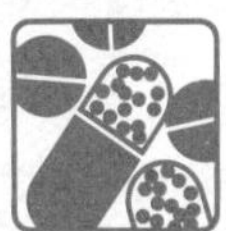

This chart lists some examples of drugs that may harm the fetus or neonate. Encourage pregnant women to avoid *all* drugs except those *essential* to maintaining the pregnancy or maternal health, administered with a doctor's approval.

CLASSIFICATION	POSSIBLE EFFECTS
ANTI-INFECTIVES	
Aminoglycosides gentamicin sulfate (Garamycin*) kanamycin sulfate (Kantrex*) streptomycin sulfate	• Hearing loss (eighth cranial nerve damage)
Miscellaneous anti-infectives chloramphenicol sodium succinate (Chloromycetin*)	• Abdominal distention, gray cyanosis, vasomotor collapse, death (gray baby syndrome)
Sulfonamides sulfamethoxazole (Gantanol*) sulfisoxazole (Gantrisin*)	• Hyperbilirubinemia, neonatal kernicterus, hemolytic anemia with G-6-PD deficiency
Tetracyclines demeclocycline hydrochloride (Declomycin*) tetracycline hydrochloride (Sumycin*)	• Permanent tooth discoloration, enamel defects, retarded bone growth
Urinary tract antiseptics nitrofurantoin macrocrystals (Macrodantin*)	• Hemolytic anemia with G-6-PD deficiency
CANCER CHEMOTHERAPEUTICS†	
Alkylating agents chlorambucil (Leukeran*) cyclophosphamide (Cytoxan*)	• Renal agenesis, multiple malformations
Antimetabolites methotrexate sodium (Mexate)	• Multiple malformations (especially skeletal)
DRUGS ACTING ON CENTRAL NERVOUS SYSTEM	
Alcohol alcoholic beverages	• Growth deficiency, microcephaly, short eye slits; possibly extremity and cardiovascular defects
Anticonvulsants phenytoin (Dilantin*)	• Congenital malformations, vitamin K deficiency
trimethadione (Tridione, Trimedone**)	• Abortion, malformations, mental retardation
Barbiturates barbital phenobarbital (Eskabarb*)	• Altered level of consciousness; possible neurologic damage; fetal asphyxia

(continued)

NURSE'S GUIDE TO SOME DRUGS WITH POSSIBLE TERATOGENIC EFFECTS *(continued)*

CLASSIFICATION	POSSIBLE EFFECTS
Narcotic analgesics	
heroin or morphine (addiction)	• Generally impaired neonatal adjustment, withdrawal symptoms, convulsions, death
Nonnarcotic analgesics	
aspirin (Bayer, Ecotrin*)	• Neonatal bleeding, coagulation defects
HORMONES AND SYNTHETIC SUBSTITUTES	
Androgens	
testosterone (Malogen*, Depo-Testosterone)	• Masculinization of female fetus: labial fusion early in pregnancy, clitoral enlargement later in pregnancy
Antidiabetic agents	
tolbutamide (Orinase*)	• Congenital anomalies, prolonged neonatal hypoglycemia
Estrogens	
diethylstilbestrol (DES, Stibilium**) esterified estrogens (Amnestrogen, Climestrone**)	• Vaginal adenocarcinoma in adolescents and young adults; nonmalignant genital changes; cervical and vaginal adenocarcinoma possible in females; testicular tumors possible in males
Progestogens	
progesterone (Progestasert*, Progestin)	• Masculinization of female fetus: labial fusion early in pregnancy, clitoral enlargement later in pregnancy
Thyroid hormone antagonists	
iodine (Potassium Iodide Solution) methimazole (Tapazole) propylthiouracil [PTU] (Propylthyracil**)	• Goiter, hypothyroidism, mental retardation
MISCELLANEOUS	
Anticoagulants	
warfarin sodium (Coumadin*)	• Fetal and neonatal hemorrhage
Antihypertensives	
chlorothiazide (Diuril*)	• Neonatal jaundice, thrombocytopenia
reserpine (Serpasil*)	• Cyanosis, neonatal nasal congestion
Vitamins	
vitamin D (Drisdol*)	• Excessive blood calcium
vitamin K analogs (Synkavite**, Synkayvite)	• Hyperbilirubinemia and toxic neonatal reactions, kernicterus

*Available in U.S. and Canada. **Available in Canada only. All other products (no symbol) available in U.S. only.

†Virtually every anticancer drug has the potential to cause teratogenic effects. Patients undergoing chemotherapy should be *strongly* encouraged to avoid pregnancy. Pregnant patients should not be given chemotherapy.

Conducting the physical examination

834 Apgar score: The first examination

Immediately after delivery, determine the neonate's Apgar score. The purpose of the Apgar scoring system is twofold: to provide an initial assessment of the neonate's physical status and to identify indications for immediate resuscitation. Check these five objective signs quickly but carefully to compile a neonate's Apgar score: heart rate, respiratory effort, muscle tone, reflex irritability, and skin color. As you evaluate each sign, assign a score of 0,1, or 2. Repeat the Apgar scoring system again at 5 minutes (see *Using the Apgar Scoring System,* page 786).

Heart rate is the most important sign, so assess this first. If the umbilical cord is still pulsating, you can palpate the neonate's heart rate by placing your fingertips at the junction of the umbilical cord and the skin. You can also place two fingers or a stethoscope over the neonate's chest at the fifth intercostal space to obtain an apical pulse.

Next, check the neonate's *respiratory effort,* the second most important Apgar sign. Assess the neonate's cry, noting its volume and vigor. Then auscultate his lungs, using a pediatric stethoscope. Assess his respirations for depth and regularity.

Determine *muscle tone* by evaluating the degree of flexion in the neonate's arms and legs and their resistance to straightening. For example, try to straighten an arm or leg and note how quickly it returns to the flexed position.

Assess *reflex irritability* by evaluating the neonate's cry for presence, vigor, and pitch. He may not cry at once, but you should elicit a cry by flicking his soles. A high-pitched or shrill cry is abnormal.

Finally, observe *skin color* for cyanosis. A neonate usually has a pink body with blue extremities. This condition, called *acrocyanosis,* appears in about 85% of normal neonates 1 minute after birth. Acrocyanosis results from decreased peripheral oxygenation caused by the transition from fetal to independent circulation. When assessing a nonwhite neonate, observe for color changes in the mucous membranes of the mouth, conjunctivae, lips, palms, and soles.

The stable neonate may be weighed at this early stage. After this preliminary assessment, you'll usually take a neonate with an acceptable Apgar score to his mother, for the first few minutes of bonding.

835 Nursery admission assessment

After the newborn infant spends some time with his mother, you'll take him to the nursery, where pertinent data concerning labor and delivery interventions should be available. Here, the evaluation continues with assessment of the neonate's vital signs, weight, length, and general characteristics.

Take the neonate's first temperature rectally (normal: 96° to 99.5° F., or 35.6° to 37.5° C.), so you can also check for anal patency. Subsequent temperatures should be axillary (normal: 97.7° to 98° F., or 36.5° to 36.7° C.), to avoid perforating the bowel. When taken for at least 3 minutes, an axillary temperature provides an approximate core temperature (it may be 1° to 2° lower) and reveals any heat or cold stress. In some nurseries, a rectal temperature is taken until it reaches normal. Use a pediatric stethoscope to determine the neonate's heart rate apically. To ensure an accurate measurement, count the pulsations for 1 minute. (The normal range is from 120 to 150 beats/minute.) Then assess his respiratory rate for at least 30 seconds. (The normal rate is 30 to 60 breaths/minute.) Also note any signs of respiratory distress, such as cyanosis, tachypnea (respiratory rate greater than 60 breaths/minute), sternal retractions, grunting, nasal flaring, or periods of apnea. Rales may be heard until fetal lung fluid is absorbed.

Measuring the neonate's length, weight, and head and chest circumference provides important baseline data and initial diagnostic information.

Even though the neonate was probably weighed in the delivery room, weigh him again on admission to the nursery. Balance the scale; then weigh the naked neonate. Most newborn infants weigh between 6 and 9 lb (2,700 and 4,000 g); the average is 7 lb 8 oz (3,400 g). Record weight in pounds and ounces as well as in grams.

Now, measure the neonate's length, from the top of the head to the heel with the leg fully extended. Normal length is 18″ to 22″ (46 to 56 cm).

Next, measure head circumference. Normal neonatal head circumference is 13″ to 14″ (33 to 35.5 cm). Remember, cranial molding or caput succedaneum from a vaginal delivery may affect this measurement, so repeat it on the second and third day and before the neonate's discharged. Measure his chest circumference at the nipple line; normal neonatal chest circumference is 12″ to 13″ (30.5 to 33 cm). Head circumference should be about 1″ (2 to 3 cm) larger than chest circumference.

Remember to observe the neonate's overall appearance, noting any obvious congenital defects or abnormalities.

836 The complete examination

During the first 24 hours of life, a neonate receives a complete physical examination. This is the third and most comprehensive step in neonatal assess-

USING THE APGAR SCORING SYSTEM

To help assess a neonate's condition, use the Apgar scoring system shown here. Make your observations within 1 minute after the neonate's delivered, then again within 5 minutes.

Notify the doctor of your findings, and document them on the neonate's chart. A neonate with a score of 10 is considered in the best possible condition. A score of 7 to 9 is considered adequate, requiring no treatment. A score of 4 to 6 requires close observation and intervention, such as suctioning. A score below 4 necessitates immediate intervention and further evaluation.

SIGN	0	1	2	Rating	
				1 min	5 min
Heart rate	Not detectable	Below 100	Over 100		
Respiratory effort	Absent	Slow, irregular	Good, crying		
Muscle tone	Flaccid	Some flexion of extremities	Active motion		
Reflex irritability (response to flick on sole)	No response	Grimace, slow motion	Cry		
Color	Blue, pale	Body pink, extremities blue	Completely pink		
Scoring system developed by Dr. Virginia Apgar			TOTAL		

ment, after the Apgar scoring in the delivery room and the examination on admission to the nursery. Make this head-to-toe assessment a priority in your care plan, because it serves as a baseline for future examinations and identifies normal and abnormal characteristics.

For this examination, you'll need the following items:
- Pediatric stethoscope
- Penlight or ophthalmoscope, and otoscope
- Infant tongue depressor
- Tape measure
- Bell (or appropriate substitute)
- Pacifier or water-filled nursing bottle
- Finger cot and catheter.

Perform the examination in a warm, well-lighted, draft-free area, keeping the neonate undressed for as short a time as possible. Lay him on a flat surface. Begin with nonstressful assessment techniques; defer those which may disturb the neonate until later in the examination. If possible, perform the examination in the presence of one or both parents (for example, by the side of the mother's bed). This affords an excellent opportunity for teaching parents about neonatal care and for answering any questions they may have.

837 Examining the neonate's head

Observe the general contour of the neonate's head. Be sure you inspect the head from different angles so you don't miss a prematurely closed suture or a flat occiput. In most vaginal vertex deliveries some cranial molding occurs, because the cranial bones haven't fused and can overlap. Next, observe and palpate the sutures and fontanelles with the neonate held upright, if possible. You can feel the sutures as slightly depressed edges. (Sometimes you can palpate an osseous ridge along the suture lines.) The anterior fontanelle is approximately 2″ (5 cm) long and 1⅛″ (3 cm) wide. You can locate the posterior fontanelle, which is less than ⅜″ (1 cm) long, by tracing the sagittal suture.

Normally, the fontanelles feel soft and either flat or slightly indented. The anterior fontanelle usually bulges when a neonate cries, coughs, or vomits. Abnormally bulging fontanelles may indicate increased intracranial pressure. Possible causes include infectious or neoplastic diseases of the central nervous system or an obstruction to ventricular circulation. A sunken fontanelle may suggest dehydration.

Observe the neonate for caput succedaneum and cephalhematoma after a vaginal vertex delivery. *Caput succedaneum* is generalized edema from prolonged pressure against the cervical os. On palpation, the scalp feels soft and edematous. This condition may appear at birth or shortly thereafter and usually resolves in a few days. In *cephalhematoma,* blood collects between the cranial bone and the periosteum. Whereas caput succedaneum appears over a large area of the neonate's scalp, cephalhematoma remains within the boundaries of the cranial bones and won't cross suture lines. Cephalhematoma may not appear for several days after birth and can take several weeks to recede.

838 Neck assessment

Observe the general appearance of the neonate's neck: It's usually short, thick, and covered with folds of tissue. Also assess the neonate's ability to use his neck muscles. He should be able to move his head from side to side and from flexion to extension. Note if he can hold his head in the midline position; this indicates that the sternocleidomastoid muscles are equal in strength. You should also observe the neonate for torticollis or for shortening of the sternocleidomastoid muscle on one side.

Gently lift the neonate, allowing some degree of hyperextension, and note the degree of his head control. Assess range of motion by eliciting the tonic neck reflex (see *Assessing Neonatal Reflexes,* pages 795 to 796). Finally, palpate the neck for abnormal masses, such as an enlarged thyroid.

839 Inspecting the neonate's eyes

Observe the neonate's eyes for symmetry of size and shape. The eyelids may be edematous for 1 or 2 days as a result of delivery and the chemical conjunctivitis caused by instillation of silver nitrate drops. Culture any purulent discharge to differentiate it from ophthalmia neonatorum caused by gonorrhea. To open a neonate's eyes for examination, gently rock him from an upright to a horizontal position, or hold him supine and gently lower his head.

The stress of delivery commonly causes subconjunctival and scleral hemorrhages. (Assure the parents that these conditions aren't pathologic.) Note the neonate's eye movements. Strabismus caused by poor neuromuscular control is normal.

Observe the color of the neonate's eyes. Light-skinned neonates usually have blue or blue-gray eyes; for darker-skinned babies, brown eyes are normal. The sclerae are usually blue-white. Redness may be caused by the instillation of silver nitrate drops. The corneas should appear clear, so note any opacity or haziness, which may be associated with congenital cataracts.

To assess a neonate's extraocular muscle movements, turn his head from side to side while observing his eye movements. A newborn infant's eyes should remain fixed (doll's eyes). An infant older than 10 days should look in the direction in which you turn. Next, gently raise the neonate to the sitting position, then quickly lower him to the supine position. If his eyes slowly drift downward, suspect cerebral dysfunction caused by kernicterus or hydrocephaly.

Next, test the red reflex of the fundus. With the diopter setting at 0, hold the ophthalmoscope 10″ (25.4 cm) from the neonate's pupils. In addition to a red reflex response, they should react to the light by constricting.

840 Nose and mouth

Because neonates are obligate nose breathers, nasal passage patency is essential. If the neonate has no difficulty breathing with his mouth closed, you can be fairly certain that his nasal passages are patent. If you suspect they aren't, try passing a #8 suction catheter. You can also assess nasal patency by blocking the neonate's mouth and one nasal passage, and noting air movement through the other canal. A neonate usually clears his nasal passages by sneezing. Nasal flaring indicates respiratory distress, so always note and report it. (A thin nasal discharge, an uncommon finding, may be cerebrospinal fluid and requires further evaluation.)

Examine the neonate's mouth for cleft palate by gently depressing his tongue when he cries. You can also palpate for cleft palate by running a clean finger along the soft and hard palates while testing the sucking reflex.

Rarely, you'll find teeth in the neonate's mouth, usually located in the lower incisor position. These are called *precocious teeth* (supernumerary teeth). If they're loose, you or the doctor should remove them to avoid the danger of aspiration. You may also see small, white epithelial cysts on the hard palate and gum margins (Epstein's pearls). These cysts are insignificant and usually disappear in a few weeks. Areas of a white, cheesy substance that don't rub off are usually from thrush or monilial infection.

Inspect the position of the frenulum; note if it's attached too closely to the tip of the tongue. Also, observe for *sucking blisters*—round, thickened areas on the neonate's lips, particularly in the center of the upper lip—which may disappear within a few weeks.

841 Examining the neonate's ears

Inspect the ears for structure, shape, and position. A full-term neonate's ears should be firm, with well-formed cartilage. The tops of the auricles should be parallel to the outer canthi of the eye. Low-set ears are associated with renal anomalies and with certain chromosomal abnormalities, especially trisomy 13, 18, and 21 (Down's syndrome). Small, preauricular skin tabs may appear just in front of the ears.

In a neonate aged less than 3 days, examine the external ear canal for patency. You can't see the eardrum because vernix caseosa covers it. To see the eardrum in a neonate aged 3 days or older, gently pull the auricle downward and inspect with an otoscope. The light reflex should be diffuse, not cone-shaped as in an infant several months old. Assess the neonate's hearing by testing for the Moro reflex (see *Assessing Neonatal Reflexes,* pages 795 to 796). Within a few hours after birth, the neonate's hearing becomes more acute, as mucus and fluid in the middle ear and eustachian tube are absorbed.

842 Assessing the neonate's skin and nails

Inspect the skin's general appearance, noting any birthmarks (see *Differentiating Common Birthmarks,* page 792). Normally, the neonate's skin appears soft and puffy immediately after delivery. After a few days, it usually looks dry and flaky—especially in the postmature neonate, whose skin may crack and peel. Skin color, of course, depends on racial and genetic characteristics. A white neonate's skin should be pink to ruddy; a black neonate should appear pink-brown. Normal variations, including acrocyanosis and circumoral cyanosis, may result from poor peripheral circulation. These skin color changes may appear immediately after delivery if the neonate is exposed to cold; they should disappear in approximately 10 days.

Assess for jaundice by blanching the tip of the neonate's nose or his gum line, preferably under natural light. If jaundice is present, the blanched area appears yellow. Jaundice in the first 24 hours after birth indicates pathology, usually hemolytic disease. Although it can also occur during the second or third day—when it may not indicate pathology—jaundice may necessitate further testing to determine the cause of elevated serum bilirubin levels and to prevent serious sequelae.

HOW TO ESTIMATE GESTATIONAL AGE

How can you tell if a neonate's full term or not? A simple, reliable way to estimate gestational age is by examining the neonate for the five characteristics listed below.

PHYSICAL CHARACTERISTICS	LESS THAN 37 WEEKS	37 TO 38 WEEKS	MORE THAN 38 WEEKS
Sole creases	Anterior transverse crease only	Some creases in anterior two thirds	Sole covered with creases
Breast nodule diameter	2 mm	4 mm	7 mm
Scalp hair	Fine and fuzzy	Fine and fuzzy	Coarse and silky
External ear	Pliable, no cartilage	Some cartilage	Stiff, with thick cartilage
Testes and scrotum	Testes in lower canal; scrotum small with few rugae	Testes in intermediate position	Testes pendulous; scrotum full with extensive rugae

A normal variation of the newborn infant's skin is erythema toxicum (newborn rash)—a pink, papular rash that appears in the first day or two after birth and spontaneously disappears after several days. You may also observe tiny white sebaceous glands (milia) on the nose and chin, which are commonly mistaken for so-called whiteheads. These disappear in a few weeks. Observe for petechiae, which may indicate a long labor, rapid delivery, intrauterine infection, or thrombocytopenia.

Immediately after birth, vernix caseosa may be found on the neonate's skin. Usually, the more premature the neonate is, the more vernix he has. Left undisturbed, vernix dries and disappears within 2 days. Lanugo—a fine, downy hair—may also be present, particularly on the arms, shoulders, back, and forehead. As with vernix, the more premature the neonate, the more abundant the lanugo.

Examine the neonate's hands and feet for normal creases (see *How to Estimate Gestational Age,* page 789). Observe for a simian crease (single horizontal palmar crease), which is associated with Down's syndrome. Then examine the neonate's nail beds, which should be pink; in acrocyanosis, they may be blue. Absent or short nails indicate prematurity; very long nails indicate postmaturity.

The breast tissue of both male and female neonates may appear engorged during the first few days of life, as the result of maternal hormone influence. The breasts may even secrete a small amount of milklike fluid. This flow usually stops within 1 or 2 weeks. Don't express this fluid from the neonate's breasts or you may introduce infection. Accessory nipples may appear, usually below and medial to normal nipples. Although their size varies, they don't contain glandular tissue. The normal breast nodule has a diameter of about 6 mm, with prominent, well-formed, symmetrical nipples.

Observe the neonate's chest for the character, rate, and pattern of his respirations. The neonate's respirations are abdominal and diaphragmatic and tend to be irregular in rate and rhythm. Apnea is a sign of respiratory distress: You should report it immediately. It may indicate a metabolic, neurologic, or infectious disorder. Differentiate between true apnea (no respirations for longer than 10 seconds) and periodic breathing (periods of apnea followed by periods of rapid respiratory rate). Other signs of respiratory distress are tachycardia (an early indication), grunting, nasal flaring, tachypnea, retractions, and cyanosis.

Auscultate the neonate's lungs with the bell of your stethoscope or a small-diaphragm stethoscope. (Remember, if the neonate's head is turned to one side, breath sounds may diminish on the other side. Also, crying produces deep breathing and enhances auscultation.) Normal breath sounds are bronchovesicular. Fine crepitant rales at the end of deep inspiration may be normal initially, until fluid is absorbed by the lungs; however, rales can indicate pneumonia or infant respiratory distress syndrome.

Next, auscultate the neonate's apical heartbeat, again using the bell or a small-diaphragm stethoscope. The apical beat is heard at the fourth or fifth intercostal space (ICS), left of the midclavicular line. If you can auscultate

IDENTIFYING HIGH-RISK NEONATES

Weight and gestational age directly affect a neonate's chance for survival. This chart shows the correlation between the neonate's weight and gestational age and infant mortality. Use it to identify high-risk neonates who require special nursing care.

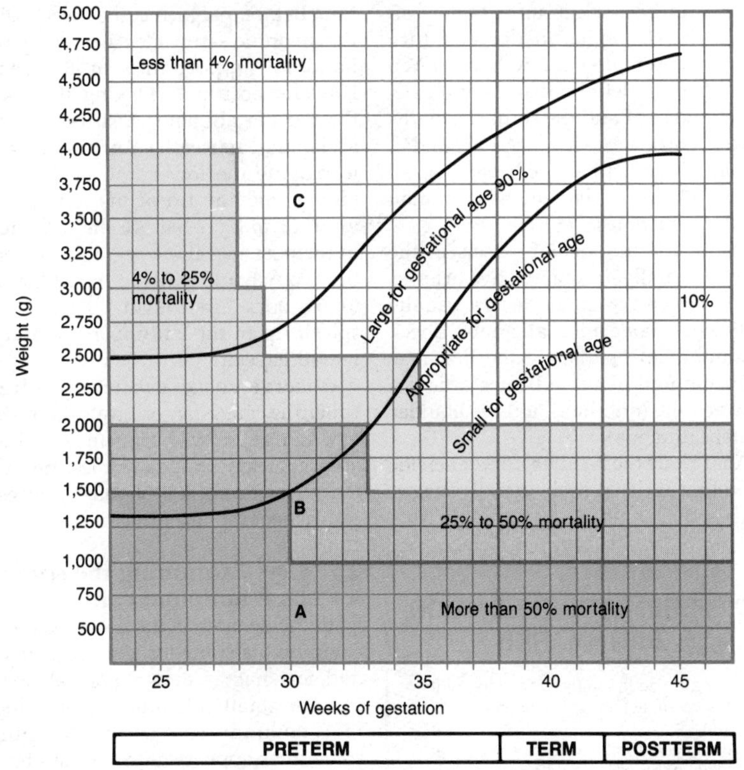

Reprinted from L.F. Whaley and D.J. Wong, *Nursing Care of Infants and Children* (2nd ed.; St. Louis: C.V. Mosby Co., 1979), and F.C. Battaglia and L.O. Lubchenco, "A Practical Classification of Newborn Infants by Weight and Gestational Ages," *Journal of Pediatrics,* 71:59, 1967, with permission of the publishers.

the apical beat on the opposite side of the neonate's chest, this may indicate a mediastinal shift. The heart rate should be 120 to 150 beats/minute; sinus arrhythmias and premature ventricular contractions are common.

Auscultate heart sounds. The first and second sounds should be clear and sharp, with the second slightly higher pitched. Remember that heart sounds in neonates are normally louder than in adults. Because of the incomplete closure of the fetal shunts, murmurs are common, especially over the heart base or at the left sternal border, near the third and fourth ICS. You should report them (see Entry 404).

Palpate the neonate's peripheral pulses, particularly the femoral, brachial, and radial pulses.

Assessment tip: A neonate's diminished or absent femoral pulse may be the only indication of coarctation of the aorta.

844 Abdominal assessment

Inspect the size and shape of the neonate's abdomen. It should be cylindrical; if it looks distended or scaphoid (sunken), report this finding immediately. A scaphoid abdomen may indicate a diaphragmatic hernia. Observe the umbilical cord; it should appear moist and blue-white immediately after birth. (It begins to dry and turn yellow-brown after a few hours.) You should see a definite demarcation between the cord and the skin. Normally, as the cord ages, the area around it becomes dry, without redness. Inspect for umbilical hernia, which is common in black neonates.

Check the number of vessels in the cord. Normally, it contains two arteries and one vein. A single artery usually indicates a congenital anomaly. Check for umbilical fistulas. Urine drainage from the umbilicus indicates a fistula between the umbilicus and the bladder (patent urachus).

Auscultate the neonate's abdomen for bowel sounds, which usually begin within a few hours after birth. Note any increase in pitch or diminishing sounds.

Palpate the abdominal quadrants for tenderness and masses. You should be able to feel the neonate's liver ⅜" to ¾" (1 to 2 cm) below the right costal margin. Before palpating the liver, relax the neonate's muscles by using one hand to support him in the semi-Fowler's position. (Flexing his knees toward his abdomen also relaxes the abdominal muscles.) You may be able to palpate the lower half of the right kidney and the tip of the left one ⅜" to ¾" (1 to 2 cm) above the umbilicus in the posterior flank region. (Remember, you should palpate the kidneys 4 to 6 hours after birth.) Palpate the spleen tip in the left upper quadrant's lateral aspect.

Observe for excessive drooling, coughing, gagging, or cyanosis during feeding. These symptoms may indicate an alteration in gastrointestinal patency (for example, esophageal atresia or tracheoesophageal fistula).

DIFFERENTIATING COMMON BIRTHMARKS

Here's a guide to the most common birthmarks you may find on the neonatal patient:

- *Mongolian spot:* a slate-blue area that appears in the gluteal and sacral regions of dark-skinned infants. It's visible at birth, then disappears in late infancy or early childhood.
- *Telangiectatic nevus* (stork bites): a small pink to red flat area that blanches easily and darkens when the patient cries. It's found on the nape of the neck, the eyelids, the upper lip, the bridge of the nose, and in the occipital area. It's visible at birth and usually disappears by age 2.
- *Nevus flammeus* (port-wine stain): a red to purple flat area that does not blanch with pressure. It's usually visible at birth and does not disappear spontaneously.
- *Nevus vascularis* (strawberry mark): a bright or dark red, raised, rough-surfaced area. It may be visible at birth but usually disappears during the 1st or 2nd month of life and usually disappears spontaneously by age 7.

845 Examining the spine and anal canal

With the neonate in the prone position, examine his spine for S-shaped curves and for masses and abnormal openings. A small pilonidal sinus, which may communicate with the spine, sometimes appears at the spine's base.

Inspect the neonate's back for any malformations of spinal canal closure. Such defects (*spina bifida*) may range from a small split in the vertebrae to the absence of several spinous processes. These malformations result from the neural tube's failure to close during the fourth month of gestation.

Unless it's already been done, check the neonate's anal opening for patency, using a rectal thermometer. Observe for fistula openings on the perineum that may be mistaken for the anus. Remember, meconium may pass through a fistula. The neonate should pass meconium in the first 24 to 48 hours. If he doesn't, he may have imperforate anus or congenital megacolon.

ASSESSING HIP DISLOCATION

Suspect hip dislocation in the neonate if you detect any of the following: asymmetrical gluteal and thigh skin folds, as shown on the left; a palpable and audible click when his affected leg is abducted (Ortolani's sign), as tested for in the top right illustration; or unequal leg lengths (Allis' sign), as shown in the bottom right illustration.

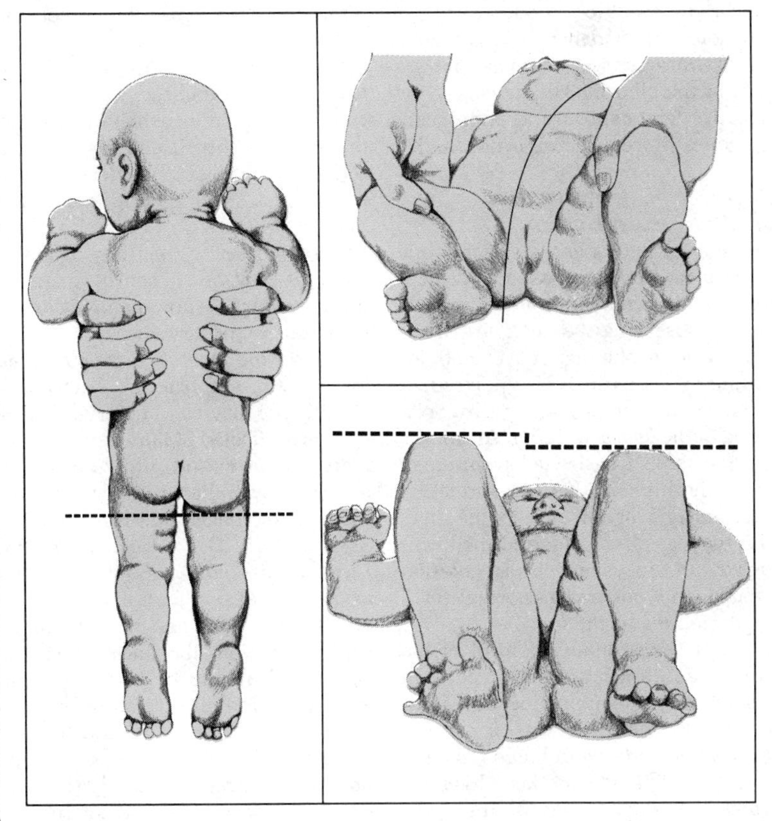

846 Genitalia assessment

Inspect the neonate's genitalia thoroughly. For a male neonate, inspect the penis for location of the urethral meatus. (Remember, the foreskin may be difficult to retract and shouldn't be forced.) Normally, the opening appears at the tip of the glans penis. Note abnormalities, such as hypospadias (meatus on the ventral surface) or epispadias (meatus on the dorsal surface). (See *Recognizing Penis Abnormalities*, page 478.) Then inspect the scrotum, which may appear edematous and proportionately large. The scrotal skin should be darkly pigmented and have distinct rugae. Palpate the scrotal sac for the testes. Hydroceles are common in males and usually disappear in a few months.

In a female neonate, the labia majora may appear edematous and cover the clitoris and the labia minora. (The genitalia are particularly edematous or bruised after a breech delivery.) A hymenal tag, which usually disappears after a few weeks, may appear at the vagina's posterior opening. You may also see a white, mucous, vaginal discharge, possibly tinged with blood (pseudomenstruation). This discharge results from the sudden withdrawal of maternal hormones. Normally, it disappears by age 2 to 4 weeks. Examine and note any evidence of ambiguous sexual characteristics, such as enlargement of the clitoris. This is caused by excessive fetal exposure to androgenic hormones (adrenogenital syndrome).

847 Neuromuscular examination

The neuromuscular examination is one of the most important aspects of neonatal assessment. First, assess muscle tone by observing the neonate's spontaneous or involuntary movements for symmetry, spasticity (hypertonia), flaccidity (hypotonia), or rigidity. Scissoring of the legs is a sign of spasticity. Observe for a frog-legged position in which the hips are held in abduction and external rotation at the same time, with the legs almost flat and the knees angled out. In a breech-presentation neonate, this position is normal for a few days after birth.

To test the neonate's control of his head, trunk, arms, and legs, hold him stomach down (supporting him with your hand under his chest). A normal, full-term neonate should hold his head at about a 45° angle and keep his back straight or slightly flexed, his arms partially extended and bent at the elbows, and his knees partially bent. A hypotonic neonate shows abnormal head lag; a limp, floppy trunk; and dangling arms and legs (floppy infant syndrome). If the neonate rapidly extends his head backward or cannot flex it on his chest, his neck muscles may be hypertonic. Next, gently straighten his arm or leg. Release it and observe whether it returns to its original position. If his extremity remains limp and in the extended position, the neonate may be hypotonic. If his extremity is difficult to straighten and rapidly flexes when released, he may be hypertonic. Observe for other signs of hypertonia, such as severely arched back, coarse tremor, or jittery extremities. Remember, some infants are normally jittery. Hypotonia may indicate hypoxia, Down's syndrome, or neurologic disorders. Hypertonia with tremors may indicate neonatal drug withdrawal. Opisthotonos, a posture in which the back is arched and the neck extended, can be normal in neonates born by face presentation, but it can also indicate serious neurologic disorders, such as meningitis. Asymmetrical muscle tone may result from paralysis or trauma. Observe for seizure activity in the neonate; it may be caused by increased intracranial pressure, meningitis, high temperature, or kernicterus.

Inspect the neonate's arms and legs for evidence of fracture or trauma. Usually the clavicle, humerus, and femur are affected. Malposition, asymmetric motion, or limited range of motion may indicate injury. Examine the hips for congenital dislocation (see *Assessing Hip Dislocation,* page 793). First, inspect the neonate for gross asymmetrical skin folds of the buttocks and thighs. With the neonate in the supine position, the knees should be flexed and able to be abducted to almost 180°. Inability to move the knee joints in this manner, an audible click during abduction (Ortolani's sign), unequal leg length (Allis' sign), or unequal gluteal or leg folds may indicate congenital dislocation.

Examine the neonate's foot position. Turned-in feet are commonly caused by intrauterine malposition. Be sure to distinguish a congenital deformity from a positional deformity by stroking the foot. This causes the positionally deformed foot to return to its normal position. Check to see if the foot and ankle align. Also, inspect the neonate's fingers and toes for polydactyly (extra toes) and syndactyly (webbing).

Test specific reflexes in the neonate, such as blinking, crying, gagging, and sneezing, as well as those involved in

ASSESSING NEONATAL REFLEXES

REFLEX	METHOD AND NORMAL RESPONSE	ABNORMAL RESPONSE SIGNIFICANCE
Blink or corneal	• Shine a bright light in neonate's face; he should blink.	• Absent or asymmetrical response may indicate blindness.
Pupillary	• Shine a bright light toward neonate's pupil; pupil should constrict.	• Fixed dilated pupil, asymmetrical reflex, or absent response is abnormal.
Sneezing, yawning	• Observe as spontaneous behavior.	• Absent or continuous yawning and sneezing seen in neonates with narcotic-addicted mother.
Cough	• Insert catheter into neonate's tracheobronchial tree; he should cough spontaneously from irritation.	• Absence is abnormal after 1 day.
Sucking	• Stroke around neonate's mouth with your fingertip, or insert finger into mouth; he should begin strong sucking movements; reflex should persist with stimulation for about 6 months, then disappear.	• Absence indicates central nervous system depression or immaturity.
Swallowing or gag	• Stimulate neonate's posterior pharynx with food or by inserting a suction catheter or feeding tube; he should swallow or gag.	• Absence may indicate damaged glossopharyngeal nerve.
Rooting	• Stroke both corners of neonate's mouth and the middle upper and middle lower lips; he should turn toward stimulus and open mouth; reflex should disappear by 4 months but may persist for 12 months.	• Absence indicates central nervous system depression or immaturity; persistence indicates prolonged immaturity of neuro-organization.
Asymmetrical tonic neck (fencing reflex)	• Quickly turn neonate's head to one side; he should extend arm and leg on this side and flex arm and leg on opposite side; reflex should disappear by 3 months and be replaced by symmetrical positioning.	• Absence or persistence may indicate central nervous system damage.
Head-raising	• Place neonate in prone position on a flat surface; he attempts to lift his head slightly; he should have more head control after 3 months.	• Absence may indicate neurologic or muscular disorder.
Galant (trunk incurvation)	• Stroke neonate's back next to spine; he should flex his trunk and move his hips toward stimulated side; reflex should disappear by 4 weeks.	• Absence may indicate spinal cord lesion.
Landau	• Hold neonate in prone position with your hand under his abdomen, letting his extremities hang; he should demonstrate some muscle tone by trying to keep spine straight.	• Absence indicates loss of muscle tone requiring further neurologic examination after 3 months.

(continued)

ASSESSING NEONATAL REFLEXES *(continued)*

REFLEX	METHOD AND NORMAL RESPONSE	ABNORMAL RESPONSE SIGNIFICANCE
Crossed extension	• Place neonate in supine position, extend one leg, and prick sole with a pin; he should extend and adduct the opposite leg; reflex should disappear after 2 months.	• Absence indicates spinal cord or nerve damage; persistence indicates pyramidal tract lesions.
Grasp (palmar, plantar)	• Touch neonate's palm and sole near base of digits; he should tightly grasp your finger and flex his toes; palmar grasp should lessen after 3 months, being replaced by voluntary movement; plantar grasp should lessen by 8 months.	• Asymmetrical flexion may indicate paralysis.
Babinski	• Stroke neonate's outer sole upward from heel and across ball of foot; his toes should fan out, his big toe should dorsiflex; reflex should disappear after age 1.	• Persistence may indicate a pyramidal tract lesion.
Moro	• Startle the neonate (with a loud noise or by jarring crib); his extremities should extend and abduct and his index finger and thumb should form a C; then, his extremities should flex and adduct; reflex should disappear after 4 months.	• Asymmetrical response may indicate brachial plexus, clavicle, or humerus injury. Decreased or absent response indicates neurologic disorder.
Placing	• Hold neonate erect and touch dorsal surface of foot or anterior portion of the leg against a hard surface; his ipsilateral leg at knee and hip should flex, lifting his foot as though to place it on surface; reflex should disappear after 1 month.	• Absence indicates neuromuscular degeneration and spinal cord injuries.
Stepping	• Hold neonate so sole touches a hard surface; simulated walking, through reciprocal flexion and extension of the leg, should result; reflex should be replaced after 3 to 4 weeks by deliberate movement.	• Persistence or recurrence indicates spinal cord injury.
Crawling	• Place neonate on abdomen; he should make crawling movements with his arms and legs; reflex should disappear after 6 weeks.	• Asymmetrical movement may indicate neuromuscular abnormality.
Deep tendon	• Tap one of neonate's tendons with your finger; his corresponding muscle should promptly contract.	• Absence of most deep reflexes is abnormal, although triceps reflex may not appear until age 6 months.

feeding, sucking, swallowing, and rooting. Then elicit responses, including the Moro, the tonic neck, and the grasping reflexes.

848 Daily assessment in the nursery

Check the neonate's vital signs and weight each day he's in the nursery.

Report any weight loss greater than 7% immediately.

Continue assessing behavior and feeding patterns, because even subtle symptoms may indicate complications. For instance, the first sign of infection in a neonate may be poor feeding or lethargy, not an elevated temperature.

Normally, neonates are breast- or bottle-fed on a 3- or 4-hour schedule. Evaluate such behavior as sucking, swallowing, rooting, and alertness as well as elimination patterns. The neonate passes meconium in the first 48 hours, commonly within the first 10 hours. Transitional stools range from green-brown to green-yellow and last from a few days to 2 weeks. At first, the neonate may pass stool with each feeding, six to eight times a day. Stools eventually become yellow. The breast-fed neonate usually has soft (or even liquid), "seedy," odorless, yellow stools. The formula-fed neonate has pasty, yellow stools. Bloody or green and watery stools are abnormal.

Formulating a diagnostic impression

849 Classifying neonatal abnormalities

During the first 28 days of extrauterine life, a neonate may suffer from many conditions that affect specific body systems or homeostasis. These conditions can be classified according to their time of onset (for more information, see *Nurse's Guide to Neonatal Disorders,* pages 798 to 803). Congenital disorders, which occur during gestation, include cardiovascular abnormalities, gastrointestinal obstructions, and infection.

During labor and delivery, abnormalities may result from birth trauma—for instance, brachial nerve palsy from head and neck traction, or splenic rupture from liver pressure during breech presentation.

The third category of conditions includes those arising after birth (postnatal). The neonate is particularly susceptible to respiratory distress syndrome, anemias, infections, and certain fluid and electrolyte imbalances.

850 Making appropriate nursing diagnoses

Common skin color changes in the neonate (cyanosis, pallor, and mottling) may result from severe peripheral vasoconstriction (an autonomic nervous system response that increases blood pressure and blood supply to major organs), a low arterial blood oxygen level caused by poor gas exchange, or a low hemoglobin level. This response results in decreased skin perfusion. Your nursing diagnoses should include *altered tissue perfusion, alterations in comfort from decreased temperature in the extremities,* and *impaired gas exchange.*

Neurologic changes—including lethargy, irritability, tetany, and seizures—may result from cerebral anoxia or electrolyte imbalance. For any of these signs and symptoms, you may make a nursing diagnosis of *impaired sleep or rest-activity patterns.* For the neonate with tetany, your nursing diagnosis may be *alterations in comfort.* If the neonate is experiencing seizures, your diagnoses include *potential for injury, potential for ineffective airway clearance,* and *decreased gas exchange.*

Respiratory distress includes dyspnea and tachypnea, a compensatory mechanism that increases oxygen supply to the tissues. Your nursing diagnoses for respiratory distress include *impaired gas exchange, ineffective breathing patterns,* and perhaps *impaired perfusion to body organs* and *irritability caused by an inability to breathe effectively.*

NURSE'S GUIDE TO NEONATAL DISORDERS

CONGENITAL DISORDERS AFFECTING BODY HOMEOSTASIS	CHIEF COMPLAINT
Galactosemia	• *Skin color changes:* jaundice • *Neurologic changes:* lethargy, irritability, seizures • *Gastrointestinal abnormalities:* vomiting and diarrhea
Phenylketonuria (PKU)	• *Neurologic changes:* microcephaly; mental deficiency in later stages
Tracheoesophageal fistula	• *Skin color changes:* cyanosis • *Neurologic changes:* agitation caused by hypoxia • *Respiratory distress:* dyspnea with aspiration of amniotic fluid, feeding, excessive saliva, or gastric secretions; or with abdominal distention; tachypnea with aspiration and hypoxia • *Altered heart rate:* tachycardia caused by hypoxia • *Gastrointestinal abnormalities:* immediate vomiting of any orally ingested fluid; abdominal distention caused by air entering stomach with each breath through fistula
Diaphragmatic hernia	• *Skin color changes:* cyanosis caused by herniation of abdominal organs into chest, displacing space for lung expansion • *Neurologic changes:* agitation followed by lethargy, caused by respiratory failure • *Respiratory distress:* dyspnea caused by herniation of abdominal organs into chest, displacing space for lung expansion • *Gastrointestinal abnormalities:* vomiting possible if stomach is distended with swallowed air
Duodenal atresia and stenosis	• *Neurologic changes:* lethargy caused by fluid and electrolyte loss • *Gastrointestinal abnormalities:* bile-stained vomitus
Pyloric stenosis	• *Skin color changes:* cyanosis with aspiration or hypoxia • *Neurologic changes:* lethargy caused by fluid and electrolyte loss • *Respiratory distress:* dyspnea with aspiration; tachypnea with hypoxia • *Altered heart rate:* rapid heart rate with hypoxia • *Gastrointestinal abnormalities:* vomiting, eventually projectile

	HISTORY	PHYSICAL EXAMINATION AND DIAGNOSTIC STUDIES
	• Congenital (recessive gene)	• Poor feeding habits; failure to gain weight; subcutaneous bleeding; dehydration (loss of skin turgor, elevated temperature, dry mucous membranes, oliguria/anuria) • Diagnostic studies include specific enzymatic screening test and urine tests, which reveal no glucose in urine.
	• Signs and symptoms not seen until disease begins to cause mental retardation; early detection is imperative to prevent brain damage. • Congenital (recessive gene)	• Diagnostic studies include blood screening (Guthrie test), performed usually during neonate's 3rd to 6th day with milk or formula feeding. Urine testing may also be performed.
	• Predisposing factors include maternal hydramnios, low birth weight.	• Fever with aspiration; choking, coughing; inability to pass a feeding tube
	• May be associated with congenital anomalies of heart, lungs, intestines.	• Mottled skin; fever with aspiration; flared nostrils; sternal retractions; no breath sounds on affected side; scaphoid abdomen
	• Predisposing factors include Down's syndrome, maternal hydramnios, vascular insufficiency. • May occur shortly following birth, or a few weeks later if obstruction is incomplete (stenosis)	• Loss of turgor and wrinkles from fluid and electrolyte loss; distended epigastrium • Diagnostic studies include abdominal roentgenography.
	• May not be discovered until a few weeks after birth • Most common in firstborn males	• Dry mucous membranes and loss of turgor from fluid loss caused by vomiting; poor feeding habits; palpable, olive-shaped lump below epigastrium (best felt after vomiting); visible peristalsis from left to right upper quadrant • Diagnostic studies reveal metabolic alkalosis caused by loss of chloride from vomiting.

(*continued*)

NURSE'S GUIDE TO NEONATAL DISORDERS *(continued)*

	CHIEF COMPLAINT
Hirschsprung's disease (congenital megacolon)	• *Skin color changes:* pallor caused by dehydration • *Neurologic changes:* irritability • *Respiratory distress:* tachypnea and grunting caused by abdominal distention • *Gastrointestinal abnormalities:* stained or fecal vomiting with severe obstruction; constipation progressing to severe diarrhea if untreated; abdominal distention
Imperforate anus	• *Gastrointestinal abnormalities:* no meconium or stool passed through rectum (may be passed through vagina if fistula is present); abdominal distention possible
Choanal atresia (upper airway obstruction)	• *Skin color changes:* cyanosis • *Respiratory distress:* lack of air exchange with absence of mouth breathing • *Neurologic changes:* irritability, agitation caused by inability to breathe
Congenital rubella	• *Skin color changes:* cyanosis; jaundice possible with hepatitis; petechiae, purpura, pallor, and mottling with cardiac and respiratory disorders • *Neurologic changes:* lethargy, irritability • *Respiratory distress:* dyspnea; tachypnea with pneumonia • *Gastrointestinal abnormalities:* enlarged liver and spleen
BIRTH INJURIES AFFECTING BODY HOMEOSTASIS	
Intracranial hemorrhage	• *Skin color changes:* cyanosis with progressive cerebral anoxia; pallor • *Neurologic changes:* lethargy, irritability, seizures; may progress rapidly to coma as intracranial pressure increases • *Respiratory distress:* periods of apnea, irregular respirations
Ruptured liver or spleen	• *Skin color changes:* pallor, jaundice • *Respiratory distress:* tachypnea • *Neurologic changes:* lethargy • *Altered heart rate:* tachycardia
POSTNATAL DISORDERS ALTERING BODY HOMEOSTASIS	
Idiopathic respiratory distress syndrome (hyaline membrane disease)	• *Skin color changes:* cyanosis, pallor • *Neurologic changes:* agitation progressing to lethargy • *Respiratory distress:* decreased air entry into lungs; tachypnea; apneic periods • *Altered heart rate:* tachycardia

HISTORY	PHYSICAL EXAMINATION AND DIAGNOSTIC STUDIES
• Predisposing factors include family history. • May be associated with other congenital defects • Most common in white males	• Loss of turgor, wrinkled skin, sunken eyes from dehydration; poor sucking and refusal to feed; possible sternal retractions with severe abdominal distention; failure to pass meconium during first 24 to 48 hours; rectal examination results in explosive release of foul-smelling gas and liquid stool. • Diagnostic studies include rectal biopsy showing absent ganglion cells.
• Congenital	• Not possible to insert rectal thermometer • Observe for small fistula openings on perineum
• Early detection less likely with only one-sided nasal obstruction	• Attempts to mouth breathe; inability to feed caused by extreme respiratory distress when swallowing; possible sternal retractions with severe respiratory distress
• Predisposing factors include maternal rubella infection, especially during first and second trimesters. • Signs and symptoms include low birth weight.	• Sternal retractions with pneumonia; decreased muscle tone in extremities; cataracts and black pigment deposits in retina may occur later.
• Predisposing factors include traumatic birth.	• Bulging fontanelle; retinal hemorrhage, unequal pupils not reactive to light; failure to suck effectively; poor muscle tone, possible paralysis, decreased or absent Moro reflex; nuchal rigidity with subarachnoid hemorrhage
• Predisposing factors include breech presentations, large size at birth. • Signs and symptoms usually evident after 2 or 3 days.	• Dehydration; poor feeding habits; palpable abdominal mass in right upper quadrant
• Predisposing factors include premature delivery, perinatal aspiration, delivery following antepartum hemorrhage, maternal diabetes.	• Possibly low body temperature; flared nostrils; frothy sputum; expiratory grunting, retractions; oliguria; peripheral edema; decreased breath sounds • Diagnostic studies reveal low Po_2 (less than 40 mmHg), high Pco_2 (greater than 40 mmHg), and acidotic pH (less than 7.36).

(*continued*)

NURSE'S GUIDE TO NEONATAL DISORDERS (*continued*)

	CHIEF COMPLAINT	
Narcotic/barbiturate withdrawal	• *Neurologic changes:* irritability, agitation, seizures • *Respiratory distress:* rapid respirations • *Altered heart rate:* tachycardia • *Gastrointestinal abnormalities:* vomiting and diarrhea	
Erythroblastosis fetalis (Rh/ABO incompatibility)	• *Skin color changes:* pallor caused by anemia; jaundice possible • *Neurologic changes:* lethargy • *Respiratory distress:* dyspnea • *Altered heart rate:* tachycardia • *Gastrointestinal abnormalities:* enlarged liver and spleen	
Kernicterus (hyperbilirubinemia with deposits of bilirubin in brain)	• *Skin color changes:* jaundice; yellow to orange within 1st week • *Neurologic changes:* lethargy; seizures progressing to coma • *Altered heart rate:* tachycardia with dehydration	
Sepsis	• *Skin color changes:* flushed, with elevated temperature or pale, cool skin; jaundice possible • *Neurologic changes:* lethargy; seizures possible with elevated temperature • *Respiratory distress:* dyspnea or tachypnea possible • *Altered heart rate:* tachycardia • *Gastrointestinal abnormalities:* distended abdomen, hepatomegaly	
Hypoglycemia	• *Skin color changes:* cyanosis, pallor • *Neurologic changes:* irritability progressing to seizures and coma • *Respiratory distress:* dyspnea	
Hyperglycemia	• *Neurologic changes:* lethargy, drowsiness, CNS depression • *Respiratory distress:* rapid respirations with hyperthermia; Kussmaul's respirations • *Altered heart rate:* tachycardia caused by dehydration	
Hypocalcemia	• *Skin color changes:* cyanosis • *Neurologic changes:* irritbility, tetany, seizures • *Gastrointestinal abnormalities:* vomiting, diarrhea	
Hypomagnesemia	• *Skin color changes:* cyanosis • *Neurologic changes:* irritability, tetany, seizures • *Gastrointestinal abnormalities:* vomiting	

HISTORY	PHYSICAL EXAMINATION AND DIAGNOSTIC STUDIES
• Predisposing factors include maternal addiction.	• Profuse perspiration; high-pitched cry; possibly chest retractions; coarse tremors; rigid, hyperreflexic extremities; incomplete Moro reflex; failure to gain weight
• Predisposing factors include Rh/ABO incompatibility. • Most common in whites	• Flared nostrils; edema of extremities • Diagnostic studies include antibody screening tests (indirect Coombs', indirect antiglobulin test).
• Predisposing factors include erythroblastosis fetalis, anoxia, infection, hypothyroidism, increased vitamin K administration.	• Loss of skin turgor with dehydration; poor feeding habits; shrill, high-pitched cry; opisthotonos position; muscle twitching, rigidity, or hypotonia; absent Moro reflex, diminished deep tendon reflexes • Diagnostic studies include serum tests for direct and indirect bilirubin and urine urobilinogen
• Predisposing factors include premature birth, premature rupture of placental membranes. • Most common in males	• Warm skin with hyperthermia; cool skin with hypothermia; wrinkled skin with dehydration; rales or rhonchi heard with respiratory tract infection (pneumonia); poor feeding habits, anorexia; bulging fontanelle and stiff neck with meningitis; purulent discharge from eyes with gonorrhea; chest retractions with respiratory distress • Diagnostic studies reveal organisms in throat, blood, and cerebrospinal fluid cultures.
• Predisposing factors include maternal diabetes, prematurity, low birth weight caused by intrauterine malnutrition. • Most common in males	• Hypothermia; abnormal eye movements; refusal to suck; shrill, high-pitched cry; hypotonia • Diagnostic studies reveal low blood glucose level.
• Predisposing factors include premature birth, I.V. glucose infusion.	• Wrinkled skin and loss of turgor from dehydration or possibly hyperthermia; sunken eyes from dehydration; increased urinary output from osmotic diuresis • Diagnostic studies reveal high blood glucose level, serum ketones, and glycosuria
• Predisposing factors include severe maternal calcium and vitamin D deficiency, maternal diabetes, premature birth, immature parathyroid, low birth weight, traumatic birth, exchange transfusion.	• Increased alertness; high-pitched cry; feeding intolerance; increased muscle tone, twitching; hyperactive reflexes • Diagnostic studies reveal low serum calcium level
• Predisposing factors include maternal malnutrition or diabetes, fetal malnutrition, multiple births.	• Increased alertness; high-pitched cry; feeding intolerance; increased muscle tone, twitching; hyperactive reflexes • Diagnostic studies reveal low serum magnesium level

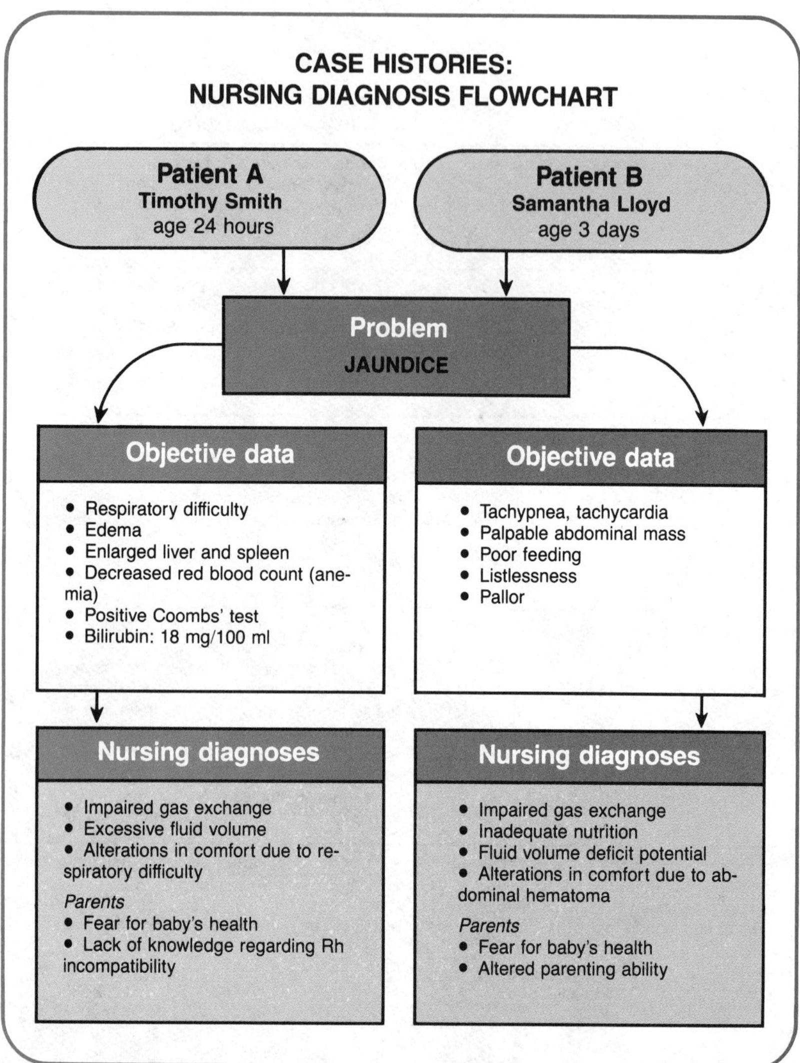

The most common heart rate alteration is tachycardia, a compensatory response to decreased tissue perfusion in which epinephrine from the autonomic nervous system tries to stimulate increased cardiac output. But as heart rate increases, tissue perfusion may actually decrease, because cardiac output diminishes as tachycardia becomes extreme and peripheral vasoconstriction occurs. Tachycardia may occur when the neonate cries or experiences discomfort. Nursing diagnoses may include *alterations in comfort, alteration in cardiac output,* and *alteration in tissue perfusion.*

Gastrointestinal changes, such as vomiting and constipation, usually result from mechanical obstruction of the neonate's alimentary or intestinal tract. Vomiting in a neonate with a diaphragmatic hernia may be caused by large amounts of air in the stomach. Appropriate nursing diagnoses include *alter-*

ations in comfort, alterations in bowel elimination, potential for aspiration, alterations in fluid and electrolyte balance, and *potential for impaired nutritional status.*

Nursing care of the neonate should focus not only on the patient but also on his parents. When you're making a nursing diagnosis for a neonate, be sure to include the effects his condition will have on his parents. Common nursing diagnoses for the neonate's parents include *impaired verbal communication, fear for the neonate's well-being, anticipatory grieving, sleep pattern disturbances, potential alterations in parenting, knowledge deficit,* and *ineffective coping.*

Selected References

Aladjem, Silvio, et al. *Clinical Perinatology,* 2nd ed. St. Louis: C.V. Mosby Co., 1979.

Bolognese, Ronald J. *Perinatal Medicine: Clinical Management of the High Risk Fetus and Neonate.* Baltimore: Williams & Wilkins Co., 1977.

Brann, A.W. "Determining Gestational Age," *Emergency Medicine* 9:51, October 1977.

Brazleton, T.B., ed. *A Neonatal Behavioral Assessment Scale.* Philadelphia: J.B. Lippincott Co., 1973.

Dubowitz, Lily M., and Dubowitz, Victor. *Gestational Age of the Newborn: A Clinical Manual.* Menlo Park, Calif.: Addison-Wesley Publishing Co., Inc., 1977.

Jensen, Margaret D., et al. *Maternity Care: The Nurse and the Family,* 2nd ed. St. Louis: C.V. Mosby Co., 1981.

Johnson, Suzanne H. *High-Risk Parenting: Nursing Assessment and Strategies for the Family at Risk.* Philadelphia: J.B. Lippincott Co., 1979.

Klaus, M., and Kennell, J. *Maternal-Infant Bonding: The Impact of Early Separation or Loss on Family Development.* St. Louis: C.V. Mosby Co., 1976.

Korones, Sheldon B. *High Risk Newborn Infants,* 3rd ed. St. Louis: C.V. Mosby Co., 1981.

Luke, Barbara. "Maternal Alcoholism and Fetal Alcohol Syndrome," *American Journal of Nursing* 77:1924, December 1977.

Malasanos, Lois, et al. *Health Assessment,* 2nd ed. St. Louis: C.V. Mosby Co., 1981.

Miller, Mary Anne, and Brooten, Dorothy. *The Childbearing Family: A Nursing Perspective.* Boston: Little, Brown & Co., 1977.

Moore, Mary L. *Newborn, Family, and Nurse.* Philadelphia: W.B. Saunders Co., 1981.

Moore, Mary L. *The Newborn and the Nurse,* 2nd ed. Philadelphia: W.B. Saunders Co., 1981.

Moore, Mary L. *Realities in Childbearing.* Philadelphia: W.B. Saunders Co., 1978.

Nelson, Waldo E. *Textbook of Pediatrics.* Philadelphia: W.B. Saunders Co., 1979.

Olds, S.B., et al. *Obstetric Nursing.* Menlo Park, Calif.: Addison-Wesley Publishing Co., Inc., 1980.

Overbach, Avrin M. "Drugs Used with Neonates and During Pregnancy: Part 3, Drugs That May Cause Fetal Damage or Cross into Breast Milk," *RN Magazine* 37:39, December 1974.

Pringle, Sheila. *Promoting the Health of Children: A Guide for Caretakers and Health Professionals.* St. Louis: C.V. Mosby Co., 1982.

Pritchard, Jack A., and MacDonald, Paul C. *Williams Obstetrics,* 16th ed. New York: Appleton-Century-Crofts, 1980.

Reeder, Sharon, et al. *Maternity Nursing.* Philadelphia: J.B. Lippincott Co., 1980.

Roberts, Florence B. *Perinatal Nursing: Care of Newborns and Their Families.* New York: McGraw-Hill Book Co., 1976.

Stevenson, R.E. *The Fetus and Newly Born Infant: Influences of the Prenatal Environment,* 2nd ed. St. Louis: C.V. Mosby Co., 1977.

Varney, Helen. *Nurse-Midwifery.* Boston: Blackwell Scientific Publications Inc., 1980.

Whaley, Lucille F., and Wong, Donna. *Nursing Care of Infants and Children.* St. Louis: C.V. Mosby Co., 1979.

Wieczorek, Rita R., and Natapoff, Janet N. *A Conceptual Approach to the Nursing of Children: Health Care from Birth through Adolescence.* Philadelphia: J.B. Lippincott Co., 1981.

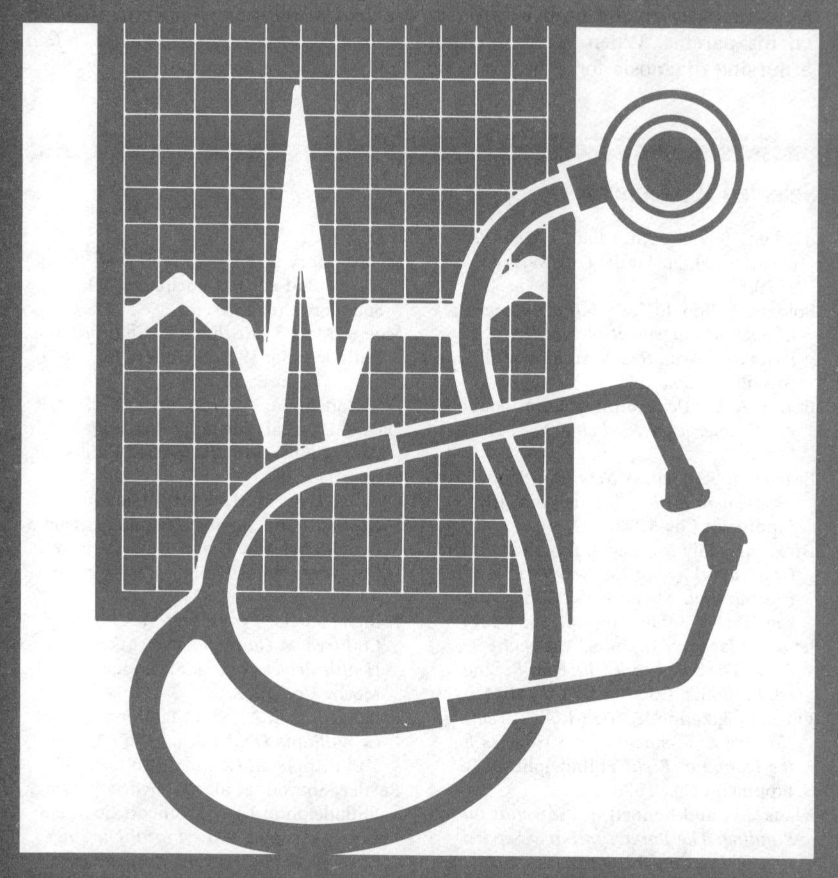

Appendices and Index

DEALING WITH POSTOPERATIVE COMPLICATIONS

Accurate preoperative and postoperative assessment depends on focused—but thorough—data collection. Prior to surgery, review the patient's history and perform a physical examination, as detailed throughout this book. Watch particularly for nutritional, respiratory, cardiovascular, and neurologic disorders. By doing this, you'll gather important baseline data—and you may uncover problems that require postponing surgery or altering intraoperative or postopera-

POSTOPERATIVE RESPIRATORY COMPLICATIONS

COMPLICATION	RESPIRATIONS	BREATH SOUNDS
Airway obstruction	• Increased rate • Limited chest expansion	• Decreased or absent • Wheezing and/or rhonchi
Hypoventilation	• No change or decreased rate; may be shallow	• Decreased or absent
Pulmonary embolus	• Increased rate or no change • Dyspnea • Possibly limited chest expansion	• Decreased rate or no change • Possibly rales, pleural rub at site
Pulmonary edema	• Increased rate • Dyspnea	• Bubbling rales
Respiratory failure	• Increased, no change, or decreased rate; shallow or deep	• Decreased • Possibly rales, rhonchi, wheezing

POSTOPERATIVE CARDIOVASCULAR COMPLICATIONS

COMPLICATION	SKIN	URINARY OUTPUT	PULSE	BLOOD PRESSURE
Hypervolemia	• No change	• Increase or no change; decrease with renal impairment	• Increased rate; bounding	• Increase or no change
Hypovolemic shock	• Cool, clammy • Cyanosis or pallor	• Decreased	• Increased rate; thready	• Decreased
Cardiogenic shock	• Cool, clammy • Cyanosis or pallor	• Decreased	• Increased rate	• Decreased

tive procedures. Accurate assessment can alert you to possible postoperative complications in time to avert or minimize them.

In postoperative assessment, again focus on the patient's respiratory, cardiovascular, and neurologic systems. Assess them as you would during a complete assessment. Then, use the charts that follow to identify possible common postoperative complications.

SKIN	MENTAL STATUS	PULMONARY ARTERY PRESSURE	OTHER
• Cyanosis	• Restlessness	• No change	• Flaring nostrils • Choking • Retractions • Use of accessory muscles
• Cyanosis	• Drowsiness	• No change	
• Cyanosis with large embolus	• Restlessness, anxiousness	• Increased or no change	• Tachycardia • Arrhythmia • Pleuritic chest pain
• Cyanosis with severe edema	• Anxiousness • Altered level of consciousness with severe edema	• Increased	• Tachycardia • Productive cough (frothy, blood-tinged) • Diastolic (S_3) gallop
• Possibly cyanosis	• Anxiousness, progressing to confusion, progressing to coma	• Increased or no change	• Possibly tachycardia or arrhythmia

HEART SOUNDS	CENTRAL VENOUS PRESSURE	PULMONARY ARTERY PRESSURE	OTHER
• No change or presence of S_3 and S_4	• Increased	• Increased	• Acute weight gain • Distended neck veins
• No change	• Decreased	• Decreased	• Tachypnea • Restlessness, apprehension, progressing to coma
• Possible presence of S_3 and S_4, or no change	• Increased or decreased	• Increased	• Tachypnea • Confusion, leading to decreased level of consciousness • Decreased cardiac output

(continued)

POSTOPERATIVE CARDIOVASCULAR COMPLICATIONS *(continued)*

COMPLICATION	SKIN	URINARY OUTPUT	PULSE	BLOOD PRESSURE
Septic shock	• Warm, flushed	• Decreased	• Increased rate	• Decreased
Congestive heart failure	• Edema or no change; cyanosis; pallor	• Decrease or no change	• Increased rate	• Decrease, no change, or increase
Myocardial infarction	• Cool, moist • Possible cyanosis or pallor	• Decrease or no change	• Increased rate • Arrhythmia possible	• Increase or decrease

POSTOPERATIVE NEUROLOGIC COMPLICATIONS

COMPLICATION	LEVEL OF CONSCIOUSNESS	PUPILS
Adverse effects of general anesthesia	• Unconsciousness • Emergence excitement • Hallucinations • Prolonged drowsiness	• Dilated during emergence excitement
Pain	• Alert (if no longer anesthetized) • Anxious	• Dilated, responsive to light
Increased intracranial pressure	• Confusion, progressing to coma	• Unequal, progressing

MISCELLANEOUS POSTOPERATIVE COMPLICATIONS

BODY SYSTEM	AREAS OF ASSESSMENT
Urinary	• Urinary color, amount • Abdominal palpation
Musculoskeletal	• Position • Movement
Psychologic	• Behavior • Verbal abilities

HEART SOUNDS	CENTRAL VENOUS PRESSURE	PULMONARY ARTERY PRESSURE	OTHER
• No change	• Decreased	• Decreased	• Fever, chills • Restlessness • Apprehension
• Possible presence of S_3 and S_4, or no change	• Increased	• Increased	• Distended neck veins • Hepatomegaly with right-sided failure; fatigue and dyspnea with left-sided failure
• Decrease • Possible presence of S_3 and S_4	• Increased or no change	• Increased	• Sudden severe chest pain • Extreme apprehension • Dyspnea • Decreased cardiac output

RESPIRATIONS	MOTOR FUNCTION	OTHER
• Depressed	• Muscle relaxation • Loss of reflexes	• Hypotension • Cardiac arrhythmias • Temperature alterations • Vomiting
• Rapid	• Restlessness • Increased muscle tension	• Tachycardia • Cool, moist skin
• Slow, dysrhythmic	• Weakened hand grasp, progressing to paralysis, progressing to hyperreflexia, progressing to decerebrate rigidity	• Papilledema • Bradycardia • Hypertension

ABNORMAL FINDINGS	COMPLICATIONS
• Oliguria or hematuria • Pain	• Renal insufficiency or failure • Ureteral trauma
• Limited movement • Painful movement • Malalignment	• Injury from surgery or positioning
• Excessive use of defense mechanisms • Anxiety, discomfort • Extreme behavior aberration • Altered level of consciousness	• Anesthetic side effects • Psychosis • Delirium tremens, withdrawal

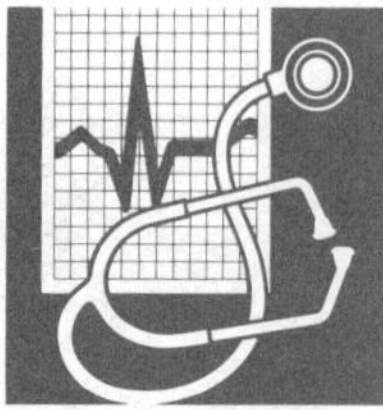

Laboratory Test Values

A

Acid phosphatase, serum
0 to 1.1 Bodansky units/ml
1 to 4 King-Armstrong units/ml
0.13 to 0.63 BLB units/ml

ACTH, plasma
< 120 pg/ml

ACTH, rapid test, plasma
Cortisol rises 7 to 18 mcg/dl above baseline, 60 minutes after injection

Activated partial thromboplastin time
25 to 36 seconds

Albumin, peritoneal fluid
50% to 70% of total protein

Albumin, serum
3.3 to 4.5 g/dl

Aldosterone, serum
1 to 21 ng/dl (standing)

Aldosterone, urine
2 to 16 mcg/24 hours

Alkaline phosphatase, peritoneal fluid
Men: > age 18, 90 to 239 units/liter
Women: < age 45, 76 to 196 units/liter; > age 45, 87 to 250 units/liter

Alkaline phosphatase, serum
1.5 to 4 Bodansky units/dl
4 to 13.5 King-Armstrong units/dl
Chemical inhibition method: Men, 90 to 239 units/dl; women < age 45, 76 to 196 units/liter; women > age 45, 87 to 250 units/liter

Alpha-fetoprotein, amniotic fluid
≤ 18.5 mcg/ml at 13 or 14 weeks

Alpha-fetoprotein, serum
Nonpregnant females: < 30 ng/ml

Amino acids, urine
50 to 200 mg/24 hours

Ammonia, peritoneal fluid
< 50 mcg/dl

Ammonia, plasma
< 50 mcg/dl

Amniotic fluid
Meconium: Absent
Lecithin/sphingomyelin ratio: > 2
Phosphatidiglycerol: Present
Bacteria: Absent

Amylase, peritoneal fluid
138 to 404 amylase units/liter

Amylase, serum
60 to 180 Somogyi units/dl

Amylase, urine
10 to 80 amylase units/hour

Antibody screening, serum
Negative

Anti–deoxyribonucleic acid antibodies, serum
< 1 mcg DNA bound/ml

Antidiuretic hormone, serum
1 to 5 pg/ml

Antiglobulin test, direct
Negative

Antimitochondrial antibodies, serum
Negative at 1:5 dilution

Antinuclear antibodies, serum
Negative at ≤ 1:32 titer

Anti–smooth-muscle antibodies, serum
Normal titer < 1:20

Antistreptolysin-O, serum
< 85 Todd units/ml

Antithyroid antibodies, serum
Normal titer < 1:100

Arterial blood gases

PaO_2:	75 to 100 mmHg
$PaCO_2$:	35 to 45 mmHg
pH:	7.35 to 7.42
O_2CT:	15% to 23%
O_2 Sat:	94% to 100%
HCO_3^-:	22 to 26 mEq/liter

Arylsulfatase A, urine
Men: 1.4 to 19.3 units/liter
Women: 1.4 to 11 units/liter

Aspergillosis antibody, serum
Normal titer < 1:8

B

B-lymphocyte count
270 to 640/mm³

Bence Jones protein, urine
Negative

Bilirubin, amniotic fluid
Absent at term

Bilirubin, serum
Adult: Direct, < 0.5 mg/dl; indirect, ≤ 1.1 mg/dl
Neonate: Total, 1 to 12 mg/dl

Bilirubin, urine
Negative

Blastomycosis antibody, serum
Normal titer < 1:8

Bleeding time
Template: 2 to 8 minutes
Ivy: 1 to 7 minutes
Duke: 1 to 3 minutes

Blood urea nitrogen
8 to 20 mg/dl

C

C-reactive protein, serum
Negative

Calcitonin, plasma
Baseline: Males, ≤ 0.155 ng/ml; females, ≤ 0.105 ng/ml
Calcium infusion: Males, 0.265 ng/ml; females, 0.120 ng/ml
Pentagastrin infusion: Males, 0.210 ng/ml; females, 0.105 ng/ml

Calcium, serum
4.5 to 5.5 mEq/liter
Atomic absorption: 8.9 to 10.1 mg/dl

Calcium, urine
Males: < 275 mg/24 hours
Females: < 250 mg/24 hours

Calculi, urine
None

Capillary fragility

Petechiae:	*Score:*
0 to 10	1 +
10 to 20	2 +
20 to 50	3 +
50	4 +

Carbon dioxide, total, blood
22 to 34 mEq/liter
Carcinoembryonic antigen, serum
< 5 ng/ml
Carotene, serum
48 to 200 mcg/dl
Catecholamines, plasma
Supine: Epinephrine, 0 to 110 pg/ml; norepinephrine, 70 to 750 pg/ml; dopamine, 0 to 30 pg/ml
Standing: Epinephrine, 0 to 140 pg/ml; norepinephrine, 200 to 1,700 pg/ml; dopamine, 0 to 30 pg/ml
Catecholamines, urine
24-hour specimen: 0 to 135 mcg
Random specimen: 0 to 18 mcg/dl
Cerebrospinal fluid
Pressure: 50 to 180 mm water
Appearance: Clear, colorless
Gram's stain: No organisms
Ceruloplasmin, serum
22.9 to 43.1 mg/dl
Chloride, cerebrospinal fluid
118 to 130 mEq/liter
Chloride, serum
100 to 108 mEq/liter
Chloride, sweat
10 to 35 mEq/liter
Chloride, urine
110 to 250 mEq/24 hours
Cholesterol, total, serum
120 to 330 mg/dl
Cholinesterase (pseudocholinesterase)
8 to 18 units/ml
Chorionic gonadotropin, serum
< 3 mIU/ml
Chorionic gonadotropin, urine
Pregnant females: First trimester, ≤ 500,000 IU/24 hours; second trimester, 10,000 to 25,000 IU/24 hours; third trimester, 5,000 to 15,000 IU/24 hours
Clot retraction
50%
Coccidioidomycosis antibody, serum
Normal titer < 1:2
Cold agglutinins, serum
Normal titer < 1:16
Complement, serum
Total: 41 to 90 hemolytic units
Cl esterase inhibitor: 16 to 33 mg/dl
C3: Males, 88 to 252 mg/dl; females, 88 to 206 mg/dl
C4: Males, 12 to 72 mg/dl; females, 13 to 75 mg/dl
Complement, synovial fluid
10 mg protein/dl: 3.7 to 33.7 units/ml
20 mg protein/dl: 7.7 to 37.7 units/ml
Copper reduction test, urine
Negative
Copper, urine
15 to 60 mcg/24 hours
Coproporphyrin, urine
Men: 0 to 96 mcg/24 hours
Women: 1 to 57 mcg/24 hours
Cortisol, free, urine
24 to 108 mcg/24 hours
Cortisol, plasma
Morning: 7 to 28 mcg/dl
Afternoon: 2 to 18 mcg/dl
Creatine phosphokinase
Total: Men, 23 to 99 units/liter; women, 15 to 57 units/liter
CPK-BB: None
CPK-MB: 0 to 7 IU/liter
CPK-MM: 5 to 70 IU/liter
Creatine, serum
Males: 0.2 to 0.6 mg/dl
Females: 0.6 to 1 mg/dl
Creatinine, amniotic fluid
> 2 mg/100 ml in mature fetus
Creatinine clearance
Men (age 20): 90 ml/minute/1.73 m^2
Women (age 20): 84 ml/minute/1.73 m^2
Creatinine, serum
Males: 0.8 to 1.2 mg/dl
Females: 0.6 to 0.9 mg/dl
Creatinine, urine
Men: 1 to 1.9 g/24 hours
Women: 0.8 to 1.7 g/24 hours
Cryoglobulins, serum
Negative
Cryptococcosis antigen, serum
Negative
Cyclic adenosine monophosphate, urine
Parathyroid hormone infusion: 3.6 to 4 μmoles increase

D

Delta-aminolevulinic acid, urine
1.5 to 7.5 mg/dl/24 hours
D-xylose absorption
Blood: Children, 730 mg/dl in 1 hour; adults, 25 to 40 mg/dl in 2 hours
Urine: Children, 16 to 33% excreted in 5 hours; adults, > 3.5 g excreted in 5 hours

E

Erythrocyte sedimentation rate
Males: 0 to 10 mm/hour
Females: 0 to 20 mm/hour
Esophageal acidity
pH > 5.0
Estriol, amniotic fluid
16 to 20 weeks: 25.7 ng/ml
Term: < 1,000 ng/ml
Estrogens, serum
Menstruating females: day 1 to 10, 24 to 68 pg/ml; day 11 to 20, 50 to 186 pg/ml; day 21 to 30, 73 to 149 pg/ml
Males: 12 to 34 pg/ml
Estrogens, total urine
Menstruating females: follicular phase, 5 to 25 mcg/24 hours; ovulatory phase, 24 to 100 mcg/24 hours; luteal phase, 12 to 80 mcg/24 hours
Postmenopausal females: < 10 mcg/24 hours
Males: 4 to 25 mcg/24 hours
Euglobulin lysis time
≥ 2 hours

F

Factor II assay
225 to 290 units/ml
Factor V assay
50% to 150% of control
Factor VII assay
65% to 135% of control
Factor VIII assay
55% to 145% of control
Factor IX assay
60% to 140% of control
Factor X assay
45% to 155% of control
Factor XI assay
65% to 135% of control
Factor XII assay
50% to 150% of control
Ferritin, serum
Men: 20 to 300 ng/ml
Women: 20 to 120 ng/ml
Fibrinogen, peritoneal fluid
0.3% to 4.5% of total protein
Fibrinogen, plasma
195 to 365 mg/dl
Fibrinogen, pleural fluid
Transudate: Absent
Exudate: Present
Fibrinogen, synovial fluid
None

Fibrin split products
Screening assay: < 10 mcg/ml
Quantitative assay: < 3 mcg/ml

Fluorescent treponemal absorption, serum
Negative

Folic acid, serum
2 to 14 ng/ml

Follicle-stimulating hormone, serum
Menstruating females: Follicular phase, 5 to 20 mIU/ml; ovulatory phase, 15 to 30 mIU/ml; luteal phase, 5 to 15 mIU//ml
Menopausal women: 5 to 100 mIU/ml
Males: 5 to 20 mIU/ml

Free fatty acids, plasma
0.3 to 1.0 mEq/liter

Free thyroxine, serum
0.8 to 3.3 ng/dl

Free triiodothyronine
0.2 to 0.6 ng/dl

G

Gamma glutamyl transferase
Males: 6 to 37 units/liter
Females: < age 45, 5 to 27 units/liter; > age 45, 6 to 37 units/liter

Gastric acid stimulation
Males: 18 to 28 mEq/hour
Females: 11 to 21 mEq/hour

Gastric secretion, basal
Males: 1 to 5 mEq/hour
Females: 0.2 to 3.8 mEq/hour

Gastrin, serum
< 300 pg/ml

Globulin, peritoneal fluid
30% to 45% of total protein

Globulin, serum
Alpha$_1$: 0.1 to 0.4 g/dl
Alpha$_2$: 0.5 to 1 g/dl
Beta: 0.7 to 1.2 g/dl
Gamma: 0.5 to 1.6 g/dl

Glucose, amniotic fluid
< 45 mg/100 ml

Glucose, cerebrospinal fluid
50 to 80 mg/100 ml

Glucose, fasting, plasma
70 to 100 mg/dl

Glucose, plasma, oral tolerance
Peak at 160 to 180 mg/dl, 30 to 60 minutes after challenge dose

Glucose, plasma, 2-hour postprandial
< 145 mg/dl

Glucose, urine
Negative

Growth hormone, serum
Men: 0 to 5 ng/ml
Women: 0 to 10 ng/ml

Growth hormone stimulation
Men: Increases to ≥ 10 ng/ml
Women: Increases to ≥ 15 ng/ml

Growth hormone suppression
0 to 3 ng/ml after 30 minutes to 2 hours

H

Haptoglobin, serum
38 to 270 mg/dl

Heinz bodies
Negative

Hematocrit
Men: 42% to 54%
Women: 38% to 46%

Hemoglobin, total
Men: 14 to 18 g/dl
Women: 12 to 16 g/dl

Hemoglobin, urine
Negative

Hemoglobins, unstable
Heat stability: Negative
Isopropanol: Stable

Hemosiderin, urine
Negative

Hepatitis-B surface antigen, serum
Negative

Heterophil agglutination, serum
Normal titer < 1:56

Hexosaminidase A and B, serum
Total: 5 to 12.9 units/liter (Hex-A is 55% to 76% of total)

Histoplasmosis antibody, serum
Normal titer: < 1:8

Homovanillic acid, urine
< 8 mg/24 hours

Hydroxybutyric dehydrogenase
Serum HBD: 114 to 290 units/ml
LDH/HBD ratio: 1.2 to 1.6:1

17-Hydroxycorticosteroids, urine
Men: 4.5 to 12 mg/24 hours
Women: 2.5 to 10 mg/24 hours

5-Hydroxyindoleacetic acid, urine
< 6 mg/24 hours

I

Immune complex assays, serum
Negative

Immunoglobulins, serum
IgG: 6.4 to 14.3 mg/ml
IgA: 0.3 to 3 mg/ml
IgM: 0.2 to 1.4 mg/ml

Insulin, serum
0 to 25 μU/ml

Inulin clearance, urine
≥ *Age 21:* 90 to 130 ml/minute

Iron, serum
Men: 70 to 150 mcg/dl
Women: 80 to 150 mcg/dl

Iron, total binding capacity, serum
Men: 300 to 400 mcg/dl (20% to 50% saturation)
Women: 300 to 450 mcg/dl (20% to 50% saturation)

Isocitrate dehydrogenase
1.2 to 7 units/liter

J, K

17-Ketogenic steroids, urine
Men: 4 to 14 mg/24 hours
Women: 2 to 12 mg/24 hours

Ketones, urine
Negative

17-Ketosteroids, urine
Men: 6 to 21 mg/24 hours
Women: 4 to 17 mg/24 hours

L

Lactic acid, blood
0.93 to 1.65 mEq/liter

Lactic dehydrogenase
Total: 48 to 115 IU/liter
LDH$_1$: 18.1% to 29%
LDH$_2$: 29.4% to 37.5%
LDH$_3$: 18.8% to 26%
LDH$_4$: 9.2% to 16.5%
LDH$_5$: 5.3% to 13.4%

Leucine aminopeptidase
< 50 units/liter

Lipase
32 to 80 units/liter

Lipids, amniotic fluid
> 20% of lipid-coated cells stain orange

Lipids, fecal
< 20% of excreted solids; < 7 g/24 hours

Lipoproteins, serum
HDL-cholesterol: 29 to 77 mg/dl
LDL-cholesterol: 62 to 185 mg/dl

Long-acting thyroid stimulator, serum
Negative

Lupus erythematosus cell preparation
Negative
Lupus erythematosus cells, synovial fluid
None
Luteinizing hormone, plasma
Menstruating females: Follicular phase, 5 to 15 mIU/ml; ovulatory phase, 30 to 60 mIU/ml; luteal phase, 5 to 15 mIU/ml
Postmenopausal females: 50 to 100 mIU/ml
Men: 5 to 20 mIU/ml
Lymphocyte transformation
60% to 90% lymphocytes respond to nonspecific antigens
Lysozyme, urine
< 3 mg/24 hours

M
Magnesium, serum
1.5 to 2.5 mEq/liter
Atomic absorption: 1.7 to 2.1 mg/dl
Magnesium, urine
< 150 mg/24 hours
Manganese, serum
0.4 to 0.85 ng/ml
Melanin, urine
Negative
Myoglobin, urine
Negative

N
5′ - Nucleotidase
2 to 17 units/liter

O
Occult blood, fecal
< 2.5 ml/24 hours
Ornithine carbamoyltransferase, serum
0 to 500 Sigma units/ml
Oxalate, urine
≤ 40 mg/24 hours

P
Para-aminohippuric acid excretion, urine
Age 20: 400 to 700 ml/minute (17 ml/minute decrease each decade after age 20)
Parathyroid hormone, serum
20 to 70 μlEq/ml
Phenylalanine, serum, screening
Negative: < 2 mg/dl
Phosphates, serum
1.8 to 2.6 mEq/liter
Atomic absorption: 2.5 to 4.5 mg/dl
Phosphates, urine
< 1,000 mg/24 hours
Phosphate, tubular reabsorption, urine and plasma
80% reabsorption
Phospholipids, plasma
180 to 320 mg/dl
Phytanic acid,, serum
< 0.3% of blood lipids
Placental lactogen, serum
Pregnant females: 5 to 27 weeks, < 4.6 mcg/ml; 28 to 31 weeks, 2.4 to 6.1 mcg/ml; 32 to 35 weeks, 3.7 to 7.7 mcg/ml; 36 weeks to term, 5 to 8.6 mcg/ml
Nonpregnant females: < 0.5 mcg/ml
Males: < 0.5 mcg/ml
Platelet aggregation
3 to 5 minutes
Platelet count
130,000 to 370,000/mm^3
Platelet survival
50% tagged platelets disappear within 84 to 116 hours
100% disappear within 8 to 10 days
Pleural fluid
Appearance: Clear (transudate); cloudy, turbulent (exudate)
Specific gravity: < 1.016 (transudate); > 1.016 (exudate)
Porphobilinogen, urine
≤ 1.5 mg/24 hours
Potassium, serum
3.8 to 5.5 mEq/liter
Pregnanediol, urine
Males: 1.5 mg/24 hours
Females: 0.5 to 1.5 mg/24 hours
Postmenopausal females: 0.2 to 1 mg/24 hours
Pregnanetriol, urine
< 3.5 mg/24 hours
Progesterone, plasma
Menstrual cycle: Follicular phase, < 150 ng/dl; lutea phase, 300 ng/dl; midluteal phase, 2,000 ng/dl
Pregnancy: First trimester, 1,500 to 5,000 ng/dl; second and third trimesters, 8,000 to 20,000 ng/dl
Prolactin, serum
0 to 23 ng/dl
Protein, cerebrospinal fluid
15 to 45 mg/dl
Protein, pleural fluid
Transudate: < 3 g/dl
Exudate: > 3 g/dl
Protein, total, peritoneal fluid
0.3 to 4.1 g/dl
Protein, total, serum
6.6 to 7.9 g/dl
Albumin fraction: 3.3 to 4.5 g/dl
Globulin levels:
Alpha$_1$–globulin, 0.1 to 0.4 g/dl; alpha$_2$–globulin, 0.5 to 1 g/dl; beta globulin, 0.7 to 1.2 g/dl; gamma globulin, 0.5 to 1.6 g/dl
Protein, total, synovial fluid
10.7 to 21.3 mg/dl
Protein, urine
≤ 150 mg/24 hours
Prothrombin consumption time
20 seconds
Prothrombin time
Males: 9.6 to 11.8 seconds
Females: 9.5 to 11.3 seconds
Pyruvate kinase
Ultraviolet: 2 to 8.8 units/g hemoglobin
Low substrate assay: 0.9 to 3.9 units/g hemoglobin
Pyruvic acid, blood
0.08 to 0.16 mEq/liter

R
Radioallergosorbent test
Negative: < 150% of control
Red blood cell count
Men: 4.5 to 6.2 million/μl venous blood
Women: 4.2 to 5.4 million/μl venous blood
Red blood cells, cerebrospinal fluid
None
Red blood cells, urine
0 to 3 per high-power field
Reticulocyte count
0.5% to 2% of total RBC count
Rheumatoid factor, serum
Negative
Rubella antibodies, serum
Titer of 1:8 or less indicates little or no immunity

S
Semen
Volume: 1.5 to 5 ml
pH: 7.3 to 7.7

Liquefaction: 30 minutes
Sperm count: 60 million to 150 million/ml
Cervical mucus: ≥ 5 motile sperm per high-power field
Spinnbarkeit: 4″ (10 cm)

Serum glutamic-oxaloacetic transaminase
8 to 20 units/liter

Serum glutamic-pyruvic transaminase
Men: 10 to 32 units/liter
Women: 9 to 24 units/liter

Sickle cell test
Negative

Sodium, serum
135 to 145 mEq/liter

Sodium, sweat
10 to 30 mEq/liter

Sodium, urine
30 to 280 mEq/24 hours

Sodium chloride, urine
5 to 20 g/24 hours

Sporotrichosis antibody, serum
Normal titers < 1:40

Sulfobromophthalein excretion
90% complete in 45 minutes

T

T-lymphocyte count
1,400 to 2,700/mm³

T_3 resin uptake
25% to 35% of T_3* binds resin

Testosterone, plasma or serum
Men: 30 to 1,200 ng/dl
Women: 30 to 95 ng/dl

Thrombin time, plasma
10 to 15 seconds

Thyroid-stimulating hormone, serum
0 to 15 μIU/ml

Thyroxine, total, serum
5 to 13.5 mcg/dl

Thyroxine-binding globulin, serum
Electrophoresis: From 10 to 26 mcg T_4 (binding capacity)/dl to 16 to 24 mcg T_4 (binding capacity)/dl (depending on the laboratory)
Radioimmunoassay: 1.3 to 2 ng/dl

Tolbutamide tolerance
Plasma glucose drops to one half fasting level for 30 minutes, recovers in 1½ to 3 hours

Transferrin, serum
250 to 390 mcg/dl

Triglycerides, serum
Ages 0 to 29: 10 to 140 mg/dl
Ages 30 to 39: 10 to 150 mg/dl
Ages 40 to 49: 10 to 160 mg/dl
Ages 50 to 59: 10 to 190 mg/dl

Triiodothyronine, serum
90 to 230 ng/dl

U

Urea, urine
Maximal clearance: 64 to 99 ml/minute

Uric acid, serum
Men: 4.3 to 8 mg/dl
Women: 2.3 to 6 mg/dl

Uric acid, synovial fluid
Men: 2 to 8 mg/dl
Women: 2 to 6 mg/dl

Uric acid, urine
250 to 750 mg/24 hours

Urinalysis, routine
Color: Straw
Odor: Slightly aromatic
Appearance: Clear
Specific gravity: 1.025 to 1.030
pH: 4.5 to 8.0
Sugars: None
Epithelial cells: Few
Casts: None, except occasional hyaline casts
Crystals: Present
Yeast cells: None

Urine concentration
Specific gravity: 1.025 to 1.032
Osmolality: > 800 mOsm/kg water

Urine dilution
Specific gravity: < 1.003
Osmolality: < 100 mOsm/kg
80% of water excreted in 4 hours

Urobilinogen, fecal
50 to 300 mg/24 hours

Urobilinogen, urine
Men: 0.3 to 2.1 Ehrlich units/2 hours
Women: 0.1 to 1.1 Ehrlich units/2 hours

Uroporphyrin, urine
Men: 0 to 42 mcg/24 hours
Women: 1 to 22 mcg/24 hours

V

Vanillylmandelic acid, urine
0.7 to 6.8 mg/24 hours

VDRL, cerebrospinal fluid
Negative

VDRL, serum
Negative

W

White blood cell count, blood
4,100 to 10,900/μl

White blood cell count, cerebrospinal fluid
0 to 5/mm³

White blood cell count, peritoneal fluid
< 300/μl

White blood cell count, pleural fluid
Transudate: Few
Exudate: Many (may be purulent)

White blood cell count, synovial fluid
0 to 200/μl

White blood cell count, urine
0 to 4 per high-power field

White blood cell differential, blood
Neutrophils: 47.6% to 76.8%
Lymphocytes: 16.2% to 43%
Monocytes: 0.6% to 9.6%
Eosinophils: 0.3% to 7%
Basophils: 0.3% to 2%

White blood cell differential, synovial fluid
Lymphocytes: 0 to 78/μl
Monocytes: 0 to 71/μl
Clasmatocytes: 0 to 26/μl
Polymorphonuclears: 0 to 25/μl
Other phagocytes: 0 to 21/μl
Synovial lining cells: 0 to 12/μl

Whole blood clotting time
5 to 15 minutes

Z

Zinc, serum
0.75 to 1.4 mcg/ml

Accepted Nursing Diagnoses

This list was accepted at the Fifth National Conference for Classification of Nursing Diagnosis, held in St. Louis, April 13-17, 1982:

Activity Intolerance
Airway Clearance, Ineffective
Anxiety
Bowel Elimination, Alterations in: Constipation
Bowel Elimination, Alterations in: Diarrhea
Bowel Elimination, Alterations in: Incontinence
Breathing Patterns, Ineffective
Cardiac Output, Alterations in: Decreased
Comfort, Alterations in: Pain
Communication, Impaired Verbal
Coping, Family: Potential for Growth
Coping, Ineffective Family: Compromised
Coping, Ineffective Family: Disabling
Coping, Ineffective Individual
Diversional Activity, Deficit
Family Processes, Alterations
Fear
Fluid Volume, Alterations in: Excess
Fluid Volume Deficit, Actual
Fluid Volume Deficit, Potential
Gas Exchange, Impaired
Grieving, Anticipatory
Grieving, Dysfunctional
Health Maintenance Alteration
Home Maintenance Management, Impaired
Injury, Potential for
Knowledge Deficit (specify)
Mobility, Impaired Physical
Noncompliance (specify)
Nutrition, Alterations in: Less Than Body Requirements
Nutrition, Alterations in: More Than Body Requirements
Nutrition, Alterations in: Potential for More Than Body Requirements
Oral Mucous Membrane, Alterations in
Parenting, Alterations in: Actual
Parenting, Alterations in: Potential
Powerlessness
Rape-Trauma Syndrome
Self-care Deficit (specify level)
Self-concept, Disturbance in
Sensory Perceptual Alterations
Sexual Dysfunction
Skin Integrity, Impairment of: Actual
Skin Integrity, Impairment of: Potential
Sleep Pattern Disturbance
Social Isolation
Spiritual Distress
Thought Processes, Alterations in
Tissue Perfusion, Alteration in
Urinary Elimination, Alteration in Patterns
Violence, Potential for

Diagnoses to be developed

Aggressive Coping Mode
Aggressive Responsive State
Cognitive Dissonance
Consciousness, Altered Levels of
Decision-making, Impaired/Ineffective
Dependent Coping Mode
Depleted Health Potential
Impulse Dominated State
Impulsive Coping Mode
Manipulative Coping Mode
Memory Deficit
Rational Anger State
Role Disturbance
Self-exaltation State
Self-harm
Social Network Support, Alteration in
Subtle Obstructive Mode
Victim Abuse Syndrome

Photo Credits

p. 188 (koilonychia) Mervyn L. Elgart, MD
pp. 188-189 © American Academy of Dermatology
p. 257 William Reifman, RN
p. 539 (1-4, 7) © American Academy of Dermatology
(5, 6) *Consultant Magazine,* Cliggott Publishing Co., Greenwich, Conn.
pp. 540-542 © American Academy of Dermatology
p. 543 (28) William C. Nyberg, RBP, Scheie Eye Institute, Philadelphia, Pa.
(29, 31, 32) Heather Boyd-Monk, Wills Eye Hospital, Philadelphia, Pa.
(30, 33) Temple University Health Sciences Center, Department of Ophthalmology, Philadelphia, Pa.
p. 544 (34, 36) Temple University Health Sciences Center, Department of Ophthalmology, Philadelphia, Pa.
(35, 37-39) Heather Boyd-Monk, Wills Eye Hospital, Philadelphia, Pa.
(40, 41) William C. Nyberg, RBP, Scheie Eye Institute, Philadelphia, Pa.
p. 545 (normal view, 42) G. Richard Bennett, MS, OD
(43-46) Temple University Health Sciences Center, Department of Ophthalmology, Philadelphia, Pa.
p. 546 William Reifman, RN
p. 549 ©Reprinted with permission. American Heart Association.
p. 551 Richard L. Miller, DDS, PhD
p. 552 United States Public Health Service, Atlanta, Ga.
p. 553 Julian C. Woodruff, JD, *Pathology of the Cervix Uteri.* New York: Famous Teachings in Modern Medicine, Medcom, Inc., 1973.
p. 554 © Arthritis Foundation, 1980.

Index

A

Italic page numbers = illustration   *c* = color illustration

B

C

D

E

F

G

H

I

Italic page numbers = illustration *c* = color illustration

M

N

O

P

Q

R

S

T

U

V

W

X

Y

Z

SAMPLE NURSING DISCHARGE SUMMARY

Cedarcrest Hospital
Springhouse, Pennsylvania

Date of Discharge *June 10, 1982* Time *11:30* A.M. ☒ P.M. ☐
Physician Discharging Patient *Max Greening M.D.*
Discharge Status: M.D. Order ☒ A.M.A. ☐ Release Signed ______
Method of Discharge: Wheelchair ☒ Litter ☐ Other ______
Accompanied By *wife*
Discharged To: Home ☒ Nursing Home ☐ Other ______

Medications

No Medications Prescribed ☐
Prescription Given: No ☐ Yes ☒ (List if "Yes")
Hydropres 25 1tab bid (9 AM and 6 PM at mealtime)

Medication Instructions Given To:

Patient ☒ Significant Other ☒ Relationship *wife*
Patient Repeats Instructions: Yes ☒ No ☐
If patient/significant other cannot repeat instructions, physician notified ☐
Comments: *Stressed to pt. and wife the importance of taking medication even when his BP is within normal limits. Both stated they understood. Reviewed side effects with pt.*

Treatments

No Treatments Prescribed ☐
Treatments Prescribed (List)
Monitor BP daily

Instructions Given To:

Patient ☒ Significant Other ☒ Relationship *wife*
Patient demonstrates treatment: Yes ☒ No ☐
If patient cannot demonstrate treatment, physician notified ☐
Comments: *Pt and wife accurately demonstrated proper use of equipment.*